Nursing Diagnosis Index

Nursing Diagnosis

Application to Clinical Practice

15TH EDITION

LYNDA JUALL CARPENITO, RN, MSN, CRNP

Family Nurse Practitioner
ChesPenn Health Services
Chester, Pennsylvania
Nursing Consultant
Mullica Hill, New Jersey

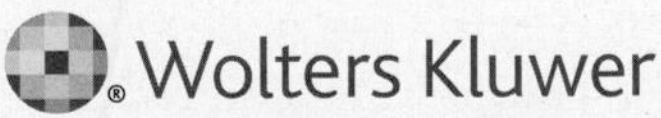

Philadelphia • Baltimore • New York • London
Buenos Aires • Hong Kong • Sydney • Tokyo

Acquisitions Editor: Natasha McIntyre
Product Development Editor: Annette Ferran
Director of Product Development: Jennifer Forestieri
Editorial Assistant: Dan Reilly
Senior Production Project Manager: Cynthia Rudy
Design Coordinator: Joan Wendt
Illustration Coordinator: Jennifer Clements
Manufacturing Coordinator: Karin Duffield
Prepress Vendor: S4Carlisle Publishing Services

15th Edition

9 8 7 6 5 4 3 2 1

Printed in China.

Library of Congress Cataloging-in-Publication Data
Names: Carpenito, Lynda Juall, editor.
Title: Nursing diagnosis : application to clinical practice / [edited by] Lynda Juall Carpenito.
Description: 15th edition. | Philadelphia, PA : Wolters Kluwer, [2017] | Includes bibliographical references and index.
Identifiers: LCCN 2016003689 | ISBN 9781496338419 (alk. paper)
Subjects: LCSH: Nursing diagnosis.
Classification: LCC RT48.6 .C39 2017 | DDC 610.73—dc23 LC record available at http://lccn.loc.gov/2016003689

LWW.com

To My Earth Angels

On December 17th, 2015, my mother, Elizabeth Julia Juall, died at 96 after living a full and healthy life. I promised her that she would have a peaceful death in her house. I kept my promise. When I was 23, my mom told me that "no matter how old you are, you are never ready to lose your mother." She was so right.

In the eighth edition of this book, I introduced the reader to Earth angels. The dictionary defines "angel" as a "spiritual being . . . an attendant spirit or guardian . . . one who aids or supports." Earth angels can be friends, strangers, adults, or children. Most often, the Earth angel does not even know the profound effects of the angelic encounter.

These Earth angels are always here, giving me permission to be imperfect, to grieve, and to heal. These are my Earth angels—Ginny, Donna, Heather, Maureen, Karen, Bob, and my formidable, caring colleagues from our local chapter of the American Association of University Women. My Earth angels continue to not be afraid of my grief or my anger, or of riding the emotional roller-coaster with me, their wings flapping in the wind. Thank you Earth angels, friends and strangers.

To Risk

By William Arthur Ward

To laugh is to risk appearing a fool,

To weep is to risk appearing sentimental,

To reach out to another is to risk involvement,

To expose feelings is to risk exposing your true self,

To place your ideas and dreams before a crowd is to risk their loss.

To love is to risk not being loved in return,

To live is to risk dying,

To hope is to risk despair,

To try is to risk failure,

But risks must be taken because the greatest hazard in life is to risk nothing.

The person who risks nothing, does nothing, has nothing, is nothing.

He may avoid suffering and sorrow,

But he cannot learn, feel, change, grow or live.

Chained by his servitude he is a slave who has forfeited all freedom.

Only a person who risks is free.

Contributors and Reviewers

Contributors

Virginia Arcangelo, PhD, RN, CRNP
Family Nurse Practitioner (Retired)
Private Practice
Berlin, New Jersey
Risks for Complications of Medication Therapy Adverse Effects

Jasmine Bhatti, MS, BSN
Clinical Nurse
Mayo Clinic
Phoenix, Arizona
Impaired Urinary Elimination

Susan Bohnenkaup, MS, RN, ACNS-BC, CCM
Clinical Nurse Specialist
University Medical Center
Tucson, Arizona
Impaired Oral Mucous Membrane

Heather Davis, BSN, IBCLC
Certified Lactation Consultant
Carondelet—St. Joseph's Hospital
Tucson, Arizona
Ineffective Breastfeeding

Colleen Galambos, PhD, MSW, ACSW, LCSW, LCSW-C
Professor
University of Missouri
Cape Girardeau, Missouri
Frail Elderly Syndrome
Risk for Frail Elderly Syndrome

Gwen Gallegos, MSN, RN, FNP, CDE
Diabetes Educator
Nurse Practitioner Family Practice
Carondelet Diabetes Care Center
El Rio Community Health Center
Tucson, Arizona
Community Nursing Diagnoses

Linda Garner, PhD, RN, APHN-BC
Assistant Professor
Southeast Missouri State University
Cape Girardeau, Missouri
Powerlessness (primary author)
Hopelessness (secondary author)

Pauline M. Green, PhD, RN, CNE
Professor
Division of Nursing
Howard University
Washington, District of Columbia
Community Contamination

Leslie Neely, BSN, RN
Pediatric Clinician
Inspira Health System
Salem, New Jersey
Pediatric Content

Laura V. Polk, PhD, RN
Professor
College of Southern Maryland
La Plata, Maryland
Community Contamination

Michele Tanz, DNP, RN, APRN
Assistant Professor
Southeast Missouri State University
Cape Girardeau, Missouri
Hopelessness (primary author)
Powerlessness (secondary author)

Teresa Wilson, MS, APRNC-OB, CNS-BC
Perinatal Clinical Nurse Specialist
Women's Care Services
Carondelet Health Network
St. Joseph's Hospital
Tucson, Arizona
Hyperbilirubinemia
Labor Pain
Reproductive Collaborative Problems
(on thePoint):
Prenatal Bleeding
Preterm Labor
Pregnancy-Associated Hypertension
Nonreassuring Fetal Status
Postpartum Hemorrhage

Ruth A. Wittmann-Price, PhD, RN, CNS, CNE, CHSE, ANEF
Dean
School of Health Science
Francis Marion University
Florence, South Carolina
Impaired Emancipated Decision Making
Risk for Impaired Emancipated Decision Making
Readiness for Enhanced Emancipated Decision Making

Donna Zazworsky, MS, RN, CCM, FAAN
Vice President of Community Health & Continuum Care
Carondelet Health Network
Tucson, Arizona
Community Nursing Diagnoses

Reviewers

Joan Boyd, MSN, MBA/HCA
Professor of Nursing
Florida State College at Jacksonville
Jacksonville, Florida

Brittny Chabalowski, MSN, RN, CNE
Director of Upper Division and Second Degree Nursing
University of South Florida
Tampa, Florida

Marci L. Dial, DNP, ARNP, NP-C, RN-BC, CHSE, LNC
Professor of Nursing
Valencia College
Orlando, Florida

Diane E. Featherston, MSN, ACNS-BC, WCC
Assistant Professor (retired)
College of Nursing
Wayne State University
Detroit, Michigan

Nancy Fleming, MAEd, RN, HBSCN
Professor/Coordinator
Lakehead University/Confederation College
Thunder Bay, Ontario, Canada

Cathryn S. Hatcher, MS, RN
Associate Professor
Reynolds Community College
Richmond, Virginia

Teri S. Hill, MSN, RN
Assistant Professor of Nursing
Mott Community College
Flint, Michigan

Damion K. Jenkins, MSN, RN
Nurse Educator
The Community College of Baltimore County
Baltimore, Maryland

Jackie L. Michael, PhD, APRN, WHNP-BC
Clinical Assistant Professor
The University of Texas at Arlington
Arlington, Texas

Jessica Morris, BSN, RN, CMSRN, WOCN
Adjunct Faculty
Arizona State University
Phoenix, Arizona

Crystal O'Connell-Schauerte, MScN
Professor of Nursing
Program Coordinator
Algonquin College
Ottawa, Ontario, Canada

Pamela K. Weinberg, MSN, RN, CNS
Nursing Instructor
Central Carolina Technical College
Sumter, South Carolina

Karla Wolsky, PhD, RN
Chair NESA BN Programs
Centre for Health and Wellness
Lethbridge, Alberta, Canada

Preface

Rapid change continues to occur in health care and in the nursing profession. Hospitals continue to decrease their nursing staffs, while the acuity of clients continues to rise. Many nurses, and even some faculty, question the usefulness of nursing diagnosis. Unfortunately, nursing diagnosis is still joined at the hip with traditional care planning. It is time to separate these conjoined twins so that they can function separately. Nursing diagnoses define the science and art of nursing and are as imperative to nurses and the nursing profession as medical diagnoses are to physicians. Nursing diagnoses organize knowledge in the literature and research, as well as in the clinician's mind. Do not underestimate the importance of this classification. A clinician with expertise in nursing diagnoses can hypothesize several explanations for an individual's anger, such as fear, anxiety, powerlessness, or spiritual distress. Without this knowledge, the individual is simply angry.

Care planning, as it is taught in schools of nursing, is an academic exercise, which is not wrong, but as the student advances in school, this academic care plan must be transformed into a clinically useful product. Endless copying from books, such as this one, does not enhance one's knowledge of nursing diagnosis and critical analysis. Students should start with a standardized document (electronically or preprinted) and then revise it according to the specific client.

Nursing diagnosis must be presented as clinically useful. Nurses who are experts in certain nursing diagnoses should be consulted, just as our medical colleagues consult other physicians for their expertise. Health-care facilities can publish a list of nursing experts in their facility for consultation. Faculty, nurse managers, administrators, and clinicians need to do their part. Change is imperative. The documentation requirements are unrealistic. There is little time to think and analyze, which the documentation mandates. Nursing must defend its right to determine its documentation requirements, just as medicine has.

If nursing continues to do business as usual, nursing as we want it—nursing as clients need it—will cease to exist. Nursing will continue to be defined by what we do and write and not by what we know. From assessment criteria to specific interventions, this book focuses on nursing. It provides a condensed and organized outline of clinical nursing practice designed to communicate creative clinical nursing. It is not meant to replace textbooks of nursing, but rather to provide nurses who work in a variety of settings with the information they need without requiring a time-consuming review of the literature. It will assist students in transferring their theoretical knowledge to clinical practice; it can also be used by experienced nurses to recall past learning and to intervene in those clinical situations that previously went ignored or unrecognized.

The author agrees that nursing needs a classification system to organize its functions and define its scope. Use of such a classification system would expedite research activities and facilitate communication between nurses, consumers, and other health-care providers. After all, medicine took more than 100 years to develop its taxonomy. Our work, at the national level, only began in 1973. It is hoped that the reader will be stimulated to participate at the local, regional, or national level in the use and development of these diagnoses.

Since the first edition was published, the use of nursing diagnosis has increased markedly throughout the United States, Canada, and internationally. Practicing nurses vary in experience with nursing diagnosis from just beginning to full practice integration for more than 40 years. With such a variance in use, questions posed by the neophyte may include the following:

- What does the label really mean?
- What kinds of assessment questions will yield nursing diagnoses?
- How do I differentiate one diagnosis from another?
- How do I tailor a diagnosis for a specific individual?
- How should I intervene after I formulate the diagnostic statement?
- How do I care-plan with nursing diagnoses?

These questions differ dramatically from those of experts:

- Should nursing diagnoses represent the only diagnoses on the nursing care plan?
- Can medical diagnoses be included in a nursing diagnosis statement?
- What are the ethical issues in using nursing diagnoses?
- What kind of problem statement should I write to describe a person at risk for hemorrhage?
- How can I efficiently use nursing diagnosis?
- What kind of nursing diagnosis should I use to describe a healthy person?
- Do I need nursing diagnoses with critical pathways?

This 15th edition of *Nursing Diagnosis: Application to Clinical Practice* seeks to continue to answer these questions.

Organization of the Text

The text is organized into three sections for ease of use.

Section 1: The Focus of Nursing Care

Section 1 sets the foundation for understanding the nursing diagnoses described in Section 2. Section 1 includes seven chapters.

Chapter 1 addresses issues and controversies. It explores arguments regarding the ethics and cultural implications of nursing diagnoses. It discusses the implications of a consistent language for nurses as members of a multidisciplinary team.

Chapter 2 focuses on the development of nursing diagnosis and the work of NANDA International (NANDA-I). The chapter explores the concepts of nursing diagnosis, classification, and taxonomic issues. It discusses the review process of NANDA-I and describes the evolving taxonomy of NANDA-I. Chapter 2 also addresses the use of non–NANDA-I-approved diagnoses and practice dilemmas associated with nursing diagnoses.

Chapter 3 differentiates among problem, risk, and possible nursing diagnoses. It also presents a discussion of wellness and syndrome diagnoses, and outlines guidelines for writing diagnostic statements and avoiding errors.

Chapter 4 describes the bifocal clinical practice model. Nursing diagnosis is outlined, differentiating what it is and what it is not. This chapter includes a more detailed discussion of nursing diagnoses and collaborative problems, covering their relationship to assessment, goals, interventions, and evaluation.

Chapter 5 describes the process of care planning and discusses various care planning systems. Topics include priority identification, collaborative goals versus individual goals, case management, and nursing accountability. The chapter differentiates interventions from nursing diagnoses and collaborative problems. It also clarifies evaluation, distinguishing evaluation of nursing care from evaluation of the condition. It presents a discussion of multidisciplinary care, along with a three-tiered care planning system aimed at increasing the clinical use of care plans without increasing writing. Samples of nursing records appear throughout the chapter.

Chapter 6 discusses putting it all together, from assessment to evaluation. The difficulty of identifying priority problems is addressed. Criteria for the selection of priority nursing diagnoses and collaborative problems are presented.

Chapter 7, new to this edition, outlines the process of transitional care from the health-care facility. Individual engagement acknowledges that clients (individuals) have an important role to play in their own health care. Strategies for engagement of the individual and families in planning and shaping health-care outcomes are described (e.g., medication reconciliation and barriers to adherence). The use of high-risk nursing diagnoses to address preventable hospital-acquired conditions is presented.

Section 2: Manual of Nursing Diagnoses

Section 2 is the heart of this text and is organized into four parts:

- Part 1: Individual Nursing Diagnoses
- Part 2: Family/Home Nursing Diagnoses
- Part 3: Community Nursing Diagnoses
- Part 4: Health Promotion/Wellness Nursing Diagnoses

Each part includes an introduction, assessment for specific population, key concepts, author's notes, and specific diagnoses for the population. Diagnoses are discussed under the following subheads:

- Definition[1]
- Defining Characteristics or Risk Factors
- Related Factors
- Author's Notes
- Errors in Diagnostic Statements
- Key Concepts, which may include:
  - Maternal Considerations
  - Pediatric Considerations
  - Geriatric Considerations
  - Transcultural Considerations
- Carp's Cues

Author's Notes and Errors in Diagnostic Statements are designed to help the nurse understand the concept behind the diagnosis, differentiate one diagnosis from another, and avoid diagnostic errors. Maternal, Pediatric, and Geriatric Considerations for all relevant diagnoses provide additional pertinent information. Transcultural Considerations strive to increase the reader's sensitivity to cultural diversity without stereotyping. Carp's Cues are notes from the author to emphasize a certain principle of care, a controversial issue, or an ethical challenge.

Goals for the care of the individual with the nursing diagnosis are provided. Related interventions are given along with rationales. These interventions represent activities in the independent domain of nursing derived from the physical and applied sciences, pharmacology, nutrition, mental health, and nursing research. If applicable, maternal, pediatric, and geriatric focus interventions and rationale are also included. One or more specific nursing diagnoses that relate to familiar clinical situations then follow.

Each nursing diagnosis includes Nursing Outcome Classification (NOC) outcome categories and Nursing Intervention Classification (NIC) major intervention categories to assist those in the development of electronic care planning. The goals, indicators, and interventions are the work of this author, not NIC or NOC.

Every attempt has been made to provide the reader with the most recent literature and research findings on the subject. Frequently, students are instructed not to use references more than 5 years old. However, occasionally, the original paper or research on a topic remains, even 10 years later, the state of science on that topic. If a subsequent author or researcher uses the original work, often his or her citation is substituted for the older one. I disagree with this practice; both citations should be listed. Therefore, throughout this book, the reader will find citations of various ages and many older than 5 years.

Section 3: Manual of Collaborative Problems

Section 3 consists of a manual of collaborative problems. In this section, each of the nine generic collaborative problems is explained under the following subheads:

- Definition
- Author's Note
- Significant Laboratory/Diagnostic Assessment Criteria

[1]Definitions designated as NANDA-I and characteristics and factors identified with a blue asterisk are from *Nursing Diagnoses: Definitions and Classification 2012–2014*. Copyright © 2012, 2009, 2007, 2003, 2001, 1998, 1996, 1994 by NANDA International. Used by arrangement with Blackwell Publishing Limited, a company of John Wiley & Sons, Inc.

Discussed under their appropriate generic problems are 54 specific collaborative problems, covering:

- Definition
- High-Risk Populations
- Collaborative Outcomes
- Interventions and Rationales

Appendices

Appendix A: Nursing Diagnoses Grouped Under Functional Health Patterns
Appendix B: Nursing Admission Baseline Assessment
Appendix C: Strategies to Promote Engagement of Individual/Families for Healthier Outcomes
Appendix D: High-Risk Assessment Tools for Preventable Hospital-Acquired Conditions

Additional Resources

Additional student resources such as assessment guides, printable handouts to give clients, such as *Getting Started to Move More*, and generic care plans are available on thePoint.

The author invites comments or suggestions from readers. Correspondence can be directed to the publisher or to the author: e-mail Juall46@msn.com

Lynda Juall Carpenito, RN, MSN, CRNP

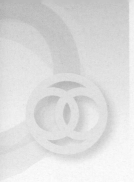

Acknowledgments

The support for this book continues nationally and internationally. It has been translated into 13 languages.

I thank the group in Detroit (Jo Ann Maklebust, Mary Sieggreen, and Linda Mondoux) for their moral support while I wrote the first edition. Rosalinda Alfaro-LeFevre recognized the need for this book in 1983 and sought me out to make it a reality.

On a personal level, my son Olen Juall Carpenito and his wife Heather have given me two special gifts—my grandsons Olen, Jr. and Aiden. They light up my world.

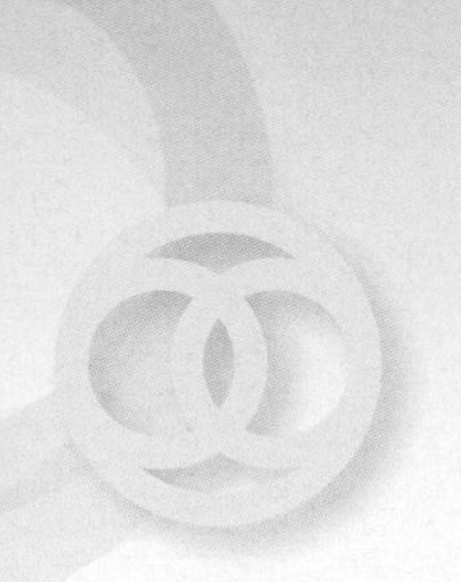

Contents

Section I

The Focus of Nursing

INTRODUCTION

Nursing is primarily assisting individuals (sick or well) with those activities contributing to health or its recovery (or to a peaceful death) that are performed unaided when they have the necessary strength, will, or knowledge. Nursing also helps individuals carry out prescribed therapy and to be independent of assistance as soon as possible (Henderson & Nite, 1960).*

All of us are constantly responding to and interacting with outside events, things, and other persons. We are also responding to what is occurring in our mind, spirit, and body. We are in a constant state of interactions and reactions.

Our *health* is a dynamic, ever-changing state influenced by past and present interaction patterns. Health is the state of wellness as the individual defines it; it is no longer defined as the presence or absence of a biologic disease or psychological disorders.

- When we seek advice or care about our health, we can choose to accept it or not.
- We define our own health.
- We are responsible for our health.
- We make choices—some healthy, some not.

Societal health needs have changed in the last few decades, and so must the nurse's view of the consumers of health care as individuals, families, or communities. An *individual* becomes a recipient of health care not only when an actual or potential problem compromises health but also when he or she desires assistance to achieve a higher level of health. The use of the term *individual* in place of *client* or *patient* to identify the health care consumer suggests an autonomous person who has freedom of choice in seeking and selecting assistance. *Family* is used to describe any persons who serve as support systems to the individual. *Community* is used to describe support systems, geographical locations (e.g., sections of a city as well as groups, such as senior citizen centers).

The definition of nursing cited earlier, now over 50 years old, is as relevant today as it was then. The services of the art and science of nursing are needed when an individual's strength, will, or knowledge are insufficient for them to participate in activities contributing to their health, recovery, or peaceful death. Nurses enable individuals, families, and communities to carry out their chosen therapies and to be independent of our assistance as soon as possible.

*We as individuals are active participants who assume responsibility for our choices.

Chapter 1

Nursing Diagnoses: Issues and Controversies

Learning Objectives

After reading the chapter, the following questions should be answered:

- Why can't we use words that we are familiar with?
- Why are student care plans different from those used in practice?
- If nursing diagnosis is so important, why is it not used more by practicing nurses?
- Do nurse practitioners, nurse anesthetists, and nurse midwives need nursing diagnoses to practice?
- Can nursing diagnoses violate confidentiality?

Nursing diagnosis arouses some emotion in almost every nurse. Responses range from apathy to excitement, from rejection to enthusiasm for scientific investigation. Although nursing diagnoses have been an accepted part of professional nursing practice for more than 40 years, some nurses continue to resist using them. This chapter explores some of the most commonly cited reasons.

Why Can't We Use the Words That We Are Familiar With?

What words have nurses always used? Diabetes mellitus? Prematurity? Pneumonia? Difficult? Cystic fibrosis? For many years, nurses used only medical diagnoses to describe the individual problems that they addressed. Gradually, however, nurses have learned that medical diagnoses do not describe many individual problems in sufficient detail to enable other nurses to provide continuing care for individuals with special needs.

The fact is that nurses have always shared with other disciplines, such as medicine, respiratory therapy, and physical therapy, a common language for certain individual problems. Examples of terms from this language include *hypokalemia*, *hypovolemic shock*, *hyperglycemia*, and *increased intracranial pressure*. Any attempt to rename labels such as these should be viewed as foolhardy and unnecessary. For instance, *dysrhythmias* should not be renamed *decreased cardiac output*, nor should *hyperglycemia* be relabeled as *altered carbohydrate metabolism*.

The author of this text believes nurses should use preestablished terminology when appropriate, whether as a collaborative problem (e.g., *Risk for Complications of Hyperglycemia*) or as a nursing diagnosis (e.g., *Risk for Pressure Ulcer*). Nursing should continue to use the terminology that clearly communicates an individual situation or problem to other nurses and other disciplines.

Having said this, let us now examine the discipline-specific language of nurses. Have nurses had a common language or set of labels for individual problems that they diagnose and treat in addition to the shared language previously discussed? Before the advent of nursing diagnoses, how did nurses describe individual problems such as

- Inability to dress self
- Difficulty selecting among treatment options
- Risk for infection
- Breastfeeding problems
- Stress in caring for an ill family member
- Spiritual dilemmas

Sometimes a nurse would use the terms listed above, but sometimes not. Often the nurse had many options available to describe a problem.

Some nurses, particularly those with more experience, want to describe individual problems in any way they wish. Although an experienced nurse may be able to decipher inconsistent terminology, how can the nursing profession teach its science to its students if each instructor, textbook, and staff nurse uses different words to describe the same situation? Consider medicine. How could medical students learn the difference between cirrhosis and cancer of the liver if "impaired liver function" was used to describe both situations?

Medicine relies on a standardized classification system to teach its science and to communicate individual problems to other disciplines. Nursing needs to do likewise.

Although nurses traditionally have had a common language for certain problems, this language has been incomplete to describe all the individual responses that nurses diagnose and treat. As nursing diagnoses are developed, nurses discover new problems that affect individual/family, these problems, now labeled as nursing diagnoses as Caregiver Role Strain, Chronic Sorrow, Dysfunctional Family Coping, Risk for Compromised Human Dignity, require professional nursing interventions. For individual/family, these diagnoses are not optional.

Why Are Student Care Plans Different From Those Used in Practice?

Students are often told by practicing nurses that the care plans they write or type are not useful in clinical nursing. It is important to distinguish between care plans of students and care plans in practice.

Students create care plans to assist them in problem solving and to prioritize and individualize their care for an individual. Student care plans are directions for a student with a particular individual. Most of these care plans are standard or expected care for a particular problem or situation. After caring for an individual, the student can then revise the plan with additions or deletions. As the student progresses in the program, these plans should emphasize additional interventions needed because of the individual's situation with less basic, standard care.

This type of care plan is not necessary in clinical practice. Predictive standard care should be known by experienced nurses on a unit. For example, if a surgical nurse is unfamiliar with the care needed for a person post hip replacement, he or she should have access to the standard care plan for the specific postoperative situation in a reference or online.

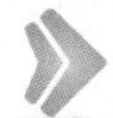

Carp's Cues

The only time a nurse should create a care plan in addition to the standard plan for another nurse to follow is when it is necessary to alert that nurse to additional care that is needed beyond the standard. The system should be easy to use to encourage these additions.

If Nursing Diagnosis Is So Important, Why Is It Not Used More by Practicing Nurses?

The majority of nursing programs identify the nursing process and nursing diagnoses as critical elements in their curricula (Carpenito-Moyet, 2010).

However, when practicing nurses were students, they most likely spent hours in the classroom listening to lectures about medical diagnoses and treatments. Unfortunately, more often than not, there was little to no discussion of nursing diagnoses. Nursing diagnosis became a documentation assignment rather than a critical concept to guide assessments and interventions.

> *Thus, in the end, medical diagnoses guide their practices after graduation, leaving nursing diagnoses as only an unpleasant memory. Nursing management of medical problems requires clinical expertise, but diagnosing a specific nursing diagnosis that causes personal suffering for a patient or family elevates that nurse's expertise. (Carpenito-Moyet, 2010)*

Practicing nurses need to understand and become experts in the pathophysiology and treatment of diabetes mellitus, cancer, and cerebral vascular accidents. However, it is just as important that they become experts in the diagnosing and treatment of *responses* to diabetes mellitus, cancer, and cerebral vascular accidents that can interfere with self-care, human dignity, and family functioning. Only with expertise in both the science of nursing and medicine, will the nurse be viewed as a professional in their own right, not as an assistant of physicians.

Do Nurse Practitioners, Nurse Anesthetists, and Nurse Midwives Need Nursing Diagnoses to Practice?[1]

Advanced nursing practice has been a hot topic of discussion in legislative forums. Many state boards of nursing have defined or are in the process of defining advanced practice.

[1]Carpenito, L. J. (1992, February). *Are nurse practitioners expert nurses?* Paper presented at the 11th Annual National Nursing Symposium, Advanced Practice Within a Restructured Health Care Environment, Los Angeles

Carp's Cues

The author of this text disagrees with the notion that nurse practitioners, nurse midwives, or nurse anesthetists are advanced practice nurses but rather they practice in an expanded role. The term advanced practice is sometimes confused with expert nursing. Expertise in nursing should not be defined by a role but rather the depth of knowledge the nurse has regardless of the role. Expert nurses have complex assessment skills and engage in rapid decision making to provide appropriate and timely care to complex individual and family health situations. Expert nurses can be staff nurses in traditional roles. Some nurses in expanded roles focus too heavily on becoming experts in medicine and not experts in nursing.

Nurse practitioners/nurse midwives diagnose and treat acute and chronic medical conditions in all ages and manage families through all stages of pregnancy, labor, delivery, and postpartum. In addition, the nurse practitioner assesses the person's overall health habits, coping patterns, and functional status. An example problem list for an individual of a nurse practitioner should include medical and nursing diagnoses.

For example, during an appointment with a 52-year-old man, the man complains of back pain, has high blood pressure, and also reports that he has blackouts from alcohol abuse. After discussing his alcohol use, it is determined that the man drinks excessively every day after work. However, he denies that he has a problem. His problem list would include the following:

- Low back pain, unknown etiology
- Hypertension (medical)
- Chronic alcoholism
- Ineffective denial (nursing)

Advanced nurses demonstrate expert nursing practice by diagnosing individual responses to varied situations (e.g., medical diagnoses or personal/maturational crises, which are nursing diagnoses). An advanced nurse would explore such questions as

- How has the individual's ability to function changed since his cerebrovascular accident?
- How has a family system changed, or how is it vulnerable because of an ill newborn who required several months of hospitalization?

Nursing has much to offer individuals and families experiencing chronic disease such as multiple sclerosis or diabetes. Individuals' most common complaints do not involve the medical care they receive, but rather focus on dissatisfaction with how their other problems are addressed. Nurses are in the optimum position to address such problems and increase individual satisfaction with health care.

Nurse practitioners, nurse anesthetists, or nurse midwives who do not formulate or treat nursing diagnoses may be too focused on medicine. To evaluate this practice, a nurse in advanced practice should ask: Do I consult with physician colleagues for complex medical problems? Do physicians consult with me for complex nursing diagnoses? If the answer is no, the nurse should explore why. Does the problem lie with the physician's attitude? Or is the nurse not overtly demonstrating diagnosis and treatment of nursing diagnoses? Or is the nurse not practicing nursing?

If nurse practitioners, nurse anesthetists, and nurse midwives do not practice as expert nurses, who diagnose and treat selected medical diagnoses using protocols, and formulate and treat nursing diagnoses, 5 years from now these nurses may still be struggling to define their roles. Carpenito (1995) uses nursing diagnoses to differentiate the discipline-specific expertise of nurse practitioners and physicians in primary care. Figure 1.1 illustrates this relationship.

The circle on the left presents the expertise of nursing. The discipline expertise of nursing is present in nurses regardless of whether they are a nurse practitioner or not. The shared expertise is where nurse practitioners differ from other nurses. Nurse practitioners diagnose and treat medical problems using their expertise in medicine.

Can Nursing Diagnoses Violate Confidentiality?

Nurses and other health professionals commonly are privy to significant personal concerns of individuals under their care. According to the American Nurses Association Code of Ethics, "the nurse safeguards the client's right to privacy by judiciously protecting information of a confidential nature." The professional mandate to apply the nursing process for all individuals, however, sometimes places the nurse in a position of conflict. Certain information recorded in assessments and diagnostic statements may compromise an individual's right to privacy, choice, or confidentiality. Nurses should never use nursing diagnostic statements to influence others to view or treat an individual, family, or group negatively. They must take great caution to ensure that a nursing diagnosis does no harm!

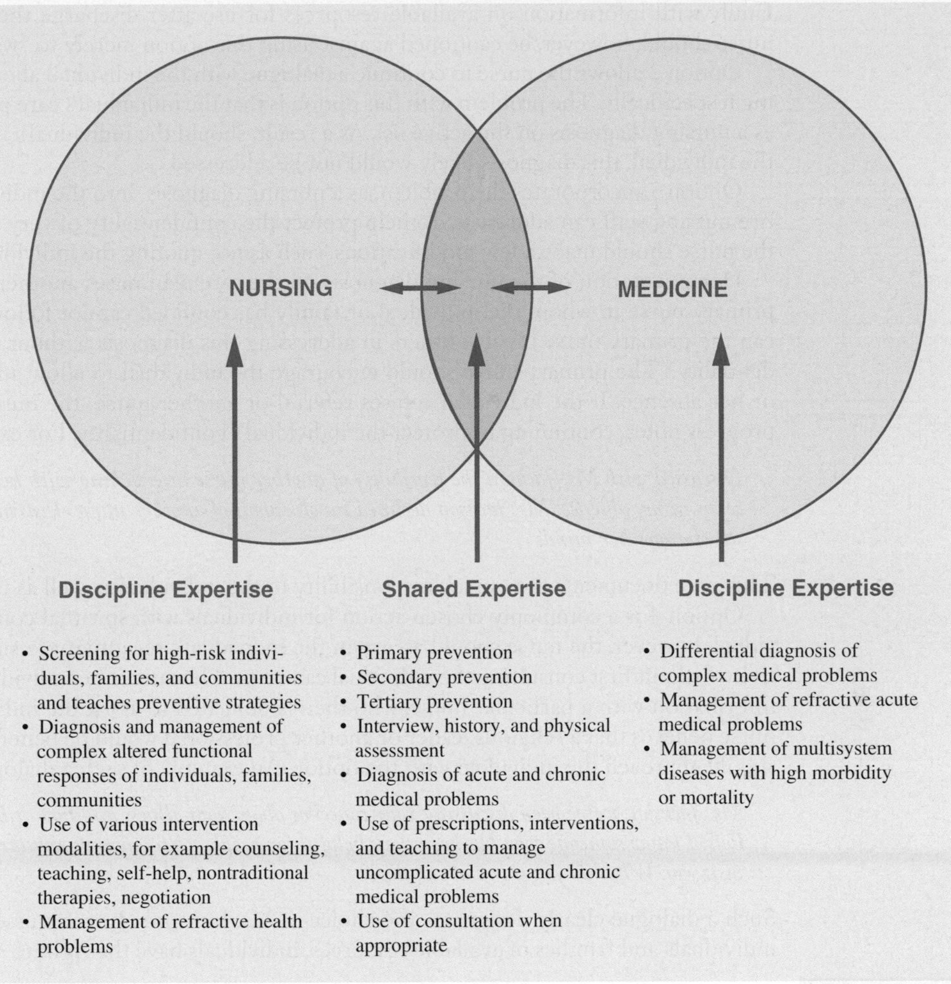

NURSING
MEDICINE
Discipline Expertise
Shared Expertise
Discipline Expertise
• Screening for high-risk individuals, families, and communities and teaches preventive strategies
• Diagnosis and management of complex altered functional responses of individuals, families, communities
• Use of various intervention modalities, for example counseling, teaching, self-help, nontraditional therapies, negotiation
• Management of refractive health problems
• Primary prevention
• Secondary prevention
• Tertiary prevention
• Interview, history, and physical assessment
• Diagnosis of acute and chronic medical problems
• Use of prescriptions, interventions, and teaching to manage uncomplicated acute and chronic medical problems
• Use of consultation when appropriate
• Differential diagnosis of complex medical problems
• Management of refractive acute medical problems
• Management of multisystem diseases with high morbidity or mortality

FIGURE 1.1 Domains of expertise of primary care nurse practitioners and primary care physicians. (©1995, 2014 by Lynda Juall Carpenito.)

Nurses have a responsibility to make nursing diagnoses and to prescribe nursing treatments. Inherent in the diagnostic process and planning of care is the responsibility to ascertain that there is permission to write, treat, or refer the diagnosis as appropriate.

When an individual shares personal information or emotions with the nurse, does this information automatically become part of the individual's record or care plan? The nurse has two basic obligations to an individual: (1) to address applicable nursing diagnoses and (2) to protect the individual's confidentiality. The nurse is *not* obligated to pass on all of an individual's nursing diagnoses to other nurses, as long as the nurse can ensure that all diagnoses are addressed.

Consider the following example: Ms. Jackson, 45 years old, is hospitalized for treatment of ovarian cancer. At one point, she states to the nurse, "The God I worship did this to me, and I hate Him for it." Further discussion validates that Ms. Jackson is disturbed about her feelings and changes in her previous beliefs. From these assessment data, the nurse develops the nursing diagnosis *Spiritual Distress* related to conflict between disease occurrence and religious faith. But what should the nurse do with the information, which Ms. Jackson makes clear she considers confidential? The nurse can assist Ms. Jackson with this nursing diagnosis through several different options:

1. Apprising her of available community resources for follow-up assistance in dealing with her spiritual distress
2. Continuing to assist her to explore her feelings and using the nurse's notes to reflect discussions (without using quotation marks to denote her actual words)
3. Recording the nursing diagnosis *Spiritual Distress* on the care plan and developing appropriate interventions
4. Referring her to an appropriate spiritual advisor

Option 1 returns the problem to the individual for management after discharge. Sometimes the nature of a problem and its priority among the individual's other problems make providing the individual or the family with information on available resources for use after discharge the most appropriate option. The nurse should, however, be cautioned against using this option merely to "wash one's hands" of a problem.

Option 2 allows the nurse to continue a dialogue with the individual about the issue, but without divulging it specifically. The problem with this option is that the individual's care plan will not reflect this problem as a nursing diagnosis on the active list. As a result, should the individual's nurse become unable to care for the individual, this diagnosis likely would not be addressed.

Option 3 incorporates the problem, as a nursing diagnosis, into the individual's care plan, where the entire nursing staff can address it. To help protect the confidentiality of very sensitive disclosed information, the nurse should make a few modifications, such as not quoting the individual's statements exactly.

Documentation of the nursing diagnosis on the care plan raises another possible dilemma. What if the primary nurse in whom the individual or family has confided cannot follow the diagnosis full time? How can the primary nurse involve others in addressing this diagnosis without violating the individual's confidentiality? The primary nurse should encourage the individual to allow another nurse to intervene in his or her absence. If the individual refuses referral or another nurse, the nurse should document this in the progress notes, continuing to protect the individual's confidentiality. For example:

Discussed with Ms. Jackson the feasibility of another nurse intervening with her regarding her spiritual concerns in my absence. Ms. Jackson declined involvement of another nurse. Instructed her on whom to contact if she changes her mind.

This note documents the nurse's responsibility to the individual as well as the nurse's accountability.

Option 4 is a commonly chosen action for individuals with spiritual conflicts. Before referring an individual, however, the nurse should ascertain the individual's receptivity to such a referral. To assume receptivity without first consulting the individual can be problematic. The individual chose to share very personal information with a particular nurse, who then is obligated to assist the individual with the problem. If the nurse believes that a religious leader or another professional would be beneficial to the individual, the nurse should approach the individual with the option. An example of such a dialogue follows:

Ms. Jackson, we've been discussing your concerns about your illness and how it has changed your spiritual beliefs. I know someone who has been very helpful for people with concerns similar to yours. I'd like to ask her to visit you. What do you think about this?

Such a dialogue clearly designates the choice as Ms. Jackson's. Just as nurses have an obligation to inform individuals and families of available resources, individuals have the right to accept or reject these resources.

SUMMARY

Unfortunately, nursing diagnosis has been maligned as not clinically useful. What is not clinically useful are the documentation systems that nurses are forced to use. These systems are repetitive and burdensome.

Nursing diagnosis provides nurses with the exact language to describe person/family responses that are unhealthy. Nursing diagnosis directs nurses to focus on problems beyond the obvious medical diagnosis or procedure. Thus, when a person is compromised post stroke, the nurse can address Risk for Caregiver Role Strain with all family members to prevent caregiver burnout. This is a powerful nursing diagnosis that can profoundly impact the individual and family members.

Professional nurses must understand the pathophysiology of medical diagnoses and the associated complications and treatments. They monitor the individual's responses, detect early changes in physiologic status, and initiate appropriate treatment and/or consultation.

Expertise in both sciences is critical for the well-being of the patients, families, and communities whose care is entrusted to a professional nurse.

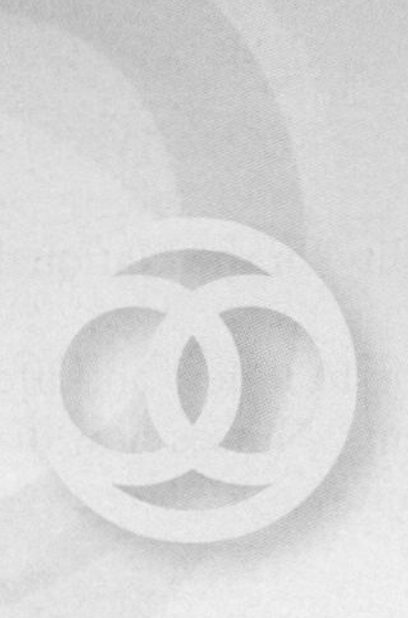

Chapter 2

Development of Nursing Diagnosis

Learning Objectives

After reading the chapter, the following questions should be answered:

- What are the benefits of a uniform language in nursing?
- What is nursing diagnosis?
- What is NANDA International?
- What is NANDA-I taxonomy?
- How are nursing diagnoses approved for clinical use?

What Are the Benefits of a Uniform Language in Nursing?

Before the development of a classification or list of nursing diagnoses, nurses used whatever word they wanted to describe client problems. For example, nurses might have described an individual recovering from surgery as "the appendectomy," another individual as "the diabetic," and another individual as "difficult." Clearly, knowing that a person has diabetes brings to mind blood sugar problems and risk for infection, so the focus is on common problems or risk factors derived from medical diagnoses. If the individual with diabetes or surgery had another problem that needed nursing attention, this problem would have gone undiagnosed. Before 1972, not only did nurses lack the terms to describe problems (except medical diagnoses), but they also did not have assessment questions to uncover such problems.

The need for a common, consistent language for medicine was identified more than 200 years ago. If physicians chose to use random words to describe their clinical situations, then

- How could they communicate with one another? With nurses?
- How could they organize research?
- How could they educate new physicians?
- How could they improve quality if they could not retrieve data systematically to determine which interventions improved the individual's condition?

For example, before the formal labeling of AIDS, defining or studying the disease was difficult, if not impossible. Often, medical records of affected individuals would show various diagnoses or causes of death, such as sepsis, cerebral hemorrhage, or pneumonia, because the AIDS diagnosis did not exist. Every physician in the world uses the same terminology for medical diagnoses. As new diagnoses are discovered, all medical clinicians can access the research using the same words.

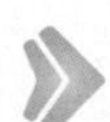

Carp's Cues

By definition, *diagnosis* is the careful, critical study of something to determine its nature. The question is not *whether* nurses can diagnose, but *what* nurses can diagnose.

What Is Nursing Diagnosis?

In 1953, Fry introduced the term *nursing diagnosis* to describe a step necessary in developing a nursing care plan. Over the next 20 years, references to nursing diagnosis appeared sporadically in the literature.

In 1973, the American Nurses Association (ANA) published its *Standards of Practice*; in 1980, it followed with its *Social Policy Statement*, which defined nursing as "the diagnosis and treatment of human response to actual or potential health problems." Most state nurse practice acts describe nursing in accordance with the ANA definition.

In March 1990, at the Ninth Conference of the North American Nursing Diagnosis Association (NANDA), the General Assembly approved an official definition of nursing diagnosis (NANDA, 1990):

> *Nursing diagnosis is a clinical judgment about individual, family, or community responses to actual or potential health problems/life processes. Nursing diagnosis provides the basis for selection of nursing interventions to achieve outcomes for which the nurse is accountable.*

This definition was revised from "the nurse is accountable" to "the nurse has accountability" at the National Conference of NANDA International in Miami (November 2009).

It is important to also emphasize that the responses called nursing diagnoses can be to illness and life events. Previously, nurses focused more on responses to medical conditions or treatments. Nurses now diagnose and treat responses to life events such as parenting, aging parents, and school failure.

What Is NANDA International?

In 1973, the first conference on nursing diagnosis was held to identify nursing knowledge and to establish a classification system suitable for computerization. From this conference developed the National Group for the Classification of Nursing Diagnosis, composed of nurses from different regions of the United States and Canada, representing all elements of the profession: practice, education, and research. In 1982, the North American Diagnosis Association (NANDA) was established.

In 2002, the organization was renamed NANDA International (NANDA-I). In addition to reviewing and accepting nursing diagnoses for addition to the list, NANDA-I also reviews previously accepted nursing diagnoses. Since the first conference, NANDA-I has grown with membership of nurses from every continent.

NANDA-I's official journal, *Nursing Diagnosis*, was first published in March 1990. The journal is now named *International Journal of Nursing Terminologies and Classifications*. This journal aims to promote the development, refinement, and application of nursing diagnoses and to serve as a forum for issues pertaining to the development and classification of nursing knowledge.

What Is NANDA-I Taxonomy?

A *taxonomy* is a type of classification, the theoretical study of systematic classifications including their bases, principles, procedures, and rules. The work of the initial theorist group at the third national conference and subsequently of the NANDA-I taxonomic committee produced the beginnings of a conceptual framework for the diagnostic classification system. This framework was named NANDA-I Nursing Diagnosis Taxonomy I, which comprised nine patterns of human response. In 2000, NANDA-I approved a new Taxonomy II, which has 13 domains, 106 classes, and 155 diagnoses (NANDA-I, 2001).

Table 2.1 illustrates the 13 domains and associated definitions. The second level, classes, may be useful as assessment criteria. The third level, diagnostic concepts, is the nursing diagnosis labels and is most useful for clinicians. Changes in terminology were made for consistency; for example, *Altered Nutrition* was changed to *Imbalanced Nutrition*. An example of one domain is

Domain 4	Activity/Rest	
Class 1	Sleep/Rest	
Diagnostic concepts	00095	Insomnia
	00096	Sleep Deprivation
	00165	Readiness for Enhanced Sleep
	00198	Disturbed Sleep Pattern

How Are Nursing Diagnoses Approved for Clinical Use?

Some believe that nursing diagnoses are created by NANDA-I. Often it is asked why NANDA-I does not have more nursing diagnoses for persons with mental illnesses. Nursing diagnoses are not developed by NANDA-I.

NANDA-I–approved nursing diagnoses can be clinically relevant only if clinical nurses are involved in their development. It is the responsibility of clinical nurses to submit missing nursing diagnoses.

The Diagnosis Development Committee (DDC) of NANDA-I is responsible for reviewing and assisting others to develop and refine their proposed diagnoses. The committee responds to submissions from nurses worldwide. After the committee determines that a submitted diagnosis meets the definition criteria for a nursing diagnosis and contains all of the required elements, the diagnosis is released for membership review and approval. Submissions can be for new nursing diagnoses or for recommendations for revisions. In addition, the DDC regularly critiques previously accepted nursing diagnoses for revision and sometimes for deletion. The process is ongoing and with the product nursing diagnosis always in refinement. Some diagnoses are retired if they are incomplete and revisions have not been submitted.

Table 2.1 TAXONOMY II DOMAINS AND DEFINITIONS

Domain 1	Health Promotion	Awareness of well-being or normality of function and the strategies used to maintain control of and enhance that well-being or normality of function
Domain 2	Nutrition	Activities of taking in, assimilating, and using nutrients for the purposes of tissue maintenance, tissue repair, and production of energy
Domain 3	Elimination and Exchange	Secretion and excretion of waste products from the body
Domain 4	Activity/Rest	Production, conservation, expenditure, or balance of energy resources
Domain 5	Perception/Cognition	Human information processing system including attention, orientation, sensation, perception, cognition, and communication
Domain 6	Self-Perception	Awareness about the self
Domain 7	Role Relationships	Positive and negative connections or associations between people or groups of people and the means by which those connections are demonstrated
Domain 8	Sexuality	Sexual identity, sexual function, and reproduction
Domain 9	Coping/Stress Tolerance	Contending with life events/life processes
Domain 10	Life Principles	Principles underlying conduct, thought, and behavior about acts, customs, or institutions viewed as being true or having intrinsic worth
Domain 11	Safety/Protection	Freedom from danger, physical injury, or immune system damage; preservation from loss; and protection of safety and security
Domain 12	Comfort	Sense of mental, physical, or social well-being or ease
Domain 13	Growth/Development	Age-appropriate increases in physical dimensions, maturation of organ systems, and/or progression through the developmental milestones

Source: NANDA International. (2012). *Nursing diagnosis: Definitions and classification 2012–2014*. West Sussex, UK: Wiley-Blackwell.

SUMMARY

A classification system for nursing diagnoses has been in continual development for the past 30 years. During this period, the initial question "Does nursing really need a classification system?" has been replaced by "How can such a system be developed in a scientifically sound manner?" The ANA has designated NANDA-I as the official organization to develop this classification system. Despite problems, through the concerted effort of many fine clinical nurses, nurse researchers, and other nursing professionals and organizations, this evolving classification system increasingly reflects both the art and science of nursing.

Chapter 3

Types and Components of Nursing Diagnoses

Learning Objectives

After reading the chapter, the following questions should be answered:

- What are the differences between problem-focused risk and possible nursing diagnoses?
- What is a health-promotion diagnosis?
- What are syndrome nursing diagnoses?
- When can a non–NANDA-I nursing diagnosis be used?
- When should unknown etiology be used?
- How can errors be avoided in diagnostic statements?

This chapter will focus on types of nursing diagnoses and writing diagnostic statements. There are five types of nursing diagnoses: problem-focused, risk, possible, health promotion, and syndrome.

Problem-Focused Nursing Diagnoses[1]

A *problem-focused nursing diagnosis* "describes human responses to health conditions/life processes that exist in an individual, family, or community. It is supported by defining characteristics (manifestations, signs, and symptoms) that cluster in patterns of related cues or inferences" (NANDA-I, 2009). This type of nursing diagnosis has four components: label, definition, defining characteristics, and related factors.

Label

The label should be in clear, concise terms that convey the meaning of the diagnosis.

Definition

The definition should add clarity to the diagnostic label. It should also help to differentiate a particular diagnosis from similar diagnoses.

Defining Characteristics

For problem-focused nursing diagnoses, defining characteristics are signs and symptoms that, when seen together, represent the nursing diagnosis. If a diagnosis has been researched, defining characteristics can be separated into major and minor designations. Table 3.1 represents major and minor defining characteristics for the researched diagnosis, *Defensive Coping* (Norris & Kunes-Connell, 1987).

- ***Major***: For researched diagnoses, at least one must be present under the 80% to 100% grouping.
- ***Minor***: These characteristics provide supporting evidence but may not be present.

Most defining characteristics listed under a nursing diagnosis are not separated into major and minor.

Related Factors

In problem-focused nursing diagnoses, related factors are contributing factors that have influenced the change in health status. Such factors can be grouped into four categories:

1. ***Pathophysiologic, Biologic, or Psychological.*** Examples include compromised oxygen transport and compromised circulation. Inadequate circulation can cause *Impaired Skin Integrity.*

[1]NANDA-I changed the name for actual nursing diagnosis to problem-focused nursing diagnosis in 2013.

Table 3.1 FREQUENCY SCORES FOR DEFINING CHARACTERISTICS OF DEFENSIVE COPING

Defining Characteristics	Frequency Scores (%)
Major (80%–100%)	
Denial of obvious problems/weaknesses	88
Projection of blame/responsibility	87
Rationalizes failures	86
Hypersensitive to slight criticism	84
Minor (50%–79%)	
Grandiosity	79
Superior attitude toward others	76
Difficulty in establishing/maintaining relationships	74
Hostile laughter or ridicule of others	71
Difficulty in testing perceptions against reality	62
Lack of follow-through or participation in treatment or therapy	56

Norris, J., & Kunes-Connell, M. (1987). Self-esteem disturbance: A clinical validation study. In A. McLane (Ed.), *Classification of nursing diagnoses: Proceedings of the seventh NANDA national conference*. St. Louis, MO: CV Mosby.

2. ***Treatment-Related.*** Examples include medications, therapies, surgery, and diagnostic study. Specifically, medications can cause nausea. Radiation can cause fatigue. Scheduled surgery can cause *Anxiety*.
3. ***Situational.*** Examples include environmental, home, community, institution, personal, life experiences, and roles. Specifically, a flood in a community can contribute to *Risk for Infection*; divorce can cause *Grieving*; obesity can contribute to *Activity Intolerance*.
4. ***Maturational.*** Examples include age-related influences, such as in children and the elderly. Specifically, the elderly are at risk for *Social Isolation*; infants are at *Risk for Injury*; and adolescents are at *Risk for Infection*.

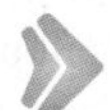

Carp's Cues

Related factors or contributing factors are the second part of a nursing diagnosis statement. Some of NANDA-I nursing diagnoses labels have the etiology in label as Death Anxiety, Labor Pain. Thus it becomes problematic when the clinician attempts to write a diagnostic statement as Labor Pain related to labor.

Problem-focused nursing diagnoses are validated by signs and symptoms (or defining characteristics). Some NANDA-I diagnoses represent signs/symptoms of that appear under other nursing diagnoses. For example, *Self-Neglect* can be associated with substance abuse, grieving, depression, confusion, homelessness and influences socialization, relationships, etc.

Anger is human response to multiple situations. Anger can be constructive or destructive. Anger can be found in the defining characteristics of many nursing diagnoses, for example, *Risk for Violence to Others, Dysfunctional Family Processes, Anxiety, Acute Confusion*. Should anger be a nursing diagnosis or it more clinically useful when with more assessments yield a more specific nursing diagnosis?

INTERACTIVE EXERCISE 3.1 To determine the presence of a problem-focused diagnosis, ask, "Are major signs and symptoms of the diagnosis in this person?"

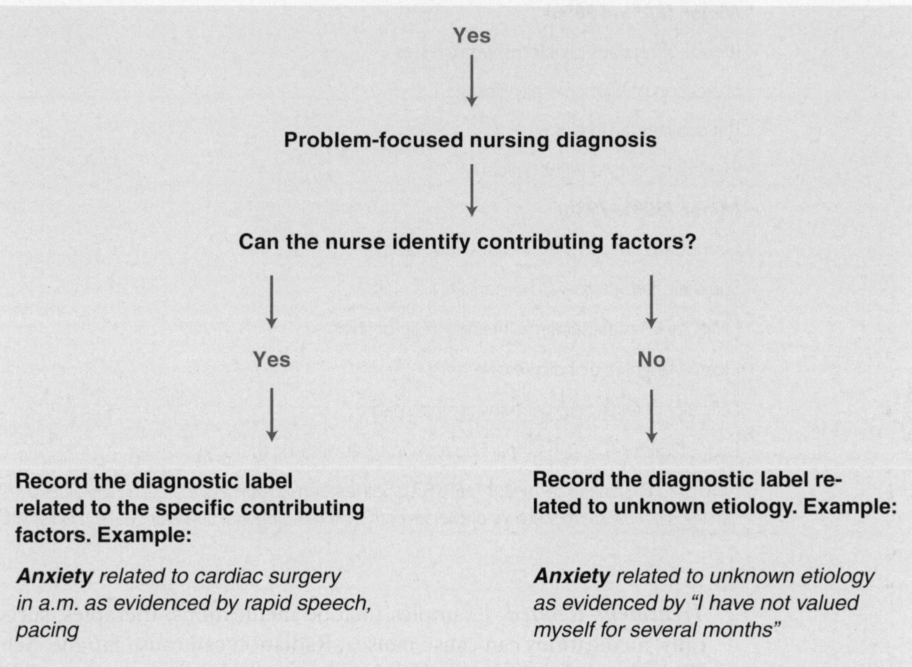
Yes
Problem-focused nursing diagnosis
Can the nurse identify contributing factors?
Yes
No
Record the diagnostic label related to the specific contributing factors. Example:
Anxiety related to cardiac surgery in a.m. as evidenced by rapid speech, pacing
Record the diagnostic label related to unknown etiology. Example:
Anxiety related to unknown etiology as evidenced by "I have not valued myself for several months"

Risk and High-Risk Nursing Diagnoses

NANDA-I defines a *risk nursing diagnosis* as "human responses to health conditions/life processes that may develop in a vulnerable individual, family, or community. It is supported by risk factors that contribute to increased vulnerability" (NANDA-I, 2009).

The concept of "at risk" is useful clinically. Nurses routinely prevent problems in people experiencing similar situations such as surgery or childbirth who are not at high risk. For example, all postoperative individuals are at risk for infection. All women postdelivery are at risk for hemorrhage. Thus, there are expected or predictive diagnoses for all individuals who have undergone surgery while on chemotherapy or with a fractured hip.

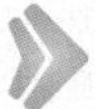

Carp's Cues

Nurses do not need to include all risk diagnoses on the individual's care plan in the hospital. In fact, it is unproductive for nurses (not students) to write text of the same predicted care repeatedly. Students are expected to identify the predicted care until they are experienced with that care. Instead, this diagnosis is part of the unit's standard of care (see Chapter 6 for a discussion of standards).

All persons admitted to the hospital are at *Risk for Infection* related to increased microorganisms in the environment, risk of person-to-person transmission, and invasive tests and therapies. Refer to Box 3.1 for an illustration of this standard diagnosis and how it is individualized to become a high-risk diagnosis. The high-risk concept is very useful for persons who have additional risk factors that make them more vulnerable for the problem to occur. In the hospital or other health care facilities, individuals should be assessed if they are at high risk for falls, infection, or delayed transition. High-risk individuals need additional preventive measures.

Box 3.1 REVISING A STANDARD SURGICAL CARE PLAN NURSING DIAGNOSIS

Standard Nursing Diagnosis

Risk for Infection related to incision and loss of protective skin barrier

Individual Nursing Diagnosis

High Risk for Infection related to incision, loss of protective skin barrier, and high blood glucose levels secondary to diabetes mellitus

Label

In a risk nursing diagnosis, the term *Risk for* precedes the nursing diagnosis label or *High Risk for* if this concept is used.

Definition

As in an actual nursing diagnosis, the definition in a risk nursing diagnosis expresses a clear, precise meaning of the diagnosis.

Risk Factors

Risk factors for risk and high-risk nursing diagnoses represent those situations that increase the vulnerability of the individual or group. These factors differentiate high-risk individuals and groups from all others in the same population who are at some risk. The validation to support an actual diagnosis is signs and symptoms (e.g., *Impaired Skin Integrity related to immobility secondary to pain as evidenced by 2-cm erythematous sacral lesion*). In contrast, the validation to support a high-risk diagnosis is risk factors (e.g., *High Risk for Impaired Skin Integrity related to immobility secondary to pain*). There is no evidence of pressure ulcers at this time, but there are risk factors.

Related Factors

The related factors for risk nursing diagnoses are the same risk factors previously explained for problem-focused nursing diagnoses. The components of a risk nursing diagnostic statement are discussed later in this chapter.

INTERACTIVE EXERCISE 3.2 To determine the presence of a risk diagnosis, ask, "Are major signs and symptoms of the diagnosis found in this person?"

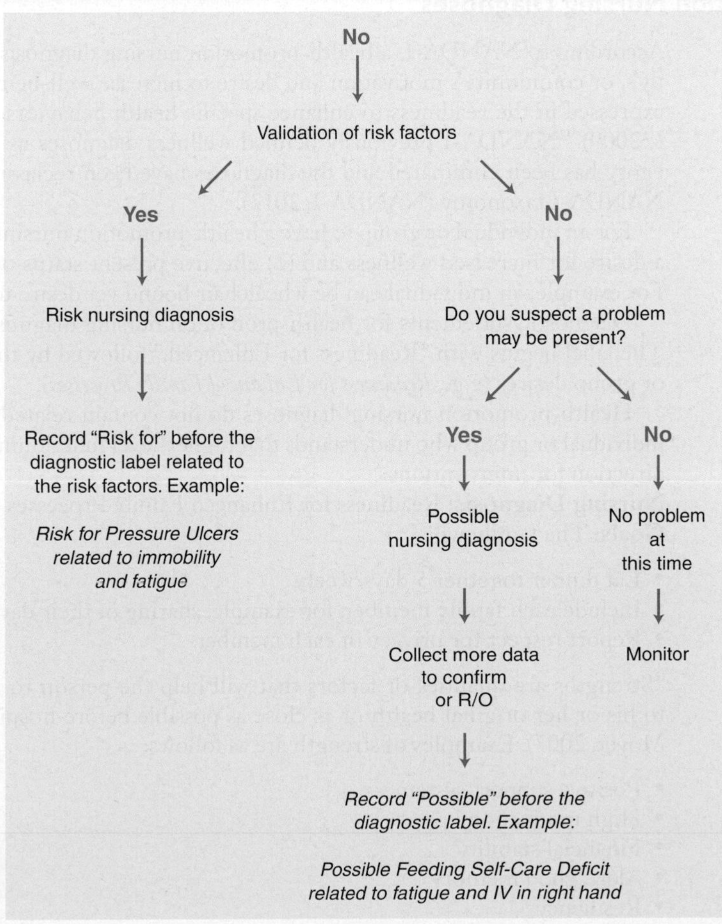

Possible Nursing Diagnoses

Possible nursing diagnoses are statements that describe a suspected problem requiring additional data. It is unfortunate that many nurses have been socialized to avoid appearing tentative. In scientific decision making, a tentative approach is not a sign of weakness or indecision, but an essential part of the process. The nurse should delay a final diagnosis until he or she has gathered and analyzed all necessary information to arrive at a sound scientific conclusion. Physicians demonstrate tentativeness with the statement *rule out (R/O)*. Nurses also should adopt a tentative position until they have completed data collection and evaluation and can confirm or R/O.

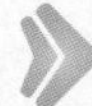

Carp's Cues

NANDA-I does not address possible nursing diagnoses because diagnoses are not a classification issue; they are an option for clinical nurses. With a possible nursing diagnosis, the nurse has some, but insufficient, data to support a problem-focused or risk diagnosis at this time.

Possible nursing diagnoses are two-part statements consisting of

1. The possible nursing diagnosis
2. The "related to" data that lead the nurse to suspect the diagnosis

An example is *Possible Disturbed Self-Concept related to recent loss of role responsibilities secondary to worsening of multiple sclerosis.*

When a nurse records a possible nursing diagnosis, he or she alerts other nurses to assess for more data to support or R/O the tentative diagnosis. After additional data collection, the nurse may take one of three actions:

1. Confirm the presence of major signs and symptoms, thus labeling a problem-focused diagnosis.
2. Confirm the presence of potential risk factors, thus labeling a risk diagnosis.
3. Rule out the presence of a diagnosis (problem-focused or risk) at this time.

Health-Promotion Nursing Diagnoses

According to NANDA-I, a health-promotion nursing diagnosis is "a clinical judgment of a person's, family's, or community's motivation and desire to increase well-being and actualize human health potential as expressed in the readiness to enhance specific health behaviors, such as nutrition and exercise (NANDA-I, 2009)." NANDA-I previously defined wellness diagnoses as a separate type of diagnosis, but this category has been eliminated and the diagnoses have been reclassified as health-promotion diagnoses in the NANDA-I taxonomy (NANDA-I, 2012).

For an individual or group to have a health-promotion nursing diagnosis, two cues should be present: (1) a desire for increased wellness and (2) effective present status or function in that specific health behavior. For example, an individual can be wheelchair bound yet desire to enhance their already good nutrition.

Diagnostic statements for health-promotion nursing diagnoses are one part, containing the label only. The label begins with "Readiness for Enhanced," followed by the higher-level wellness that the individual or group desires (e.g., *Readiness for Enhanced Family Processes*).

Health-promotion nursing diagnoses do not contain related factors. Inherent in these diagnoses is an individual or group who understands that higher-level functioning is available. The related goals would give direction for interventions:

Nursing Diagnosis: Readiness for Enhanced Family Processes
Goals: The family will

- Eat dinner together 5 days/week.
- Include each family member, for example, sharing of their day, family decisions.
- Report respect for privacy of each member.

"Strengths are qualities or factors that will help the person to recover, cope with stressors, and progress to his or her original health or as close as possible before hospitalization, illness, or surgery" (Carpenito-Moyet, 2007). Examples of strength are as follows:

- Positive support system
- High motivation
- Financial stability
- Alert, good memory
- Resiliency

Table 3.2 FUNCTIONAL HEALTH PATTERNS AND ASSOCIATED POSITIVE FUNCTIONING ASSESSMENT STATEMENTS

Functional Health Pattern	Positive Functioning Assessment Statements
1. Health perception–health management pattern	1. Positive health perception effective health management
2. Nutritional–metabolic pattern	2. Effective nutritional–metabolic pattern
3. Elimination pattern	3. Effective elimination pattern
4. Activity–exercise pattern	4. Effective activity–exercise pattern
5. Sleep–rest pattern	5. Effective sleep–rest pattern
6. Cognitive–perceptual pattern	6. Positive cognitive–perceptual pattern
7. Self-perception pattern	7. Positive self-perception pattern
8. Role–relationship pattern	8. Positive role–relationship pattern
9. Sexuality–reproductive pattern	9. Positive sexuality–reproductive pattern
10. Coping–stress intolerance pattern	10. Effective coping–stress tolerance pattern
11. Value–belief pattern	11. Positive value–belief pattern

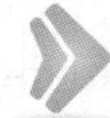

Carp's Cues

Strengths are different from health-promotion diagnoses. Table 3.2 lists statements that describe strengths for each of the 11 functional health patterns. When the nurse and individual conclude that there is positive functioning in a functional health pattern, this conclusion is an assessment conclusion, but by itself is not a nursing diagnosis. The nurse uses these data, for example strong religious beliefs can enhance coping with Death Anxiety to plan interventions for altered or at risk for altered functioning.

One could incorporate positive functioning assessment statements under each functional health pattern on the admission assessment tool, as illustrated by sleep–rest pattern (Box 3.2).

Syndrome Nursing Diagnoses

Syndrome nursing diagnoses are an interesting development in nursing diagnosis. They comprise a cluster of predicted actual or high-risk nursing diagnoses related to a certain event or situation. For example, Carlson-Catalino (1998) used an exploratory qualitative study of post–acute-phase battered women to identify 24 nursing diagnoses in all the subjects. This research supports a diagnosis of *Battered Woman Syndrome*. In medicine, syndromes cluster signs and symptoms, not diagnoses. In nursing, a cluster of signs and symptoms represents a single nursing diagnosis, not a syndrome nursing diagnosis.

Nurses should approach the development of syndrome diagnosis carefully. They must also dialogue with individuals to determine other nursing diagnoses indicating the need for individual–nurse interventions. The clinical advantage of a syndrome diagnosis is that it alerts the nurse to a "complex clinical condition requiring expert nursing assessments and interventions" (McCourt, 1991).

Frail elderly syndrome was accepted as a NANDA-I nursing diagnosis in 2013. The defining characteristics are other nursing diagnoses, which is consistent with the concept of a syndrome nursing diagnosis.

Diagnostic Statements

Nursing diagnostic statements can have one, two, or three parts. One-part statements contain only the diagnostic label, as in health-promotion and syndrome nursing diagnoses. Two-part statements contain the label and the factors that have contributed or could contribute to a change in health status, as in risk and possible diagnoses. Three-part statements contain the label, contributing factors, and signs and symptoms of the diagnosis, as in problem-focused diagnoses. Box 3.3 lists diagnostic statements with examples.

Box 3.2 SLEEP–REST PATTERN

Habits: ____ 8 hr/night ____ <8 hr __✓__ >8 hr ____ AM nap ____ PM nap

Feel rested after sleep __✓__ Yes ____ No

Problems: __✓__ None ____ Early waking ____ Insomnia ____ Nightmares

☒ Effective Sleep-Rest Pattern

Box 3.3 TYPES OF DIAGNOSTIC STATEMENTS

One-Part Statement

- Health-promotion nursing diagnoses (e.g., *Readiness for Enhanced Parenting, Readiness for Enhanced Nutrition*)
- Syndrome nursing diagnoses (e.g., *Disuse Syndrome, Rape-Trauma Syndrome*)

Two-Part Statement

- Risk nursing diagnoses (e.g., *Risk for Injury* related to lack of awareness of hazards)
- Possible nursing diagnoses (e.g., Possible *Disturbed Body Image* related to isolating behaviors postsurgery)

Three-Part Statement

- Problem-focused nursing diagnoses (e.g., *Impaired Skin Integrity* related to prolonged immobility secondary to fractured pelvis, as evidenced by a 2-cm lesion on back)

Writing Diagnostic Statements

Three-part diagnostic statements (problem-focused nursing diagnoses) contain the following elements:

Problem		Etiology		Symptom
Diagnostic label	*related to*	Contributing factors	*as evidenced by*	Signs and symptoms

In two-part and three-part diagnostic statements, *related to* reflects a relationship between the first and second parts of the statement. The more specific that the second part of the statement is, the more specialized the interventions can be. For example, the diagnosis *Noncompliance* stated alone usually conveys the negative implication that the individual is not cooperating. When the nurse relates the noncompliance to be contributing factors, however, this diagnosis can transmit a very different message:

- *Noncompliance related to negative side effects of a drug (reduced libido, fatigue), as evidenced by "I stopped my blood pressure medicine."*
- *Noncompliance related to inability to understand the need for weekly blood pressure measurements, as evidenced by "I don't keep my appointments if I'm busy."*

Using "Unknown Etiology" in Diagnostic Statements

If the defining characteristics of a nursing diagnosis are present, but the etiologic and contributing factors are unknown, the statement can include the phrase *unknown etiology* (e.g., *Fear related to unknown etiology, as evidenced by rapid speech, pacing, and "I'm worried."*). The use of *unknown etiology* alerts the nurse and other members of the nursing staff to assess for contributing factors as they intervene for the current problem.

Syndrome diagnoses contain the related factors or etiology in the label. Rape Syndrome is caused by rape, Disuse Syndrome is caused by disuse, thus no related factors are needed. As more specific diagnoses evolve, it may become unnecessary for the nurse to write *related to* statements. Instead, many future nursing diagnoses may be one-part statements, such as *Functional Incontinence* or *Death Anxiety*.

Avoiding Errors in Diagnostic Statements

As with any other skill, writing diagnostic statements takes knowledge and practice. To increase the accuracy and usefulness of diagnostic statements (and to reduce frustration), nurses should avoid several common errors. See Table 3.3 for examples of errors to avoid.

Nursing diagnostic statements should not be written in terms of:

- Cues (e.g., crying, hemoglobin level)
- Goals (e.g., should perform own colostomy care)
- Individual needs (e.g., needs to walk every shift; needs to express fears)
- Nursing needs (e.g., change dressing, check blood pressure)

Nurses should avoid legally inadvisable or judgmental statements, such as

- *Fear related to frequent beatings by husband*
- *Ineffective Family Coping related to mother-in-law's continual harassment of daughter-in-law*
- *Risk for Impaired Parenting related to low IQ of mother*

Table 3.3 EXAMPLES OF ERRORS TO AVOID WHEN WRITING DIAGNOSTIC STATEMENTS

Incorrect	Correct
Medical Diagnoses	
Risk for Infection related to diabetes mellitus	*Risk for Infection related to increased microorganism activity with hyperglycemia*
Treatments or Equipment	
Imbalanced Nutrition related to feeding tube	*Impaired Comfort related to irritation of feeding tube*
Medication Side Effects	
Risk for Infection related to chemotherapy	*Risk for Infection related to decreased white blood cells secondary to chemotherapy*
Diagnostic studies	
Cardiac catheterization	*Anxiety related to scheduled cardiac cauterization*
Situations	
Dying	*Powerlessness related to his course of terminal illness*

Carp's Cues

A nursing diagnosis should not be related to a medical diagnosis, such as *Disturbed Self-Concept related to multiple sclerosis* or *Anxiety related to myocardial infarction*. If the use of a medical diagnosis adds clarity to the diagnosis, the nurse can link it to the statement with the phrase *secondary to* (e.g., *Disturbed Self-Concept related to recent losses of role responsibilities secondary to multiple sclerosis, as evidenced by "My mother comes every day to run my house,"* or *"I can no longer be the woman in charge of my house."*)

INTERACTIVE EXERCISE 3.3 Examine the following diagnostic statements and determine whether they are written correctly or incorrectly.

1. Anxiety related to AIDS
2. Chronic Sorrow related to crying and episodes of inability to sleep
3. Risk for Injury related to dizziness secondary to high blood pressure
4. Impaired Parenting related to frequent screaming at child
5. Risk for Functional Constipation related to reports of bowel movements once a week

SUMMARY Nursing has been and continues to be defined by what we do not know as much as by what we know. The lack of consistent terminology or use of medical diagnoses exclusively contributes to this misrepresentation of professional nursing. Nursing diagnosis provides the terminology to distinguish the unique knowledge of nursing from other health care professionals.

Integrating nursing diagnosis into practice is a collective and personal process. Collectively, the nursing profession has to develop a documentation system that presents the predictive care (standardized care plan) and allows the nurse to add to this plan, instead of requiring each nurse to select the expected care needed over and over.

Each nurse has a responsibility to assess individuals/families for problems beyond those outlined in the standardized plan. Diagnosing and intervening with nursing diagnoses such as *Grieving* or *Caregiver Role Strain* will enhance individual and family coping. Collectively and individually, these struggles will continue, but in the end the nursing profession and those in their care will benefit from nursing diagnosis.

Chapter 4

Nursing Diagnosis: What It Is, What It Is Not

Learning Objectives

After reading the chapter, the following questions should be answered:

- What is the bifocal clinical practice model?
- How do nursing diagnoses differ from collaborative problems?
- How are collaborative problems written?
- Is monitoring an intervention?

As discussed in Chapter 2, the official NANDA-I definition of nursing diagnosis reads, "Nursing diagnosis is a clinical judgment about an individual, family, or community response to actual or potential health problems or life processes. Nursing diagnosis provides the basis for selection of nursing interventions to achieve outcomes for which the nurse has accountability" (NANDA-I, 2009). But what about other clinical situations—those that nursing diagnosis does not cover, those that necessitates nursing intervention and medical interventions? Where do they fit within the scope of nursing practice? What about clinical situations in which both the nurses and physicians must prescribe interventions to achieve outcomes?

Collaboration With Other Disciplines

The practice of nursing requires three different types of nursing responsibilities:

1. Assessing for and validating nursing diagnoses, providing interventions for treatment, and evaluating progress
2. Monitoring for physiologic instability and collaborating with physicians/physician assistants and nurse practitioners, who determine medical treatment
3. Consulting with other disciplines (physical therapy, occupational therapy, social service, respiratory therapy, pharmacology) to increase the nurse's expertise in providing care to a particular individual

When nurses collaborate with other disciplines such as physical therapy, nutrition, respiratory therapy, and social service, they may offer recommendations for the management of a problem. These recommendations can be either made informally to the nurse and added to the care plan at the discretion of the nurse or ordered by the discipline on the order record according to the institutional policies.

Carp's Cues

Other disciplines should not add interventions to the care plan unless it is a multidiscipline care plan. These interventions on a multidiscipline care plan would indicate what discipline is prescribing and providing care. When the care plan is not multidisciplinary and a physical therapist has recommendations for nursing interventions for an individual, the nurse and the physical therapist will determine whether these interventions are to be added to the care plan. This is the same as when a physician requests a specialist to see an individual. The specialist usually does not write orders for the individual but instead communicates recommendations in a consultation report.

Bifocal Clinical Practice Model

In 1983, Carpenito introduced a model for practice that describes the clinical focus of professional nurses in addition to NANDA-I nursing diagnoses. This *bifocal clinical practice model* identifies the two clinical situations in which nurses intervene: one as primary prescriber and the other in collaboration with medicine. This model not only organizes the focus of nursing practice, but also helps distinguish nursing from other health-care disciplines (Fig. 4.1).

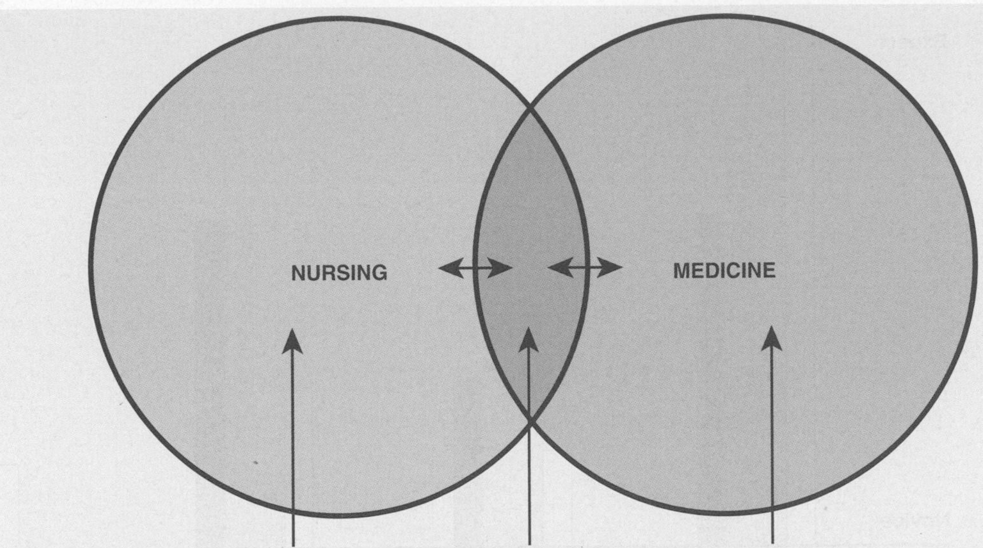

Nursing Discipline Expertise

- Interview, history, and physical assessment
- Screening for high risk individuals, families, and communities
- Teaching preventive strategies
- Diagnosis and management of compromised, problematic responses of individuals, families, and communities
- Use of various intervention modalities (e.g., counseling, teaching, self-help, nontraditional therapies, negotiations)
- Management of refractive health problems

Collaborative Nursing Expertise

- Monitoring for early detection of physiologic complications of medical diagnosis, treatment
- Initiating nurse-prescribed interventions and physician/NP/PA-prescribed interventions to prevent morbidity and mortality

Medical Discipline Expertise

- Interview, history, and physical assessment
- Diagnosis of acute and chronic medical problems
- Use of prescriptions, interventions, and teaching to manage acute and chronic medical conditions
- Differential diagnosis of complex medical problems
- Management of refractive medical problems
- Management of multisystem diseases with high mortality and morbidity
- Use of consultation when appropriate

FIGURE 4.1 Domains of expertise of professional nurses and physicians.

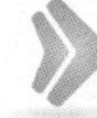

Carp's Cues

Collaborative problems are specifically defined as physiological; problems that are at risk to occur or have occurred that require both medicine and nursing interventions to treat. Collaboration with other disciplines (e.g., physical therapy, nutrition, respiratory therapy, and the use of nursing diagnosis) is discussed earlier.

Nursing derives its knowledge from various disciplines, including biology, medicine, pharmacology, psychology, nutrition, and physical therapy. Nursing differs from other disciplines in its broad range of knowledge. Figure 4.2 illustrates the varied types of this knowledge as compared with other disciplines. Certainly, the nutritionist has more expertise in the field of nutrition, and the pharmacist in the field of therapeutic pharmacology, than any nurse has. But every nurse brings knowledge of nutrition and pharmacology to individual interactions that is appropriate for most clinical situations. (Note that when a nurse's knowledge is insufficient, nursing practice calls for consultation with appropriate disciplines.)

No other discipline has this wide knowledge base, possibly explaining why past attempts to substitute other disciplines for nursing have proved costly and ultimately unsuccessful. For this reason, any workable model for nursing practice must encompass all the varied situations in which nurses intervene while also identifying situations in nursing that nonnursing personnel must address.

Nursing prescribes for and treats individual and group *responses* to situations. These situations can be organized into five categories:

1. Pathophysiologic (e.g., myocardial infarction, borderline personality, burns)
2. Treatment-related (e.g., anticoagulant therapy, dialysis, arteriography)

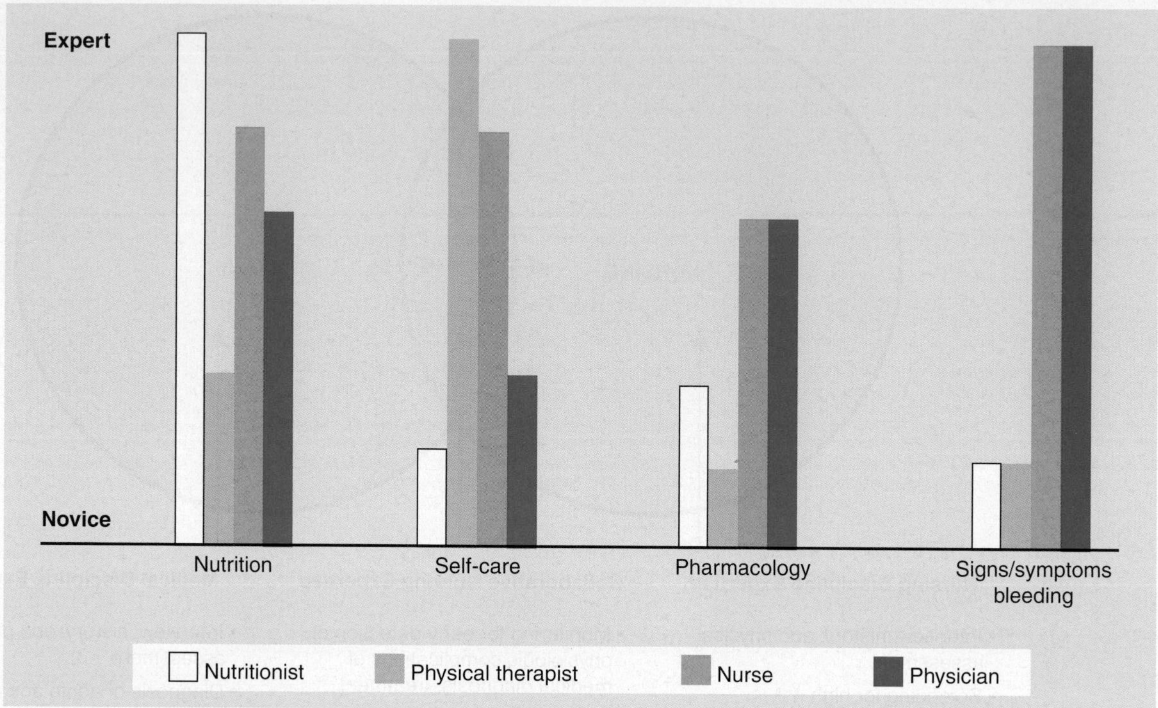

FIGURE 4.2 Comparison of types of knowledge by discipline.

3. Personal (e.g., dying, divorce, relocation)
4. Environmental (e.g., overcrowded school, no handrails on steps, rodents)
5. Maturational (e.g., peer pressure, parenthood, aging)

The bifocal clinical practice model, diagrammed in Figure 4.3, identifies these responses as either *nursing diagnoses* or *collaborative problems*. Together, nursing diagnoses and collaborative problems represent the

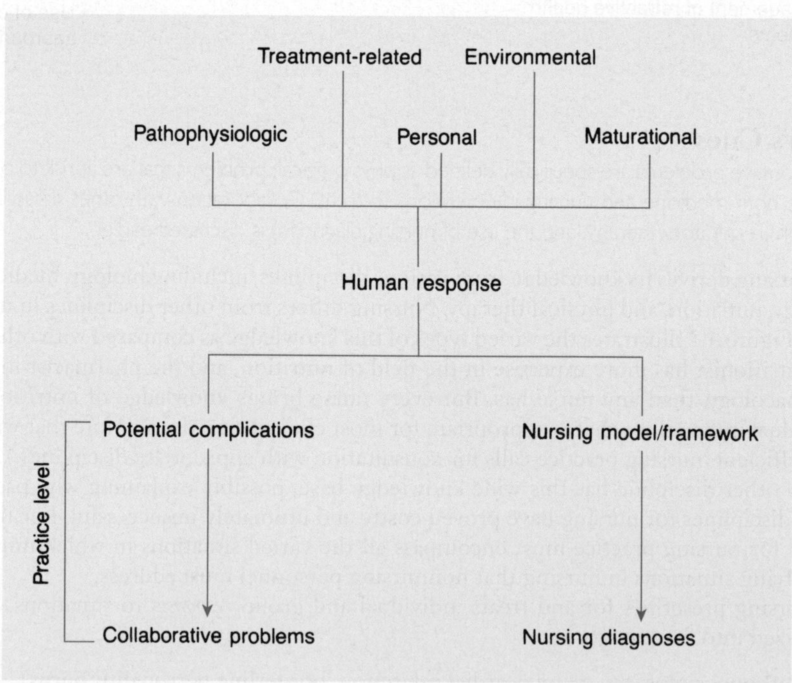

FIGURE 4.3 Bifocal clinical nursing model. (© 1985 by Lynda Juall Carpenito.)

range of conditions that necessitate nursing care. The major assumptions in the bifocal clinical practice model are as follows:

1. **Client**[1]
   - Has the power for self-healing
   - Continually interrelates with the environment
   - Makes health decisions according to individual priorities
   - Is a unified whole, seeking balance
   - Has individual worth and dignity
   - Is an expert on own health
2. **Health**
   - Is a dynamic, ever-changing state
   - Is defined by the individual
   - Is an expression of optimum physical, spiritual, and psychosocial well-being
   - Is the responsibility of the individual and the health-care system
3. **Environment**
   - Represents external factors, situations, and people who influence or are influenced by the individual
   - Includes physical and ecologic environments, life events, and treatment modalities
4. **Nursing**
   - Is accessed by the individual when he or she needs assistance to improve, restore, or maintain health or to achieve a peaceful death (Henderson & Nite, 1960)
   - Ensures the individual has the needed information for an informed consent
   - Supports the right of the individual to refuse recommendations
   - Engages the individual to assume responsibility in self-healing decisions and practices
   - Reduces or eliminates factors that can or do cause compromised functioning, for example, effects of diseases, relationship problems, comprehension barriers, financial issues

Understanding Collaborative Problems

Carpenito (1999) defines collaborative problems as

Certain physiologic complications that nurses monitor to detect onset or changes in status. Nurses manage collaborative problems using physician-prescribed and nursing-prescribed interventions to minimize the complications of the events.

The designation *certain* clarifies that all physiologic complications are not collaborative problems. If the nurse can prevent the onset of the complication or provide the primary treatment for it, then the diagnosis is a nursing diagnosis. For example:

Nurses can prevent	**Nursing diagnosis**
Pressure ulcers	*Risk for Pressure Ulcers*
Complications of immobility	*Disuse Syndrome*
Aspiration	*Risk for Aspiration*
Nurses can treat	**Nursing diagnosis**
Stage I or II pressure ulcers	*Impaired Skin Integrity*
Swallowing problems	*Impaired Swallowing*
Ineffective cough	*Ineffective Airway Clearance*
Nurses cannot prevent	**Collaborative problems**
Seizures	*Risk for Complication of Seizures*
Bleeding	*Risk for Complication of Bleeding*
Dysrhythmias	*Risk for Complication of Dysrhythmias*

Prevention versus Detection

Nurses can prevent some physiologic complications, such as pressure ulcers, infection from invasive lines. Prevention differs from detection. Nurses do not prevent hemorrhage or seizure; instead, they monitor to detect its presence early to prevent greater severity of complication or even death. Physicians cannot

[1]The term client can be an individual, a family, significant others, a group, or a community.

treat collaborative problems without nursing's knowledge, vigilance, and judgment. For collaborative problems, nurses institute orders, such as position changes, individual teaching, or specific protocols, in addition to monitoring for early signs/symptoms of physiologic deterioration, which require medical interventions.

Unlike medical diagnoses, however, nursing diagnoses represent situations that are the primary responsibility of nurses, who diagnose onset and implement interventions to manage changes in status. For a collaborative problem, nursing focuses on monitoring for onset or change in status of physiologic complications and on responding to any such changes with physician-prescribed and nurse-prescribed nursing interventions. The nurse makes independent decisions for both collaborative problems and nursing diagnoses. The difference is that for nursing diagnoses, nursing prescribes the definitive treatment to achieve the desired outcome and will change nursing interventions as needed; in contrast, for collaborative problems, prescription for definitive treatment comes from both nursing and medicine.

Even though a nurse cannot prevent bleeding, early detection will prevent hemorrhage. Thus, for collaborative problems, nurses can detect onset of a physiologic problem such as urinary bleeding or decreased urine output. The nurse can also monitor for changes in an existing problem such as high blood pressure or pneumonia.

Collaborative Problem Diagnostic Statements

The 13th edition of this book changed the label for all collaborative problems to *Risk for Complications (RC) of (RC of)*. For example:

- *RC of Renal Failure*
- *RC of Peptic Ulcer*
- *RC of Asthma*

This label indicates that the nursing focus is to reduce the severity of certain physiologic factors or events. For example, *RC of Hypertension* alerts the nurse that the individual either is experiencing or is at high risk for hypertension. In either event, the nurse will receive a report on the status of the collaborative problem or will proceed to evaluate the individual's blood pressure. Trying to have different terminology to distinguish whether the individual is actually hypertensive or simply at risk is not necessary or realistic, given the fluctuating condition of most individuals. The following illustrates this difference.

Situation:	A man admitted post myocardial infarction experiencing cardiogenic shock	A man admitted post myocardial infarction in normal sinus rhythm
	↓	↓
Diagnosis:	*RC of Cardiogenic Shock*	*RC of Cardiogenic Shock*
	↓	↓
Nursing Focus:	To monitor the status and manage episodes of cardiogenic shock	To monitor for onset and manage episodes as necessary

If the nurse is managing a cluster or group of complications, he or she may record the collaborative problems together:

- *RC of Cardiac Dysfunction*
- *RC of Pacemaker Insertion*

The nurse can also word the collaborative problem to reflect a specific cause, as in *RC of Hyperglycemia related to long-term corticosteroid therapy*. In most cases, however, such a link is unnecessary.

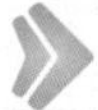

Carp's Cues

When writing collaborative problem statements, the nurse must make sure not to omit the stem *Risk for Complications of*. This stem designates that nurse-prescribed interventions are required for treatment. Without the stem, the collaborative problem could be misread as a medical diagnosis, in which case nursing involvement becomes subordinate to medicine, the discipline primarily responsible for the diagnosis and treatment of medical conditions.

Differentiating Nursing Diagnoses From Collaborative Problems

Both nursing diagnoses and collaborative problems involve all steps of the nursing process: assessment, diagnosis, planning, implementation, and evaluation. Each, however, requires a different approach from the nurse.

Assessment and Diagnosis

For nursing diagnoses, assessment involves data collection to identify signs and symptoms of actual nursing diagnoses or risk factors for high-risk nursing diagnoses. For collaborative problems, assessment focuses on determining physiologic stability or risk for instability. The nurse identifies a collaborative problem when certain situations increase the individual's vulnerability for a complication or the individual has experienced one.

Collaborative problems are not medical diagnoses, although sometimes a medical diagnosis, such as pneumonia, can be a collaborative problem as *Risk for Complication of Pneumonia*. An individual with pneumonia has a medical diagnosis, while an individual with chronic bronchitis would be at risk for pneumonia postsurgery as *Risk for Complication of Pneumonia*.

Medical diagnoses are not useful problem statements for nurses. For example, diabetes mellitus is not the problem focus. Instead, hypoglycemia or hyperglycemia is used. Sometimes the medical diagnosis and the collaborative problem use the same terminology, such as seizures or hyperkalemia. The key is, "Can the nurse monitor the condition?" The nurse monitors for hyperglycemia or hypoglycemia, not diabetes mellitus.

Collaborative problems usually are associated with a specific pathology or treatment. For example, all individuals who have undergone abdominal surgery are at some risk for such problems as hemorrhage and urinary retention. Expert nursing knowledge is required to assess a particular individual's specific risk for these problems and to identify them early to prevent complications and death. Table 4.1 illustrates the difference.

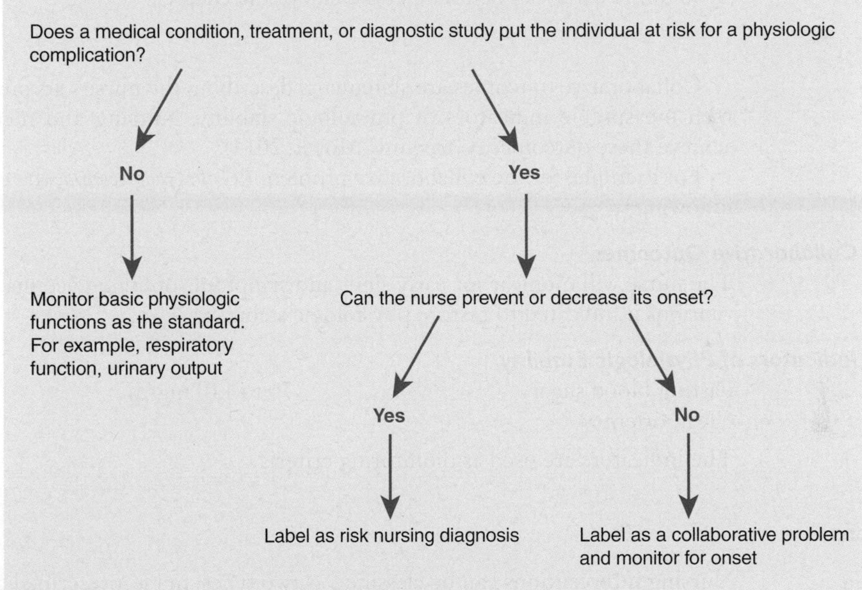

Table 4.1 NURSING DIAGNOSES AND COLLABORATIVE PROBLEMS

	Nursing Diagnoses	Collaborative Problems
Assessment	Requires data collection of risk factors (risk dx) or sign/symptoms of problem nursing diagnoses	No specific assessment is needed because certain collaborative problems will be addressed when specific medical conditions, treatments of diagnostic studies make the individual high-risk for a physiologic complication to occur
Focus of Interventions	Institute nursing interventions to prevent risk nursing diagnosis Institute nursing interventions to reduce or eliminate an actual nursing diagnosis	Monitoring for physiologic instability Institute nursing interventions to minimize the severity of the complication Consult with medicine for medical orders for the individual

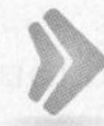

Carp's Cues

Because of each individual's uniqueness, identifying nursing diagnoses is often more difficult than identifying collaborative problems. This does not mean, however, that nursing diagnoses are more important, just different.

Goals

Nursing diagnoses and collaborative problems have different implications for goals. Bulechek and McCloskey (1985) define *goals* as "guideposts to the selection of nursing interventions and criteria in the evaluation of nursing interventions." They continue by saying that "readily identifiable and logical links should exist between the diagnoses and the plan of care, and the activities prescribed should assist or enable the client to meet the identified expected outcome." Thus, goals and interventions can be critical to differentiating nursing diagnoses from collaborative problems that nurses treat.

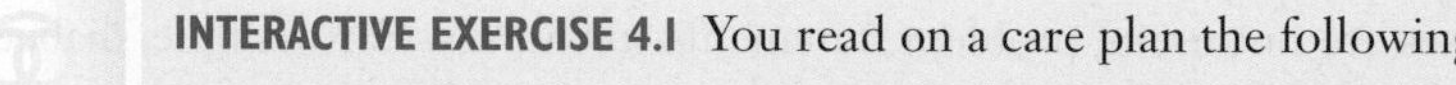

INTERACTIVE EXERCISE 4.1 You read on a care plan the following:

Risk for Deficient Fluid Volume related to loss of fluids during surgery and possible hemorrhage postoperatively
Goal: The individual will demonstrate BP and pulse within normal limits and no bleeding.
Interventions:

1. Monitor intake of IV fluids.
2. Monitor vital signs every hour.
3. Inspect dressing for sign/symptoms of bleeding.
4. Monitor urine output hourly.
5. Notify physician with changes as needed.

During your care of this individual, his urine output decreases and his pulse increases. What would you do? Answer can be found at the end of the chapter.

Collaborative outcomes are statements describing the nurse's accountability for collaborative problems, with measurable indicators of physiologic stability. Nursing and medical interventions are required to achieve these outcomes (Carpenito-Moyet, 2014).

For example, for the collaborative problem *RC of Hypoglycemia*, the collaborative outcomes would be the following:

Collaborative Outcomes

The nurse will monitor for early signs and symptoms of hypoglycemia and will receive collaborative interventions if indicated to restore physiologic stability.

Indicators of Physiologic Stability

Fasting blood sugar 70 to 110 mg/dL
Clear, oriented

The indicators are used as monitoring criteria.

Interventions

Nursing interventions can be classified as two types: nurse-prescribed and physician-prescribed (*delegated*). Regardless of type, all nursing interventions require astute nursing judgment because the nurse is legally accountable for intervening appropriately.

For both nursing diagnoses and collaborative problems, the nurse makes independent decisions concerning nursing interventions. The nature of these decisions differs, however. For nursing diagnoses, the nurse independently prescribes the primary treatment for goal achievement. In contrast, for collaborative problems, the nurse confers with a physician and implements physician-prescribed as well as nurse-prescribed nursing interventions.

Primary treatment describes those interventions that are most responsible for successful outcome achievement. Nevertheless, these are not the only interventions used to treat the diagnosed condition. For example, interventions for an individual with the nursing diagnosis *Impaired Physical Mobility related to incisional pain* might include the following:

- Explain the need for moving and ambulation.
- Teach the individual how to splint the incision before coughing, deep breathing, sitting up, or turning in bed.
- If pain relief medication is scheduled PRN, instruct the individual to request medication as soon as the pain returns.

- Evaluate whether pain relief is satisfactory; if not, contact the physician for increased dosages or decreased interval between doses.
- Schedule activities, bathing, and ambulation to correspond with times when the individual's comfort level is highest.
- Discuss and negotiate ambulation goals with the individual.

All of these are nurse-prescribed interventions. A physician-prescribed intervention for this individual might be Oxycodone-5. This medication is important to manage the individual's postoperative pain; however, it alone cannot be considered a primary treatment.

The difference between a nursing diagnosis and a collaborative problem is illustrated below.

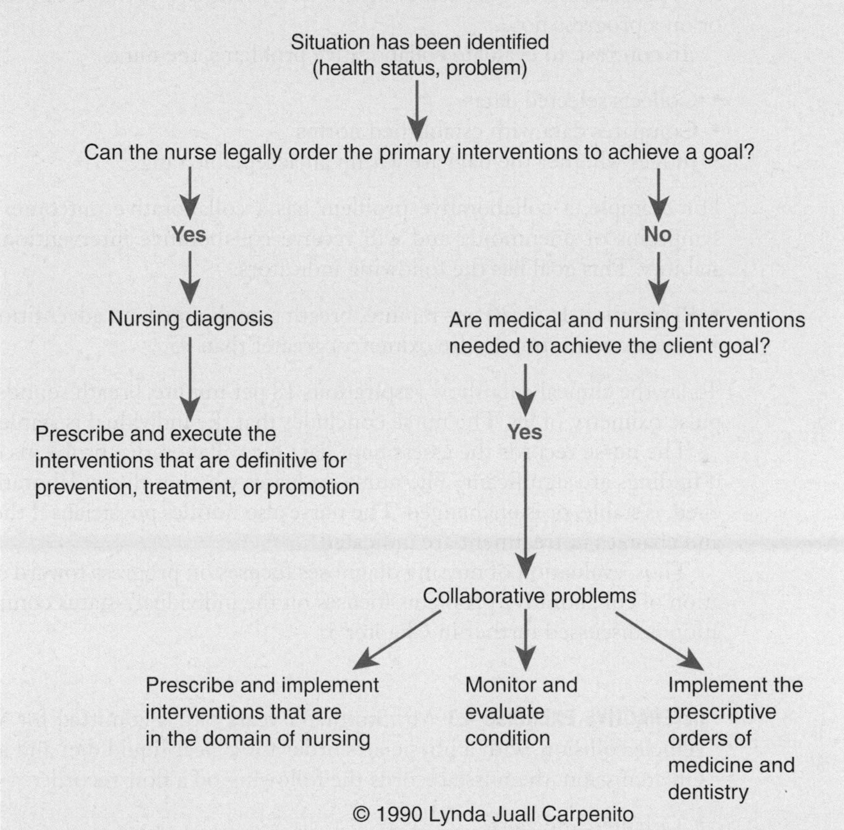

INTERACTIVE EXERCISE 4.2 Refer to Section 3 under collaborative problem *RC of GI Bleeding*. Review the interventions, and label each one as nurse-prescribed or physician-prescribed.

Monitoring versus Prevention

Is monitoring an intervention? Interventions are directed as improving a person's condition or preventing a problem. *Monitoring* involves continually collecting selected data to evaluate whether the individual's condition has changed (improved, deteriorated, not improved, or remained within a normal range). Monitoring does not improve an individual's health status or prevent a problem; rather, it provides information necessary to determine *whether* or *what type* of interventions are needed. Monitoring detects problems. It is associated with every type of nursing diagnosis and collaborative problem:

- For actual nursing diagnosis, monitor the individual's condition for improvement.
- For risk nursing diagnosis, monitor the individual for signs of the problem.
- For wellness nursing diagnosis, monitor the individual's participation in lifestyle changes.
- For collaborative problems, monitor for onset or change in status of a problem.

Although monitoring does not qualify as an intervention, it is an activity. For convenience, monitoring is included with the interventions in Sections 2 and 3.

Evaluation

The nurse evaluates an individual's status and progress differently for nursing diagnoses and collaborative problems. When evaluating nursing diagnoses, the nurse:

- Assesses the individual's status
- Compares this response to the goals
- Concludes whether the individual is progressing toward outcome achievement

For example, an individual has the following goal: "Will walk 25 feet with assistance by discharge." Two days before the projected discharge date, the individual walked 20 feet with assistance. The nurse concludes that he is progressing to goal achievement by discharge. The nurse can record this evaluation on a flow record or on a progress note.

In contrast, to evaluate collaborative problems, the nurse

- Collects selected data
- Compares data with established norms
- Judges whether the data are within an acceptable range

For example, a collaborative problem has a collaborative outcome: "The nurse will detect early signs/symptoms of pneumonia and will receive collaborative interventions if indicated to restore physiologic stability. This goal has the following indicators:

- Respiration 16 to 20 per minute, breath sounds equal, no adventitious sounds
- Oxygen saturation (pulse oximetry) greater than 95

Today the clinical data show respirations 18 per minute, breath sounds equal, no adventitious sounds, and a pulse oximetry of 98. The nurse concludes that the individual is stable.

The nurse records the assessment data for collaborative problems on flow records or on progress notes if findings are significant. The nurse evaluates whether the collaborative problem has improved, has worsened, is stable, or is unchanged. The nurse also notifies physicians if the individual's condition has worsened and changes in treatment are indicated.

Thus, evaluation of nursing diagnoses focuses on progress toward achieving client goals, whereas evaluation of collaborative problems focuses on the individual's status compared with established norms. Evaluation is discussed further in Chapter 5.

INTERACTIVE EXERCISE 4.3 Mr. Smith, 35 years old, is admitted for a possible concussion after a motor vehicle collision, with a physician's order for a clear liquid diet and a neurologic assessment every hour. On admission, the nurse records the following on a flow record:

- Oriented and alert
- Pupils 6 mm, equal, and reactive to light
- BP 120/72, pulse 84, resp 20, temp 99° F

Two hours later, the nurse records the following on the nurse's or progress note:

- Vomiting
- Restlessness
- Pupils 6 mm, equal, with a sluggish response to light
- BP 140/60, pulse 65, resp 12, temp 99° F

Problem: Possible increased intracranial pressure (ICP)

Now, apply the following criteria questions:

- Can the nurse legally order the primary interventions to achieve the client goal (which would be a reversal of the increasing ICP)?
- Are medical and nursing interventions needed for goal achievement?

INTERACTIVE EXERCISE 4.4 Mr. Green, 45 years old, has a cholecystectomy incision (10 days postop) that is not healing and has continual purulent drainage. The nursing care consists of the following:

- Inspecting and cleansing the incision and the surrounding area q8h
- Applying a drainage pouch
- Promoting optimal nutrition and hydration to enhance healing

Problem: Adjacent skin at risk for erosion

Now apply the following criteria question:

- Can the nurse legally order the definitive interventions to achieve the goals (which would be continued intact surrounding tissue)?

SUMMARY According to Wallace and Ivey (1989), "Understanding which nursing diagnoses are most effective and the situations in which the term collaborative problem is best applied helps group the mass of data the nurse must consider." The bifocal clinical practice model provides a structure for forming this understanding. In doing so, it uniquely distinguishes nursing from other health-care professions while providing nurses with a logical description of the focus of clinical nursing.

Chapter 5

Planning Care With Nursing Diagnosis

Learning Objectives

After reading the chapter, the following questions should be answered:

- What are functional health patterns?
- How are priority nursing diagnoses identified?
- What is the difference between goals for nursing diagnoses and collaborative problems?
- How is evaluation different for nursing diagnoses and collaborative problems?
- What are standardized care plans?

Because individuals require nursing care 7 days a week and 24 hours a day, nurses must rely on each other and nonlicensed nursing personnel to help individuals achieve outcomes of care. Clearly, some system of communication is necessary. For more than 30 years, this system consisted of handwritten care plans or verbal reports, neither of which was very useful. This chapter addresses the various methods that nurses use today to communicate an individual's care to other caregivers.

Assessment: Data Collection Formats

Data collection usually consists of two formats: the nursing baseline or screening assessment and the focus or ongoing assessment. The nurse can use each alone or together. As discussed in Chapter 4, nurses encounter, diagnose, and treat two types of response: nursing diagnoses and collaborative problems. Each type requires a different assessment focus.

Initial, Baseline, or Screening Assessment

An initial, baseline, or screening assessment involves collecting a predetermined set of data during initial contact with the individual (e.g., on admission, first home visit). This assessment serves as a tool for "narrowing the universe of possibilities" (Gordon, 1994). During this assessment, the nurse interprets data as significant or insignificant. This process is explored later in this chapter.

The nurse should have an assessment tool that permits the initial assessment to be systematic and efficient. Appendix B illustrates an assessment form with checking or circling options, which can be in an electronic medical record. The nurse always can elaborate with additional questions and comments. Open-ended questions are better for assessment of certain functional areas, such as fear or anxiety. Nurses should view assessment formats as guides, not as mandates. Before requesting information from an individual, nurses should ask themselves, "What am I going to do with the data?" If certain information is useless or irrelevant for a particular individual, then its collection is unnecessary and potentially distressing for the individual. For example, asking a terminally ill individual how much he or she smokes is unnecessary unless the nurse has a specific goal. If an individual will be NPO, collecting data about eating habits is probably unnecessary at this time. Such assessment will be indicated if the individual resumes eating.

If an individual is extremely stressed, the nurse should collect only necessary data and defer the assessment of functional patterns to another time.

Functional Health Patterns

As discussed earlier, nursing assessment focuses on collecting data that validate nursing diagnoses. Gordon's (1994) system of functional health patterns provides an excellent, relevant format for nursing data collection to determine an individual's or group's health status and functioning. For over 20 years, Functional Health Patterns have served to direct the nurse to assess for the effects of illness and disabilities on daily functioning of individuals and their significant others. After data collection is complete, the nurse and individual can determine positive functioning, altered functioning, or at risk for altered functioning. Altered functioning is defined as functioning that the client (individual or group) perceives as negative or undesirable. Refer to Box 5.1 for functional health patterns.

Box 5.1 FUNCTIONAL HEALTH PATTERNS

1. **Health Perception–Health Management Pattern**
   - Perceived pattern of health, well-being
   - Knowledge of lifestyle and relationship to health
   - Knowledge of preventive health practices
   - Adherence to medical, nursing prescriptions
2. **Nutritional–Metabolic Pattern**
   - Usual pattern of food and fluid intake
   - Types of food and fluid intake
   - Actual weight, weight loss or gain
   - Appetite, preferences
3. **Elimination Pattern**
   - Bowel elimination pattern, changes
   - Bladder elimination pattern, changes
   - Control problems
   - Use of assistive devices
   - Use of medications
4. **Activity–Exercise Pattern**
   - Pattern of exercise, activity, leisure, recreation
   - Ability to perform activities of daily living (self-care, home maintenance, work, eating, shopping, cooking)
5. **Sleep–Rest Pattern**
   - Patterns of sleep, rest
   - Perception of quality, quantity
6. **Cognitive–Perceptual Pattern**
   - Vision, learning, taste, touch, smell
   - Language adequacy
   - Memory
   - Decision-making ability, patterns
   - Complaints of discomforts
7. **Self-Perception–Self-Concept Pattern**
   - Attitudes about self, sense of worth
   - Perception of abilities
   - Emotional patterns
   - Body image, identity
8. **Role–Relationship Patterns**
   - Patterns of relationships
   - Role responsibilities
   - Satisfaction with relationships and responsibilities
9. **Sexuality–Reproductive Pattern**
   - Menstrual, reproductive history
   - Satisfaction with sexual relationships, sexual identity
   - Premenopausal or postmenopausal problems
   - Accuracy of sex education
10. **Coping–Stress Tolerance Patterns**
    - Ability to manage stress
    - Knowledge of stress tolerance
    - Sources of support
    - Number of stressful life events in last year
11. **Value–Belief Pattern**
    - Values, goals, beliefs
    - Spiritual practices
    - Perceived conflicts in values

Refer to Appendix A for a sample initial assessment organized according to functional health patterns. It is designed to assist the nurse in gathering subjective and objective data. Should questions arise concerning a pattern, the nurse would gather more data about the diagnosis using the focus assessment under the diagnosis.

When collecting data according to the functional health patterns, the nurse questions, observes, and evaluates the individual or family. For example, under the Cognitive–Perceptual Pattern, the nurse asks the individual whether he or she has difficulty hearing, observes whether the individual is wearing a hearing aid, and evaluates whether the individual understands English.

Physical Assessment

In addition to functional health pattern assessment, the nurse also collects data related to body system functioning. Physical assessment, the collection of objective data concerning the individual's physical status, incorporates head-to-toe examination with a focus on the body systems. The techniques that can be used include inspection, palpation, percussion, and auscultation.

Appendix B lists those areas of physical assessment in which nurse generalists should be proficient. Physical assessment by nurses should be clearly "nursing" in focus. By examining their philosophy and definition of nursing, nurses should seek to develop expertise in those areas that will enhance their nursing practice.

Keeping in mind that separation of functional health patterns from physical assessment is done for organizational purposes only. No useful nursing assessment framework can restrict actual data collection in such a manner. Because humans are open systems, a problem in one functional health pattern invariably influences body system functioning or functioning in another functional health pattern. Anxiety can affect appetite; sleep problems can increase coping difficulties.

Focus Assessment

Focus assessment is the acquisition of selected or specific data as determined by the individual's condition or by the nurse and the individual or family (Carpenito, 1986). The nurse who assesses the vital signs, surgical

INTERACTIVE EXERCISE 5.1 Mr. Gene, 61, is admitted for neurologic surgery. He has a history of peripheral vascular disease and Parkinson's disease. The nurse's initial assessment reveals the following under the functional health pattern Activity–Exercise and physical assessment of musculoskeletal function:

ACTIVITY–EXERCISE PATTERN

SELF-CARE ABILITY:

0 = Independent 1 = Assistive device 2 = Assistance from others
3 = Assistance from person and equipment 4 = Dependent/unable

	0	1	2	3	4
Eating/drinking	✓				
Bathing			✓		
Dressing/grooming			✓		
Toileting			✓		
Bed mobility			✓		
Transferring			✓		
Ambulating		✓			
Stair climbing	✓				
Shopping					✓
Cooking					✓
Home maintenance					✓

ASSISTIVE DEVICES: ______ None ______ Crutches ______ bedside commode__✓__Walker __✕__
______ Cane ______ Splint/brace ______ Wheelchair ______ Other ______

PHYSICAL ASSESSMENT

MUSCULAR–SKELETAL

Range of motion: __✓__ Full ______ Other ______________

Balance and gait: ______ Steady __✓__ Unsteady

Hand grasps: __✓__ Equal __✓__ Strong ______ Weakness/paralysis (______ Right ______ Left)

Leg muscles: ______ Equal ______ Strong __✓__ Weakness/paralysis (__✓__ Right __✕__ Left)

Examine the above assessment data. What data are significant?

site, bowel function/sounds, hydration, comfort of a new postoperative individual, for example, is performing a focus assessment. These assessments are ongoing during the hospitalization.

The nurse can also perform a focus assessment during the initial interview if collected data suggest a possible problem that the nurse must validate or rule out. For example, during the baseline interview, the individual reports a problem with occasional constipation. The nurse then collects additional data (focus assessment) to confirm a problem or risk nursing diagnosis or rule out a constipation problem.

Planning: The Care Planning Process

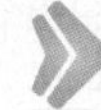

Carp's Cues

Care plans serve a function, which is to communicate to the nurse who is caring for an individual the care needed to achieve positive outcomes and transition. If an individual has had a total hip replacement, this care can be predetermined in an electronic or paper care plan. It is unnecessary for a nurse to create a so called "individualized care plan." What is necessary for the nurse to determine whether all the elements on the electronic or paper care plan are relevant to her or his individual. If the individual also has Diabetes Mellitus, then *Risk for Complications of Hypo/Hyperglycemia* must be added to the problem list.

Today, the methods used to communicate individual care between nurses and other caregivers vary. Critical pathways, electronic health systems, and preprinted standardized care plans have replaced handwritten care plans. Later in this chapter, types of care planning systems will be discussed.

Critical pathways, electronic health systems, and preprinted standardized care plans reflect the expected diagnoses and associated goals and interventions commonly related to an individual's medical or surgical problem. This type of system frees nurses from the repetitive, unnecessary writing of routine care. The care outlined on the standardized plan or critical pathway should represent the responsible care to which the individual is entitled.

Before discussing the care planning process, the nurse must identify the type, as well as the duration, of needed care. People receiving nursing care for less than 8 hours, as in the emergency department, short-stay surgery, or recovery room, have a specific medical diagnosis or need a specific procedure. Nursing care is derived from standardized plans or protocols. In nonacute settings such as long-term care, community or home care, or assisted-living and rehabilitation units, nurses will supplement predetermined standardized plans with personalized care plans. The longer the nurse–individual relationship, the more data there is available to individualize the plan. Care plans represent the planning, not the delivery, of care. This planning phase of the nursing process has three components:

1. Establishing a priority set of diagnoses
2. Designating client goals and collaborative goals
3. Prescribing nursing interventions

Establishing a Priority Set of Diagnoses

Realistically, a nurse cannot address all, or even most, of the nursing diagnoses and collaborative problems that can apply to an individual, family, or community during an encounter or length of stay. By identifying a priority set—a group of nursing diagnoses and collaborative problems that take precedence over others—the nurse can best direct resources toward goal achievement. Differentiating priority diagnoses from nonpriority diagnoses is crucial.

- ***Priority diagnoses*** are those nursing diagnoses or collaborative problems that, if not managed now, will deter progress to achieve outcomes or will negatively affect functional status.
- ***Nonpriority diagnoses*** are those nursing diagnoses or collaborative problems for which treatment can be delayed without compromising present functional status.

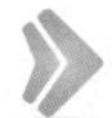

Carp's Cues

Numbering the diagnoses on a problem list does not indicate priority; rather, it shows the order in which the nurse entered them on the list. Assigning absolute priority to nursing diagnoses or collaborative problems can create the false assumption that number one is automatically the first priority. In the clinical setting, priorities can shift rapidly as the individual's condition changes. For this reason, the nurse must view the entire problem list as the priority set, with priorities shifting within the list periodically.

Priority Diagnoses

In an acute care setting, the individual enters the hospital for a specific purpose, such as surgery or other treatments for acute illness. In such a situation, certain nursing diagnoses or collaborative problems requiring specific nursing interventions often apply, which can be found on the standardized plan (electronic, paper). Carpenito (1995) uses the term *diagnostic cluster* to describe such a group; this cluster can appear in a critical pathway or standardized plan of care. For example, Box 5.2 is a diagnostic cluster for a person having abdominal surgery.

All of these diagnoses in the diagnostic cluster are priority diagnoses. When should additional diagnoses (other than in the diagnostic cluster) be added to the problem list or care plan?

- Are there additional collaborative problems associated with coexisting medical conditions that require monitoring (e.g., hypoglycemia)?
- Are there additional nursing diagnoses that, if not managed or prevented now, will deter recovery or affect the individual's functional status (e.g., *High Risk for Constipation*)?
- What problems does the individual perceive as priority?

Additional nursing diagnoses and/or collaborative problems can be added to an electronic care plan or written on the problem/care plan.

Box 5.2 DIAGNOSTIC CLUSTER

Preoperative

Nursing Diagnosis

- *Anxiety/Fear related to surgical experience, loss of control, unpredictable outcome, and insufficient knowledge of preoperative routines, postoperative exercises and activities, and postoperative changes and sensations*

Postoperative

Collaborative Problems

- *RC of Hemorrhage*
- *RC of Hypovolemia/Shock*
- *RC of Evisceration/Dehiscence*
- *RC of Paralytic Ileus*
- *RC of Infection (Peritonitis)*
- *RC of Urinary Retention*
- *RC of Thrombophlebitis*

Nursing Diagnoses

- *Risk for Ineffective Respiratory Function related to immobility secondary to post anesthesia sedation and pain*
- *Risk for Infection related to a site for organism invasion secondary to surgery*
- *Acute Pain related to surgical interruption of body structures, flatus, and immobility*
- *Risk for Imbalanced Nutrition: Less Than Body Requirements related to increased protein and vitamin requirements for wound healing and decreased intake secondary to pain, nausea, vomiting, and diet restrictions*
- *Risk for Constipation related to decreased peristalsis secondary to immobility and the effects of anesthesia and opioids*
- *Activity Intolerance related to pain and weakness secondary to anesthesia, tissue hypoxia, and insufficient fluid and nutrient intake*
- *Risk for Self-Health Management related to insufficient knowledge of care of operative site, restrictions (diet, activity), medications, signs and symptoms of complications, and follow-up care.*

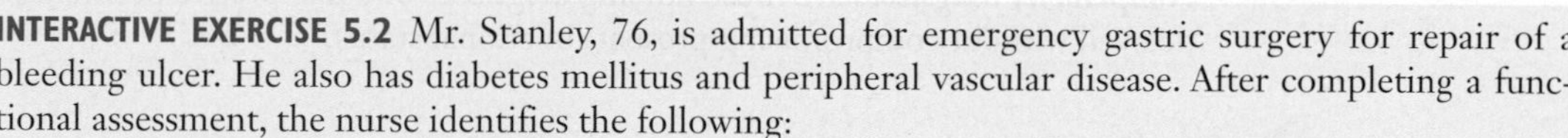

INTERACTIVE EXERCISE 5.2 Mr. Stanley, 76, is admitted for emergency gastric surgery for repair of a bleeding ulcer. He also has diabetes mellitus and peripheral vascular disease. After completing a functional assessment, the nurse identifies the following:

- Compromised gait
- Occasional incontinence when walking to the bathroom
- Wife complaining of many caregiver responsibilities and an unmotivated husband

Examine the data above and begin to formulate nursing diagnoses and collaborative problems that need nursing interventions. Refer to the three questions above to assist with this analysis and to determine whether Mr. Stanley and his family have other diagnoses that require nursing interventions. Mr. Stanley's priority list (diagnostic cluster) follows.

From Postoperative Standard of Care (Diagnostic Cluster):

- *RC of Urinary Retention*
- *RC of Hemorrhage*
- *RC of Hypovolemia/Shock*
- *RC of Pneumonia (stasis)*
- *RC of Peritonitis*
- *RC of Thrombophlebitis*
- *RC of Paralytic ileus*
- *Risk for Infection related to destruction of first line of defense against bacterial invasion*
- *Risk for Impaired Respiratory Function related to postanesthesia state, postoperative immobility, and pain*
- *Impaired Physical Mobility related to pain and weakness secondary to anesthesia, tissue hypoxia, and insufficient fluids/nutrients*
- *Risk for Imbalanced Nutrition: Less Than Body Requirements related to increased protein/vitamin requirements for wound healing and decreased intake secondary to pain, nausea, vomiting, and diet restrictions*
- *Risk for Compromised Human Dignity related to multiple factors associated with hospitalization (standard to all hospitalized persons)*
- *Risk for Ineffective Self-Health Management related to insufficient knowledge of home care, incisional care, signs and symptoms of complications, activity restriction, and follow-up care*

From Medical History of Diabetes Mellitus:

- *RC of Hypo/Hyperglycemia*

From Medical History of Peripheral Vascular Disease and Reported Prolonged Immobility:

- *High Risk for Injury related to altered gait and deconditioning secondary to peripheral vascular disease and decreased motivation*

From Nursing Admission Assessment:

- Possible *Functional Incontinence related to reports of occasional incontinence when walking to bathroom. Refer to Primary provider for evaluation after transition.*
- *High Risk for Caregiver Role Strain (wife) related to multiple caregiver responsibilities and progressive deterioration of husband. Refer to Home Health Nurse for evaluation after transition.*

Nonpriority Nursing Diagnoses

Nonpriority diagnoses that are identified are referred for management after discharge. For example, for an individual who is 50 lb overweight and hospitalized after myocardial infarction, the nurse would eventually want to explain the effects of obesity on cardiac function and refer the individual to a weight-reduction program after discharge. Documentation would reflect the teaching and referral; a nursing diagnosis related to weight reduction would not need to appear on the problem list.

The individual probably has many other important but nonpriority nursing diagnoses; however, because of the limited length of stay, nursing resources must be directed toward those problems that will deter progress at this time. The nurse can discuss important diagnoses with the individual and family, with recommendations for future attention (e.g., referral to a community agency).

Designating Client Goals and Collaborative Outcomes

Client goals (outcome criteria) and collaborative outcomes are standards or measures used to evaluate the individual's progress (outcome) or the nurse's performance (process) (Carpenito-Moyet, 2014). According to Alfaro (2014), client *goals* are statements describing a measurable behavior of the individual, family, or group that denotes a favorable status (changed or maintained) after the delivery of nursing care. Collaborative outcomes are statements describing the nurse's accountability for collaborative problems, with measurable indicators of physiologic stability. Nursing and medical interventions are required to achieve these outcomes (Carpenito-Moyet, 2014). As discussed in Chapter 4, nursing diagnoses have individual goals, whereas collaborative problems have collaborative outcomes.

Certain situations may call for involvement from several disciplines. For example, for an individual experiencing extreme anxiety, the physician may prescribe an antianxiety medication, an occupational therapist may provide diversional activities, and a nurse may institute nonpharmacologic anxiety-reducing measures, such as listening, coaching in relaxation exercises. According to Gordon (1994), "Saying a nursing diagnosis is a health problem a nurse can treat does not mean that non nursing consultants cannot be used. The critical element is whether the nurse-prescribed interventions can achieve the outcome established with the client."

INTERACTIVE EXERCISE 5.3 Examine the following outcomes:

The individual will

- Demonstrate stable vital signs
- Have electrolytes within normal range
- Have cardiac rhythm and rate within normal limits
- Have blood loss within acceptable limits after surgery

While you are caring for this individual, his cardiac rhythm becomes abnormal and his surgical wound begins to bleed. What would you do?

- Change the nursing interventions.
- Revise the goal.
- Change the diagnosis.
- Call the doctor for physician-prescribed interventions.

Reevaluating the Goal for Nursing Diagnoses

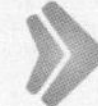

Carp's Cues

Reevaluating goals is a process usually more appropriate in long-term care or home care setting.

If a client goal is not achieved or progress toward achievement is not evident, the nurse must reevaluate the attainability of the goal or review the nursing care plan, asking the following questions (Carpenito, 1999):

- Is the diagnosis correct?
- Has the goal been set mutually? Is the individual participating?
- Is more time needed for the plan to work?
- Does the goal need to be revised?
- Does the plan need to be revised?
- Are physician-prescribed interventions needed?

Goals for Collaborative Problems

As discussed earlier, identifying client goals for collaborative problems is inappropriate and can imply erroneous accountability for nurses. Rather, collaborative problems involve collaborative outcomes that reflect nursing accountability in situations requiring physician-prescribed and nurse-prescribed interventions. This accountability includes (1) monitoring for physiologic instability, (2) consulting standing orders and protocols or a physician to obtain orders for appropriate interventions, (3) performing specific actions to manage and to reduce the severity of an event or situation, and (4) evaluating individual responses.

Nursing goals for collaborative problems can be written as "The nurse will manage and minimize the problem." The following are examples of goals for collaborative problems

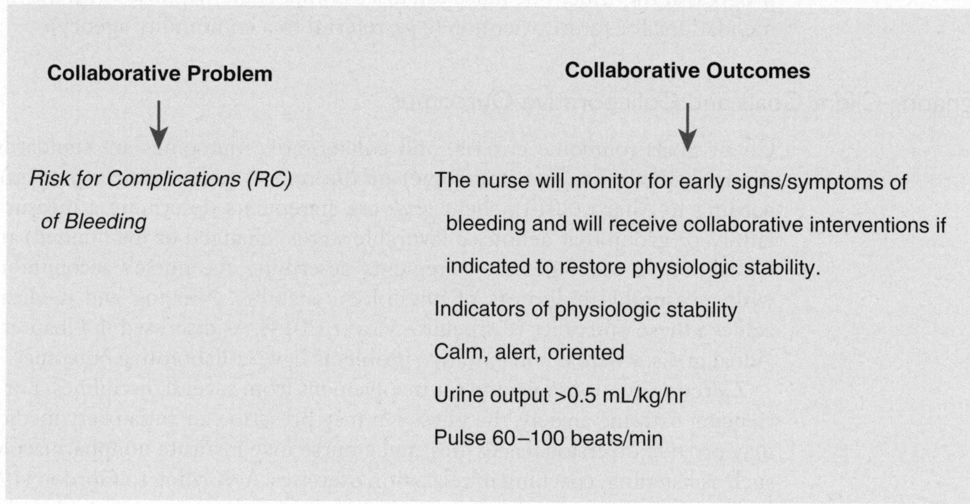

Collaborative Problem
Collaborative Outcomes
Risk for Complications (RC) of Bleeding
The nurse will monitor for early signs/symptoms of bleeding and will receive collaborative interventions if indicated to restore physiologic stability.
Indicators of physiologic stability
Calm, alert, oriented
Urine output >0.5 mL/kg/hr
Pulse 60–100 beats/min

Goals for Nursing Diagnoses

Client goals can represent predicted resolution of a problem, evidence of progress toward resolution of a problem, progress toward improved health status, or continued maintenance of good health or function. Nurses and individuals use these goals to direct interventions to achieve desired changes or maintenance and to measure the effectiveness and validity of interventions. Nurses can formulate goals/outcome criteria to direct and measure positive results or to prevent complications. Goals (outcome criteria) seek to direct interventions to provide the individual with

- Improved health status by increasing comfort (physiologic, psychological, social, spiritual) and coping abilities (e.g., the individual will discuss relationship between activity and carbohydrate requirements and walk unassisted to end of hall four times a day)
- Maintenance of present optimal level of health (e.g., the individual will continue to share fears)
- Optimal levels of coping with significant others (e.g., the individual will relate an intent to discuss with her husband her concern about returning to work)
- Optimal adaptation to deterioration of health status (e.g., the individual will visually scan the environment to prevent injury while walking)
- Optimal adaptation to terminal illness (e.g., the individual will compensate for periods of anorexia and nausea)

- Collaboration and satisfaction with health care providers (e.g., the individual will ask questions concerning the care of his colostomy)

Alternatively, goals seek to direct interventions to prevent negative alterations in the individual, such as:

- Complications (e.g., the individual will not experience the complications of imposed bed rest as evidenced by continued intact skin; full range of motion, no calf tenderness, and clear lung fields)
- Disabilities (e.g., the individual will elevate left arm on pillow and exercise fingers on sponge ball to reduce edema)
- Unwarranted death (e.g., the infant will be attached to an apnea monitor at night)

Components of Goals for Nursing Diagnoses

The essential characteristics of goals are as follows:

- Long-term and/or short-term
- Measurable behavior
- Specific in content and time
- Attainable

A *long-term goal* is an objective that the individual is expected to achieve over weeks or months. A *short-term goal* is an objective that the individual is expected to achieve in a few days or as a stepping stone toward a long-term goal. Long-term goals are appropriate for all individuals in long-term care facilities and for some individuals in rehabilitation units, mental health units, community nursing settings, and ambulatory services. For an individual with a nursing diagnosis of *Risk for Suicide* (Varcarolis, 2011):

Long-Term Goal	Individual will state that she wants to live.
Short-Term Goals	Individual will discuss painful feelings.
	Individual will make no-suicide contract with nurse by end of first session.

Measurable behavior is expressed by use of measurable verbs, or verbs that describe the exact action that the nurse expects the individual to display when he or she has met the goal. The action or behavior must be such that the nurse can validate it through seeing or hearing. (The nurse may occasionally use touch, taste, and smell to measure goal achievement.) If the verb does not describe a result that can be seen or heard (e.g., the individual *will experience* less anxiety), the nurse can change it to a behaviorally measurable one (e.g., the individual *will report* less anxiety).

INTERACTIVE EXERCISE 5.4 Evaluate the following goals:

The individual will

- Accept the death of his wife
- State the signs and symptoms of high blood glucose
- Know the signs and symptoms of low blood glucose
- Administer insulin correctly
- Understand the importance of a low-fat diet

Which goals can you evaluate by seeing or hearing?

Nurses can make measuring goal achievement easier by

- Using the phrase *as evidenced by* to introduce measurable evidence of reduced signs and symptoms (e.g., the individual will experience less anxiety, as evidenced by reduced pacing; the individual will demonstrate tolerance to activity, as evidenced by a return to resting pulse of 76 within 3 minute after activity)
- Adding the phrase *within normal limits* (WNL) (e.g., the individual will demonstrate healing WNL)

A student may be asked to define what WNL is. For example, the individual will demonstrate healing WNL as evidenced by intact, approximate wound edges and no or little abnormal drainage. The process of writing measurable goals is below.

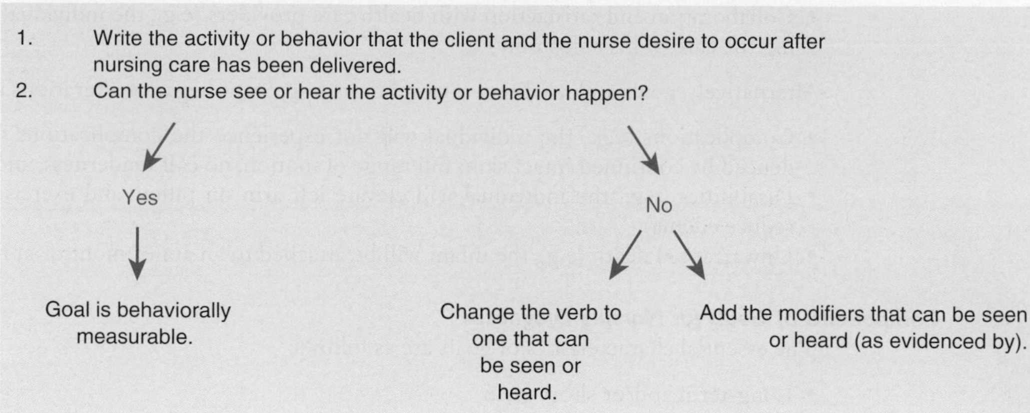

1. Write the activity or behavior that the client and the nurse desire to occur after nursing care has been delivered.
2. Can the nurse see or hear the activity or behavior happen?
Yes
No
Goal is behaviorally measurable.
Change the verb to one that can be seen or heard.
Add the modifiers that can be seen or heard (as evidenced by).

Goals should be *specific in content and time*. Three elements add to the specificity of a goal: (1) content, (2) modifiers, and (3) achievement time. The *content* indicates what the individual is to do, experience, or learn (e.g., drink, walk, cough, verbalize). *Modifiers* add individual preferences to the goal and are usually adjectives or adverbs explaining what, where, when, and how. Nurses can add the *time for achievement* to a goal using one of three options:

1. By discharge (e.g., the individual will relate intent to discuss fears regarding diagnosis with wife at home)
2. Continued (e.g., the individual will demonstrate continued intact skin)
3. By date (e.g., the individual will walk half the length of the hallway with assistance by Friday morning)

Finally, a goal must be *attainable*, meaning that the individual must be able to achieve the goal based on his or her age, condition, mental status, and motivation.

Goals for Possible Nursing Diagnoses

It is inappropriate for nurses to formulate client goals for collaborative problems and possible nursing diagnoses because they have not been confirmed. Consider the following possible nursing diagnosis and associated goal:

- **Nursing diagnosis:** *Possible Feeding Self-Care Deficit related to IV in right hand*
- **Goal:** The individual will feed himself.

Possible nursing diagnoses do not have goals until they are confirmed. How can the nurse write a client goal for a diagnosis that has not been confirmed or ruled out yet?

Prescribing Nursing Interventions

As previously discussed in Chapter 4, the two types of nursing interventions are nurse-prescribed and physician-prescribed (delegated). *Nurse-prescribed interventions* are those that nurses formulate for themselves or other nursing staff to implement. *Physician-prescribed (delegated) interventions* are prescriptions for individuals that physicians formulate for nursing staff to implement. Physicians' orders are not orders for nurses; rather, they are orders for individuals that nurses implement if indicated.

Both types of interventions require independent nursing judgment, because legally the nurse must determine whether it is appropriate to initiate the action, regardless of whether it is independent or delegated. Box 5.3 shows a sample nursing care plan with both types of interventions.

Note that nurses can and should consult with other disciplines, such as social workers, nutritionists, and physical therapists, as appropriate. Nevertheless, doing so is consultative only; if interventions for nursing diagnoses result from such consultation, the nurse writes these orders on the nursing care plan for other nursing staff to implement. A discussion of other disciplines and their role in nursing care plans is included later in this chapter.

Bulechek and McCloskey (1989) define nursing interventions as "any direct care treatment that a nurse performs on behalf of a client. These treatments include nurse-initiated treatments resulting from nursing diagnoses, physician-initiated treatments resulting from medical diagnoses, and performance of essential daily functions for the client who cannot do these." Their definition links all nursing interventions with nursing diagnoses. This author links all nursing interventions with nursing diagnoses and collaborative

Box 5.3 NURSE-PRESCRIBED AND DELEGATED INTERVENTIONS

Standard of Care

RC of Increased Intracranial Pressure

NP1. Monitor for signs and symptoms of increased intracranial pressure.
- Pulse changes: slowing rate to 60 or below; increasing rate to 100 or above
- Respiratory irregularities: slowing rate with lengthening periods of apnea
- Rising blood pressure or widening pulse pressure with moderately elevated temperature
- Temperature rising
- Level of responsiveness: variable change from baseline (alert, lethargic, comatose)
- Pupillary changes (size, equality, reaction to light, movements)
- Eye movements (doll's eyes, nystagmus)
- Vomiting
- Headache: constant, increasing in intensity; aggravated by movement/standing
- Subtle changes: restlessness, forced breathing, purposeless movements, and mental cloudiness
- Paresthesia, paralysis

NP2. Avoid:
- Carotid massage
- Prone position
- Neck flexion
- Extreme neck rotation
- Valsalva maneuver
- Isometric exercises
- Digital stimulation (anal)

NP3. Maintain a position with slight head elevation.
NP4. Avoid rapidly changing positions.
NP5. Maintain a quiet, calm environment (soft lighting).
NP6. Plan activities to reduce interruptions.
NP7. Intake and output; use infusion pump to ensure accuracy.
NP8. Consult for stool softeners.
Del9. Maintain fluid restrictions as ordered (may be restricted to 1,000 mL/day for a few days).
Del10. Administer fluids at an even rate as prescribed.
Del11. Administer medications (osmotic diuretics [e.g., mannitol] and corticosteroids [e.g., dexamethasone, methylprednisolone if administered]).

Del = Delegated; NP = Nurse-prescribed.

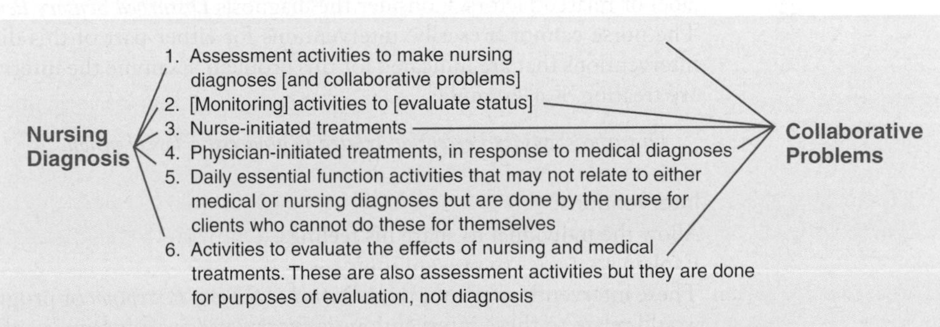

FIGURE 5.1 Relationship of nursing interventions to nursing diagnosis and collaborative problems. *Brackets* indicate the changes made by the author. (From Bulechek, G., & McCloskey, J. (1989). Nursing interventions: Treatments for potential nursing diagnoses. In R. M. Carroll-Johnson (Ed.), *Classification of nursing diagnoses: Proceedings of the eighth national conference*. Philadelphia, PA: J. B. Lippincott.)

problems. Figure 5.1 lists the six basic types of nursing interventions identified by Bulechek and McCloskey (1989), with this author's changes.

Focus of Nursing Interventions

As discussed in Chapter 3, the major focus of interventions differs for problem, risk, and possible nursing diagnoses and collaborative problems.

For *problem nursing diagnoses*, interventions seek to

- Reduce or eliminate contributing factors or the diagnosis
- Promote wellness
- Monitor and evaluate status

For *risk nursing diagnoses*, interventions seek to

- Reduce or eliminate risk factors
- Prevent the problem
- Monitor and evaluate status

For *possible nursing diagnoses*, interventions seek to

- Collect additional data to rule out or confirm the diagnosis

For *collaborative problems*, interventions seek to

- Monitor for changes in status
- Manage changes in status with nurse-prescribed and physician-prescribed interventions
- Evaluate response

Integral to the prevention or treatment of both nursing diagnoses and collaborative problems is the ongoing teaching that nurses provide individuals and family. Appendix C addresses teaching strategies as Teach Back and adapting to individuals with low literacy.

Nursing Orders

When the nurse adds additional directions for other nurses to implement, they consist of the following:

- Date
- Directive verb
- What, when, how often, how long, where
- Signature

What If the Nurse Cannot Treat the Contributing Factors?

Sometimes, nursing interventions cannot reduce or eliminate the related factors for the nursing diagnosis. Some literature has specified that nurses direct interventions toward reducing or eliminating etiologic or contributing factors. Specifically, if the nurse cannot treat the contributing factors, then the nursing diagnosis is considered incorrect. This is problematic. As the diagnostic labels evolve into more specific labels, nurses may encounter nursing diagnoses with contributing factors that nursing cannot treat. Consider, for example, *Risk for Infection related to compromised immune system*. The nurse does not prescribe for a compromised immune system but can prevent infection in some individuals with this problem. In some instances, the label directs the interventions, and the etiologic or contributing factors are not involved.

To be correct, the nurse must be able to provide the definite interventions for the nursing diagnosis label or related factors. Consider the diagnosis *Disturbed Sensory Perception related to progressive loss of vision.* The nurse cannot prescribe interventions for either part of this diagnosis. When this happens, write the interventions that are indicated for this problem. Examine the interventions and decide what problems they are treating. For example:

Disturbed Sensory Perception related to progressive loss of vision.

Interventions:
Allow the individual to share his feelings.
Explain strategies to prevent injury.
These interventions do not treat *Disturbed Sensory Perception* or progressive loss of vision. The diagnosis that would relate to these interventions is *Fear related to progressive loss of vision*.

Implementation

The implementation component of the nursing process involves applying the skills that nurses need to implement the nursing interventions. The skills and knowledge necessary for implementation usually focus on

- Performing the activity for or assisting the individual
- Performing nursing assessments to identify new problems or to monitor the status of existing problems
- Teaching to help individuals/significant others gain new knowledge concerning their own health or the management of a disorder
- Assisting individuals to make decisions about their own health care
- Consulting with and referring to other health-care professionals to obtain appropriate direction
- Providing specific treatment actions to remove, reduce, or resolve health problems

- Assisting individuals to perform activities themselves or their significant others.
- Assisting individuals/significant others to identify risks or problems and to explore options available, for example, referrals

Carp's Cues

Nurses not only must possess these skills, but they also must assess, teach, and evaluate them in all nursing personnel that they manage. Often, the nurse is responsible for planning, but not actually implementing, care. This requires the management skills of delegation, assertion, evaluation, and knowledge of change.

Evaluation

Evaluation involves three different considerations:

1. Evaluation of the individual's status
2. Evaluation of the individual's progress toward goal achievement
3. Evaluation of the care plan's status and currency (longer care settings such as rehabilitation, long-term care, home care)

The nurse is responsible for evaluating the individual's status regularly. Some individuals require daily evaluation; others, such as those with neurologic problems, need hourly or continuous evaluation. The nurse approaches evaluation differently for nursing diagnoses and collaborative problems.

Evaluating Nursing Diagnoses

Nurses need client goals (outcome criteria) to evaluate a nursing diagnosis. After providing care, the nurse will (1) assess the individual's status, (2) compare this response with the outcome criteria, and (3) conclude whether the individual is progressing toward outcome achievement. Figure 5.2 and the example that follows illustrate this evaluation process.

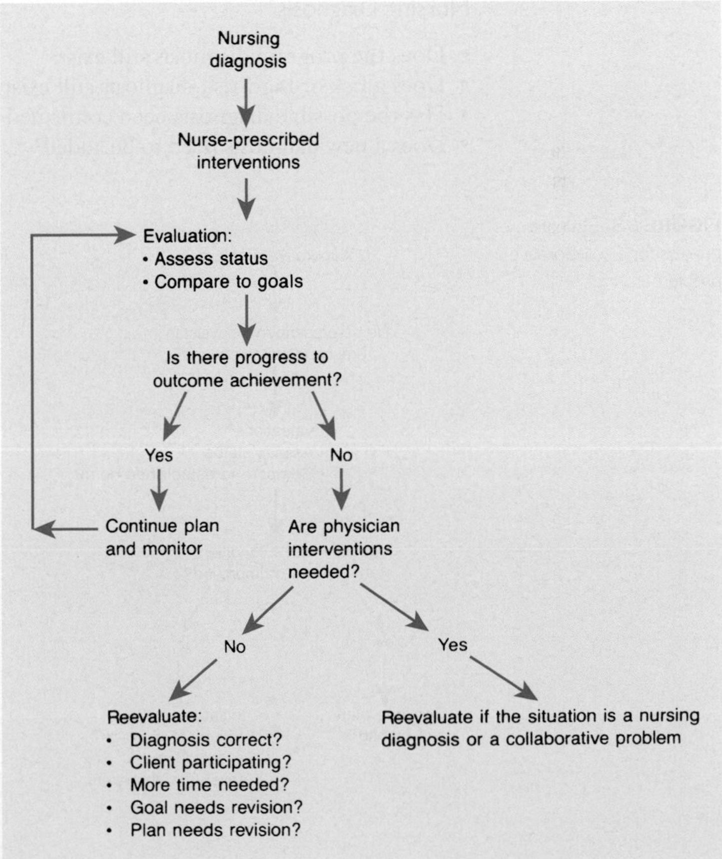

FIGURE 5.2 Evaluation process for a nursing diagnosis.

If a goal is "The individual will walk unassisted half the length of the hall," the nurse would observe the individual's response to interventions, asking, "How far did the individual walk?" and "Did he or she need assistance?" The nurse then would compare the individual's response after interventions with the established goals.

The nurse can record the individual's response on flow charts or progress notes. Flow charts record clinical data, such as vital signs, skin condition, any side effects, and wound assessments. Progress notes record specific responses that are not appropriate for flow charts, such as response to counseling, response of family members to the individual, and any unusual responses.

Evaluating Collaborative Problems

Because collaborative problems have collaborative outcomes, the nurse evaluates them differently from nursing diagnoses. For collaborative problems, the nurse will (1) assess the individual's physiologic status, (2) compare the data with established norms, (3) judge whether the data fall within acceptable ranges, and (4) conclude if the individual's condition is stable, improved, unimproved, or worse. See Figure 5.3.

For example, for *RC of Hypertension*, the nurse takes a blood pressure reading and compares the finding against the normal range. If it falls within the range, the nurse concludes that the individual exhibits normal blood pressure. If the blood pressure is outside the normal range, the nurse checks the individual's previous blood pressure readings. If this is a recent change, consult with a physician/physician assistant or nurse practitioner.

The nurse can record the assessment data for collaborative problems on flow records and use progress notes for significant or unusual findings, along with nursing response to the situation.

Evaluating the Care Plan in Extended/Long-Term Care

This type of evaluation depends on the conclusions derived from the evaluation of the individual's progress or condition in extended and long-term settings, for example, hospice, rehabilitation centers, long-term care settings, home care. After examining the individual's response, the nurse should ask the following questions:

Nursing Diagnosis

- Does the program diagnosis still exist?
- Does a risk or high-risk diagnosis still exist?
- Has the possible diagnosis been confirmed or ruled out?
- Does a new diagnosis need to be added?

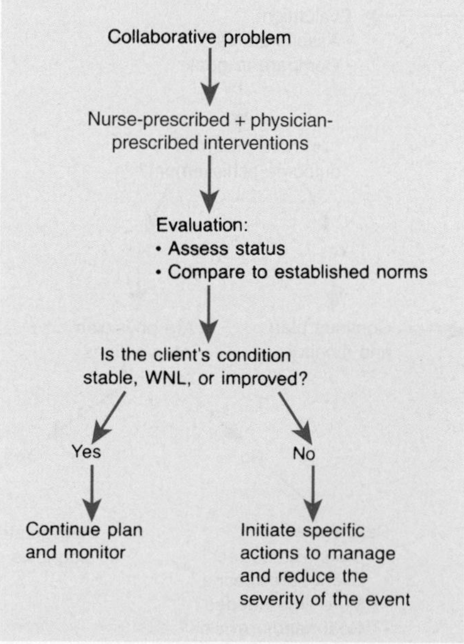

FIGURE 5.3 Evaluation process for a collaborative problem.

Goals

- Have they been achieved?
- Do they reflect the present focus of care?
- Can more specific modifiers be added?
- Are they acceptable to the individual?

Interventions

- Are they acceptable to the individual/significant others?
- Are they specific to the individual?
- Do they provide clear instructions to the nursing staff?

Collaborative Problems

- Is continuing monitoring indicated?

In reviewing the problems and interventions in long-term settings, the nurse records one of the following decisions in the evaluation column or in the progress notes at the time prescribed for evaluation:

- ***Continue.*** The diagnosis is still present, and the goals and interventions are appropriate.
- ***Revised.*** The diagnosis is still present, but the goals or nursing orders require revision. The revisions are then recorded.
- ***Ruled Out/Confirmed.*** Additional data collection has confirmed or ruled out a possible diagnosis. Goals and nursing orders are written.
- ***Achieved.*** The goals have been achieved, and that portion of the care plan is discontinued.
- ***Reinstate.*** A diagnosis that had been resolved returns.

The nurse caring for or directing the individual's care can make minor revisions on a care plan daily. On paper, the nurse can use a yellow felt-tip marker (highlighter) to mark those areas no longer in use. Because it is still possible to read through the yellow marking, the nurse can refer to previous planning. In addition, the marking will not interfere with photocopying. Examples of evaluation documentation are presented later in this chapter. In electronic systems, changes are tracked and visible.

Multidisciplinary Care Planning

Commonly, multiple disciplines provide the care of individuals, families, or groups. Good coordination of this care is critical for optimal use of resources and to prevent duplication. Given overall knowledge level and time spent with individuals, nurses typically are in the best position to coordinate this care. The case management model subscribes to this philosophy.

Agencies take various steps to promote coordinated multidisciplinary planning:

- Conducting regular multidisciplinary planning conferences
- Creating multidisciplinary problem lists
- Creating multidisciplinary care plans

Some of these strategies, however, can be problematic for nurses. As discussed in this chapter, care plans serve as directions for nursing staff in providing individual care. Should staff from other disciplines—physical therapy, social services, nutrition—write on nursing care plans? If so, should they write interventions for nurses to follow or only add interventions specific to their discipline?

Physician-prescribed or nurse practitioner-prescribed interventions are transferred from the chart to appropriate documents, such as medication administration records, treatment records, and Kardexes. It is not necessary to enter physician-prescribed interventions on nursing care plans.

A nurse is accountable for following the interventions that other professional nurses prescribe. If a nurse disagrees with another nurse's care plan, the two nurses should consult and discuss the problem. If doing so is impossible, then the disagreeing nurse can delete or revise the existing nursing orders. Professional courtesy dictates that the nurse should leave a note to the previous nurse explaining the change, if it could be problematic.

Should other disciplines add interventions for nursing staff to the nursing care plan?

When a discipline other than nursing or medicine has suggestions for nursing management of a nursing diagnosis, the nurse should view these suggestions as expert advice. The nurse may or may not incorporate

Box 5.4 SAMPLE MULTIDISCIPLINARY CARE PLAN FOR AN INDIVIDUAL AFTER TOTAL HIP REPLACEMENT

Nursing Diagnosis:

Impaired Physical Mobility related to pain, stiffness, fatigue, restrictive equipment, and prescribed activity restrictions

Goal:

The individual will increase activity to walking with walker for 15 min tid and demonstrate proper positioning and transfer techniques.

Interventions:

PT	1. Establish an exercise program tailored to the individual's ability.
	2. Implement exercises at regular intervals.
PT/Nsg	3. Teach body mechanics and transfer techniques.
	4. Encourage independence.
PT/Nsg	5. Teach and supervise use of ambulatory aids.

such advice into the nursing care plan. This situation is similar to that of a consulting physician/nurse practitioner, who may make recommendations but does not write medical orders for another physician's individual.

When a nurse enters an intervention on the care plan based on a suggestion from another discipline, the nurse credits the order to that discipline. For example:

Gently perform passive ROM to arms after meals and at 8 to 9 PM, per consult with C. Levy, RPT.

Historically, nurses exclusively have used nursing diagnoses and collaborative problems to describe the focus of nursing care. But nursing diagnoses and collaborative problems also can describe the focus of care for other nonphysician disciplines, such as physical therapy, respiratory therapy, social service, occupational therapy, nutritional therapy, and speech therapy. Other disciplines could add their discipline-specific interventions to standardized care plans with the designation that the interventions are prescribed and provided by that discipline (not nursing). These disciplines would also be encouraged to revise or add to care plans for their interventions. Box 5.4 illustrates a multidisciplinary care plan. Note that all nursing diagnoses or collaborative problems do not have non–nurse-prescribed interventions.

Multidisciplinary conferencing provides an excellent way to review and evaluate the status and progress of the individual, family, or group. In longer-term settings, such conferencing is required for all applicable individuals.

Care Planning Systems

Standards of care are detailed electronic or paper guidelines that represent the predicted care for specific situations. They do not direct nurses to provide medical interventions; rather, they provide an efficient method for retrieving predicted generic nursing interventions for medical conditions or procedures. Standards of care identify a set of problems (actual or at risk) that typically occur in a particular situation—a diagnostic cluster. An efficient, professional, and useful care planning system encompasses standards of care, individual problem lists, and standardized and addendum care plans.

Standardization

Like any concept or system, standardized care planning forms have both advantages and disadvantages. Advantages include the following:

- Eliminate the need to write routine nursing interventions
- Illustrate to new or part-time employees the unit standard of care
- Direct nursing staff to selected documentation requirements
- Provide the criteria for a quality improvement program and resource management
- Allow the nurse to spend more time delivering than documenting care

Disadvantages are as follows:

- May replace a needed individualized intervention
- May encourage nurses to focus on predictable problems instead of additional problems

Some nurses experienced these disadvantages when standardized care plans were introduced into their clinical setting. In such cases, the solution was to eliminate standardized care plans. Follow-up care plan audits revealed that the nurses were writing what previously was contained on the standard of care (e.g., *turn q2h, administer pain relief medication*).

Keep in mind that standards of care should represent the care that nurses are responsible for providing, not an ideal level of care. Unrealistic, ideal standards merely frustrate nurses and hold them legally accountable for care that they cannot provide.

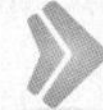

Carp's Cues

Nurses also have been socialized to view standardization as mediocre and unprofessional care. ***Standards of care or standardized care plans should represent responsible nursing care predicted for certain situations.*** Nurses should view these predictions as scientific. When problems arise with the misuse of standardized forms, the solution is not to eliminate the forms but to address their misuse.

Levels of Care

As discussed earlier, the nurse cannot hope to address all—or, usually, even most—of an individual's problems. Rather, the nurse must focus on the individual's most serious, or priority, problems. The nurse should refer problems that will not be addressed in the health-care facility to both the individual and the family for interventions after discharge. Referrals to community agencies, such as weight loss or smoking cessation programs and psychological counseling, may be indicated after discharge. Nurses must create realistic standards based on individual acuity, length of stay, and available resources.

A care planning system can be structured with three tiers or levels of care:

1. Level I—generic unit standard of care
2. Level II—diagnostic cluster or single-diagnosis standardized care plan
3. Level III—addendum care plans

Level I—Unit Standards of Care

Level I standards of care represent the predicted generic care required for all or most individuals on a unit. These standards contain nursing diagnoses or collaborative problems (the diagnostic cluster) applicable to the specific situation. Box 5.5 presents a sample diagnostic cluster for standards of care in a general medical unit. Each unit—orthopedics, oncology, pediatrics, surgical, postanesthesia, neonatal, emergency, mental health, postpartum, and so on—should have a generic unit standard of care.

Box 5.5 GENERIC DIAGNOSTIC CLUSTER FOR HOSPITALIZED ADULTS WITH MEDICAL CONDITIONS

Collaborative Problems

- *RC of Cardiovascular*
- *RC of Respiratory*

Nursing Diagnosis

- *Anxiety related to unfamiliar environment, routines, diagnostic tests and treatments, and loss of control*
- *Risk for Injury related to unfamiliar environment and physical/mental limitations secondary to condition, medications, therapies, and diagnostic tests*
- *Risk for Infection related to increased microorganisms in environment, the risk for person-to-person transmission, and invasive tests and therapies*
- *Self-Care Deficit related to pain, sensory, cognitive, mobility, endurance, or motivation problems*
- *Risk for Imbalanced Nutrition: Less Than Body Requirements related to decreased appetite secondary to treatments, fatigue, environment, and changes in usual diet, and increased protein/vitamin requirements for healing*
- *Risk for Constipation related to change in fluid/food intake, routine and activity level, effects of medications, and emotional stress*
- *Disturbed Sleep Patterns related to unfamiliar, noisy environment, change in bedtime ritual, emotional stress, and change in circadian rhythm*
- *Risk for Spiritual Distress related to separation from religious support system, lack of privacy, or inability to practice spiritual rituals*
- *Interrupted Family Process related to disruption of routines, change in role responsibilities, and fatigue associated with increased workload and visiting hour requirements*
- *Risk for Compromised Human Dignity related to multiple factors associated with hospitalization*
- *Risk for Self-Health Management related to complexity and cost of therapeutic regimen, self-care deficits, barriers to comprehension (e.g., anxiety, language skills, cognitive deficits and insufficient knowledge of treatments, restrictions (diet, activity), medications, signs and symptoms of complications, and follow-up care*

Level I standards can be laminated and placed in each individual care area as a reference for nurses. Because these standards apply to all individuals, the nurse does not have to write these nursing diagnoses or collaborative problems on an individual client's care plan. Instead, institutional policy can specify that the generic standard will be implemented for all individuals if indicated.

The concept of high risk is not useful at the unit standard level. At this level, all or most individuals are at risk, but not at *high* risk. For example, after surgery all individuals are at risk for infection, but not all are at high risk.

To document Level I standards of care, the nurse should use flow chart notations unless he or she finds unusual data or significant incidents occur. Although standards of care do not have to be part of the individual's record, the record should specify what standards have been selected for the individual. The problem list, representing the priority nursing diagnoses and collaborative problems for an individual client can serve this purpose.

Level II—Standardized Care Plans

Preprinted care plans that represent care to provide for an individual, family, or group in addition to the Level I unit standards of care, Level II standardized care plans are supplements to the generic unit standard. Thus, an individual admitted to a medical unit will receive nursing care based on both the Level I unit standards and the Level II standardized care plan for the specific condition that led to admission.

A Level II standardized care plan contains either a diagnostic cluster or a single nursing diagnosis or collaborative problem, such as *High Risk for Impaired Skin Integrity* or *RC of Fluid/Electrolyte Imbalances*. Box 5.6 presents a Level II standardized care plan for the collaborative problem *RC of Hypo/Hyperglycemia.*

A diagnostic cluster Level II standard would contain additional nursing diagnoses and collaborative problems that are predicted to be present and prior because of a medical condition, surgical intervention,

Box 5.6 LEVEL II STANDARDIZED CARE PLAN FOR RC OF HYPO/HYPERGLYCEMIA

RC of Hypo/Hyperglycemia

Collaborative Outcome:

The nurse will monitor for early signs/symptoms of hypo/hyperglycemia and will receive collaborative interventions if indicated to restore physiologic stability.

Indicators of Physiologic Stability

No ketones in urine

Fasting blood glucose 70–130 mg/dL

Clear, oriented

Warm, dry skin

The nurse will manage and minimize hypo- or hyperglycemia episodes.

1. Monitor for signs and symptoms of hypoglycemia:
   - Blood glucose less than 70 mg/dL
   - Pale, moist, cool skin
   - Tachycardia, diaphoresis
   - Jitteriness, irritability
   - Headache, slurred speech
   - Incoordination
   - Drowsiness
   - Visual changes
   - Hunger, nausea, abdominal pain
2. Follow protocols when indicated, for example, concentrated glucose (oral, IV) insulin sliding scale
3. Monitor for signs and symptoms of ketoacidosis:
   - Blood glucose greater than 300 mg/dL
   - Positive plasma ketone, acetone breath
   - Headache, tachycardia
   - Kussmaul's respirations, decreased BP
   - Anorexia, nausea, vomiting
   - Polyuria, polydipsia
   - If ketoacidosis occurs, follow protocols, for example, initiation of IV fluids, insulin IV.
   - If episode is severe, monitor vital signs, urine output, specific gravity, ketones, blood glucose electrolytes q30 min or PRN.
   - Document blood glucose findings and other assessment data on flow record. Document unusual events or responses on progress notes.

or therapy. For example, the following presents a problem list of the individual who is 1 day after total hip replacement surgery and the source of the care.

Problem list	Source
RC of Dislocation of Joint *RC of Neurovascular Compromise* *RC of Emboli (fat, blood)* *Impaired Physical Mobility* *High Risk for Pressure Ulcers* *High Risk for Falls* *High Risk for Ineffective Self-Health Management*	Individual's problem list from Level II Standard—Post 1 Total Hip Replacement

If this individual also had diabetes mellitus, the nurse would add the following single diagnosis standard to the problem list: *RC of Hypo/Hyperglycemia*.

After the nursing staff are well oriented to the details of the unit standard, the diagnoses on the Level I unit standard can be omitted from individual problem lists or care plans. Policy would indicate that this standard would apply to all the individuals on the unit.

Level III—Addendum Care Plans

An addendum care plan lists additional interventions beyond the Levels I and II standards that an individual requires. These specific interventions may be added to a standardized care plan or may be associated with additional priority nursing diagnoses or collaborative problems not included on the Level II standardized care plan or Level I unit standards.

For many hospitalized individuals, the nurse can direct initial care responsibility using standards of care. Assessment information obtained during subsequent nurse–individual interactions may warrant specific additions to the individual's care plan to ensure outcome achievement. The nurse can add or delete from standardized plans or handwrite or free-text (by computer) an addendum diagnosis with its applicable goals and interventions.

The documentation of implementation does not take place on a care plan but on flow charts, graphic charts, or nursing progress notes, depending on the types of data being recorded.

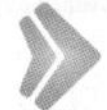

Carp's Cues

The uniqueness of all persons predicts that the nurse can always add additional nursing diagnoses to every client problem list. However, given the shortened length of stay of hospitalized persons, the nurse must determine if the additional diagnoses are priority. The standardized care plan should address most of the priority nursing diagnoses. It is important to note that the nurse can always individualize interventions for standardized nursing diagnoses for each individual as needed.

Problem List/Care Plan

As discussed earlier, a problem list represents the priority set of nursing diagnoses and collaborative problems that the nursing staff will manage for a particular individual. When appropriate, the term *diagnostic* can be used in place of *problem* (i.e., diagnosis list/care plan) to accommodate wellness diagnoses.

The problem list is a permanent chart record that identifies both the nursing diagnoses and the collaborative problems receiving nursing management and also the source for interventions: standard of care, standardized care plan, or addendum care plan. Figure 5.4 illustrates a sample nursing problem list/care plan for an individual with a history of type 1 diabetes mellitus who is admitted to a medical unit for treatment of pneumonia. This sample includes the individual's priority set of diagnoses as well as the addendum interventions that the nurse has added to the standardized care plan under the diagnosis *Acute Pain*.

Carp's Cues

Problem lists are an excellent method to communicate the specific nursing focus for an individual. They can easily cross reference to a standardized plan or addendum individualized plan.

FIGURE 5.4 Sample problem list/care plan.

Nursing Problem List/Care Plan

Nursing Diagnosis/ Collaborative Problem	Status	Standard	Addendum	Evaluation of Progress				
Med Unit Standard	9/20 A	✔		9/21 P/LJC	9/22 P/Pw	9/23 P-GA		
RC of Hyperthermia	9/20			S/LJC	S/Jw	S-GA		
RC of Hyper/Hypoglycemia	9/20 A	✔						
Acute Pain	9/20 A	✔	✔					

STATUS CODE: A = Active R = Resolved RO = Ruled-out
EVALUATION CODE: S = Stable, I = Improved, *W = Worsened, U = Unchanged, *P = Not Progressing, P = Progressing

Reviewed With Client/Family 9/21 LJC, ______, ______, (Date)

Addendum Care Plan

Nsg Dx/ Coll Prob	Client/Nursing Goals	Date/ Initials	Interventions
Acute Pain	–	9/23 LJC	1. Provide a gentle back rub in
			evening
			2. Leave blanket at foot of bed for
			easy access

Initials/Signature			
1. LJC Lynda J. Carpenito	3.	5.	7.
2. Pw Poti Wychoff	4. G. Arcangelo	6.	8.

SUMMARY The repetitive writing or selecting of routine care items in an electronic record of the same care predicted to be present because of a particular medical condition or surgical procedure continues today.

It is a waste of nurses' time.
It consumes time better spent with individuals and families.
It deters nurses from writing individualized plans when needed.

All nursing units can provide care using standardized care plans and can be more motivated to individualize this care when the needless writing is eliminated.

Chapter 6

Eleven Steps to Putting It All Together With or Without Concept Mapping

Learning Objectives

After reading the chapter, the following questions should be answered:

- What is concept mapping?
- How should you focus your assessment for a particular individual?
- How do you write a care plan if you have not met the individual?
- What additional information should you add to the care plan?
- After providing care, how do you evaluate the individual's progress?

What Is Concept Mapping?

"Concept mapping is a technique that can help you organize data for analysis. It uses diagrams to demonstrate the relationship of one concept or piece of information to other concepts or pieces of information" (Carpenito-Moyet, 2007). This is useful for students and others, who are new to care planning and nursing diagnoses.

Concept mapping can help you

- Explain relationships of data
- Identify both strengths and risk factors in individuals
- Determine whether there is sufficient data to support your diagnosis

The concept map is composed of a center circle with a ring of outer circles that are connected to the center circle. This is the diagram that you can use to map clinical data on the individual.

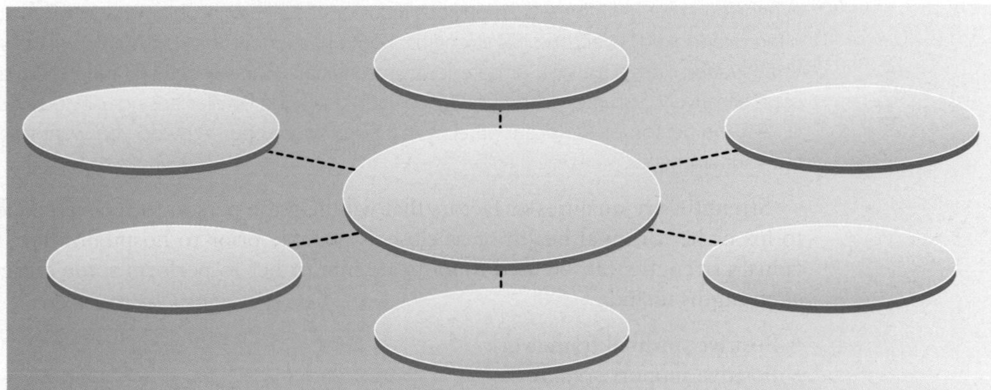

Sample concept maps for an individual are shown below and on the following pages. The individual's strengths are mapped below:

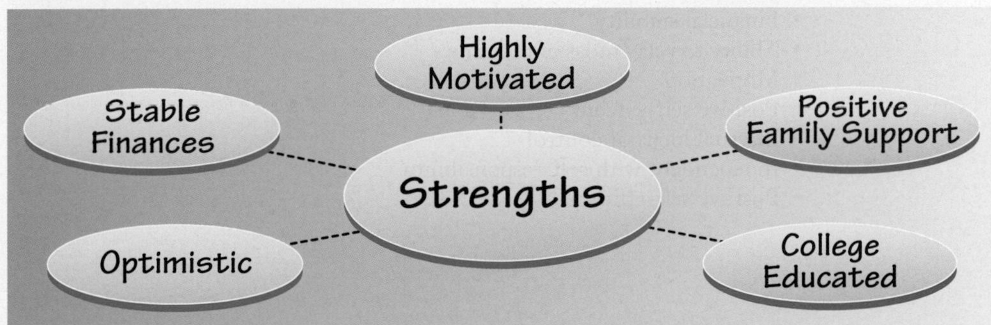
Highly Motivated
Stable Finances
Positive Family Support
Strengths
Optimistic
College Educated

His risk factors are mapped below:

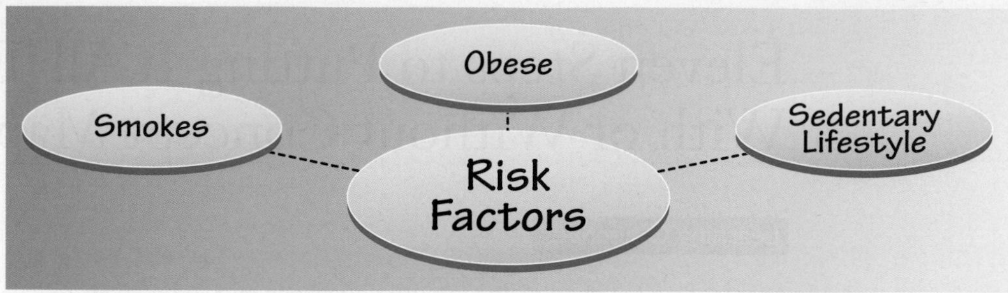

Throughout the 11 steps you can use concept mapping to help organize the data.

Now you have learned the five steps in the nursing process in Chapter 5, you will have the tools to create a plan of care (or care plan) for the individual.

Step 1: Assessment

Transitional Risk Assessment Plan

On admission, the individual needs to be assessed for their vulnerability for infection, pressure ulcers, falls, and delayed transition. Use the evidence-based assessment tools in Appendix D.

If you need to write a care plan before you can interview the individual, go to Step 2 now. If you interview the individual before you write your care plan, complete your assessment using the form recommended by your faculty.

After you complete your assessment, you will need to identify

- Strengths
- Risk factors
- Problems in one or more Functional Health Patterns

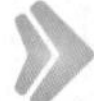

Carp's Cues

When someone is ill, there is an obvious focus on the illness, problems, and risk factors. Unfortunately, strengths are often overlooked. Everyone has strengths. Some have more than others. Our strengths help us through hard times. With sudden illness, trauma, or deteriorating conditions, the strengths of the individual and family can be mobilized to cope effectively. Sometimes the strength of individuals and families are not obvious. Search for them!

Ask the person or significant other: What gives your hope? Why do you want to get better? Nurse/Student. What are your strengths?

Strengths are qualities or factors that will help the person to recover, cope with stressors, and progress to his or her original health or as close as possible prior to hospitalization, illness, or surgery. The individual's strengths can be used to motivate him or her to perform some difficult activities. Some examples of strengths include

- Positive spiritual framework
- Positive support system
- Ability to perform self-care
- No eating difficulties
- Effective sleep habits
- Alertness and good memory
- Financial stability
- Ability to relax most of the time
- Motivation
- Positive self-esteem
- Internal locus of control
- Independent with self-responsibility
- Positive self-efficacy

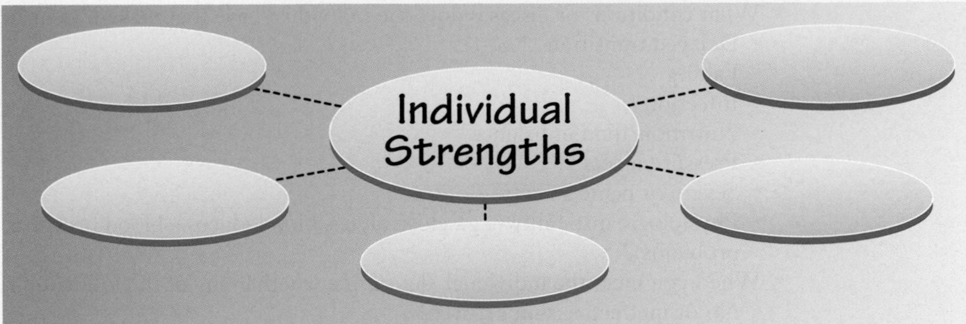

Write a list of the individual's strengths or use a concept map with strengths as the center.

Risk factors are situations, personal characteristics, disabilities, or medical conditions that can hinder the person's ability to heal, cope with stressors, and progress to his or her original health prior to hospitalization, illness, or surgery. Examples of risk factors are as follows:

- No or ineffective support system
- Substance abuse (alcohol, tobacco, drugs)
- No or little regular exercise
- Inadequate or poor nutritional habits
- Learning difficulties
- Denial
- Poor coping skills
- Communication problems
- Obesity
- Fatigue
- Limited ability to speak or understand English
- Memory/comprehension problems
- Hearing problems
- Self-care problems before hospitalization
- Difficulty walking
- Financial problems
- Negative self-efficacy

Write a list of risk factors for the individual or create a concept map of risk factors.

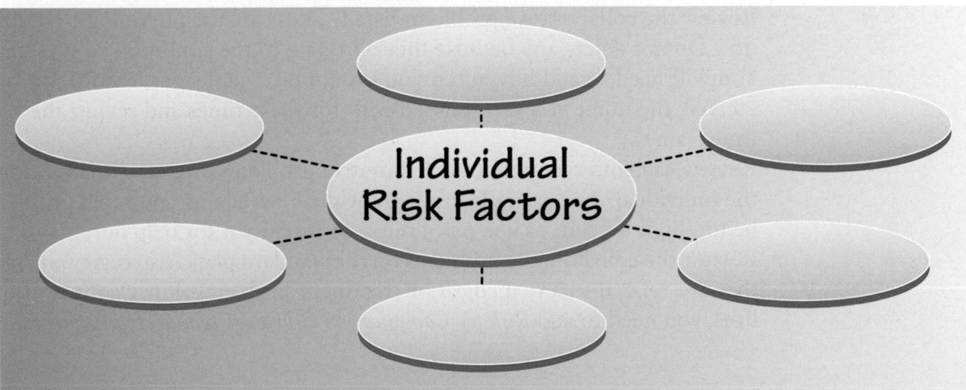

Step 2: Same-Day Assessment

If you have not completed a screening assessment of the individual, determine the following as soon as you can by asking the individual, family, or nurse assigned to the individual.

- Before hospitalization:
  - Could the individual perform self-care?
  - Did the individual need assistance?
  - Could the individual walk unassisted?
  - Did the individual have memory problems?
  - Did the individual have hearing problems?
  - Did the individual smoke cigarettes?

- What conditions or diseases does the individual have that make him or her more vulnerable to
  - Delayed transition
  - Falling
  - Infection
  - Nutrition/fluid imbalance
  - Pressure ulcers
  - Severe or panic anxiety
  - Physiologic instability (e.g., electrolytes, blood glucose, blood pressure, respiratory function, healing problems)
- When you meet the individual, determine whether any of the following risk factors are present:
  - No or ineffective support system
  - Obesity
  - Communication problems/learning difficulties
  - Movement difficulties
  - Inadequate nutritional status
  - Recent or ongoing stress (e.g., financial, death in family)
  - Substance abuse (alcohol, tobacco, drugs)

Write significant data on an index card. Go to Step 3.

Step 3: Create Your Initial Care Plan

If the individual is in the hospital for a medical problem, refer to the generic medical care plan online (thePoint®). If the individual is in the hospital for a surgical condition, refer to the generic surgical care plan B, also online. These generic care plans reflect the usual predicted care an individual needs.

Ask your instructor if you can use them and revise them electronically for the individual.

You can also refer to *Handbook of Nursing Diagnoses*, 15th edition (Carpenito-Moyet, 2017) for examples of nursing diagnoses and collaborative problems associated with medical and surgical conditions.

For specific care plans for 76 medical conditions, surgical interventions or diagnostic/therapeutic situations, refer to *Nursing Care Plans: Transitional Patient & Family Centered Care*, 6th edition (Carpenito-Moyet, 2014).

A diagnostic cluster for an individual post general surgery can be found in Box 5.2 in Chapter 5.

Step 4: Review the Collaborative Problems on the Generic Plan

- Review the collaborative problems listed. These are the physiologic complications that you need to monitor. Do not delete any because they all relate to the condition or procedure that the individual has had. You will need to add how often you should take vital signs, record intake and output, change dressings, etc. Ask the nurse you are assigned with for these times and review the Kardex, which also may have the time frames.
- Review each intervention for collaborative problems. Are any interventions unsafe or contraindicated for the individual? For example, if the individual has edema and renal problems, the fluid requirements may be too high for him or her. Ask a nurse or instructor for help here.
- Review the collaborative problems on the standard plan. Also review all additional collaborative problems that are related to any medical or treatment problems. For example, if the individual has diabetes mellitus, you need to add *Risk for Complication of Hypoglycemia/Hyperglycemia.*

Step 5: Review the Nursing Diagnoses on the Standard Plan

Review each nursing diagnosis on the plan.

- Does it apply to the individual?
- Does the individual have any risk factors that could make this diagnosis worse (see your index card)?

An example on the Generic Medical Care Plan is *Risk for Injury related to unfamiliar environment and physical or mental limitations secondary to condition, medication, therapies, or diagnostic tests*.

Now look at your list of risk factors for the individual. Can any factors listed contribute to the individual's sustaining an injury? For example, is he or she having problems walking or seeing? Is he or she experiencing dizziness?

If the individual has an unstable gait related to peripheral vascular disease (PVD), you would add the following: *unstable gait secondary to peripheral vascular disease secondary to Risk for Injury related to unfamiliar environment.* Review the goals listed for the nursing diagnosis:

- Are they pertinent to the individual?
- Can the individual demonstrate achievement of the goal on the day you provide care?
- Do you need more time?
- Do you need to make the goal more specific for the individual?

Delete goals that are inappropriate for the individual. If the individual will need more time to meet the goal, add "by discharge." If the individual can accomplish the goal this day, write "by (insert date)" after the goal.

Using the same diagnosis *Risk for Injury related to unfamiliar environment and physical and mental limitations secondary to the condition, therapies, and diagnostic tests*, consider this goal: The individual will request assistance with activities of daily living (ADLs).

Indicators

- Identify factors that increase risk of injury.
- Describe appropriate safety measures.

If it is realistic for the individual to achieve all the goals on the day of your care, you should add the date to all of them.

If the individual is confused, you can add the date to the main goal, but you would delete all the indicators because the person is confused. Or you could modify the goal by writing "Family member will identify factors that increase the individual's risk of injury."

Review each intervention for each nursing diagnosis:

- Are they relevant for the individual?
- Will you have time to provide them?
- Are any interventions not appropriate or contraindicated for the individual?
- Can you add any specific interventions?
- Do you need to modify any interventions because of risk factors (see index card)?

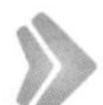

Carp's Cues

Remember that you cannot individualize a care plan for an individual until you spend time with him or her, but you can add or delete interventions based on your preclinical knowledge of the individual (e.g., medical diagnosis, coexisting medical conditions).

Step 6: Prepare the Care Plan (Electronic, Written, or Printed)

You can prepare the care plan by

- Typing the online generic care plan into your word processor, then deleting or adding specifics for the individual (use another color or a different type font for additions/deletions)
- Photocopying a section from this book, then adding or deleting specifics for the individual
- Writing the care plan

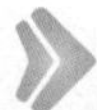

Carp's Cues

Ask your faculty person what options are acceptable. Using different colors or fonts allows him or her to clearly see your analysis. Be prepared to provide rationales for why you added or deleted items.

Step 7: Initial Care Plan Completed

Now that you have a care plan of the collaborative problems and nursing diagnoses for the primary condition that initiated hospitalization, are there any risk factors or other medical problems present that are priority? Confusion? Diabetes Mellitus?

Step 8: Additional Risk Factors

If the individual has risk factors (on the index card) that you identified in Steps 1 and 2, evaluate if these risk factors make the individual more vulnerable to develop a problem.

The following questions can help to determine whether the individual or family has additional diagnoses that need nursing interventions:

- Are additional collaborative problems associated with coexisting medical conditions that require monitoring (e.g., hypoglycemia)?
- Are there additional nursing diagnoses that, if not managed or prevented now, will deter recovery or affect the individual's functional status (e.g., *Risk for Constipation*)?
- What problems does the individual perceive as priority?
- What nursing diagnoses are important but treatment for them can be delayed without compromising functional status?

Carp's Cues

You can address nursing diagnoses not on the priority list by referring the individual for assistance after discharge (e.g., counseling, weight loss program). Limited time and resources mandate that these problems be referred back to the individual for management after discharge. Do not create a care plan that is impossible for you to provide to the individual and family.

Priority identification is a very important but difficult concept. Because of shortened hospital stays and because many individuals have several chronic diseases at once, nurses cannot address most of the nursing diagnoses for every individual. Nurses must focus on those for which the individual would be injured, experience more anxiety or not make progress if they were not addressed. Ask your clinical faculty to review your list. Be prepared to provide rationales for your selections.

Step 9: Evaluate the Status of the Individual (After You Provide Care)

Collaborative Problems

Review the collaborative goals for the collaborative problems:

- Assess the individual's status.
- Compare the data with established norms (indicators).
- Judge if the data fall within acceptable ranges.
- Conclude if the individual is stable, improved, unimproved, or worse.

Is the individual stable or improved?

- If yes, continue to monitor the individual and to provide interventions indicated.
- If not, has there been a dramatic change (e.g., elevated blood pressure and decreased urinary output)? Have you notified the physician or advanced practice nurse? Have you increased your monitoring of the individual? Communicate your evaluations of the status of collaborative problems to your clinical faculty and to the nurse assigned to the individual.

Nursing Diagnoses

Review the goals or outcome criteria for each nursing diagnosis.

- Did the individual demonstrate or state the activity defined in the goal?
- If yes, then communicate (document) the achievement on your plan.
- If not and the individual needs more time, change the target date.
- If time is not the issue, evaluate why the individual did not achieve the goal.

Was the goal

- Not realistic because of other priorities?
- Not acceptable to the individual?

Review the Interventions for each nursing diagnosis.

- Are they acceptable to the individual?
- Can you make them more specific?
- Are there any interventions that should be revised or deleted?

Step 10: Document the Care

Document the care in the electronic health record, the agency's forms, flow records, and progress notes.

Step 11: Evaluate the Care Plan

After each day of caring for the individual, go back to Step 9 and repeat the evaluation and make revisions to the plan if needed.

SUMMARY

More than one nurse has told you that care planning is a useless, waste of time. Probably this nurse has experienced care planning systems that require mindless writing or repetitive data selection on an electronic charting system.

As a student of nursing, it is important for you to learn the standard of care that is expected to be needed in many clinical situations.

Some clinical examples are as follows:

- Postabdominal surgery
- Newborn care
- Postpartum care
- Individual with pneumonia
- Individual after a stroke (CVA)
- Individual postmyocardial infarction

After you have experienced giving care to several individuals after abdominal surgery, you will know the care that is indicated. This will allow you to focus on other possible nursing diagnoses. You need first to become an expert in the standard of care. Care planning that does not require you to write the same care repeatedly will allow you more opportunities to individualize the care. Learning the nursing process by writing can help you to understand this type of scientific problem solving.

Chapter 7

Transitional Individual/Family Centered-Care[1]

Learning Objectives

After reading this chapter, the following questions should be answered:

- Why is referring to a person or family as noncompliant not clinically useful?
- How does transition of a person from a hospital differ from discharge of a person from a hospital?
- What is a nurse assessing for when completing a medication reconciliation?
- Name three occurrences in the hospital that are labeled "never events?"

Engagement of Individual and/or Families in Planning and Shaping Their Health Care

"Patient activation" refers to a patient's knowledge, skills, ability, and willingness to manage his or her own health and care. "Patient engagement" is a broader concept that combines patient activation with interventions designed to increase activation and promote positive patient behavior, such as obtaining preventive care or exercising regularly. Patient engagement is one strategy to achieve the "triple aim" of improved health outcomes, better patient care, and lower costs (James, 2013, p. 1).

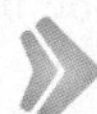

Carp's Cues

The concept of "engagement" implies a two-way process; whereas terms such as "noncompliance" and "nonadherance" imply that the individual or family is not cooperating with care. It targets the individual/family as problematic, rather than focusing on whether the process used was problematic. Thus the nursing diagnosis Noncompliance should be revised to one labeled as Nonengagement or Risk for Nonengagement. The clinical focus would be on related or risk factors that are barriers to engagement.

Coulter (2012) reports, "Patient engagement acknowledges that patients have an important role to play in their own health care. This includes reading, understanding and acting on health information (health literacy), working together with clinicians to select appropriate treatments or management options (shared decision making), and providing feedback on health-care processes and outcomes (quality improvement)."

Strategies are focused on supporting and strengthening the individual's determinations of their health-care needs and self-care efforts with improved health. These strategies can attract an individual/family by focusing on their priorities and individualizing the interactions that are appropriative and comfortable (e.g., health literacy, readiness for change, accessible, affordable).

This is a very large culture change. Previously, the professional would approach health teaching with a list of what to teach and proceed to teach the contents of the list. It was concluded that the individual/family has learned. Without an understanding of the individual/family readiness or ability to learn, this "one size fits all" concludes with little understanding or motivation to change health behaviors, with a probable outcome of increased anxiety for those involved.

To engage individuals/families, health professionals focus on listening not talking, and increased question asking, to assess the specific concerns and barriers to change. The desired outcomes are increased comfort to ask questions, enhance confidence with better support, more informed, more discriminating about the effects of medical treatment, and more opportunities for participation (Coulter, 2012).

Evidence of effective engagement strategies can be (Barnsteiner, Disch, & Walton, 2014; Coulter, 2012):

- Choosing healthier lifestyle
- Understanding the causes of disease and behaviors to prevent onset or exacerbation of the disease
- Self-diagnosing and treating minor conditions
- Knowing when to seek advice and professional help

[1]Portions of this chapter can be found in Carpenito-Moyet, L. J. (2014). *Nursing care plans/patient and family centered care* (6th ed.). Philadelphia: Lippincott Williams & Wilkins.

- Choosing appropriate health-care providers
- Accessing the appropriate care site, for example, primary care, urgent care, emergency room, and specialists
- Coping with the effects of chronic illness and self-managing their care
- Monitoring symptoms and treatment effects; knowing what is problematic
- Determining their own end-of-life decisions
- Decreased nonparticipations in health-care decisions; decreased onset or exacerbations of disorders and related care costs

Refer to Appendix D Strategies to Promote Engagement of Individual/Families for Healthier Outcomes in varied health-care settings, for example, primary/specialty care, acute care, long term.

Discharge versus Transition

In the last 5 years, hospitals and skilled and long-term care facilities have reorganized under the "transitional health-care model." Previously, discharge was an event. Dramatic reengineering has changed the concept of discharge, from an event to transition as a process. Discharge was episodic and often unexpected; transition is planned and anticipated.

Transition to home or another care facility is a proactive, collaborative process among medicine, nursing, social service, physical therapy, occupational therapy, and nutritionist with each other, with community-based professionals (primary providers, specialists, home care professionals), and with the ill individual and his/her support system.

This collaborative process requires effective communication, early identification of transition date, daily review of status and early identification of barriers, clinicians responsible 7 days a week, and timely access to services in the community.

This complex process takes place in a health-care setting with extreme pressure to discharge or transfer individuals, shorter length of stays, and penalties if individuals are readmitted.

Nurses may view this new emphasis on a safe, timely transition as a means "to save finances" for the health-care institution or the third-party payer. When health-care funds dwindle, the recipients, unfortunately, suffer the most.

Buerhaus and Kurtzman (2008, p. 30) wrote:

Most hospital nurses are salaried; hospitals consider those salaries a cost of doing business. In most hospitals, nurses represent about 40% of the direct-care budget. By contrast, physicians are revenue generators because hospitals charge the CMS and other payers for the costs of the resources used to produce medical care provided by or ordered by physicians. Until now, there hasn't been a mechanism under Medicare payment policies for measuring nurses' specific economic contribution to hospitals. CMS-1533-FC offers a mechanism for doing so; to the degree that nursing care prevents costly complications, hospitals will not lose money. In this way, the new Medicare payment rule has the potential to more clearly demonstrate nurses' economic value to hospitals.

Each day an individual stays in the hospital, the following effects occur:

- Sleep deprivation
- Deconditioning
- Increase in infections
- Family disruption
- Sensory overload
- Nutritional deficits

Early Identification of High-Risk Individuals and/or Family

On admission, all individuals will have a nursing assessment of vital signs, functional health patterns, and body systems (e.g., skin, respiratory, cardiac) using the Nursing Admission Assessment Base. Refer to Appendix B for an example.

After the initial assessment, determine the likelihood that the individual will have an uncomplicated complex transition. For the majority of individuals, the transition will be uncomplicated, as described as:

- Will usually return to their own home or someone else's for a short stay
- Having care needs that can be managed by the individual or support system and do not require complex planning, teaching, or referrals

Uncomplicated transition individuals should be told prior to admission how long they can expect to be in hospital and the time of day they can expect to be discharged, so that they can plan with their support persons.

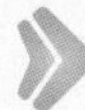

Carp's Cues

Individuals/families that were providing good care at home for long-term chronic conditions may be able to resume this care with little help. Keep in mind that a change in the individual's status or support system situation can change a transition process to uncomplicated from complex.

To differentiate between a predicted uncomplicated and complex transition, the following assessments are indicated:

- Medication reconciliation and barriers to adherence
- Factors that are barriers to effective transition to home care
- Factors that increase the individual's risk for injury, falls, pressure ulcers, and/or infection during hospitalization

Medication Reconciliation and Barriers to Adherence

Medication errors occur 46% of the time during transitions, admission, transfer, or discharge from a clinical unit or hospital. Almost 60% of individuals have at least one discrepancy in their medication history completed on admission (Cornish et al., 2005). "The most common error (46.4%) was omission of a regularly used medication. Most (61.4%) of the discrepancies were judged to have no potential to cause serious harm. However, 38.6% of the discrepancies had the potential to cause moderate to severe discomfort or clinical deterioration" (Cornish et al., 2005, p. 424).

Medication reconciliation on admission to the health-care facilities often entails the following:

- Name of medication (prescribed, over the counter)
- Prescribed dose
- Frequency (daily, bid, tid, as needed)

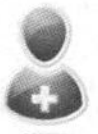

Clinical Alert A list of medications that have been prescribed by a provider does not represent a process of medication reconciliation. As an example, a family member took an older relative to the ER with chest pain. A typed list of her medications was given to the ER nurse. No discussion occurred about her medication.

One of two hypertension medications the patient regularly took was not entered in the electronic health record. Since her blood pressure was elevated on admission and persisted, another antihypertensive medication was ordered. After two days, another medication was added with good results.

The first medication that was added was the medication she was already taking prior to admission. So essentially, no new medication was added as a result of the error. She spent three unnecessary days in the hospital with increased costs to Medicare and would have definitely rather been home eating her own food and having a good night sleep in her own bed.

According to the Joint Commission (2010, p. 1),

> *Medication reconciliation is the process of comparing a client's medication orders to all of the medications that the patient has been taking. This reconciliation is done to avoid medication errors such as omissions, duplications, dosing errors, or drug interactions. It should be done at every transition of care in which new medications are ordered or existing orders are rewritten. Transitions in care include changes in setting, service, practitioner, or level of care. The process comprises five steps: (1) develop a list of current medications; (2) develop a list of medications to be prescribed; (3) compare the medications on the two lists; (4) make clinical decisions based on the comparison; and (5) communicate the new list to appropriate caregivers to the patient.*

Table 7.1 outlines a comprehensive list of medications to review during medication reconciliations.

Critical to acquiring a list of medications authorized in Table 7.1 are the additional assessment questions, which are the defining elements for medication reconciliation: *versus a list of medications reported to be taking.*

The individual/family member is asked the following:

For each medication reported ask:

- What is the reason you are taking each medication?
- Are you taking the medication as prescribed? Specify once a day, twice a day, etc.

Table 7.1 SOURCES OF MEDICATION HISTORY

The medication history can be obtained from a variety of sources:
- The individual
- A list the patient may have
- The medications themselves, if brought in from home
- A friend or family member
- A medical record
- The individual's pharmacy

- Are you skipping any doses? Do you sometimes run out of medications?
- How often are you taking the medication prescribed "if needed as a pain medication?"
- Have you stopped taking any of these medications?
- How much does it cost you to take your medications?
- Are you taking anybody else's medication?

Factors that increase are barriers to effectively transition to home.

Individuals, on admission to an acute care setting, necessitate an assessment to determine the presence of barriers to a timely transition to home care (or a community health setting).

Barriers that effectively transition from acute care setting are:

- Personal
- Support system
- Home environment

Personal Barriers

Determine if any of these barriers to self-care are responsible for this admission. Access the appropriate resource in the institution as early as possible to initiate resolving or reducing barriers (e.g., social service, home care).

Individuals are assessed for disabilities and compromised functioning at admission. Assess if the individual:

- Is homeless
- Has no medical insurance
- Is unable to live alone
- Is physically impaired
- Is mentally compromised
- Can read, and at what level of comprehension
- Understand English
- Is abusing drugs, alcohol

Support System Barriers

Preparing family members/support persons for home care is addressed through care plans (such as those presented in Unit III of *Nursing Care Plans: Transitionals and Family Centered Care Plans* [Carpenito-Moyet, 2017]). If a support system is not present, nonexistent, or incapable of providing home care, refer to the appropriate resource in the institution as early as possible (e.g., social service, home care agency).

Determine the present status of a support system. Assess:

- What kind of assistance is needed for home care 24/7 (e.g., daily visits, phone calls, etc.)?
- Is there a support system? Who?
- Are they willing/available to provide assistance?
- Will they arrange for assistance from others?
- Are they capable of providing needed care at home (e.g., elderly spouse)?

Home Environment

If there are barriers to home care due to the environment, refer to the appropriate resource in the institution as early as possible (e.g., social service, home health agency).

Determine the status of the home environment. Assess:

- Where does the person live? Home alone? Shelter? Homeless? With others?
- Can equipment for home care be accessed? Insurance coverage? Home barriers?
- Is the person capable accessing home/apartment? Stairs?
- Is there access to a bathroom without using stairs?
- If there is a temporary alternative (e.g., family member's home)?

Factors That Increase the Individual's Risk of Injury, Falls, Pressure Ulcers, and/or Infection During Hospitalization and Preventable Hospital-Acquired Conditions

The Centers for Medicare and Medicaid Services (CMS) in 2008 published "Roadmap for Implementing Value Driven Healthcare in the Traditional Medicare Fee-for-Service-Program."

CMS objective is "to improve the accuracy of Medicare's payment under the acute care hospital inpatient prospective payment system . . . while providing additional incentives for hospitals to engage in quality improvement efforts" (CMS, 2008).

Of equal importance is that additional payments will be denied for the treatment of the following 14 hospital-acquired conditions (CMS, 2008):

- Stages II and IV pressure ulcers
- Falls and trauma such as fractures, dislocations, intracranial injuries, crushing injuries, burns, and other injuries
- Manifestations of poor glycemic control (e.g., ketoacidosis, hyperosmolar coma, hypoglycemic coma, secondary diabetes with ketoacidosis, or hyperosmolarity)
- Catheter-associated urinary tract infections
- Vascular catheter-associated infections
- Surgical-site infection, mediastinitis, following coronary artery bypass graft (CABG)
- Surgical-site infection following bariatric surgery for obesity (laparoscopic gastric bypass, gastroenterostomy, laparoscopic gastric restrictive surgery)
- Surgical-site infection following certain orthopedic procedures (spine, neck, shoulder, elbow)
- Surgical-site infection following cardiac implantable electronic device (CIED)
- Foreign objects retained after surgery
- Deep vein thrombosis (DVT) and pulmonary embolism (PE) following certain orthopedic procedures (total knee replacement, hip replacement)
- Iatrogenic puemothorax with venous catheterization
- Air embolism
- Blood incompatibility

A white paper[2] on Preventing Never Events/Evidence-Based Practice reported the following (Leonardi, Faller, & Siroky, 2011, p. 8):

- 1 in 25 individuals suffer injury at a cost of $17 to $29 billion per year (Agency for Healthcare Research and Quality [AHRQ], 2010)
- 1.5 million injuries occurred in 2008 from medical errors at an average cost $13,000/injury or a total of $19.5 billion (Shreve et al., 2010)
- 7% of admissions had some type of medical injury according to inpatient billing records (Shreve et al., 2010)
- 42,243 individuals (0.2% of inpatients) developed a hospital-acquired infection
- Approximately 1.7 million hospital-acquired infections, the most common complications of hospital care (McGlynn, 2009), occur each year in hospitals, leading to about 100,000 deaths (AHRQ, 2010)

High-Risk Nursing Diagnoses for Preventable Hospital-Acquired Conditions

The Bifocal Clinical Practice Model (described in Chapter 5) can be used to identify high-risk individuals for the eight conditions identified by CMS. Using evidence-based guidelines, the following can be accessed:

- Nursing diagnoses that represent prevention of infection, falls, pressure ulcers, and delayed discharge
- Collaborative problems that identify individuals at high risk for air emboli, deep vein thrombosis, sepsis

[2]A white paper in nursing is an authoritative report of research or expert opinion to understand an issue, solve a problem, or make a decision.

Table 7.2 EXAMPLES OF PREVENTION OF HOSPITAL-ACQUIRED CONDITIONS OR DETECTION OF COMPLICATIONS

Nursing Diagnoses

- Risk for surgical site infection
- Risk for catheter site infection
- Risk for pressure ulcers

Collaborative Problems

- Risk for complication of deep vein thrombosis
- Risk for complications of fat embolism
- Risk for complications of sepsis

- Medical condition, postsurgical care, and treatment plan specifically identify adverse events that are associated with clinical diagnoses or situations
- Standardized risk assessment tools for falls, infection, and pressure ulcers that are incorporated in every care plan

Table 7.2 illustrates examples of prevention of hospital-acquired conditions or detection of complications.

SUMMARY

Nurses have been the primary health-care professionals in all health-care facilities for decades. Unfortunately, the impact of scientific caring nursing has eluded measurement and thus has been invisible. Individuals are admitted to hospitals for medical or surgical care that requires professional nursing. If professional nursing was not indicated, their medical condition would be managed by the primary care provider or specialist in an ambulatory setting. If professional nursing care is not indicated past a surgical procedure, it completed as a same-day surgery. The reason an individual is admitted to an intensive care unit is for specialized nursing care. The reason individuals are transitioned to their home is that they no longer need professional nursing care in the hospital. The reason an individual transfers to a skilled care facility is that he or she needs a type of professional and skilled nursing care. The assumption that individuals are admitted to hospitals primarily for medical care is erroneous. They need professional nursing expertise in order for medical management to be successful.

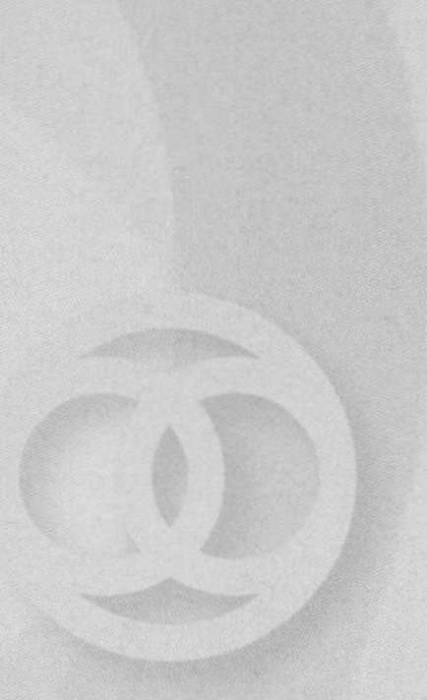

Section 2

Manual of Nursing Diagnoses

INTRODUCTION

The *Manual of Nursing Diagnoses* consists of nursing diagnoses.[1] This 15th edition has 25 new NANDA-I-approved nursing diagnoses. In addition, the following changes were instituted by NANDA-I:

- Actual Nursing Diagnoses are now named "Problem Focused"
- Risk Nursing Diagnoses have a change in definition from "at risk for" to "vulnerable to"
- Health Promotion Diagnoses have a change in definition and in most definitions of specific health promotion diagnoses

This section has been divided into four parts with the diagnoses placed in the appropriate categories:

- Part 1—Individual Nursing Diagnoses
- Part 2—Family/Home Nursing Diagnoses
- Part 3—Community Nursing Diagnoses
- Part 4—Health Promotion/Nursing Diagnoses

They are described with the three NANDA-I–required elements first:

- Definition
- Defining characteristics, signs and symptoms, or risk factors of the diagnosis
- Related factors or risk factors organized according to pathophysiologic, treatment related, situational, and maturational, that may contribute to or cause the actual diagnosis

Additional components include the following:

- Author's Note, which clarifies the concept and clinical use of the diagnosis
- Errors in Diagnostic Statements, which explain common mistakes in formulating diagnoses and ways to correct them
- Key Concepts, which list scientific explanations about the diagnosis and interventions, categorized as General, Pediatric, Maternal, Geriatric, and Transcultural Considerations
  - Carp's Cues: additional commentary similar to "did you know? "or "What if?"
  - Goals: represent statements that can be utilized to measure resolution of the problem, progress toward improved health, or continuance of good health and function.
  - Interventions: are actions that reduce or eliminate contributing factors or the diagnosis, prevent nursing diagnoses, and promote wellness; in addition, monitoring to evaluate onset of a nursing diagnosis or status of a nursing diagnosis.

[1]Definitions designated as NANDA-I and characteristics and factors identified with an asterisk are from *Nursing Diagnoses: Definitions and Classification 2012–2014*. Copyright © 2015, 2012, 2009, 2007, 2003, 2001, 1998, 1996, 1994 by NANDA International. Used by arrangement with Blackwell Publishing Limited, a company of John Wiley & Sons, Inc.

Part I

Individual Nursing Diagnoses

ACTIVITY INTOLERANCE

Activity Intolerance

Related to Insufficient Knowledge of Adaptive Techniques Needed Secondary to COPD
Related to Insufficient Knowledge of Adaptive Techniques Needed Secondary to Impaired Cardiac Function

NANDA-I Definition

Insufficient physiologic or psychological energy to endure or complete required or desired daily activities

Defining Characteristics

Major (Must Be Present)

An altered physiologic response to activity

Respiratory

Exertional dyspnea*
Excessively increased rate
Shortness of breath
Decreased rate

Pulse

Weak
Excessively increased
Rhythm change
Decreased
Failure to return to preactivity level after 3 minutes
EKG changes reflecting arrhythmias or ischemia*

Blood Pressure

Abnormal blood pressure response to activity
Failure to increase with activity
Increased diastolic pressure greater than 15 mm Hg

Minor (May Be Present)

Verbal report of weakness*
Pallor or cyanosis
Verbal reports of vertigo
Verbal report of fatigue*
Confusion

Related Factors

Any factors that compromise oxygen transport, physical conditioning, or create excessive energy demands that outstrip the individual's physical and psychological abilities can cause activity intolerance. Some common factors follow.

Pathophysiologic

Related to deconditioning secondary to prolonged immobilization and pain

Related to imbalance between oxygen supply/demand*

Related to compromised oxygen transport system secondary to:

Cardiac

- Cardiomyopathies
- Dysrhythmias
- Myocardial infarction (MI)
- Congenital heart disease
- Congestive heart failure
- Angina
- Valvular disease

Respiratory

- Chronic obstructive pulmonary disease (COPD)
- Bronchopulmonary dysplasia
- Atelectasis

Circulatory

- Anemia
- Hypovolemia
- Peripheral arterial disease

Related to increased metabolic demands secondary to:

- Acute or chronic infections
- Viral infection
- Endocrine or metabolic disorders
- Pain
- Mononucleosis
- Hepatitis

Chronic Diseases

- Renal
- Inflammatory
- Neurologic
- Hepatic
- Musculoskeletal

Related to inadequate energy sources secondary to:

- Obesity
- Malnourishment
- Inadequate diet

Treatment Related

Related to increased metabolic demands secondary to:

- Malignancies
- Diagnostic studies
- Surgery
- Treatment schedule/frequency

Related to compromised oxygen transport secondary to:

- Hypovolemia
- Bed rest* (related to inactivity secondary to assistive equipment [walkers, crutches, braces])
- Immobility*

Situational (Personal, Environmental)

Related to inactivity secondary to:

- Depression
- Inadequate social support
- Sedentary lifestyle*

Related to increased metabolic demands secondary to:

- Climate extremes (especially hot, humid climates)
- Air pollution (e.g., smog)
- Atmospheric pressure (e.g., recent relocation to high-altitude living)
- Environmental barriers (e.g., stairs)

Related to inadequate motivation secondary to:

- Fear of falling
- Depression
- Obesity
- Pain
- Dyspnea
- Generalized weakness*

Maturational

Older adults may have decreased muscle strength and flexibility, as well as sensory deficits. These factors can undermine body confidence and may contribute directly or indirectly to activity intolerance.

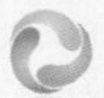

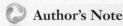

Author's Note

Activity Intolerance is a diagnostic judgment that describes an individual with compromised physical conditioning. This individual can engage in therapies to increase strength and endurance. *Activity Intolerance* is different from *Fatigue; Fatigue* is a pervasive, subjective draining feeling. Rest does treat *Fatigue*, but it can also cause tiredness. Moreover, in *Activity Intolerance*, the goal is to increase tolerance and endurance to activity; in *Fatigue*, the goal is to assist the individual to adapt to the fatigue, not to increase endurance.

Errors in Diagnostic Statements

***Activity Intolerance* related to dysrhythmic episodes in response to increased activity secondary to recent MI**

The current goals would be to monitor cardiac response to activity and to prevent decreased cardiac output, not to increase tolerance to activity. This situation would be labeled more appropriately as a collaborative problem: *Risk for Complications of Decreased Cardiac Output*.

***Activity Intolerance* related to fatigue secondary to chemotherapy**

Rest does not relieve fatigue associated with chemotherapy, nor is such fatigue amenable to interventions to increase endurance. The correction would be *Fatigue related to anemia and chemical changes secondary to toxic effects of chemotherapy*.

Key Concepts

General Considerations

- "Consensus Guidelines for Physical Activity and Public Health from the American Heart Association and American College of Sports Medicine call for at least 150 minutes per week of moderate ET or 75 minutes per week of vigorous ET in the general adult population. Those guidelines also suggest that larger doses of ET may be necessary in some groups, such as those with or at risk for CHD (30 to 60 minutes daily), adults trying to prevent the transition to overweight or obesity (45 to 60 minutes per day), and formerly obese individuals trying to prevent weight regain (60 to 90 minutes per day). These guidelines also caution that high-intensity ET increases risk of musculoskeletal injuries and adverse CV events" (*Haskell et al., 2007; La Gerche, Robberecht, & Kuiperi, 2010).
- The effects of bed rest and the supine position are illustrated in Figure II.1.
- The effects of bed rest deconditioning develop rapidly and may take weeks or months to reverse. All people confined to bed are at risk for activity intolerance as a result of bed rest-induced deconditioning.
- Early mobility has been linked to decreased morbidity and mortality as inactivity has a profound adverse effect on the brain, skin, skeletal muscle, pulmonary, and cardiovascular systems (Zomorodi, Darla Topley, & McAnaw, 2012).
- Delirium, decubitus ulcers, muscular atrophy, and deconditioning may occur in the immobile patient, as a result of atelectasis, pneumonia, orthostatic hypotension, and deep venous thrombosis (Zomorodi et al., 2012).
- *Endurance* is the ability to continue a specified task; *fatigue* is the inability to continue a specified task. Conceptually, endurance and fatigue are opposites. Nursing interventions, such as work simplification, aim to delay task-related fatigue by maximizing efficient use of the muscles that control motion, movement, and locomotion.
- The ability to maintain a given level of performance depends on *personal factors*, strength, coordination, reaction time, alertness, and motivation, and on *activity-related factors*, frequency, duration, and intensity.
- "Emerging data suggest that chronic training for and competing in extreme endurance events such as marathons, ultramarathons, ironman distance triathlons, and very long distance bicycle races, can cause transient acute volume overload of the atria and right ventricle, with transient reductions in right ventricular ejection fraction and elevations of cardiac biomarkers, all of which return to normal within 1 week. Over months to years of repetitive injury, this process, in some individuals, may lead to patchy myocardial fibrosis, particularly in the atria, interventricular septum, and right ventricle, creating a substrate for atrial and ventricular arrhythmias" (O'Keefe et al., 2012, p. 588).

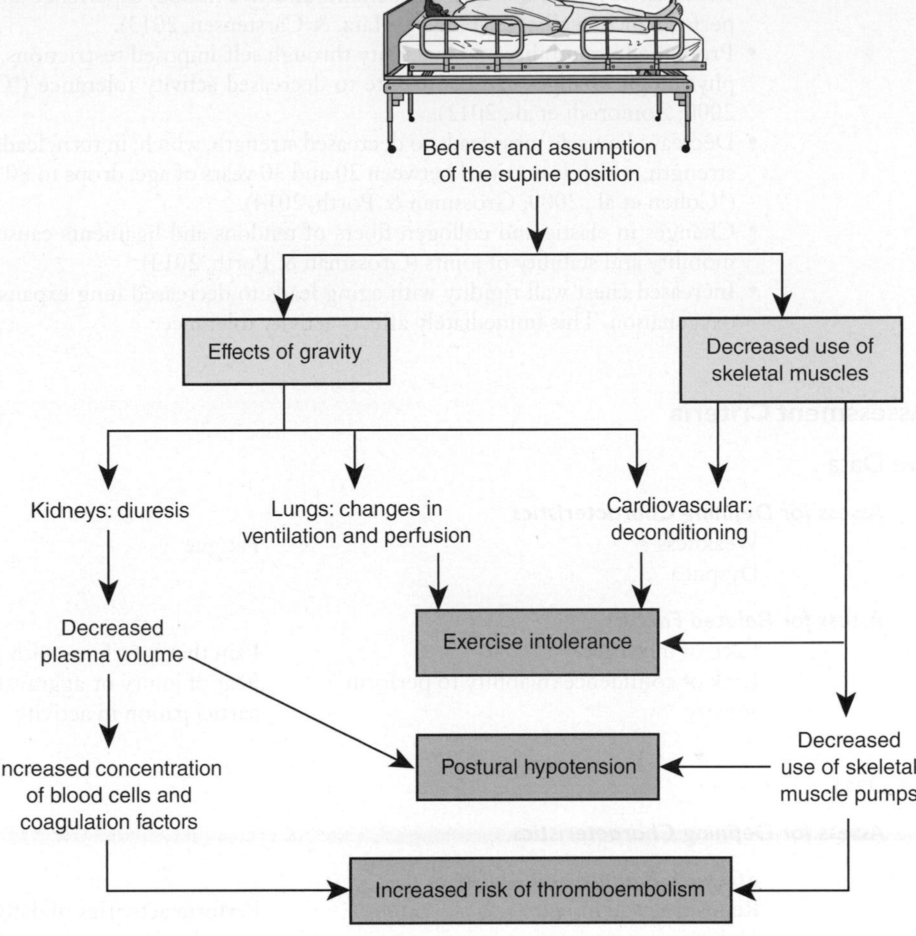

FIGURE II.1 Effects of Bedrest on Body Systems

Pediatric Considerations

- Children at special risk for activity intolerance include those with respiratory conditions, cardiovascular conditions, anemia, and chronic illnesses (Hockenberry & Wilson, 2015).
- "It is important to recognize that most children with congenital heart defects are relatively sedentary and that the physical and psychosocial health benefits of physical activity are important for this population, which is at risk for exercise intolerance, obesity, and psychosocial morbidities. Therefore, counseling to encourage daily participation in appropriate physical activity should be a core component of every child/parent encounter" (Longmuir et al., 2013).
- Research shows that supervised exercise training at moderate intensity is safe and produces significant beneficial changes in hemodynamics and exercise time in children with cardiac disease (*Balfour, 1991; Longmuir et al., 2013).

Geriatric Considerations

- Decreased cardiac output in older adults has been attributed to disease-related, not age-related, processes (Miller, 2015). Fleg (*1986) found no age-related changes in resting cardiac output in a study of healthy people between 30 and 80 years of age.
- Studies have demonstrated an average decline of 5% to 15% per decade in maximum oxygen consumption VO_2 (max) from 25 to 75 years of age. Very athletic people have declines in VO_2 max; however, it is only half of the 10% per decade decline that less athletic people exhibit. There seems to be either decreased efficiency in mobilizing blood to exercising muscles or increased difficulty for muscles to extract and use oxygen because of decreased muscle mass (Grossman & Porth, 2014).

- Researchers report that exercise benefits affective (mood) experience and cognitive (processing, memory) performance in all ages (Hogan, Mata, & Carstensen, 2013).
- Prolonged immobility and inactivity through self-imposed restrictions, mental status changes, or pathophysiologic changes can contribute to decreased activity tolerance (*Cohen, Gorenberg, & Schroeder, 2000; Zomorodi et al., 2012).
- Decreased muscle mass leads to decreased strength, which, in turn, leads to decreased endurance. Muscle strength, which is maximal between 20 and 30 years of age, drops to 80% of that value by 65 years of age (*Cohen et al., 2000; Grossman & Porth, 2014).
- Changes in elastic and collogen fibers of tendons and ligaments cause decreased flexibility and loss of mobility and stability of joints (Grossman & Porth, 2014).
- Increased chest wall rigidity with aging leads to decreased lung expansion, resulting in decreased tissue oxygenation. This immediately affects activity tolerance.

Focus Assessment Criteria

Subjective Data

Assess for Defining Characteristics

Weakness
Dyspnea
Fatigue

Assess for Related Factors

Lack of incentive
Lack of confidence in ability to perform activity
Pain that interferes with performance of activities
Fear of injury or aggravating disease as a result of partici pation in activity

Objective Data

Assess for Defining Characteristics

Strength Balance and Ability to
Reposition self in bed
Maintain erect posture
Rise to standing position
Perform activities of daily living (ADLs)
Ambulate
Assume and maintain sitting position

Assess for Related Factors

Refer to Related Factors.

Goals

NOC
Activity Intolerance

The individual will progress activity to (specify level of activity desired), evidenced by these indicators:

- Identify the factors that aggravate activity intolerance.
- Identify the methods to reduce activity intolerance.
- Maintain blood pressure within normal limits 3 minutes after activity.

Interventions

Explain the Benefits and Risks of Inactivity

R: *Mobilization is prescribed to exploit the benefits on the cardiovascular, respiratory, hematological, renal, as well as the musculoskeletal and neurologic systems to support increasing levels of physiologic work demands (*Stiller, 2007).*

NIC
Activity Tolerance, Energy Management, Exercise Promotion, Sleep Enhancement, Mutual Goal Setting

Elicit From the Individual Their Personal Goals to Improve Their Health

R: *In particular, the use of mutual goal setting (MGS) as a nursing intervention was found to significantly enhance and sustain perceptions of mental health and QOL in HF participants. stents (*Scott, Setter-Kline, & Britton, 2004).*

Table II.1 PHYSIOLOGIC RESPONSE TO ACTIVITY (EXPECTED AND ABNORMAL)

	Pulse	Blood Pressure	Respiration
Resting			
Normal	60–90	<140/90	<20
Abnormal	>100	>140/90	>20
Immediately After Activity			
Normal	↑Rate ↑Strength	↑Systolic	↑Rate ↑Depth
Abnormal	↑Rate (excessive) ↑Strength Irregular rhythm	Decrease or no change in systolic	Excessive ↓Rate or ↑Rate
3 Minutes After Activity			
Normal	Within 6 beats of resting pulse		
Abnormal	>7 beats of resting pulse		

Monitor the Individual's Response to Activity and Record Response

- Starting with preactivity assessment, establish baseline "at rest" measurements of vital signs (Table II.1): pulse (rate, rhythm, quality), respirations (rate, depth, effort), and blood pressure.
- Have the individual perform the activity. If pathology is known in a particular organ system (e.g., exertional dyspnea in pulmonary disease, angina in cardiac disease, increased spasticity in neuromuscular disease), then during activity focus on the signs and symptoms indicating intolerance in that system.
- Take vital signs immediately after the activity.
- Have the individual rest for 3 minutes; take vital signs again. Compare finding with resting vital signs (Table II.1).
- Assess for pallor, cyanosis, chest pain, confusion, vertigo, and use of accessory muscles.
- During postactivity evaluation, assess recovery time—the time required for blood pressure, pulse, and respiration to return to preactivity levels—which reflects physiologic tolerance for activity.

R: *The cardiopulmonary responses to activity involve the circulatory functions of the heart and blood vessels and the gas exchanges in the respiratory system (Grossman & Porth, 2014). Response to activity can be evaluated by comparing preactivity blood pressure, pulse, and respiration with postactivity results. These, in turn, are compared with recovery time.*

R: *Strenuous activity may increase the pulse by 50 beats. This rate is still satisfactory as long as it returns to resting pulse within 3 minutes.*

- Discontinue the activity if the individual responds with
  - Complaints of chest pain, vertigo, or confusion
  - Decreased pulse rate
  - Failure of systolic blood pressure to increase
  - Decreased systolic blood pressure
  - Increased diastolic blood pressure by 15 mm Hg
  - Decreased respiratory response
- Reduce the intensity or duration of the activity if
  - The pulse takes longer than 3 to 4 minutes to return to within 6 beats of the resting pulse.
  - The respiratory rate increase is excessive after the activity.

R: *Clinical responses that require discontinuation or reduction in the activity level are evidence of compromised cardiac or respiratory ability (Grossman & Porth, 2014).*

Promote a Sincere "Can-Do" Attitude

- Identify factors that undermine the individual's confidence, such as fear of falling, perceived weakness, and visual impairment.

- Explore possible incentives with the individual and the family; consider what the individual values (e.g., playing with grandchildren, returning to work, going fishing, performing a task or craft).
- Allow the individual to set the activity schedule and functional activity goals. If the goal is too low, negotiate (e.g., "Walking 25 feet seems low. Let's increase it to 50 feet. I'll walk with you.").
- Plan a purpose for the activity, such as sitting up in a chair to eat lunch, walking to a window to see the view, or walking to the kitchen to get some juice.
- Help the individual to identify progress. Do not underestimate the value of praise and encouragement as effective motivational techniques. In selected cases, assisting the individual to keep a written record of activities may help to demonstrate progress.

R: *Nursing interventions for activity intolerance promote participation in activities to achieve a level of activity desired by the individual for the therapeutic regimen. Strategies that are individualized can increase motivation.*

Increase the Activity Gradually

- Increase tolerance for activity by having the individual perform the activity more slowly, for a shorter time, with more rest pauses, or with more assistance.
- Minimize the deconditioning effects of prolonged bed rest and imposed immobility.
- Reduce the amount of time lying prone. Position sitting in bed and if possible in a chair.

R: *"Sitting upright for example shifts circulating blood volume dependently, and facilitates diaphragmatic motion and lung volumes and capacities and reducing closing volume of the dependent airways. Body positioning studies often use more than one body position, usually a more erect position" (*Stiller, 2007).*

- Begin active range of motion (ROM) at least twice a day. For the individual who is unable, passive ROM is indicated.
- Encourage isometric exercise.
- Encourage the individual to turn and lift self actively unless contraindicated.
- Promote optimal sitting balance and tolerance by increasing muscle strength.
- Increase tolerance gradually starting with 15 minutes the first time out of bed.
- Have the individual get out of bed three times a day, increasing the time out of bed by 15 minutes each day.
- Practice transfers. Have the person do as much active movements as possible during transfers.
- Promote ambulation with or without assistive devices.
- Provide support when the person begins to stand.
- If the person cannot stand without buckling the knees, he or she is not ready for ambulation; help the individual to practice standing in place with assistance.
- Choose a safe gait. (If the gait appears awkward but stable, continue; stay close by and give clear coaching messages, e.g., "Look straight ahead, not down.")
- Prior to ambulation agree on the distance. Allow the person to gauge the rate of ambulation.
- Provide sufficient support to ensure safety and prevent falling.
- Encourage the person to wear comfortable walking shoes (slippers do not support the feet properly).

R: *Activity tolerance develops cyclically through adjusting frequency, duration, and intensity of activity until the desired level is achieved. Increasing activity frequency precedes increasing duration and intensity (work demand). Increased intensity is offset by reduced duration and frequency. As tolerance for more intensive activity of short duration develops, frequency is once again increased (Grossman & Porth, 2014).*

Determine Adequacy of Sleep (See Disturbed Sleep Pattern for More Information)

- Plan rest periods according to the individual's daily schedule. (They should occur throughout the day and between activities.)
- Encourage the individual to rest during the first hour after meals. (Rest can take many forms: napping, watching TV, or sitting with legs elevated.)

R: *Rest relieves the symptoms of activity intolerance. The daily schedule is planned to allow for alternating periods of activity and rest and is coordinated to reduce excess energy expenditure.*

Initiate Health Teaching as Indicated

Explain the components of a regular exercise program that contributes to increase endurance, reduction of falls, and increase well-being. Consult with primary care provider prior to initiating any exercise program. Start slowly.

- *Aerobic exercise*: walking and cycling (20 to 30 min, 3 to 5 times/week)
- *Strengthening exercise*: arm/legs muscles (weights 3 repetitions of 10) and trunk muscles (core stability [sit-ups] 2 to 3 times/week)
- *Flexibility exercise*: range of motion of arm. legs, shoulder, neck, spine (3 to 5 times/week)

Activity Intolerance • Related to Insufficient Knowledge of Adaptive Techniques Needed Secondary to COPD

Goals

NOC

Activity Intolerance

The individual will progress the activity to (specify level of activity desired), evidenced by these indicators:

- Demonstrate methods of controlled breathing to conserve energy.
- Demonstrate ability to perform controlled coughing.

Interventions

NIC

Same as for General, Smoking Cessation Assistance, Nutrition Management, Respiratory Monitoring, Teaching: Prescribed Activity/Exercise

The following interventions apply to people experiencing *Activity Intolerance* resulting from a known cause: COPD. Nurses use these interventions in conjunction with the generic interventions identified for *Activity Intolerance*.

Eliminate or Reduce Contributing Factors

- Elicit from the individual their personal goals for improved quality of life.

R: *In particular, the use of mutual goal setting as a nursing intervention was found to significantly enhance and sustain perceptions of mental health and QOL (*Scott et al., 2004).*

Lack of Knowledge

- Assess understanding of prescribed therapeutic regimen; proceed with health teaching using simple, clear instructions; include family members.
- Specifically assess the knowledge of pulmonary hygiene and adaptive breathing techniques.

R: *Pulmonary rehabilitation can decrease anxiety and depression associated with breathlessness.*

Inadequate Pulmonary Hygiene Routine

- Explain the importance of adhering to daily coughing schedule for clearing the lungs and that doing so is a lifetime commitment.
- Teach the proper method of controlled coughing:
  - Breathe deeply and slowly while sitting up as upright as possible.
  - Use diaphragmatic breathing.
  - Hold the breath for 3 to 5 seconds; then slowly exhale as much of this breath as possible through the mouth. (Lower rib cage and abdomen should sink down with exhaling.)
  - Take a second deep breath, hold, and cough forcefully from deep in the chest (not from the back of the mouth or throat); use two short, forceful coughs.
- Rest after coughing sessions.
- Instruct the individual to practice controlled coughing four times a day: 30 minutes before meals and at bedtime. Allow 15 to 30 minutes of rest after coughing session and before meals.
- Consider use of inhaled humidity, postural drainage, and chest clapping before coughing session. Assess for use of prescribed aerosol bronchodilators to dilate airways and thin secretions.

R: *Clearing and defense of the airways are of utmost importance in meeting tissue demands for increased oxygen during periods of rest and periods of increased activity.*

Suboptimal Breathing Techniques

- Beginning instruction in physical and mental relaxation techniques is helpful before teaching controlled breathing.

R: *Techniques of physical relaxation minimize muscle tension. Relaxation is an essential preliminary step in teaching controlled breathing to eliminate wasteful and unproductive motions of the upper chest, shoulders, and neck.*

- Instruct by demonstrating the desired breathing technique; then direct him or her to mimic your breathing pattern.
- Pursed-lip breathing: Have the individual breathe in through the nose, then breathe out slowly through partially closed lips while counting to seven and making a "pu" sound. (Often, people with progressive lung disease learn this naturally.)
  - Pursed-lip breathing slows breathing down thus keeping airways open longer so trapped air can be exhaled. This improves the exchange of oxygen and carbon dioxide (COPD Foundation, 2015).
- Diaphragmatic breathing:
  - Place your hands on the individual's abdomen below the base of the ribs and keep them there while he or she inhales.
  - To inhale, the individual relaxes the shoulders, breathes in through the nose, and pushes the stomach outward against your hands. The individual holds the breath for 1 to 2 seconds to keep the alveoli open, then exhales.
  - To exhale, the individual breathes out slowly through the mouth while you apply slight pressure at the base of the ribs.
  - Have the individual practice this breathing technique several times with you; then, the individual should place his or her own hands at the base of the ribs to practice alone.
  - Once the technique has been learned, have the individual practice it a few times each hour.

R: *The diaphragm is the main muscle of breathing. In individual with COPD, when the diaphragm weaken, the muscles in the neck, shoulders, and back are used instead (COPD Foundation, 2015).*
Therapeutic efforts to improve respiratory muscle function need to be tailored to each individual, according to the muscle group most likely to benefit. In the early stages of COPD, treatment should focus on the diaphragm, whereas for more advanced disease, the focus must shift to the inspiratory muscles of the rib cage and of exhalation.

Insufficient Activity Level

- Assess current activity level. Consider:
  - Current pattern of activity/rest
  - Distribution of energy demand over the course of the day
  - Perceptions of the most demanding required activities
  - Perceptions of the areas for which the individual desires or requires increased participation
  - Efficacy of current adaptive techniques
- Identify physical barriers at home and work (e.g., number of stairs) that seem insurmountable or limit participation in activities.
- Identify ways to reduce the work demand of frequently performed tasks (e.g., sitting, rather than standing, to prepare meals; keeping frequently used utensils on a countertop to avoid unnecessary overhead reaching or bending).
- Identify ways of alternating periods of exertion with periods of rest to overcome barriers (e.g., place a chair in the bathroom near the sink so the individual can rest during daily hygiene).
- Keep in mind that a plan including frequent, short rest periods during an activity is less demanding and more conducive to completing the activity than a plan that calls for a burst of energy followed by a long period of rest.

R: *Symptom-limited endurance training has been shown effective for improving performance and reducing perceived breathlessness (*Punzal, Ries, Kaplan, & Prewitt, 1991). The minimal duration and frequency of exercise required to improve performance appears to be 20 to 30 minutes three to five times/week. Not all people, however, are candidates for exercise reconditioning. A pulmonologist should be consulted.*

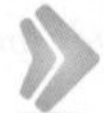

Carp's Cues

Smokers know that smoking is harming their health. Everyone tells them to quit. This implies quitting is in fact easy. Addiction to tobacco is stronger than addiction to heroin. About 70% of smokers say they want to quit and about half try to quit each year, but only 4% to 7% succeed without help. This is because smokers not only become physically dependent on nicotine, but also have a strong psychological dependence (Centers for Disease Control and Prevention [CDC], 2014).

Nicotine reaches the brain within seconds after taking a puff. Nicotine alters the balance of chemicals in your brain. It mainly affects chemicals called dopamine and noradrenaline. Nicotine induces pleasure and reduces stress and anxiety. Smokers use it to modulate levels of arousal and to control mood (CDC, 2014).

On average, women metabolize nicotine more quickly than men, which may contribute to their increased susceptibility to nicotine addiction and may help to explain why, among smokers, it is more difficult for women to quit (CDC, 2014).

Tobacco Use

- During hospitalization, focus on the individual's readiness to quit, and clarify misinformation. Ask the individual the following questions:
  - How smoking has affected their health?
  - Have they ever tried to quit?
  - How long did they stop?
  - Do they want to quit?

R: *Focusing the discussion on the person's experiences and perceptions may provide insight into assisting the person to quit.*

- While in the hospital, discuss the effects of smoking on the cardiovascular, respiratory, circulatory, and musculoskeletal systems. Specifically related chronic or episodic complaints that are specific to the individual (e.g., frequent infections, leg cramps, worsening of COPD, cardiac problems)

R: *"Hospitalization can provide multiple opportunities for smoking cessation counseling from a range of health care providers, removing the barriers of time and travel that often limit participation in formal programs" (*Sciamanna et al., 2000).*

- Assess the likelihood of quitting with the question, "How likely is it that you will stay off cigarettes after you leave the hospital?"

R: *Sciamanna et al. (*2000) found that a high predictor of successful cessation of smoking was if the person responded likely or very likely. The researches not quit in the long-term may prompt heath care professionals to address other health risk factors (e.g., nutrition, obesity, physical activity) during the hospital stay or consider referring to a different or more intensive smoking cessation intervention in the community.*

- Explain that there is no such thing as "a few cigarettes a day."

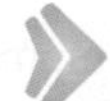

Carp's Cues

Every year, smoking kills more than 5 million people globally, including 440 000 people in the United States, where the long-term decline in smoking prevalence has slowed (McAfee, Davis, Alexander, Pechacek, & Bunnell, 2013). More deaths are caused by cigarette smoking than by all deaths from HIV, illegal drug use, alcohol use, motor vehicle accidents, suicide, and murders combined (CDC, 2015).

- Provide smokers (individual, family) with these services: 1-800-QUIT-NOW quitline or www.smokefree.gov.
- Refer to *Tobacco Use* in index for more interventions.
- Refer to Getting Started to Quit Smoking on the Point at http://thePoint.lww.com/Carpenito6e

Monitor the Individual's Response to Activity

- Refer to Generic Interventions under *Activity Intolerance*.

Increase Activity Gradually

- Reassure the individual that some increase in daily activity is possible.
- Encourage to use controlled breathing techniques to decrease work of breathing during activities.
- After the individual masters controlled breathing in relaxed positions, begin to increase activity.
- Teach to maintain a controlled breathing pattern while sitting or standing and progress to maintaining controlled breathing during bed-to-chair transfers and walking.
- Some individuals can learn to maintain rhythmic breathing during walking by using a simple 2:4 ratio: two steps during inspiration and four steps during expiration.

R: *People with COPD can benefit from specific breathing exercises, which involve retraining of breathing patterns, and from general exercise programs that support normal daily activities.*

Encourage Discussion of Sexuality

- Encourage the individual to discuss the effects of the condition on sexual function.
- Refer to *Ineffective Sexuality Patterns.*

Initiate Health Teaching

- Teach to observe sputum; note changes in color, amount, and odor; seek professional advice if sputum changes.
- Instruct the individual to wear warm, dry clothing; avoid crowds, heavy smoke, fumes, and irritants; avoid exertion in cold, hot, or humid weather; and balance work, rest, and recreation to regulate energy expenditure.
- Emphasize the importance of maintaining a nutritious diet (high calorie, high vitamin C, high protein, and 2 to 3 quarts of liquid a day, unless on fluid restriction).

R: *Individuals with COPD are susceptible to infection and must detect symptoms early and consult with primary care provider for treatment (frequently, early antibiotic therapy is necessary). Strategies to increase resistance to infection include immunizations (influenza, pneumovax, prenar 13), avoiding environmental irritants and crowds, and maintaining optimal nutrition and hydration.*

- "Explain that the tripod position, in which the patient sits or stands leaning forward with the arms supported, forces the diaphragm down and forward and stabilizes the chest while reducing the work of breathing. If the patient reports increased dyspnea when performing activities of daily living (ADLs), especially when raising the arms above the head, recommend supporting the arms during ADLs, as by resting the elbows on a surface. Point out that this reduces competing demands of the arm, chest, and neck muscles needed for breathing" (Bauldoff, 2015; *Bauldoff et al., 1996; *Breslin, 1992).
- Teach how to increase unsupported arm endurance with lower extremity exercises performed during the exhalation phase of respiration (*Bauldoff et al., 1996; *Breslin, 1992).

R: *The physiologic demands of unsupported arm tasks lead to both exercise-induced increases in respiratory muscle work and nonventilatory recruitment of respiratory muscles to maintain chest wall position (*Breslin, 1992). Research has shown that arm support during performance of arm tasks reduces diaphragmatic recruitment, increases respiratory endurance, and increases arm exercise endurance. Providing arm support (e.g., resting elbows on a tabletop while shaving or eating) may enhance independence and improve functional capacity (Bauldoff, 2015; *Bauldoff et al., 1996).*

- Evaluate the individual's knowledge of the care, cleansing, and use of inhalator equipment.

R: *Inhalator equipment can harbor microorganisms and must be disinfected properly.*

Make Referrals as Indicated

- Refer to a community nurse for follow-up if indicated.
- Consult a physical therapist for a comprehensive exercise program, especially for people with COPD.

Activity Intolerance • Related to Insufficient Knowledge of Adaptive Techniques Needed Secondary to Impaired Cardiac Function

Goals

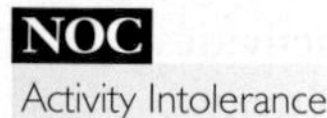

Activity Intolerance

The individual will demonstrate tolerance for increased activity by maintaining pulse, respirations, and blood pressure within predetermined ranges, evidenced by the following indicators:

- Identify factors that increase cardiac workload.
- Describe adaptive techniques needed to perform ADLs.
- Identify cues for stopping activity: fatigue, shortness of breath, chest pain.

Interventions

Elicit From the Individual Their Personal Goals to Improve Their Health

R: *In particular, the use of MGS as a nursing intervention was found to significantly enhance and sustain perceptions of mental health and QOL (*Scott et al., 2004).*

NIC
Same as for General, Smoking Cessation Assistance, Weight Reduction Assistance, Knowledge: Illness Care, Teaching: Prescribed Activity/ Exercise, Nutrition Management

Assess Knowledge and Behavior Related to the Four "E's": Eating, Exertion, Exposure, and Emotional Stress (Adapted from *Day, 1984)

Eating

- Assess knowledge of restricted diet.
- Explain importance of adhering to prescribed salt-restricted diet.
- Explore alternatives to salt for seasoning foods to taste using natural herbs and spices.
- Encourage a light meal in the evening to promote a more comfortable night's rest.

Exertion

- Teach to modify approaches to activities to regulate energy expenditure and reduce cardiac workload (e.g., take rest periods during activities, at intervals during the day, and for 1 hour after meals; sit rather than stand when performing activities; when performing a task, rest every 3 minutes for 5 minutes to allow the heart to recover; stop an activity if exertional fatigue or signs of cardiac hypoxia occur, such as markedly increased pulse rate, dyspnea, or chest pain).
- Instruct to avoid certain types of exertion: isometric exercises (e.g., using arms to lift self, carry objects) and Valsalva maneuver (e.g., bending at the waist in a sit-up fashion to rise from bed, straining during a bowel movement).

Exposure

- Instruct the individual to avoid unnecessary exposure to environmental extremes and exertion during hot, humid weather or extreme cold weather, which places additional demands on the heart.
- Instruct the individual to dress warmly during cold weather (e.g., create a barrier to cold weather by wearing layers of clothing).

Emotional Stress

- Assist to identify emotional stressors (e.g., at home, at work, socially).
- Discuss usual responses to emotional stress (e.g., anger, depression, avoidance, discussion).
- Explain the effects of emotional stress on the cardiovascular system (increased heart rate, blood pressure, respirations).
- Discuss various methods for stress management/reduction (e.g., deliberate problem solving, relaxation techniques, yoga or meditation, biofeedback, regular exercise).

R: *An integrated program of medically supervised exercise, dietary restriction, stress management, and limited exposure to environmental extremes maximizes activity tolerance.*

Tobacco Use

Carp's Cues

Smokers know that smoking is harming their health. Everyone tells them to quit. This implies quitting is in fact easy. Addiction to tobacco is stronger than addiction to heroin. About 70% of smokers say they want to quit and about half try to quit each year, but only 4% to 7% succeed without help. This is because smokers not only become physically dependent on nicotine, but also have a strong psychological dependence (CDC, 2014).

Nicotine reaches the brain within seconds after taking a puff. Nicotine alters the balance of chemicals in your brain. It mainly affects chemicals called dopamine and noradrenaline. Nicotine induces pleasure and reduces stress and anxiety. Smokers use it to modulate levels of arousal and to control mood (CDC, 2014).

On average, women metabolize nicotine more quickly than men, which may contribute to their increased susceptibility to nicotine addiction and may help to explain why, among smokers, it is more difficult for women to quit (CDC, 2014).

"Every year, smoking kills more than 5 million people globally, including 440 000 people in the USA, where the long-term decline in smoking prevalence has slowed" (McAfee et al., 2013). More deaths are caused by cigarette smoking than by all deaths from HIV, illegal drug use, alcohol use, motor vehicle accidents, suicide, and murders combined (CDC, 2015).

- Advise that smoking is one of the three principle nonhereditary risk factors for coronary heart disease; the others being raised cholesterol and high blood pressure.

R: *Tobacco is a potent vasoconstrictor that increases the workload of the heart, damages lung tissue, damages blood vessels, and decreases circulation to muscles and bones.*

- Emphasize that "giving up smoking dramatically reduces the risk of a heart attack and is particularly important for those who have other risk factors such as high blood pressure, raised blood cholesterol levels, and are diabetic or overweight and physically inactive" (National Institute of Health and Care Excellence, 2010).

R: *"Within a year of giving up, the risk of a heart attack halves compared to that of an active smoker and declines gradually thereafter. After 15 years of no smoking, the risk of a heart attack is the same for non-smokers as for those who formally quit" (National Institute of Health and Care Excellence, 2010).*

- Refer to the previous nursing diagnosis: *Activity Intolerance—Related to Insufficient Knowledge of Adaptive Techniques Needed Secondary to COPD* for interventions addressing smoking cessation.
- Provide smokers (individual, family) with these services: 1-800-QUIT-NOW quitline or www.smokefree.gov.
- Refer to *Tobacco Use* in index for more interventions.
- Refer to THE POINT to "Getting Started to quit smoking" PRINT and give to individuals.

Address Overweight/Obesity (Specifically Focus on the Effects of Overweight/Obesity Have on Cardiovascular System)

- Continuous pressure overload, increased blood viscosity, obesity-related hypertension, and left ventricular hypertrophy (LVH) increasing the risk of heart failure and cardiac arrhythmias. Atrial fibrillation can cause stokes (Reilly & Kelly, 2011).
- Increased values of fibrinogen, factor VII, factor VIII (von Willebrand factor), and plasminogen activator inhibitors, as well as decreased levels of anti-thrombin III and circulating fibrinolysis activity. When combined with decreased mobility and venous stasis, place obese individuals at increased risk for thromboembolic disease, especially deep vein thrombosis and pulmonary embolism (*Garrett, Lauer, & Christopher, 2004; Reilly & Kelly, 2011).

Monitor Response to Activity (see Interventions) and Teach Self-Monitoring Techniques

- Take resting pulse.
- Take pulse during or immediately after activity.
- Take pulse 3 minutes after cessation of activity.
- Instruct the individual to stop activity and report:
  - Decreased pulse rate during activity
  - Pulse rate greater than 112 beats per minute
  - Irregular pulse
  - Pulse rate that does not return to within 6 beats of resting pulse after 3 minutes
  - Dyspnea
  - Chest pain
  - Palpitations
  - Perceptions of exertional fatigue

R: *Response to activity can be evaluated by comparing preactivity blood pressure, pulse, and respiration with postactivity blood pressure, pulse, and respiration. Refer to Table II.1 for the norms of physiologic responses to Activity.*

Increase the Activity Gradually

- Allow for periods of rest before and after planned periods of exertion, such as treatments, ambulation, and meals.
- Encourage gradual increases in activity and ambulation to prevent a sudden increase in cardiac workload.
- Assess the individual's perceived capability for increased activity.
- Assist the individual in setting short-term activity goals that are realistic and achievable.
- Reassure the individual that even small increases in activity will lift spirits and restore self-confidence.

R: *An exercise program that is monitored can increase maximal oxygen consumption by the muscle tissues, which will allow for increased activity at a lower heart rate and blood pressure (Grossman & Porth, 2014).*

Initiate Health Teaching and Referrals as Indicated

- Instruct the individual to consult his or her primary care provider for a long-term exercise program.
- Explain dietary restrictions to both individual and family. Give them written instructions or refer them to pertinent literature or websites for information on nutrition.

R: *Specific instructions will be needed for management of condition and treatments.*

INEFFECTIVE ACTIVITY PLANNING

Ineffective Activity Planning

Risk for Ineffective Activity Planning

NANDA-I Definition

Inability to prepare for a set of actions fixed in time and under certain conditions

Defining Characteristics*

Verbalization of fear toward a task to be undertaken
Verbalization of worries toward a task to be undertaken
Excessive anxieties toward a task to be undertaken
Failure pattern of behavior
Lack of plan
Lack of resources
Lack of sequential organization
Procrastination
Unmet goals for chosen activity

Related Factors*

Compromised ability to process information
Defensive flight behavior when faced with proposed solution
Hedonism
Lack of family support
Lack of friend support
Unrealistic perception of events
Unrealistic perception of personal competence

Author's Note

This newly accepted NANDA-I nursing diagnosis can represent a problematic response that relates to many existing nursing diagnoses such as *Chronic Confusion, Self-Care Deficit, Anxiety, Ineffective Denial, Ineffective Coping, and Ineffective Health Management.* This author recommends that *Ineffective Activity Planning* should be seen as a sign or symptom. The questions are as follows:

- What activities are not being planned effectively? Self-care? Self-health management?
- What is preventing effective activity planning? Confusion? Anxiety? Fear? Denial? Stress overload? Examples:
  - *Stress Overload related to unrealistic perception of events as evidenced by impaired ability to plan . . .* (specify activity)
  - *Ineffective Health Management related to lack of plan, lack of resources, lack of social support as evidenced by impaired ability to plan . . .* (specify activity)
  - *Anxiety related to compromised ability to process information and unrealistic perception of personal competence as evidenced by impaired ability to plan . . .* (specify activity)

Risk for Ineffective Activity Planning

NANDA-I Definition

Vulnerable to an inability to prepare for a set of actions fixed in time and under certain conditions which can compromise functioning.

Risk Factors*

Compromised ability to process information
Defensive flight behavior when faced with proposed solution
Hedonism
History of procrastination
Ineffective support system
Insufficient support system
Unrealistic perception of events
Unrealistic perception of personal competence

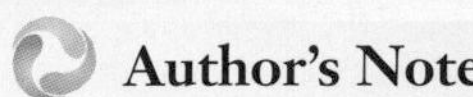

Author's Note

Refer to *Ineffective Activity Planning*.

RISK FOR ADVERSE REACTION TO IODINATED CONTRAST MEDIA

NANDA-I Definition

Vulnerable to noxious or unintended reaction associated with the use of iodinated contrast media (ICM) that can occur within seven (7) days after contrast agent injection, which may compromise health

Risk Factors

Pathophysiologic

For Acute Reaction
History of asthma
Prior reaction to contrast
Atropy (typically associated with heightened immune responses to common allergens, especially inhaled allergens and food allergens)

For Delayed Reaction
Prior reaction to contrasts
Those being treated with interleukin 2
Sun exposure

For Contrast-Induced Nephropathy
Preexisting renal dysfunction
Concurrent use of renotoxic drugs
Use of a high-osmolality contrast agent
High volumes of contrast agent
Hypertension
Heart failure
Hemodynamic instability
ACE inhibitors
Dehydration
Diabetes mellitus
Poor renal perfusion
Myocardial infarction
Underlying disease (e.g., heart disease, pulmonary disease, blood dyscrasias, endocrine disease, renal disease, pheochromocytoma, autoimmune disease)*
Collagen vascular disease
Sickle cell disease
Myeloma
Polycythemia
Paraproteinemia syndrome/disease (e.g., multiple myeloma)
History of a kidney transplant, renal tumor, renal surgery, or single kidney
History of end-stage liver disease
Dehydration*
Elevated creatinine levels
Recent history (1 month) of (Robbins & Pozniak, 2010):

Major infection (e.g., pneumonia, sepsis, osteomyelitis)
Vascular ischemia of extremities (e.g., amputation, arterial thrombosis)
Venous or arterial thrombosis
Major surgery or vascular procedure (e.g., amputation, transplantation, CABG)
Multiorgan system failure

Treatment Related

Greater than 20-mg iodine
Chemotherapy or amino glycoside within past month
Concurrent use of medications (e.g., ACE inhibitors, beta-blockers, interleukin 2, metformin, nephrotoxic medications* NSAIDs, aminoglycosides)
Fragile veins (e.g., prior or actual chemotherapy treatment or radiation in the limb to be injected, multiple attempts to obtain intravenous access, indwelling intravenous lines in place for more than 24 hours, previous axillary lymph node dissection in the limb to be injected, distal intravenous access sites: hand, wrist, foot, ankle)*
Physical and chemical properties of the contrast media (e.g., iodine concentration, viscosity, high osmolality, ion toxicity, unconsciousness)*

Situational (Personal, Environmental)

Females > males
Anxiety*
Generalized debilitation*
History of previous adverse effect from iodinated contrast media*

Maturational

Older than 60 years
Extremes of age*

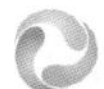

Author's Note

This NDA-I nursing diagnosis represents a clinical situation in which iodinated contrast media are infused for radiographic diagnostic tests. Complications of intravascular injection of iodinated contrast include anaphylactoid contrast reaction, contrast-induced nephropathy, and contrast media extravasation (Pasternak & Williamson, 2012). Reactions can be mild and self-limiting (e.g., scattered urticaria, nausea) to severe and life-threatening (e.g., cardiac arrhythmias, seizures). Nurses caring for individuals scheduled for these tests must be aware of individuals who are at higher risk for adverse events. Nurses in radiology departments are responsible for assessing for high-risk individuals, reviewing renal function status of the individual prior to the procedure, monitoring for early signs or reactions, and using protocols when indicated.

This clinical situation can be described with this nursing diagnosis. In contrast, *Risk for Complications of Contrast Media* is more appropriate as a collaborative problem, since interventions required are nurse and physician prescribed with protocols for treatment of adverse events. The interventions included with this diagnosis can be used with *Risk for Adverse Reaction to Iodinated Contrast Media* or *Risk for Complications of Contrast Media*.

Key Concepts

- The risk for ICM-related reactions are separated into three categories: (1) those with increased risk for idiosyncratic reactions, (2) those with increased risk for contrast agent-induced nephropathy, and (3) those with increased risk for nonidiosyncratic reactions (Siddiqi, 2011).
- The incidence of any adverse reaction to ICM is reported to be about 15% (Siddiqi, 2011). Persons with asthma have 1.2 to 2.5 times the risk for an adverse reaction, and their reaction can be more severe (more than 5 to 9 times greater than in nonasthmatic persons). Persons with allergies (e.g., hay fever) have 1.5 to 3.0 times higher risk for an adverse reaction (Siddiqi, 2011).
- Adverse reactions to ICM are classified as idiosyncratic (anaphylactic) and nonidiosyncratic. Idiosyncratic reactions are not true hypersensitivity reactions; Immunoglobin E (IgE) is not involved. These anaphylactic reactions do not require previous sensitivity, nor do they consistently recur in an individual with a prior reaction. Reactions can be mild, moderate, or severe. Nonidiosyncratic reactions are

nonanaphylactic and are thought to be related to the media changing the homeostasis of the body, particularly blood circulation. This results in disruption of electrical charges for neural and cardiac function and changes in osmolality, which causes fluid shifts (Siddiqi, 2011).

- Prophylaxis for adverse reactions to ICM is indicated for persons with a history of moderate or severe reactions (e.g., methyl prednisone and H_1 antihistamines with H_2 histamine-receptor blockers; Siddiqi, 2011).
- Individuals who have renal insufficiency before the administration of contrast material are 5 to 10 times more likely to develop contrast-induced renal failure than the general population (Pasternak & Williamson, 2012).
- Extravasation of ICM into soft tissues during injection can cause tissue damage from the direct toxicity of the contrast agent. The reaction can be self-limiting (edema, pain, erythema) to compartmental syndrome, which may require surgical intervention (Siddiqi, 2011) (Table II.2).

Focus Assessment Criteria

Subjective Data

Assess for Risk Factors

Currently or recently used medications (prescribed, OTC such as NSAIDs)
Pregnancy status
Previous contrast administration (e.g., reactions, date of procedure)
Serum creatinine level or clearance

Goals

NOC

Vital Signs, Coping, Medication Response, Peripheral Vascular Access, Allergic Response, Symptom Severity, Risk Detection

The individual will report risk factors for adverse reaction and any symptoms experienced during infusion, evidenced by the following indicators:

- State risk factors for adverse reactions.
- Report any sensations that are felt during and after infusion.
- Describe delayed reactions and the need to report.

Table II.2 CONTRAST MEDIUM REACTIONS

Idiosyncratic		
Mild Reactions (Self-limited)		
Limited cutaneous edema	Transient flushing	"Scratchy" sore throat
Scattered urticaria	Limited itching	Nasal congestion
Limited nausea/vomiting	Anxiety	Chills
Sneezing	Mild hypertension	Dizziness
Moderate Reactions		
Persistent nausea/vomiting	Diffuse urticaria/pruritus	Wheezing/bronchospasm
Facial edema, no dyspnea	Tachycardia	Hypertension urgency
Palpitations	Throat tightness/hoarseness	Abdominal cramps
Vasovagal reaction (bradycardia, fainting) that requires and is responsive to treatment		
Severe Reactions[a]		
Bronchospasm, significant hypoxia	Anaphylactic shock (hypotension + tachycardia)	Overt bronchospasm
Life-threatening arrhythmias	Laryngeal edema	Syncope
Pulmonary edema	Seizures	Hypertensive emergency
Nonidiosyncratic		
Bradycardia	Hypotension	Vasovagal reactions
Neuropathy	Cardiovascular reactions	Extravasation
Delayed oral reaction	Sensations of warmth	Metallic taste in mouth
Nausea/vomiting		

[a]Signs and symptoms are often life-threatening and can result in permanent morbidity or death if not managed appropriately.

Sources: Siddiqi, N. (2015). Contrast medium reactions. In *Medscape*. Retrieved from http://emedicine.medscape.com/article/422855-overview; American College of Radiology Committee on Drugs and Contrast Media. (2013). *ACR manual on contrast media: Version 9*. Reston, VA: American College of Radiology. Retrieved from www.acr.org/quality-%20safety/resources/~/media/37D84428BF1D4E1B9A3A2918DA9E27A3.pdf/.

Interventions

NIC

Teaching: individual, Vital Sign Monitoring Venous Access Device, Maintenance, Anxiety Reduction, Circulatory Precautions, Peripheral Sensation Management, Preparatory Sensory Information: Procedure, Allergy Management, Risk Identification, Surveillance

Assess for Factors That Increase Risk for Contrast Medium Adverse Reactions

- Refer to Risk Factors.
- Review with the individual/significant others previous experiences with contrast media infusions.
- Consult with radiologist if indicated.

R: *Depending on the type of previous reaction, specific prophylaxis may be indicated (Pasternak & Williamson, 2012)*

Prep are the Individual for the Procedure

On Unit

- Explain the procedure (e.g., administration, sensations that may be felt such as mild, warm flushing at site of injection, which may spread over body and may be more intense in perineum, metallic taste).
- Evaluate level of anxiety. Consult with prescribing physician and/or NP if anxiety is high.
- Ensure that the individual is well hydrated prior to procedure. Consult with physician and/or NP for additional hydration if indicated.
- For individuals who can drink: administer 500 mL prior to procedure and 2,500 mL over 24 hours after the procedure.
- Intravenous: 0.95 OR 0, 45% saline, 100 mL/hr beginning 4 hours prior to the procedure and continuing for 24 hours after the procedure UNLESS contraindicated.

R: *Hydration minimizes or decreases the incidence of renal failure induced by contrast media (Pasternak & Williamson, 2012).*

- Assure serum creatinine/clearance results are documented. Consult with radiologist if abnormal.

R: *Preexisting renal insufficiency can contribute to acute renal failure following ICM administration (Siddiqi, 2011).*

- Assess whether the individual has received metformin or other oral hyperglycemic agents before. Withhold metformin for 48 hours after the procedure.

R: *Metformin and other oral hyperglycemic agents have been associated with the development of severe lactic acidosis following administration of ICM (Pasternak & Williamson, 2012).*

- Determine when the last contrast media was infused.

R: *If multiple studies are required, 5 days should be allotted between the studies to allow for the kidneys to recover (Siddiqi, 2011).*

- Consult with radiologist/physician/NP if needed.

In Radiology Department

- Ensure that emergency equipment and medications are available:
  - EKG machine
  - Respiratory equipment (oxygen, bag-valve mask, airways)
  - Emergency medications
  - Crash cart
  - IV fluids
- Ensure that the individual is well hydrated prior to procedure.

R: *Hydration minimizes or decreases the incidence of renal failure induced by contrast media (Pasternak & Williamson, 2012).*

- Explain the procedure (e.g., administration, sensations that may be felt such as mild, warm flushing at site of injection, which may spread over body, may be more intense in perineum, metallic taste).
- Evaluate level of anxiety. Consult with prescribing physician, PA, or NP if anxiety is high.
- Encourage continuous conversation and feedback from the individual during the procedure (Singh & Daftary, 2008).

R: *Concrete, objective information decreases distress during the procedure (*Maguire, Walsh, & Little, 2004). There is anecdotal evidence that severe adverse effects to contrast media or to procedures can be mitigated at least in part by reducing anxiety (American College of Radiology Committee, 2013).*

- Follow protocol for administration of contrast media (e.g., site preparation, rate of infusion, warming of ICM).

R: *Too rapid infusion has been associated with adverse reactions. Warming ICM to body temperature reduces viscosity and may reduce discomfort during infusion (Siddiqi, 2011).*

- Monitor the individual's emotional and physiologic response continuously during infusion.
- Refer to Table II.2 for signs/symptoms of adverse reactions.
- Monitor for extravasation of contrast by assessing for swelling, erythema, and pain that usually abate with no residual problems.
- If extravasation is suspected (Robbins & Pozniak, 2010):
  - Discontinue injection/infusion.
  - Notify responsible physician.
  - Elevate the affected extremity above the heart.
  - Provide brief compression for no more than 1 minute.
  - Follow agency protocol for documentation and reporting.
  - Consult with plastic surgeon if swelling or pain progresses, decreased capillary refill is present, sensation alters, and/or skin ulcers or blisters.

R: *These interventions reduce the absorption of the contrast into the tissues and seek to identify early signs of extravasation.*

Explain Delayed Contrast Reactions

- Advise the individual/family that a delayed contrast reaction can occur anytime between 3 hours and 7 days following the administration of contrast.
- Advise to avoid direct sun exposure for 1 week.
- Explain that delayed reaction can be cutaneous xanthem, pruritus without urticaria, nausea, vomiting, drowsiness, and headache.
- Advise them to report signs/symptoms to responsible physician/NP.
- Advise to go to ER if symptoms increase or difficulty swallowing or breathing occurs (Siddiqi, 2011).

R: *Most delayed reactions are self-limiting, but some can be serious (e.g., anaphylactic, Stevens–Johnson syndrome) (Robbins & Pozniak, 2010).*

RISK FOR ALLERGY RESPONSE

NANDA-I Definition

Vulnerable to an exaggerated immune response or reaction to substances, which may compromise health.

Risk Factors

Treatment Related

Pharmaceutical agents (e.g., penicillin*, sulfa)
Adhesive tape
Latex

Situational (Personal, Environmental)

Chemical products (e.g., bleach*, solvents, paint, glue)
Animals (e.g., dander)
Environmental substances* (e.g., mold, dust mites, hay)
Food (e.g., peanuts, shellfish, mushrooms*, citrus fruits, sulfites)
Insect stings*
Repeated exposure to environmental substances*
Down pillows, quilts
Cosmetics*, lotions, creams, perfumes
Nickle
Plants (e.g., tomato, poison ivy)
Maturational
Genetic predisposition to atopic disease

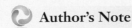

Author's Note

This new NANDA-I diagnosis can represent a diagnosis with the nursing assessments and educational interventions that can assist individuals and families with the prevention of allergic responses. The collaborative problem in Section 3 *Risk for Complications of Allergic Reaction* is indicated when nursing and medical interventions are needed for an allergic reaction.

Key Concepts

- "Between 20 and 30 percent of people report food allergy in themselves or their children. However, only 6 to 8 percent of children under the age of five and 3 to 4 percent of adults have a true food allergy" (Burks, 2014).
- An allergic reaction is a manifestation of tissue injury resulting from a reexposure between an antigen and an antibody. This immune response can cause tissue injury and disease. Immediate hypersensitivity can occur in minutes or a few hours (Porth, Gaspard, & Noble, 2010).
- The clinical manifestations of type I reactions are attributed to the effects of histamine on a large number of mast cells in targeted tissue in GI tract, the skin, and the respiratory tract.
- There is a genetic predisposition to develop some allergies. If one parent has atopic disease, there is a 40% incidence in their children. If both parents have atopic disease, the incidence increase is 80% (Grossman & Porth, 2014).
- Anaphylaxis is a rapid and severe response, which can be systemic (generalized) or local (cutaneous). Symptoms of systemic anaphylaxis include itching, erythema, diarrhea, vomiting, abdominal cramps, and breathing difficulties. Severe reactions cause laryngeal edema and vascular collapse, and can progress to hypotension, shock, respiratory distress, and death (Grossman & Porth, 2014).

Focus Assessment Criteria

For use with individuals who have experienced some allergic symptoms

Allergic symptoms experienced:

Eyes

Pruritus
Swelling
Burning
Lacrimation
Injection
Discharge

Ears

Pruritus
Fullness
Popping
Frequent infections

Nose

Sneezing
Rhinorrhea
Obstruction
Pruritus
Mouth-breathing
Purulent drainage

Throat

Soreness
Postnasal drip
Palatal pruritus
Mucus in the morning

Chest

Cough
Pain
Wheezing
Sputum description
Dyspnea associated with (specify)

Skin

Dermatitis
Eczema
Urticaria
Family allergies
Previous skin testing

Bothered by:

Alcohol
Insecticides
Newspapers
Adhesive tape
Heat
Cosmetics
Muggy weather
Cold
Latex
Hair spray
Perfume
Air-conditioning
Weather changes
Paints
Chemicals
Animals

Do symptoms occur around?

Old leaves
Summer homes
Lawn mowing
Hay
Dry attic
Other
Lakeside
Damp basement
Barns
Animals

Do symptoms occur after eating?

Cheese	Mushrooms	Beer	Melons
Bananas	Fish	Nuts	Citrus fruits
Shellfish	Wine	Sulfites	

What is done when symptoms occur?

What medications administered such as Benadryl, prednisone, Epi-pen (specify) Emergency Room visits? When?

Home environment

Type of carpets, pillows, quilts
Type of heating/cooling systems
Pets (type, owned for how long?)

Goals

NOC

Immune Hypersensitivity Control, Allergic Response: Localized, Allergic Response: Systemic, Symptom Severity

The individual will report fewer or no allergy symptoms as evidenced by the following indicators:

- Describe strategies to avoid exposure.
- Describe methods to reduce environmental exposure.
- Describe pharmaceutical management of a reaction.

Interventions

NIC

Risk Identification. Surveillance, Allergy Management Environmental Risk Protection, Teaching,

For Food Allergies

- Explain that symptoms of a food allergy can vary from mild to severe or even life-threatening. It is not possible to predict how severe the reaction will be as compared with previous reactions. Reactions are not necessarily worse after each exposure.

R: *It is not advisable for the individual or family to ignore a reaction associated with food, which can become life-threatening even without a prior severe reaction (Burks, 2014).*

Instruct to go to ER if One or More of the Following Symptoms Occur After Eating (Burks, 2014)

- Nausea or vomiting
- Cramping, abdominal pain, or diarrhea, especially if there is blood or mucus in the stool
- Itching or raised red welts on the skin
- Flushed (reddened, warm) skin
- Swelling of the lips, mouth, face, or throat
- Wheezing, coughing, or difficulty breathing
- Lightheadedness or passing out

R: *The above reaction can be from food intolerance or allergy; a medical evaluation is warranted (Burks, 2014).*

Refer the Individual to Allergy Specialist for Testing and Treatment if the Individual Has Food Allergies

R: *Individual /families can be instructed in the use of antihistamines and corticosteroids to prevent or manage a reaction. Skin testing may be indicated. Desensitization may be initiated to prevent IgE-mediated HSRs (Burks, 2014).*

Instruct the Individual on How to Reduce Allergens in Home

- Refer individual/family to the Asthma and Allergy Foundation of America, at www.aafa.org (Asthma and Allergy Foundation of America, 2011; Mayo Clinic Staff, 2011).

Develop Weekly/Monthly Cleaning Routine

- Damp-mop wood or linoleum flooring and vacuum carpeting. Use a vacuum cleaner with a small-particle or a high-efficiency particulate air (HEPA) filter.
- Use a damp cloth to clean other surfaces, including the tops of doors, windowsills, and window frames.

R: *These actions will reduce moisture and mold.*

- Vacuum weekly with a vacuum cleaner that has a small-particle or HEPA filter. Wash area rugs and floor mats weekly. Shampoo wall-to-wall carpets periodically.
- If you have allergies, either wear a dust mask while cleaning, or ask someone who does not have allergies to do the cleaning.
- Change or clean heating and cooling system filters once a month.
- Use HEPA filters in your whole house central air system, or in room air cleaning devices. Replace filters regularly.

R: *Ordinary house dust actually makes up a collection of all types of allergens—pollen from outdoors, pet and human dander, mites, dirt, insect droppings, mold, and more—all of which can trigger a frightening asthma attack in people with allergic asthma and other allergic responses.*

Bedroom
- Encase pillows, mattresses, and box springs in dust-mite–proof covers.
- Wash sheets once a week in 130° hot water to kill mites and their eggs.
- Replace mattresses every 10 years.
- Replace pillows every 5 years.
- Remove, wash, or cover comforters. Choose bedding made of synthetic materials, not down.

R: *These actions kill dust mites and their eggs.*

Kitchen
- Refer to Asthma and Allergy Foundation of America, at www.aafa.org, for specific methods to reduce sources of allergic responses in the kitchen (e.g., install and use a vented exhaust fan). Most stovetop hoods simply filter cooking particulates without venting outside.

R: *These methods can reduce moisture, mold, and insects and their excreta. Cockroach droppings and even their microscopic shedding can trigger allergic responses. Moisture can lead to mold. Mold also finds its way into the kitchen, frequently turning up under the sink, refrigerator, and dishwasher, which are damp spaces where mold thrives.*

Bathroom
- Refer to Asthma and Allergy Foundation of America, at www.aafa.org, for methods to reduce moisture and mold.

R: *These actions will reduce moisture and mold. Warm, damp environments are the breeding ground for mold. As in the kitchen, you can often find it under the bathroom sink, as well as in the shower and on shower doors, towels, floor mats, and tiles.*

Windows/Doors
- Close windows, and rely on air-conditioning during pollen season. Clean mold and condensation from window frames and sills. Use double-paned windows if you live in a cold climate.
- Use washable curtains made of plain cotton or synthetic fabric. Replace horizontal blinds with washable roller-type shades.

R: *These actions decrease pollen and mold.*

Humidity
- Vent clothes dryer outside.
- Choose an air filter that has a small-particle or HEPA filter. Try adjusting your air filter so that it directs clean air toward your head when you sleep.
- Maintain temperature at 70° F (21° C), and keep relative humidity no higher than 50%. Clean or replace small-particle filters in central heating and cooling systems and in room air-conditioners at least once a month.

R: *Hot, humid houses are breeding grounds for dust mites and mold.*

Pets
- Never allow pets on the bed.
- Keep pet sleeping areas and/or bird cages out of bedrooms.
- Bathe pets at least twice a week as this may reduce the amount of allergen in the dander they shed.

R: *Pets can bring in mold and pollen from outdoors. Pet dander (little flakes off their skin and coats) settles on bed linen and becomes food for dust mites.*

Fireplaces
- Avoid use of wood-burning fireplaces or stoves.

R: *Smoke and gases can worsen respiratory allergies. Most natural gas fireplaces won't cause this problem.*

Kid's Room

- Refer to Asthma and Allergy Foundation of America, at www.aafa.org, for methods that reduce allergens.

R: *Allergens can hide in the most unlikely places: on stuffed animals, in drawers, and under rugs. Dust mites, mold, and pet dander accumulate in and on children's toys, especially when pets play with them, and can trigger allergic asthma symptoms. Damp clothes, carelessly tossed aside after play, become a home for mold and mites in drawers and other dark places. The space underneath wall-to-wall carpeting is another refuge for mold.*

Living Room

- Refer to Asthma and Allergy Foundation of America, at www.aafa.org, for methods that reduce dust mites in living rooms, for example, vacuum furniture and curtains/drapes once a week.

R: *Dust mites find their way into furniture as easily as they do into beds. They lay eggs in upholstery and leave droppings and shedding that can trigger allergic asthma symptoms. Mold can grow on upholstered furniture, as well as on curtains and drapes. Cockroaches are drawn to crumbs.*

Basement

- Refer to Assthma and Allergy Foundation of America, at www.aafa.org, for methods that reduce dust mites in basements.

R: *Cockroaches and rats find their way into the basement, where they leave their usual shedding and droppings. Mold also easily grows in dark, damp atmospheres, especially around beams and pipes. It releases spores that can trigger allergic symptoms.*

Instruct on Treatments at Home if Symptoms Occur

- Instruct to consult with allergist, primary care provider (physician, NP) regarding medical management of symptoms at home (e.g., Benadryl).
- Ensure that the individual has an Epi-pen, knows when and how to use it, and has transportation to the ER.
- Advise of the need to check expiration dates.

R: *Early pharmaceutical interventions can reduce adverse responses.*

Do Not Allow Smoking Anywhere Inside Your House

R: *Secondary smoke and smoke on clothes can trigger allergic responses.*

Seek Immediate Emergency Care If

- Facial edema occurs.
- Change in voice.
- Difficulty breathing or swallowing.

R: *Bronchospasm can lead to respiratory arrest.*

Call 911; Do Not Drive to the ER

R: *Emergency response teams have medications and equipment to prevent anaphylaxis.*

Wear an Allergy ID Bracelet, Carry a List of Allergies, and/or Store a List of Allergies in Cell Phone in Designated Site

ANXIETY

Anxiety

Death Anxiety

NANDA-I Definition

Vague uneasy feeling of discomfort or dread accompanied by an autonomic response (the source often unspecific or unknown to the individual); a feeling of apprehension caused by anticipation of danger. It is an alerting signal that warns of impending danger and enables the individual to take measures to deal with threat.

Defining Characteristics

Major (Must Be Present)

Manifested by symptoms from each category—physiologic, emotional, and cognitive; symptoms vary according to level of anxiety (*Whitley, 1994).

Physiologic

Increased pulse[2]
Increased respiration[2]
Diaphoresis[2]
Voice quivering[2]
Palpitations
Urinary frequency, hesitancy, urgency[2]
Insomnia[2]
Facial flushing[2] or pallor
Body aches and pains (especially chest, back, neck)
Paresthesias
Increased blood pressure[2]
Pupil dilation[2]
Trembling, twitching[2]
Nausea[2]
Diarrhea[2]
Fatigue[2]
Dry mouth[2]
Restlessness[2]
Faintness[2]/dizziness
Anorexia[2]

Emotional

Individual states feeling:

Apprehensive[2]
Jittery[2]
Loss of control
Persistent increased helplessness[2]
Vigilance[2]
Tension or being "keyed up"
Anticipation of misfortune

Individual exhibits:

Irritability[2]/impatience
Crying
Startle reaction
Withdrawal
Self-deprecation
Angry outbursts
Tendency to blame others[2]
Criticism of self and others
Lack of initiative
Poor eye contact[2]

Cognitive

Impaired attention[2]; difficulty concentrating[2]
Forgetfulness[2]
Orientation to past
Hyperattentiveness
Diminished ability to learn[2]
Lack of awareness of surroundings
Rumination[2]
Blocking of thoughts (inability to remember)
Preoccupation[2]
Confusion*

Related Factors

Pathophysiologic

Any factor that interferes with physiologic stability.

Related to respiratory distress secondary to:

Chest pain
Mind-altering drugs
Cancer diagnosis

Treatment Related

Related to (examples):

Impending surgery
Effects of chemotherapy
Invasive procedure

[2]The items represent the results of concept analysis research of anxiety by Georgia Whitley in 1994.

Situational (Personal, Environmental)

Related to threat to self-concept secondary to:

Change in or threat to role status/function[1] and prestige
Failure (or success)
Ethical dilemma (Halter, 2014; Varcarolis, 2011)
Exposure to phobic object or situation
Intrusive, unwanted thoughts
Flashbacks
Lack of recognition from others
Loss of valued possessions
Fear of panic attack
Unmet needs
Cessation of ritualistic behavior

Related to loss of significant others secondary to:

Threat of death[1]
Cultural pressures
Temporary or permanent separation
Divorce
Moving
Death

Related to threat to biologic integrity secondary to:

Dying
Invasive procedures
Assault
Disease (specify)

Related to change in environment secondary to:

Hospitalization
Retirement
Environmental pollutants
Moving
Safety hazards
Incarceration
Natural disasters
Refugee issues
Military or political deployment
Airline travel

Related to change in socioeconomic status secondary to:

Unemployment
Promotion
New job
Displacement

Related to idealistic expectations of self and unrealistic goals (specify)

Maturational

Infant/Child

Related to separation

Related to unfamiliar environment, people

Related to changes in peer relationships

Related to death of (specify) with unfamiliar rituals and grieving adults

Adolescent

Related to death of (specify)

Related to threat to self-concept secondary to:
Sexual development
Academic failure
Peer relationship changes

Adult

Related to threat to self-concept secondary to:
Pregnancy
Career changes
Parenting
Effects of aging

Related to previous pregnancy complications, miscarriage, or fetal death

Related to lack of knowledge of changes associated with pregnancy

Related to lack of knowledge about labor experience

Older Adult

Related to threat to self-concept secondary to:

Sensory losers
Motor losses
Financial problems
Retirement changes

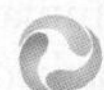

Author's Note

Several researchers have examined the nursing diagnoses of *Anxiety* and *Fear* (*Jones & Jakob, 1984; *Taylor-Loughran, O'Brien, LaChapelle, & Rangel, 1989; *Whitley, 1994; *Yokom, 1984). Differentiation of these diagnoses focuses on whether the threat can be identified. If so, the diagnosis is *Fear;* if not, it is *Anxiety* (NANDA, 2002). This differentiation, however, has not proved useful for clinicians (*Taylor-Loughran et al., 1989).

Anxiety is a vague feeling of apprehension and uneasiness in response to a threat to one's value system or security pattern (*May, 1977). The individual may be able to identify the situation (e.g., surgery, cancer), but actually the threat to self relates to the enmeshed uneasiness and apprehension. In other words, the situation is the source of, but is not itself, the threat. In contrast, fear is feelings of apprehension related to a specific threat or danger to which one's security patterns respond (e.g., flying, heights, snakes). When the threat is removed, fear dissipates (*May, 1977). Anxiety is distinguished from fear, which is feeling afraid or threatened by a clearly identifiable external stimulus that represents danger to the person. "Anxiety affects us at a deeper level . . . invades the central core of the personality and erodes feelings of self-esteem and personal worth" (Halter, 2014, p. 279; Varcarolis, 2011). Anxiety is unavoidable in life and can serve many positive functions by motivating the person to take action to solve a problem or to resolve a crisis (*Varcarolis, Carson, & Shoemaker, 2005).

Clinically, both anxiety and fear may coexist in a response to a situation. For example, an individual facing surgery may be fearful of pain and anxious about possible cancer. According to Yokom (*1984), "Fear can be allayed by withdrawal from the situation, removal of the offending object, or by reassurance. Anxiety is reduced by admitting its presence and by being convinced that the values to be gained by moving ahead are greater than those to be gained by escape."

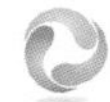

Errors in Diagnostic Statements

Fear **related to upcoming surgery**

Anticipated surgery can be a source of many threats, including threats to security patterns, health, values, self-concept, role functioning, goal achievement, and relationships. These threats can produce vague feelings ranging from mild uneasiness to panic. Identifying a threat as merely surgery is too simplistic; personal threats also are involved. Moreover, although some uneasiness may be attributed to fear (which teaching can eliminate), the remaining feelings relate to anxiety. Because this situation is inescapable, the nurse must assist the individual with coping mechanisms for managing anxiety and fear.

Key Concepts

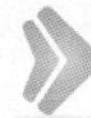

Carp's Cues

Frequent workplace stress can impact the physical and mental well-being of health professionals, resulting in burnout. This will also impact the ability to practice effectively and with empathy with individuals and their significant others (McCann et al., 2013).

McCann et al. (2013) conducted a review of literature on resilience in health care professionals. Factors that were identified in nurses that relate to increased resilience are self-reflection, insight, self-efficacy, positive self-talk/attitude, positive reflection, hope/optimism, and beliefs/spiritual. Contextual factors in nursing that contribute to resilience are partner, family, and friend support, organizational support, colleague support, and mentors.

General Considerations

- Lyon (*2002) has identified five factors that contribute to stressful lifestyles: idealistic expectations of self, unrealistic goals, toxic thoughts, negative self-talk, and procrastination.
- Anxiety refers to feelings aroused by a nonspecific threat to an individual's self-concept that impinges on health, assets, values, environment, role functioning, needs fulfillment, goal achievement, personal

relationships, and sense of security (Miller, 2015). It varies in intensity depending on the severity of the perceived threat and the success or failure of efforts to cope with the feelings.

- Anxiety and fear produce a similar sympathetic response: cardiovascular excitation, pupillary dilation, sweating, tremors, and dry mouth. Anxiety also involves a parasympathetic response of increased gastrointestinal (GI) activity; in contrast, fear is associated with decreased GI activity. Behaviorally the fearful person exhibits increased alertness and concentration, with avoidance, attack, or decreasing the risk of threat. Conversely, the anxious person experiences increased tension, general restlessness, insomnia, worry, and helplessness and vagueness concerning a situation that cannot be easily avoided or attacked (Halter, 2014).
- *Interpersonal patterns* of coping include the following:
  - Acting out: converting anxiety into anger (either overtly or covertly expressed)
  - Paralysis or retreating behaviors: withdrawing or being immobilized by anxiety
  - Somatizing: converting anxiety into physical symptoms
  - Constructive action: using anxiety to learn and to solve problems (includes goal setting, learning new skills, and seeking information)
- Defense mechanisms lower anxiety and protect self-esteem. People develop a range of coping behaviors, both maladaptive and adaptive. Maladaptive coping mechanisms are characterized by the inability to make choices, conflict, repetition, rigidity, alienation, and secondary gains.
- Anxiety can be classified as normal, acute (state), and chronic (trait) (Halter, 2014; Varcarolis, 2011).
  - Normal anxiety is necessary for survival. It prompts constructive behaviors, such as being on time or studying for a test.
  - Acute, or state, anxiety is the response to an imminent loss or change that disrupts one's sense of security. Examples include apprehension before a speech or the death of a close relative or friend.
  - Chronic, or trait, anxiety is anxiety that one lives with daily. In children, chronic anxiety may manifest as permanent apprehension or overreaction to unexpected stimuli. In adults, chronic anxiety may manifest as poor concentration, insomnia, relationship problems, and chronic fatigue.
- The effects of anxiety on an individual's abilities vary with degree (Halter, 2014; Varcarolis, 2011).
  - Mild
    - Heightened perception and attention; alertness
    - Ability to integrate past, present, and future experiences
    - Effective problem-solving ability
    - Mild tension-relieving behaviors (nail biting, hair twisting)
    - Restlessness, impatience
  - Moderate
    - Slightly narrowed perception; selective inattention, which can be directed
    - Slight difficulty concentrating; learning requires more effort
    - Poor concentration
    - Voice/pitch changes
    - Increased respiratory and heart rates
    - Tremors, shakiness, pacing
    - Somatic complaints (urinary frequency, headache, insomnia)
  - Severe
    - Significantly reduced and distorted perception; focus on scattered details; inability to attend to more even when instructed
    - Severely impaired learning; high distractibility and inability to concentrate
    - Problem solving "seems impossible"
    - Confusion, diaphoresis
    - Hyperventilation, tachycardia, headache, dizziness, nausea
    - Loud, rapid speech, threats, demands
  - Panic
    - Unable to process what is happening
    - Cannot problem solve
    - Cannot make choices or decisions
    - Inability to function; usually increased motor activity or unpredictable responses to minor stimuli; communication not understandable
    - Feelings of impending doom (terror, delusion, hallucinations, panic)
    - Somatic complaints (dyspnea, dizziness/faintness, palpitations, trembling, choking, paresthesia, hot/cold flashes, sweating)

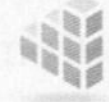

Pediatric Considerations

Anxiety

- Signs of anxiety in children vary greatly depending on developmental stage, temperament, past experience, and parental involvement (Hockenberry & Wilson, 2015). The most common sign in children and adolescents is increased motor activity. Signs of anxiety can be viewed developmentally and may be reflected in the following ways:
  - *Birth to 9 months:* Disruption in physiologic functioning (e.g., sleep disorders, còlic)
  - *9 months to 4 years:* Major source is loss of significant others and loss of love. Therefore, anxiety may be seen as anger when parents leave; somatic illnesses; motor restlessness; regressive behaviors (thumb sucking, rocking); regression in toilet training.
  - *4 to 6 years:* Major source is fear of body damage; belief that bad behavior causes bad things (e.g., illness); somatic complaints of headache, stomachache. In addition, anxiety related to starting school, separation from parent(s), and/or lack of adult supervision (latchkey status) (Pillitteri, 2014).
  - *6 to 12 years:* Excessive verbalization, compulsive behavior (e.g., repeating tasks)
  - *Adolescence:* Similar to 6 to 12 years, plus negativistic behavior
- Separation from parents, change in usual routines, strange environments, painful procedures, and parental anxiety may heighten anxiety (Hockenberry & Wilson, 2015). Assess for alterations in the functional health patterns to detect anxiety.
- Sources of anxiety for children and adolescents are related to school (e.g., performance, peer pressure), separation, social situations, and family.
- Refer children who manifest disorders of avoidance, over anxiousness, severe separation anxiety, and school phobia to mental health experts.

Responses to Death

- A child's concept of death has three stages:
  - *Younger than 5 years:* Death is reversible, seen as asleep or unable to move.
  - *5 to 9 years:* Death is perceived as a person (angel or monster) carrying away people. Believes own death can be avoided.
  - *After 9 or 10 years:* Death is final and inevitable.
- A child's involvement in funeral rituals should be encouraged if age-appropriate. Shielding children from these rituals does not promote a healthy adaptation to the reality of death.
- An adolescent inexperienced with death and wanting to appear in control may not openly grieve. He or she may continue in usual actions such as online activities and meeting friends as if nothing has happened (Hockenberry & Wilson, 2015).

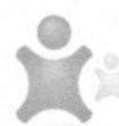

Maternal Considerations

- Multiple sources of anxiety are fear for personal or fetal well-being, previous miscarriages or complications, anticipated labor, responsibilities of parenthood, and relationship with partner (Pillitteri, 2014).

Geriatric Considerations

- Yochim, Mueller, June, and Segal (2011) reported the prevalence of anxiety in community-living elders from 15% to 52%.
- Blay and Marinko (2012) reported that "Late life anxiety disorder is defined as a persistent condition of excessive anxiety that interferes with daily life and leads to serious physical and mental disorders" (Miller, 2015, p. 215).
- Additional signs and symptoms of anxiety are pacing, fidgeting, changes in sleeping or eating patterns, and complaints of fatigue, pain, insomnia, or GI upsets (Miller, 2015).
- Anxiety that starts for the first time in late life is frequently associated with another condition such as depression, dementia, physical illness, or medication toxicity or withdrawal. Phobias, particularly agoraphobia, and generalized anxiety disorder are the most common late-life disorders (Halter, 2014; Varcarolis, 2011).

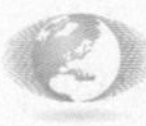

Transcultural Considerations

- Individuals and families from different cultures face many challenges when they seek health care in the dominant culture's health care delivery systems. In addition to usual sources of anxiety (e.g., unfamiliar people, unknown prognosis), they may be anxious about language difficulties, privacy, separation from support systems, and cost (Andrews & Boyle, 2008).

- Members of cultures who depend on family for caring will expect more humanistic kinds of nursing care and less scientific-technologic care (Andrews & Boyle, 2011).

Focus Assessment Criteria

Subjective Data

Assess for Defining Characteristics

Palpitations, Dyspnea, Dry Mouth, Nausea, Diaphoresis
Precipitating factors
Frequency
Duration

Feelings

Extreme sadness and worthlessness	Rejection or isolation
Guilt	Inability to cope/falling apart
Apprehension	Racing thoughts

Usual Coping Behavior
"What did you usually do when you face a difficult situations?"
"Is your response effective?

Subjective and Objective Data

Assess for Defining Characteristics

General Appearance
Facial expression (e.g., sad, hostile, expressionless)
Dress (e.g., meticulous, disheveled, seductive, eccentric)

Interaction Skills

With Nurse, with significant others

Appropriate	Hostile
Shows dependency	Relates well
Demanding/pleading	Withdrawn/preoccupied with self

Refer to Key Concepts to differentiate mild, moderate, severe, and panic levels of anxiety.

Goals

NOC
Anxiety Level, Social Anxiety Level, Coping, Anxiety Self-Control

The individual will relate increased psychological and physiologic comfort, evidenced by the following indicators:

- Describes own anxiety and coping patterns.
- Identifies two strategies to reduce anxiety.

Interventions

NIC
Anxiety Reduction, Impulse Control Training, Anticipatory Guidance, Calming Enhancement, Relaxation Therapy

Nursing interventions for *Anxiety* can apply to any individual with anxiety regardless of etiologic and contributing factors.

Assist the Individual to Reduce Present Level of Anxiety

- Assess the level of anxiety (see Key Concepts): mild, moderate, severe, or panic.
  - Provide reassurance and comfort. Ensure someone stays with the person with severe or panic levels of anxiety.
  - Support present coping mechanisms (e.g., allow the individual to talk, cry); do not confront or argue with defenses or rationalizations.
  - Speak slowly and calmly.

- Be aware of your own concern and avoid reciprocal anxiety.
- Convey empathic understanding (e.g., quiet presence, touch, allowing crying, talking).
- Provide reassurance that a solution can be found.
- Remind the individual that feelings are not harmful.
- Respect personal space.

R: *Nursing strategies differ depending on the level of anxiety (*Tarsitano, 1992).*

- If anxiety is at severe or panic level:
  - Do not make demands or ask the person to make decision.
  - Provide a quiet, nonstimulating environment with soft lighting.
  - Remain calm in your approach.
  - Use short, simple sentences; speak slowly.
  - Give concise directions.
  - Focus on the present.
  - Remove excess stimulation (e.g., take the individual to a quieter room); limit contact with others who are also anxious (e.g., other individuals, family).
  - Avoid suggesting the individual to "relax." Do not leave the individual alone.
  - Provide assistance with all tasks during acute episodes of dyspnea.
  - During an acute episode, do not discuss preventive measures.
  - During nonacute episodes, teach relaxation techniques (e.g., tapes, guided imagery).
  - Consult a physician, PA, or NP for possible pharmacologic therapy, if indicated.

R: *The severely anxious individual tends to overgeneralize, assume, and anticipate catastrophe. Resulting cognitive problems include difficulty with attention and concentration, loss of objectivity, and vigilance. Providing emotional support and relaxation techniques and encouraging sharing may help an individual clarify and verbalize fears, allowing the nurse to give realistic feedback and reassurance. Exercise helps to dispel some anxiety.*

If the Individual is Hyperventilating or Experiencing Dyspnea, Have Him or Her to Breathe into a Paper Bag or Ask the Individual to Breathe With you, For Example, Slow Abdominal Breathing Rhythm

R: *One technique involves breathing in CO_2, which will slow the rate of breathing. The other technique focuses on a slow rhythmic breathing, which with practice can distract and provide relaxation.*

When Anxiety Diminishes, Assist the Individual in Recognizing Anxiety and Causes

- Help to see that mild anxiety can be a positive catalyst for change and does not need to be avoided.
- Assist in reevaluation of perceived threat by discussing the following:
  - Were expectations realistic? Too idealistic?
  - Was it possible to meet expectations?
  - Where in the sequence of events was change possible?

R: *Verbalization allows sharing and provides an opportunity to correct misconceptions.*

- "Keep focused on manageable problems; define them simply and concretely" (Halter, 2014; Varcarolis, 2011).

R: *Simply defined problems can result in concrete interventions (Halter, 2014; Varcarolis, 2011).*

With Individuals with Cancer, Explore Sources of Anxiety/Fear

- Pain, dyspnea, uncontrolled symptoms, loss of function, dying
- Dependence on others
- Loss of control
- Feeling associated with the end of a therapy (radiation, chemotherapy) (Berger, Shuster, & Van Roenn, 2013)

R: *The loss of the routine of therapy, close supervision, and support may provoke worry and distress about losing these positive aspects of therapy . If the therapy is discontinued for adverse effects or nontherapeutic response, can increase feeling of dread and fear of unknown (Berger et al., 2013).*

- Teach anxiety interrupters to use when the individual cannot avoid stressful situations:
  - Look up. Lower shoulders.
  - Control breathing.
  - Slow thoughts. Alter voice.

- Give self-directions (out loud, if possible).
- Exercise.
- "Scruff your face"—changes facial expression.
- Change perspective: imagine watching a situation from a distance (*Grainger, 1990).

R: *Relaxation techniques help the person switch the autonomous system from the fight-or-flight response to a more relaxed response (Varcarolis, 2011).*

Reduce or Eliminate Problematic Coping Mechanisms

- Depression, withdrawal (see *Ineffective Coping*)
- Violent behavior (see *Risk for Other-Directed Violence*)
- Denial
  - Develop an atmosphere of empathic understanding.
  - Assist in lowering the level of anxiety.
  - Focus on the present situation.
  - Give feedback about current reality; identify positive achievements.
  - Have the individual describe events in detail; focus on specifics of who, what, when, and where.

R: *Denial can be an effective defense mechanism when the situation is too stressful to cope.*

- Numerous physical complaints with no known organic base (*Maynard, 2004; Videbeck, 2014)
  - Talk to the individual each shift with a focus on expression of feelings.

R: *This will demonstrate consistent interest and does not require the individual to complain about something to have the nurse's attention.*

- Give positive feedback when the individual is symptom free.
- Acknowledge that symptoms must be burdensome.
- Encourage interest in the external environment (e.g., volunteering, helping others).
- Listen to complaints, but minimize the amount of time or attention given to complaints. Consult with physician, PA, or NP to explain new complaint.

R: *"If physical complaints are unsuccessful in gaining attention, they should decrease in frequency over time" (Videbeck, 2014, p. 417).*

- Consult significant others to explain the dynamics of hypochondriacal behavior, underlying issues, and the secondary gains. Stress this behavior does have psychological origins.

R: *Discussion with family can help to interrupt the cycle.*

- Engage in discussions not related to symptoms.

R: *The conversion of emotional distress into physical symptoms is called somatization. Psychological concepts that may underlie somatization are amplification of body sensations, the need to be sick and the attention the complaints receive (*Maynard, 2004; Videbeck, 2014).*

- Anger (e.g., demanding behavior, manipulation; with adults, see *Ineffective Coping*)
- Unrealistic expectations of self (*Lyon, 2002; Videbeck, 2014)
  - Help to set realistic goals with short-term daily or weekly goals.
  - Allow for setbacks.
  - Use positive self-talk.
  - Practice "thought stopping" with toxic thinking.

R: *Unrealistic expectations will heighten the expectations of self and increase anxiety. Participating in decision making can give an individual a sense of control, which enhances coping ability. Perception of loss of control can result in a sense of powerlessness, then hopelessness (*Courts, Barba, & Tesh, 2001).*

- Toxic thoughts (*Lyon, 2002)
  - Avoid assigning negative meaning to an event.
  - Avoid "reading someone else's mind."
  - Avoid all-or-nothing, black-or-white thinking.
  - Avoid making the worst of a situation.
  - Attempt to fix the problem; avoid assigning blame.

R: *Toxic thoughts can confuse the situation, increase anxiety, and reduce effective coping (Varcarolis, 2011).*

- Teach to recognize that certain autonomic thinking can trigger anxiety (e.g., should, never, always). Role-play alternative thinking (Varcarolis, 2011).

R: *Words that are more neutral and objective can reduce anxiety (e.g., sometimes, "I can now") (Varcarolis, 2011).*

Promote Resiliency

- Avoid minimizing positive experiences.
- Gently encourage humor.
- Encourage optimism.
- Encourage discussion with significant others.
- Encourage the individual to seek spiritual comfort through religion, nature, prayer, meditation, or other methods.

R: *Resilience is a combination of abilities and characteristics that interact to allow an individual to bounce back, cope successfully, and function above the norm in spite of significant stress or adversity (*Tusaie & Dyer, 2004). For professionals, McCann et al. (2013, p. 61) defined "resilience as the ability to maintain personal and professional well-being in the face of on-going work stress and adversity." Environmental factors that favor resilience are perceived social support or a sense of connectedness.*

Initiate Health Teaching and Referrals as Indicated

- Refer people identified as having chronic anxiety and maladaptive coping mechanisms for ongoing mental health counseling and treatment.
- Instruct in nontechnical, understandable terms regarding illness and associated treatments.

R: *Simple and repeating explanations are needed because anxiety may interfere with learning.*

- Instruct (or refer) the individual for assertiveness training.

R: *Assertiveness training helps one ask for what he or she wants, learn how to say no, and reduce the stress of unrealistic expectations of others.*

- Instruct the individual to increase exercise and reduce TV watching (refer to *Risk-Prone Health Behavior* for specific interventions).

R: *Studies show that exercise is very effective at reducing fatigue, improving alertness and concentration, and enhancing overall cognitive function (Centers for Disease Control and Prevention [CDC], 2013).*

R: *Exercise can effectively reduce anxiety. Exercise is an effective method for reducing state anxiety in breast cancer survivors (*Blanchard, Courneya, & Laing, 2001).*

- Instruct in use of relaxation techniques (e.g., aromatherapy [orange, lavender], hydrotherapy, music therapy, massage).
- Explain the benefits of foot massage and reflexology (*Grealish, Lomasney, & Whiteman, 2000; Rahbar et al., 2011; *Stephenson, Weinrich, & Tavakoli, 2000).

R: *Complementary therapies such as massage, aromatherapy, and hydrotherapy are useful in managing stress and anxiety (*Lehrner, Marwinski, Lehr, Johren, & Deecke, 2005; *Mok & Woo, 2004; *Wong, Lopez-Nahas, & Molassiotis, 2001; *Yilmaz et al., 2003).*

R: *Music therapy is an effective nursing intervention in decreasing anxiety (*Wong et al., 2001).*

- Provide telephone numbers for emergency intervention: hotlines, psychiatric emergency room, and on-call staff if available.

R: *Providing access to help in the community can reduce feelings of aloneness and powerlessness.*

Pediatric Interventions

- Explain events that are sources of anxiety using simple, age-appropriate terms and illustrations, such as puppets, dolls, and sample equipment.

R: *Explanations that are age-appropriate can reduce anxiety.*

- Allow child to wear underwear and have familiar toys or objects.

R: *Any strategy that increases comfort and familiarity can reduce anxiety.*

- Assist the child to cope with anxiety (Hockenberry & Wilson, 2015):
  - Establish a trusting relationship.
  - Minimize separation from parents.
  - Encourage expression of feelings.
  - Involve the child in play.
  - Prepare the child for new experiences (e.g., procedures, surgery).
  - Provide comfort measures.
  - Allow for regression.
  - Encourage parental involvement in care.
  - Allay parental apprehension and provide them information.

R: *The presence of parents provides a familiar, stabilizing support. Parental anxiety influences the child's anxiety.*

- Assist a child with anger.
  - Encourage the child to share anger (e.g., "How did you feel when you had your injection?").
  - Tell the child that being angry is okay (e.g., "I sometimes get angry when I can't have what I want.").
  - Encourage and allow the child to express anger in acceptable ways (e.g., loud talking, running outside around the house).

R: *Children need opportunities and encouragement to express anger in a controlled, acceptable way (e.g., choosing not to play a particular game or with a particular person, slamming a door, voicing anger). Unacceptable expressions of anger include throwing or breaking objects and hitting others. Children who are not permitted to express anger may develop hostility and perceive the world as unfriendly.*

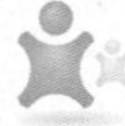

Maternal Interventions

- Discuss expectations and concerns regarding pregnancy and parenthood with the woman alone, her partner alone, and then together as indicated.

R: *Some fears are based on inaccurate information, which accurate data can relieve.*

- Acknowledge anxieties and their normality (*Lugina, Christensson, Massawe, Nystrom, & Lindmark, 2001):
  - *1 week postpartum:* worried about self (e.g., feeling tired and nervous about breasts, perineum, and infection)
  - *1 week postpartum:* worried about baby's health (e.g., baby's eyes, respirations, temperature, safety, and crying)
  - *6 weeks postpartum:* worried about partner's reaction to her and baby

R: *Providing emotional support and encouraging sharing may help an individual clarify and verbalize fears, allowing the nurse to give realistic feedback and reassurance. If there was a previous fetal or neonatal death, provide opportunities for both mother and father to share their feelings and fears.*

R: *Partners of women with a previous pregnancy loss or neonatal death are often expected to appear strong to support their partner. Research reported that men who experience this very personal tragedy need as much emotional support and opportunities to share their grief as the mother (*McCreight, 2004).*

Death Anxiety

NANDA-I Definition

Vague uneasy feeling of discomfort or dread generated by perceptions of a real or imagined threat to one's existence

Defining Characteristics*

Individual reports:
Worry about the impact of one's own death on significant others
Feeling powerless over dying
Fear of loss of mental abilities when dying

Fear of pain related to dying
Fear of suffering related to dying
Deep sadness
Fear of the process of dying
Concerns of overworking the caregiver
Negative thoughts related to death and dying
Fear of prolonged dying
Fear of premature death
Fear of developing a terminal illness

Related Factors

A diagnosis of a potentially terminal condition or impending death can cause this diagnosis. Additional factors can contribute to death anxiety.

Situational (Personal, Environmental)

Related to discussions on topic of death*

Related to near death experience*

Related to perceived proximity of death*

Related to uncertainty of prognosis*

Related to anticipating suffering*

Related to confronting reality of terminal disease*

Related to observations related to death

Related to anticipating pain*

Related to nonacceptance of own mortality*

Related to uncertainty about life after death*

Related to uncertainty about an encounter with a higher power*

Related to uncertainty about the existence of a higher power*

Related to experiencing the dying process*

Related to anticipating impact of death on others*

Related to anticipating adverse consequences of general anesthesia*

Related to personal conflict with palliative versus curative care

Related to conflict with family regarding palliative versus curative care

Related to fear of being a burden

Related to fear of unmanageable pain

Related to fear of abandonment

Related to unresolved conflict (family, friends)

Related to fear that one's life lacked meaning

Related to social disengagement

Related to powerlessness and vulnerability

Author's Note

The inclusion of *Death Anxiety* in the NANDA-I classification creates a diagnostic category with the etiology in the label. This opens the NANDA-I list to many diagnostic labels with etiology (e.g., separation anxiety, failure anxiety, and travel anxiety). Many diagnostic labels can take this same path: fear as claustrophobic fear, diarrhea as traveler's diarrhea, decisional conflict as end-of-life decisional conflict.

Specifically end-of-life situations create multiple responses in individuals and significant others. Some of these are shared and expected of those involved. These responses could be described with a syndrome diagnosis as end-of-life syndrome. This author recommends its development by nurses engaged in palliative and hospice care.

Errors in Diagnostic Statements

Death anxiety related to terminal illness

This diagnosis reflects multiple issues and responses to terminal illness as fear, pain, powerlessness, grieving, interrupted family processes, etc. Without a syndrome diagnosis, the nurse must assess for problematic responses and use specific nursing diagnoses such as *Pain, Grieving.*

Reserve death anxiety for those related factors that will inhibit the individual to a peaceful death psychologically and spiritually (e.g., an unresolved conflict with a friend).

Key Concepts

- In a research study of the reactions of 153 rehabilitation counselors to possible individual death, 22% reported they preferred not to work with individuals with life-threatening illnesses. Death anxiety scores were higher in younger respondents (younger than 44 years of age). Educational programs and support groups help reduce death anxiety in health care workers (Hunt & Rosenthal, 2000).
- In response to the difficult situation of attempting to help an individual understand the seriousness of metastatic cancer, Campbell (*2008) reports, "When cancer has spread from where it has started to somewhere else in the body, it means it is metastatic and cannot be cured. That means that while we can treat your cancer, hopefully lengthening your life and controlling symptoms, we can never make it go away. And because you are otherwise healthy, it means it's likely you will one day die from this cancer." When the prognosis is very poor, Campbell (*2008) reports, "I am afraid you are dying".
- The detrimental impact of untreated, persistent anxiety was demonstrated in one multicenter study of over 600 patients with advanced cancer that evaluated associations between anxiety disorders and multiple endpoints, including physician—patient relationships. Patients with anxiety disorders had less trust in their clinicians compared to those without anxiety (Alici & Levin 2010; Irwin, & Hirst, 2014).
- Yun, Watanabe, and Shimojo (2012) reported a majority of patients (58.0%) and caregivers (83.4%) were aware of the patient's terminal status. However only 30% of patients and 50% of caregivers were told directly by a physician. "For approximately 28% of patients and 23% of caregivers reported that they guessed it from the patient's worsening condition. The patient group was more likely than the caregiver group (78.6% vs. 69.6%) to prefer that patients be informed of their terminal status."

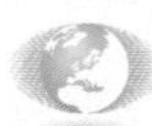

Transcultural Considerations

Truth-telling is critical to the dominant culture of Americans and Canadians to preserve individual autonomy. Other cultures may not value truth-telling if it disrupts family solidarity. Refer to *Spiritual Distress* for a review of religious beliefs and rituals regarding death.

Focus Assessment Criteria

See *Anxiety* and *Grieving*.

Goals

NOC

Dignified Life Closure, Comfortable Death, Coping, Suffering Severity, Fear Level, Self-Control, Individual Satisfaction, Decision-Making, Family Coping

The individual will report diminished anxiety or fear, as evidenced by the following indicators:

- Share feelings regarding dying.
- Identify specific requests that will increase psychological comfort.

Interventions

Carp's Cues

"Does fear of death impact on nurses' caring for patients at the end of life and if so, what steps should be taken to improve the quality of care?" (Peters, Cant, & Payne, 2012) All people have personal, cultural, social, and philosophical belief systems that shape their conscious or unconscious behaviors of their own attitudes towards death. These attitudes can enhance or impede empathetic, therapeutic care to dying individual and their significant others (Peters et al., 2012), giving rise to anxiety and unease.

"In particular, the primary work of critical care, intensive care and emergency doctors and nurses is to rescue patients from medical crises. It is also complicated by the clinical environments in these areas that are designed to allow for intervention and observation, are rarely private for the patient or their family and are always in high demand. Thus, time for caring is limited. There is also a real conflict for nurses who have the competing demands of caring for a dying patient along with an acute or 'rescuable' patient group" (Peters et al., 2012).

Some nurses are perceived as being comfortable and confident when caring for individuals and/or their significant others dealing with impending death. Tell them you notice their expertise and share your interest in learning from them.

NIC

Anxiety Reduction, Patient Rights Protection, Family Support, Dying Care, Coping Enhancement, Active Listening, Emotional Support, Spiritual Support

For an Individual With New or Early Diagnosis of a Potentially Terminal Condition

- Explore your own feelings regarding your dying or those you love. Examine if you or your nurse/physician colleagues engage in "death avoidance" (Braun, Gordon, & Uziely, 2010).
- Braun et al. (2010) found that nurses' attitudes toward caring for dying patients were related to personal attitudes toward death. Those demonstrating positive attitudes reported more engagement with dying individuals. A mediating role was found for death avoidance, suggesting some may use avoidance to cope with fear of death. Culture and religion may be key to attitudes (most were Jewish).
- Allow the individual and family separate opportunities to discuss their understanding of the condition. Correct misinformation.
- Access valid information regarding condition, treatment options, and stage of condition from primary provider (physician, nurse practitioner).
- Ensure a discussion of the prognosis if known.
  - Individuals with high anxiety reported being (Alici & Levin 2010; Irwin, & Hirst, 2014)
  - Less comfortable asking questions about their health
  - Less likely to understand the clinical information
  - More likely to believe that their clinicians would offer them futile therapies
  - Less certain that they would have adequate symptom control at the end of life

R: *With a diagnosis of a potential terminal illness, individuals and families should be given opportunities to talk about treatments, cures, and goals regarding quality of life (e.g., curative vs. symptomatic comfort care).*

For the Individual Experiencing a Progression of a Terminal Illness

- Explore his or her understanding of the situation and feelings. Encourage the sharing of fears about what their death will look like and what events will lead up to it.

R: *It is important to determine the person's understanding of the situation and personal preferences or requests.*

- Ensure that the primary physician, physician assistant, or nurse practitioner has initiated a discussion regarding the situation and options desired by the individual.

R: *These discussions provide insight into the individual's understanding and direct treatment decisions. Research reports that only 31% of persons with terminal conditions reported end-of-life discussions with a physician (*Wright, 2008).*

- Discuss with family and individual palliative care and strategies that can be used for dyspnea, pain, and other discomforts (Yarbro, Wujcik, & Gobel, 2013).

R: *During the final stage of life, anxiety for the individual and the family is highly correlated with the presence or fear of other symptoms such as dyspnea, pain, and fear of the unknown (Yarbro et al., 2013).*

- Elicit from the individual and individual's family specific requests for end-of-life care.

R: *Persons with advanced cancer identified their priorities as protection of dignity, sense of control, pain control, inappropriate prolongation of dying, and strengthening relationships (Singer, Salvator, Guo, Collin, Lilien, & Baley, 1999; Volker & Wu, 2011).*

- Provide family with an explanation of changes in their loved one that may occur as death nears (e.g., death rattle, anorexia, nausea, weakness, withdrawal, decreased perfusion in extremities) (Yarbro et al., 2013).

R: *Clear, direct discussions can reduce the family's anxiety when these signs and symptoms occur (Yarbro et al., 2013).*

- Avoid giving a specific time for the expected time of death. "It is helpful to give a range of time, such as 'hours to days,' 'days to weeks,' or 'weeks to months'" (Yarbro et al., 2013).

R: *Family members and friends will be able to better plan their time spent with their loved one with this information (Yarbro et al., 2013).*

- Provide opportunities for the person to discuss end-of-life decisions. Be direct and empathetic.

R: *Clover, Browne, MsErwin, and Vanderberg (*2004) found that a person's readiness to participate in end-of-life decisions depends on the skills of the professional nurse to encourage the individual to divulge his or her wishes.*

- Encourage the individual to reconstruct his or her world view:
  - Allow the individual to verbalize feelings about the meaning of death.
  - Advise the individual that there are no right or wrong feelings.
  - Advise the individual that responses are his or her choice.
  - Acknowledge struggles.
  - Encourage dialogue with a spiritual mentor or close friend.

R: *When an individual is facing death, reconstructing a world view involves balancing thoughts about the painful subject with avoiding painful thoughts.*

- Allow significant others opportunities to share their perceptions and concerns. Advise them that sadness is expected and normal.

R: *Clarification is needed to determine if their concerns regarding end-of-life care is consistent with the individual. "It is normal and healthy to feel sad at the end of life, to grieve the impending loss of everything a person holds dear" (*Coombs-Lee, 2008, p. 12).*

- Discuss the value of truthful conversations (e.g., sorrow, mistakes, disagreements).

R: *"Avoiding truthful conversations does not bring hope and comfort: it brings isolation and loneliness" (*Coombs-Lee, 2008).*

- To foster psychospiritual growth, open dialogue with the individual specifically (*Yakimo, 2011):
  - If your time is indeed shortened, what do you need to get done?
  - Are there people whom you need to contact to resolve feelings or unfinished business?
  - What do you want to do with the time you have left?
- If appropriate, offer to help the individual contact others to resolve conflicts (old or new) verbally or in writing. Validate that forgiveness is not a seeking reconciliation, "but a letting go of a hurt" (*Yakimo, 2011).

R: *"Asking for or providing forgiveness is a powerful healing tool" (*Yakimo, 2011).*

- Respect the dying individual's wishes (e.g., few or no visitors, modifications in care, no heroic measures, food or liquid preferences).

R: *If the individual is ready to release life and die and others expect him or her to want to continue to live, the individual's own depression, grief, and turmoil are increased (*Yakimo, 2011).*

- Encourage the individual to
  - Tell life stories and reminisce
  - Discuss leaving a legacy: donation, personal articles, or taped messages

R: *Strategies that help the individual find meaning in failures and successes can reduce anxiety and depression.*

- Encourage reflective activities, such as personal prayer, meditation, and journal writing.
- Return of the gift of love to others by listening, praying for others, sharing personal wisdom gained from illness, and creating legacy gifts.

R: *Promoting and restoring interests, imagination, and creativity enhance quality of life (*Brant, 1998).*

- Aggressively manage unrelieved symptoms (e.g., nausea, pruritus, pain, vomiting, fatigue).

R: *Serious unrelieved symptoms can cause a distressing death and needless added suffering for families (*Nelson Walsh, Behrens, Zhukovsky, Lipnickey, & Brady, 2000). Fatigue and pain consume excess energy and reduce energy needed for optimal dialogue (*Matzo & Sherman, 2001).*

- Initiate referrals and health teaching as indicated to explain palliative care (Miller, 2015):
  - Ensure the primary focus is on comfort, psychosocial, and spiritual well-being, rather than on improving physical function.
  - Physical exercise may prove beneficial, even among the seriously ill. Exercise can decrease worry and anxiety, while improving overall functioning. Exercise may also serve an important role in providing a sense of autonomy, control, or success.
  - Individuals who are bedbound can engage in activities that provide exercise, even it if is only practicing passive range of motion.
  - Manage distressing symptoms (e.g., pain, thirst, nausea, dyspnea, constipation, dry mouth).
  - Educate and support family and significant others.
  - Consult, educate, and support professional caregivers.

R: *Palliative care is a holistic approach to caring for persons with advanced progressive illness. Palliative care can be provided at any point during the course of an illness. Palliative care will always be a part of hospice care, but it can be provided to persons not in a hospice program (Miller, 2015).*

- Initiate referrals and health teaching as indicated to explain hospice care:
  - Hospice has designated caregivers, nurses, social service, physicians, and nurse practitioners in the program.
  - Hospice provides palliative care in homes and health care settings.
  - Refer to educational resources (e.g., National Hospice and Palliative Care Organization, www.nhpco .org).

Pediatric Interventions

- Educate parents about the need to explain honestly and age-appropriately the child's impending death; consult with experts as needed.

R: *Chronically ill children with poor prognoses or terminal illnesses often know more about death than adults may think. "Children are harmed by what they do not know, by what they are not told, and by their misconceptions" (*Yakimo, 2011).*

- In cases where death is likely however not definite:
  - Educate the family that involving a palliative care team does not equal a death sentence for the child.
  - Explain that such an approach can be beneficial for those who may recover, as the ultimate goal of palliative care is improvement in the quality of life for the child who is dying or seriously ill/injured.
  - It is not beneficial, however, to give false hope; always be honest about the seriousness of the child's condition.

R: *Palliative care should be considered early on, once a terminal diagnosis is made. It refers to the interdisciplinary team who specialize in educating the child and their family about the process and prognosis. They can also advocate for measures to relieve symptoms and anxieties surrounding the dying process (Ball, Bindler, & Cowen, 2015).*

- In situations where the child is a candidate for organ donation:
  - In a gentle and compassionate manner, raise the possibility of organ donation.

R: *It is encouraged that the possibility of donation be discussed with end-of-life planning, not only once death has occurred (Ball et al., 2015).*

  - If the child is of an age to understand and participate in the end-of-life planning process, the child's opinion on organ donation should be considered and taken seriously.
  - Once the child is officially a candidate for donation, contact the Organ Procurement Organization.

R: *Designated members of staff should carry out communications with the family regarding the process.*

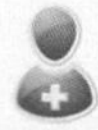

Clinical Alert Sudden unexpected death of the infant (SUID) occurs between 1 month and 1 year of age typically. It is usually a result of risk factors, but can also have no apparent cause. These cases are referred to the medical examiner for further investigation and autopsy. Child abuse/filicide should be considered in the differential diagnosis, but it should be kept in mind that only an estimated 1% to 5% of SIDS cases are considered infanticide (Corwin, Michael, McClain, & Mary, 2014).

- When someone else or a pet is dying or has died (*Yakimo, 2011)
  - Explain what is happening or what has happened
  - Ask the child how he or she feels
  - Have a funeral for the pet
  - Be specific that the child is not responsible for the death
  - Explain the funeral service and discuss if the child will attend
  - Explain that adults will be sad and crying. Limit exposure.
- Do not
  - Associate death with sleep
  - Force a young child to attend the funeral
  - Tell the child not to cry
  - Give a long, detailed explanation beyond the child's level of understanding

R: *Explanations regarding death need to be age-appropriate and factual to avoid misconceptions and escalation of fears. Shielding older children from death and funerals does not prepare them for the reality of death (Hockenberry, Wilson, & Winkelstein, 2013).*

- For the child who has, or is about to, experience the death of a loved one (Ball et al., 2015; Muriel, 2013):
  - Always be honest and explain what is happening in terms the child will understand.
  - Encourage the child to talk about their feelings as well as open communication about the death process.
  - Explain the funeral process. The family should discuss whether or not it would be appropriate for the child to attend the funeral based on the child's emotional development.
  - Children may become more distant or overly attached to the person who is about the die in a form of anticipatory grief.
- Infants and toddlers (0 to 2 years of age):
  - They will feel separation and distress over change in routine as well as be affected by the emotional stress of those grieving around them.
- Preschoolers (3 to 5 years):
  - These children will not comprehend the finality of death. Avoid describing death as something the child may regard as reversible or that they may develop a fear of the same thing happening to them. For example, do not refer to death as sleep.
  - This age group is also egocentric; they may need frequent reassurance that they were not the cause of the death/loss or why others are grieving.
- School-age (6 to 12 years):
  - At this age, school has become a major part of the child's life. It should be considered that certain school staff be made aware of the death for purposes of support.
  - Encouraging children at this age to continue their normal daily routines may help facilitate the notion that life goes on after the loss.
- Adolescents (13 to 18 years):
  - A normally developing adolescent is by nature self-involved, and it should be kept in mind as opposed to considering them aloof or selfish in their grief.

R: *Explanations regarding death need to be age-appropriate and factual to avoid misconceptions and escalation of fears. Shielding older children from death and funerals does not prepare them for the reality of death (Hockenberry & Wilson, 2015).*

RISK FOR BLEEDING

See also *Risk for Complications of Bleeding* in Section 3.

NANDA-I Definition

At risk for a decrease in blood volume that may compromise health

Risk Factors*

Aneurysm
Circumcision

Deficient knowledge
Disseminated intravascular coagulopathy
History of falls
Gastrointestinal disorders (e.g., gastric ulcer disease, polyps, varices)
Impaired liver function (e.g., cirrhosis, hepatitis)
Inherent coagulopathies (e.g., thrombocytopenia)
Postpartum complications (e.g., uterine atony, retained placenta)
Pregnancy-related complications (e.g., placenta previa, molar pregnancy, placenta abruptio [placental abruption])
Trauma
Treatment-related side effects (e.g., surgery, medications, administration of platelet-deficient blood products, chemotherapy)

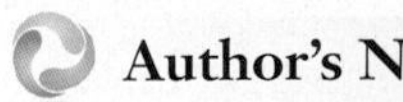

Author's Note

This NANDA-I diagnosis represents several collaborative problems.

Goals/Interventions

Refer to Section 3 for the specific collaborative problems such as *Risk for Complications of Hypovolemia*, *Risk for Complications of Bleeding*, *Risk for Complications of GI Bleeding*, *Risk for Complications of Prenatal Bleeding*, *Risk for Complications of Postpartum Hemorrhage*, or *Risk for Complications of Anticoagulant Therapy Adverse Effects*.

RISK FOR UNSTABLE BLOOD GLUCOSE LEVEL

See also *Risk for Complications of Hypo/Hyperglycemia* in Section 3.

NANDA-I Definition

At risk for variation of blood glucose/sugar levels from the normal range that may compromise health

Risk Factors*

Deficient knowledge of diabetes management (e.g., action plan)
Developmental level
Dietary intake
Inadequate blood glucose monitoring
Lack of acceptance of diagnosis
Lack of adherence to diabetes management (e.g., adhering to action plan)
Lack of diabetes management (e.g., action plan)
Medication management
Physical activity level
Physical health status
Pregnancy
Rapid growth periods
Stress
Weight gain
Weight loss

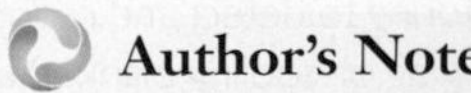

Author's Note

This nursing diagnosis represents a situation that requires collaborative intervention with medicine. This author recommends that the collaborative problem *Risk for Complications of Hypo/Hyperglycemia* be used instead. Students should consult with their faculty for advice about whether to use *Risk for Unstable Blood Glucose Level* or *Risk for Complications of Hypo/Hyperglycemia.* Refer to Section 3 for interventions for these specific diagnoses. In addition, the nursing diagnosis of *Ineffective Health Management* relates to insufficient knowledge of blood glucose monitoring, dietary requirements of diabetes mellitus, need for exercise and prevention of complications, and risk for infection. Refer to Section 2 Part I under *Ineffective Health Management* for more information.

RISK FOR IMBALANCED BODY TEMPERATURE

Risk for Imbalanced Body Temperature

Hyperthermia
Hypothermia
Ineffective Thermoregulation
Ineffective Thermoregulation • Related to Newborn Transition to Extrauterine Environment

NANDA-I Definition

At risk for failure to maintain body temperature within normal range

Risk Factors

Treatment Related

Related to cooling effects of:

Parenteral fluid infusion/blood transfusion
Cooling blanket
Dialysis
Operating suite

Situational (Personal, Environmental)

Related to:

Consumption of alcohol
Exposure to extremes of environmental temperature*
Inappropriate clothing for environmental temperature*
Inability to pay for shelter, heat, or air conditioning
Extremes of weight*
Dehydration*/malnutrition
Newborn birth environment exposure

Maturational

Related to ineffective temperature regulation secondary to extremes of age* (e.g., newborn, older adult)

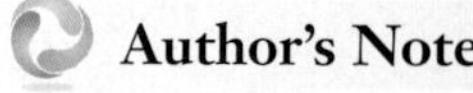

Author's Note

Risk for Imbalanced Body Temperature includes those at risk for *Hyperthermia, Hypothermia, Ineffective Thermoregulation*, or all of these. If the individual is at risk for only one (e.g., *Hypothermia* but not *Hyperthermia*), then it is more useful to label the problem with the specific diagnosis (*Risk for Hypothermia*). If the individual is at risk for two or more, then *Risk for Imbalanced Body Temperature* is more appropriate. The focus of nursing care is preventing abnormal body temperatures by identifying and treating those with normal temperature who demonstrate risk factors that nurse-prescribed interventions (e.g., removing blankets, adjusting environmental temperature) can control. If the imbalance is related to a pathophysiologic complication that requires nursing and medical interventions, then the problem should be labeled as a collaborative problem (e.g., *Risk for Complications of Severe Hypothermia related to hypothalamus injury, Risk for Complications of Neuroleptic Malignant Syndrome*). The focus of concern then becomes monitoring to detect and report significant temperature fluctuations and implementing collaborative interventions (e.g., a warming or cooling blanket) as ordered. See also Author's Note for *Hyperthermia* and *Hypothermia*.

Key Concepts

General Considerations

- *Conduction:* Direct transfer of heat from the body to cooler objects without motion (e.g., from cells and capillaries to skin to clothing)
- *Convection:* Transfer of heat by circulation (e.g., from warmer core areas to peripheral areas and from air movement next to the skin)
- *Radiation:* Transfer of heat between the skin and the environment
- *Evaporation:* Transfer of heat when skin or clothing is wet and heat is lost through moisture into the environment
- Heat production occurs in the core, which is innervated by thermoreceptor stimulation from the hypothalamus.
- Instead of 98.6° F as the norm for body temperature, Waalen and Buxbaum (2011) reported the results of a large study (>18,000) that normal temperature for healthy adults is 98.2° F and older adults is 97° F.
- Heat loss and gain vary in individuals and are influenced by body surface area, peripheral vasomotor tone, and quantity of subcutaneous tissue. Shivering, the body's physiologic attempt to generate heat, produces profound physiologic responses:
  - Increased oxygen consumption two to five times the normal rate
  - Increased metabolic demand to as much as 400% to 500%
  - Increased myocardial work, carbon dioxide production, cutaneous vasoconstriction, and eventual lactic acid production
- Temperature reliability depends on accurate temperature-taking technique, minimization of variables affecting the temperature measurement device, and site chosen for measurement.
  - Oral temperature readings may be unreliable (from such variables as poor contact between the thermometer and mucosa, air movement, and smoking or drinking before temperature taking); oral temperatures measure 0.5° F (0.3° C) below core temperature (*Giuliano , Giuliano, Scott, & MacLachlan, 2000; Grossman & Porth, 2014).
  - Rectal temperature readings, which have fewer affecting variables, are more reliable than oral readings; rectal temperatures measure 1° F (0.6° C) *higher* than oral temperature readings, with normal as 99.6° F (37.6° C).
  - Axillary temperature readings are reliable only for skin temperature; they measure 1° F (0.6° C) *lower* than oral temperature readings, with normal as 97.6° F (36.4° C).
  - Smitz, Van De Winckel, and Smitz (2009) reported that ear-based thermometry can predict rectal temperatures in afebrile and febrile older adults.

Hyperthermia

- The body responds to hot environments by increasing heat dissipation through increased sweat production and dilation of peripheral blood vessels.
- Increased metabolic rate increases body temperature and vice versa (increased body temperature increases metabolic rate).
- Fever is a major sign of onset of infection, inflammation, and disease. Treatment with aspirin or acetaminophen without medical consultation may mask important symptoms that should receive medical attention.
- Blood is the body's cooling fluid: low blood volume from dehydration predisposes one to fever.

Hypothermia

- The body responds to cold environments with mechanisms aimed at preventing heat loss and increasing heat production, such as
  - Muscle contraction
  - Increased heart rate
  - Shivering and vasodilatation
  - Peripheral vasoconstriction
  - Dilation of blood vessels in muscles
  - Release of thyroxine and corticosteroids
- Severe hypothermia can cause life-threatening arrhythmias and requires immediate interventions.
- Without safe and effective rewarming, hypothermia (a core temperature <95° F [35° C]) in the postoperative period has profound negative effects (decreased myocardial and cerebral functions, respiratory

acidosis, impaired hematologic and immunologic functions, and cold diuresis). Hypothermia also reduces blood pressure and contributes to shock.

- Therapeutic hypothermia (82.4° F to 89.6° F) can be used after brain injury, cardiac arrest, and during certain surgeries to reduce brain metabolism and decrease inflammation.

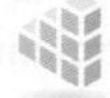

Pediatric Considerations

- Almost every child experiences a fever of 100° F to 104° F (37.8° C to 40° C) at some time. Usually, this does not harm normal children. Only approximately 4% of febrile children are susceptible to convulsions.
- Nonshivering thermogenesis is a heat production mechanism located in brown fat (highly vascular adipose tissue) found only in infants. When skin temperature begins to drop, thermal receptors transmit impulses to the central nervous system (CNS). The following sequence illustrates this mechanism:
  - CNS → stimulates sympathetic nervous system → release of norepinephrine from adrenal gland and at nerve endings in brown fat → heat production
  - Thermoregulation is controlled by the hypothalamus. Untreated hypothermia can result in newborn weight loss, glucose utilization, metabolic hypoxemia, hypoxia, and death.
- Treating all fevers in children is unnecessary. Fevers related to heat stroke can be treated with tepid or cold sponging. Fevers (less than 104° F or 40° C) in previously well children with no history of febrile convulsions and without a threatening illness can be left untreated or, if desired, treated with acetaminophen. Sponging increases the child's discomfort. Tepid sponging instead of antipyretic drugs is indicated for very young infants and children with severe liver disease or a history of hypersensitivity to antipyretic drugs.

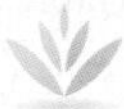

Geriatric Considerations

- Older adults can become hypothermic or hyperthermic in moderately cold or hot environments, compared with younger adults, who require exposure to extremely cold or hot temperatures (Miller, 2015).
- Age-related changes that interfere with the body's ability to adapt to cold temperatures include inefficient vasoconstriction, decreased peripheral circulation, decreased ability to acclimatize to heat, decreased cardiac output, decreased subcutaneous tissue, and delayed and diminished sweating (Miller, 2015).
- Older adults have a higher threshold for onset and decreased efficiency of sweating, as well as a dulled perception of cold and warmth and thus may lack the stimulus to initiate protective actions. Additionally, the thirst mechanism becomes less efficient with aging, as does the kidney's ability to concentrate urine, increasing the risk of heat-related dehydration (Miller, 2015).
- Inactivity and immobility increase susceptibility to hypothermia by suppressing shivering and reducing heat-generating muscle activity.
- Seventy percent of all victims of heat stroke are older than 60 years.
- Older adults may present no sign of fever with infection due to normally low body temperature (*Güneş & Zaybak, 2008).
- Most elderly people of age 80 and older do not show signs of shivering until their core temperature drops to 95.3° F (35.1° C) (*Güneş & Zaybak, 2008).

Focus Assessment Criteria

Subjective Data

Assess for Defining Characteristics

History and onset of symptoms (abnormal skin temperature, altered mentation, headaches, nausea, lethargy, vertigo)

Assess for Related Factors

Hyperthermia
Dehydration
Recent exposure to communicable disease without known immunity (e.g., measles without vaccine or previous illness)
Recent overexposure to or overactivity in sun, heat, humidity
Radiation/chemotherapy/immunosuppression
Caffeine
Impaired judgment
Home environment

Adequate ventilation?
Automobile environment?
Air conditioning?
Room temperature?

Medications
Diuretics
Antidepressants
Anticholinergics
Beta-blockers, angiotensin-converting enzyme inhibitors
Vasoconstrictors
How often taken?
Last dose taken when?

Hypothermia
Recent exposure to cold/dampness
Inactivity
Apathy
Impaired judgment
Slurred speech
Arrhythmias
Vasodilators
CNS depressants
Home environment
Heating, blankets
Clothing (e.g., socks, hat, gloves)
Shelter

Objective Data

Assess for Defining Characteristics

Vital Signs
Temperature <97.0°, >99.5°
Abnormal vital signs
Change in mental status
Malaise/fatigue/weakness
Skin: cool, pallor*, piloerection*
Shivering*
Slow capillary
Signs of dehydration: parched mouth/furrowed tongue/dry lips
Increased urine specific gravity

Goals

NOC
Thermoregulation, Hydration, Risk Detection

The individual will demonstrate a temperature within normal limits (WNL) for age evidenced by the following indicators:

- Reports measures to prevent temperature fluctuations
- Reports episodes of chills, diaphoresis, shivering, cool skin

Interventions

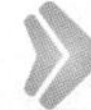

Carp's Cues

Hypothermia and heat-related illness are serious events for older adults (Miller, 2015).

Noe, Jin, and Wolken (2012) reported that hyperthermia-related hospital visits (n = 10,007) were more frequent than hypothermia-related visits (n=8,761) for years 2004 and 2005. In comparison, hypothermia-related visits resulted in more deaths (359 vs. 42), higher mortality rates (0.50/100,000 vs. 0.06/100,000), higher inpatient rates (5.29/100,000 vs. 1.76/100,000), longer hospital stays (median days=4 vs. 2), and higher total health care costs ($98 million vs. $36 million). It is unfortunate that most, if not all, of these events could have been prevented.

NIC
Temperature Regulation, Temperature Regulation: Intraoperative, Environmental Management

- Monitor temperature as needed (1 to 4 hours). Use continuous temperature monitoring for vulnerable individuals (e.g., critically ill adults, neonates, infants).

R: *Continuous temperature monitoring will provide early detection of temperature changes to prevent cardiovascular complications (*Smith, 2004).*

- Use oral thermometers if possible.

R: *The oral route is more reliable than tympanic or axillary.*

- Maintain consistent room temperature of 72° F (22.2° C). Avoid drafts.

R: *This temperature will prevent heat loss through radiation.*

- During bathing, expose only small sections of the body. After washing, cover the area with absorbent blanket.

R: *These interventions will reduce heat loss from evaporation.*

- Ensure that optimal nutrition and hydration is achieved.

R: *Dehydration can decrease body temperature by reducing fluid volume. Increased calories are needed to maintain metabolic functioning during fever (*Edwards, 1999).*

R: *Although using a mercury thermometer under the tongue remains the most popular way to check body temperature, a rectal temperature is considered the most accurate for obtaining a core temperature (*Moran & Mendal, 2002).*

- Refer to *Ineffective Thermoregulation* for interventions for newborns.
- Refer to *Hypothermia* or *Hyperthermia* for interventions to prevent body temperature disruptions.

Hyperthermia

NANDA-I Definition

Body temperature elevated above normal range

Defining Characteristics

Major (Must Be Present)

Temperature higher than 100° F (37.8° C) orally or 101° F (38.8° C) rectally

Minor (May Be Present)

Flushed skin*
Tachycardia*
Tachypnea*
Shivering/goose pimples
Warm to touch*
Malaise/fatigue/weakness
Loss of appetite
Specific or generalized aches and pains (e.g., headache)

Related Factors

Treatment Related

Related to decreased ability to perspire* secondary to (specify)

Situational (Personal, Environmental)

Related to:

Exposure to hot environment*
Inappropriate clothing* for climate
No access to air conditioning
Newborn hospital environment warming equipment

Related to decreased circulation secondary to:

Extremes of weight
Dehydration*

Related to insufficient hydration for vigorous activity*

Maturational

Related to ineffective temperature regulation secondary to age (refer to **Ineffective Thermoregulation*****)***

Author's Note

The nursing diagnoses *Hypothermia* and *Hyperthermia* represent the condition in people with temperature below and above normal, respectively. Some of these states are treatable by nursing interventions, such as correcting external causes (e.g., inappropriate clothing, exposure to elements [heat or cold], and dehydration). Nursing care centers on preventing or treating mild hypothermia and hyperthermia. As life-threatening situations that require medical and nursing interventions, severe hypothermia and hyperthermia represent collaborative problems and should be labeled *Risk for Complications of Hypothermia* or *Risk for Complications of Hyperthermia.*

Temperature elevation from infections, other disorders (e.g., hypothalamic), or treatments (e.g., hypothermia units) requires collaborative treatment. If desired, the nurse could use the nursing diagnosis *Impaired Comfort* and the collaborative problem *Risk for Complications of Hypothermia* or *Risk for Complications of Hyperthermia*.

Errors in Diagnostic Statements

***Hyperthermia* related to intraoperative pharmacogenetic hypermetabolism**

This situation describes malignant hyperthermia, a life-threatening, inherited disorder resulting in a hypermetabolic state related to the use of anesthetic agents and depolarizing muscle relaxants. *Risk for Complications of Malignant Hypertension* would more appropriately describe this situation, which necessitates rapid detection and treatment by both nursing and medicine.

***Hyperthermia* related to effect of circulating endotoxins on hypothalamus secondary to sepsis**

Nursing for people with elevated temperature in acute care focuses on monitoring and managing the fever with nursing and physician orders or promoting comfort through nursing orders. *Impaired Comfort* would more appropriately describe a situation that nurses treat, with *Risk for Complications of Sepsis* representing the physiologic complication that nurses monitor for and manage with nurse-prescribed and physician-prescribed interventions.

Focus Assessment Criteria

See *Risk for Imbalanced Body Temperature.*

Goals

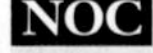

Thermoregulation, Hydration, Risk Detection

The individual will maintain body temperature as evidenced by the following indicators:

- Identifies risk factors for hyperthermia
- Reduces risk factors for hyperthermia

Interventions

Remove or Reduce Contributing Risk Factors Dehydration

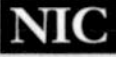

Fever Treatment, Temperature Regulation, Environmental Management, Fluid Management

- Monitor intake and output and provide favorite beverage. Teach the importance of maintaining adequate fluid intake (at least 2,000 mL a day of cool liquids unless contraindicated by heart or kidney disease).
- Explain the importance of not relying on thirst sensation as an indication of the need for fluid.
- Monitor amount and color of urine.

R: *A good indicator of hydration is to drink enough fluid so that the body does not feel physically thirsty and so that it produces regular, light-colored urine.*

- Recommended fluid replacement for moderate activities in hot weather (*DeFabio, 2000) is as follows:
  - 78° F to 84.9° F (25.6° C to 29.4° C) 16 oz/hr
  - 85° F to 89.9° F (29.4° C to 32.2° C) 24 oz/hr
  - Greater than 90° F (32.2° C) 32 oz/hr

See also *Deficient Fluid Volume*.

R: *Strategies are used to maintain balance between intake and output.*

Environmental Warmth/Exercise

- Instruct to assess whether clothing or bedcovers are too warm for the environment or planned activity.
- Remove excess clothing or blankets (remove hat, gloves, or socks, as appropriate) to promote heat loss. Encourage wearing loose cotton clothing.

R: *Adding clothes or blankets inhibits the body's natural ability to reduce body temperature; removing clothes or blankets enhances the body's natural ability to reduce body temperature.*

R: *Exposure of the head, face, hands, and feet can affect body temperature greatly. Heat is conducted from the blood vessels of these vascular areas to the skin and from the skin to the air. Cold is conducted from the air to the skin and from the skin to the blood vessels.*

- Provide air conditioning, dehumidifiers, fans, or cool baths or compresses as appropriate.
- Explain factors that increase the risk of hypo/hyperthermia in older adults (Miller, 2015):
  - Medical conditions (hyperthyroidism, cardiovascular disease, electrolyte imbalances, Parkinson's disease)
  - Medications (diuretics, anticholinergics, beta-blockers, angiotensin-converting enzyme inhibitors, selective serotonin reuptake inhibitors antidepressants, proton pump inhibitors)
  - Excess alcohol intake
  - Personal (older than 75), extreme climate-temperature variation, substandard living conditions (no air conditioning, poor ventilation)

Initiate Health Teaching as Indicated

- Instruct on precautions to take when engaging in activities outside in hot weather to prevent dehydration and heat stroke.

R: *It is recommended that men consume around 13 cups of total fluids a day and women consume about 9 cups, which includes water from other beverages as well as high-water containing foods. A good indicator of hydration is to drink enough fluid so that the body does not feel physically thirsty and so that it produces regular, light-colored urine.*

- To replace lost fluids during outdoor activity
  - Drink 8 oz of water prior to going out in heat.
  - Drink cool, not cold water, as cool water is more readily absorbed.
  - Avoid caffeinated, protein, and alcoholic drinks (e.g., colored soda, coffee, tea).
  - Drink 4 to 8 oz every 30 minutes to 1 hour depending on heat index.
  - Do not wait to be thirsty to drink water.
  - Avoid sports drinks unless exercising over 1 hour in hot weather and sweating a lot.

R: *During hot weather activities/exercising, dehydration occurs more frequently and has more severe consequences. Drink early and at regular intervals. The perception of thirst is a poor index of the magnitude of fluid deficit.*

- Consider the following:
  - Avoid the midday sun by exercising before 10 AM or after 6 PM, if possible.
  - Use a sunscreen with a rating of SPF-15 or lower depending on skin type. Ratings above SPF-15 can interfere with the skin's thermal regulation.
  - Wear light-weight and breathable clothing.
  - If you experience weakness, headache, dizziness muscle cramps, nausea, or vomiting
    - Stop and get out of heat.
    - Drink water, wet your skin.
    - Call 911 if you are feeling faint, weak, or confused or have someone take you for medical care.

R: *Severe heat stroke is a medical emergency and can result in death if untreated.*

- Teach the early signs of hyperthermia or heat stroke:
  - Flushed skin
  - Fatigue
  - Headache/confusion
  - Loss of appetite
  - Nausea/vomiting
  - Muscle cramps

Hypothermia

NANDA-I Definition

Body temperature below normal range

Defining Characteristics[3]

Body temperature below normal range*
Cool skin*
Piloerection*
Shivering*

Hypertension*
Pallor*
Slow capillary refill*
Tachycardia*

Related Factors

Situational (Personal, Environmental)

Related to:

Exposure to cool environment* (e.g., surgical suite)
Evaporation from skin in cool environment* (e.g., during bathing, surgery)
Inappropriate clothing*
Inability to pay for shelter or heat
Malnutrition*

Related to decreased circulation secondary to:

Extremes of weight
Consumption of alcohol*
Dehydration
Inactivity*

Maturational

Related to ineffective temperature regulation secondary to age (e.g., neonate, older adult)

Author's Note

Because more serious hypothermia (temperatures below 95° F or 35° C rectally) can cause severe pathophysiologic consequences, such as decreased myocardial and respiratory function, the nurse must report low readings to the physician. This is a collaborative problem: *Risk for Complications of Hypothermia*. Nurses most often initiate nurse-prescribed interventions for mild hypothermia (temperatures between 95° F [35° C] and 97° F [36° C] rectally) to prevent more serious hypothermia. Nurses are commonly responsible for identifying and preventing *Risk for Hypothermia*. See also *Risk for Imbalanced Body Temperature*.

Errors in Diagnostic Statements

See *Risk for Imbalanced Body Temperature* and *Hyperthermia*.

Focus Assessment Criteria

See *Risk for Imbalanced Body Temperature*.

Goals

NOC

Thermoregulation, Hydration, Risk Detection

The individual will maintain body temperature WNL evidenced by the following indicators:

- Identifies risk factors for hypothermia
- Reduces risk factors for hypothermia

Interventions

NIC

Hypothermia Treatment, Temperature Regulation, Temperature Regulation: Intraoperative, Environmental Management

Assess for Risk Factors

- Refer to Related Factors.

Reduce or Eliminate Causative or Contributing Factors, If Possible

Prolonged Exposure to Cold Environment

- Assess room temperatures at home.
- Teach to keep room temperatures at 70° F to 75° F (21.1° C to 23.9° C) or to layer clothing.

[3]Adapted from Carroll, S. M. (1989). Nursing diagnosis: Hypothermia. In R. M. Carroll-Johnson (Ed.), *Classification of nursing diagnosis: Proceedings of the eighth conference*. Philadelphia: J. B. Lippincott.

- Explain the importance of wearing a hat, gloves, warm socks, and shoes to prevent heat loss.
- Discourage going outside when temperatures are very cold.
- Acquire an electric blanket, warm blankets, or down comforter and flannel sheets for the bed.
- Teach to wear close-knit undergarments to prevent heat loss.
- Explain that more clothes may be needed in the morning, when body metabolism is lowest.

R: *Individuals can rewarm themselves even when extremely hypothermic (*Nicoll, 2002).*

- Consult with social services to identify the sources of financial assistance, warm clothing, blankets, and shelter.
- Teach the importance of preventing heat loss before body temperature is actually lowered (e.g., warm socks, sweaters, gloves, and hats).

R: *Minimizing evaporation, convection, conduction, and radiation can prevent significant heat losses.*

Neurovascular/Peripheral Vascular Disease

- Keep room temperature at 70° F to 74° F (21.1° C to 23.3° C).
- Assess for adequate circulation to the extremities (i.e., satisfactory peripheral pulses).
- Instruct the individual to wear warm gloves and socks to reduce heat loss.
- Teach the individual to take a warm bath if he or she cannot get warm.

R: *Decreased circulation causes cold extremities.*

Initiate Health Teaching If Indicated

- Teach the signs of hypothermia (National Institutes of Health, 2010):
  - Early
    - Cool skin
    - Pallor
    - Blanching
    - Redness
    - Slurred speech
    - Confusion (*Nicoll, 2002)
  - Later
    - Confusion or sleepiness
    - Slowed, slurred speech, or shallow breathing
    - Weak pulse
    - Change in behavior or in the way a person looks
    - Severe shivering or no shivering; stiffness in the arms or legs
    - Poor control over body movements or slow reactions
- Explain the need to drink 8 to 10 glasses of water daily unless instructed to limit fluid intake and to consume frequent, small meals with warm liquids.
- Explain the need to avoid alcohol during periods of very cold weather.

R: *Early detection of hypothermia can prevent tissue damage.*

- For additional information on preventing hypothermia, refer older adults and their family to www.nia.nih.gov/health/publication/hypothermia#signs
- Low-income home energy assistance program, National Energy Assistance Referral Hotline (NEAR), 1-866-674-6327 (toll-free), www.acf.hhs.gov/programs/ocs/liheap

Pediatric and Geriatric Interventions

For Extremes of Age (Newborns, Older Adults)

- Maintain room temperature at 70° F to 74° F (21.1° C to 23.3° C).
- Instruct the adult individual to wear hat, gloves, and socks if necessary to prevent heat loss.
- Explain to family members that newborns, infants, and older adults are more susceptible to heat loss (see also *Ineffective Thermoregulation*).

R: *Older adults can become hypothermic or hyperthermic in moderately cold or hot environments, compared with younger adults, who require exposure to extreme cold or heat (Miller, 2015).*

R: *Infants are vulnerable to heat loss because of large body surface area relative to body mass, increased basal metabolic rate, and less adipose tissue for insulation (Pillitteri, 2014).*

Ineffective Thermoregulation

NANDA-I Definition

Temperature fluctuation between hypothermia and hyperthermia

Defining Characteristics

Refer to Defining Characteristics for *Hypothermia* and *Hyperthermia*

Related Factors

Situational (Personal, Environmental)

Related to:
Fluctuating environmental temperatures
Cold or wet articles (clothes, cribs, equipment)
Inadequate housing
Wet body surface
Inadequate clothing for weather (excessive, insufficient)

Maturational

Related to limited metabolic compensatory regulation secondary to age (e.g., neonate, older adult)

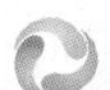

Author's Note

Ineffective Thermoregulation is a useful diagnosis for people with difficulty maintaining a stable core body temperature over a span of environmental temperatures. This diagnosis most commonly applies to older adults and newborns. Thermoregulation involves balancing heat production and heat loss. Nursing care focuses on manipulating external factors (e.g., clothing and environmental conditions) to maintain body temperature WNL and on teaching prevention strategies.

Errors in Diagnostic Statements

Ineffective Thermoregulation **related to effects of a hypothalamic tumor**

Hypothalamic tumors can affect the temperature-regulating centers, resulting in body temperature shifts. This situation requires constant surveillance and rapid response to changes with appropriate nursing and medical treatments. Thus, this situation would be better described as a collaborative problem: *Risk for Complications of Hypo/Hyperthermia*.

Ineffective Thermoregulation **related to temperature fluctuations**

Temperature fluctuations represent a manifestation of the diagnosis, not a related factor. If the fluctuations result from age-related limited compensatory regulation, the diagnosis would be written as *Ineffective Thermoregulation related to decreased ability to acclimatize to heat or cold secondary to age*, as evidenced by temperature fluctuations.

Focus Assessment Criteria

Objective Data

Assess for Defining Characteristics

Skin
Color
Temperature
Nailbeds
Rashes

Temperature
Environment (home, infant [ambient, radiant warmer; Isolette])
Body (adult, child [rectal, oral], newborn [axillary])

Respiration
Rate
Any retractions
Rhythm
Breath sounds
Heart rate

Ineffective Thermoregulation • Related to Newborn Transition to Extrauterine Environment

Goals

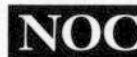

NOC

Thermoregulation, Hydration, Risk Detection

- The infant will have a temperature between 97.5° F and 98.6° F (36.4° C and 37° C).
- The parent will explain techniques to avoid heat loss at home.

Indicators

- List situations that increase heat loss.
- Demonstrate how to conserve heat during bathing.
- Demonstrate how to take an infant's temperature.
- State appropriate newborn attire for various outdoor and indoor climates.

Interventions

NIC

Temperature Regulation, Environmental Management, Newborn Monitoring, Vital Sign Monitoring

Assess for Contributing Factors

- Environmental sources of heat loss
- Lack of knowledge (caregivers, parents)

Reduce or Eliminate Sources of Heat Loss

- Evaporation (loss of heat when water on skin changes to vapor)
    - In the delivery room, quickly dry skin and hair with a heated towel and place infant in a prewarmed heated environment.
    - When bathing, provide a warm environment or bath under heat source.
    - Wash and dry the infant in sections to reduce evaporation.
    - Limit time in contact with wet diapers or blankets.
- Convection (loss of heat when cool air flows over skin)
    - Reduce drafts in the delivery room.
    - Place the sides of the radiant warmer bed up at all times.
    - Use only portholes for infant access in the Isolette whenever possible.
    - Avoid drafts on the infant (air conditioning, fans, windows, open portholes on Isolette).
- Conduction (transfer of heat when skin surface is in direct contact with a cool surface)
    - Warm all articles for care (stethoscopes, scales, hands of caregivers, clothes, bed linens, cribs).
    - Place the infant very close to the mother to conserve heat (and foster bonding).
    - Warm or cover any equipment that may come in contact with the infant's skin.
- Radiation (transfer of heat between the skin and the environment)
    - Place the infant next to the mother in the delivery room.
    - Reduce objects in the room that absorb heat (metal).
    - Place the crib or Isolette as far away from walls (outside) or windows as possible.
    - Preheat incubator.

R: *The newborn loses heat through evaporation, convection, radiation, and conduction (Hockenberry & Wilson, 2015).*

R: *Newborns have a larger body surface to body weight ratio when compared to that of an adult; therefore, they may lose more heat (Pillitteri, 2014).*

Monitor Temperature of Newborn to Maintain Axillary Temperature at 97.8° F (36.5° C)

- Assess axillary temperature initially every 30 minutes until stable, then every 4 to 8 hours.

R: *Axillary temperatures should be measured for 5 minutes. In infants and children the axillary route is preferred. Rectal thermometers should be avoided in newborns because of the risk of damaging rectal mucosa (Pillitteri, 2014).*

- If temperature is less than 97.3° F (36.3° C)
  - Wrap infant in two blankets.
  - Put stockinette cap on.
  - Assess for environmental sources of heat loss.
  - Notify a physician (if hypothermia persists over 1 hour).
  - Assess for complications of cold stress: hypoxia, respiratory acidosis, hypoglycemia, fluid and electrolyte imbalances, and weight loss.

R: *Significant heat losses the first few moments after birth can drop the newborn's temperature. Drying, heated blankets, and swaddling can reduce these losses (*Varda & Behnke, 2000).*

R: *Premature or low–birth-weight infants are more susceptible to heat loss because of the reduced metabolic reserves available (e.g., glycogen), increased brown adipose tissue, increased total body water, and thin skin.*

- If temperature is greater than 98.6° F (37° C)
  - Loosen blanket.
  - Remove cap, if on.
  - Assess environment for thermal gain.
  - Notify a physician (if hyperthermia persists over 1 hour).

R: *Exposure of the head, face, hands, and feet can affect body temperature greatly. Heat is conducted from blood vessels of these vascular areas to the skin and from the skin to the air. Cold is conducted from the air to the skin and from the skin to the blood vessels.*

Initiate Health Teaching

- Teach caregiver why infant is vulnerable to temperature fluctuations (cold and heat).
- Explain the sources of environmental heat loss.
- Demonstrate how to reduce heat loss during bathing.
- Instruct that it is not necessary to check the infant's temperature at home routinely.

R: *Parents are taught to prevent heat loss via evaporation, convection, conduction, and radiation during infant care and in home environment (Hockenberry & Wilson, 2015).*

- Teach to check temperature if infant is hot, sick, or irritable. Use axillary or skin route. Never use a rectal thermometer.

R: *Tympanic devices are not effective in newborns due to the presence of vernix in ears. Rectal thermometers should be avoided in newborns because of the risk of damaging fragile rectal mucosa (Pillitteri, 2014).*

BOWEL INCONTINENCE

NANDA-I Definition

Change in normal bowel habits characterized by involuntary passage of stool

Defining Characteristics*

Constant dribbling of soft stool
Fecal odor
Fecal staining of bedding
Fecal staining of clothing
Inability to delay defecation
Urgency

Inability to recognize urge to defecate
Inattention to urge to defecate
Recognizes rectal fullness but reports inability to expel formed stool
Red perianal skin
Self-report of inability to recognize rectal fullness

Related Factors

Pathophysiologic

Related to rectal sphincter abnormality secondary to:

Anal or rectal surgery
Anal or rectal injury
Obstetric injuries
Peripheral neuropathy

Related to overdistention of rectum secondary to chronic constipation

Related to loss of rectal sphincter control* secondary to:

Progressive neuromuscular disorder
Spinal cord compression
Cerebral vascular accident
Spinal cord injury
Multiple sclerosis

Related to impaired reservoir capacity* secondary to:

Inflammatory bowel disease
Chronic rectal ischemia

Treatment Related

Related to impaired reservoir capacity* secondary to:

Colectomy
Radiation proctitis

Situational (Personal, Environmental)

Related to inability to recognize, interpret, or respond to rectal cues secondary to:

Depression
Impaired cognition*

Errors in Diagnostic Statements

Bowel Incontinence related to oozing of stool

Oozing of stool does not cause bowel incontinence; rather, it is evident that an individual may be bowel incontinent. If the etiology is unknown, the diagnosis should be written as *Bowel Incontinence related to unknown etiology*, as evidenced by oozing of stool. When the etiology is known, the diagnosis should reflect this (e.g., *Bowel Incontinence related to relaxed anal sphincter secondary to S4 lesion as evidenced by oozing of stool*).

Key Concepts

General Considerations

- The incidence of fecal incontinence is reported as 36.2% in individuals aged 65 and older (Markland & Tobin, 2010).
- Bowel incontinence has three major causes: underlying disease of the colon, rectum, or anus; long-standing constipation or fecal impaction; and neurogenic rectal changes.

- Complete spinal cord injury, spinal cord lesions, neurologic disease, or congenital defects that interrupt the sacral reflex arc (at the sacral segments S2, S3, S4) result in an areflexic (autonomous) or flaccid bowel. Flaccid paralysis at this level, known as an LMN lesion, results in loss of the defecation reflex, loss of sphincter control (flaccid anal sphincter), and no bulbocavernosus reflex.
- Because of an interrupted sacral reflex arc and a flaccid anal sphincter, bowel incontinence can occur without rectal stimulation whenever stool is in the rectal vault. The stool may leak out if it is too soft or remain (if not extracted), predisposing the individual to fecal impaction or constipation. Some intrinsic contractile abilities of the colon remain, but peristalsis is sluggish, leading to stool retention with contents in the rectal vault.
- Complete CNS lesions or trauma above sacral cord segments S2, S3, S4 (T12–L1–L2 vertebral level) results in an areflexic neurogenic bowel. They interrupt the ascending sensory signals between the sacral reflex center and the brain, resulting in the inability to feel the urge to defecate. They also interrupt descending motor signals from the brain, causing loss of voluntary control over the anal sphincter. Because the sacral reflex center is preserved, it is possible to develop a stimulation–response bowel evacuation program using digital stimulation or digital stimulation devices.

Geriatric Considerations

- Age-related changes in the large intestines include reduced mucus production, decreased elasticity of the rectal wall, and diminished perception of rectal wall distention (Miller, 2015).
- These age-related changes require a larger rectal volume to perceive the urge to defecate and may predispose the individual to constipation (Miller, 2015).

Focus Assessment Criteria

See *Constipation*.

Goals

NOC

Bowel Continence, Tissue Integrity Bowel Elimination

The individual will evacuate a soft, formed stool every other day or every third day:

- Relates bowel elimination techniques
- Describes fluid and dietary requirements

Interventions

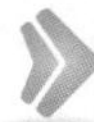

Carp's Cues

The diagnosis of fecal incontinence (FI) must be differentiated from diarrhea. Individuals with FI may inaccurately report diarrhea as the presenting problem. Conversely, diarrhea can be mislabeled as primary FI. Many of the causes of acute and chronic diarrhea in the older adult are treatable as adverse effects of medications, tube feedings, lactose intolerance, celiac disease, microscopic colitis, ischemic colitis, radiation proctitis, hypersecretory tumors, and diabetic diarrhea (Shah, Chokhavatia, & Rose, 2012).

NIC

Bowel Incontinence Care, Bowel Training, Bowel Management, Self-Care Assistance: Toileting Skin Surveillance

Assess Contributing Factors

- Refer to Related Factors.

Assess the Individual's Ability to Participate in Bowel Continence

- Ability to reach toilet
- Control of rectal sphincter
- Intact anorectal sensation
- Orientation, motivation

R: *To maintain bowel continence, an individual must have access to a toileting facility, be able to contract puborectalis and external anal sphincter muscles, have intact anorectal sensation, be able to store feces consciously, and must be motivated.*

R: *Cognitive impairments can impede recognition of bowel cues. Another cause of bowel incontinence is rectal sphincter abnormalities.*

Plan a Consistent, Appropriate Time for Elimination

- Institute a daily bowel program for 5 days or until a pattern develops, then move to an alternate-day program (morning or evening).
- Provide privacy and a nonstressful environment.
- Offer reassurance and protect from embarrassment while establishing the bowel program.

R: *Long-standing constipation or fecal impaction causes overdistention of the rectum by feces. This causes continuous reflex stimulation which reduces sphincter tone. Incontinence will be either diarrhea leaking around the impaction or leaking of feces from a full rectum.*

- Implement prompted voiding program.

R: *Research has shown prompted voiding results in an increase in bowel continence (*Demata, 2000).*

Teach Effective Bowel Elimination Techniques

- Position a functionally able individual upright or sitting. If he or she is not functionally able (e.g., quadriplegic), place the individual in left side-lying position.

R: *Techniques that facilitate gravity and increase intra-abdominal pressure to pass stool enhance bowel elimination.*

- For a functionally able individual, use assistive devices (e.g., dil stick, digital stimulator, raised commode seat, lubricant, gloves) as appropriate.

R: *Digital stimulation results in reflex peristalsis and evacuation.*

- For an individual with impaired upper extremity mobility and decreased abdominal muscle function, teach bowel elimination facilitation techniques as appropriate:
  - Abdominal massage
  - Forward bends
  - Pelvic floor exercises
  - Sitting push-ups
  - Valsalva maneuver

R: *These techniques increase intra-abdominal pressure to aid in stool evacuation. Pelvic floor exercises can increase the strength of the puborectalis and external anal sphincter muscles.*

- Maintain an elimination record or a flow sheet of the bowel schedule that includes time, stool characteristics, assistive methods used, and number of involuntary stools, if any.

R: *This record will assist in planning an individualized bowel schedule.*

Explain Fluid and Dietary Recommendations to Decrease FI (Shah et al., 2012)

- Avoid artificial sugars and caffeine.

R: *Intake of these substances can decrease colonic transit time, leading to FI.*

- Evaluate the effects of fatty foods on FI.

R: *FI is triggered by fatty foods in some individuals.*

- Add more fiber to diet.

R: *Psyllium fiber can improve stool consistencies and decrease the number of incontinent stools. Stool consistency and volume are important for continence. Large volumes of loose stool overwhelm the continence mechanism. Small, hard stools that do not distend or stimulate the rectum do not alert the individual of the need to defecate (*Bliss, Savik, Jung, Whitebird, & Lowry, 2011).*

Explain Effects of Activity on Peristalsis

- Assist in determining the appropriate exercises for the individual's functional ability.

R: *Exercise increases gastrointestinal motility and improves bowel function.*

Initiate Health Teaching, as Indicated

- Explain the effects of stool on the skin and ways to protect the skin. Refer to *Diarrhea* for interventions.
- Explain the hazards of using stool softeners, laxatives, suppositories, and enemas.

R: *Laxatives cause unscheduled bowel movements, loss of colon tone, and inconsistent stool consistency. Enemas can overstretch the bowel and decrease tone. Stool softeners are not needed with adequate food or fluid intake.*

- Explain the signs and symptoms of fecal impaction and constipation. Refer to *Dysreflexia* for additional information.
- Initiate teaching of a bowel program before discharge. If the individual is functionally able, encourage independence with the bowel program; if not, incorporate assistive devices or attendant care, as needed.

INEFFECTIVE BREASTFEEDING

NANDA-I Definition

Dissatisfaction or difficulty a mother, infant, or child experiences with the breastfeeding process

Defining Characteristics

Unsatisfactory breastfeeding process*
Perceived inadequate milk supply*
Infant inability to latch on to maternal breast correctly*
Observable signs of inadequate infant intake*; poor weight gain, voids, or stools
No observable signs of oxytocin release*
Nonsustained or insufficient opportunity for suckling at the breast*
Persistence of sore nipples beyond the first week of breastfeeding
Infant exhibiting fussiness and/or crying within the first hour after breastfeeding*, unresponsive to other comfort measures*
Infant arching or crying at the breast, resisting latching on*

Related Factors (Evans, Marinelli, Taylor, & The Academy of Breastfeeding Medicine, 2014)

Physiologic

Related to difficulty of neonate to attach or suck* secondary to:

Poor infant sucking reflex*
Prematurity*, late preterm
Low birth weight
Sleepy infant
Oral anatomic abnormality (cleft lip/palate, tight frenulum, microglossia)
Infant medical problem (hypoglycemia, jaundice, infection, respiratory distress)
Previous breast surgery*
Flat, inverted, or very large nipples
Extremely or previously sore nipples
Previous breast abscess
Inadequate let-down reflex
Lack of noticeable breast enlargement during puberty or pregnancy

Situational (Personal, Environmental)

Related to maternal fatigue

Related to peripartum complication

Related to maternal anxiety*

Related to maternal ambivalence*

Related to multiple birth

Related to inadequate nutrition intake

Related to inadequate fluid intake

Related to previous history of unsuccessful breastfeeding*

Related to nonsupportive partner/family*

Related to knowledge deficit*

Related to interruption in breastfeeding* secondary to ill mother, ill infant

Related to work schedule and/or barriers in the work environment

Related to infant receiving supplemental feedings with artificial nipple*

Related to maternal medications

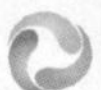

Author's Note

In managing breastfeeding, nurses strive to reduce or eliminate factors that contribute to *Ineffective Breastfeeding* or factors that can increase vulnerability for a problem using the diagnosis *Risk for Ineffective Breastfeeding.*

In the acute setting after delivery, little time will have elapsed for the nurse to conclude that there is no problem in breastfeeding, unless the mother is experienced. For many mother–infant dyads, *Risk for Ineffective Breastfeeding related to inexperience with the breastfeeding process* would represent a nursing focus on preventing problems in breastfeeding. *Risk* would not be indicated for all mothers.

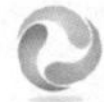

Errors in Diagnostic Statements

Ineffective Breastfeeding **related to reports of no symptoms of let-down reflex**

When a mother reports or the nurse observes no signs of let-down reflex, *Ineffective Breastfeeding* is validated. If contributing factors are unknown, the diagnosis could be written as *Ineffective Breastfeeding related to unknown etiology*, as evidenced by reports of no symptoms of let-down reflex and mother's anxiety regarding feeding.

If the nurse has validated contributing factors, he or she can add them. The nurse should assess for various possible contributing factors, rather than prematurely focusing on a common etiology that may be incorrect for the specific situation.

Key Concepts (American Academy of Pediatrics [AAP], 2012; AWHONN, 2015; Hale, 2012; Walker, 2013)

General Considerations

- Lactation results from complex interactions among the mother's health and nutrition status, the infant's health status, and breast tissue development under the influence of estrogen and progesterone.
- Prolactin and oxytocin are pituitary hormones that control milk production and are stimulated by infant sucking and maternal emotions.
- Many medications are excreted in breast milk. Some are harmful to the infant. Advise the mother to consult with a health care professional (nurse, physician, or pharmacist) before taking any medication (prescribed or over-the-counter).
- The benefits for the infant of receiving breast milk are as follows:
    - Easier to digest, less constipation
    - Meets nutritional needs
    - Reduces allergies and asthma
    - Provides antibodies and macrophages for early immunization
    - Reduces risk for gastrointestinal diseases (celiac disease, inflammatory bowel disease)
    - Improves tooth alignment
    - Reduces childhood respiratory and ear infections throughout childhood if nursing continues for 1 year
    - Up to a 30% reduction in the incidence of type 1 diabetes mellitus and a 40% reduction in type 2 diabetes mellitus in infants who exclusively breastfed for at least 3 months
    - Reduces incidence of sudden infant death syndrome
    - Decreases incidence of necrotizing enterocolitis in preterm infants in NICU
    - Improves neurodevelopmental outcomes in preterm infants
    - Gives bowel movements a pleasant odor
    - Does not smell sour or stain clothing in vomitus

- The benefits of breastfeeding for the mother are as follows:
  - Decreases postpartum blood loss and more rapid uterine involution
  - Allows more time to rest during feedings
  - Requires less preparation and decreased costs
  - Promotes faster bonding
  - Quickens postpartum weight loss
  - Reduces risks for breast, ovarian, and uterine cancers
  - May decrease occurrence of osteoporosis and rheumatoid arthritis
  - Reduces hypertension, hyperlipidemia, cardiovascular disease, and diabetes in women with a cumulative lactation history of 12 to 23 months
- The disadvantage of breastfeeding is an alternate person cannot substitute for the mother.
- Breastfeeding is a learned process for the mother and the baby. It requires about 4 to 6 weeks of commitment to adjust to and learn the skills of breastfeeding and for the milk to thoroughly regulate to the baby's needs.
- Breast milk is nearly completely digested; therefore, intestinal emptying is faster, and the newborn may need to feed more often than with formula.

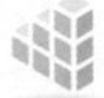

Pediatric Considerations

Physical and psychosocial pressure influence an adolescent's eating habits, which may put the teenage mother and her infant at risk during the breastfeeding period.

Focus Assessment Criteria (AAP, 2012; AWHONN, 2015; BFAR, 2010; Evans et al., 2014; Riordian & Wombach, 2009)

Subjective Data

Assess for Related Factors

History of breastfeeding (self, sibling, friend)
Supportive people (partner, friend, sibling, parent)
Daily intake of infant and mother
Calories—400 to 500 extra per day
Basic food groups—be aware that high consumption of dairy by the mother may contribute to fussiness, diarrhea, bloody stools, or rash.
Calcium
Fluids
Vitamin supplements—the mother should continue taking prenatal vitamins during breastfeeding. Consult physician and/or pharmacist.
History of breast surgery—length of time between reduction and breastfeeding may allow recanalization of milk ducts. The mother may not have full milk supply, so watch for voids and stools. A lactation consultant should follow up (AAP, 2009; BFAR, 2010).

Objective Data

Assess for Defining Characteristics

Breast condition (soft, firm, engorged)
Nipples (cracked, sore, inverted, dense nipple tissue is a barrier to feeding)
All are related to latch.

Goals

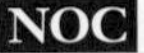

NOC
Breastfeeding Establishment: Infant, Breastfeeding Establishment: Maternal, Breastfeeding Management, Knowledge: Breastfeeding

The mother will report confidence in establishing satisfying, effective breastfeeding. The mother will demonstrate effective breastfeeding independently.

- Identify factors that deter breastfeeding.
- Identify factors that promote breastfeeding.
- Demonstrate effective positioning.

Infant shows signs of adequate intake, evidenced by the following indicators: Wet diapers, weight gain, relaxed, feeding.

Interventions (Amir & ABM, 2014; AZDHS, 2012; Evans et al., 2014; Lawrence & Lawrence, 2010)

Assess for Causative or Contributing Factors

- Lack of knowledge
- Lack of role model or support (partner, physician, family)
- Discomfort
- Engorgement
  - Milk leakage from engorgement or oversupply
- Nipple soreness
- Embarrassment
- Attitudes and misconceptions of mother
- Social pressure against breastfeeding
- Change in body image
- Change in sexuality
- Feelings of being tied down
- Stress
- Lack of conviction regarding decision to breastfeed
- Sleepy, unresponsive infant
- Infant with hyperbilirubinemia
- Fatigue
- Separation from infant (premature or sick infant, sick mother)
- Barriers in workplace

Promote Open Dialogue

- Assess knowledge
  - Has the woman taken a class in breastfeeding?
  - Has the woman attended a breastfeeding support group prior to delivery?
  - Has she read anything on the subject?
  - Does she have friends who are breastfeeding their babies?
  - Did her mother breastfeed?
- Explain myths and misconceptions. Ask the mother to list anticipated difficulties. Common myths include the following:
  - My breasts are too small.
  - My breasts are too large.
  - My mother couldn't breastfeed.
  - How do I know my milk is good?
  - How do I know the baby is getting enough?
  - The baby will know that I'm nervous.
  - I have to go back to work, so what's the point of breastfeeding for a short time?
  - I'll never have any freedom.
  - Breastfeeding will cause my breasts to sag.
  - My nipples are inverted, so I can't breastfeed.
  - My husband won't like my breasts anymore.
  - I'll have to stay fat if I breastfeed.
  - I can't breastfeed if I have a cesarean section.
  - You cannot get pregnant when breastfeeding.

R: *Listening to the mother's and the partner's concerns can help prioritize them.*

- Build on the mother's knowledge.
  - Clarify misconceptions.
  - Explain the process of breastfeeding.
  - Offer literature.
  - Show video.
  - Discuss advantages and disadvantages.
  - Bring breastfeeding mothers together to talk about breastfeeding and their concerns.
  - Discuss contraindications to breastfeeding.
- Support mother's decision to breastfeed or bottlefeed.

R: *Consistent positive feedback is essential for an inexperienced mother. The decision to breastfeed is very personal and should not be made without adequate information.*

Assist Mother During First Feedings

- Promote relaxation.
  - Position comfortably, using pillows (especially cesarean-section mothers). The use of breastfeeding support pillows will also promote comfort in bringing the infant up to her to feed.
  - Use a footstool or phone book to bring knees up while sitting.
  - Use relaxation breathing techniques. Encourage relaxing and opening/pulling shoulders back to promote oxygenation and blood flow to the breast tissue (physical therapy).

R: *Inadequate let-down reflex can result from a tense or nervous mother, pain, insufficient milk, engorgement, or inadequate sucking position or motions. Note that 20% of lactating women will not or may not feel the milk ejection reflex. Encourage all mothers to observe for swallowing in infants.*

- Demonstrate different positions and rooting reflex.
  - Sitting
  - Lying
  - Football hold
  - Skin-to-skin
- Instruct the mother to place a supporting hand on the baby's bottom and turn the body toward her (promotes security in infant).
- Show the mother how she can help the infant latch on. Tell her to look at where the infant's nose and chin are on her breast and to compress her breast with her thumb and middle finger behind these contact points.
- Skin-to-skin
  - Use of skin-to-skin contact for a minimum of 60 minutes per session one to two times a day has been shown to bring the mother's milk in an average of 18 hours faster.
  - Skin-to-skin contact allows infant vital signs to be regulated.
  - It allows for infant to be colonized by beneficial bacteria from mother.
  - Infants will cry less; breasts will warm or cool depending on needs of baby's body temperature.
  - Maintain skin-to-skin contact between attempts at the breast.
  - The more skin-to-skin contact in the first few days will help extend the breastfeeding experience.
- Show the mother how to grasp her breast with her fingers under the breast and her thumbs on the top; this way she can roll the nipple toward the roof of baby's mouth (avoid scissors hold, which constricts milk flow). This will aid in a deeper latch.
- Make sure the baby grasps a good portion of the areola, not just the nipple.
- Observe gliding action of the jaw, which indicates proper latch-on and suck.
- The infant should not be chewing or simply sucking with the lips.
- Listen for swallowing or observe the chin as it drops slightly during a swallow.
- Observe for bruising, creasing, or beveling of nipple tip after feeding.

R: *Successful breastfeeding is dependent on the ability of the infant to latch on.*

Promote Successful Breastfeeding

- Advise the mother to increase feeding times gradually.
  - Allow infant to finish the first breast before moving to the second.
  - Allow the infant unrestricted, unlimited access to the breast.
  - Average feeding time may be 5 to 45 minutes on each side (*Walker, 2006).
- Instruct the mother to offer both breasts at each feeding.
  - Alternate the beginning side each time.
  - Demonstrate how to support the infant's head at the nape of the neck to allow the chin to contact the underside of the areola, and allow the infant to latch with nose touching breast (explain that nose may touch breast). This will change the position of the nipple in the infant's mouth.
  - Demonstrate how the mother can place her finger in the infant's mouth to break the seal before removing from the breast.
  - Demonstrate ways to awaken the infant, which may be necessary before offering the second breast (e.g., change diaper, massage infant). Do not use a cold, wet wash cloth to wipe over the infant.
- Discuss burping.
  - Inform the mother that burping may be unnecessary with breastfed infants but to always attempt.
  - If the infant grunts and seems full between breasts, the mother should attempt to burp the infant, and then continue feeding.

R: *Successful breastfeeding depends on both physical and emotional support. Physical support includes promotion of comfort and proper technique.*

Provide Follow-Up Support During Hospital Stay

- During the hospital stay, develop a care plan so other health team members are aware of any problems or needs. Tell the mother to be flexible as the plan of care may change throughout the day and over the next few days and weeks as the infant's feeding behaviors change.
- Allow for flexibility of feeding schedule; avoid scheduling feedings. Strive for 10 to 12 feedings every 24 hours according to the infant's size and need (frequent feedings help prevent or reduce breast engorgement). Feeding on demand will aid in milk supply increasing. Allow the infant unlimited, unrestricted access to the breasts.
- Try not to use artificial nipples and pacifiers until breastfeeding is well established, usually about 3 to 4 weeks.
- Ensure that the mother has resources for breastfeeding assistance when leaving the hospital.
- Encourage exclusive breastfeeding and do not encourage the use of artificial baby milk unless medically indicated.
- Encourage latching the baby during the first hour after birth.
- Promote rooming-in.
- Allow for privacy during feedings.
- Be available for questions.
- Be positive even if the experience is difficult.
- Reassure the mother that this is a learning time for her and the infant. They will develop together as the days pass.
- Ice, heat, and massage prior to each feeding throughout the engorgement phase will help to reduce painful engorgement

R: *Mothers need continuous support to enhance the breastfeeding experience.*

Teach the Ways to Control Specific Nursing Problems (May Need Assistance of Lactation Consultant)

- Engorgement
  - Wear correct-fitting support brassiere day and night.
  - Apply ice compresses for 10 minutes, then warm compresses with firm massage for a few minutes before breastfeeding.
  - Nurse frequently (on demand).
  - Use hand expression, hand pump, or electric pump to tap off some of the tension before putting the infant to the breast.
  - Massage breasts and apply a warm washcloth before expression.
  - Encourage rooming-in and feeding on demand.

R: *The above strategies prevent breast tissue compression and encourage frequent and more complete emptying.*

- Sore nipples
  - Keep nipples warm and dry.
  - If nipple pain is too great, pumping breast milk for 24 to 36 hours instead of the infant breastfeeding may be needed to allow healing. Suggest alternate positions to rotate the infant's grasps. Allow the breasts to dry after each feeding.
  - Keep nursing pads dry.
  - Coat the nipples with breast milk (which has healing properties) and allow to air dry.
  - A lactation consultant should be seen prior to using nipple shields as improper use may result in a decrease in milk supply.
  - Explain that nipple soreness usually resolves within 7 to 10 days as long as the latch has been corrected.

R: *Nipple shields diminish milk supply and should not be recommended routinely. The newborn may develop a nipple shield preference. Nipple shields can cause damage if not used properly. The mother should observe for voids and stools, swallowing (an indicator of milk transfer), and milk in the tip of the shield.*

- Stasis, mastitis
  - If one area of the breast is sore or tender, apply moist heat before each breastfeeding session.
  - Gently massage the breast from the base toward the nipple before beginning to breastfeed and during feeding.
  - Breastfeed frequently and change the infant's position during feeding.
  - Rest frequently.
  - Monitor for signs and symptoms of mastitis: chills, body aches, fatigue, and fever above 100.4° F.

- Consult primary care provider if painful area accompanied by signs and symptoms of mastitis does not resolve within 24 to 48 hours. Observe for signs of abscess.

R: *Early self-management may prevent complications.*

- Difficulty with baby grasping nipple. Consult with a lactation specialist if indicated.
  - Cup the breast with the fingers underneath.
  - Position the baby for the mother's and infant's comfort (turn the baby's abdomen toward the mother's body).
  - Stroke the infant's lips gently with the nipple tip.
  - Hand-express some milk into the infant's mouth.
  - Roll nipples to bring them out before feeding. Use a nipple shell between feedings to help extend inverted nipples. Remove shield after let-down.
  - Assess the infant's suck—the baby may need assistance in the development of suck. Suck training may be needed.

R: *The infant at the breast must be in a relaxed, correct alignment (ear, shoulder, hip), have correct tongue and areolar placement, have sufficient motion for areolar compression, and demonstrate audible swallowing.*

Encourage Verbal Expression of Feelings Regarding Changes in Body

- Many women dislike leaking and lack of control. Explain that this is temporary.
- Demonstrate the use of a nursing pad. To prevent irritation from the use of a disposable pad, the individual should not use the waterproof backing; cotton (washable) pads seem to reduce irritation. Must keep nipples clean, cool, and dry.
- Breasts change from "sexual objects" to "implements of nutrition," which can affect the sexual relationship. Sexual partners will get milk if they suck on the woman's nipples, and orgasm releases milk. Infant suckling is "sensual" and may cause guilt or confusion in the woman. Encourage discussion with other mothers. Include the partner in at least one discussion to assess his or her feelings and how they affect the breastfeeding experience.
- Explore the woman's feelings about self-consciousness during feedings.
  - Where?
  - Around whom?
  - What is the partner's reaction to when and where she breastfeeds?
  - Demonstrate the use of a shawl for modesty, allowing breastfeeding in public.
  - Remind the mother that what she is doing is normal and natural.

R: *Dialogue can alienate fears which can deter breastfeeding.*

Assist the Family With the Following

- Sibling reaction
  - Explore feelings and anticipation of problems. An older child may be jealous of contact with the baby. Mother can use this time to read to the older child.
  - The older child may want to breastfeed. Allow him or her to try; usually, the child will not like it.
  - Stress the older child's attributes: freedom, movement, and choices.
- Fatigue and stress
  - Explore the situation.
  - Encourage the mother to make herself and the infant a priority.
  - Encourage her to limit visitors for the first 2 weeks to allow optimum bonding and learning to breastfeed for mother and baby.
  - Emphasize that the mother will need support and assistance during the first 4 weeks. Encourage the support person to help as much as possible.
  - Encourage the mother not to try to be "superwoman," but to ask directly for help from friends or relatives or to hire someone.
- Feelings of being enslaved
  - Allow the mother to express feelings.
  - Encourage her to seek assistance and to pump milk to allow others to feed the baby at 3 to 4 weeks of age.
  - Advise her that she can store harvested breast milk for 8 hours at room temperature, 6 to 7 days in the refrigerator, and 6 months in the freezer. (*Note:* Tell the woman never to microwave frozen breast milk, as doing so destroys its immune properties and may cause uneven heating which may burn the infant's mouth.)

- Remember that time between feedings will get longer (every 2 hours for 4 weeks, then every 3 to 4 hours for 3 months), but this is not definite. Feeding patterns will change as the infant ages and goes through growth spurts.

R: *Mothers who are prepared for possible problems at home will have more confidence and be more likely to continue breastfeeding.*

Initiate Referrals, as Indicated

- Refer to lactation consultant if indicated by
  - Lack of confidence
  - Ambivalence
  - Problems with infant suck and latch-on
  - Infant weight drop or lack of urination
  - Barriers in the workplace
  - Prolonged soreness
  - Hot, tender spots on the breast
- Refer to La Leche League and community resources.
- Refer to childbirth educator and childbirth class members.
- Refer to other breastfeeding mothers.

R: *Referrals to community resources can provide continued support and information.*

R: *Company-sponsored lactation programs enable employed mothers to continue breastfeeding as long as they desire).*

INTERRUPTED BREASTFEEDING

NANDA-I Definition

Break in the continuity of the breastfeeding process as a result of inability or inadvisability to put baby to breast for feeding

Defining Characteristics*

Infant receives no nourishment at the breast for some or all feedings
Maternal desire to eventually provide breast milk for child's nutritional needs
Maternal desire to maintain breastfeeding for child's nutritional needs

Related Factors*

Maternal or infant illness
Prematurity
Maternal employment
Contraindications (e.g., drugs, true breast milk, jaundice)
Need to wean infant abruptly
Lack of education

Author's Note

This diagnosis represents a situation, not a response. Nursing interventions do not treat the interruption but, instead, its effects. The situation is interrupted breastfeeding; the responses can vary. For example, if continued breastfeeding or use of a breast pump is contraindicated, the nurse focuses on the loss of this breastfeeding experience using the nursing diagnosis *Grieving*.

If breastfeeding continues with expression and storage of breast milk, teaching, and support, the diagnosis will be *Risk for Ineffective Breastfeeding related to continuity problems secondary to (specify) (e.g., maternal employment)*. If difficulty is experienced, the diagnosis would be *Ineffective Breastfeeding related to interruption secondary to (specify) and lack of knowledge*.

INSUFFICIENT BREAST MILK

NANDA-I Definition

Low production of maternal breast milk

Defining Characteristics*

Infant
Constipation
Does not seem satisfied after sucking
Frequent crying
Voids small amounts of concentrated urine (less than four to six times a day)
Long breastfeeding time
Wants to suck very frequently
Refuses to suck
Weight gain is lower than 500 g in a month (comparing two measures)

Related Factors

Infant
Ineffective latching on
Rejection of breast
Ineffective sucking
Short sucking time
Insufficient opportunity to suckle

Mother
Alcohol intake
Medication side effects (e.g., contraceptives, diuretics)
Malnutrition
Tobacco smoking/use
Pregnancy
Fluid volume depletion (e.g., dehydration, hemorrhage)
Lack of education

Author's Note

In managing breastfeeding, nurses strive to reduce or eliminate factors that contribute to *Ineffective Breastfeeding* or factors that can increase vulnerability for a problem using the diagnosis *Risk for Ineffective Breastfeeding*.

In the acute setting after delivery, too little time will have lapsed for the nurse to conclude that there is no problem in breastfeeding, unless the mother is experienced. For many mother–infant dyads, *Risk for Ineffective Breastfeeding related to inexperience with the breastfeeding process* would represent a nursing focus on preventing problems in breastfeeding. Risk would not be indicated for all inexperienced mothers.

Insufficient Breast Milk is a new NANDA-I accepted diagnosis that represents a more specific diagnosis under *Ineffective Breastfeeding*. When this specific etiology can be identified with *Ineffective Breastfeeding*, the nurse can use either one.

Focus Assessment Criteria

Refer to *Ineffective Breastfeeding*.

Goals/Interventions

Refer to *Ineffective Breastfeeding*.

DECREASED CARDIAC OUTPUT

See also *Risk for Complications of Decreased Cardiac Output* in Section 3.

NANDA-I Definition

Inadequate blood pumped by the heart to meet the metabolic demands of the body

Defining Characteristics*

Altered heart rate/rhythm (e.g., arrhythmias, bradycardia, EKG changes, palpitations, tachycardia)
Altered preload (e.g., edema, decreased central venous pressure, decreased pulmonary artery wedge pressure [PAWP])
Altered contractility
Altered afterload
Behavioral/emotional (anxiety, restlessness)

Related Factors*

Altered heart rate
Altered rhythm
Altered stroke volume
Altered afterload
Altered contractility
Altered preload

Author's Note

This nursing diagnosis represents a situation in which nurses have multiple responsibilities. People experiencing decreased cardiac output may display various responses that disrupt functioning (e.g., activity intolerance, disturbed sleep–rest, anxiety, fear). Or they may be at risk for developing such physiologic complications as arrhythmias, cardiogenic shock, and heart failure.

When *Decreased Cardiac Output* is used clinically, associated goals usually are written:

- Systolic blood pressure is greater than 100
- Urine output is greater than 30 mL/hr
- Cardiac output is greater than 5
- Cardiac rate and rhythm are within normal limits

These goals do not represent parameters for evaluating nursing care, but for evaluating the individual's status. Because they are monitoring the criteria that the nurse uses to guide implementation of nurse-prescribed and physician-prescribed interventions, students consult with faculty to determine which diagnosis to use: *Decreased Cardiac Output* or *Risk for Complications of Decreased Cardiac Output*. Refer to *Activity Intolerance—Related to Insufficient Knowledge of Adaptive Techniques Needed Secondary to Impaired Cardiac Function* and *Risk for Complications of Decreased Cardiac Output* in Section 3 for specific interventions.

CAREGIVER ROLE STRAIN

Caregiver Role Strain

Risk for Caregiver Role Strain

Definition

Difficulty in performing family/significant other caregiver role (NANDA-I)

A state in which a person is experiencing physical, emotional, social, and/or financial burden(s) in the process of giving care to a significant other.[4]

Defining Characteristics

Expressed or Observed

Insufficient time or physical energy
Difficulty performing required caregiving activities
Conflicts between caregiving responsibilities and other important roles (e.g., work, relationships)
Apprehension about the future for the care receiver's health and ability to provide care
Apprehension about care receiver's care when caregiver is ill or deceased
Feelings of depression or anger
Feelings of exhaustion and resentment

Related Factors

Pathophysiologic

Related to unrelenting or complex care requirements secondary to:

Addiction*
Chronic mental illness
Cognitive problems*
Debilitating conditions (acute, progressive)
Disability
Progressive dementia
Unpredictability of illness course*

Treatment Related

Related to 24-hour care responsibilities*

Related to time-consuming activities (e.g., dialysis, transportation)

Related to complexity of activities*

Related to increasing care needs*

Situational (Personal, Environmental)

Related to years of caregiving*

Related to unpredictability of care situation or illness course*

Related to inadequate informal support*

Related to unrealistic expectations of caregiver by care receiver, self, or others*

Related to pattern of impaired individual coping (e.g., abuse, violence, addiction)*

Related to compromised physical or mental health of caregiver*

Related to history of poor relationship* or family dysfunction*

Related to history of marginal family coping*

Related to duration of caregiving required

Related to isolation

Related to insufficient respite

Related to insufficient finances*

[4]This definition has been added by Lynda Juall Carpenito, the author, for clarity and usefulness.

Related to inadequate community resources*

Related to no or unavailable support

Related to insufficient resources

Related to inexperience with caregiving*

Related to deficient knowledge about community resources*

Maturational

Infant, Child, and Adolescent

Related to unrelenting care requirements secondary to:

Developmental delay
Mental disabilities (specify)
Physical disabilities (specify)

Author's Note

Caregiver Role Strain and *Risk for Caregiver Role Strain* are two nursing diagnoses that when addressed by nurses will provide support and education to individuals and their caregivers, which can profoundly influence factors that bond families, not destroy them.

"Health care policies that rely on caregiver sacrifice can be made to appear cost-effective only if the emotional, social, physical, and financial costs incurred by the caregiver are ignored" (*Winslow & Carter, 1999, p. 285). Worldwide, family caregivers provide most care for dependent persons of all ages whether living in developing countries or developed countries (AARP, 2009). The care receivers have physical and/or mental disabilities, which can be temporary or permanent. Some disabilities are permanent but stable (e.g., blindness); others signal progressive deterioration (e.g., Alzheimer's disease).

Caring and caregiving are intrinsic to all close relationships. They are "found in the context of established roles such as wife–husband, child–parent" (*Pearlin, Mullan, Semple, & Skaff, 1990, p. 583). Under some circumstances, caregiving is "transformed from the ordinary exchange of assistance among people standing in close relationship to one another to an extraordinary and unequally distributed burden" (*Pearlin et al., 1990, p. 583). It becomes a dominant, overriding component occupying the entire situation (*Pearlin et al., 1990).

Caregiver Role Strain represents the burden of caregiving on the physical and emotional health of the caregiver and its effects on the family and social system of the caregiver and care receiver. *Risk for Caregiver Role Strain* can be a very significant nursing diagnosis because nurses can identify those at high risk and assist them to prevent this grave situation.

Chronic sorrow has been associated with caregivers of people with mental illness and children with chronic illness. See *Chronic Sorrow* for more information.

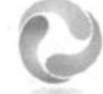

Errors in Diagnostic Statements

Caregiver Role Strain related to depression and anger at family as evidenced by unrealistic expectations of caregiver for self and by others

Too often, caregivers with multiple, unrelenting responsibilities are reluctant to admit they need help. Others may interpret this reluctance as not needing help. The caregiver is further isolated, feeling no one really cares or appreciates the work involved, which can contribute to depression and anger. Thus, this diagnosis must be rewritten to reflect the unrealistic expectations as the *Related Factors* and the resulting symptoms as evidence. It is helpful to quote the data if relevant: *Caregiver Role Strain related to unrealistic expectations of caregiver for self and by others, as evidenced by depressed feelings and anger at family who "don't understand my burden."*

Key Concepts

General Considerations

- According to the National Women's Health Information Center (2011), 52 million persons provide care for someone else, 13% are older than 65, and 52% are women.

- Nearly one-third of young adults of age 18 to 44 suffer from a chronic illness, and there has been an increase in the survival of low birth weight and premature infants with an increase of caregiving responsibilities for their family members (National Center for Health Statistics, 2011).
- "Quality of life is affected by four major characteristics of a care giving situation: (1) high caregiving demands, (2) loss of physical health for the caregiver, (3) psychological distress, and (4) interference with life roles" (Yarbro, Wujcik, & Gobel, 2013). Chronic sorrow has been associated with caregivers of people with mental illness and children with chronic illness. See *Chronic Sorrow* for more information.
- Smith, Smith, and Toseland (*1991) reported the following problems (by priority) identified by family caregivers:
  - Improving coping skills (e.g., time management, stress management)
  - Family issues (sibling conflict, other role conflicts)
  - Responding to care receiver's needs (emotional, physical, financial)
  - Eliciting formal and informal support
  - Guilt and feelings of inadequacy
  - Long-term planning
  - Quality of relationship with care receiver

Grandparents as Caregivers

- "Recent estimates from a nationally representative sample of 13,626 grandparents found that 28% of grandparents provided at least 50 hours or care per year for grandchildren with whom they did not live" (Luo et al., 2012, p. 1153; in Yahirun, 2012, p. 37).
- Miller (2015, p. 17 from Numkung, 2016) reported that, "about 6.5 million children (8.8%) live with at least one grandparent, with 1.6 million children living in households headed by grandparents with no parent present".
- AAUP (2014) reported findings from a collaboration with several organizations that 72% of grandparents take care of their grandchildren on a regular basis and 13% are primary caregivers.
- Yahirun (2012, p. 44) wrote

> *That the family safety net is still functioning is evident in grandmothers' willingness to become primary caregivers to grandchildren whose parents cannot look after them. Even though custodial grandmothers have more health problems and experience higher rates of poverty than other grandmothers who live with a grandchild, they continue to care for the youngest generation. This is a dramatic example of the important role that older persons play in the family safety net.*

Pediatric Considerations

- Children considered candidates for home care services are those
  - Who depend on mechanical ventilation
  - Who need prolonged intravenous nutritional or drug therapy
  - Who have a terminal illness
  - Who require nutritional support (e.g., tube feedings) or respiratory support (e.g., tracheostomy, suctioning)
  - Who need daily or near-daily nursing care for apnea monitoring, dialysis, urinary catheters, or colostomy pouches
- Parents with caregiving responsibilities for children with chronic conditions have (in addition to the usual parenting responsibilities) to the following concomitant burdens (Cousino & Hazen, 2013):
  - Medical and therapy appointments
  - Treatments
  - Schooling issues frequent hospitalizations
  - Witnessing their child suffering
  - Balancing the parenting responsibilities for their other children

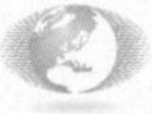

Transcultural Considerations

- *Grandparents in the Filipino family are viewed as an integral family member, not a burden.* Grandparents are frequently caregivers and live with their grandchildren in African-American, Hispanic, and Asian ethnic groups (Giger, 2013).
- Dilworth-Anderson, Williams, and Gibson (*2002) reported that ethnic minority families accessed fewer formal services but instead used more informal family member support for family caregiving activities.

Focus Assessment Criteria

Subjective Data

Assess for Defining Characteristics

How well do you manage your
- Caregiving responsibilities?
- Household responsibilities?
- Life outside caregiving?
- Work responsibilities?
- Family responsibilities?
- Social life?

On a scale from 0 to 10 (0 = not tired, peppy to 10 = total exhaustion), rate the fatigue you usually feel.
Does it change during the day or week? If so, why?

What do you do when you are overly stressed?

What are you most concerned about? For the present? For the future?

Assess for Related Factors

Caregiver History

Lifestyle

Health

Ability to perform activities of daily living
Chronic conditions

Family Members in household

Parents, spouse, children
Grandparents—extended family
In-laws

Economic Resources

Sources
Adequacy

Care Receiver Characteristics

Cognitive Status (e.g., Memory, Speech)

History of Relationship With Caregiver

Problematic Behaviors (*Pearlin et al., 1990)

Wanders
Threatens
Uses foul language
Incontinence
Suspicious
Sexually inappropriate
Cries easily
Repeats questions and requests
Clings
Depressed
Insomnia
Substance abuse

Support System

Who? (family, friends, clergy, agency, group)
What? (visits, respite, chores, empathy)
How often?
What have you lost because of your caregiver responsibilities?

Goals

NOC

Caregiver Well-Being, Caregiver Lifestyle Disruption, Caregiver Emotional Health, Caregiver Home Care: Readiness, Caregiver Role Endurance Potential, Family Coping, Family Integrity

The caregiver will report a plan to decrease caregiver's burden:

- Share frustrations regarding caregiving responsibilities.
- Identify one source of support.
- Identify two changes that would improve daily life if implemented.

The family will establish a plan for weekly support or help

- Relate two strategies to increase support.
- Convey empathy to caregiver regarding daily responsibilities.

Interventions

NIC

Caregiver Support, Respite Care, Coping Enhancement, Family Mobilization, Mutual Goal Setting, Support System Enhancement, Anticipatory Guidance

Assess for Causative or Contributing Factors

- Refer to Related Factors.

For a New Caregiver (Smith & Segal, 2015)

- Learn as much as you can about your family member's illness and about how to be a caregiver.
- Seek out other caregivers for mutual sharing and support.
- If some advice is questionable, ask for more discussion.
- Encourage your loved one to do as much as they can. This will promote their self-esteem independence.
- Know your limits. Be realistic about how much of your time and yourself you can give. Set clear limits, and communicate those limits to doctors, family members, and other people involved.

Explore With the Caregivers the History and Quality of Their Relationship With Their Family Member and How They Feel About Being a Caregiver (Smith & Segal, 2015)

- Anxiety about their ability, fears related to future
- Anger toward the person, not receiving help, other family members, about daily responsibilities
- Guilt for not doing more, not being a "better" caregiver or having more patience, accepting your situation with more equanimity, or in the case of long-distance caregiving, not being available more often.
- **Grief** for the "many losses that can come with caregiving (the healthy future you envisioned with your spouse or child; the goals and dreams you've had to set aside)." In addition, if your loved one is terminally ill, grieving is present.

Provide Empathy and Promote a Sense of Competency

- Allow caregiver to share feelings.
- Emphasize the difficulties of the caregiving responsibilities.
- If indicated encourage the caregiver opportunities to share the positive aspects of their caregiving.

R: *Sharing their personal positive aspects as personal gratification, social approval, giving back to parent can add clarity and meaning, which may mediate the burdens of caregiving (Shim, Barroso, Giles, & Davis, 2013).*

- Evaluate the effects of caregiving periodically (depression, burnout).

R: *Lindgren (*1990) reported that burnout in caregivers was related to emotional exhaustion and a low sense of accomplishment. Caregivers who were commended for their accomplishments reported lower levels of burnout.*

R: *Caregiving to a chronically ill family member or friend with many behavioral problems is the most stressful situation one can encounter.*

Promote Insight Into the Situation

- Ask the caregiver to describe a typical day
    - Caregiving and household tasks
    - Work outside the home
    - Role responsibilities
- Ask the caregiver to describe
    - At-home leisure activities (daily, weekly)
    - Outside-the-home social activities (weekly)

- Engage other family members in discussion, as appropriate.
- Caution the caregiver about the danger of viewing helpers as less competent or less essential.

R: *Caregiver stress is not an event but "a mix of circumstances, experiences, responses, and resources that vary considerably among caregivers and that consequently vary in their impact on caregivers' health and behavior" (Pearlin et al., 1990).*

Assist Caregiver to Identify the Activities for Which He or She Desires Assistance

- Advise to (list of caregiving needs; Smith & Segal, 2015)
  - Laundry
  - House cleaning
  - Meals
  - Shopping, errands
  - Transportation
  - Appointments (primary care providers, specialists, tests, hairdresser)
  - Yard work
  - House repairs
  - Respite (hours per week)
  - Money management
  - Go over list with family members one at a time. Ask the individual what areas can he or she help with. (Take responsibility for something themselves, pay for respite.)
  - Emphasize that their help is both beneficial for you and your loved one.

R: *Shields (*1992) reported a primary source of conflict among family members and the caregiver as unsatisfied needs. The caregiver wishes for others to affirm the burden, when, in fact, the family responds to the caregiver's complaints with problem-solving techniques. The caregiver appears to reject suggestions, which annoys the family. The results are a "caregiver feeling unappreciated, unsupported, and depressed, and family members feeling angry and rejected toward the caregiver."*

Stress the Importance of Taking Care of Self

- Rest–exercise balance
- Effective stress management (e.g., yoga, relaxation training, creative arts)
- Low-fat, high–complex-carbohydrate diet
- Supportive social networks
- Appropriate screening practices for age
- Maintain a good sense of humor; associate with others who laugh
- Advise caregivers to initiate phone contacts or visits with friends or relatives rather than waiting for others to do it.

R: *Caregivers must maintain their own health in order to be successful with coping with caregiving responsibilities.*

Engage Family to Appraise Situation (Apart From Caregiver) (Shields, 1992)

- Allow the family to share frustrations.
- Share the need for the caregiver to feel appreciated.
- Discuss the importance of regularly acknowledging the burden of the situation for the caregiver.
- Differentiate the types of social support (emotional, appraisal, informational, instrumental).
- Emphasize the importance of emotional and appraisal support, and identify sources of this support (e.g., regular phone calls, cards, letters, visits).
- Stress "that in many situations, there are no problems to be solved, only pain to be shared" (*Shields, 1992).
- Discuss the need to give the caregiver "permission" to enjoy self (e.g., vacations, day trips).
- Advise them to ask the caregiver "How can I help you?"

R: *Numerous researchers have identified consistent social supports as the single most significant factor that reduces or prevents caregiver role strain (*Clipp & George, 1990; *Pearlin et al., 1990; *Shields, 1992).*

Assist With Accessing Informational and Instrumental Support

- Provide information that is needed with problem-solving strategies.
- Provide information that is needed for skill-building.

Role Play How to Ask for Help With Activities

- For example: "I have three appointments this week, could you drive me to one?" "I could watch your children once or twice a week in exchange for you watching my husband."
- Identify all possible sources of volunteer help: family (siblings, cousins), friends, neighbors, church, and community groups.

R: *Skill-building interventions improve optimism and success in providing care.*

- Discuss how most people feel good when they provide a "little help."

R: *The number of people in a household influences how many secondary, informal caregivers assist the primary caregiver. Spouse primary caregivers are less likely to have secondary caregivers to help them with care activities. Older people cared for by spouses received about 15% to 20% fewer person-days of help than those cared for by adult children.*

Initiate Health Teaching and Referrals, if Indicated

- Explain the benefits of sharing with other caregivers.
  - Support group
  - Individual and group counseling
  - Telephone buddy system with another caregiver

R: *It has been reported that individual and group counseling increased the number of support persons and decreased caregiver stress (*Roth et al., 2005; Halter, 2014).*

- Access information online, for example, two good sources include the website for the Office on Women's Health, where one can find the publication: "Caregiver stress fact sheet"; and through the website HelpGuide.Org, look for the article, "Caregiving Support and Help: Tips for Making Family Caregiving Easier and More Rewarding."
- Identify community resources available (e.g., counseling, social service, day care).
- Arrange a home visit by a professional nurse or a physical therapist to provide strategies to improve communication, time management, and caregiving.
- Engage others to work actively to increase state, federal, and private agencies' financial support for resources to enhance caregiving in the home.

R: *These strategies emphasize the need for the caregiver to protect their health with a balance of work, sleep, leisure, and support and to identify sources of help in the community.*

Pediatric Interventions

- Determine parents' understanding of and concerns about child's illness, course, prognosis, and related care needs.
- Elicit the effects of caregiving responsibility on
  - Personal life (work, rest, leisure)
  - Marriage (time alone, communication, decisions, attention)

R: *Strategies to promote family cohesiveness reduce isolation or aloneness.*

- Assist parents to meet the well siblings' needs for
  - Knowledge of sibling's illness and relationship to own health
  - Sharing feelings of anger, unfairness, embarrassment
  - Discussions of future of ill sibling and self (e.g., family planning, care responsibilities)

R: *Addressing the developmental tasks of the ill child and the well siblings provides opportunities to grow, develop, gain independence, and master effective coping skills.*

- Discuss strategies to help siblings adapt.
  - Include in family decisions when appropriate.
  - Keep informed about ill child's condition.
  - Maintain routines (e.g., meals, vacations).
  - Prepare for changes in home life.
  - Promote activities with peers.
  - Avoid making the ill child the center of the family.
  - Determine what daily assistance in caregiving is realistic.
  - Plan for time alone.

R: *Strategies to promote family cohesiveness and individual family needs can enhance effective stress management (Williams, 2000).*

- Advise teachers of home situation.
- Address developmental needs. See *Delayed Growth and Development*.
- Advise that caregiving activities produce fatigue that can increase over time (Williams, 2000).

Risk for Caregiver Role Strain

NANDA-I Definition

At risk for caregiver vulnerability for felt difficulty in performing the family caregiver role

Risk Factors

Primary caregiver responsibilities for a recipient who requires regular assistance with self-care or supervision because of physical or mental disabilities in addition to one or more of the related factors for *Caregiver Role Strain*

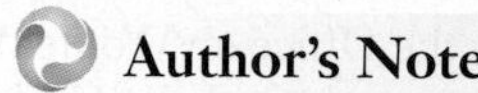

Author's Note

Refer to *Caregiver Role Strain*.

Errors in Diagnostic Statements

Refer to *Caregiver Role Strain*.

Key Concepts

Refer to *Caregiver Role Strain*.

Focus Assessment Criteria

Refer to *Caregiver Role Strain*.

Goals

NOC

Refer to *Caregiver Role Strain*.

The individual will relate a plan for how to continue social activities despite caregiving responsibilities.

- Identify activities that are important for self.
- Relate intent to enlist the help of at least two people weekly.

Interventions

NIC

Refer to *Caregiver Role Strain*.

Explain the Causes of Caregiver Role Strain

- Refer to Related Factors for *Caregiver Role Strain*.

Teach Caregiver and Significant Others to be Alert for Danger Signals (*Murray, Zentner, & Yakimo, 2009)

- No matter what you do, it is never enough.
- You believe you are the only individual in the world doing this.
- You have no time or place to be alone for a brief respite.
- Family relationships are breaking down because of the caregiving pressures.
- Your caregiving duties are interfering with your work and social life.
- You are in a "no-win situation" and will not admit difficulty.
- You are alone because you have alienated everyone who could help.

- You are overeating, under eating, abusing drugs or alcohol, or being harsh and abusive with others.
- There are no more happy times. Love and care have given way to exhaustion and resentment. You no longer feel good about yourself or take pride in what you are doing.

R: *Danger signals must be addressed to preserve health and relationships and to prevent abuse.*

Explain the Four Types of Social Support to All Involved

- Emotional (e.g., concern, trust)
- Appraisal (e.g., affirms self-worth)
- Informational (e.g., useful advice, information for problem solving)
- Instrumental assistance (e.g., caregiving) or tangible assistance (e.g., money, help with chores)

R: *Identifying the various sources of social support can help the caregiver seek out*

Stress the Importance of Daily Health Promotion Activities

- Rest–exercise balance
- Effective stress management
- Low-fat, high–complex-carbohydrate diet
- Supportive social networks
- Appropriate screening practices for age
- Maintain a good sense of humor; associate with others who laugh.
- Advise caregivers to initiate phone contacts or visits with friends or relatives rather than waiting for others to do it.

R: *Caregivers must maintain their own health in order to be successful with coping with caregiving responsibilities.*

Assist Caregiver to Identify the Activities for Which He or She Desires Assistance

- Refer to *Caregiver Role Strain.*

Assist with Accessing Informational and Instrumental Support

- Refer to *Caregiver Role Strain.*

Initiate Health Teaching and Referrals, if Indicated

- Refer to *Caregiver Role Strain.*

INEFFECTIVE CHILDBEARING PROCESS

Ineffective Childbearing Process

Risk for Ineffective Childbearing Process

NANDA-I Definition

Pregnancy and childbirth process and care of the newborn that does not match the environmental context, norms, and expectations

Defining Characteristics*

During Pregnancy

Does not access support systems appropriately

Does report appropriate physical preparations

Does not report appropriate prenatal lifestyle (e.g., nutrition, elimination, sleep, bodily movement, exercise, personal hygiene)

Does not report availability of support systems

Does not report managing unpleasant symptoms in pregnancy

Does not report realistic birth plan

Does not seek necessary knowledge (e.g., labor and delivery, newborn care)
Failure to prepare necessary newborn care items
Inconsistent prenatal health visits
Lack of prenatal visits
Lack of respect for unborn baby

During Labor and Delivery
Does not access support systems appropriately
Does not report lifestyle (e.g., diet, elimination, sleep, bodily movement, personal hygiene) that is appropriate for the stage of labor
Does not report availability of support systems
Does not demonstrate attachment behavior to the newborn
Does not respond appropriately to onset of labor
Lacks proactivity during labor and delivery

After Birth
Does not access support systems appropriately
Does not demonstrate appropriate baby feeding techniques
Does not demonstrate appropriate breast care
Does not demonstrate attachment behavior to the newborn
Does not demonstrate basic baby care techniques
Does not provide safe environment for the baby
Does not report appropriate postpartum lifestyle (e.g., diet, elimination, sleep, bodily movement, exercise, personal hygiene)
Does not report availability of support systems

Related Factors

Deficient knowledge (e.g., of labor and delivery, newborn care)
Domestic violence
Inconsistent prenatal health visits
Lack of appropriate role models for parenthood
Lack of cognitive readiness for parenthood
Lack of maternal confidence
Lack of a realistic birth plan
Lack of sufficient support systems
Maternal powerlessness
Suboptimal maternal nutrition
Substance abuse
Unplanned pregnancy
Unsafe environment

Author's Note

This new NANDA-I diagnosis represents numerous situations and factors that can compromise the well-being of a mother and her relationship with her infant during labor and delivery and after birth. It can be used to organize a standard of care for all pregnant women during the process of labor and delivery and after birth.

Embedded in this broad diagnosis is a multitude of specific actual or risk problematic responses; some examples are as follows:
Risk for Dysfunctional Family Processes
Interrupted Family Processes
Altered Nutrition
Risk-Prone Health Behavior
Ineffective Coping
Powerlessness
Ineffective Health Management
Risk for Ineffective Childbearing Process would be the standard of care on the appropriate units.

If *Ineffective Childbearing Process* is validated, it may be more clinically useful to use a more specific nursing diagnosis. However, if there are multiple related factors complicating the childbearing process, this diagnosis would be useful.

Due to the extensive art and science of nursing that is related to this specialty diagnosis, the author refers the reader to *Maternal-Child Nursing* literature for goals, interventions, and rationale.

Risk for Ineffective Childbearing Process

NANDA-I Definition

Risk for a pregnancy and childbirth process and care of the newborn that does not match the environmental context, norms, and expectations

Risk Factors*

Deficient knowledge (e.g., of labor and delivery, newborn care)
Domestic violence
Inconsistent prenatal health visits
Lack of appropriate role models for parenthood
Lack of cognitive readiness for parenthood
Lack of maternal confidence
Lack of prenatal health visits
Lack of a realistic birth plan
Lack of sufficient support systems
Maternal powerlessness
Maternal psychological distress
Suboptimal maternal; nutrition
Substance abuse
Unsafe environment
Unplanned pregnancy

Author's Note

Refer to Author's Note under *Ineffective Childbearing Process*.

IMPAIRED COMFORT[5]

Impaired Comfort*

Acute Pain
Chronic Pain
Chronic Pain Syndrome
Labor Pain
Nausea

NANDA-I Definition

Perceived lack of ease, relief, and transcendence in physical, psychospiritual, environmental, cultural, and social dimensions

Defining Characteristics

The client reports or demonstrates discomfort.
Autonomic response in acute pain
Increased blood pressure

[5]This diagnosis was developed by Lynda Juall Carpenito.

- Increased pulse
- Increased respirations
- Diaphoresis
- Dilated pupils

Guarded position
Facial mask of pain
Crying, moaning
Inability to relax*
Irritability*
Reports*

- Abdominal heaviness
- Anxiety
- Being cold or hot
- Being uncomfortable
- Lack of privacy
- Malaise
- Nausea
- Pruritus
- Treatment-related side effects (medications, radiation)
- Disturbed sleep pattern
- Itching
- Vomiting

Related Factors

Any factor can contribute to impaired comfort. The most common are listed below.

Biopathophysiologic

Related to uterine contractions during labor

Related to trauma to perineum during labor and delivery

Related to involution of uterus and engorged breasts

Related to tissue trauma and reflex muscle spasms secondary to:

Musculoskeletal Disorders

Fractures
Contractures
Spasms
Arthritis
Spinal cord disorders
Fibromyalgia

Visceral Disorders

Cardiac
Renal
Hepatic
Intestinal
Pulmonary

Cancer

Vascular Disorders

Vasospasm
Occlusion
Phlebitis
Vasodilation (headache)

Related to inflammation of, or injury:

Nerve
Tendon
Bursa
Joint
Muscle
Juxta-articular structures

Related to fatigue, malaise, or pruritus secondary to contagious diseases:

Rubella
Hepatitis
Pancreatitis
Chicken pox
Mononucleosis

Related to abdominal cramps, diarrhea, and vomiting secondary to:

Gastroenteritis
Gastric ulcers
Influenza

Related to inflammation and smooth muscle spasms secondary to:

Gastrointestinal infections
Renal calculi

Treatment Related

Related to tissue trauma and reflex muscle spasms secondary to:

Accidents
Burns
Diagnostic tests (venipuncture, invasive scanning, biopsy)
Surgery

Related to nausea and vomiting secondary to:

Anesthesia
Chemotherapy
Side effects of (specify)

Situational (Personal, Environmental)

Related to fever

Related to immobility/improper positioning

Related to overactivity

Related to pressure points (tight cast, elastic bandages)

Related to allergic response

Related to chemical irritants

Related to unmet dependency needs

Related to severe repressed anxiety

Maturational

Related to tissue trauma and reflex muscle spasms secondary to:

Infancy: Colic
Infancy and early childhood: Teething, ear pain
Middle childhood: Recurrent abdominal pain, growing pains
Adolescence: Headaches, chest pain, dysmenorrhea

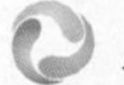

Author's Note

A diagnosis not on the current NANDA-I list, *Impaired Comfort* can represent various uncomfortable sensations (e.g., pruritus, immobility, NPO status). For a client experiencing nausea and vomiting, the nurse should assess whether *Impaired Comfort, Risk for Impaired Comfort or Risk for Imbalanced Nutrition* is appropriate. Short-lived episodes of nausea, vomiting, or both (e.g., postoperatively) are best described with *Impaired Comfort related to effects of anesthesia or analgesics*. When nausea/vomiting may compromise nutritional intake, the appropriate diagnosis may be *Risk for Imbalanced Nutrition related to nausea and vomiting secondary to (specify)*. *Impaired Comfort* also can be used to describe a cluster of discomforts related to a condition or treatment, such as radiation therapy.

Errors in Diagnostic Statements

Impaired Comfort related to immobility

Although immobility can contribute to impaired comfort, the nursing diagnosis *Disuse Syndrome* describes a cluster of nursing diagnoses that apply or are at high risk to apply as a result of immobility. *Impaired Comfort* can be included in *Disuse Syndrome*; thus, the diagnosis should be written as *Disuse Syndrome*.

Impaired Comfort related to nausea and vomiting secondary to chemotherapy

Nausea and vomiting represent signs and symptoms, not contributing factors, of impaired comfort. *Impaired Comfort* can be used to describe a cluster of discomforts associated with chemotherapy, such as *Impaired Comfort related to the effects of chemotherapy on bone marrow production and irritation of emetic center*, as evidenced by complaints of nausea, vomiting, anorexia, and fatigue.

Key Concepts

General Considerations

- Refer also to General Considerations under *Acute* and *Chronic Pain*.
- Pruritus (itching) is the most common skin complaint and can occur in response to an allergen or a sign or symptom of a systemic disease, such as cancer, liver disease, renal dysfunction, or diabetes.
- Pruritus, described as a tickling or tormenting sensation, originates exclusively in the skin and provokes the urge to scratch.
- Although the same neurons are likely to transmit signals for itching as for pressure, pain, and touch, each sensation is perceived and mediated differently (Grossman & Porth, 2014).
- Pruritus arises from subepidermal nerve stimulation by proteolytic enzymes, which the epidermis releases as a result of either primary irritation or secondary allergic responses (Grossman & Porth, 2014).
- The same unmyelinated nerves that act for burning pain also serve for pruritus. As a pruritic sensation increases in intensity, it may become burning (Grossman & Porth, 2014).

Geriatric Considerations

- Asteatosis (excessive skin dryness) is the most common cause of pruritus in older adults. Its incidences range from 40% to 80%, as a result of varying criteria and climate differences. With scratching, small breaks in the epidermis can increase the risk of infection owing to age-related changes in the immune system (Miller, 2015).

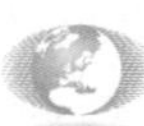

Transcultural Considerations

- Pain is a universally recognized "private experience that is greatly influenced by cultural heritage" (*Ludwig-Beymer, 1989).
- US nurses are preponderantly white, middle-class women socialized to believe "that in any situation self-control is better than open displays of strong feelings" (Ludwig-Beymer, 1989). Nurses should not stereotype members of a particular culture, but instead accept a range of pain expressions (Ludwig-Beymer, 1989).
- The nurse's own cultural background influences interpretation of an individual's pain (*Lovering, 2006).
- To be honest and forthcoming regarding pain, clients must attain a level of trust with their practitioners, which may be difficult in specific environments, (such as the ED), leaving health-care providers an additional barrier to overcome in treating pain (*Johnson, Fudala, & Payne, 2005).
- Families transmit to their children cultural norms related to pain (Ludwig-Beymer, 1989).
- Zborowski (*1952), in his classic studies on the influence of culture on the pain experience, found that the pain event, its meaning, and responses are culturally learned and specific. He reported the following cultural variations in interpretation and responses to pain: Campbell and Edwards (2012) has added to this work.
  - *Third-generation Americans:* Unexpressive; concerned with implications; controlled emotional response
  - *Jewish:* Concerned about the implication of the pain; readily seek relief; frequently express pain to others
  - *Irish:* See pain as private; unexpressive; unemotional
  - *Italian:* Concerned with immediate pain relief; present oriented
  - *Japanese:* Value self-control; will not express pain or ask for relief, fear addiction, which is a strong taboo

- *Hispanic:* Present oriented; use folk medicine frequently; view suffering as a positive spiritual experience, may be outspoken in expressing pain
- *Chinese:* May ignore symptoms and describe an imbalance between Yin and Yang use of alternative health practices, for example, massages, elixir, relaxation, oil
- *Black Americans:* May respond stoically because of dominant culture pressure; can believe that pain is God's will, suffering is inevitable, and prayer can relieve suffering
- Chinese women believe they will dishonor themselves and their family if they are loud.
- Women from many South and Central American cultures believe the more intense the expression of pain during labor, the stronger the love toward the infant (*Weber, 1996).

Focus Assessment Criteria

This nursing assessment of pain is designed to acquire data for assessing adaptation to pain, not for determining the cause or existence of pain.

Subjective Data

Assess for Defining Characteristics

Pain

"Where is your discomfort located; does it radiate?" (Ask child to point the place.)

"When did it begin?"

"Can you relate the cause of this discomfort?" or "What do you think has caused your discomfort?"

"Describe the discomfort and its pattern."

Time of day

Frequency (constant, intermittent, transient)

Duration

Quality/intensity

Ask the client to rate the pain: At its best, after pain-relief measures, and at its worst. Use consistent scale, language, or set of behaviors to assess pain.

For adults, use an oral or visual analogue scale of 0 to 10 (0 = no pain, 10 = excruciating). For someone who may not understand the 0 to 10 scale, try to elicit past painful experiences from the individual and assist him/her to attach a number to it. If the 0 to 10 pain scale was drawn as a thermometer (vertically) it may represent what a 10 means versus a horizontal picture.

For children, select a scale appropriate for developmental age: A scale for assessed age or younger can be used; include the child in selection:

3 years and older: Use drawings or photographs of faces (Oucher scale), ranging from smiling to frowning to crying with numeric scale.

4 years and older: Use four white poker chips to ask the child how many pieces of hurt he or she feels (no hurt = no chips).

6 years and older: Use a numeric scale, 0 to 5 or 0 to 10 (verbally or visually); use blank drawing of body, front and back, asking the child to use three different crayons to color places with a little pain, medium pain, and a lot of pain (Eland Color Tool).

"Are there any other symptoms associated with your discomfort (nausea, vomiting, numbness)?"

Ask what effect pain has had or is anticipated to have on the following patterns:

Work/activity (work/home activities, leisure/play)
Relationships/relating (wanting to be alone, with people)
Sleep (difficulty falling asleep/staying asleep)
Eating (appetite, weight gain/loss)
Elimination (bowel, constipation/diarrhea, bladder)
Menses
Sex (libido, function)

Assess for Cultural Influences on Pain

Country of origin
Time in United States
Native language
Ability to understand/speak English
Availability of interpreter
Religious practices (blood transfusion, specific clothing, male attendants)

Food, beverage preferences
Hygiene practices

Pruritus
Onset
Precipitated by what
Site(s)
Relieved by what
History of allergy (individual, family)

Nausea/Vomiting
Onset, duration
Vomitus (amount, appearance)
Frequency, severity
Relief measures

Objective Data (Acute/Chronic Pain)

Assess for Defining Characteristics

Behavioral Manifestations

Mood
Calmness
Moaning
Crying
Grimacing
Pacing
Restlessness
Oriented to time and place
Withdrawn

When the behaviors associated with pain are not present, it should not be assumed that pain is absent (Pasero & McCaffery, 2011).

Musculoskeletal Manifestations

Mobility of Painful Part

Muscle Tone

Dermatologic Manifestations
Color (redness)
Moisture/diaphoresis
Temperature
Edema

Cardiorespiratory Manifestations

Sensory Alterations
Paresthesia
Dysesthesias

Developmental Manifestations

Infant
Irritability
Changes in eating or sleeping
Inconsolability
Generalized body movements

Toddler
Irritability
Changes in eating or sleeping
Aggression (kicking, biting)
Rocking
Sucking
Clenched teeth

Preschool
Irritability
Changes in eating or sleeping
Aggression
Verbal expressions of pain

School-Aged
Changes in eating or sleeping
Change in play patterns
Verbal expressions of pain
Denial of pain

Adolescent
Mood changes
Behavior extremes (“acting out”)
Verbal expressions when asked
Changes in eating or sleeping

For clients unable to provide self-report (e.g., coma, confusion), one Pain Assessment Checklist for individual with limited ability to communicate (PACSLAC) addresses (*Fuchs-Lacrelle & Hadjistavropoulos, 2004) the following:
Facial expression
Activity/Body movements
Social/Personality/Mood
Other behaviors (physiological changes, eating, sleeping changes, voice behaviors)

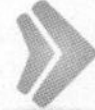

Carp's Cues

The assessment of pain in individuals who cannot communicate verbally their pain, severity and site is extremely difficult and frustrating. The PACSLAC is one example of a tool to achieve the assessment. The above adapted scale is presented as a reference only. Access the exact tool, the scoring guideline, and permission to utilize this scale through the office of Thomas Hadjistavropoulos at the University of Regina, Canada.

Principles of Assessing Individual With Cognitive Deficits or Comatose (Miller, 2015)

Assess individual in several types of conditions as resting, walking, during activities of daily living, different times in day.
Observe for nonverbal indicators (e.g., increased confusion, withdrawal, resistance/combativeness).
Observations from family, other caregivers

Goals

NOC
Symptom Control, Comfort Status, Pain Level

The individual will report acceptable control of symptoms as evidenced by the following indicators:

- Describe factors that increase symptoms.
- Describe measures to improve comfort.

Interventions

NIC
Pruritus Management, Fever Treatment, Environmental Management: Comfort, Sleep Enhancement

Assess for Sources of Discomfort

- Pruritus
- Prolonged bed rest
- Fever

Explain Aggravating Factors Should be Avoided, Including the Following
(National Cancer Institute, 2011)

- Fluid loss secondary to fever, diarrhea, nausea and vomiting, or decreased fluid intake.
- Use of ointments (e.g., petroleum, mineral oil).
- Bathing with hot water.
- Use of soaps that contain detergents.
- Frequent bathing or bathing for longer than half an hour.
- Adding oil early to a bath.
- Genital deodorants or bubble baths.
- Dry environment.
- Sheets and clothing laundered with detergent.
- Tight restrictive clothing or clothing made of wool, synthetics, or other harsh fabric.
- Emotional stress.

Maintain Hygiene Without Producing Dry Skin

- Encourage frequent baths:
  - Use cool water when acceptable.
  - Use mild soap or soaps made for sensitive skin (Castile, lanolin) or soap substitute.
  - Blot skin dry; do not rub.

Prevent Excessive Dryness (National Cancer Institute, 2011)

- Lubricate skin with a moisturizer or emollients, unless contraindicated; pat on with hand or gauze.
- Apply ointments/lotions with gloved or bare hand, depending on type, to lightly cover skin; rub creams into skin.

- Use frequent, thin applications of ointment, rather than one thick application.
- Apply emollient creams or lotions at least two or three times daily and after bathing. Recommended emollient creams include Eucerin or Nivea or lotions such as Lubriderm, Alpha Keri, or Nivea.
- Avoid skin products containing alcohol and menthol.
- Avoid petroleum products on irradiated skin.

R: *Petrolatum is poorly absorbed by irradiated skin and is not easily removed. A thick layer could produce an undesired bolus effect when applied within a radiation treatment field.*

- Limiting bathing to half an hour daily or every other day.
- Adding oil at the end of a bath or adding a colloidal oatmeal treatment early to the bath.
- Avoid topical agents including talcum powders, perfumed powders, bubble baths, and cornstarch.

R: *They can irritate the skin and cause pruritus.*

- Use of cornstarch to areas of irradiated skin following bathing.

R: *"Cornstarch has been an acceptable intervention for pruritus associated with dry desquamation related to radiation therapy, but it should not be applied to moist skin surfaces, areas with hair, sebaceous glands, skin folds or areas close to mucosal surfaces" (National Cancer Institute, 2011)*

- Avoid underarm deodorants or antiperspirants during radiation therapy.

R: *Agents with metal ions (i.e., talcum and aluminum used in antiperspirants) enhance skin reactions during external beam radiation therapy and should be avoided throughout the course of radiation therapy.*

- Apply lubrication after bath, before skin is dry, to encourage moisture retention.
- Apply wet dressings continuously or intermittently. Provide 20- to 30-minute tub soaks of 32° F to 38° F; water can contain oatmeal powder, Aveeno, cornstarch, or baking soda.

R: *Hydration will relieve itching and remove crusts and exudates.*

- Avoid excessive warmth or dryness; create a humid environment (e.g., humidifier).

R: *"Heat increases cutaneous blood flow and may enhance itching. Heat also lowers humidity, and skin loses moisture when the relative humidity is less than 40%. A cool, humid environment may reverse these processes" (National Cancer Institute, 2011).*

- Avoid perfumes, cosmetics, deodorants, rough fabrics, fatigue, stress, and monotony (lack of distractions) (Yarbro, Wujcik, & Gobel, 2013).

R: *Pruritus is aggravated by conditions that stimulate nerve endings.*

Promote Comfort and Prevent Further Injury

- Advise against scratching; explain the scratch–itch–scratch cycle.

R: *The Scratch–Itch–Scratch Cycle. Itch produces scratching which increases inflammation and causes excitation of nerve fibers, leading to more itching and scratching (Grossman & Porth, 2014).*

- Teaching to apply a cool washcloth or ice over the site may be useful. Firm pressure at the site of itching, at a site contralateral to the site of itching, and at acupressure points may break the neural pathway.

R: *These techniques can break the stimulation of neural pathway (Scratch–Itch–Scratch) (National Cancer Institute, 2011).*

- Secure order for topical corticosteroid cream for local inflamed pruritic areas; apply sparingly and occlude area with plastic wrap at night to increase effectiveness of cream and prevent further scratching.
- Secure an antihistamine order if itching is unrelieved, increased doses at bedtime.
- Use mitts (or cotton socks), if necessary, on children and confused adults.
- Maintain trimmed nails to prevent injury; file after trimming.
- Remove particles from bed (food crumbs, caked powder).
- Use old, soft or cotton sheets and avoid wrinkles in bed; if bed protector pads are used, place sheet over them to eliminate direct contact with skin.

R: *Anything that scratches the skin will stimulate itching.*

- Washing of sheets, clothing, and undergarments in mild soaps for infant clothing (e.g., Dreft, Purrex). Avoid use of fabric softeners. Double rinse or add 1 teaspoon of white vinegar per quart of water to rinse water (National Cancer Institute, 2011).

R: *Residue left by detergents and other washing additives, for example, softeners, antistatic may aggravate pruritus. Detergent residue can be neutralized by the addition of vinegar (1 teaspoon per quart of water) to rinse water.*

- Wearing of loose-fitting clothing and clothing made of cotton or other soft fabrics.

R: *Dryness increases skin sensitivity by stimulating nerve endings.*

Proceed With Health Teaching, When Indicated

- Explain causes of pruritus and possible prevention methods.
- Explain factors that increase symptoms (e.g., low humidity, heat).
- Explain interventions that relieve symptoms (e.g., fluid intake of 3,000 mL/day unless contraindicated).
- Teach about medications, such as diuretics, that decrease skin moisture.
- Advise about exposure to sun and heat and protective products.
- Teach the client to avoid fabrics that irritate skin (wool, coarse textures).
- Teach to wear protective clothing (rubber gloves, apron) when using chemical irritants.
- Refer for allergy testing, if indicated.
- Provide opportunity to discuss frustrations.

R: *Refer to preceding rationales.*

For a Client on Bed Rest (Refer Also to *Disuse Syndrome* for Specific Interventions)

- Vary position at least every 2 hours unless other variables necessitate more frequent changes.
- Use small pillows or folded towels to support limbs.
- Vary positions with flexion and extension, abduction, or adduction.
- Use prone position if tolerable.

R: *Frequent position changes maintain musculoskeletal function and prevent contractures.*

Pediatric Interventions

- Refer also to Interventions above.
- Explain to children why they should not scratch.
- Dress the child in long sleeves, long pants, or a one-piece outfit to prevent scratching.
- Avoid overdressing the child, which will increase warmth.
- Give the child a tepid bath before bedtime; add two cups of cornstarch to bath water.
- Apply Caladryl lotion to weeping pruritic lesions; apply with small paintbrush.
- Use cotton blankets or sheets next to skin.
- Remove furry toys that may increase lint and pruritus.
- Teach the child to press or (if permitted) put a cool cloth on the area that itches, but not to scratch.

R: *See rationales for Interventions.*

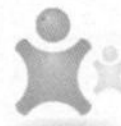

Maternal Interventions

- Explain changes in breast expected during pregnancy:
  - Increase in size, firmness, and tenderness.

R: *Milk glands and fat tissue will enlarge as your blood supply increases. Your nipples can also darken, and sometimes a thick fluid called colostrum may leak from your breasts. All of these changes are normal.*

  - Bluish veins, darkened nipples

R: *This is caused by increase blood supply.*

  - Thick fluid from nipples

- Instruct to
  - Wear a firm support bra big enough not to irritate nipples (e.g., maternity or nursing bra).
  - Choose cotton bras or those made from natural fibers.
  - Try wearing a bra during the night.
  - If breast are leaking, use breast pads or gauze pads.
  - Wash your breasts with warm water only. Don't use soap or other products that can cause dryness.

R: *Good support and protection of nipples can prevent discomfort and nipple skin irritation.*

- Explain fatigue in early pregnancy is related to the increased metabolic needs of the growing fetus and/ or anemia
- Advise a short rest period every day, for example, ½ hour to 1 hour with legs elevated

R: *Even though pregnancy is not an illness, this fatigue can prevent proper nutrition and increase nausea. Elevating legs can help prevent varicosities and reduce the risk of thrombophlebitis (Pillitteri, 2014).*

- Explain the sources of muscle discomforts in pregnancy:
  - Pressure across some joints is increased up to twofold.
  - Exaggerated lordosis of the lower back
  - Joint laxity in the ligaments of the lumbar spine creates more instability.
  - Widening and increased mobility of the sacroiliac joints and pubic symphysis in preparation for the fetus' passage through the birth canal

R: *During pregnancy, women gain 25 to 35 pounds, on average, and undergo multiple hormonal changes and biomechanical alterations that strain the axial skeleton and pelvis (Bermas, 2014).*

- Teach the following to prevent or manage strain on back muscles:
  - Avoid heavy lifting or get assistance; use leg muscles, not back muscles.
  - Place one foot higher than the other when standing for prolonged periods.
  - Wear low heeled shoes with good arch support, but not flat.
  - Place a board between the mattress and box spring if your bed is too soft.
    - Squat down, bend knees and keep the back straight when lifting.
    - Sit in chairs with good back support, or use a small pillow to provide support.
    - Sleep on the side with pillows between the knees for support.
    - Apply heat, cold, or massage to the painful area.
  - Practice pelvic rocking or tilt throughout the day.
    - Apply heat or cold to back two or three times daily.
- If leg cramps occur and are not caused by thrombophlebitis, teach the client to flex or bend foot and not massage. Instruct the client to stretch calf muscles before going to bed.

R: *Lowered serum calcium and increased phosphate levels are thought to increase neuromuscular irritability and leg cramps (Pillitteri, 2014)*

- Advise to consult with their pregnancy provider if acetaminophen is an option.

R: *Acetaminophen (Tylenol) is considered safe and effective during pregnancy (Pillitteri, 2014).*

Acute Pain

NANDA-I Definition

Unpleasant sensory and emotional experience arising from actual or potential tissue damage or described in terms of such damage (International Association for the Study of Pain); sudden or slow onset of any intensity from mild to severe with anticipated or predictable end and a duration of <6 months

Defining Characteristics

Appetite changes
Physiologic responses (e.g., mean arterial pressure [MAP], heart rate [HR], respiratory rate [RR], transcutaneous oxygen saturation [SpO_2], and end-tidal CO_2)
Diaphoresis
Distraction behavior (e.g., pacing, seeking out other people and/or activities, repetitive activities)
Expressive behavior (e.g., restlessness, moaning, crying)
Facial expressions of pain (e.g., eyes lack luster, beaten look, fixed or scattered movement, grimace)
Guarding behavior
Hopelessness
Narrowed focus (e.g., altered time perception, impaired thought processes, reduced interaction with people and environment)

Narrowed focus (e.g., altered time perception, impaired thought processes, reduced interaction with people and environment)
Observed evidence of pain using standardized pain behavior checklists
For those unable to verbally communicate (e.g., Behavioral Pain Scale, Neonatal Infant Pain Scale, Pain Assessment Checklist for seniors with limited ability to communicate)
Positioning to avoid pain
Protective gestures
Proxy reporting of pain and behavior/activity changes (e.g., family members, caregivers)
Pupillary dilation
Self-focusing
Self-report of intensity using standardized pain intensity scales (e.g., Wong–Baker FACES scale, visual analogue scale, numeric rating scale)
Self-report of pain characteristics (e.g., aching, burning, electric shock, pins and needles, shooting, sore/tender, stabbing, throbbing) using standardized pain scales (e.g., McGill Pain Questionnaire, Brief Pain Inventory

Related Factors

See *Impaired Comfort.*

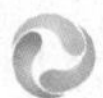 Author's Note

Nursing management of pain presents specific challenges. Is acute pain a response that nurses treat as a nursing diagnosis or collaborative problem? Is acute pain the etiology of another response that better describes the condition that nurses treat? Does some cluster of nursing diagnoses represent a pain syndrome or CPS (e.g., *Fear, Risk for Ineffective Family Coping, Impaired Physical Mobility, Social Isolation, Ineffective Sexuality Patterns, Risk for Colonic Constipation, Fatigue*)? McCaffery and Beebe (*1989) cite 18 nursing diagnoses that can apply to people experiencing pain. Viewing pain as a syndrome diagnosis can provide nurses with a comprehensive nursing diagnosis for people in pain to whom many related nursing diagnoses could apply.

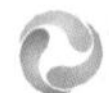 Errors in Diagnostic Statements

Acute Pain related to surgical incision

For a client who has undergone surgery, the nurse focuses on reducing pain to permit increased participation in activities and to reduce anxiety, as described by the nursing diagnosis *Acute Pain related to surgical manipulation of body structures, flatus, and progressive need for increased activity*

Acute Pain related to cardiac tissue ischemia

The nurse has several responsibilities for a client experiencing chest pain: Evaluating cardiac status, reducing activity, administering PRN medication, and reducing anxiety. Before discharge, the nurse teaches self-monitoring, self-medication, signs and symptoms of complications, follow-up care, and necessary lifestyle modifications. *Acute Pain related to cardiac tissue ischemia* is correct, however other diagnoses are needed evaluation and management of chest pain involves nurse-prescribed and physician-prescribed interventions, so this situation should be described as the collaborative problem *Risk for Complications of Decreased Cardiac Output*. This collaborative problem encompasses various cardiac complications (e.g., dysrhythmias, acute coronary syndrome cardiogenic shock, and angina).

CLINICAL ALERT There is an ethical duty to relieve pain (*Johnson, Fudala, Payne, 2005). Nurses should be as aggressive in advocating for effective pain relief for their individuals as they would be if the individual was their child, mother, partner, or best friend. Those most in need for effective pain relief may be the poor, uneducated, substance abuser, and others who are voiceless in the health-care system.

The research reports the following:

- **Under treatment of pain in the elderly has been described by Denny and Guido (2012).**
- **Greco et al. (2014) reported that pain management of cancer has improved since last reported in 2008 but 1/3 of individuals "still do not receive pain medication proportional to their pain intensity."**

- Deandrea et al. (2010) reported that 40% of individuals with cancer pain are undertreated.
- Undertreatment of pain management in children undergoing painful procedures has been reported to occur over 2/3 of the time by Stevent et al. (2011).
- "All neonates in the Neonatal Intensive Care Unit (NICU) or during the first days of life undergo painful and stressful procedures. Epidemiologic studies have shown that pain induced by these procedures is not effectively prevented or is inadequately treated" (Walter-Nicole, Annequin, Biran, Mitanchez, & Tourniaire, 2010).
- Mosset (2011) reported, "Racial/ethnic minorities consistently receive less adequate treatment for acute and chronic pain than non-Hispanic whites, even after controlling for age, gender, and pain intensity. Pain intensity underreporting appears to be a major contribution of minority individuals to pain management disparities. The major contribution by physicians to such disparities appears to reflect limited awareness of their own cultural beliefs and stereotypes regarding pain, minority individuals, and use of narcotic analgesics." In addition the researcher reported, "there is consistent evidence that racial/ethnic minority individuals are overrepresented among those who experience such pain and whose pain management is inadequate".

Key Concepts

General Considerations

- All pain is real, regardless of its cause. Pure psychogenic pain is probably rare, as is pure organic pain. Most bodily pain is a combination of mental events (psychogenic) and physical stimuli (organic).
- Pain has two components: Sensory, which is neurophysiologic, and perceptual or experiential, which has cognitive and emotional origins. The interaction of these two components determines the amount of suffering (Grossman & Porth, 2014).
- Pain tolerance means the duration and intensity of pain that a client is willing to endure. It differs among individual, cultures, and may vary in one client in different situations, for example, time of day, level of stress, fatigue.
- Pain threshold is the point at which a client reports that a stimulus is painful (Pasero & McCaffery, 2011).
- Pain can be classified as acute or chronic, according to cause and duration, not intensity.
  - *Acute pain* can last for 1 second to less than 6 months. The cause is usually organic disease or injury. With healing, the pain subsides and eventually disappears.
  - *Chronic pain* lasts for 3 to 6 months or longer. It can be described as limited, intermittent, or persistent.
  - *Limited pain* results from a known physical lesion, but pain will end (e.g., burns).
  - *Intermittent pain* provides the client with pain-free periods. The cause may or may not be known (e.g., headaches).
  - *Persistent pain* usually occurs daily. The cause may or may not be known and is usually not a threat to life (e.g., low back pain).
- The individual may respond to acute pain physiologically by diaphoresis and increased blood pressure and heart and respiratory rates and behaviorally by crying, moaning, or showing anger.
- The individual with chronic pain usually has adapted to it, both physiologically and behaviorally. Thus, he or she may not show visible signs of the pain.
- Price (*1999) defined pain as "a somatic perception containing (as cited in Rosenquist, 2015):
  - a bodily sensation with qualities like those reported during tissue-damaging stimulation,
  - an experienced threat associated with this sensation, and
  - a feeling of unpleasantness or other negative emotion based on this experienced threat."

The American Society of Anesthesiologists (2010) defines "chronic pain as pain of any etiology not directly related to neoplastic involvement, extending in duration beyond the expected temporal boundary of tissue injury and normal healing and adversely affecting the function or well-being of the individual."

Placebos

- Studies have shown that diagnosed physiologic pain can respond to placebos, so a positive response to placebo cannot be used to diagnose pain as psychogenic. Placebos are inappropriate to use except in approved clinical studies for the following reasons (Pasero & McCaffery, 2011):
  - Placebos may be effective for one client at one time and not at another.
  - Placebos often are used to prove a client wrong.
  - "Deceit is harmful to both patients and health-care professionals."
  - "Literature review shows no basis for the assumption that placebo pain medication is useful to patients." The use of placebos constitutes "liability for fraud, malpractice, breach of contract, and medical negligence."

Carp's Cues

"While the under treatment of pain is a recognized issue amongst pain researchers, we argue that the concept of 'pseudoaddiction' is problematic because it ultimately relies on a clinical judgment that attempts to separate out 'bad' drug seeking addicts from 'good 'undertreated pain patients in the face of behaviors that are *virtually indistinguishable*" (Bell & Salmon, 2009).

In the practice of this author as a family nurse practitioner, I encounter weekly requests for controlled medications. After careful assessments, if I am still uncertain if the request is due to undertreated pain or abuse, I will prescribe the medication at this visit for 14 days. On the next visit with additional assessment, I can better differentiate the origins of the request, I can differentiate the legitimate request from those that are not. This practice has caused me to sometimes prescribe once for a drug-seeking addict or street entrepreneur. But most importantly, I did not deprive a person with creditable pain the medication for relief of their pain. I can live with both outcomes.

Drug Tolerance, Drug Dependence, Addiction

- "Because the prescription of opiate drugs is central to its clinical practice, pain medicine has developed a definition of addiction which does not implicate drugs as the primary agents of addictive disorder. Instead it constructs addiction as a psychological disorder recognizable by the addict's out of control behavior, her drug-focused lifestyle and her destructive patterns of drug use. The prevention of addiction in the pain clinic therefore centers on the identification of certain 'at risk' and predisposed individuals, including those with a past history of substance abuse. These risky patients require extra-vigilant monitoring and surveillance if they are to be prescribed opiate drugs. Clinicians must be alert to any aberrant or suspicious behavior such as noncompliance, aggression, erratic appointments, doctor-shopping and stories of lost and stolen medication which may indicate the development of addiction" (American Society of Addiction Medicine, 2015).
- Addiction is a primary, chronic disease of brain reward, motivation, memory, and related circuitry. Dysfunction in these circuits leads to characteristic biological, psychological, social, and spiritual manifestations. This is reflected in an individual pathologically pursuing reward and/or relief by substance use and other behaviors (American Society of Addiction Medicine, 2015).
- Addiction is characterized by inability to consistently abstain, impairment in behavioral control, craving, diminished recognition of significant problems with one's behaviors and interpersonal relationships, and a dysfunctional emotional response. Like other chronic diseases, addiction often involves cycles of relapse and remission. Without treatment or engagement in recovery activities, addiction is progressive and can result in disability or premature death (American Society of Addiction Medicine, 2015).
- "Addiction is a chronic or relapsing condition for many individuals. Yet the traditional treatment model for addiction has emphasized episodic intensive treatment for medically supervised substance withdrawal and/or stabilization, followed by time-limited outpatient care" (Bell & Salmon, 2009).
- "In the context of pain treatment, opiates are not dangerous illicit substances but effective and safe analgesics appropriate for long-term use in selected individuals."
- "At its core, addiction isn't just a social problem or a moral problem or a criminal problem. It's a brain problem whose behaviors manifest in all these other areas" (Bell & Salmon, 2009).
- Pseudoaddiction is a term that has been used to describe patient behaviors that may occur when pain is undertreated. Patients with unrelieved pain may become focused on obtaining medications, may "clock watch," and may otherwise seem inappropriately "drug-seeking." Even such behaviors as illicit drug use and deception can occur in the patient's efforts to obtain relief (American Psychiatric Association [APA], 2014).
- Pseudoaddiction can be distinguished from true addiction in that the behaviors resolve when pain is effectively treated (Bell & Salmon, 2009).
- Drug tolerance occurs when the person no longer responds to the drug in the way that person initially responded. Higher doses are required for an effective response. There is no compulsive use of the drug but withdrawal symptoms can occur (National Institute of Drug Abuse, 2007).
- Drug dependence syndrome as being a cluster of physiological, behavioral, and cognitive phenomena in which the use of a substance or a class of substances takes on a much higher priority for a given individual than other behaviors that once had greater value (Hockenberry & Wilson, 2015; WHO, 2015).
- The drug is needed for the individual to function normally (National Institute of Drug Abuse, 2007).
- *Multimodal therapy (balanced analgesia)* involves the use of two or three classes of analgesics (nonsteroidal anti-inflammatory agents, opioids, and local anesthetics). This approach allows for lower doses of each drug in the plan. The use of one or two classes can prevent both inflammatory and neuropathic pain. Lower doses of several analgesics reduce the likelihood of significant side effects from a single agent or method (Pasero & McAffery, 2011).

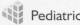

Pediatric Considerations

- Studies have shown that, when adults and children undergo the same surgery, children are undermedicated (Hockenberry & Wilson, 2015). In one study, 52% of the children received no analgesic postoperatively, whereas the remaining 48% received predominately aspirin or acetaminophen.
- Despite continual evaluation and advances in treatment options for pain management in children, children and adolescents continue to suffer from inadequately treated pain (Hockenberry & Wilson, 2015).
- Always use the appropriate pain scale with consideration to the patient's developmental age (e.g., FLACC, rFLACC, FACES, Numeric) and be consistent with that scale's use.
- Maturational and chronologic age, cause of pain, coping style, parental response, culture, past pain experiences, and whether pain is acute or chronic influence the child's response to pain and therefore influence the team's approach to pain management.

Infant

- Cries
- Will respond physically to source of pain (e.g., local reflex withdrawal from source of pain and generalized stiffening)
- Cries loudly and makes verbal protests long after the stimulus is withdrawn, but will console with comfort from parent
- May exhibit poor feeding

Toddler

- Fears body intrusion
- Does not understand rationale for pain or have ability to conceptualize the duration of the experience even if told
- Will respond more deliberately to avoid source of pain (e.g., pushing away from pain source or attempt to cling to parent)
- Seeks out parental figures as a source of comfort

Preschooler

- Engages in magical thinking or fantasies (e.g., believes something they thought or did may have caused the pain)
- Uses increased verbal skills to communicate pain but also cries and screams
- Still responds physically and deliberately with more purpose to avoid pain (e.g., kicking, thrashing, pushing away)
- After pain passes, talks to toys or other children/family about the pain experience
- Is able to experience anticipation anxiety of painful procedure
- Denies pain, especially if he or she associates it with adverse consequences (e.g., injection as a punishment for bad behavior)

School-Aged

- Fears body injury
- Can describe the cause, type, quality, and severity of pain
- May display time-wasting behavior, stalling
- Attempts to relate the pain experience to previous events and gain control over actions
- Denies pain, especially if he or she associates it with adverse consequences
- May be influenced by presence of parents in expressing pain

Adolescent

- Considers body image as very important
- Will typically display less verbal and physical resistance
- May use overconfidence to compensate for fear
- May use more "socially acceptable" behavioral responses to pain than do younger children, but fear and anxiety may not necessarily be decreased
- May also be influenced by presence of parents in verbalizing their assessment of their pain

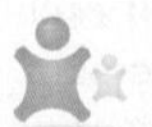

Maternal Considerations

- Refer to *Labor Pain.*

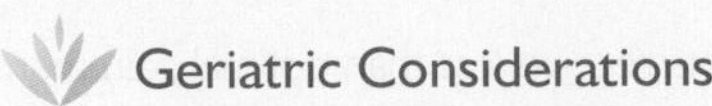

Geriatric Considerations

- "The results of the study indicated that >90% of the elderly living in the community experienced pain within the past month, with 41% reporting discomforting, distressing, horrible, or excruciating pain." Over 28% of those with moderate or severe pain reported they experience continuous pain (Brown, Kirkpatrick, Swanson, & McKenzie, 2011).
- "Musculoskeletal pain (92%) was found to be the most predominant pain, and inactivity was the most effective strategy used to lessen pain" (Brown et al., 2011).
- "For a variety of reasons, older adults may be more hesitant than younger individuals to report pain. Some 'barriers' to discussing pain include: perception that pain simply is a concomitant of aging; reluctance to 'bother' their clinician with complaints of pain; not wanting to detract the clinician's attention away from other 'medical' complaints. Older adults also may use different descriptive terms for their pain (aching, soreness, hurting, discomfort), including some that are not included in commonly used pain instruments" (Rosenquist, 2015).
- Pain is omnipresent in older adults and may be accepted by them and professionals as a normal and unavoidable accompaniment to aging. Unfortunately, many chronic diseases that are common in older adults, such as osteoarthritis and rheumatoid arthritis, may not receive adequate pain management (Brown et al., 2011; Denny & Guido, 2012; Pasero & McCaffery, 2011).
- Older adults may not demonstrate objective signs and symptoms of pain because of years of adaptation and increased pain tolerance. They may eventually accept the pain, thereby lowering expectations for comfort and mobility. Pain-coping mechanisms cultivated throughout life are important to identify and reinforce in pain management. Effective pain management can greatly improve overall physical functioning and emotional well-being (Miller, 2015).
- The effects of narcotic opioid analgesics are prolonged in older adults because of decreased metabolism and clearance of the drug. Also, side effects seem to be more frequent and pronounced, especially anticholinergic effects, extrapyramidal effects, and sedation. For older adults, it is advised that drugs be started at a lower dosage. Because older adults often take multiple drugs, drug interactions should be monitored (Arcangelo & Peterson, 2016).

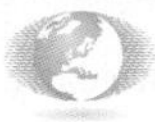

Transcultural Considerations

- See *Impaired Comfort*.

Focus Assessment Criteria

See *Impaired Comfort*.

Goals

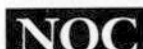

NOC

Comfort Level, Pain Control, Knowledge: Acute Illness Management

The client will experience a satisfactory relief measure as evidenced by (specify):

- Reporting a pain score that was determined to be acceptable by him/her
- Increased participation in activities of recovery
- Reduction in pain behaviors (specify)
- Improvement in mood, coping

Interventions

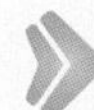

Carp's Cues

"This tendency to feel that one's own cultural norms are correct and to evaluate others' beliefs in light of them is known as ethnocentrism. Most everyone is ethnocentric. Most of us tend to believe that attitudes and behaviors that match our own are correct and those that don't are abnormal, wrong, or inferior" (Narayan, 2010).

Researchers from the American Pain Society reported that disparities in pain management are evident over a wide variety of conditions and types of pain, including acute bone fractures, metastatic cancer, and postsurgical and chronic pain, and across multiple treatment settings (EDs, hospitals, long-term care facilities, home health care, palliative care, and others) (*Green, 2002).

NIC
Pain Management, Medication Management, Emotional Support, Teaching: Individual, Hot/Cold Application, Simple Massage, Anxiety Reduction, Relaxation Therapy

"As distasteful as it is to consider, nurses must examine whether some patients receive less than optimal pain management because of prejudicial stereotypes or negative judgments based on race or ethnicity" (Narayan, 2010[6]).

Explore the Individual's/Families' Pain Experience and the Influences of Their Culture (Narayan, 2010)

R: *To determine how best to help a person with pain, nurses must first discern how he/she thinks and feels about the pain experience (Narayan, 2010).*

- Language and interpretation problems.
- Reluctance to share personal complaints.

R: *Some cultural groups tend to instill in their members self-efficacy—a sense of control over life, including how to respond to and manage pain.*

- Believe they can exert little influence over the future, for example, fatalistic
- Pain is viewed as something to be tolerated or deserved as a punishment.
- Confusion over nonverbal behaviors
- Reluctance to use pain medications, for example, fears of misuse, cultural taboos

R: *Effective communication is essential for valid pain assessments. Many nonverbal cues such as facial expression, body posture, and activity level can also vary among cultures and thus be misinterpreted. Culture beliefs can present as barriers to this assessment.*

Reduce or Eliminate Factors That Increase Pain

Disbelief From Others

R: *Trying to convince health-care providers that he or she is experiencing pain will cause the client anxiety, which compounds the pain. Both are energy depleting.*

- Establish a supportive accepting relationship:
  - Acknowledge the pain.
  - Listen attentively to their discussion of their pain.
  - Convey that you are assessing pain because you want to understand it better (not determine if it really exists).
- Assess the family for any misconceptions about pain or its treatment:
  - Explain the concept of pain as an individual experience.
  - Discuss factors related to increased pain and options to manage.
  - Encourage family members to share their concerns privately (e.g., fear of addiction).

Lack of Knowledge/Uncertainty

- Explain the cause of the pain, if known.
- Relate the severity of the pain and how long it will last, if known.
- Explain diagnostic tests and procedures in detail by relating the discomforts and sensations that the individual will feel; approximate the duration.

R: *People who are prepared for painful procedures by explanations of the actual sensations experience less stress than those who receive vague explanations.*

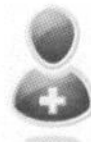

Clinical Alert Support the individual in addressing specific questions regarding diagnosis, risks, benefits of treatment, and prognosis. Consult with the specialist or primary care provider. If there are barriers to full disclosure, refer to *Risk for Compromised Human Dignity*.

Fear of Addiction

- Provide accurate information to reduce fear of addiction.
  - Explore reasons for the fear.
  - Explain the difference between drug tolerance, dependence, and addiction (see Key Concepts).
- Explain the taking prescribed opioids for pain is not the cause of addiction. In the context of pain treatment, opiates are not dangerous illicit substances but effective and safe analgesics appropriate for use in selected individuals.

[6]Narayan has published excellent article on cultural influences on managing pain with a focus on the client's culture and the nurses with Self-Assessment Questions to Help Nurses Determine Their Cultural Norms Concerning Pain. The reader is referred to the Narayan, M. C. (2010). Culture's effects on pain assessment and management. *The American Journal of Nursing, 110*(4), 38–47. Accessed at http://www.nursingcenter.com/lnc/cearticle?tid=998868#sthash.VV2KzGeo.dpuf

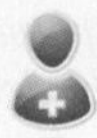

CLINICAL ALERT "In the context of pain treatment, opiates are not dangerous illicit substances but effective and safe analgesics appropriate for long-term use in selected individuals." "At its core, addiction isn't just a social problem or a moral problem or a criminal problem. It's a brain problem whose behaviors manifest in all these other areas" (Bell & Salmon 2009).

R: *Addiction is a psychological syndrome characterized by compulsive drug-seeking behavior generally associated with a desire for drug administration to produce euphoria or other effects, not pain relief. There is no evidence that adequate administration of opioids for pain produces addiction (Pasero & McCaffery, 2011).*

- Assist in reducing fear of losing control.
  - Include the individual in setting a realistic pain goal and in adopting strategies for pain control which are congruent with his or her beliefs and experiences.
  - Provide privacy for the client's pain experience.
  - Attempt to limit the number of health-care providers who provide care.
  - Allow the client to share intensity of pain; express how well he or she tolerated it.

R: *One's overt responses to pain can be embarrassing and unacceptable for some.*

Fatigue

- Determine the cause of fatigue (sedatives, analgesics, sleep deprivation).
- Explain that pain contributes to stress, which increases fatigue.
- Assess present sleep pattern and the influence of pain on sleep.
- Provide opportunities to rest during the day and with periods of uninterrupted sleep at night (must rest when pain is decreased).
- Consult with physician for an increased dose of pain medication at bedtime.
- Refer to *Insomnia* for specific interventions to enhance sleep.

R: *Relaxation and guided imagery effectively manage pain by increasing sense of control, reducing feelings of helplessness and hopelessness, providing a calming diversion, and disrupting the pain–anxiety–tension cycle (Rosenquest, 2015; *Sloman, 1995).*

Explore Nonpharmacological Treatments for Pain.

- Refer to *Chronic Pain* for interventions.

Provide Optimal Pain Relief With Prescribed Analgesics

R: *Analgesics should be initiated at the lowest effective dose, and titrated to achieve pain control with minimal adverse effects; this requires frequent reassessment of patients for pain relief and side effects as doses are adjusted. Localized use of medication (e.g., joint injections, trigger point injections) may be preferable to systemic medications (e.g., oral analgesics) when applicable (Galicia-Castillo & Weiner, 2014).*

- Use oral route when feasible, intravenous or rectal routes if needed with permission.
- Avoid intramuscular routes due to erratic absorption and unnecessary pain.

R: *Oral administration is preferred when possible. Liquid medications can be given to those who have difficulty swallowing.*

R: *If frequent injections are necessary, the IV route is preferred because it is not painful and absorption is guaranteed. Side effects (decreased respirations and blood pressure), however, may be more profound.*

R: *Intramuscular injections are less effective at offering pain control than PCA administration (*Chang et al., 2004).*

- Assess vital signs, especially respiratory rate, before administration.
- Consult with pharmacist for possible adverse interactions with other medications (e.g., muscle relaxants, tranquilizers).
- Use the around the clock (ATC) approach, not PRN.

R: *Paice, Noskin, Vanagunas (*2005) reported the results of comparing the use of ATC scheduled opioid doses with PRN opioid doses in medical inpatients and found that those who received ATC doses had lower pain intensity ratings. "As might be expected, a significantly greater percentage of the prescribed opioid was administered when it was given ATC (70.8%) compared with PRN (38%); however, there were no differences in adverse effects between the two groups" (Pasero, 2010).*

R: *The preventive approach may increase the total 24-hour dose compared with the PRN approach. The ATC approach will provide a constant therapeutic blood level of the drug, reducing cravings for the drug, and reducing the anxiety of having to ask and wait for PRN relief*

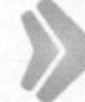

Carp's Cues

Pain management should be aggressive and individualized to eliminate unnecessary pain with drugs administered on a regular schedule rather than PRN. If resistance from prescribers is met, emphasize the benefits, especially if the individual's pain is being undertreated. Address myths of increased sedation side effects, not indicated for older adults. Bernhofer and Sorrell (2014) reported that barriers to optimal pain management were difficulties in nurse/physician communication and lack of pain education.

- Determine with the individual/family if the person should be awakened for a nighttime dose. Consider:
  - how well the person sleeps without it
  - what is the reported intensity of the pain if the nighttime dose is not given or delayed

R: *Since there is no research for direction, the nurse must assess each situation and determine the appropriate action (Pasero, 2010).*

R: *"The routine treatment of breakthrough pain is considered, in general, to be conventional practice in populations for which opioid therapy is the mainstay for the long-term management of moderate to severe pain—specifically those with active cancer or other types of advanced medical illness" (Pasero, 2010, p. 38).*

- Neuropathic pain is described as burning, stabbing, stinging, electric, pins and needles, shooting, or numbness.

R: *Nociceptive pain can be somatic and visceral. Somatic pain results from the activation of peripheral nociceptors as in muscle, joints, bone, or connective tissue. Visceral pain results from activation of nociceptors in the abdomen or thoracic cavity (McMenamin, 2011).*

- Nociceptive pain from nerve damage is responsive to anticonvulsants (gabapentin, pregabalin), selective serotonin reuptake inhibitors (SSRIs), tricyclic antidepressants (TCAs), clonidine, Lidoderm patches, and *N*-methyl-D-aspartate receptor antagonists (NMDAs) such as ketamine or methadone *(McMenamin, 2011).*

R: *Neuropathic pain results when there is abnormal processing of input by the peripheral or central nervous system (McMenamin, 2011).*

Assess the Individual's Response to the Pain-Relief Medication

- After administration, return in 30 minutes to assess effectiveness.
- Ask to rate severity of pain before the medication and amount of relief received.
- Ask to indicate when the pain began to increase. How long it has been since the last pain medication? After a certain activity (e.g., ambulation, dressing change)?
- Advise the client to request pain medication earlier. Plan pain-relief measures prior to activities.
- Consult with prescriber if a dosage or interval change is needed; the dose may be increased by 50% until effective (Pasero & McCaffery, 2011).
- Collaborate with the prescriber to multimodal analgesia.

R: *Multimodal analgesia, which uses two or three classes of analgesics, can be more effective than one class only. The combined lower doses of each class are more effective than higher doses of one class with less side effects (Pasero & McCaffery, 2013).*

Reduce or Eliminate Common Side Effects of Opioids

Sedation

- Identify risk factors for oversedation and respiratory depression include (Myers-Glower, 2013; Pasero & McCafferty, 2011):
  - First 24 hours of opioid therapy
  - Prolonged surgery
  - Thoracic surgery
  - Bolus injection of neuraxial morphine
  - Continuous opioid infusion in opioid-naïve persons
  - Use of benzodiazepines, antihistamines, diphenhydramine, sedatives, or other central nervous depressants

- Age older than 60 (the risk is 2.8 times greater from ages 61 to 70, 5.4 times greater from ages 71 to 80, and 8.7 greater times after age 80)
- Lack of recent opioid use
- Higher opioid dosage requirement or opioid habituation
- Sleep apnea
- Sleep disorders
- Pulmonary disorders
- Morbid obesity (BMI > 35) with an associated high risk of sleep apnea
- History of snoring
- History of smoking

- Carefully monitor individuals who are taking sedating medications and opioid analgesics for respiratory failure every hour for first 12 hours on opioids (Myers-Glower, 2013).
- Pulse oximetry, blood pressure, respiratory rate

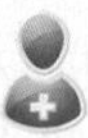

Clinical Alert If the person is receiving oxygen, pulse oximetry also may not provide accurate information. Oxygen saturation is a measure of gas exchange in the lung rather than a direct indicator of ventilatory efficacy.

- Signs and symptoms of hypercapnia (flushed skin, (early) full pulse, tachypnea, dyspnea, muscle twitches, hand flaps, reduced neural activity, and possibly increased blood pressure

R: *Significant hypercapnia may arise before oxygen desaturation occurs (Myers-Glower, 2013).*

- When individual appears to be sleeping, arouse him/her to differentiate between sleeping and sedation (Pasero & McCaffery, 2011).
  - Sleep—awake, alert, or slightly drowsy and easy to arouse
  - Sedation—arousable, increasing drowsiness, falls asleep during assessment, sombulent, little or no response to arousal attempts
  - Notify the prescriber or anesthesiologist for a reduction of opioid dose or if somnolent and difficult to arouse—stop opioid and intervene immediately, for example, rapid response team, diluted IV naloxone.
- Assess whether the cause is the opioid, fatigue, sleep deprivation, or other drugs (e.g., sedatives, antiemetic).
- Advise to ask for assistance to avoid injury (e.g., falls).

Constipation

For individuals with predisposing factors (advanced age, immobility, poor diet, intra-abdominal pathology, on other constipating medications) (Portenoy, Mehta, & Ahmed, 2015)

- Consider prophylactic laxative therapy, for example, senna 2 tablets at bedtime with or without a stool softener
- Increased fiber with increased fluids

R: *Opioids cause constipation reducing bowel motility and increased GI transit time, which causes excessive water and electrolyte reabsorption (Portenoy et al., 2015).*

Nausea and Vomiting (Refer to *Nausea*)

R: *Opioids cause nausea and vomiting due to its direct effect on chemoreceptor trigger, increases vestibular sensitivity, and delayed gastric emptying (Portenoy et al., 2015).*

Dry Mouth (Refer also to *Impaired Oral Mucous Membranes*)

- Explain that opioids decrease saliva production.
- Instruct the client to rinse mouth often, suck on sugarless sour candies, eat pineapple chunks or watermelon (if permissible), and drink liquids often.
- Explain the necessity of good oral hygiene and dental care.

R: *Opioid use can lower the amount of saliva in the mouth. Saliva helps flush out bacteria and prevent tooth decay.*

Assist Family to Respond Optimally to the Individual's Pain Experience

- Assess family's knowledge of pain and response to it.
- Give accurate information to correct misconceptions (e.g., addiction, doubt about pain).
- Provide each family member with opportunities to discuss fears, anger, and frustrations privately; acknowledge the difficulty of the situation.
- Incorporate family members in the pain-relief modality, if possible (e.g., stroking, massage).
- Praise their participation and concern.

R: *Helping the family to understand the pain experience can enhance positive coping (Pasero & McCafferty, 2011).*

Initiate Health Teaching, as Indicated

- Discuss with the individual and family noninvasive pain-relief measures (e.g., relaxation, distraction, massage, music).
- Teach the techniques of choice to the client and family.
- Explain the expected course of the pain (resolution) if known (e.g., fractured arm, surgical incision).
- Provide the client with written guidelines for weaning from pain medications when the acute event is relieved.

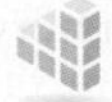

Pediatric Interventions

Assess the Child's Pain Experience

- Determine the child's concept of the cause of pain, if feasible.
- Ask the child to point to the area that hurts. See Focus Assessment Criteria under *Impaired Comfort*.
- Determine the intensity of the pain at its worst and best. Use a pain scale appropriate for the child's developmental age. Use the same scale the same way each time and encourage its use by parents and other health-care professionals. Indicate on the care plan which scale to use and how (introduction of scale, language specific for child); attach copy if visual scale (Hockenberry & Wilson, 2015).
- Ask the child what makes the pain better and what makes it worse.
- Include the parents' rating of their child's pain in assessment. Parents and nurses can rate a child's pain differently. The parents' observation is often more accurate (Kyle & Carman, 2013).
- Assess whether fear, loneliness, or anxiety is contributing to pain.
- Assess effect of pain on sleep and play. Note: A child who sleeps, plays, or both can still be in pain (sleep and play can serve as distractions).
- With infants, assess crying, facial expressions, body postures, and movements. Infants exhibit distress from environmental stimuli (light, sound) as well as from touch and treatments.
- Use tactile and vocal stimuli to comfort infants while assessing the effects of comfort measures and individualized interventions.
- Evaluate for potential cultural barriers/differences in regards to pain management. Families of different beliefs may have different opinions on pain management techniques and consequences of pain overall (Hockenberry & Wilson, 2015).
- Explain the pain source to the child, as developmentally appropriate, using verbal and sensory (visual, tactile) explanations (e.g., perform treatment on doll, allow the child to handle equipment). Explicitly explain and reinforce to the child that he or she is not being punished.

Assess the Child and Family for Misconceptions About Pain or Its Treatment

- Explain to the parents the necessity of good explanations to promote trust.
- Do not lie to parents, or especially the child, that something will not hurt if there is possibility that it likely will for the sake of easing the child's anxiety about pain. Doing this breeds mistrust between family/patient and the medical team.
- Explain to the parents that the child may cry more openly when they are present, but that their presence is important for promoting trust.
- Parents and older children may have misconceptions about analgesia and may fear narcotic use/abuse. Emphasize that narcotic use for moderate or severe pain that is prescribed by physicians and monitored by medical professionals would not lead to addition.

R: *Assessment of pain in children consists of three parts: the nature of the pain-producing pathology, the anatomic responses of acute pain, and the child's behaviors. It never should be based on only behavior.*

R: *Nurses, physicians, and the parents should identify and use consistent pain assessment criteria (e.g., assessment scale, specific behaviors) to assess pain in a child (Hockenberry & Wilson, 2015).*

Promote Security With Honest Explanations and Opportunities for Choice

Promote Open, Honest Communication

- Tell the truth; explain:
    - How much it will hurt
    - How long it will last
    - What will help with the pain

- Do not threaten (e.g., do not tell the child, "If you don't hold still, you won't go home.")
- Explain to the child that the procedure is necessary so he or she can get better and that holding still is important so it can be done quickly *and possibly with less pain.*
- Discuss with parents the importance of truth-telling. Instruct them to
  - Tell the child when they are leaving and when they will return.
  - Relate to the child that they cannot take away pain, but that they will be with him or her (except in circumstances when parents are not permitted to remain).
- Allow parents opportunities to share their feelings about witnessing their child's pain and their helplessness.

R: *Anxiety, fear, and separation can increase pain.*

Prepare the Child for a Painful Procedure

- Discuss the procedure with the parents; determine what they have told the child.
- Explain the procedure in words suited to the child's age and developmental level (see *Delayed Growth and Development* for age-appropriate needs).
- Relate the likely discomforts (e.g., what the child will feel, taste, see, or smell). "You will get an injection that will hurt for a little while and then it will stop."
- Be sure to explain when an injection will cause two discomforts: the prick of the needle and the injection of the drug.
- Encourage the child to ask questions before and during the procedure; ask the child to share what he or she thinks will happen and why.
- Share with the older child that:
  - You expect them to hold still and that it will please you if he or she can.
  - It is all right to cry or squeeze someone's hand if it hurts.
- Find something to praise after the procedure, even if the child could not hold still.
- Arrange to have the parents present for procedures (especially for young children) and explain to them what to expect before the procedure. Give them a role during the procedure such as holding child's hand or talking to them.

R: *Verbal communication usually is not sufficient or reliable to explain pain or painful procedures with younger children. The nurse can explain by demonstrating with pictures, dolls, or actual equipment as case-appropriate. The more senses that are stimulated in explanations to children, the greater the communication. When possible, parents should be included in preparation.*

Reduce the Pain During Treatments When Possible

- If restraints must be used, have sufficient clientele available so the procedure is not delayed *and so restraints are applied smoothly as not to increase anxiety/discomfort.*
- If injections are ordered, try to obtain an order for oral or IV analgesics instead. If injections must be used:
  - Expect the older child to hold still, however have extra staff available to assist with holding the younger child still to minimize increased pain or possible injury to staff or patient.
  - Consider use of topical analgesics prior to injections (e.g., LET/L-M-X4/EMLA gels and creams or vapocoolant sprays).
  - Have the child participate by holding the Band-Aid for you.
  - Tell the child how pleased you are that he or she helped.
  - Pull the skin surface as taught as possible for injections.
  - Comfort the child after the procedure, *or leave room so that parents can comfort child in the event that staff's presence continues to upset child.*
- Tell child step-by-step what is going to happen right before it is done.
- Offer the child, as age-appropriate, the option of learning distraction techniques for use during procedure. (The use of distraction without the child's knowledge of the impending discomfort is not advocated because the child will learn to mistrust.)
  - Tell a story with a puppet.
  - Use a cell phone, hand-held gaming device, and/or electronic tablet.
  - Blow a party noisemaker, pinwheels, or bubbles.
  - Ask the child to name or count objects in a picture.
  - Ask the child to look at the picture and to locate certain objects (e.g., "Where is the dog?").
  - Ask the child to tell you a story or about something from their lives.
  - Ask the child to count your blinks.

- Avoid rectal thermometers in preschoolers; if possible, use other methods such as tympanic, temporal, or oral (if tolerated) as allowed by the medical institution's guidelines and protocols.
  - Provide the child with privacy during the painful procedure; use a treatment room rather than the child's bed.
  - The child's bed should be a "safe place."
  - No procedures should be done in the playroom or schoolroom.

R: *School-aged children can understand why a procedure needs to be done. Assessments tools can be used.*

Provide the Child Optimal Pain Relief With Prescribed Analgesics

- Medicate child before painful procedure or activity (e.g., dressing change, obtaining x-ray of fractured limb, ambulation, injection/PIV placement).
- Consult with physician for change of the IM route to the IV route when appropriate.
- Assess appropriateness of medication, dose, and schedule for cause of pain, child's weight, and child's response, not age.
- Along with using pain assessment scales, observe for behavioral signs of pain (because the child may deny pain); if possible, identify specific behaviors that indicate pain in an individual child.
- Assess the potential for use of patient-controlled analgesia (PCA), which provides intermittent controlled doses of IV analgesia (with or without continuous infusion) as determined by the child's need. Children as young as 5 years can use PCA. Parents of children physically unable can administer it to them. PCA has been found to be safe and to provide superior pain relief compared with conventional-demand analgesia (Ball, Bindler, & Cowen, 2015).
- Consult with physician about the use of epidural infusion of morphine for treatment of postoperative pain. Epidural morphine infusion has been used safely in both adults and children in nonintensive care settings.
- Conscious sedation can be used for longer or more invasive procedures or treatments. It refers to a medically induced, depressed level of consciousness through a combination of drugs including, benzodiazepines (e.g., Versed), hypnotics/barbiturates (Pentobarbital), and dissociatives (Ketamine) (Ball et al., 2015). When under appropriate level of conscious sedation, the child will not require intubation; however, close monitoring is required with emergency equipment being readily available.
- Use of regional blocks with Lidocaine for invasive emergent procedures can be considered. In these cases, the Lidocaine can be buffered with sodium bicarbonate to decrease discomfort caused by injection of the Lidocaine (Ball et al., 2015).

R: *Assessment of pain in children consists of three parts: (1) the nature of the pain-producing pathology, (2) the autonomic response of acute pain, and (3) the child's behaviors. Assessment should never be based on behavior alone.*

R: *Nurses, physicians, and parents should identify and use consistent pain assessment criteria (e.g., assessment scale, specific behaviors) to assess pain in a child.*

Reduce or Eliminate the Common Side Effects of Opioids

Sedation

- Assess whether the cause is the opioid, fatigue, sleep deprivation, or other drugs (sedatives, antiemetics).
- If drowsiness is excessive, consult with physician about reducing dose.

Constipation

- Explain to older children why pain medications cause constipation.
- Increase fiber containing foods and water in diet.
- Instruct the child to keep a record of exercises (e.g., make a chart with a star sticker placed on it whenever the exercises are done).
- Refer to *Constipation* for additional interventions.

Dry Mouth

- Explain to older children that narcotics decrease saliva production.
- Instruct the child to rinse mouth often, suck on sugarless sour candies, eat pineapple chunks and watermelon, and drink liquids often.
- Explain the necessity of brushing teeth after every meal.
- Discontinue medications/treatments that are causing symptoms as soon as appropriate.

R: *Management of side effects will increase comfort and use of medications.*

Assist Child with the Aftermath of Pain

- Tell the child when the painful procedure is over. Allow the child to have contact with parent or person whom they find comforting.

- Encourage the child to discuss pain experience (draw or act out with dolls).
- Encourage the child to perform the painful procedure using the same equipment on a doll under supervision.
- Praise the child for his or her endurance and convey that he or she handled the pain well regardless of actual behavior (unless the child was violent to others).
- Reward for good behavior, such as sticker, ice pop, or other prize.
- Teach the child to keep a record of painful experiences and to plan a reward each time he or she achieves a behavioral goal, such as a *sticker* (reward) for each time the child holds still (goal) during an injection. Encourage achievable goals; holding still during an injection may not be possible for every child, but counting or taking deep breaths may be.
- Consult with Child Life Specialists for assistance in teaching coping techniques, providing distraction, and modifying behavior in cases where the child is receiving repetitive, unpleasant treatments (e.g., child who has difficulty with frequent, routine blood draws).

R: *Provides an opportunity to discuss experience.*

Collaborate With Child to Initiate Appropriate Noninvasive Pain-Relief Modalities

- Encourage mobility as much as indicated, especially when pain is lowest.
- Discuss with the child and parents activities that they like and incorporate them in daily schedule (e.g., clay modeling, drawing/coloring).
- Discuss with older children that thinking about something else can decrease the pain (e.g., guided imagery and/or progressive muscle relaxation).
- Consider the use of transcutaneous electrical nerve stimulation (TENS) for procedure, acute, and chronic pain. TENS has been studied and used effectively in children with postoperative pain, headache, and procedural pain, without adverse effects.
- L-M-X4/EMLA/LET gels and cream can be applied to injection sites prior to actual injection or needlestick site. It serves to numb the outer dermal layers to decrease procedure discomfort. These applications require application some time before the actual procedure is to take place (Ball et al., 2015).
- Vapocoolant sprays are applied topically and can be applied just prior to procedure, requiring only a minute of contact with intact skin (Ball et al., 2015).
- Distraction measures can include listening to music, watching video, or blowing bubbles. Keep in mind that even if child seems adequately distracted, the child could still be experiencing pain (Ball et al., 2015).
- Sucrose solutions have been found to be very effective in the infant population for pain control in that it is believed to activate the endogenous opioid system through taste. Effects generally last between 3 and 5 minutes (Ball et al., 2015).
- Refer to guidelines for noninvasive pain-relief measures.

R: *Pharmacologic measures combined with noninvasive techniques provide the most effective means of treating pain in children.*

Assist Family to Respond Optimally to Child's Pain Experience

- Assess family's knowledge of and response to pain (e.g., do parents support the child who has pain?).
- Assure parents that they can touch or hold their child, if feasible (e.g., demonstrate that touching is possible even with tubes and equipment).
- Give accurate information to correct misconceptions (e.g., the necessity of the treatment even though it causes pain).
- Provide parents opportunities to discuss privately their fears, anger, and frustrations.
- Acknowledge the difficulty of the situation.
- Incorporate parents in the pain-relief modality if possible (e.g., stroking, massage, distraction).
- Praise their participation and concern.
- Negotiate goals of pain management plan; reevaluate regularly (e.g., goal of decreased pain/increased comfort is being pain-free is an unrealistic goal).

Initiate Health Teaching and Referrals, if Indicated

- Provide child and family with ongoing explanations.
- Use the care plan to promote continuity of care for hospitalized child.
- Use available mental health professionals, if needed, for assistance with guided imagery, progressive relaxations, and hypnosis.
- Use available pain service (pain team) at pediatric health-care centers for an interdisciplinary and comprehensive approach to pain management in children.
- Refer parents to pertinent literature for themselves and children (see Bibliography).

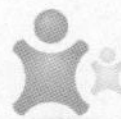

Maternal Interventions

- Refer to *Labor Pain*.

Chronic Pain

NANDA-I Definition

Unpleasant sensory and emotional experience arising from actual or potential tissue damage or described in terms of such damage (International Association for the Study of Pain); sudden or slow onset of any intensity from mild to severe, constant or reoccurring without an anticipated or predictable end and a duration of greater than three(>3) months

Defining Characteristics

Reports that pain has existed for more than 3 months (may be the only assessment data present)
Evidence of pain using standardized pain behavior checklist for those unable to communicate verbally (e.g., Neonatal Infant Pain Scale, Pain Assessment Checklist for those with limited ability to communicate)
Discomfort
Anger, frustration, depression because of situation
Facial mask of pain
Anorexia, weight loss
Insomnia
Guarded movement
Muscle spasms
Redness, swelling, heat
Color changes in affected area
Reflex abnormalities

Related Factors

See *Impaired Comfort*.

Author's Note

In the United States, at least 116 million adults in 2011 report living with chronic pain (Institute of Medicine, 2011). "No matter what the cause or pattern of the pain, its chronicity causes physiologic and psychological stress that wears on the patient (and their loved ones[7]) physically and emotionally" (D'Arcy, 2008).

The real tragedy of experiencing chronic pain is the failure of health-care professionals to understand the lived experience or perhaps worse project disbelief or commendation toward those who suffer.

Utilizing epidemiological studies prior to 1996, the associated relationship of pain and depression is explored and validated, but the reason is unknown (*Von Korff & Simon, 1996). "Thus pain and psychological illness should be viewed as having a reciprocal psychological and behavioral effects involving both processes of illness expression and adaption, as well as pain having specific effects on emotional state and behavioral function" (*Von Korff & Simon, 1996). The researchers asked "Is depression evident before the onset of the pain problem, early in the natural history, or only after pain has become chronic?"

Errors in Diagnostic Statements

See *Impaired Comfort*.

Key Concepts

Refer to *Acute Pain*.

[7]Parentheses added by this author

Focus Assessment Criteria

See *Impaired Comfort*.

Goals

NOC

Pain Control, Pain Level, Pain: Disruptive Effects, Pain Control, Depression Control, Pain: Adverse Psychological Response

The client will relate improvement of pain and increased daily activities as evidenced by the following indicators:

- Relate that others validate that their pain exists.
- Practice selected noninvasive pain-relief measures.

The child will demonstrate coping mechanism for pain, methods to control pain and the pain cause/disease, as evidenced by increased play and usual activities of childhood, and the following indicators:

- Communicate improvement in pain verbally, by pain assessment scale, or by behavior (specify).
- Maintain usual family role and relationships throughout pain experience, as evidenced by (specify).

Carp's Cues

"While the under treatment of pain is a recognized issue amongst pain researchers, we argue that the concept of 'pseudoaddiction' is problematic because it ultimately relies on a clinical judgment that attempts to separate out 'bad' drug seeking addicts from 'good 'undertreated pain patients in the face of behaviors that are virtually indistinguishable" (Bell & Salmon, 2009).

In the practice of this author as a family nurse practitioner, I encounter weekly requests for controlled medications. After careful assessments, if I am still uncertain if the request is due to undertreated pain or abuse, I will prescribe the medication at this visit for 14 days. On the next visit with additional assessment, I can better differentiate the origins of the request, I can differentiate the legitimate request from those that are not. This practice has caused me to sometimes prescribe once for a drug-seeking addict or street entrepreneur. But most importantly, I did not deprive a person with creditable pain the medication for relief of their pain. I can live with both outcomes.

Interventions

NIC

Pain Management, Medication Management, Exercise Promotion, Mood Management, Coping Enhancement, Acupressure, Heat/Cold Application, Distraction.

Explore the Individual's/Families' Pain Experience and the Influences of Their Culture (Narayan, 2010)

R: *To determine how best to help a person with pain, nurses must first discern how he/she thinks and feels about the pain experience (Narayan, 2010).*

- Language and interpretation problems.
- Reluctance to share personal complaints.

R: *Some cultural groups tend to instill in their members self-efficacy—a sense of control over life, including how to respond to and manage pain.*

- Believe they can exert little influence over the future, for example, fatalistic
- Pain is viewed as something to be tolerated or deserved as a punishment.
- Confusion over nonverbal behaviors
- Reluctance to use pain medications, for example, fears of misuse, cultural taboos.

R: *Effective communication is essential for valid pain assessments. Many nonverbal cues such as facial expression, body posture, and activity level can also vary among cultures and thus be misinterpreted. Culture beliefs can present as barriers.*

Discuss With the Individual and Family the Effects of Chronic Pain on the Individual's Life

- Last week, how many days could you not do what you wanted to, for example, work, chores, shopping, meal preparation.
- What do you/family do for fun or socialization? How often?
- Last week, how well did you sleep? Naps?
- How does pain interfere with your mood, relationships?
- How would you describe your health?
- What could your family, friends do to improve your life?
- What would your family say you could do to improve your life?

R: *The client with chronic pain may respond with withdrawal, depression, anxiety, anger, frustration, and dependency, all of which can affect the family in the same way. Fifty percent of clients with chronic pain have depression or anxiety disorders (Weisberg & Boatwright, 2007). Interventions focus on helping families understand pain's effects on roles and relationships.*

Explore the Individual/Families Understanding of the Causes of the Pain and Related Treatments/Diagnostic Studies

- What is their understanding of the causes?
- Clarify misunderstandings or access a physician/PA/NP to provide the information.
- Relate the severity of the pain and how long it will last, if known.

R: *If clarification is needed on information they have received, it can be provided. If the individual/family have not received an explanation, access physician/PA/NP.*

- Explain diagnostic tests and procedures in detail by relating the discomforts and sensations that the individual will feel; approximate the duration.

R: *People who are prepared for painful procedures by explanations of the actual sensations experience less stress than those who receive vague explanations.*

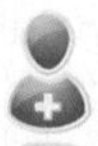

Clinical Alert Support the individual in addressing specific questions regarding diagnosis, risks, benefits of treatment, and prognosis. Consult with the specialist or primary care provider. If there are barriers to full disclosure, refer to *Risk for Compromised Human Dignity*.

Specifically identify positive aspects/events in the individual's life, for example, social events, children, grandchildren. Address reasons or barriers to socialization.

R: *"Depression can occur secondary to impaired social role performance and reduce activity levels" thus resulting in learned helplessness (*Von Korff & Simon, 1996).*

Collaborate With the Individual About Possible Methods to Reduce Pain Intensity

- See *Acute Pain*.

Provide Pain Relief With Prescribed Analgesic. Use the Around the Clock (ATC) Approach, not PRN

R: *Paice et al. (*2005) reported the results of comparing the use of ATC scheduled opioid doses with PRN opioid doses in medical inpatients and found that those who received ATC doses had lower pain intensity ratings. "As might be expected, a significantly greater percentage of the prescribed opioid was administered when it was given ATC (70.8%) compared with PRN (38%); however, there were no differences in adverse effects between the two groups" (Pasero, 2010). The preventive approach may increase the total 24-hour therapeutic blood level of the drug, reducing cravings for the drug, and reducing the anxiety of having to ask and wait for PRN relief*

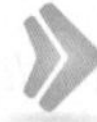

Carp's Cues

Pain management should be aggressive and individualized to eliminate unnecessary pain with drugs administered on a regular schedule rather than PRN. If resistance from prescribers is met, emphasize the benefits, especially if the individual's pain is being undertreated. Ensure the home pain management regimen continues in the hospital.

- Tylenol, NSAIDS, for example, ibuprofen
- Topical agents, for example, capsaicin, EMLA, Lidocaine gel, patch
- Opioids (transdermal, oral, parenteral)
- Anticonvulsants, for example, gabapentin (Neurontin)
- Antidepressants, for example, duloxetine, SSRI, MAO inhibitors

If Indicated, Consider the PRN Approach for Breakthrough Pain. Consult with Prescriber. Instruct Individual/Family to

- Request the PRN medication
- Emphasize to "stay on top of pain" by requesting medication prior to pain becoming severe

R: *Breakthrough pain (sometimes called pain flare, episodic pain, or transient pain) is defined as a transitory exacerbation of pain in a person who has relatively stable and adequately controlled baseline pain (Pasero, 2011).*

Discuss Fears (Individual, Family) of Addiction and Undertreatment of Pain

- Explain tolerance versus addiction. Refer to Key Concepts.

R: *Control of pain effectively requires clarifying misconception about addiction and overdose. Opioid tolerance and physical dependence are expected with long-term opioid treatment. Addiction is different and not usual in clients who use opioids for pain management (Pasero & McCafferty, 2011).*

Reduce or Eliminate Common Side Effects of Opioids (e.g., Constipation, Nausea, Dry Mouth)

- See *Acute Pain.*

Assist Family to Respond Optimally to the Client's Pain Experience

- See *Acute Pain.*
- Encourage family to seek assistance if needed for specific problems, such as coping with chronic pain: family counselor; financial and service agencies (e.g., American Cancer Society).

Explain the Various Noninvasive Pain-Relief Methods to the Client and Family and Why They are Effective

- Explain the therapeutic uses of menthol preparations, massage, and vibration
- Training in mindfulness meditation

R: *Ziedan et al. (2012) reported a review of the research and concluded that "training in mindfulness meditation improves anxiety, depression, stress, cognition and provides pain relief." Mindfulness-related health benefits are associated with enhancements in cognitive control, emotion regulation, positive mood, and acceptance, each of which has been associated with pain modulation.*

R: *Nonpharmacologic interventions provide a major treatment approach for pain, specifically chronic pain. They provide clients with an increased sense of control, promote active involvement, reduce stress and anxiety, elevate mood, and raise the pain threshold (*McGuire, Sheidler, & Polomano, 2000).*

- Relaxation, for example, yoga, breathing exercises, guided imagery

R: *Studies have shown that relaxation promotes the human brain to secrete endorphins, which have opiate-like properties that relieve pain. The release of endorphins may be responsible for the positive effects of placebos and noninvasive pain-relief measures (Pasero & McCafferty, 2011).*

- Music

R: *Evidence suggests that music-based interventions can have a positive impact on pain, anxiety, mood disturbance, and quality of life in cancer patients (Archie, Bruera, & Cohen, 2013; Beebe & Wyatt 2009).*

- Discuss the use of heat applications,* their therapeutic effects, indications, and related precautions. Apply dry heat to the area for 20 to 30 minutes every 2 hours for as many days as directed.
  - Hot water bottle
  - Warm tub
  - Hot summer sun
  - Electric heating pad
  - Moist heat pack
  - Thin plastic wrap over painful area to retain body heat (e.g., knee, elbow)

R: *Heat dilates blood vessels, which increases blood flow, which increases oxygen and nutrients to the area. The therapeutic effects of heat increase the flexibility of collagen tissues, decreasing joint stiffness; reducing pain; relieving muscle spasms; reducing inflammation, and edema. Dry heat is more effective than moist heat (Grossman & Porth, 2014). Heat also can distract the person from feeling the pain (Yarbro et al., 2013).*

- Discuss the use of cold applications, their therapeutic effects, indications, and related precautions. Use an ice pack[8] or put crushed ice in a plastic bag. Cover it with a towel and place it on the area for 15 to 20 minutes every hour as directed.
  - Cold towels (wrung out)
  - Ice bag
  - Ice massage
  - Cold water immersion for small body parts
  - Cold gel pack

---

[8]Ice pack should be soft (e.g., gel) to conform to painful site. Homemade gel packs are made with 1 cup of water to ¼ cup rubbing alcohol (can double or triple the quantities for larger ice packs) and poured into a Ziploc bag sealed and placed in another bag to prevent leaking. Place in freezer.

R: *Cold slows down blood flow to an injury, thereby reducing pain and swelling. Cold therapy slows circulation, reducing inflammation, muscle spasm, and pain. It should be used if the area is swollen or bruised.*

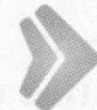

Carp's Cues

"The characteristics that most strongly predict depression are diffuseness of pain and the extent to which pain interferes with activities" (*Von Korff & Simon, 1996). Figure II.2 represents the cycle of inactivity, pain and depression.

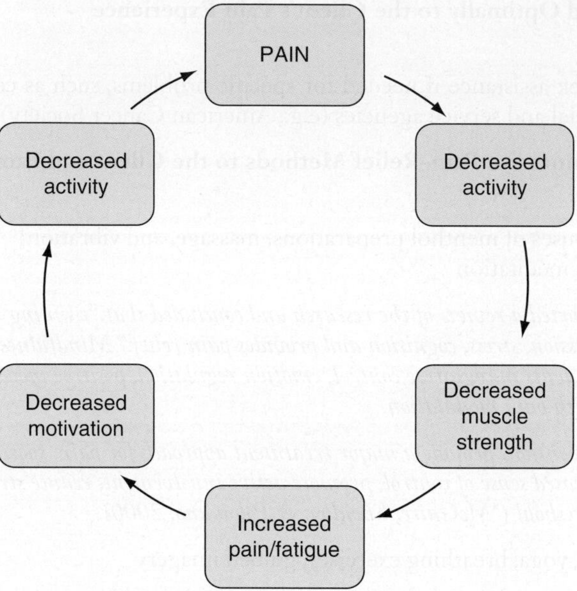

FIGURE II.2 The relationship of inactivity, pain and depression.

Promote Optimal Mobility With a Discussion of its Value

- Discuss the value of increased activity
  - Stress management
  - Increase endorphins
  - Increased flexibility, muscle strength
  - Boosts brain function
  - Increased sense of control
- Review with the individual options as yoga, stretching, stationary bike, walking at a comfortable pace, water aerobics. Suggest TV exercise programs if desired.
- Plan daily activities when pain is at its lowest level.

R: *Exercise also increases concentrations of norepinephrine, a chemical that can moderate the brain's response to stress. The benefits of increased activity are the rationale for doing.*

Initiate Health Teaching and Referrals as Indicated

- Discuss with the individual and family the various treatment modalities available:
  - Family therapy
  - Behavior modification
  - Hypnosis
  - Exercise program
  - Group therapy
  - Biofeedback
  - Acupuncture

Geriatric Interventions

Assess Cognitive Status (e.g., Dementia, Delirium), Mental State (e.g., Anxiety, Agitation, Depression), and Functional Status

- If there is evidence of cognitive impairment, refer to Focus Assessment Criteria.
- Pain Assessment Checklist for individual with limited ability to communicate (PACSLAC)
- Explore the impact of chronic pain on the functionality of the individual within the community, including shopping, home chores, and socialization, as well as the ability to perform ADLs.

R: *Brown et al. (2011) reported that community-living older adults reported that pain had negative decline in their relationships (8%), Concentration (9%), and overall enjoyment of life (15%).*

- Discuss the value of increased activity:
  - Stress management
  - Increased endorphins
  - Increased flexibility, muscle strength
  - Boosts brain function
  - Increased sense of control
- Review with the individual options as yoga. chair exercises, stretching, stationary bike, walking at a comfortable pace, water aerobics. Suggest TV exercise programs if desired.
- Plan daily activities when pain is at its lowest level.

R: *Older adults are at higher risk for functional consequences of chronic pain and inactivity. Brown et al. (2011) reported that community-living older adults reported functional consequences in walking (36%), general activity (22%), and sleeping (14%).*

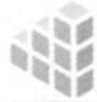

Pediatric Interventions

- Assess pain experiences by using developmentally appropriate assessment scales and by assessing behavior. Incorporate child and family in ongoing assessment. Identify potential for secondary gain for reporting pain (e.g., companionship, attention, concern, caring, distraction); include strategies for meeting identified needs in plan of care.
- Set short-term and long-term goals for pain management with child and family and evaluate regularly (e.g., totally or partially relieve pain, control behavior or anxiety associated with pain).
- Promote normal growth and development; involve family and available resources, such as occupational, physical, and child life therapists.
- Promote the "normal" aspects of the child's life: play, school, family relationships, physical activity.
- Promote a trusting environment for child and family.
- Believe the child's pain.
- Encourage child's perception that interventions are attempts to help.
- Provide continuity of care and pain management by health-care providers (nurse, physician, pain team) and in different settings (inpatient, outpatient, emergency department, home).
- Use interdisciplinary team for pain management as necessary (e.g., nurse, physician, child life therapist, mental health therapist, occupational therapist, physical therapist, nutritionist).
- Identify myths and misconceptions about pediatric pain management (e.g., IM analgesia, narcotic use and dosing, assessment) in attitudes of health-care professionals, child, and family; provide accurate information and opportunities for effective communication.
- Provide parents and siblings with opportunities to share their experiences and fears.

R: *See rationales for Acute Pain.*

R: *Parents of a child with pain report unendurable pain, helplessness, total commitment, feeling the pain physically, being unprepared, agony, terror, and wishing for death in cases of terminal illness (*Ferrell, 1995). Interventions attempt to elicit these feelings and experiences.*

R: *Assessing the child's cognitive level and age is important to provide appropriate explanations.*

R: *Preschoolers assume their pain has resulted from bad deeds. Nurses must attempt to reduce their sense of blame.*

Chronic Pain Syndrome

Definition

Unpleasant sensory and emotional experience associated with acute or potential tissue damage, or described in terms of such damage (International Association for the Study of Pain); sudden or slow onset of any intensity from mild to severe, constant or recurring without an anticipated or predictable end and a duration of greater than three (>3) months.

Defining Characteristics

Alteration in ability to continue previous activities
Alteration in sleep pattern
Anorexia
Evidence of pain using standardized pain behavior checklist for those unable to communicate verbally (e.g., Neonatal Infant Pain Scale, Pain Assessment Checklist for seniors with limited ability to communicate)
Facial expression of pain (e.g., eyes lack luster, beaten look, fixed or scattered movement, grimace)
Proxy report of pain behavior/ activity changes (e.g., family member caregiver)
Self-focused
Self-report of intensity using standardized pain scale (e.g., Wong–Baker FACES scale, visual analogue scale, numeric rating scale)
Self-report of pain characteristics using standardized pain instrument (e.g., McGill Pain Questionnaire, Brief Pain Inventory)

Related Factors

Age >50
Alteration in sleep pattern
Chronic musculoskeletal condition
Contusion
Crush injury
Damage to the nervous system
Emotional distress
Fatigue
Female gender
Fracture
Genetic disorder
History of abuse (e.g., physical, psychological, sexual)
History of genital mutilation
History of overindebtedness
History of static work postures
History of substance abuse
History of vigorous exercise
Imbalance of neurotransmitters, neuromodulators, and receptors
Immune disorder (e.g., HIV-associated neuropathy, varicella-zoster virus)
Impaired metabolic functioning
Increase in body mass index
Ineffective sexuality pattern
Injury agent*
Ischemic condition
Malnutrition
Muscle injury
Nerve compression
Posttrauma related condition (e.g., infection, inflammation)
Prolonged increase in cortisol level
Repeated handling of heavy loads
Social isolation
Rheumatoid arthritis
Tumor infiltration
Whole-body vibration
May be present, but is not required; pain may be of unknown etiology

Author Note

Chronic Pain Syndrome is a newly accepted NANDA-I nursing diagnosis. This "syndrome" is problematic as approved as a nursing diagnosis. As one reviews the "defining characteristics," they represent *Chronic Pain*. As one reviews the list of "related factors," they represent causative or contributing factors for *Chronic Pain*.

"It is important to distinguish between CHRONIC PAIN and a CHRONIC PAIN SYNDROME. The pathophysiology of chronic pain syndrome (CPS) is multifactorial and complex and still is poorly understood. A chronic pain syndrome differs from chronic pain in that people with a chronic pain syndrome, over time, develop a number of related life problems beyond the sensation of pain itself. It is important to distinguish between the two because they respond to different types of treatment" (Singh, 2014; Grossman & Varcarolis, 2014).

Treatment of chronic pain syndrome (CPS) must be tailored for each individual patient. The treatment should be aimed at interruption of reinforcement of the pain behavior and modulation of the pain response. The goals of treatment must be realistic and should be focused on restoration of normal function (minimal disability), better quality of life, reduction of use of medication, and prevention of relapse of chronic symptoms.

A self-directed or therapist-directed physical therapy (PT) program, individualized to the patient's needs and goals and provided in association with occupational therapy (OT), has an important role in functional restoration for patients with CPS.

The goal of a PT program is to increase strength and flexibility gradually, beginning with gentle gliding exercises. Patients usually are reluctant to participate in PT because of intense pain.

PT techniques include hot or cold applications, positioning, stretching exercises, traction, massage, ultrasonographic therapy, TENS, and manipulations.

Key Concepts

- Many health-care professionals fail to recognize the complexity of pain and believe that it can be dichotomized based on the presence or absence of physical findings, secondary gain, or prior emotional problems. As a result, countless individuals have been informed that "The pain is all in your head". And if these same individuals react with anger and hurt, we (health-care staff) are ready to compound the problem by labeling the individual as hostile, demanding, or aggressive.
- The paradigm of thinking of that pain can be either "medically explained" or is psychogenic pain is outdated and harmful to individuals experiencing pain (Von Korff & Simon, 1996). The Diagnostic Statistical Manual of Mental Disorders (DSM 5; APA, 2014) has replaced Somatoform Disorders with Somatic Symptom Disorders. One component of somatic disorder is psychological factors affecting medical condition.
- "Chronic Pain Syndrome has been described learned behavioral syndrome that begins with a noxious stimulus that causes pain. This pain behavior then is rewarded externally or internally. Thus, this pain behavior is reinforced, and then it occurs without any noxious stimulus. Internal reinforces are relief from personal factors associated with many emotions (e.g., guilt, fear of work, sex, responsibilities). External reinforces include such factors as attention from family members and friends, socialization with the health-care providers, medications, compensation, and time off from work" (Singh, 2014).
- Most individuals with chronic pain (estimates are about 75% nationally) do not develop the more complicated and distressful CPS. Although they may experience the pain for the remainder of their lives, their responses to pain in their daily activities, family relationships, work, or other life components are usually adaptive (D'Arcy, 2008; *Hayes et al., 2002; Humphreys, Cooper, & Miaskowski, 2010; Price, 1999; Rosenquist, 2015; Singh, 2014; *Von Korff & Simon, 1996).
- Somatic symptom disorder is characterized by (APA, 2014; Grossman & Varcarolis, 2014):
  - Somatizing individuals can also be recognized by a pattern that began in their early 20s
  - with the multiple unexplained symptoms, vague and
  - inconsistent history, and
  - underlying sense of anguish,
  - lack of factors that exacerbate or alleviate symptoms,
  - lack of positive findings on physical examination.
  - they often have witnessed this behavior as a child in their family. They often elicit negative feelings from their clinician and are viewed as difficult patients (Barsky, 2014; Singh, 2014).
- Symptoms are distressing, unexplainable, and excessive.
- Symptoms cannot be explained by with significant physical findings or medical diagnoses.
- Symptoms are authentic, not intentionally produced and overly exaggerated.
- Individuals report high levels of functional impairments.
- Individuals are "sicker than sick."
- Somatic Symptom Disorder is not Factitious Disorder or Malingering (Boyd, 2012; Greenberg, 2015; Grossman & Varcarolis, 2013):
  - Factitious Disorder (a somatic disorder) is intentionally faking symptoms to assume a "sick role" and have their emotional needs met. The contrived illness can be physical or psychiatric, for example, hypoglycemia, seizures, cancer, HIV. Intentionally infecting wounds.

- Malingering (not a specific mental illness) is intentionally faking or exaggerating symptoms for a desire for material or external benefit, for example, money, housing, medications, disability compensation, evade military service insurance fraud. Malingering is a behavior, not a psychiatric disorder. Some behaviors are demanding specific medications, referred by an attorney for evaluation, nonadherence with diagnostic evaluation/treatment, inconsistencies in history, vague responses, dramatically describing symptoms and using technical medical terms.
- Individual with physical complaints must be afforded appropriate diagnostic investigation, for example, history and physical, laboratory tests, imaging, consultations with specialists to rule out serious or life-threatening conditions, for example, multiple sclerosis, systemic lupus (Greenberg, 2015).
- In addition, a psychiatric evaluation is imperative to evaluate for depression, panic disorder, substance abuse disorder, anxiety disorder, and other psychiatric conditions.
- Somatic symptom syndrome (CPS) is a constellation of syndromes that usually do not respond to the medical model of care. This condition is managed best with a multidisciplinary approach, requiring good integration and knowledge of multiple organ systems. Extreme care should be taken during diagnostic testing for CPS. Carefully review prior testing to eliminate unnecessary repetition.
- In addition, a good psychosocial or psychosexual history is needed when organic diseases are excluded or coexisting psychiatric disorders are suggested. Obtain sufficient history to evaluate depression; anxiety disorder; somatization; physical or sexual abuse; drug abuse/dependence; and family, marital, or sexual problems (Singh, 2014).
- "The diagnostic label of somatoform disorder, or any of the subtype labels, appeared to contribute to negative stereotyping rather than being used as a tool to assist in increasing knowledge and understanding of clients and their family. This reinforces the need for the development of honest, transparent and non-threatening approaches to informing clients and their families about the somatoform disorder diagnosis" (*Dickson, Hay-Smith, & Dean, 2009, pp. 120–121).
- There is further work required to develop honest and transparent approaches to informing clients and their families about the somatoform disorder diagnosis, which are nonthreatening. All clients have the "right to be fully informed" about their diagnosis.
- "Psychological interventions, in conjunction with medical interventions, PT, and OT, increase the effectiveness of the treatment program. Family members are involved in the evaluation and treatment processes" (*Dickson et al., 2009, p. 120).
- Individual with these syndromes have overinclusive or unrealistic concept of good health, increased attention to bodily processes to detect possible signs of illness, catastrophic interpretations of bodily sensations, lack of external stimulation, expectations, operant conditioning, and difficulty with information processing (Boyd, 2012; Halter, 2014; O'Malley et al., 1999).
- Treatment of CPS must be tailored for each individual. The treatment should be aimed at interruption of reinforcement of the pain behavior and modulation of the pain response.
- The goals of treatment must be realistic and should be focused on restoration of normal function (minimal disability), better quality of life, reduction of use of medication, and prevention of relapse of chronic symptoms (Boyd, 2011; Halter, 2014).
- Treatment of CPS must be tailored for each individual. The treatment should be focused on (Singh, 2014):
  - Interruption of reinforcement of the pain behavior
  - Reducing the intensity of their pain response
  - Setting realistic goals with the individual
  - Restoration of normal function (minimal disability) with a better quality of life
  - Reduction of use of medication
  - Prevention of relapse of chronic symptoms
- Treatment encompasses primary care intervention, psychological intervention (by primary care provider or mental health professions), physical therapy, occupational therapy. Family members are involved in the evaluation and treatment processes. Family therapy may be indicated.
- An endless array of conditions, injuries or surgical procedures can be the origin(s) of a somatic symptom syndrome (CPS). It is not the medical condition that triggers somatic symptom syndrome (CPS). For example, since every individual with back pain or osteoarthritis do not develop Somatic Symptom Disorder, then why do some?
- Singh (2014) identified over 70 conditions that can be associated with somatic symptom syndrome (or CPS). These associated conditions are musculoskeletal disorders, neurologic disorders. urologic disorders, gastrointestinal disorders, reproductive disorders (extrauterine), reproductive disorders (uterine), and psychological disorders.

Focus Assessment Criteria

Refer Focus Assessment Criteria under *Impaired Comfort.*

Note: This nursing assessment focuses on the individual's pain at point of care. It does not replace a Comprehensive Pain Assessment with a specific psychological component to address co-morbidities.

Goals

NOC

Pain Control, Pain Level, Pain: Disruptive Effects, Pain Control, Depression Control, Pain: Adverse Psychological Response, Coping, Stress Level

The client will experience a satisfactory relief measure as evidenced by (specify):

- Increased participation in activities of recovery
- Reduction in pain behaviors (specify)
- Improvement in mood, coping

Interventions

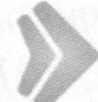

Carp's Cues

"Given the large burden of human suffering that occurs when pain and psychological illness coincide, there is a pressing need to understand the interplay of pain and psychological illness with research of individual early in the development of their comorbidity" (*Von Korff & Simon, 1996). Written almost 20 years ago, how far have we advanced the care of these individuals? Currently in my practice setting, these individuals are shunned, overly tested, and referred to multiple specialists, who further test them only to have them return to our primary care office with the same complains as in their initial office visit.

NIC

Pain Management, Medication Management, Exercise Promotion, Mood Management, Coping Enhancement, Acupressure, Heat/Cold Application, Distraction.

- Refer to *Chronic Pain* for interventions related to the individual's pain management.

The Interventions to Follow are Strategies, Utilizing Basic-Level Principles of Cognitive–Behavioral Therapy That a Professional Nurse can Utilize to (Grossman & Varcarolis, 2014)

- Create a therapeutic relationship with the individual.
- Promote positive self-esteem.
- Reward nonillness related behaviors.

Carefully Evaluate Your Beliefs or Biases That can be Barriers to Providing Empathetic, Ethical, Professional Nursing Care to This Individual

R: *Since Somatic Symptom Disorder is an extremely complex disorder, confirmations of this diagnoses requires an extensive work-up and interactive therapeutic sessions. Until this syndrome has been systematically ruled out, the nurse should provide intervention indicated for the syndrome.*

Individuals With this Syndrome are not Faking, They do Experience the Symptoms (Refer to Key Concepts for the Differentiation of Factious Disorder and Malingering)

- Do you believe?
  - Somatic Symptom Disorder is not valid for this person?
  - You can correctly differentiate between "deserving pain patients" and "undeserving addicts."
  - This person is faking?
  - This person is drug-seeking?
  - This person is wasting your time?
  - Most people who chronically take opioids are addictive.

R: *Dickson et al. (*2009) interviewed professionals working in rehabilitation units in regard to their feelings when providing care to individuals with somatic symptom syndrome. They reported unpredictability of the situation, uncomfortable, and uncertainty of what interventions should be provided, Individuals with this diagnosis are "Demonized" and are "too hard." Enmeshed in this clinical situation, is that majority of individuals are not told of their diagnosis and the goals of treatment (Dickson et al., 2009).*

- As one examines one's biases, keep in mind. "There are no such things as bad thoughts only bad actions."
- Attempt limiting the number of nurses assigned to person.

R: *This can prevent manipulation and allow for consistent intervention. It can prevent the need "to tell their story" over and over, which reinforces illness behaviors.*

- Specifically validate that you believe his/her symptoms are real. Share this with other staff.

R: *The psychogenic symptoms are real to the person. They represent an excessive response to symptoms (Grossman & Varcarolis, 2014). Attempts to prove the person wrong will only result in more symptoms "to prove" it.*

- Specifically explore what makes her/him feel less stressed or anxious.

R: *Encourages the person to engage in this behavior, reinforce strengths and problem-solving abilities and enhances self-esteem (Grossman & Varcarolis, 2013).*

- "Listen to understand rather than listening to respond" (Procter, Hamer, McGarry, Wilson, & Froggatt, 2014, p. 93) especially in nonillness related discussions.

R: *When one listens to respond, one is thinking of their response. "Withholding one's reactions to what is being said, hearing what is being said, and then exploring the person's perspective with curious questioning, rather than launching into one's own agenda, leads one to develop a more balance and inclusive appraisal of the person's situation" (Proctor et al., 2014, p. 93).*

- Stop by his/her room when the person has not called with a request or comfort.

R: *This rewards nonillness related behavior and reinforces the person does not have to complain for the nurse's attention. This can minimize sick role behaviors (Greenberg, 2015; Grossman & Varcarolis, 2014).*

Reduce Anxiety About Illness (Boyd, 2012)

- Explain diagnostic tests that have been ordered.

R: *This can help to decrease anxiety.*

- Do not advise that specific diagnostic testing may be needed.

R: *"Often persons with Somatic Symptom Disorder have had numerous diagnostic studies (some repetitive) and specialist consultations in response to their complaints. The primary care provider must remain the responsible caregiver, and the psychiatrist's advice reduces diagnostic uncertainty and potentially harmful procedures and interventions" (Greenberg, 2015).*

Explain the Various Noninvasive Stress-Relief Methods to the Individual and Family and Why They are Effective

- Explain the therapeutic uses of menthol preparations, massage, and vibration
- Training in mindfulness meditation

R: *Ziedan et al. (2012) reported a review of the research and concluded that "training in mindfulness meditation improves anxiety, depression, stress, cognition and provides pain relief. Mindfulness-related health benefits are associated with enhancements in cognitive control, emotion regulation, positive mood, and acceptance, each of which have been associated with pain modulation".*

R: *Nonpharmacologic interventions provide a major treatment approach for pain, specifically chronic pain (*McGuire et al., 2000). They provide individuals with an increased sense of control, promote active involvement, reduce stress and anxiety, elevate mood, and raise the pain threshold (Grossman & Varcarolis, 2013; *McGuire et al., 2000).*

- Relaxation, for example, yoga, breathing exercises, guided imagery

R: *Studies have shown that relaxation promotes the human brain to secrete endorphins, which have opiate-like properties that relieve pain. The release of endorphins may be responsible for the positive effects of placebos and noninvasive pain-relief measures (Pasero & McCafferty, 2011).*

- Music

R: *Evidence suggests that music-based interventions can have a positive impact on pain, anxiety, mood disturbance, and quality of life in cancer patients (Archie et al., 2013; Beebe & Wyatt 2009).*

Initiate Health Teaching and Referrals as Indicated

- Clarify with the individual/family what follow-up has been recommended

Labor Pain

NANDA-I Definition

Sensory and emotional experience that varies from pleasant to unpleasant, associated with labor

Sensory and emotional experience that varies from cramping to severe pain and intense pressure which can be highly variable, associated with labor and childbirth (T. Wilson, Personal Communication).

Defining Characteristics

Altered muscle tension
Altered neuroendocrine function
Altered urinary function
Change in blood pressure
Change in heart rate
Change in respiratory rate
Diaphoresis
Distraction behavior
Expressive behavior
Facial mask
Increased appetite
Lack of appetite
Narrowed focus
Nausea
Noted evidence of contractions
Observed evidence of contractions
Perineum pressure sensation
Positioning to avoid pain
Protective gesture
Pupillary dilation
Reports pressure[9]
Reports pain
Requests pain relief interventions[9]
Self-focused
Sleep pattern disturbance
Vomiting

Related Factors

Physiologic

Related to dilation period (uterine contractions, cervical stretching, and dilation and distention of lower uterine segment)

Related to transition and expulsion period (uterine contractions and distension of pelvic floor, vagina, and perineum, pressure on pelvic nerves)

Situational (Personal, Environmental)

Related to:

Fear
Anxiety
Emotional stress
Anticipation of pain
No prenatal education
Absent labor support
Fatigue
Anemia
Previous experience with pain
History of perinatal loss
History of neonatal death
History of neonatal health problems
Fetal position
Prior surgical procedures
Language barriers
Substance abuse (history, present)
History of abuse
History of sexual abuse/violence
History of trauma
Sexual orientation

Maturational

Adolescent
Developmental delay

Author's Note

This new NANDA-I nursing diagnosis contains the etiology of the pain in the diagnostic statement. What is problematic are what the related factors are when a woman is experiencing normal labor pain. The experience of labor can be

[9]Added by T. Wilson, contributor.

complicated when the mother is 14 years old or has a history of perinatal loss. Labor pain is complicated by fear and anxiety; thus, this nursing diagnosis should be added with the related factors that reflect why this labor experience may be more difficult and necessitates additional nursing individuals.

Labor Pain may be more clinically useful as *Labor Syndrome*, which would include *Acute Pain*, *Impaired Comfort*, *Fear*, *Anxiety*, *Interrupted Family Processes*, and others.

Key Concepts

Physiologic Considerations (Blackburn, 2013)

- The woman in labor experiences two types of pain: visceral and somatic.
  - Visceral pain is related to contraction of the uterus and dilation and stretching of the cervix. Uterine pain during the first stage of labor results from ischemia caused by constriction and contraction of the arteries supplying the myometrium. Visceral pain is experienced primarily during the first stage of labor.
  - Somatic pain is caused by pressure of the presenting part on the birth canal, vulva, and perineum. Somatic pain is experienced during transition and the second stage and is more intense and localized.
- Pain from uterine contractions and dilation of the cervix during the first stage of labor is transmitted by afferent fibers to the sympathetic chain of the posterior spinal cord at T10 to T12, and L1. In early labor, pain is transmitted primarily to T11 to T12.
- Pain during the first stage may be referred, that is, the nerve impulses from the uterus and cervix stimulate spinal cord neurons, innervating both the uterus and the abdominal wall. As a result the woman experiences pain over the abdominal wall between the umbilicus and symphysis pubis, around the iliac crests to the gluteal area, radiating down the thighs, and in the lumbar and sacral regions.
- During transition and the second stage, somatic pain impulses from distention of the birth canal, vulva, and perineum by the presenting part are transmitted by the pudendal nerves through the posterior roots of the parasympathetic chain at S2, S3, and S4.
- The corpus of the uterus is relatively denervated by late pregnancy while the cervix remains densely innervated. This suggests that the cervical area may be the major site of pain in labor.
- Near term numbers of nerve cells and fibers in the sensory area of the spinal column decrease accompanied by increased excitability of mechanosensitive afferents in the cervix.
- The pain threshold may be altered in late pregnancy, enhanced by elevated β-endorphins, leading to a proposed "pregnancy-induced hypoanalgesia."
- Pain during the intrapartum period may be modulated by endogenous opiate peptides such as β-endorphins and enkephalins. These modulating factors are produced by the placenta as well as the mother and may include an opioid-enhancing factor.
- Endogenous opioids alter the release of neurotransmitters from afferent nerves and interfere with efferent pathways from the spinal cord to the brain. In addition to their analgesic role, they may also alter mood during pregnancy and have a role in regulation of secretion of pituitary hormones.
- Other modulating factors include analgesia induced by mechanical stimulation of the hypogastric (uterine mechanical stimulation) and pelvic (vaginal distention) nerves.
- Exogenous modification of labor pain includes both pharmacologic interventions and nonpharmacologic cognitive, behavioral, and sensory techniques.
- The perception of pain is influenced by physiologic, psychological, and cultural factors.
- Pain can lead to anxiety and influence maternal physiologic responses and the course of labor. For example, physical manifestations of anxiety may include muscular tension, hyperventilation, increased sympathetic activity, and norepinephrine release, which can lead to increased cardiac output, blood pressure, metabolic rate, and oxygen consumption and impaired uterine contractility.
- Anxiety can also increase fear and tension, reducing pain tolerance, which decreases uterine contractility.
- Relaxation techniques such as progressive muscle relaxation, touch, breathing, imagery, and autosuggestion help reduce anxiety and prevent or stop this cycle (Blackburn, 2013).
- Women identify labor support as a continuous presence by another, emotional support (reassurance, encouragement, and guidance), physical comforting, providing information, and guidance for the woman and her partner regarding decision making, facilitating of communication, anticipatory guidance, and explanation of procedures (*Simkin & Bolding, 2004).
- Providing for physician comfort includes offering a variety of nonpharmacologic and pharmacologic interventions.
- Emotional support includes behaviors such as giving praise, encouragement, and reassurance; being positive; appearing calm and confident; assisting with breathing and relaxation; providing explanations about labor progress; identifying ways to include family members in the experience; and treating women with respect (Burke, 2014).

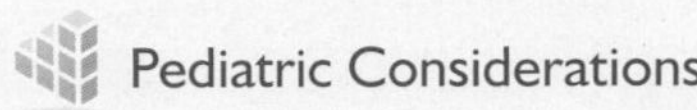

Pediatric Considerations

Adolescents

- In 2013, there were 26.6 births for every 1,000 adolescent females ages 15 to 19, or 274,641 babies born to females in this age group (U.S. Department of Health and Human Services Office of Adolescent Health, 2014).
- Nearly eighty-nine percent of these births occurred outside of marriage.
- The 2013 teen birth rate indicates a decline of 10% from 2012 when the birth rate was 29.4 per 1,000 (U.S. Department of Health and Human Services Office of Adolescent Health, 2014).
- About 77% of teen pregnancies are unplanned (U.S. Department of Health and Human Services Office of Adolescent Health, 2014). Adolescents' needs appear to focus on pain relief, nonjudgmental nursing care, and emotional support.
- Middle adolescents wanted supportive care that focused on affirmation of themselves, while late adolescents wanted pain relief (Sauls, 2004). Because adolescents have less life experience, they may also have fewer resources to cope with labor and delivery.
- Many adolescents do not tolerate pain well and may need anesthesia and analgesia. They may not be able to concentrate or may not wish to concentrate on breathing or relaxation techniques.
- Maternal–infant attachment may also be facilitated by a positive birth experience.
- Adolescents have many emotional needs during the intrapartum period.
- Adolescents may have an intense fear of pain and worry about how they will manage life after the baby arrives.
- Nonjudgmental care and simple instructions are essential to caring for the pregnant adolescent (*Montgomery, 2002).

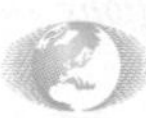

Transcultural Considerations

- Cultural factors that influence labor pain (Mattson, 2011):
  - Appropriate setting/environment for labor and birth
  - Degree and kind of interventions during labor and birth
  - Role of support persons and health-care providers
  - Those who may attend the woman during labor and birth
  - Expectations of the length of labor
  - Positioning, moving, and massage during labor
  - Culturally appropriate expression of pain
  - Vocalization during labor
  - Dietary recommendations during labor
  - Environmental noise level during labor and birth
  - Acceptability of pharmacologic and nonpharmacologic interventions

Focus Assessment Criteria

See *Impaired Comfort*.

Subjective

Assess for Defining Characteristics

Pain
Effects of pain
Management of pain

Assess for Other Related Factors That Can Negatively Affect Labor Pain

Length of labor
Frequency and intensity of uterine contractions
Administration of oxytocin to induce or augment labor
Presence of support person

Objective

Assess for Defining Characteristics

Behavioral manifestations (See *Impaired Comfort*)
Labor progress

Goals

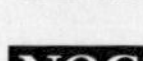
NOC
Refer to Acute Pain.

The mother will report or exhibit satisfactory pain level as evidenced by

- Reduction in pain behaviors (specify)
- Increased relaxation between contractions
- Improved coping skills

Interventions

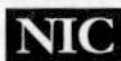
NIC
Refer to Acute Pain.

Refer to nursing diagnosis Acute Pain for basic pain management interventions.

Assess Progress in Labor

- Uterine contraction pattern
- Cervical dilation
- Fetal position and station

R: *Location and intensity of pain varies with phase or stage of labor.*

Assess Support Person's Readiness to Participate

Determine effect of

- Age and developmental status
- Culture and religion on expectations

R: *Perception and expression of pain is influenced by life experience, developmental stage, and cultural or religious norms.*

Provide Comfort Measures

- Gown and linen changes as needed
- Frequent pericare
- Cool, damp cloth to forehead, neck, or upper back

Provide Labor Support

- Labor support ideally is continuous and provided by a variety of individuals.
- Labor support should begin in early labor and continue through delivery.
- Assist the woman to cope with pain, build her self-confidence, and maintain a sense of mastery and well-being.
- Encourage verbalizations of feelings, pain, or pressure.
- Be supportive of patient's choices and wishes for her birth experience.
- Reassure, guide, and encourage the woman.
- Provide acceptance of her coping style.
- Reinforce positive coping mechanisms.
- Introduce and demonstrate new methods for coping with pain.

R: *The element that best predicts a woman's experience of labor pain is her level of confidence in her ability to cope with labor (*Simkin & Bolding, 2004).*

R: *Women who are provided continuously available support during labor have improved outcomes compared with women who do not have one-to-one continuously available support.*

R: *For women in labor, continuous support can result in the following:*

- Shorter labor
- Decreased use of analgesia/anesthesia
- Decreased operative vaginal births or cesarean births
- Decreased need for oxytocin/uterotonics
- Increased likelihood of breastfeeding
- Increased satisfaction with childbirth experience

R: *Many of the mother's childbirth outcomes listed above also benefit the neonate (Association of Women's Health, Obstetric and Neonatal Nurses [AWHONN], 2011).*

- Encourage Adequate Intake of Oral Fluids by Monitoring Oral and IV Intake and by Offering
- Ice chips

- Popsicles
- Jell-O
- Suckers
- Wet washcloths

Encourage Woman to Void at Least Every 2 Hours If No Urinary Catheter

- Catheterize patient as indicated.

R: *Bladder distention can interfere with fetal descent and increase uterine contraction pain.*

Guide and Support Woman and Her Support Person in Using Self-Comforting Techniques

Demonstrate and Encourage Support Person to Assist With Supportive Techniques as Needed

R: *Qualitative research has demonstrated that one of the most significant aspects of the experience of labor for women is the presence of one or more support persons. Postpartum women report that one of the things contributing to a positive labor experience was the presence of a family member or friend in the room (Burke, 2014).*

Encourage Rest and Promote Relaxation Between Contractions

Encourage and Support Nonpharmacologic Pain Relief Measures

R: *Achieving a state of relaxation is the basis of all nonpharmacologic interventions during labor. Relaxation enhances the effectiveness of nonpharmacologic and pharmacologic pain management strategies (Burke, 2014).*

- Relaxation techniques
- Patterned breathing techniques

R: *Breathing techniques are used as a distraction during labor to decrease pain and promote relaxation (Burke, 2014).*

- Discourage supine position to prevent supine hypotension or vena cava syndrome.
- Patterned physical movement, frequent position changes, and ambulation:
  - Leaning or leaning forward with support
  - Sitting
  - Standing
  - Side-lying
  - Pillows to help with positioning
  - Squatting
  - Hands and knees
  - Rocking chair
  - Birthing ball

R: *Women naturally choose positions of comfort and are more likely to change positions in early labor (Burke, 2014).*

R: *The birthing ball provides support for the woman's body as she assumes a variety of positions during labor. This may enhance maternal comfort. A birthing ball helps the woman use pelvic rocking, promotes mobility, and helps to provide support for the woman in the upright position (AWHONN, 2008a, b).*

- Biofeedback
- Hypnosis
- Attention focusing—focal point or imagery
- Music
- Aromatherapy
- Hydrotherapy
  - Shower, pool, or tub

R: *With appropriate attention to water temperature, duration of the bath, and safety considerations, baths in labor are effective in reducing pain and suffering during labor (*Simkin & Bolding, 2004).*

- Touch
  - Massage, effleurage, and counterpressure
  - Application of heat or cold
  - Therapeutic touch and healing touch

R: *Various forms of touch can convey to the woman a sense of caring, reassurance, understanding, or nonverbal support (Simkin & Ancheta, 2011). Purposeful use of massage is employed during labor as a relaxation and* *stress-reduction technique that functions as a distraction, may stimulate cutaneous nerve fibers that block painful impulses, and stimulates the local release of endorphins (Burke, 2014).*

- Transcutaneous electrical nerve stimulation decreases pain perception by providing alternate sensation

R: *Transcutaneous electrical nerve stimulation provides modest pain relief benefits and is a satisfying option for most women who use it (*Simkin & Bolding, 2004).*

- Acupuncture/Acupressure

R: *Acupuncture provides an effective alternative to pharmacologic pain relief (*Simkin & Bolding, 2004).*

- Intradermal injections of sterile water

R: *Intradermal injections of sterile water decrease lower back pain in most laboring women without any identified side effects on the fetus or mother (*Simkin & Bolding, 2004).*

Offer/Encourage Pharmacologic Pain Relief Measures Including (Burke, 2014)

- Sedatives and hypnotics
- Barbiturates—pentobarbital (Nembutal), secobarbital sodium (Seconal), zolpidem tartrate (Ambien)
- H_1-receptor antagonists—promethazine hydrochloride (Phenergan), hydroxyzine hydrochloride (Vistaril, Atarax)

R: *Barbiturates*

- *Provide sedation or sleep*
- *Depress the central nervous system*
- *Decrease anxiety*
- *Are rarely used in modern-day obstetrics because of long half-life*
- *Historically, women experiencing prolonged latent labor were thought to benefit from the brief period of therapeutic rest or sleep following administration of barbiturates.*

R: *H_1-receptor antagonists may be administered with narcotics during labor to*

- *Decrease anxiety*
- *Increase sedation*
- *Decrease nausea and vomiting*

- Analgesics
  - Opioids—morphine and meperidine
  - Synthetic opioids—fentanyl (Sublimaze) and remifentanil
  - Opioid agonist–antagonists—butorphanol (Stadol) and nalbuphine (Nubain)

R: *Analgesics allow women to relax and rest between contractions by*

- *Blunting effect with increase in pain threshold*
- *Decreased perception of pain*
- *Somnolence*
- Neuraxial analgesia
  - Epidural or spinal
  - Combined spinal–epidural (CSE)
  - Patient-controlled epidural analgesia (PCEA)

R: *Neuraxial analgesia in labor*

- *Provides superior pain relief*
- *Provides sufficient analgesia effect with as little motor block as possible*
- *Is flexible and effective method of pain relief*
- *Results in less central nervous system depression of mother and neonate than other pharmacologic methods*

- Regional anesthesia (rarely used in modern obstetrics)
  - Pudendal block—provides vaginal, vulvar, and perineal anesthesia via injection of anesthetic agent through lateral walls into area of pudendal nerve
  - Paracervical block—injection of anesthetic agent around the cervix

Discuss the Maternal–Fetal–Neonatal Side Effects of Pharmacologic Pain Relief Measures (Burke, 2014)

- Sedatives and hypnotics can
  - Potentiate respiratory depression in mother and neonate
- H_1-receptor antagonists can cause
  - Drowsiness and sedation in mother and neonate
  - Anticholinergic effects
  - Dry mouth
  - Respiratory depression
- Opioids can cause
  - Nausea and vomiting
  - Respiratory depression in mother and neonate
  - Decreased fetal heart rate variability
  - Neonatal respiratory depression at birth
  - Neonate exhibiting decreased muscle tone and alertness
  - Inhibited neonatal suckling at the breast
- Maternal side effects of neuraxial analgesia:
  - Hypotension
  - Inadequate, one-sided, or failed block
  - Pruritus
  - Nausea/vomiting
  - Fever
  - Urinary retention
  - Back pain
  - Postdural headache
- Major complications of neuraxial analgesia:
  - Intravascular injection of epinephrine and local anesthetic agent into an epidural vein
  - High spinal block due to inadvertent placement of epidural catheter and local anesthetic agent in the intrathecal space
  - Epidural hematoma due to bleeding within the spinal neuraxis
  - Respiratory depression
  - Neuraxial infection (meningitis)

R: *Intravascular injection of epinephrine and local anesthetic agent can result in*

- Systemic toxicity leading to
  - Immediate maternal heart rate
  - Palpitations
  - Elevated BP
  - Numbness around the tongue or mouth
  - Metallic taste
  - Tinnitus
  - Slurred speech
  - Jitteriness or agitation
  - Seizures
  - Cardiac arrest

R: *High spinal block can result in*

- Anesthetic agent ascends intrathecally into the brain stem, leading to
  - Respiratory paralysis
  - Total autonomic blockage
  - Loss of consciousness

R: *Epidural hematoma can result in*

- Severe pain
- Progressive sensory or motor blockade
- Deteriorating function of the lower extremities and bowel and bladder

R: *Signs and symptoms of meningitis may occur within 12 hours to a few days following birth and include*

- Fever
- Severe unrelenting headache
- Nick stiffness
- Sensitivity to light
- Nausea and vomiting
- Drowsiness
- Confusion
- Seizures

Monitor and Evaluate Effects of Pain Management Interventions on Mother and Fetus

- Assess comfort level before and after pain management interventions.
- Monitor fetal heart rate for nonreassuring characteristics (Refer to Nonreassuring Fetal Status in *Risk for Complications of Reproductive Dysfunction*).

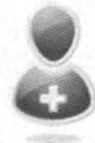

CLINICAL ALERT Notify the anesthesia provider if any of the following occurs:

- Hypotension
- High sensory-level block
- Bradycardia
- Respiratory compromise
- Apnea
- Arm/hand numbness or paralysis
- Nausea
- Anxiety
- Decreasing level of consciousness

Initiate Health Teaching as Indicated

- Instruct mother and her family on labor process.
- Explain physiology of pain in labor.
- Provide information about analgesia/anesthesia measures, side effects, and potential complications.
- Provide information about procedures to the mother and her family.

Nausea

NANDA-I Definition

A subjective phenomenon of an unpleasant feeling in the back of the throat and stomach that may or may not result in vomiting

Defining Characteristics*

Aversion toward food
Gagging sensation
Increased salivation
Increased swallowing
Reports nausea
Reports sour taste in mouth

Related Factors

Biopathophysiologic

Related to tissue trauma and reflex muscle spasms secondary to:

Acute gastroenteritis
Peptic ulcer disease
Irritable bowel syndrome
Pancreatitis
Infections (e.g., food poisoning)

Drug overdose
Renal calculi
Uterine cramps associated with menses
Motion sickness

Treatment Related

Related to effects of chemotherapy, theophylline, digitalis, antibiotics, iron supplements

Related to effects of anesthesia

Situational (Personal, Environmental)*

Anxiety
Noxious odors, taste
Fear
Pain
Psychological factors
Unpleasant visual stimulation

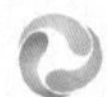

Errors in Diagnostic Statements

Refer to *Impaired Comfort*.

Key Concepts

General Considerations

- Nausea results from stimulation of the medullary vomiting center in the brain by the visceral and vagal afferent pathways (Grossman & Porth, 2014).
- Nausea and vomiting, when determined to have emotional origins, may result from developmental adjustment and adaptation. A child learns that vomiting is unacceptable and thus learns to control it. He or she receives approval for not vomiting. Should childhood situations or conflicts resurface, the adult may experience nausea and vomiting.
- Nausea is the third most common side effect of chemotherapy after alopecia and fatigue.
- Nausea and vomiting associated with chemotherapy can be classified as acute, delayed, and anticipatory, which occur as follows (Yarbro et al., 2013):
  - Acute—1 to 2 hours after treatment resolving in 24 hours.
  - Delayed—persist or develop 24 hours after treatment.
  - Anticipatory—a conditioned response 12 hours prior to treatment.

Maternal Considerations

- Approximately 50% to 90% of women report some nausea and vomiting in early pregnancy (Pillitteri, 2014).
- Lacroix, Eason, and Melzack (2000) reported "Although commonly termed 'morning sickness,' only 17% of women report being affected only in the morning. In a prospective study in which 160 women provided daily diaries in early pregnancy, 74% reported nausea with a mean duration of 34.6 days, 'morning sickness' occurred in only 1.8%, and 80% reported nausea lasting all day. Only half of women reported relief by 14 weeks, but 90% had relief by 22 weeks" (*King & Murphy, 2009).
- The etiology of nausea during pregnancy has not been validated. Nausea may be related to fatigue, stress, decreased gastric motility, high estrogen or progesterone levels, vitamin B_6, lower maternal blood sugar, and/or sensitivity to a high level of chorionic gonadotropin hormones.
- Nausea during pregnancy is usually time-limited, with onset about the fifth week after the last menstrual period (LMP), a peak at 8 to 12 weeks, and resolution by 16 to 18 weeks for most women. Approximately 5% of women will have symptoms throughout pregnancy (*King & Murphy, 2009; Pillitteri, 2014; *Sherman & Flaxman, 2002).
- There is evidence that ginger produces an anticoagulant effect and might increase the risk of bleeding, especially postdelivery or with premature separation of placenta (Tiran, 2012).

Focus Assessment Criteria

Subjective Data

Onset/duration
Time of day, pattern
Frequency
Vomitus (amount, time of day)
Associated with
- Medications
- Activity
- Specific foods
- Pain
- Position
- Relief measures

Goals

NOC

Comfort Status: Physical, Nutrition Status, Hydration, Nausea and Vomiting Control, Appetite

The client will report decreased nausea as experienced by the following indicators:

- Name foods or beverages that do not increase nausea.
- Describe factors that increase nausea.
- Describe one nonpharmacological measure to reduce nausea.

Interventions

NIC

Medication Management, Nausea Management, Fluid/Electrolyte Management, Nutrition Management, Relaxation therapy, Vomiting Management

Take Measures to Prevent Treatment-Related Nausea

- Aggressive management before, during, and after chemotherapy can prevent nausea. Follow protocols (Yarbro et al., 2013).
- Aggressively prevent nausea and vomiting in those with risk factors (Pasero & McCaffery, 2011):
  - Female gender
  - Nonsmoker
  - History of motion sickness/postoperative nausea/vomiting
- Use of volatile anesthetics within 0 to 2 hours, Nitrous oxide and or intraoperative and postoperative opioids.
- Duration of surgery
- Type of surgery (e.g., laparoscopic, ENT, neurosurgery, breast, plastic surgery)

R: *The presence of one risk factor increases the incidence to 10% to 20%. Two or more risk factors increases the incidence to 39% to 78% (*Apfel et al., 1999).*

- Consult with anesthesia specialist to prevent postoperative nausea and vomiting intraoperatively and postoperatively (Pasero & McCaffery, 2011).

R: *Postoperative nausea and vomiting can cause aspiration, tension on sutures, increased intracranial or intraocular pressure, and fluid and electrolyte imbalances (Pasero & McCaffery, 2011).*

Promote Comfort During Nausea and Vomiting

- Protect those at risk for aspiration (immobile, children).
- Address the cleanliness of the client and environment.
- Provide an opportunity for oral care after each episode.
- Apply a cool, damp cloth to the client's forehead, neck, and wrists.

R: *Comfort measures also reduce the stimuli for vomiting.*

Reduce or Eliminate Noxious Stimuli

Pain

- Plan care to avoid unpleasant or painful procedures before meals.
- Medicate clients for pain 30 minutes before meals according to physician/NP's orders.

- Provide a pleasant, relaxed atmosphere for eating (no bedpans in sight, do not rush); try a "surprise" (e.g., flowers with meal).
- Arrange the plan of care to decrease or eliminate nauseating odors or procedures near mealtimes.

Fatigue

- Teach or assist the client to rest before meals.
- Teach the client to spend minimal energy preparing food (cook large quantities and freeze several meals at a time, request assistance from others).

Odor of Food

- Teach to avoid cooking odors—frying food, brewing coffee—if possible (take a walk; select foods that can be eaten cold).
- Suggest using foods that require little cooking during periods of nausea. Try cold foods.
- Suggest trying sour foods.

R: *Unpleasant sights or odors can stimulate the vomiting center.*

Decrease Stimulation of the Vomiting Center

- Reduce unpleasant sights and odors. Restrict activity.
- Provide good mouth care after vomiting.
- Teach to practice deep breathing and voluntary swallowing to suppress the vomiting reflex.
- Instruct to sit down after eating, but not to lie down.
- Encourage to eat smaller meals and to eat slowly.
- Restrict liquids with meals to avoid overdistending the stomach; also, avoid fluids 1 hour before and after meals.
- Loosen clothing.
- Encourage to sit in fresh air or use a fan to circulate air.
- Advise to avoid lying flat for at least 2 hours after eating. (An individual who must rest should sit or recline so the head is at least 4 inches higher than the feet.)
- Advise to listen to music.
- Offer muscle relaxation and distraction techniques, for example, music.

R: *Evidence suggests that music-based interventions can have a positive impact on pain, anxiety, mood disturbance, and quality of life in cancer patients (Archie et al., 2013).*

R: *Both muscle relaxation and distraction techniques have been found to decrease nausea and vomiting in adults receiving chemotherapy (Miller & Kearney, 2004; Yarbro et al., 2013).*

- Teach acupressure at pressure points on his or her inner wrist (Sloan Kettering Cancer Center, 2013).
  - The location of the pressure point is shown in Figure II.3A.
  - To find pressure point P-6, place the first three fingers of your opposite hand across your wrist. Then, place your thumb on the point just below your index finger (see Fig. II.3B). You should be able to feel two large tendons under your thumb.
  - Press on this point with your thumb or forefinger and apply a circular motion for 2 to 3 minutes. The pressure should be firm but not cause discomfort.
  - Repeat the process on your other wrist.
  - Another option is wearing a acupressure band on wrist.

R: *Acupressure has been proven to be effective for nausea after some surgeries, and discomforts related to cancer and treatments (Doran & Halm, 2010, Sloan Kettering Cancer Center, 2013; *Streitberger et al., 2004).*

- Consider:
  - Small amounts of clear fluids and foods and beverages with ginger.

R: *Ginger as a treatment for nausea has been studied numerous times, with mixed results (Jiyeon & Heeyoung, 2013). Many anecdotal reports suggested the benefits of ginger ale (made from real ginger) to be soothing to GI disturbances and nausea reduction. Drinking large amounts of ginger ale that contains real ginger can cause some blood thinning. This blood thinning can be dangerous in patients who are already taking medications that prevent blood clotting, including aspirin, warfarin, or heparin*

  - Slice a lemon in half on plate and slowly inhale the aroma.

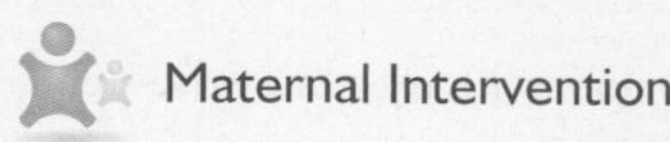

Maternal Interventions

Explain the Frequency, Causes and Course of Nausea in Pregnancy, Refer to *Maternal Considerations* for Specific Information

Teach That Various Interventions Have Been Reported to Help Control Nausea During Pregnancy (Pillitteri, 2014)

- Assure her that nausea is common during pregnancy.
- Avoid fatigue and sudden movements.

R: *Fatigue has been reported to precipitate such nausea/vomiting (*Voda & Randall, 1982).*

- Avoid greasy, high-fat foods, spicy foods. Avoid even smelling or cooking these types of foods.
- Eat high-protein meals and a snack before retiring.

R: *This will allow breakfast to be delayed (Pillitteri, 2014).*

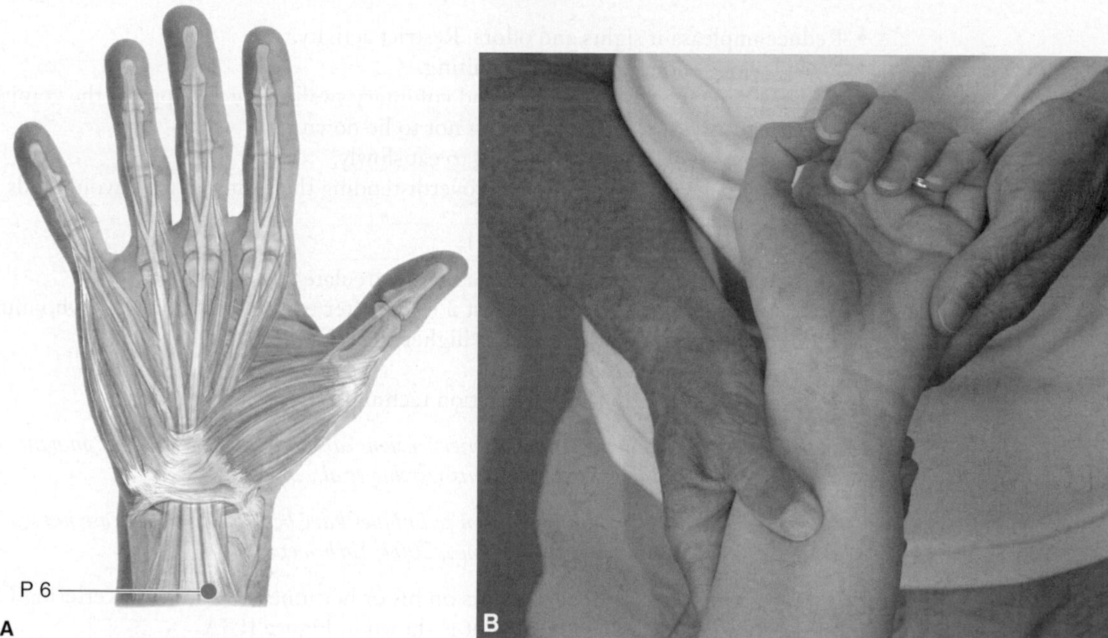

FIGURE II.3 Acupressure Points to Relieve Nausea

R: *Voda and Randall (1982) reported that eating a high-protein snack before going to bed at night decreases morning nausea in some pregnant women and prevents hypoglycemia.*

- Chew gum or suck hard candies.
- Eat carbohydrates (e.g., crackers, toast, sour ball candy) on arising; delay eating breakfast until nausea passes.
- Delay a meal until nausea passes.
- Eat immediately when hungry.
- Do not go longer than 12 hours without eating.
- If nauseated, sip/consume carbonated beverages (e.g., Coke syrup, orange juice, ginger ale, and herbal teas such as ginger).
- Try deep breaths of fresh air.
- Lie down to relieve symptoms.

R: *The goal of interventions is to reduce nausea and prevent nutritional and fluid imbalances.*

Use Acupressure (Refer to Description Under General Interventions for *Nausea*).

R: *Multiple studies have shown acupressure to be effective for nausea in pregnancy (*Ezzo, Streitberger, & Schneider 2006; Forouhari et al., 2014; *King & Murphy, 2009).*

Explain Ginger as a Treatment for Nausea/Vomiting During Pregnancy. Consult with OB Provider if Small Amounts of Ginger Ale (real ginger) are Permissible.

R: *Ginger has been found to be beneficial for relieving nausea. (*King & Murphy, 2009) Ginger can cause some blood thinning. This could be fatal if placenta separates, which would result in hemorrhage (Pillitteri, 2014; Tiran, 2012).*

Instruct the Pregnant Woman to Try One Food or Beverage Type at a Time (e.g., High-Protein Meals/Bedtime Snack)

- If nausea is not relieved, try another measure.
- Explain use of acupressure and acupuncture. Refer to resources.

R: *Acupressure and acupuncture have proven effective for nausea and vomiting in pregnancy.*

Advised to Notify Health-Care Provider if she (Pillitteri, 2014)

- Vomits more than once daily.
- Is losing weight.
- Is not eating enough during the day.
- Has decreased urine or darker yellow colored urine.
- Must alter her lifestyle, for example, work schedule.

R: *Nausea that does no resolve at some time during the day or excessive vomiting can negatively impact the woman's nutritional and hydration status. Pharmacological interventions may be indicated.*

IMPAIRED COMMUNICATION[10]

Impaired Communication

Related to Effects of Hearing Loss
Related to Effects of Aphasia on Expression or Interpretation
Related to Foreign Language Barrier
Impaired Verbal Communication

Definition

The state in which a person experiences, or is at risk to experience, difficulty exchanging thoughts, ideas, wants, or needs with others

Defining Characteristics

Major (Must Be Present)

Inappropriate or absent speech or response
Impaired ability to speak or hear

Minor (May Be Present)

Incongruence between verbal and nonverbal messages
Stuttering
Slurring
Word-finding problems
Weak or absent voice
Statements of being misunderstood or not understanding
Dysarthria
Aphasia
Language barrier

[10]This diagnosis is not presently on the NANDA-I list but has been added for clarity and usefulness.

Related Factors

Pathophysiologic

Related to disordered, unrealistic thinking secondary to:

Schizophrenic disorder
Psychotic disorder
Delusional disorder
Paranoid disorder

Related to impaired motor function of muscles of speech secondary to:

Cerebrovascular accident ("Brain attack")
Oral or facial trauma
Brain damage (e.g., birth/head trauma)
Central nervous system (CNS) depression/increased intracranial pressure
Tumor (of the head, neck, or spinal cord)
Chronic hypoxia/decreased cerebral blood flow
Nervous system diseases (e.g., myasthenia gravis, multiple sclerosis, muscular dystrophy, Alzheimer's disease)
Vocal cord paralysis/quadriplegia

Related to impaired ability to produce speech secondary to:

Respiratory impairment (e.g., shortness of breath)
Laryngeal edema/infection
Oral deformities
- Cleft lip or palate
- Missing teeth
- Malocclusion or fractured jaw
- Dysarthria

Related to Auditory Impairment

Treatment Related

Related to impaired ability to produce speech secondary to:

Endotracheal intubation
Surgery of the head, face, neck, or mouth
CNS depressants
Tracheostomy/tracheotomy/laryngectomy
Pain (especially of the mouth or throat)

Situational (Personal, Environmental)

Related to decreased attention secondary to fatigue, anger, anxiety, or pain

Related to no access to or malfunction of hearing aid

Related to psychological barrier (e.g., fear, shyness)

Related to lack of privacy

Related to unavailable interpreter

Maturational

Infant/Child
Related to inadequate sensory stimulation

Older Adult (Auditory Losses)
Related to hearing impairment

Related to cognitive impairments secondary to (specify)

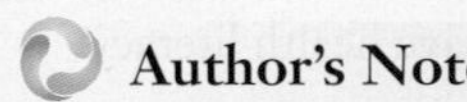

Author's Note

Impaired Communication is clinically useful with individuals with communication receptive deficits and language barriers. *Impaired Communication* may not be useful to describe communication problems that are a manifestation of psychiatric illness or coping problems. If nursing interventions focus on reducing hallucinations, fear, or anxiety, *Confusion*, *Fear*, or *Anxiety* would be more appropriate.

Errors in Diagnostic Statements

***Impaired Communication* related to failure of staff to use effective communication techniques**

This diagnostic statement should not be used as a vehicle to reveal a problem resulting from incorrect or insufficient nursing intervention. Instead, the diagnosis should be *Impaired Verbal Communication related to effects of tracheotomy on ability to talk.* The care plan should specify the communication techniques to use.

Key Concepts

General Considerations

- Messages are sent more by body language and tone of voice than by words.
- Speech represents the fundamental way for humans to express needs, desires, and feelings. If only one person expresses information without any feedback from a listener, effective communication has not occurred.
- Any of the following can cause problems with *sending* information:
  - Inability or failure to send messages that the listener can clearly understand (e.g., language or word-meaning problems, failure to speak when listener is ready)
  - Fear of being overheard, judged, or misunderstood (e.g., lack of privacy, confidentiality, trust, or nonjudgmental attitude)
  - Concern over response (e.g., "I don't want to hurt or anger anyone.")
  - Use of words that "talk down" to the receiver (e.g., talking to an elderly or handicapped person as if he or she were a child)
  - Failure to allow sufficient time for listening or providing feedback
  - Physical problems (e.g., noise, lack of privacy that interfere with the ability to see, talk, or move)
- Any of the following can cause problems with *receiving* information:
  - Too much information being given at one time
  - More than one person talking at once
  - Person talking too fast or with a strong accent
  - Language or vocabulary problems
  - Fatigue, pain, fear, anxiety, distractions, attention span problems
  - Not realizing the importance of the information
  - Problems that interfere with the ability to see or hear
- Dysarthria is a disturbance in the voluntary muscular control of speech. It is caused by conditions such as Parkinson's disease, multiple sclerosis, myasthenia gravis, cerebral palsy, and CNS damage. The same muscles are used in eating and swallowing.

Types of Literacy

- Low health literacy, cultural barriers, and limited English proficiency have been coined the "triple threat" to effective health communication by The Joint Commission (Schyve, 2007)
- Functional illiteracy
  - Functional illiteracy is when someone who has minimal reading and writing skills does not have the capacity for health literacy to manage ordinary everyday needs and requirements of most employments.
  - Individuals who are illiterate (who cannot read or write) are easier to identify than someone who is functionally illiterate.
- Health literacy
  - Health literacy is the capacity to obtain, process, and understand basic health information and services needed to make appropriate health decisions (*Ratzan, 2001) and to follow instructions for treatment (White & Dillow, 2005). In 2003, the National Assessment of Adult Literacy (NAAL)

reported that 9 out of 10 English-speaking adults in the United States do not have health literacy (*Kutner, Greenberg, Jiny, & Paulsen, 2006).

- A large study on the scope of health literacy at two public hospitals found the following (*Williams et al., 1995):
  - Half of English-speaking patients could not read and understand basic health education material.
  - 60% could not understand a routine consent form.
  - 26% could not understand the appointment card.
  - 42% failed to understand directions for taking their medications.
- The AMA's (*1999) committee of health literacy found inadequate health literacy was most prevalent in the elderly and individuals who report poor overall health . The report concluded that individuals who reported "the worst health status have less understanding about their medical conditions and treatment" (AMA, 1999, p. 57).

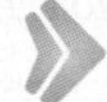

Carp's Cues

"Social and educational levels have little relationship to health literacy" (Speros, 2005, p. 638). Individuals will hide the literacy problems if allowed. Many individuals are at risk of understanding, but it is hard to identify them (DeWalt et al., 2010).

Aphasia

- Stroke is a leading cause of death in the United States, killing nearly 130,000 Americans each year (Centers for Disease Control and Prevention, 2015).
- Deficits post stroke include "altered level of consciousness, confusion, behavioral disturbances, cognitive deficits in higher functions such as memory and ability to learn, motor deficits, disturbance in balance and coordination, somatosensory deficits, disorders of vision, unilateral neglect, speech and language deficits, swallowing disorder (dysphagia), and affective disorder" (Summers, Leonard, & Wentworth, 2009, p. 2913).
- The most common cause of aphasia is cerebrovascular disease, specifically cerebral infarction (stroke). Aphasia occurs in 15% to 38% of ischemic strokes. Other causes of aphasia are structural pathologies (infection, trauma, neoplasm) and certain neurodegenerative diseases (primary progressive aphasia) (Clark, 2015).
- The different types of aphasia affect one's ability to form words or to write. Other types affect the person's ability to understand speech or to read. Some of the types of aphasia are as follows (Clark, 2012; Grossman & Porth, 2014):
  - *Broca's aphasia* (also called nonfluent aphasia or expressive aphasia): This type of aphasia affects one's ability to speak but the person usually can understand well.
  - *Wernicke's aphasia* (also called fluent aphasia): This type of aphasia affects one's ability to form speech, but there is no difficulty understanding it. They can produce a lot of speech that doesn't make sense.
  - *Global aphasia*: With this type of aphasia, individuals cannot speak or understand written or spoken language.
  - *Anomic aphasia*: With this aphasia, individuals have difficulty naming specific objects; even though they might still be able to speak, they cannot recall what different things are called.
  - *Alexia*: This type of aphasia affects one's ability to read.
- People with aphasia communicated with fewer friends and had smaller social networks (Davidson, Worrall, & Hickson).
- *Expressive aphasia* is a disturbance in the ability to speak, write, or gesture understandably.
- *Receptive aphasia* is a disturbance in the ability to comprehend written and spoken language. Those with receptive aphasia may have intact hearing, but cannot process or are unaware of their own sounds.
- Understanding of and respect for differences in personality and thinking styles are essential for communicating in ways that enhance interpersonal relations.

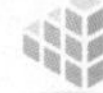

Pediatric Considerations

- There are four major ways in which hearing loss affects children—American Speech-Language-Hearing Association
  - It causes delay in the development of receptive and expressive communication skills (speech and language).
  - The language deficit causes learning problems that result in reduced academic achievement.
  - Communication difficulties often lead to social isolation and poor self-concept.
  - It may have an impact on vocational choices.

- Although most verbal communication occurs between the nurse and the parents, the adults should not ignore the child's input. Nurses should assess writing, drawing, play, and body language (facial expressions, gestures).
- Play therapy can be invaluable in establishing rapport and communicating true feelings.
- The child with hearing loss may exhibit alterations in the following responses:
  - Orientation (e.g., lack of startle reflex to a loud sound)
  - Vocalizations and sound production (e.g., lack of babbling by 7 months of age)
  - Visual attention (e.g., responding more to facial expression than to verbal explanation)
  - Social emotional behavior (e.g., becomes irritable at inability to make self understood)
- "Children with severe to profound hearing losses often report feeling isolated, without friends, and unhappy in school, particularly when their socialization with other children with hearing loss is limited" (American Speech-Language-Hearing Association, 2014).
- These social problems appear to be more frequent in children with a mild or moderate hearing loss than in those with a severe to profound loss (American Speech-Language-Hearing Association, 2014).
- For deaf infants, visual and tactile modalities are particularly important for communicating, interacting, and gaining information about the environment (Joint Committee on Infant Hearing, 2007).
- Early detection is critical. Failure to detect hearing deficits can lead to life-long deficits and delays in development (*Storbeck & Calvert-Evers, 2008).

Geriatric Considerations

- Approximately one in three people between the ages of 65 and 74 have hearing loss, and nearly half of those older than 75 have difficulty hearing (National Institute on Deafness and Other Communication Disorders, 2013).
- Impacted cerumen (wax) is the leading cause of hearing loss in older adults (Miller, 2015). This occurs in 57% of older adults living in nursing homes (Roland et al., 2008).
- Social isolation is a common side effect of hearing impairment. Individuals and loved ones should be educated on effective communication techniques which can help prevent social isolation (e.g., hearing aids, reducing background noise and distraction, facing the hearing-impaired person when talking). Sensitivity to the needs by loved ones and caretakers and communication of the needs by the client are keys to success.

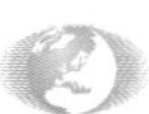

Transcultural Considerations

- Studies have shown that patients with limited English proficiency have less access to care, poorer adherence to treatment regimens, and consequently contribute to increased health disparities. This issue is of particular importance for nurses due to the intimate contact and need for frequent and lengthy patient interactions. A majority of nurses reported that language barriers are a significant impediment to quality care and a source of stress in the workplace. Incomplete nursing assessments, misunderstood medical information, and the lack of therapeutic relationships between providers and patients are problems encountered when patients have limited English proficiency. Nursing students are the future of the nursing profession; therefore, it is important to address the impact of language barriers on health-care disparities in the nursing curriculum (Houle, 2010).
- All cultures have rules about who touches whom, when, and where.
- Touch is a strong form of communication with many meanings and interpretations. There are cultural standards regarding touch, in some are strict as touching someone's head, who is of Chinese descent is considered a serious breach of etiquette (Giger, 2013).
- The dominant US culture tends to conceal feelings and is considered (Giger, 2013).
- Cultural uses of touch vary, with touch between same-sex people considered as taboo in some cultures but expected in others (Giger, 2013).
- English and German cultures do not encourage touching.
- Some highly tactile cultures are Spanish, Italian, French, Jewish, and South American.
- In some cultures, a nod is a polite response meaning "I heard you, but I do not necessarily understand or agree" (Giger, 2013).
- The dominant US culture views eye contact as an indication of a positive self-concept, openness, and honesty. It views lack of eye contact as low self-esteem, guilt, or lack of interest. Some cultures are not accustomed to eye contact, including Filipino, Native American, and Vietnamese (Giger, 2013).

- The individual and family should be encouraged to communicate their interpretations of health, illness, and health care (Giger, 2013) within the context of their specific culture.
- People from certain ethnic or racial backgrounds may speak English with varied geographic dialects. For example, certain syllables or consonants may be pronounced differently (e.g., pronouncing *th* as *d*, as in "*des*" for "these"). These different pronunciations should not be viewed as substandard or ungrammatical. In addition, some slang words may have different meanings—for example, "the birth of my daughter was a real bad experience." The person may mean it was unique and positive (Giger, 2013).
- Mexican-Americans speak Spanish, which has more than 50 dialects; thus, a nurse who speaks Spanish may have difficulty understanding a different dialect. Both men and women may be modest and restrict self-disclosure to those whom they know well. The culture considers direct confrontation and arguments rude; thus, agreeing may be a courtesy, not a commitment. A folk illness called *mal ojo* (evil eye) is thought to harm a child when the child is admired, but not touched, by a person thought to have special powers. When interacting with children, touch them lightly to avoid *mal ojo*. These clients may view kidding as rude and deprecating.
- Chinese-Americans value silence and avoid disagreeing or criticizing. Whereas many Americans of other cultural backgrounds naturally raise the voice to make a point, Chinese-Americans associate raising the voice with anger and loss of control. They rarely use "no," and "yes" can mean "perhaps" or "no." Touching the head is a serious breach of etiquette. Hesitation, ambiguity, and subtlety dominate Chinese speech (Giger, 2013).

Focus Assessment Criteria

Subjective Data

Assess for Defining Characteristics

Note the usual pattern of communication as described by the person or family:

Very verbal
Sometimes verbal
Uses sign language
Only writes
Responds inappropriately
Does not speak/respond
Speaks only when spoken to gestures only

Does the person feel he or she is communicating normally today?
If not, what does the individual feel may help him or her to communicate better?
Does the person have trouble hearing?

Hearing problem
Both ears or one?
How long? Gradual? Sudden?
Has his or her ears been examined for cerumen (wax)?
Use of a hearing aid
Family history of hearing loss
History of exposure to loud noises

Ask the individual/caregiver to

Rate the ability to communicate on a scale of 0 to 10, with 0 signifying "completely unable to communicate" and 10 signifying "communicates well"
Describe factors that aid communication

Assess for Related Factors

Can the person identify barriers that interfere with his or her ability to communicate?

Objective Data

Assess for Defining Characteristics

Describe Ability to Speak, Ability to Comprehend (Note: Individual May Need More Time to Process and Respond)

Follows simple commands or ideas
Can follow complex instructions or ideas

Sometimes can follow instructions or ideas
Follows commands and ideas only if the hearing aid is working
Follows commands and ideas only if he or she can see the speaker's mouth (lip-reads)

What Is the Developmental Age?

Describe Ability to Form Sentences

Is Eye Contact Maintained?

Hearing Loss (Check Each Ear Separately)

External Ear
Deformities
Lesions
Lumps or tenderness

Middle and Inner Ear
Cerumen
Discharge
Redness
Swelling

Auditory Acuity
Can hear ticking watch or whispered words

Hearing Aid?
Left ear
Right ear

Assess for Related Factors

Barriers—refer to Related Factors

Goals

NOC
Communication, Communication: Receptive, Communication: Expressive

The person will report improved satisfaction with ability to communicate as evidenced by the following indicators:

- Demonstrates increased ability to understand
- Demonstrates improved ability to express self
- Uses alternative methods of communication, as indicated

Interventions

NIC
Communication Enhancement: Speech, Communication Enhancement: Hearing Deficit, Communication Enhancement: Speech Deficit, Communication Enhancement: Visual Deficit, Active Listening, Socialization Enhancement, Touch, Presence, Validation Therapy

Therapeutic Communication Begins With

- Presenting yourself with *unconditional positive regard* or genuine warmth to the person being helped by
  - Introducing yourself and your position (e.g., RN assigned to him/her)
  - Using age and/or culturally appropriate titles of respect as Mr., Mrs., Miss, Ms., Senora, Senor, Dr., Reverend
  - Asking the person how he or she wants to be addressed. If needed, ask them to pronounce their name.
  - Slowing your walking pace as you enter the room
- If the topic is serious, bring a chair to the bedside and sit, face to face, even if only for a few minutes.

R: *Sitting at eye level with the person increases the message that you are ready to engage in dialogue and provides a more comforting position than standing over the person.*

R: *Therapeutic communication encompasses a capacity for empathic understanding of the person's internal frame of reference. This means working to understand how the person really feels and remaining unbiased.*

Practice "Listening to Understand Rather Than Listening to Respond" (Proctor, Hammer, McGarry, & McLane, 2014, p. 93), **Especially in Nonillness-Related Discussions**

- Quieting your mind caring about the other person and being free of judgment of what he or she thinks or feels

R: *When one listens to respond, one is focused on the response. "Withholding one's reactions to what is being said, hearing what is being said, and then exploring the person's perspective with curious questioning, rather than* *launching into one's own agenda, leads one to develop a more balance and inclusive appraisal of the person's situation" (Proctor et al., 2014, p. 93).*

Identify a Method to Communicate Basic Needs

- Assess ability to comprehend, speak, read, and write.
- Provide alternative methods of communication.
  - Use a computer, pad and pencil, hand signals, eye blinks, head nods, and bell signals.
  - Make flash cards with pictures or words depicting frequently used phrases (e.g., "Wet my lips," "Move my foot," "I need a glass of water," or "I need a bedpan").
  - Encourage the person to point, use gestures, and pantomime.
- Establishing an alternative form of communication is imperative for all individuals to prevent heightened anxiety, isolation, and alienation, which will promote a sense of control; and enhance a sense of security (Boyd, 2012; Miller, 2015).

Identify Factors That Promote Communication

- Provide a nonrushed environment.
- Use techniques to increase understanding:
  - Face the client and establish eye contact if possible.
  - Look at the client when speaking, enunciate words, and speak slowly.
  - Use uncomplicated one-step commands and directives.
  - Have only one person talk (following a conversation among multiple parties can be difficult).
  - Speak clearly, not loudly.
  - Encourage the use of gestures and pantomime.
  - Match words with actions; use pictures.
  - Terminate the conversation on a note of success (e.g., move back to an easier item).
  - Do not ask the person/family if they understand. Instead ask a question about something you just said (e.g., "So how are you going to take this medicine at home?").
  - Give information in writing to reinforce.

R: *Communication is the core of all human relations. Impaired ability to communicate spontaneously is frustrating and embarrassing. Nursing actions should focus on decreasing tension and conveying understanding of how difficult the situation must be for the individual (Miller, 2015).*

Initiate Health Teaching and Referrals, If Needed

- Seek consultation with a speech or audiology specialist.

R: *Specialists may be needed after discharge.*

Pediatric Interventions

- Use age-appropriate words and gestures.
- Initially talk to the parent and allow the child to observe. Gradually include the child.
  - Approach the child slowly and speak in a quiet, unhurried, confident voice.
  - Assume an eye-level position.
  - Use simple words and short sentences.
  - Talk about something not related to the present situation (e.g., school, toy, hair, clothes).
- Offer choices as much as possible.
- Encourage the child to share concerns and fears.
- Allow the child an opportunity to touch and use articles (e.g., stethoscope, tongue blade).

R: *Communication with children must be based on developmental stage, language abilities, and cognitive level.*

R: *In children, receptive language is always more advanced than expressive language; children understand more than they can articulate.*

Impaired Communication • Related to Effects of Hearing Loss

Goals

NOC
Communication, Communication: Receptive, Communication: Expressive

The person will relate/demonstrate an improved ability to communicate as evidenced by the following indicators:

- Wears functioning hearing aid if appropriate
- Communicates through alternative methods

Interventions

NIC
Active Listening, Communication Enhancement: Hearing Deficit

Ask the Person What Mode of Communication He or She Desires

Record on Care Plan the Method to Use (May Be Combination of the Following):

- Writing
- Speech-reading (or lip-reading)
- Speaking
- Gesturing
- Sign language

R: *Successful interaction with deaf or hearing-impaired clients requires knowing background issues, including age of onset, choice of language, cultural background, education level, and type of hearing loss.*

Assess Ability to Receive Verbal Messages

If Individual Can Hear With a Hearing Aid, Make Sure That It Is on and Functioning

- Check batteries by turning volume all the way up until it whistles. If it does not whistle, insert new batteries.
- Make sure that the volume is at a level that enhances hearing. (Many people with hearing aids turn the volume down occasionally for peace and quiet.)
- Make a special effort to ensure the individual wears the hearing aid during off-the-unit visits (e.g., special studies, the operating room).

If Individual Can Hear With Only One Ear, Speak Slowly and Clearly Directly Into the Good Ear. It Is More Important to Speak Distinctly Than Loudly

- Place bed in a position so the person's good ear faces the door.
- Stand or sit on the side on which the client hears the best (e.g., if left ear is better, sit on the left).

R: *Many older adults with hearing impairments do not wear hearing aids. Those who wear them must be encouraged to use them consistently, clean and maintain them, and replace batteries. Encourage the person to be assertive in letting significant others know about situations and environmental areas in which they experience difficulty because of background noise.*

If the Person Can Speech-Read, Do Not Call It Lip-Reading (*Bauman & Gell, 2000; Office of Student Disabilities Services, 2014)

- Look directly at the person; even a slight turn of your head can obscure the speech-reading view and
  - Speak slowly and clearly.
  - Do not yell, exaggerate, or overenunciate.

R: *It is estimated that only 3 out of 10 spoken words are visible on the lips. Overemphasis of words distorts lip movements and makes speech-reading more difficult.*

- Try to enunciate each word without force or tension. Short sentences are easier to understand than long ones.
- Do not place anything in your mouth when speaking.
- Mustaches that obscure the lips and putting your hands in front of your face can make lip-reading difficult.
- If the person looks surprised/perplexed/bemused, stop and clarify.

R: *Studies show that only 23% of hard of hearing people become effective speech-readers.*

- Avoid standing in front of light—have the light on your face so the person can see your lips.

R: *The bright background and shadows created on the face make it almost impossible to speech-read.*

- Minimize distractions that may inhibit the person's concentration.

R: *Another downside of speech-reading is that there is so much of time spent just trying to understand the words the person is saying that the person can easily miss the meaning of what someone is trying to communicate.*

- Maintain eye contact even if an interpreter is present; speak directly to the person. He or she will turn to the interpreter as needed.

R: *Eye contact conveys the feeling of direct communication. Avoid standing in front of a light source, such as a window or bright light. The bright background and shadows created on the face make it almost impossible to speech-read (Office of Student Disabilities Services, 2014).*

- Minimize conversations if the person is fatigued, or use written communication.
- Use open-ended questions, which must be answered by more than "yes," or "no."

R: *Open-ended questions ensure that your information has been communicated (Office of Student Disabilities Services, 2014).*

- Reinforce important communications by writing them down.

R: *Only 40% of the English language is visible. Speech-reading is difficult and fatiguing in the hospital. Unfamiliar terminology, anxiety, and poor lighting can contribute to errors. Even the best speech-reader catches only about 25% to 30% of what is said. However, be aware that about 10% of the population move their lips in such a way that it is absolutely impossible to speech-read even one word they say.*

If Individual Can Read and Write, Provide Pad and Pencil at All Times. If the Person Can Understand Only Sign Language, Have an Interpreter With Him or Her as Much as Possible

- Address all communication to the person, not to the interpreter (e.g., do not say, "Ask Mrs. Jones"). Record name and phone number of interpreter(s) on the care plan or per hospital policy.
- If in a group setting (e.g., diabetes class), place the client at front of the room near the instructor or send interpreter with him or her.
- Carefully evaluate the person's understanding of required knowledge.
- Give information in writing.

R: *When using an interpreter, some things may be omitted or misunderstood. Whenever possible, give information in writing as well as through the interpreter.*

- Validate the person's understanding by asking questions that require more than "yes" or "no" answers. Avoid asking, "Do you understand?"

R: *Hearing aids magnify all sounds. Therefore, extraneous sounds (e.g., rusting of papers, minor squeaks) can inhibit understanding of voiced messages.*

R: *Available to assist clients with hearing impairment is DEAFNET, a computer system that allows clients to type messages to a computer at the phone company, which a voice synthesizer translates verbally.*

Initiate Referrals as Needed

- Seek consultation with a speech or audiology specialist for assistance with communication.
- Telecommunication devices for the deaf (known as TDD) that operate by communicating electronically, messages that are typed, infrared systems, computers, voice amplifiers, amplified telephones, low-frequency doorbells and telephone ringers, closed-caption TV decoders, flashing alarm clocks, flashing smoke detectors, hearing aids, and lip-reading and signing instruction
- Deaf service centers available in most communities to help with housing, job seeking, travel arrangements, recreation, and adult education opportunities

R: *Under the Rehabilitation Act of 1973 and the Americans with Disabilities Act (ADA) of 1990, hospitals must offer reasonable accommodations for hearing-impaired individuals. For example, they must provide qualified interpreters and auxiliary tools, such as teletype machines, unless doing so imposes an undue financial or other burden.*

Impaired Communication • Related to Effects of Aphasia on Expression or Interpretation

Aphasia is a communication impairment—a difficulty in expressing, in understanding, or a combination of both—resulting from cerebral impairments.

Goals

NOC

Communication: Expressive

The person will report decreased frustration with communication as evidenced by the following indicators:

- Demonstrates increased ability to understand
- Demonstrates improved ability to express ideas, thoughts, and needs

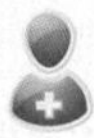

CLINICAL ALERT Individuals with poststroke aphasia are likely to experience some improvement after the initial event. The prognosis for full recovery is greatest when patients have milder degrees of aphasia at the onset.

Interventions

NIC

Communication Enhancement: Speech Deficit, Active Listening, Anxiety Reduction

Identify the Ability of the Individual to Express and Receive Information

R: *The ability of persons poststroke to communicate is influenced by their spatial orientation, their hearing and vision, and their level of communication impairment (McGilton et al., 2012).*

- Establish the specifics of the person's ability to send and receive communication. Consult with speech therapist.
- Hear, see, need for glasses, hearing aids.
- Read, write, use phone.
- Understand others.
- Speak appropriately.
- Point to objects that are named, or name objects.
- Presence of emotional variability, emotions not consistent with situation
- Specifically communication abilities and barriers to all caregivers. Use visual reminders, care plan.

Initiate the Dialogue. Make a Concerted Effort to Understand the Individual

- At the start of the conversation, check if the person is comfortable and there are no problems. If they normally wear glasses, a hearing aid, or dentures, make sure these are available.
- Provide sufficient light and remove distractions.
- Speak when the person is ready to listen.
- Achieve eye contact, if possible.
- Gain the person's attention by a gentle touch on the arm and a verbal message of "Listen to me" or "I want to talk to you."

R: *Deliberate actions can improve speech. As speech improves, confidence increases and the individual will make more attempts at speaking (McGilton et al., 2012).*

Use Techniques That Enhance Understanding

- Allow person time to respond; do not interrupt; supply words only occasionally.
  - Watch for when they are finished, or when they are looking for help. Ask if your help is needed before giving it.
  - Try to keep conversation natural and meaningful to them.

Modify Your Speech

- Speak slowly; enunciate distinctly.
- Use common adult words.
- Do not use slang or sayings: Say what you mean.
- Do not change subjects or ask multiple questions in succession.
- Repeat or rephrase requests.

- Do not increase volume of voice unless person has a hearing deficit.
- Match your nonverbal behavior with your verbal actions to avoid misinterpretation (e.g., do not laugh with a coworker while performing a task).
- Try to use the same words with the same task (e.g., bathroom vs. toilet, pill vs. medication).
- Rephrase messages aloud to validate what was said.
- Acknowledge when you understand, and do not be concerned with imperfect pronunciation at first.
- Ignore mistakes and profanity.
- Do not pretend you understand if you do not.
- Observe nonverbal cues for validation (e.g., answers yes and shakes head no).
- Focus on one topic at a time using short sentences. For example, instead of saying, "Your wife called and she will be here at 4 PM to pick you up and take you home," say: "Your wife called." (pause) "She will be here at 4 PM." (pause) "You can go home then." (Stroke Association, 2012)
- Use all forms of communication to help reinforce what you are saying, such as clear gestures, drawing and communication aids.
- Allow enough time to listen.

R: *Improving the individual's comprehension can help decrease frustration and increase trust. Individuals with aphasia can correctly interpret tone of voice.*

- Learn what this person's interests were prior to stroke and utilize this in your conversations.
- Have family bring in pictures of family, vacations.
- Identify an activity that may be meaningful to watch or engage in (e.g., knitting, singing).
- Look at a photo album together and talk about the places visited and the people in the photos. Have family engage in this activity.

R: *"When providing care knowing what interests them helps to limit the patient's behavioral symptoms. Topics of interest (i.e., hobbies, families, etc.) for conversations that will engage the patient in meaningful interactions are obtained from the individual and family"* (McGilton et al., 2012).

Acknowledge Client's Frustration and Improvements

- Verbally address frustration over inability to communicate and explain that both nurse and client need to use patience.
- Maintain a calm, positive attitude (e.g., "I can understand you if we work at it.").
- Use reassurance (e.g., "I know it's difficult, but you'll get it."); use touch if acceptable.
- Maintain a sense of humor.
- Allow tears (e.g., "It's OK. I know it's frustrating. Crying can let it all out.").
- Give the person opportunities to make care-related decisions (e.g., "Would you rather have orange juice or prune juice?").
- Provide alternative methods of self-expression:
  - Humming/singing (Magee & Baker, 2009)
  - Dancing/exercising/walking
  - Writing/drawing/painting/coloring
  - Helping (tasks such as opening mail, choosing meals)

R: *Good communicators are also good listeners, who listen for both facts and feelings.*

- Just being present and available, even if one says or does little, can effectively communicate caring to another.

Teach Techniques to Improve Speech

- Ask to slow speech down and say each word clearly while providing the example.
- Encourage the client to speak in short phrases.
- Explain that the individual's words are not clearly understood (e.g., "I can't understand what you are saying.").
- Suggest a slower rate of talking or taking a breath before beginning to speak.
- Ask the client to write down message or to draw a picture if verbal communication is difficult. (Note: It is not uncommon for clients with aphasia to be unable to write words.)

- Focus on the present; avoid controversial, emotional, abstract, or lengthy topics.

R: *Poor communication can cause frustration, anger, hostility, depression, fear, confusion, and isolation.*

Use Multiple Methods of Communication

- Use pantomime.
- Point.
- Use flash cards.
- Show what you mean (e.g., pick up a glass).
- Write key words on a card, so the individual can practice them while you show the object (e.g., paper).

R: *Using alternative forms of communication can help to decrease anxiety, isolation, and alienation (McGilton et al., 2012).*

Explain the Benefits of Daily Speech Practice. Consult With Speech Therapist for Specific Exercises.

R: *Daily exercises help improve the efficiency of speech musculature and increase rate, volume, and articulation. Research shows comprehensive care during the first 4 weeks after a stroke improves overall morbidity and mortality (Clark, 2012).*

Show Respect When Providing Care

- Avoid discussing the person's condition in his or her presence; assume the individual can understand despite deficits.
- Monitor other health-care providers for adherence to plan of care.
- Talk to the person whenever you are with him or her.

R: *After survival, perhaps the most basic human need is to communicate with others. Communication provides security by reinforcing that individuals are not alone and that others will listen. Poor communication can cause frustration, anger, hostility, depression, fear, confusion, and isolation.*

Initiate Health Teaching and Referrals, If Indicated

- Explain the reasons for labile emotions and profanity.

R: *Emotional lability (swings between crying and laughing) is common in people with aphasia. This behavior is not intentional and declines with recovery.*

- Refer to *Caregiver Role Strain.*
- Continue consultation with a speech pathologist after transition from acute-care center.

R: *Speech represents the fundamental way for humans to express needs, desires, and feelings. If only one person expresses information without any feedback from a listener, effective communication cannot be said to have happened. Research shows comprehensive care during the first 4 weeks after a stroke improves overall morbidity and mortality (Clark, 2012).*

- National Aphasia Association. www.aphasia.org/Aphasia%20Facts/aphasia_faq.html. Accessed August, 2012.

Impaired Communication • Related to Foreign Language Barrier

Goals

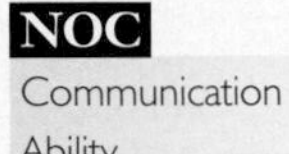

Communication Ability

The person will communicate needs and concerns (through interpreter if needed) as evidenced by the following indicators:

- Demonstrates ability to understand information
- Relates feelings of reduced frustration and isolation

Interventions

NIC

Culture Brokerage, Active Listening, Communication Enhancement

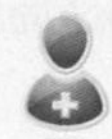

Clinical Alert Low health literacy, cultural barriers, and limited English proficiency have been coined the "triple threat" to effective health communication by The Joint Commission (Schyve, 2007). "At a practical level, nurses must be cognizant that culture affects individual and collective experiences that are directly and indirectly related to health. Examples of cultural influences on patient health beliefs and behaviors can be found in patients' perceptions of locus of control, preferences, communication norms, and prioritization of needs, as well as in their understanding of physical and mental illness and of the roles of the individual, family, and community" (Singleton & Krause, 2009).

R: *The culturally bound beliefs, values, and preferences a person holds influence how a person interprets health-care messages. Knowing about a patient's language and culture is key for knowing how health literate the person is in a given situation.*

Assess Ability to Communicate in English

- Assess language the individual speaks best.
- Assess the individual's ability to read, write, speak, and comprehend English.
- Assess for red flags literacy, health literacy (DeWalt et al., 2010).
- Frequently missed appointments
- Incomplete registration forms
- Noncompliance with medication
- Unable to name medications, explain purpose, or dosing
- Identifies pills by looking at them, not reading label
- Unable to give coherent, sequential history
- Asks fewer questions
- Lack of follow-through on tests or referrals

R: *The Institute of Medicine (2011) has reported that 58% of Black and 66% of Hispanic adults exhibited "basic" or "below basic" health literacy compared to only 28% of white adults.*

- Do not evaluate understanding based on "yes" or "no" responses.

R: *An answer of "yes" may be an effort to please, rather than a sign of understanding.*

Identify Factors That Promote Communication Without a Translator

- Face the person and give a pleasant greeting in a normal tone of voice.
- Talk clearly and somewhat slower than normal (do not overdo it).

R: *An attempt on the nurse's part to communicate over a language barrier encourages the individual to do the same.*

R: *People should overcome the human tendency either to ignore or to shout at people who do not speak the dominant language.*

- If the person does not understand or speak (respond), use an alternative communication method:
  - Write message.
  - Use gestures or actions.
  - Use pictures or drawings.
  - Make flash cards that translate words or phrases.
- Encourage the client to teach others some words or greetings of his or her own language (helps to promote acceptance and willingness to learn).
- Do not correct an individual or family's pronunciation.
- Clarify the exact meaning of an unclear word.
- Use medical terms and the slang word when indicated (e.g., vomiting/throwing up).

R: *Be aware that, when one learns a language, one usually learns only one meaning for a word. Some words in English have more than one meaning, such as "discharge" and "pupil."*

R: *During the initial assessment, start with general questions. Allow time for the person to talk even if it is not related. Use nondirect, open-ended questions when possible. Delay asking very personal questions, if possible.*

Be Cognizant of Possible Cultural Barriers

- Be careful when touching the person; some cultures may consider touch inappropriate.
- Be aware of different ways the culture expects men and women to be treated (cultural attitudes may influence whether a man speaks to a woman about certain matters or vice versa).

R: *Communicating through touch or holding varies among cultures. Some cultures view touch as an extremely familiar gesture, some shy away from touching a given part of the body (a pat on the head may be offensive), and some consider it appropriate for men to kiss one another and for women to hold hands (Giger, 2013).*

- Make a conscious effort to be nonjudgmental about cultural differences.

R: *Nurses must have transcultural sensitivity, understand how to impart knowledge, and know how to advocate to represent the individual's needs. Interpreting with cultural sensitivity is much more complex than simply putting words in another language (Giger, 2013).*

- Make note of what seems to be a comfortable distance from which to speak.

R: *Appropriate distance between communicators varies across cultures. Some normally stand face to face, whereas others stand several feet apart to be comfortable.*

For Comprehension to Occur, the Nurse Must Accept That There is Limited Time and That the Use of This Time is Enhanced by (Carpenito-Moyet, 2014)

- Using every contact time to teach something
- Creating a relaxed encounter
- Using eye contact
- Slowing down—break it down into short statements
- Limited content—focus on 2 or 3 concepts
- Using plain language (refer to Box 4.1)
- Engaging individual/family in discussion
- Using graphics
- Explaining what you are doing to the individual/family and why
- Asking them to tell you about what you taught. Tell them to use their own words.

Initiate Referrals, When Needed

R: *Sixty-one percent reported that NASNs never or rarely called the interpreter.*

- Use a *fluent* translator when discussing important matters (e.g., taking a health history, signing an operation permit). Reinforce communications through the translator with written information. (Many hospitals require a "Certified Translator" to be used at least once per day. This should be documented in the medical record per hospital policy.)
- If possible, allow the translator to spend as much time as the person wishes (be flexible with visitors' rules and regulations).
- If a translator is unavailable, plan a daily visit from someone who has some knowledge of the person's language. (Many hospitals and social welfare offices keep a "language" bank with names and phone numbers of people who are willing to translate.)
- Use a telephone translating system when necessary.

R: *Effective communication is critical and must be ensured with persons who do not speak or understand English.*

Impaired Verbal Communication

NANDA-I Definition

Decreased, delayed, or absent ability to receive, process, transmit, and/or use a system of symbols

Defining Characteristics

Difficulty or inability to speak words but can understand others
Articulation or motor planning deficits

Related Factors

See *Impaired Communication.*

Key Concepts

See *Impaired Communication.*

Focus Assessment Criteria

See *Impaired Communication.*

Goals

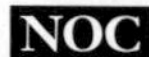

Communication: Expressive Ability

The person will demonstrate improved ability to express self as evidenced by the following indicators:

- Relates decreased frustration with communication
- Uses alternative methods as indicated

Interventions

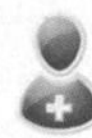

CLINICAL ALERT It has been reported that 40% of intubated individuals' rate their communication with nurses as somewhat or extremely difficult (Khalaila, Zbidat, & Anwar, 2011).

Identify a Method for Communicating Basic Needs

- See *Impaired Communication* for general interventions.

Identify Factors That Promote Communication

For Clients With Dysarthria

- Reduce environmental noise (e.g., radio, TV) to increase the caregiver's ability to listen to words.
- Do not alter your speech or messages, because the client's comprehension is not affected; speak on an adult level.
- Encourage the client to make a conscious effort to slow down speech and to speak louder (e.g., "Take a deep breath between sentences.").
- Ask the client to repeat unclear words; observe for nonverbal cues to help understanding.
- If the client is tired, ask questions that require only short answers.

R: *Simple questions that can be answered with yes or no enhance communication and reduce energy expenditure (Grossbach, Stranberg, & Chlan, 2011).*

- If speech is unintelligible, teach use of gestures, written messages, and communication cards.

R: *Dysarthria is a disturbance in the voluntary muscular control of speech. People with dysarthria usually do not have problems with comprehension.*

For Those Who Cannot Speak (e.g., Endotracheal Intubation, Tracheostomy)

R: *Research reported that individuals treated with mechanical ventilation experience a moderate to extreme level of psychoemotional distress because they cannot speak and communicate their needs (Khalaila et al., 2011).*

- Reassure that speech will return, if it will. If not, explain available alternatives (e.g., esophageal speech, sign language).
- Do not alter your speech, tone, or type of message; speak on an adult level.
  - Use gestures, head nods, mouthing of words, writing, use of letter/picture boards and common words or phrases tailored to meet individualized patients' needs (Grossbach et al., 2011).

R: *Every attempt must be made for successful communication. Each patient used about three communications while unable to speak, including squeezing hands (92%), shaking or nodding the head (86%), lip-reading (83%), facial expressions (83%), pen and paper (57%), word or picture charts (17%), alphabet boards (6%), and electronic voice output (5%).*

Utilize Stress-Reducing and Comfort Interventions With Every Encounter

R: *Research has supported that interventions to prevent emotional distress among individuals with mechanical ventilation should target those with communication difficulties (Khalaila et al., 2011).*

- Touch.
- "It must be frightening to be in your situation. Is there anything I can do to make you feel better, safer?
- Ensure the call bell system is always visible and available.
- Verbally address frustration over inability to communicate. Explain that both nurse and client must use patience.
- Maintain a calm, positive attitude (e.g., "I can understand you if we work at it.").
- Use reassurance (e.g., "I know it's difficult, but you'll get it.").
- Maintain a sense of humor.
- Allow tears (e.g., "It's OK. I know it's frustrating. Crying can let it all out.").
- For the client with limited speaking ability (e.g., can make simple requests, but not lengthy statements), encourage letter writing or keeping a diary to express feelings and share concerns.
- Anticipate needs and ask questions that need a simple yes or no answer.

R: *After survival, perhaps the most basic human need is to communicate with others. Communication provides security by reinforcing that clients are not alone and that others will listen. Researches have reported that "difficulty in communication was a positive predictor of patients' psychological distress, and length of anesthesia was a negative predictor." Fear and anger were also positively related to difficulty in communication (Khalaila et al., 2011).*

Provide Anxiety-Reducing and Comfort Interventions (e.g., Explain Exactly What You Are Doing, How It Will Feel and How Long It Will Take During)

- Suctioning
- Dressing changes
- Moving to a stretcher
- Getting out of bed

R: *Researchers found "that negative experiences, such as pain or discomfort associated with suctioning via the endotracheal tube, interference with sleep, thirst, and difficulty swallowing, also increase emotional distress. These findings indicate that purposive interventions designed to affect emotional distress in patients treated with mechanical ventilation should focus on the preventable stressful experiences associated with use of an endotracheal tube" (Khalaila et al., 2011).*

Maintain a Specific Care Plan

- Write the method of communication that is used (e.g., "Uses word cards," "Points for bedpan," alphabet board, picture board writing materials).
- Record directions for specific measures (e.g., allow him to keep a urinal in bed).

R: *Written directions will help to reduce communication problems and frustration.*

Initiate Health Teaching and Referrals, as Indicated

- Teach communication techniques and repetitive approaches to significant others.
- Encourage the family to share feelings concerning communication problems.

R: *After survival, perhaps the most basic human need is to communicate with others. Communication provides security by reinforcing that clients are not alone and that others will listen. Poor communication can cause frustration, anger, hostility, depression, fear, confusion, and isolation.*

Pediatric Interventions

- Ensure that the family and child are connected to services for hearing impaired.

R: *Recent research indicates that children identified with a hearing loss who begin services early may be able to develop language (spoken and/or signed) on a par with their hearing peers.*

- Establish a method of communication appropriate for age.

R: *The ability to communicate with people in the environment increases the child's independence, self-esteem, and self-actualization and decreases fear.*

- If a young child is deprived of vocalization, teach basic language gestures (e.g., time, food, family relationships, emotions, animals, numbers, frequent requests).

R: *Children who cannot vocalize are at risk for delays in receptive and expressive language development (i.e., vocal speech, voice production).*

- Consult with a speech pathologist for ongoing assistance.
- Discuss with parents or caregivers the importance of providing the child with a method of communication.

R: *Communication promotes bonding and attachment with the child's caregiver as the primary source of support. NIC*

ACUTE CONFUSION

NANDA-I Definition

Abrupt onset of reversible disturbances of consciousness, attention, cognition, and perception that develop over a short period of time

Defining Characteristics

Major (Must be Present)

Abrupt onset of:
Fluctuation in cognition*
Fluctuation in level of consciousness*

Fluctuation in psychomotor activity*
Increased agitation*
Reduced ability to focus
Disorientation
Increased restlessness*
Hypervigilance
Incoherence
Fear
Anxiety
Excitement

Symptoms are worse at night or when fatigued or in new situations.

Minor (May Be Present)

Illusions
Hallucinations*
Delusions
Misperceptions*

Related Factors

Factors that increase the risk for delirium and confusional states can be classified into those that increase baseline vulnerability (e.g., underlying brain diseases such as dementia, stroke, or Parkinson's disease) and those that precipitate the disturbance (e.g., infection, sedatives, immobility) (Francis & Young, 2012).

Related to abrupt onset of cerebral hypoxia or disturbance in cerebral metabolism secondary to (Miller, 2015):

Fluid and Electrolyte Disturbances

Dehydration
Acidosis/alkalosis
Hypercalcemia/hypocalcemia
Hypokalemia
Hyponatremia/hypernatremia
Hypoglycemia/hyperglycemia

Nutritional Deficiencies

Folate or vitamin B_{12} deficiency
Anemia
Niacin deficiency
Magnesium deficiency

Cardiovascular Disturbances

Myocardial infarction
Congestive heart failure
Dysrhythmias
Heart block
Temporal arteritis
Subdural hematoma

Respiratory Disorders

Chronic obstructive pulmonary disease: tuberculosis and pneumonia
Pulmonary embolism

Infections

Sepsis
Meningitis, encephalitis
Urinary tract infection (especially elderly)

Metabolic and Endocrine Disorders

Hypothyroidism/hyperthyroidism: hypoadrenocorticism/hyperadrenocorticism
Hypopituitarism/hyperpituitarism: postural hypotension, hypothermia/hyperthermia
Parathyroid disorders: hepatic or renal failure

Central Nervous System Disorders

Cerebral vascular accident
Multiple infarctions
Tumors
Normal-pressure hydrocephalus
Head trauma
Seizures and postconvulsive states

Treatment Related

Related to a disturbance in cerebral metabolism secondary to:

Surgery
Therapeutic drug intoxication
  Neuroleptics: opioids
  General anesthesia
Side effects of medication:

Diuretics
Digitalis
Propranolol
Atropine
Oral hypoglycemics
Anti-inflammatories
Antianxiety agents
Phenothiazines
Benzodiazepines
Barbiturates
Methyldopa
Disulfiram
Lithium
Phenytoin
Over-the-counter cold, cough, and sleeping preparations
Ciprofloxacin
Metronidazole
Acyclovir
H_2 receptor antagonists
Anticholinergics
Over-the-counter cold, cough, and sleeping preparations
Sulfa drugs

Situational (Personal, Environmental)

Related to disturbance in cerebral metabolism secondary to:

Withdrawal from alcohol, opioids, sedatives, hypnotics
Heavy metal or carbon monoxide intoxication

Related to:

Pain
Bowel impaction
Immobility
Depression
Unfamiliar situations

Related to chemical intoxications or medications (specify):

Alcohol
Cocaine
Methadone
Methamphetamines
PCP
Opioids (e.g., heroin)

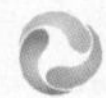

Author's Note

"Confusion" is a term nurses use frequently to describe an array of cognitive impairments. "Identifying a person as confused is just an initial step" (*Rasin, 1990;*Roberts, 2001). Confusion is a behavior that indicates a disturbance in cerebral metabolism.

Acute confusion (delirium) can occur in any age group. This can develop over a period of hours to days (Grossman & Porth, 2014). Factors that increase the risk for delirium and confusional states can be classified into those that increase baseline vulnerability (e.g., underlying brain diseases such as dementia, stroke, or Parkinson's disease) and those that precipitate the disturbance (e.g., infection, sedatives, immobility) (Francis & Young, 2012). The disturbance is typically caused by a medical condition, substance intoxication, or medication side effect (Francis & Young, 2012).

"Chronic confusion (dementia) is a syndrome of acquired, persistent, impairment in several domains of intellectual function, including memory, language, visuospatial ability, and cognition" (Grossman & Porth, 2014, p. 65).

Individuals with dementia can experience acute confusion (delirium). Nurses need to determine prehospital function and confer with family to observe for deterioration.

The addition of *Acute Confusion* and *Chronic Confusion* to the NANDA-I list provides the nurse with more diagnostic clarity than *Confusion* or *Disturbed Thought Processes. Acute Confusion* has an abrupt onset with fluctuating symptoms, whereas *Chronic Confusion* describes long-standing or progressive degeneration. *Disturbed Thought Processes* is also a disruption of cognitive processes; however, the causes are related to coping problems or personality disorders.

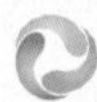

Errors in Diagnostic Statements

Acute Confusion related to advanced age

This diagnosis does not represent an understanding of confusion, aging, and its effects on cognition. An aged person who is confused could have various reasons for confusion (e.g., electrolytic imbalance, fever, cerebral infarctions, Alzheimer's disease). He or she needs a medical and nursing assessment. If the duration is known and causes are unknown, this diagnosis can be stated as *NIC Acute Confusion related to unknown etiology* or *Chronic Confusion related to unknown etiology.*

Key Concepts

General Considerations

- Delirium is defined (American Psychiatric Association, 2014; Francis & Young, 2012) as:
  - Disturbance of consciousness with reduced ability to focus, sustain, or shift attention.
  - Change in cognition or the development of a perceptual disturbance that is not better accounted for by a preexisting, established, or evolving dementia.
  - The disturbance develops over a short period of time (usually hours to days) and tends to fluctuate during the course of the day.
  - There is evidence from the history, physical examination, or laboratory findings that the disturbance is caused by a medical condition, substance intoxication, or medication side effect.
- Nearly 30% of older medical patients experience delirium at some time during hospitalization (Francis & Young, 2014).

Geriatric Considerations

- Moderate-to-severe cognitive impairment in older adults can result from dementia, delirium, or depression. Nurses must approach their assessment carefully and cautiously; they should not base the diagnosis on a single symptom or physical finding.
- "Delirium is an acute disorder of attention and cognition in elderly people (i.e., those aged 65 years or older) that is common, serious, costly, under-recognized, and often fatal" (Inouye, Westendorp, & Saczynski, 2013, p. 1). A formal cognitive assessment and history of acute onset of symptoms are necessary for diagnosis. In view of the complex multifactorial causes of delirium, multicomponent nonpharmacological risk factor approaches are the most effective strategy for prevention. No convincing evidence shows that pharmacological prevention or treatment is effective. Drug reduction for sedation and analgesia and nonpharmacological approaches are recommended.
- Infection is one of the most common causes of changes of mental status in seniors (e.g., urinary, respiratory) (Bishop, 2006; Caljouw, den Elzen, Cools, & Gussekloo, 2011).

Table II.3 AGE-RELATED CHANGES THAT MAY INFLUENCE MEDICATION CONCENTRATIONS

Age-Related Changes	Effect on Some Medications
Decreased body water, decreased lean tissue, increased body fat	Increased or decreased serum concentration
Decreased serum albumin	Increased amount of the active portion of protein-bound medications
Decreased renal and liver functioning	Increased serum concentration
Decreased gastric acid, increased gastric pH	Altered absorption of medications that are sensitive to stomach pH
Altered homeostatic mechanisms	Increased potential for adverse effects
Altered receptor sensitivity	Increased or decreased therapeutic effect

Source: Miller, C. (2009). *Nursing for wellness in older adults* (5th ed.). Philadelphia, PA: Lippincott Williams & Wilkins.

- With age, intelligence does not alter (perhaps until the very later years), but the older person needs more time to process information. Reaction time increases as well. There may be some difficulty in learning new information because of increased distractibility, decreased concrete thinking, and difficulty solving new problems. Older adults usually compensate for these deficiencies by taking more time to process the information, screening out distractions, and using extreme care in making decisions. Marked cognitive decline usually is attributed to disease processes such as atherosclerosis, loss of neurons, and other pathologic changes (Miller, 2015).
- Most older adults exhibit no cognitive impairment (Miller, 2015). Research has reported that brain maturation and related cognitive functions continue to mature through adulthood and into older adults (Aine et al., 2011).
- Age-related changes can influence medication actions and produce negative consequences. See Table II.3.
- Dementia describes impairments of intellectual, not behavioral, functioning. It refers to a group of symptoms, not a disease (Miller, 2015). Alzheimer's disease, the fourth leading cause of death in adults, is one type of dementia.
- Late-life depression is reported to be 14%. It is also reported that 40% to 50% of elders in nursing homes suffer from depression (Centers for Medicare and Medicaid Services, 2012).

Focus Assessment Criteria

From the individual and significant others.

Subjective Data

History of the Individual

Lifestyle

Interests
Past and present coping
Previous functioning
Strengths and limitations
Education
Previous handling of stress
Work history
Use of alcohol/drugs

Support System (Availability)

History of Medical Problems and Treatments (Medications)

Activities of Daily Living (ADLs; Ability and Desire to Perform)

Knowledge of Individual of the Diagnosis

History of Symptoms (Onset and Duration)

Acute or chronic
Downward progression
Time of day
Continuous or intermittent
Sudden or gradual

Assess for Fears

Harm from others
Being held prisoner
Thoughts racing
Being unable to cope
Falling apart
Assess for hallucinations (visual, olfactory, auditory)
Tactile (includes objective component)

Assess for Behaviors Associated with Depression, Dementia, and Delirium (Francis & Young, 2012; Halter, 2014)

Depression
- Sudden or gradual onset
- Sleep difficulties
- Slowed motor behavior
- Sadness, loss of interest and pleasure
- Memory intact

Dementia
- Gradual, insidious onset
- May sleep less; restlessness
- Wandering behavior
- Defensiveness
- Gradual loss of ability to remember

Delirium
- Sudden, acute onset
- Behavior worsens at night
- Hypo/hyperarousal
- Hallucinations and illusions in attention
- Fluctuating performance

Objective Data (Includes a Subjective Component)

General Appearance

- Facial expression (alert, sad, hostile, expressionless)
- Dress (meticulous, disheveled, seductive, eccentric)

Behavior During Interview

- Withdrawn
- Cooperative
- Attention/concentration
- Level of anxiety
- Apathetic
- Negativism
- Hostile
- Quiet

Communication Pattern

- Appropriate
- Sexual preoccupations
- Denying problem
- Delusions
- Obsessions
- Suspicious
- Suicidal ideas
- Rambling
- Homicidal plans
- Worthlessness

Speech Pattern

- Appropriate
- Topic jumping
- Loose connections
- Circumstantial
- Blocking (cannot finish idea)
- Cannot reach a conclusion

Rate of Speech

- Appropriate
- Pressured
- Reduced
- Excessive

Affect

- Blunted
- Appropriate to content
- Sad
- Congruent with content
- Flat
- Bright
- Inappropriate to content

Interaction Skills

With Nurse
- Inappropriate
- Hostile
- Demanding/pleading
- Withdrawn/preoccupied
- Relates well

With Significant Others
- Relates with all (some) family members
- Does not seek interaction
- Hostile toward all (some) family members
- Does not have visitors

Activities of Daily Living

- Capable of self-care (observed, reported)

Nutrition–Hydration Status

Appetite, weight, eating patterns

Sleep–Rest Pattern

Sleeps too much or too little	Early wakefulness	Cycle reversed
Insomnia	Fragmented sleep	

Personal Hygiene

Cleanliness, grooming

Motor Activity

Within normal limits	Agitated	Decreased/stuporous

Goals

NOC

Cognition, Cognitive Orientation, Distorted Thought Self-Control

The person will have diminished episodes of delirium as evidenced by the following indicators:

- Be less agitated
- Participates in ADLs
- Be less combative

Interventions

Assess for Causative and Contributing Factors

- Refer to Related Factors.

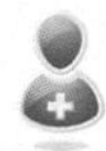

Clinical Alert "Nearly 30 percent of older patients experience delirium at some time during hospitalization; the incidence is higher in intensive care units. Among older patients who have had surgery, the risk of delirium varies from 10 to greater than 50 percent" (Francis & Young, 2012).

NIC

Delirium Management, Calming Technique, Reality Orientation, Environmental Management: Safety

Assess for Early Signs of Acute Confusion (Francis & Young, 2012)

- A change in the level of awareness and the ability to focus, sustain, or shift attention
- Family members or caregivers who report that a patient "isn't acting quite right"
- Is distracted during conversations, not focused
- Tangential or disorganized speech

R: *The above behaviors must not be attributed to age, dementia, or fatigue until it is validated that this is this person's norm before hospitalization (Francis & Young, 2012).*

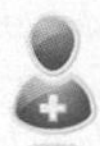

Clinical Alert Notify responsible physician, physician assistant, or nurse practitioner of these observed changes.

Assess Personal and Environmental Factors That Contribute to or Cause Acute Confusion

R: *In addition to the medical and psychiatric conditions that can cause or contribute to acute confusion (delirium), there are personal and environmental factors that are contributory as follows (Godfrey et al., 2013):*

- Hearing or visual deficits
  - Ensure glasses and/or hearing aids are worn during the day and in working condition.
- Inadequate sleep
  - Use nightlights or dim lights at night
  - Use indirect lighting and turn on lights before dark.
  - Establish care routines that reduce waking the person (e.g., vital signs, meds, high-stimulus activity [e.g., crowds] or images [e.g., frightening pictures or movies]).
  - Provide earplugs.

- Refer to *Disturbed Sleep Pattern* for additional interventions.

R: *Rompaey, Elseviers, Van Drom, Fromont, & Jorens (2012) found that the use of earplugs at night was associated with a lower incidence of confusion in individuals in ICU.*

- Disoriented, time, place
  - Provide large wall clocks.
  - Reduce abrupt changes in schedule or relocation.
  - Keep the client oriented to time and place.
  - Refer to time of day and place each morning.
  - Provide the client with a clock and calendar large enough to see.
  - Provide the client with the opportunity to see daylight and dark through a window, or take the client outdoors.
  - Single out holidays with cards or pins (e.g., wear a red heart for Valentine's Day).

R: *Sensory input is carefully planned to promote orientation.*

Insufficient Cognitive Stimulation

- Encourage visitors, but caution against having too many at once.

R: *This could result in overstimulation or visitors talking among themselves versus to the individual.*

- Discuss current events, seasonal events (snow, water activities); share your interests (travel, crafts).
- Attempt to obtain information for conversation (likes, dislikes; interests, hobbies; work history).
- Solicit the aid of volunteers to spend meaningful time with individuals, who have insufficient visitors.
- Encourage the family to bring in familiar objects from home (e.g., photographs with nonglare glass, afghan).
- Ask the client to tell you about the picture.
- Focus on familiar topics.
- Immobility
  - Provide position changes as needed.
  - Out of bed in to a chair, use wheel chair to provide another environment for socialization.
  - Ambulate if possible.
  - Have the client eat meals out of bed, unless contraindicated.
- Pain
  - Refer to *Acute Pain* for interventions.

R: *It is important to balance the benefits of using opioids to treat significant pain with the potential for an opioid-related delirium.*

- Dehydration
  - Refer to *Fluid Volume Deficit*

R: *Francis and Young (2014) described a classic study by Inouye et al. (2014) which utilized standardized protocols to screen and control for six risk factors for delirium in 852 hospitalized patients aged 70 or older: cognitive impairment, sleep deprivation, immobility, visual impairment, hearing impairment, and dehydration. The risk factors were targeted with nursing interventions. The results showed a significant reduction in the number of delirium episodes compared with usual care (62 vs. 90) and in the total number of days with delirium (105 vs. 161); subsequent papers and randomized studies have confirmed that such multicomponent interventions can reduce the incidence of delirium and/or related complication (American Geriatrics Society, 2015; Deschodt et al., 2012; Godfrey et al., 2013).*

- Psychoactive medications
  - Discuss with physician, physician assistant, or nurse practitioner the prescribed psychoactive drugs (e.g., anticholinergics, sedatives or hypnotics, opioids); to discontinue, lower dosages or avoid required dosing.
  - Use nonpharmacological approaches for sleep and anxiety, including music, massage, relaxation techniques.

R: *In vulnerable individuals, those with underlying dementia and multimorbidity, a dose of a sedative–hypnotic drug might be enough to precipitate delirium. "Thus, in vulnerable patients, such as those with underlying dementia and multimorbidity, a seemingly benign insult—eg, a dose of a sedative–hypnotic drug—might be enough to precipitate delirium" (Inouye et al., 2013, p. 2).*

- Infection

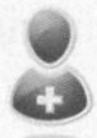

Clinical Alert The incidence of urinary tract infections is common in older adults with 12% to 29% in community settings and between 44% and 58% in long-term care facilities (Caljouw et al., 2011). "Yet, multiple studies show that between 21% and 55.7% of urinary catheters are placed in patients who do not have an appropriate indication and, therefore, may not even need a catheter" (Meddings et al., 2014). In long-term care facilities, almost 100% of individuals with a catheter for 30 days or longer will develop a UTI (Andreessen, Wilde, & Herendeen, 2012).

R: *Mild infections (e.g., urinary, respiratory) can cause acute confusion in older adults. More serious infections, for example, sepsis, can cause confusion at any age (Francis & Young, 2012; Miller, 2015).*

- Refer to *Risk for Infection* for specific interventions to prevent infections in health-care settings.

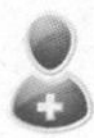

Clinical Alert In one large cluster-randomized control study based in nursing homes, implementation of a computerized system to identify the use of problematic medications triggered a medication review. The incidence of delirium was reduced when the medication in question was discontinued or a dose reduction made (Clegg, Siddiqi, Heaven, Young, & Holt, 2014).

Nurses can identify the use of problematic medications in residents and address their concerns to the prescribing professions regardless of having the computerized system or not.

Ensure That a Thorough Diagnostic Workup has Been Completed

Laboratory
- CBC and electrolytes
- TSH, T4
- Vitamin B_{12} and folate, thiamine
- Serum thyroxine and serum-free thyroxine
- Rapid plasma reagin (RPR)
- Calcium and phosphate
- Na and K
- Creatinine, blood urea nitrogen
- AST, ALT, and bilirubin
- Serum glucose and fasting blood sugar
- Urinalysis

Diagnostic
- EEG
- CT scan
- Chest X-ray
- ECG

Psychiatric Evaluation
- Evaluate for depression

Educate Family, Significant Others, and Caregivers About the Situation and Coping Methods

- Explain the cause of the confusion.
- Explain that the individual does not realize the situation.
- Explain the need to remain patient, flexible, and calm.
- Stress the need to respond to the client as an adult.
- Explain that the behavior is part of a disorder and is not voluntary.

R: *Differentiating between acute (reversible) and chronic (irreversible) confusion is important for family and caregivers (Miller, 2015).*

- Provide respect and promote sharing.
  - Pay attention to what the individual says.
  - Pick out meaningful comments and continue talking.
  - Call the client by name and introduce yourself each time you make contact; use touch if welcomed.
  - Use the name the client prefers; avoid "Pops" or "Mom," which can increase confusion and is unacceptable.

- Convey to the client that you are concerned and friendly (through smiles, an unhurried pace, humor, and praise; do not argue).
- Focus on the feeling behind the spoken word or action.

R: *This demonstrates unconditional positive regard and communicates acceptance and affection to a person who has difficulty interpreting the environment (Hall, 1994).*

R: *"Functional or baseline behavior is likely to occur when the external demands (stressors) on the individual are adjusted to the level to which the person has adapted" (*Hall, 1991).*

- In teaching a task or activity—such as eating—break it into small, brief steps by giving only one instruction at a time.
  - Remove covers from food plate and cups.
  - Locate the napkin and utensils.
  - Add sugar and milk to coffee.
  - Add condiments to food (sugar, salt, pepper).
  - Cut foods.
  - Offer simple explanations of tasks.
  - Allow the individual to handle equipment related to each task.
  - Allow the individual to participate in the task, such as washing his face.
  - Acknowledge that you are leaving, and say when you will return.

R: *Memory loss and diminished intellectual functioning create a need for consistency.*

R: *Sensory input is carefully planned to reduce excess stimuli, which increase confusion (Miller, 2015).*

Promote a Wellness Role and Protect the Integrity of the Individual at All Times

- Allow former habits (e.g., reading in the bathroom).
- Encourage the wearing of dentures.
- Ask the individual/significant other about his usual grooming routine and encourage him to follow it.
- Provide privacy at all times; when it is necessary to expose a body surface, take precautions to cover all other areas (e.g., if washing a back, use towels or blankets to cover legs and front torso).
- Provide for personal hygiene according to preferences (hair grooming, showers or bath, nail care, cosmetics, deodorants, fragrances).
- Discourage the use of nightclothes during the day; have the client wear shoes, not slippers.
- Promote socialization during meals (e.g., set up lunch for four individuals in the lounge).
- Plan an activity each day to look forward to (e.g., bingo, ice cream sundae gathering).
- Encourage participation in decision making (e.g., selecting what he wishes to wear).

R: *Strategies that emphasize normalcy can contribute to positive self-esteem and reduce confusion.*

Do Not Endorse Confusion

- Do not argue with the client.
- Determine the best response to confused statements.
- Sometimes the confused individual may be comforted by a response that reduces his or her fear; for example, "I want to see my mother," when his or her mother has been dead for 20 years. The nurse may respond with, "I know that your mother loved you."
- Direct the client back to reality; do not allow him or her to ramble.
- Adhere to the schedule; if changes are necessary, advise the client of them.
- Avoid talking to coworkers about other topics in the client's presence.
- Provide simple explanations that cannot be misinterpreted.
- Remember to acknowledge your entrance with a greeting and your exit with a closure ("I will be back in 10 minutes").
- Avoid open-ended questions.
- Replace five- or six-step tasks with two- or three-step tasks.

R: *Unconditional positive regard communicates acceptance and affection to a person who has difficulty interpreting the environment. Careful listening is critical to evaluate responses to prevent escalation of anxiety and to detect physiologic discomforts (Miller, 2015).*

Prevent Injury to the Individual

- Refer to *Risk for Falls* for preventive interventions.

Initiate Referrals, as Needed

- Refer caregivers to appropriate community resources.

R: *Additional community services may be needed for management at home.*

CHRONIC CONFUSION

NANDA-I Definition

Irreversible, long-standing, and/or progressive deterioration of intellect and personality characterized by decreased ability to interpret environmental stimuli; decreased capacity for intellectual thought processes; and manifested by disturbances of memory, orientation, and behavior

Defining Characteristics

Normal level of consciousness
Irreversible, long-standing, and/or progressive:

Alteration in interpretation
Alteration in long-term memory
Alteration in personality
Alteration in short-term memory
Alteration in cognitive functioning
Chronic cognitive impairment
Impaired social functioning
Organic brain disorder
Alteration in response to stimuli

Related Factors

Pathophysiologic (Farlow, 2015)
Alzheimer's disease*
Multi-infarct dementia (MID)*
Vascular dementia (damaged areas of brain because of reduced blood flow, e.g., from chronic high blood pressure, uncontrolled diabetes mellitus)
Cumulative damage to the brain (e.g., chronic alcoholism) or repeated head injuries (e.g., former professional boxers or football players)
Frontotemporal dementia (formerly called Pick's disease)
Inflammatory and autoimmune diseases (e.g., multiple sclerosis, systemic lupus erythematosis, encephalitis)
Toxic substance injection
Brain tumors
Infectious diseases (e.g., HIV-associated neurocognitive disorder [HAND], herpes encephalitis, neurosyphilis)
End-stage diseases (e.g., AIDS, cirrhosis, cancer, renal failure, cardiac failure, chronic obstructive pulmonary disease)
Creutzfeldt–Jakob disease
Degenerative neurologic disease
Huntington's chorea
Psychiatric disorders
Dementia with Lewy bodies is a form of dementia caused by abnormal protein structures called *Lewy bodies.*

Author's Note

Refer to *Acute Confusion*.

Errors in Diagnostic Statements

Refer to *Acute Confusion*.

Key Concepts

- See *Acute Confusion.*
- Progressive dementing illnesses have four clusters of symptoms (*Hall, 1991).
- Both depression and dementia cause cognitive impairments. Differentiating the underlying cause is critical, because depression is treatable (Miller, 2015).
- Chronic confusion affects one's ability to function in numerous ways. Some are as follows:
  - Intellectual losses
    - o Loss of memory (recent initially)
    - o Inability to make choices
    - o Loss of sense of time
    - o Altered ability to identify visual or auditory stimuli
    - o Inability to solve problems and reason
    - o Loss of expressive and receptive language
  - Affective personality losses
    - o Loss of affect
    - o Emotional lability
    - o Decreased attention span
    - o Loss of tact
    - o Decreased inhibitions
    - o Increased self-preoccupation
  - Cognitive or planning losses
    - o Loss of ability to plan
    - o Loss of energy reserves
    - o Loss of instrumental functions (e.g., money management, mail, shopping)
    - o Motor apraxia
    - o Frustration, refusal to participate
    - o Functional losses (e.g., bathing, choosing clothes)
  - Progressively lowered stress threshold
    - o Confused or agitated night awakening
    - o Violent, agitated, anxious behavior
    - o Purposeful wandering
    - o Compulsive repetitive behavior

Disclosure of Diagnosis of Alzheimer's disease

- "It's unfortunate I waited a year to get a diagnosis because that meant an additional year of worry, concern and hiding my issues from family and friends. I was exhausting myself needlessly when getting a diagnosis actually simplified and improved my life greatly"—Lou B., an individual living with Alzheimer's disease (Alzheimer's Association, 2015a).
- "People can overprotect you, which robs you of your independence much quicker."—Person with dementia (Alzheimer's Association, 2015a).
- Gibson and Anderson (2011) reported that 58% of caregivers reported that a definitive diagnosis still took 3 months or longer, with 12% waiting more than 1 year. Caregivers also reported a sense of reluctance among doctors to disclose the diagnosis.
- "While negative reactions to disclosure, such as depression, loss of hope, psychological distress and suicide have been cited as reasons for withholding the diagnosis, catastrophic reactions are rare. These potentially negative consequences are offset by a range of positive consequences and many people with dementia are able to cope with their diagnosis particularly when adequate support is available. Furthermore, the majority of people to whom a diagnosis of dementia was disclosed have positive attitudes to disclosure" (Lecouturier et al., 2008).
- Findings disclosed that disclosure cannot be viewed as a single encounter, but rather is a complex process, far more "than simply naming the illness" (Lecouturier et al., 2008).
- Eight distinct categories of behaviors were identified: preparing for disclosure; integrating family members; exploring the patient's perspective; disclosing the diagnosis; responding to patient reactions; focusing on quality of life and well-being; planning for the future; and communicating effectively (Lecouturier et al., 2008).

Carp's Cues

Of the eight categories, the first is critical to convincing professionals, family, and others that disclosure is a right that an individual can choose or not.

- Preparing for disclosure includes (Lecouturier et al., 2008):
  - Prediagnostic counseling such as establishing individual's preferences for disclosure and raising the possibility that dementia may be a possible diagnosis (e.g., Presently we are seeking causes of your symptoms. If the cause is the beginning of deterioration in your brain from a disease, do you want to be told this?)
- This predisclosure discussion can help in identifying the approach most suited to the individual (Lecouturier et al., 2008).
  - The researchers of the Alzheimer's Europe—Value of Knowing (2011) noted, "Gaining knowledge and developing a treatment plan, individuals may realize that they can take an active role in managing the illness, enhancing a sense of self-efficacy where before they might have felt helpless."
- The research cited above offers important findings for professional working with individuals and families with dementia. The researchers sought to identify a comprehensive list of behaviors in disclosure by conducting a literature review, interviewing people with dementia and informal caregivers, and using a consensus process involving health and social care professionals. Content analysis of the full list of behaviors was carried out, resulting in eight distinct categories of behaviors recommended for the process of disclosure (Lecouturier et al., 2008).
- Numerous studies[11] have found benefits to promptly and clearly explaining a diagnosis of dementia to the affected person and to that person's caregiver(s) (Alzheimer's Association, 2015a):
  - Better diagnosis: Knowledge of their diagnosis can promote seeking other medical opinions or the advice of specialists.
  - Better decision making: When individuals are fully aware of their diagnosis in the early stages of the disease, they are involved in the decision-making process, which can increase their participation in the treatment plan.
  - Better medical care: "Studies have shown that when patients understand their diagnosis and are active participants in, the quality of care they receive is better than the care received by uninformed patients" (p. 65).
  - Respect for the patient's wishes: Despite limited studies, the evidence indicates that most individuals with mild dementia want to be told their diagnosis.

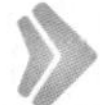

Carp's Cues

Fundamentally, each person should be afforded the respect for their autonomy. Even though we may think we know what is best for someone we love, are you willing to accept others making the life-altering decisions for you? Secrets build walls: barriers to sharing. Barriers to sharing build walls to caring. So, all are left to suffer alone.

  - Planning for the future: Prompt disclosure allows individuals and caregivers to get legal and financial affairs in order.
  - Understanding changes: Fear of the unknown is a very powerful fear. Knowing why they feel their symptoms does provide the answer and can propel the person to active decision making.
  - Coping: "Although the initial disclosure can be shocking, distressing or embarrassing, being aware of the diagnosis gives patients and their caregivers the opportunity to express their fears and grief and to adopt positive strategies for coping" (p. 66).
  - Access to services: Knowing the diagnosis can prompt individual/ family to access information about a variety of support services.
  - Safety: Knowledge of the diagnosis allows all involved to evaluate and plan for a safe home environment.
  - Social support: Informed individuals can make decisions on what/who is important to them and can plan activities, vacations, etc.

Focus Assessment Criteria

Refer to *Acute Confusion*.

[11] The entire document with the research support can be accessed at http://www.alz.org/facts/downloads/facts_figures_2015.pdf

Goals

NOC

Decision-Making, Cognitive Ability, Cognitive Orientation, Distorted Thought Self-Control, Surveillance: Safety, Emotional Support, Environmental Management, Fall Prevention, Calming Technique

The person will participate to the maximum level of independence in a therapeutic milieu as evidenced by the following indicators:

- Decreased frustration
- Diminished episodes of combativeness
- Increased hours of sleep at night
- Stabilized or increased weight

Interventions

NIC

Validation Therapy, Decision-Making Support, Patient Rights Protection, Dementia Management: Multisensory Therapy, Cognitive Stimulation, Calming Technique, Reality Orientation, Environmental Management: Safety

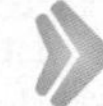

Carp's Cues

"An estimated 5.3 million Americans of all ages have Alzheimer's disease in 2015. This number includes an estimated 5.1 million people age 65 and older and approximately 200,000 individuals under age 65 who have younger-onset Alzheimer's. Approximately 473,000 people age 65 or older will develop Alzheimer's disease in the United States in 2015" (Alzheimer's Association, 2015b, p. 16). A recent study of caregivers' experience with the diagnostic process reported that it took >2 years after the initial physician visit for some patients to receive a dementia diagnosis. Caregivers also reported a sense of reluctance among doctors to disclose the diagnosis (Gibson & Anderson, 2011).

Literature Reviews Continue to Show That Clinicians Who Suspect Dementia Often Do Not Disclose or Document a Formal Diagnosis (*Bamford et al., 2004; *Carpenter & Dave, 2004)

- A large five-country survey (France, Germany, Poland, Spain, and the United States) examined public attitudes about Alzheimer's disease. It reported the following (Harvard School of Public Health, 2011):
  - More than 80% of all adults ($N = 2,678$) and 89% of US adults ($N = 639$) responded that if they had memory or confusion symptoms, they would go to a doctor to determine if the cause was Alzheimer's disease. This US finding is consistent with previously published reports over the last two decades.
  - Of the US respondents, 65% said that even if they were asymptomatic, they would likely or somewhat likely be interested in getting a medical test that would determine if they would get Alzheimer's disease in the future (if one becomes available).

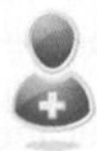

Clinical Alert The decision to disclose a diagnosis of Alzheimer's disease continues to be debated with speculation of what the individual would want to know. This uncertainty allows caregivers and family to justify their silence.

Refer to the Key Concepts for a discussion of the research findings on disclosure.

Refer to Interventions Under Acute Confusion

- Determine if individual is unaware of diagnosis. If the individual is unaware of the diagnosis and is capable of cognitively understanding, initiate a dialogue with the appropriate physician, physician assistant, or nurse practitioner.

SBAR

Situation: In caring for Mr. Smith, in room 330, I became aware that he does not know his diagnosis. He has expressed concerns about his memory problems and what is happening to him.

Background: Mr. Smith is 68 years old and has acute coronary syndrome. He is clinically stable and scheduled for transition to home in 2 days.

Assessment: In my review of his records, there are references to Alzheimer's disease. He appears to be in the early phase of Alzheimer's disease.

Recommendation: Are you aware of this situation? Is there a plan to disclose his diagnosis to him? Are there any reasons why this has not occurred? Family resistance?

R: *"Practitioners show great variations in practice, with only around 50% of clinicians regularly telling patients with dementia their diagnosis. The majority of caregivers also appear to prefer the diagnosis to be withheld from the patient with dementia. However, most practitioners and caregivers would wish to know themselves if they had* *the illness" (Pinner & Bouman, 2002, p. 127). As a result, approximately 50% of patients with dementia have no documentation of diagnosis in their medical record (Bradford, Kunik, Schulz, Williams, & Singh, 2009).*

- If the family is preventing disclosure and the individual capable of understanding, engage in a discussion with family if they are preventing disclosure.

R: *Refer to Key Concepts for specifics regarding barriers and benefits to disclosure.*

Observe to Determine Baseline Behaviors

- Best time of day
- Response time to a simple question
- Amount of distraction tolerated
- Judgment
- Insight into disability
- Signs/symptoms of depression
- Routines

R: *Baseline behavior can be used to assess for early signs of an exacerbation.*

Promote the Individual's Sense of Integrity (Miller, 2015)

Assess Who the Person Was Before the Onset of Confusion

- Educational level, career
- Hobbies, lifestyle
- Coping styles

R: *Assessing the individual's personal history can provide insight into current behavior patterns and communicates the nurse's interest. Specific personal data can improve individualization of care (*Hall, 1994).*

Adapt Communication to the Person's Level

- Avoid "baby talk" and a condescending tone of voice.
- Use simple sentences and present one idea at a time.
- If the individual does not understand, repeat the sentence using the same words.
- Use positive statements; avoid "don'ts."
- Unless a safety issue is involved, do not argue.
- Avoid general questions, such as, "What would you like to do?" Instead, ask, "Do you want to go for a walk or work on your rug?"
- Be sensitive to the feelings the individual is trying to express.
- Avoid questions you know the individual cannot answer.
- If possible, demonstrate to reinforce verbal communication.
- Use touch to gain attention or show concern unless a negative response is elicited.
- Maintain good eye contact and pleasant facial expressions.
- Determine which sense dominates the individual's perception of the world (auditory, kinesthetic, olfactory, or gustatory). Communicate through the preferred sense.

R: *Alzheimer's disease-related dementia affects communication abilities (i.e., receptive and expressive; *Hall, 1994).*

Promote the Individual's Safety (Miller, 2015)

- Check the placement, access, and height of furniture are safe for the individual.
- Provide bright lights in room during the day.
- Ensure path to bathroom is barrier free and/or that the call bell is accessible.
- Adapt the environment so the person can pace or walk if desired.
- Keep the environment uncluttered.
- Refer to *Risk for Falls* for additional interventions.

R: *Confused persons are at high risk for injury.*

Intravenous Therapy

- Camouflage tubing with loose gauze.
- Consider an intermittent access device instead of continuous IV therapy.
- If dehydration is a problem, institute a regular schedule for offering oral fluids.
- Use the least restrictive sites.

Urinary Catheters

- Evaluate causes of incontinence.
- Institute a specific treatment depending on type. Refer to *Impaired Urinary Elimination*.
- Avoid indwelling catheters if at all possible.
- Place urinary collection bag at the end of the bed with catheter between rather than draped over legs. Velcro bands can hold the catheter against the leg.
- Refer to *Risk for Infection* regarding catheter use.

Gastrointestinal Tubes

- Check frequently for pressure against nares.
- If the individual is pulling out tubes, use mitts instead of wrist restraints.
- Evaluate if restlessness is associated with pain. If analgesics are used, adjust dosage to reduce side effects.

R: *Treatments and equipment can increase confusion and agitation.*

If Combative, Determine the Source of the Fear and Frustration

Fatigue

R: *Fatigue is the most frequent cause of dysfunctional episodes. Physical stressors can precipitate a dysfunctional episode (e.g., urinary tract infections, caffeine, and constipation) (American Geriatrics Society, 2015a; *Foreman, Mion, Tyrostad, & Flitcher, 1999).*

- Misleading or inappropriate stimuli
- Change in routine, environment, caregiver
- Pressure to exceed functional capacity
- Physical stress, pain, infection, acute illness, discomfort
- Engaging them in singing, rhythm playing, dancing, physical exercise, and other structured music activities can diffuse this behavior and redirect their attention.

R: *Nonverbal individuals in late dementia often become agitated out of frustration and sensory overload from the inability to process environmental stimuli. Engaging them in singing, rhythm playing, dancing, physical exercise, and other structured music activities can diffuse this behavior and redirect their attention (Clair & Tomaino, 2015).*

If a Dysfunctional Episode Occurs (Boyd, 2012)

- Address the individual by surname. Quiet the environment.
- Get his or her attention with a soft voice, tell them they are safe.
- Assume a dependent position by sitting down.
- Do not ask him or her to something, simplify the activity, and reduce the need to make choices.
- Distract from hallucinations, if possible.
- Distract the individual with cues that require automatic social behavior (e.g., "Mrs. Smith, would you like some juice now?").
- After the episode has passed, discuss the episode with the person, if indicated.
- Document what occurred to precipitate the behavior, behavior observed, and consequences.

R: *The threshold for stress is lowered in persons with Alzheimer's disease (Boyd, 2012). These strategies can reduce aggression and may prevent future episodes with careful recording of the episode.*

Address Sundowner Syndrome

- Geriatric clinicians have frequently observed that some demented individuals show increased agitation, restlessness, and confusion in late afternoon, evening, or night.

R: *Sundowner syndrome is an exacerbation of existing daytime behavioral abnormalities and new symptoms occurring primarily in the late afternoon. It has a rate of 20%. Sundowning is not a disease, but a group of symptoms that occur at a specific time of the day that may affect people with dementia (Bliwise & Lee, 1993; Khachiyants, Trinkle, Son, & Kim, 2011).*

- Factors that may aggravate late-day confusion include
  - Fatigue
  - Low lighting
  - Increased shadows
  - Disruption of the body's "internal clock"
  - Difficulty separating reality from dreams

- Tips for reducing sundowning:
  - A variety of treatment options have been found to be helpful to ameliorate the neuropsychiatric symptoms associated with this phenomenon: bright light therapy, melatonin, acetylcholinesterase inhibitors.
- Try to maintain a predictable routine for bedtime, waking, meals, and activities.
- Allow for light exposure in the early morning to help set internal clock.
- Discourage daytime napping to regulate sleep cycle.
- Plan for activities and exposure to light during the day to encourage nighttime sleepiness.
- Limit daytime napping.
- Limit caffeine and sugar to morning hours.
- Among many factors, Khachiyants indicated that low lighting and increased shadows may aggravate late-day confusion and sundowning.
- Keep a night light on to reduce agitation that occurs when surroundings are dark or unfamiliar.
- In the evening, try to reduce background noise and stimulating activities, including TV viewing, which can sometimes be upsetting.
- In a strange or unfamiliar setting, bring familiar items—such as photographs—to create a more relaxed, familiar setting.
- Play familiar gentle music in the evening or relaxing sounds of nature, such as the sound of waves.
- Talk with your loved one's doctor if you suspect an underlying condition, such as a urinary tract infection or sleep apnea, might be worsening sundowning behavior.

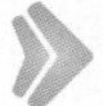

Carp's Cues

Some research suggests that a low dose of melatonin—a naturally occurring hormone that induces sleepiness—alone or in combination with exposure to bright light during the day may help ease sundowning (*Haffmans, Sival, Lucius, Cats, & van Gelder, 2001).

Some research suggests that sundowning may be related to changes to the brain's circadian pacemaker. That's a cluster of nerve cells that keeps the body on a 24-hour clock.

Studies in mice suggest that chemical changes in the brain that are characteristic of Alzheimer's disease may play a role. Researchers found that older mice make more of an enzyme that's associated with anxiety and agitation before they go to sleep than middle-aged mice do.

"The middle-aged mice had a distinct pattern of activity, with three peaks of activity during their waking hours," Bedrosian said. "But the aged mice had a flattened rhythm in which they showed the same level of activity throughout their active period." That means that in the evening, when the middle aged mice would slow down compared to their peak activity levels, the aged mice kept going.

Ensure Physical Comfort and Maintenance of Basic Health Needs

- Refer to *Self-Care Deficits*.

Select Modalities Involving the Five Senses (Hearing, Sight, Smell, Taste, and Touch) That Provide Favorable Stimuli for the Individual

R: *Multisensory stimulation with or without a specially designed room has shown to increase interest in newspapers, motivation, energy levels, smiling, and personal cleanliness as well as decreased wandering, anxiety, hostility, and incontinence (Lykkeslet, Gjengedal, Skrondal, & Storjord).*

Music Therapy

R: *Familiar music can stimulate memory recall, improve mood, opportunities to interact socially with others, heighten arousal in patients with AD, allowing better attention and improved memory, and increase stimulation that promotes interest (Chatterton, Baker, & Morgan, 2010; Hulme Wright, Crocker, Oluboyede, & House 2010; Simmons-Stern, Budson, & Ally, 2010; Wollen, 2010). Music therapy at least 30 minutes before the individual's usual peak level of agitation can reduce agitation (*Gerdner, 1999).*

- Determine the individual's preferences. Play this music before the usual level of agitation for at least 30 minutes; assess response.
- Evaluate response, as some music can agitate individuals.
- Provide soft, soothing music during meals.
- Arrange group songfests with consideration to cultural/ethical orientation.
- Play music during other therapies (physical, occupational, and speech).
- Have the individual exercise to music.
- Organize guest entertainment.
- Use client-developed songbooks (large print and decorative covers).

Recreation/Exercise Therapy (Ahlskog, Geda, Graff-Radford, & Petersen, 2011; Cohen-Mansfield et al., 2012; Hattori, Hattori, Hokao, Mizushima, & Mase, 2011; Scherder, Bogen, Eggermont, Hamers, & Swaab, 2010; Wollen, 2010)

- Encourage arts and crafts
- Suggest creative writing
- Provide puzzles
- Organize group games
- Group or individual exercises

Doll Therapy

R: *Doll therapy is a nonpharmacological intervention aimed at reducing behavioral and psychological disorders in institutionalized patients with dementia. Researchers cited that the use of doll therapy promotes clinically significant improvements in the ability to relate with the surrounding world (Pezzati et al., 2014).*

Carp's Cues

Mitchell (2014) presents a thought-provoking discussion of the pros and cons of doll therapy. He writes, "Healthcare professionals who care for people with dementia find themselves in a difficult position when considering doll therapy. There are ethical positions that support engagement and disengagement with dolls (Mitchell, 2014). Practitioners should keep the person with dementia at the heart of their decision making by asking the question: Will the individual with dementia benefit from doll therapy" (Mitchell, 2014, p. 27).

- Consider giving the person something to hold (e.g., stuffed animal, doll) (Mitchell, 2014, p. 25).

R: *An increasing body of evidence suggests the use of dolls can have a positive impact on people with dementia in residential care and suggest that the use of doll therapy promotes clinically significant improvements in the ability to relate with the surrounding world (Higgins, 2010; Pezzati et al., 2014).*

- Inform family and health-care professionals in the unit before introduction of dolls.
- Use a different doll for each individual involved.
- Avoid dolls that eyes close or cry.
- Do not remove doll without permission. Use a reason that would be appropriate for a real baby (e.g. nap, bath).
- Handle the doll gently and have a place to put the doll that is perceived as comfortable and safe.

R: *Providing a doll to someone with dementia has been associated with a number of benefits which include a reduction in episodes of distress, an increase in general well-being, improved dietary intake, and higher levels of engagement with others (Mitchell, 2014).*

- Reduced agitation and aggression
- Reduced tendency to wander
- Increased well-being
- Increased interaction with staff and family members
- Reduction in use of psychotropic drugs

Remotivation Therapy

R: *While the aim of reality orientation is to help any confused person adjust to his surroundings, the focus of remotivation therapy is to recreate interest in life by focusing on strengths. It is a restorative modality to success dormant cognitive function beneath an illness. It can also delay or prevent loss of function (Stotts & Dyer, 2013).*

- Organize group sessions into five steps (*Dennis, 1984; Stotts & Dyer, 2013):
  Step 1: Create a climate of acceptance (approx. 5 minutes).
  - Maintain a relaxed atmosphere; introduce leaders and participants.
  - Provide large-letter name tags and names on chairs.
  - Maintain assigned places for every session.

  Step 2: Create a bridge to reality (approx. 15 minutes).
  - Use a prop (visual, audio, song, picture, object, poem) to introduce the theme of the session.

  Step 3: Share the world we live in (approx. 15 minutes).
  - Discuss the topic as a group.
  - Promote stimulation of senses.

Step 4: Appreciate the work of the world (approx. 20 minutes).
- Discuss how the topic relates to their past experiences (work, leisure).

Step 5: Create a climate of appreciation (approx. 5 minutes).
- Thank each member individually.
- Announce the next session's topic and meeting date.
- Use associations and analogies (e.g., "If ice is cold, then fire is..?" "If day is light, then night is..?").

- Choose topics for remotivation sessions based on suggestions from group leaders and group interests. Examples are pets, bodies of water, canning fruits and vegetables, transportation, and holidays.

Sensory Training (Wollen, 2010)
- Stimulate vision (with brightly colored items of different shape, pictures, colored decorations, kaleidoscopes).
- Stimulate smell (with flowers, soothing aromas from lavender or scented lotion).
- Stimulate hearing (play music with soothing sounds such as ocean or rain).
- Stimulate touch (massage, vibrating recliner, fuzzy objects, velvet, silk, stuffed animals).
- Stimulate taste (spices, salt, sugar, sour substances).

Reminiscence Therapy
- Consider instituting reminiscence therapy on a one-to-one or group basis. Discuss the purpose and goals with the client care team. Prepare well before initiating.

R: *These therapies can focus the person and can reduce confusion.*

Implement Techniques to Lower the Stress Threshold (Boyd, 2012; *Hall & Buckwalter, 1987; Miller, 2015)

- Refer also to *Acute Confusion* under Assess Personal and Environmental Factors That Contribute to or Increase Confusion.

Plan and Maintain a Consistent Routine
- Attempt to assign the same caregivers.
- Elicit from family members specific methods that help or hinder care.
- Arrange personal care items in order of use (e.g., clothes, toothbrush, mouthwash, etc.).
- Determine a daily routine with the individual and family.
- Write down the sequence for all caregivers.
- Reduce the stress when change is anticipated:
  - Keep the change as simple as possible (minimal holiday decorations).
  - Ensure the individual is well rested.
  - Institute change during the individual's best time of day if possible.

R: *Consistency can reduce confusion and increase comfort.*

Focus on the Individual's Ability Level
- Do not request performance of function beyond ability.
- Express unconditional positive regard for the individual.
- Modify environment to compensate for ability (e.g., use of Velcro fasteners, loose clothing, elastic waistbands).
- Use simple sentences; demonstrate activity.
- Do not ask questions that the individual cannot answer.
- Avoid open-ended questions (e.g., "What do you want to eat?" "When do you want to take a bath?").
- Avoid using pronouns; name objects.
- Offer simple choices (e.g., "Do you want a cookie or crackers?").
- Use finger foods (e.g., sandwiches) to encourage self-feeding.

R: *Attempting to perform functions that exceed cognitive capacity will result in fear, anger, and frustration (Boyd, 2012; *Hall, 1994).*

Minimize Fatigue (Ahlskog et al., 2011; *Hall, 1994)
- Provide rest periods twice daily.
- Choose a rest activity with the individual, such as reading or listening to music.
- Encourage napping in recliner chairs, not in bed.
- Plan high-stress or fatiguing activities during the best time of day for the individual.

- Allow the person to cease an activity at any time.
- Incorporate regular exercise in the daily plan.
- Be alert to expressions of fatigue and increased anxiety; immediately reduce stimuli.

R: *Fatigue can increase confusion by interfering with cognitive processing of incoming stimuli.*

Initiate Health Teaching and Referrals, as Needed

- Support groups
- Community-based programs (e.g., day care, respite care)
- Alzheimer's association (www.alz.org)
- Long-term care facilities

CHRONIC FUNCTIONAL CONSTIPATION

Chronic Functional Constipation

Perceived Constipation

Definition

Infrequent or difficult evacuation of feces, which has been present for at least three of the prior 12 months.

Defining Characteristics

Abdominal distention

Adult: Presence of ≥2 of the following symptoms on Rome III classification system:

- Lumpy or hard stools in ≥25% defecations
- Straining during ≥25% of defecations
- Sensation of incomplete evacuation for ≥25% of defecations
- Sensation of anorectal obstruction/blockage for ≥25% of defecations
- Manual maneuvers to facilitate ≥25% of defecations (digital manipulation, pelvic support)
- ≤3 evacuations per week

Child ≤4 years: Presence of ≥2 criteria on Roman III Pediatric classification system for ≥1 month:

- ≤2 defecations per week
- ≥1 episode of fecal incontinence per week
- Stool retentive posturing
- Painful or hard bowel movements
- Presence of large fecal mass in the rectum
- Large diameter stools that may obstruct the toilet

Child ≥4 years: Presence of ≥2 criteria on Roman III Pediatric classification system for ≥2 months:

- ≤2 defecations per week
- ≥1 episode of fecal incontinence per week
- Stool retentive posturing
- Painful or hard bowel movements
- Presence of large fecal mass in the rectum
- Large diameter stools that may obstruct the toilet

Fecal impaction

Fecal incontinence (in children)

Leakage of stool with digital stimulation

Pain with defecation

Palpable abdominal mass

Positive fecal occult blood test

Prolonged straining

Type 1 or 2 on Bristol Stool Chart

Related Factors

Pathophysiologic

Related to defective nerve stimulation, weak pelvic floor muscles, and immobility secondary to:
Spinal cord lesions
Spinal cord injury
Spina bifida
Cerebrovascular accident (stroke)
Neurologic diseases (multiple sclerosis, Parkinson's)
Dementia

Related to decreased metabolic rate secondary to:
Obesity
Pheochromocytoma
Hypothyroidism
Hyperparathyroidism
Uremia
Hypopituitarism
Diabetic neuropathy

Related to decreased response to urge to defecate secondary to:
Affective disorders

Related to pain (on defecation):
Hemorrhoids
Back injury

Related to decreased peristalsis secondary to hypoxia (cardiac, pulmonary)

Related to motility disturbances secondary to irritable bowel syndrome

Related to failure to relax anal sphincter or high resting pressure in the anal canal secondary to:
Multiple vaginal deliveries
Chronic straining

Treatment Related

Related to side effects of (specify):
Analgesic nonsteroidal anti-inflammatory agents
Antidepressants (e.g., monoamine-oxidase inhibitors tricyclic: amitriptyline)
Antacids (calcium, aluminum)
Iron
Barium
Aluminum
Phenothiazines
Anticonvulsants
Calcium channel blockers
Calcium
Anticholinergics (e.g., Pepto-Bismol)
Antihistamines (e.g., diphenhydramine [Benadryl and others])
Muscle relaxants (e.g., cyclobenzaprine [Flexeril], metaxolone [Skelaxin])
Phenothiazines (e.g., sedative-hypnotic phenobarbital [Luminal], zolpidem [Ambien], other)
Anesthetics
Narcotics (e.g., codeine, morphine)
Diuretics
Anti-Parkinson agents (e.g., carbamazepine [Equetro and others], levodopa [Dopar])

Aspirin
Chemotherapy
Lipid lowering drugs (e.g., cholestyramine [Prevalite], pravastatin [Pravachol]), simvastatin (e.g., Zocor)

Related to effects of anesthesia and surgical manipulation on peristalsis

Related to habitual laxative use

Related to mucositis secondary to radiation

Situational (Personal, Environmental)

Related to decreased peristalsis secondary to:

Immobility
Pregnancy
Stress
Lack of exercise

Related to irregular evacuation patterns

Related to cultural/health beliefs

Related to lack of privacy

Related to inadequate diet (lack of roughage, fiber, thiamine) or fluid intake

Related to fear of rectal or cardiac pain

Related to faulty appraisal

Related to inability to perceive bowel cues

Author's Note

Yearly, more than 2.5 million Americans see their health care provider for relief from constipation (Wald, 2015). Constipation occurs in 15% to 30% of older adults living in the community and 75% to 80% living in institutional settings (Miller, 2015).

Constipation results from delayed passage of food residue in the bowel because of factors that the nurse can treat and teach the individual (e.g., dehydration, insufficient dietary roughage, immobility). Often constipation is reported and with further assessment it is the person's misunderstanding of normal defecation patterns (Erichsén, Milberg, Jaarsma, & Friedrichsen, 2015). *Perceived Constipation* refers to a faulty perception of constipation with self-prescribed overuse of laxatives, enemas, and/or suppositories.

Errors in Diagnostic Statements

Constipation related to reports of infrequent hard, dry feces

A report of infrequent hard, dry feces validates constipation—it is not a contributing factor. If the nurse does not know the cause, he or she can write: *Constipation related to unknown etiology, as evidenced by reports of infrequent hard, dry feces.*

Key Concepts

General Considerations

- Constipation occurs in as many as 70% of individuals taking opioid analgesics (Yarbro, Wujcik, & Gobel, 2013).
- Irritable bowel syndrome affects 10% to 20% of the US population to some degree and can include constipation, diarrhea, and pain. Constipation is a predominant symptom in many individuals with irritable bowel syndrome (Lehrer, 2015).

Table 11.4 COMPONENTS FOR NORMAL BOWEL ELIMINATION AND CORRESPONDING BARRIERS

Components	Barriers
Daily diet of fiber (15–25 g)	Lack of access to fresh foods
	Financial constraints
	Insufficient knowledge[a]
8–10 glasses of water a day	Mobility problems
	Fear of incontinence
	Impaired thought process[a]
	Low motivation
Daily exercise	Minimal activity level
	Pain, fatigue
	Fear of falling
Cognitive appraisal	Impaired thought process
	Faulty appraisal
Toileting routine	Low motivation
	Change in routine
	Stress
Response to rectal cues	Mobility problems
	Decreased awareness
	Environmental constraints
	Self-care deficits

[a]These barriers can impede all the components.

- Bowel elimination is controlled primarily by muscular and neurologic activity. Undigested food or feces passes through the large intestine propelled by involuntary muscles within the intestinal walls. At the same time, water that was needed for digestion is reabsorbed. The feces passes through the sigmoid colon, which empties into the rectum. At some point, the amount of stool in the rectum stimulates a defecation reflex, which causes the anal sphincter to relax and defecation to occur (Grossman & Porth, 2014). Table II.4 illustrates the components needed for normal bowel elimination and the conditions that impede them.
- Chronic and disorders of defecatory or rectal evacuation (Grossman & Porth, 2014). Bowel patterns are culturally or family determined. Range of normal varies from three times a day to once every 3 days (Miller, 2015).
- Undigested fiber absorbs water, which adds bulk and softness to the stool, speeding its passage through the intestines. Fiber without adequate fluid can aggravate, not facilitate, bowel function (Miller, 2015).
- Laxatives and enemas are not components of a bowel management program. They are for emergency use only (Miller, 2015).
- Chronic use of stool softeners can cause fecal incontinence and is not recommended for treatment of chronic constipation in nonambulatory individuals.

Pediatric Considerations

- Unlike adults, constipation in children is not defined by frequency, but by the character of stool. Passage of firm or hard stool with symptoms of difficulty in expulsion, blood-streaked bowel movements, and abdominal discomfort characterize constipation in children.
- As the infant ages, the stomach enlarges to hold more food, and the peristaltic activity of the gastrointestinal (GI) tract slows. Thus, stools change in color, consistency, and frequency (Hockenberry & Wilson, 2015).

- Voluntary withholding (functional constipation) is the most common cause of constipation beyond the neonatal period. Conflicts in toilet training or pain on defecation may lead to stool retention (Hockenberry & Wilson, 2012).
- Encopresis is fecal soiling or incontinence secondary to constipation. Previously toilet-trained children with encopresis should be evaluated psychologically.
- Children with functional constipation associate defecation with discomfort. When the sensation of relaxation of the internal anal sphincter occurs, the child contracts the external sphincter to prevent the expulsion of stools. Eventually the rectum dilates, resulting in more stool retention and diminished sensory response.

Maternal Considerations

- Constipation in pregnancy results from (Pillitteri, 2014)
  - Displacement of the intestines
  - Increased water absorption from colon
  - Hormonal influences
  - Prolonged intestinal time
  - Use of iron supplements
- Postpartum causes of constipation are
  - Relaxed abdominal tone
  - Decreased peristalsis
  - Food and fluid restrictions during labor

Geriatric Considerations

- Constipation occurs in 15% to 30% of older adults living in the community and 75% to 80% living in institutional settings (Miller, 2015).
- Age-related factors are not responsible for constipation in older adults. Risk factors are diminished mobility, metabolic conditions (e.g., hypothyroidism), obesity, lower socioeconomic status, adverse medication effects, misuse of laxatives, and inadequate dietary intake of water and fiber (Miller, 2015).
- Sensory dysfunction in the anorectal area of older adults can reduce the ability to sense rectal distention (defecation cues).

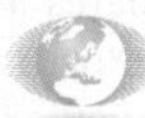

Transcultural Considerations

- Some cultures have folk medicine for elimination problems. For example, Mexican Americans differentiate diarrhea as hot or cold. If the stool is green or yellow, it is hot and treated with cold tea. If white, the stool is cold and treated with hot tea (Giger, 2013).

Focus Assessment Criteria

Subjective Data

Assess for Defining Characteristics

Ask the person how often they think they should have a bowel movement

Elimination pattern: usual, present
What frequency is considered normal?
Laxative/enema use: type, how often
Episodes of diarrhea: how often, frequency, duration
Precipitated by what?
Associated symptoms/complaints of: headache, thirst, weakness, pain, lethargy, cramping, anorexia, weight loss/gain, awareness of bowel cues

Assess for Related Factors

Lifestyle
Activity level, Occupation
Exercise: type, how often
Nutrition (recall intake [food, fluids] for 3 days)

Current drug therapy
Medical–surgical history
Present conditions

24-hour recall of foods and liquids taken
Usual 24-hour intake: carbohydrates, fat, protein, fiber, liquids

Past conditions
Surgical history: colostomy, ileostomy

Objective Data

Assess for Defining Characteristics

Stool
Color
Consistency
Components: blood, parasites, mucus, undigested food, pus

Bowel Sounds
High-pitched, gurgling
Weak and infrequent
High-pitched, frequent, loud, pushing (5 minutes)
Absent

Assess for Related Factors

Nutrition
Food intake: type, amounts
Fluid intake: type, amounts

Perianal Area/Rectal Examination
Hemorrhoids
Fissures
Control of rectal sphincter (presence of anal wink, bulbocavernosus reflex)
Irritation
Impaction
Stool in rectum

Goals

NOC
Bowel Elimination, Hydration, Knowledge: Healthy Diet, Exercise Participation

The individual will report bowel movements at least every 2 to 3 days as evidenced by the following indicators:

- Describe components for effective bowel movements.
- Explain lifestyle change(s) needed and why.

Interventions

NIC
Bowel Management, Fluid Management, Nutrition Management, Constipation/Impaction Management

Assess Contributing Factors

- Refer to Related Factors.

Evaluate Medications for Side Effects of Constipation

- Refer to Related Factors for specific medications.

Promote Corrective Measures

Regular Time for Elimination

- Review daily routine.
- Advise to include time for defecation as part of his or her daily routine.
- Discuss a suitable time (based on responsibilities, availability of facilities, etc.).
- Provide a stimulus to defecation (e.g., coffee, prune juice).
- Advise to attempt to defecate about 1 hour or so after meals and that remaining in the bathroom for a suitable length of time may be necessary.
- Avoid straining.

R: *The gastrocolic and duodenocolic reflexes stimulate mass peristalsis two or three times a day, most often after meals.*

Adequate Exercise

- Review the current exercise pattern.
- Provide for frequent moderate physical exercise (if not contraindicated).

- Provide frequent ambulation of the hospitalized client when tolerable. Refer to *Impaired Physical Mobility*.
- Perform range-of-motion exercises for those who are bedridden.
- For individuals who are unable to walk or are restricted to bed rest (McCay, Fravel, & Scanlon, 2012):
  - While lying down, raise lower limbs, keeping knees straight.
  - Turn and change positions in bed, lifting hips.
  - Teach, chair, or bed exercises such as pelvic tilt, low trunk rotation, and single leg lifts.
  - Lift knees alternately to the chest, stretching arms out to side and up over the head.
  - Contract abdominal muscles several times throughout the day.
  - Remind to do for 15 to 20 minutes at least twice per day.

R: *Regular physical activity promotes muscle tonicity needed for fecal expulsion. It also increases circulation to the digestive system, which promotes peristalsis and easier feces evacuation (Grossman & Porth, 2014).*

Balanced Diet

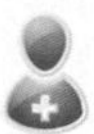

Clinical Alert "A diet high in fiber is not recommended for individuals who are immobile or who do not consume at least 1,500 mL of fluids per day" (McCay et al., 2012).

- Review list of foods high in fiber:
  - Fresh fruits, fruit juices, and vegetables with skins
  - Beans (navy, kidney, lima), nuts, and seeds
  - Whole-grain breads, cereal, and bran
- Consider financial limitations (encourage the use of fruits and vegetables in season).
- Discuss dietary preferences.
- Consider any food intolerances or allergies.
- Include approximately 800 g of fruits and vegetables (about four pieces of fresh fruit and large salad) for normal daily bowel movement. Avoid cooked fruits.
- Suggest moderate use of bran at first (may irritate GI tract, produce flatulence, cause diarrhea, or blockage).
- Gradually increase bran as tolerated (may add to cereals, baked goods, etc.). Explain the need for fluid intake with bran.
- Suggest 30 to 60 mL daily of a recipe of 2 cups of all-bran cereal, 2 cups of applesauce, and 1 cup of prune juice.
- Explain Pajala Porridge as a cooked mixture of flax seeds, prunes (chopped), apricots (chopped), raisins, water, rolled oats , and oat bran.

R: *Wisten and Messner (*2005), reported that individuals "in the porridge group had a daily defecation without laxatives on average 76% of the time compared with 23% of the time for those not eating the porridge."*

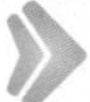

Carp's Cues

A diet high in fiber is not recommended for individuals who are immobile or who do not consume at least 1,500 mL of fluids per day.

For the Recipe for "Pajala Porridge"

- Refer to https://gettingtothebottomofit.wordpress.com/tag/pajala-porridge/. Consult with primary care provider prior to using.

R: *Fiber results in bulkier and softer stools. Waste then moves through the body more quickly, allowing easier and more regular bowel movements (McCay et al., 2012).*

R: *Three tablespoons of bran daily increases dietary fiber by 25% to 40% and eliminates constipation in 60% of individuals (*Shua-Haim, Sabo, & Ross, 1999).*

Adequate Fluid Intake

- Encourage intake of at least 2 to 3 L (8 to 13 glasses) unless contraindicated by cardiac and/or renal disorders (Lutz & Przytulski, 2011).
- Teach the person to monitor hydration by the color of their urine.

R: *Optimal hydration will produce light colored urine.*

- Discuss fluid preferences.
- Set up regular schedule for fluid intake.

- Recommend drinking a glass of hot water 30 minutes before breakfast, which may stimulate bowel evacuation.
- Advise avoiding grapefruit juice, coffee, tea, cola, and chocolate drinks as daily fluid intake.

R: Sufficient fluid intake, at least 2 to 3 L daily, is necessary to maintain bowel patterns and to promote proper stool consistency.

Optimal Position

- Provide privacy (close door, draw curtains around the bed, play the television or radio to mask sounds, have a room deodorizer available).
- Use the bathroom instead of a bedpan if possible. Allow suitable position (sitting and leaning forward, if not contraindicated).
- Elevate the legs on a footstool when on the toilet.
- Assist the client onto the bedpan if necessary; elevate the head of the bed to high Fowler's position or elevation permitted.

R: *Flexing the hip pulls the anal canal open, which decreases resistance of feces movement. An upright position uses gravity to promote feces movement. Elevating the legs can increase intra-abdominal pressure (*Shua-Haim et al., 1999).*

Conduct Health Teaching, as Indicated

- Explain the relationship of lifestyle changes to constipation.

R: *Sedentary lifestyle, inadequate fluid intake, inadequate dietary fiber, and stress can contribute to constipation.*

- Instruct when to call primary care provider (Wald, 2015). When the constipation
  - Is new (i.e., represents a change in your normal pattern)
  - Lasts longer than 3 weeks
  - Is severe
  - Is associated with any other concerning features such as blood on the toilet paper, weight loss, fevers, or weakness

R: *A recent change in bowel habits, blood in the stool, weight loss, or a family history of colon cancer. Testing may include blood tests, x-rays, sigmoidoscopy, colonoscopy, or more specialized testing if needed.*

- Encourage increased intake of high-roughage foods and increased fluid intake as an adjunct to iron therapy (e.g., fresh fruits and vegetables with skins, bran, nuts, seeds, whole-wheat bread).
- Encourage early ambulation, with assistance if necessary, to counter effects of anesthetic agents.
- Advise the client about medications that cause constipation. Refer to list under Related Factors.
- Discuss laxative abuse (see *Perceived Constipation*).

R: *Laxatives upset a bowel program because they cause much of the bowel to empty and can cause unscheduled bowel movements. With constant use, the colon loses tone and stool retention becomes difficult. Chronic use of bowel aids can lead to problems in stool consistency, which interferes with the scheduled bowel program and bowel management. Stool softeners may not be necessary if diet and fluid intake are adequate. Enemas lead to an overstretched bowel and loss of bowel tone, contributing to further constipation.*

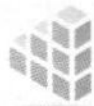

Pediatric Considerations

R: *Most contributing factors causing constipation in children are preventable. Several factors contribute to constipation:*

- Insufficient roughage or bulk
- A bland diet, too high in dairy products, which results in reduced colonic motility
- Insufficient oral intake of fluids, which allows the normal reabsorption of water from the colon to dehydrate the feces too much, or dehydration stemming from any activities that increase fluid loss from sweating
- Fecal retention by the child
- Medications (e.g., narcotics or anticonvulsants)
- The child's emotional state
- If bowel movements are infrequent with hard stools:
  - With infants, add corn syrup to feeding or fruit to diet. Avoid apple juice or sauce.
  - With children, add bran cereal, prune juice, and fruits and vegetables high in bulk.

- Refer cases of persistent constipation for medical evaluation.
- Explain to adolescents the effects of fluids, fiber, and exercise on bowel function.

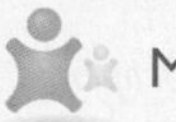

Maternal Considerations

- Explain the risks of constipation in pregnancy and postpartum:
  - Decreased gastric motility
  - Prolonged intestinal time
  - Pressure of enlarging uterus
  - Distended abdominal muscles (post)
  - Relaxation of intestines (post)
  - Iron supplements

R: *Iron supplements provide the iron stored for the fetus for growth and development (Pillitteri, 2014).*

- Explain aggravating factors for hemorrhoid development (straining at defecation, constipation, prolonged standing, wearing constrictive clothing).
- If woman has a history of constipation, discuss use of bulk-producing laxatives to soften bowels postdelivery.
- Assess abdomen (bowel sounds, distention, presence of flatus).
- Assess for hemorrhoids and perineal swelling.
- Provide relief of rectal or perineal pain.
- Instruct the client to take sitz baths and use cool, astringent compresses for hemorrhoids.

R: *Explaining the causes of constipation during pregnancy and the postpartum period can increase participation in behaviors that decrease or prevent constipation.*

- Refer to Interventions for preventing constipation.

Perceived Constipation

NANDA-I Definition

Self-diagnoses of constipation combined with abuse of laxatives, enemas, and/or suppositories to ensure a daily bowel movement

Defining Characteristics

Expectation of a daily bowel movement*
Overuse of laxatives, enemas, and/or suppositories*
Expectation of passage of stool at same time, every day*

Related Factors

Pathophysiologic

Related to faulty appraisal* secondary to:

Obsessive–compulsive disorders
Deterioration of the CNS
Depression
Impaired thought processes*

Situational (Personal, Environmental)

Related to inaccurate information secondary to:

Cultural health beliefs*
Family health beliefs*

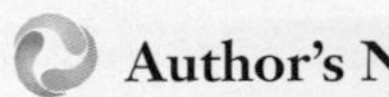

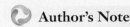

Author's Note

Refer to Author's Note under *Constipation*.

Key Concepts

Refer to Key Concepts under *Constipation*.

Focus Assessment Criteria

Refer to Focus Assessment Criteria under *Constipation*.

Goals

NOC

Bowel Elimination, Health Beliefs: Perceived Threat

The client will verbalize acceptance of a bowel movement every 1 to 3 days as evidenced by the following indicators:

- The client will not use laxatives regularly.
- The client will relate the causes of constipation.
- The client will describe the hazards of laxative use.
- The client will relate an intent to increase fiber, fluid, and exercise in daily life as instructed.

Interventions

NIC

Bowel Management, Health Education, Behavior Modification, Fluid Management, Nutrition Management

Assess Causative or Contributing Factors

- Cultural/familial belief
- Faulty appraisal

Explain That Bowel Movements Are Needed Every 2 to 3 Days, Not Daily (Erichsén et al., 2015)

- Be sensitive to the client's beliefs.
- Be patient.

R: *Lifetime habits and beliefs can be corrected with teaching.*

Explain the Hazards of Regular Laxative Use

- They provide only temporary relief and can promote constipation by interfering with peristalsis.
- They can interfere with absorption of vitamins A, D, E, and K.
- They can cause diarrhea.

R: *Regular laxative interferes with the defecation reflex and can cause an inability to have a bowel movement without laxatives (Grossman & Porth, 2014).*

- Refer to *Chronic Constipation* for interventions to promote optimal elimination.

INEFFECTIVE COPING

Ineffective Coping

Defensive Coping

Ineffective Impulse Control

Ineffective Denial

Ineffective Denial • Related to Impaired Ability to Accept the Consequences of Own Behavior as Evidenced by Lack of Acknowledgment of an Addiction (Substance Abuse/Dependency: Pathological Gambling, Kleptomania, Pyromania, Compulsive Buying, Compulsive Sexual Behavior)

Labile Emotional Control

Impaired Mood Regulation

NANDA-I Definition

Inability to form a valid appraisal of the stressors, inadequate choices of practiced responses, and/or inability to use available resources

Defining Characteristics

Verbalization of inability to cope or ask for help*
Inappropriate use of defense mechanisms
Inability to meet role expectations*
Chronic worry, anxiety
Sleep disturbance*
Fatigue*
High illness rate*
Reported difficulty with life stressors
Poor concentration*
Difficulty organizing information*
Decreased use of social support*
Inadequate problem-solving*
Impaired social participation
Use of forms of coping that impedes adaptive behavior*
Risk taking*
Lack of goal-directed behavior*
Destructive behavior toward self or others*
Change in usual communication patterns*
High incidence of accidents
Substance abuse*

Related Factors

Pathophysiologic

Related to chronicity of condition

Related to biochemical changes in brain secondary to:

Bipolar disorder
Chemical dependency
Schizophrenia
Personality disorder
Attention-deficient disorders

Related to complex self-care regimens

Related to neurologic changes in brain secondary to:

Stroke
Alzheimer's disease
Multiple sclerosis
End-stage diseases

Related to changes in body integrity secondary to:

Loss of body part
Disfigurement secondary to trauma

Related to altered affect caused by changes secondary to:

Body chemistry
Tumor (brain)
Intake of mood-altering substance
Mental retardation

Treatment Related

Related to separation from family and home (e.g., hospitalization, nursing home)

Related to disfigurement caused by surgery

Related to altered appearance from drugs, radiation, or other treatment

Situational (Personal, Environmental)

Related to poor impulse control and frustration tolerance

Related to disturbed relationship with parent/caregiver

Related to disorganized family system

Related to ineffective problem-solving skills

Related to increased food consumption in response to stressors

Related to changes in physical environment secondary to:

War
Homelessness
Seasonal work
Poverty
Relocation
Natural disaster
Inadequate finances

Related to disruption of emotional bonds secondary to:

Death
Desertion
Jail
Institutionalization
Separation or divorce
Educational institution
Relocation
Orphanage/foster care

Related to unsatisfactory support system

Related to sensory overload secondary to:

Factory environment
Urbanization: crowding, noise pollution, excessive activity

Related to inadequate psychological resources secondary to:

Poor self-esteem
Excessive negative beliefs about self
Negative role modeling
Helplessness
Lack of motivation to respond

Related to culturally related conflicts with (specify):

Premarital sex
Maturational
Abortion

Maturational

Child/Adolescent
Related to:

Inconsistent methods of discipline
Poor social skills
Peer rejection
Parental rejection
Fear of failure

Adolescent
Related to inadequate psychological resources to adapt to:

Physical and emotional changes
Educational demands
Sexual awareness
Sexual relationships
Independence from family
Career choices

Young Adult
Related to inadequate psychological resources to adapt to:

Career choices
Parenthood
Marriage
Leaving home
Educational demands

Middle Adult

Related to inadequate psychological resources to adapt to:

Physical signs of aging
Social status needs
Problems with relatives
Child-rearing problems
Career pressures
Aging parents

Older Adult

Related to inadequate resources (psychological, social support, financial, instrumental) to adapt to:

Daily stressors
Physical changes
Retirement
Changes in residence
Changes in financial status

Author's Note

Margaret O's son Nicholas, age 26, diagnosed with schizophrenia, died on a psychiatric unit of mixed drug toxicity. Margaret wrote to students in mental health, "To care for people with mental illness in times of crisis with insight and compassion . . . these are my hopes for you" (Proctor, Hamer, McGarry, Wilson, & Froggatt, 2014, p. vii).

World Health Organization (WHO, 2014) defines mental health "as a state of well-being in which every individual realizes his or her own potential, can cope with the normal stresses of life, can work productively and fruitfully, and is able to make a contribution to her or his community." In addition, WHO has described mental health and illness as follows:

- Mental health is an integral part of health; indeed, there is no health without mental health.
- Mental health is more than the absence of mental disorders.
- Mental and substance use disorders are the leading cause of disability worldwide.
- Mental disorders increase the risk of getting ill from other diseases such as HIV, cardiovascular disease, diabetes, and vice-versa.
- Stigma and discrimination against patients and families prevent people from seeking mental health care.
- Human rights violations of people with mental and psychosocial disability are routinely reported in most countries.

Ineffective Coping describes a person who is experiencing difficulty adapting to stress. *Ineffective Coping* can be a recent, episodic problem, or a chronic problem. Usual coping mechanisms may be inappropriate or ineffective, or the person may have a poor history of coping with stressors.

If the event is recent, *Ineffective Coping* may be a premature judgment. For example, a person may respond to overwhelming stress with a grief response such as denial, anger, or sadness, making a *Grieving* or *Fear* or *Anxiety* diagnosis appropriate.

Impaired Adjustment may be more useful than *Ineffective Coping* in the initial period after a stressful event. *Ineffective Coping* and its related diagnoses may be more applicable to prolonged or chronic coping problems, such as *Defensive Coping* for a person with a long-standing pattern of ineffective coping.

Errors in Diagnostic Statements

***Ineffective Coping* related to perceived effects of breast cancer on life goals, as evidenced by crying and refusal to talk**

If the diagnosis of breast cancer was recent, the person's response of crying and refusal to talk would be normal. Thus, the proper diagnosis would be *Grieving related to perceived effects of breast cancer on life goals.* If this response was prolonged with no evidence of adaptive behaviors (e.g., initiation of social activities), a new assessment is indicated.

Ineffective Coping related to reports of substance abuse

Substance abuse is a reportable or observable cue validating a diagnosis. If the person acknowledged the abuse and desires assistance, the diagnosis would be *Ineffective Coping related to inability to manage stressors without drugs.* If the substance abuse is validated but the person denied it or denied that it was a problem, the diagnosis would be *Ineffective Denial related to unknown etiology, as evidenced by lack of acknowledgment of drug dependency.*

Key Concepts

General Considerations

- Negative attitudes about mental illness often underlie stigma, which can cause affected persons to deny symptoms; delay treatment; be excluded from employment, housing, or relationships; and interfere with recovery (Centers for Disease Control and Prevention [CDC], 2010).

- The CDC (2010) reported:
  - 57% of all adults believed that people are caring and sympathetic to persons with mental illness.
  - Only 25% of adults with mental health symptoms believed that people are caring and sympathetic to persons with mental illness.
- Lazarus (*1985) defines coping as "constantly changing cognitive and behavioral efforts to manage specific external and/or internal demands that are taxing or exceeding the resources of the person."
- "Coping mechanisms are often confused and interchanged with defense mechanisms due to their similarities. Both processes are activated in times of adversity. Defense mechanisms and coping strategies reduce arousal of negative emotions. Furthermore, both processes aim at achieving adaptation only the means to the end differ" (Galor & Hentschel, 2012).
- Defense mechanisms help by distorting reality and coping strategies attempt to change the reality by solving the problem (*Cramer, 1998).
- Coping behaviors fall into two broad categories (*Lazarus & Folkman, 1984):
  - *Problem-focused:* These are behaviors that attempt to improve the situation through change or taking action. Examples include making an appointment with one's boss to discuss a pay raise, creating and following a schedule for homework, and seeking help.
  - *Emotion-focused:* These are thoughts or actions that relieve emotional distress. They do not alter the situation, but they help the person feel better. Examples include going for a walk, denying anything is wrong, using food to relax, and joking.
- Defense mechanisms are "unconscious measures that people use to defend their personal stability and protect against anxiety and threat" (Halter, 2014). Defense mechanisms can be very useful, but can be dysfunctional if they interfere with overall coping. Some examples are as follows:
  - *Projection, displacement*, and *suppression of anger* are when a person attributes anger to or expresses it toward a less threatening person or thing. Doing so may reduce the threat enough to allow the person to deal with it. Distortion of reality and disturbance of relationships may result, which further compound the problem. Suppressed anger may become dysfunctional when it results in stress-related physical symptoms or injures relationships.
  - *Anticipatory preparation* is the mental rehearsal of possible consequences or outcomes of behavior or stressful situations. It provides an opportunity to develop perspective as well as to prepare for the worst. It becomes dysfunctional when it creates unmanageable stress, as, for example, in anticipatory mourning.
  - Denial can help with the initial reporting of tragedy. Refusing to recognize a reality may be harmful as with denial of addictive behavior or a loved one's death.
- Splitting is the inability to identify the positive and negative qualities of oneself or others into a cohesive image. An example is your partner has no positive qualities. This is always maladaptive.
- Selye (*1974) defined stress as the nonspecific response of the body to any demand. Responses to stress vary according to personal perceptions. Both positive and negative life events may initiate a stress response.
- People with chronic mental illness experience low self-esteem and a lack of confidence, competence, and sense of efficacy. Altered perceptions, attention deficits, cognitive confusion, and labile emotions interfere with decision making, problem-solving, and interpersonal relationships (*Finkelman, 2000; Halter, 2014).
- The fight-or-flight response is more characteristic of males. Females respond to stress with the tend-and-befriend theory (Lee & Harley, 2012).
- A recent study identified the SRY gene, which is located on the Y chromosome and may promote aggression and other traditionally male behavioral traits, resulting in the fight-or-flight reaction to stress (Lee & Harley, 2012).
- In response to stress, the SRY gene and its proteins may contribute to the release of large amounts of norepinephrine with an increase in blood pressure and motor activity, thus evoking a "fight" response. Women do not have the SRY gene. Responses to stress in woman are regulated by other genes and other physiological changes involving estrogen hormones, oxytocin, and endorphins. These physiological changes, in turn, facilitate the expression of the tend-and-befriend response (Lee & Harley, 2012).

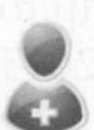

CLINICAL ALERT This biological difference does not justify aggressive behavior in males and passive behavior in females. Both need to learn more productive responses to stress.

Coping With Caregiving Responsibilities

- Uren and Graham (2013) explored the emotional experiences of caregivers of individuals in palliative home care using an interpretative, phenomenological paradigm.

- The following are factors related to coping, which "are significant in that they are able to influence one another, having a cumulative effect on the caregivers' well-being" (Uren & Graham, 2013).
  - Finding a Right Support Person
  - Surviving the High Workload
  - Seeking Alternative Means of Support
  - Juggling Home and Work Difficulties
  - Potentially Failing to Cope
  - Disillusionment versus Acceptance
- "Caregivers reiterated their need for someone to confide in, but felt that support was not easily found or was coupled with a fear of occupational repercussions" (Uren & Graham, 2013). Ineffective coping often led to the accumulation of stressors, with a considerable impact on the caregiver and their working abilities. This highlighted the importance of coping, and the necessity to support caregivers and to put measures in place to prevent burnout and stress (Uren & Graham, 2013).
- Refer to *Risk for Caregiver Role Strain* for specific interventions.

Carp's Cues

The reader is encouraged to access this study online to fully appreciate these caregivers' lived experience, when caring for a family member in palliative care.

Pediatric Considerations

- Inborn traits, social support, and family coping affect a child's ability to cope (Hockenberry & Wilson, 2015).
- As children mature, they develop and expand their coping strategies.
- The prevalence of depression is estimated to be 9.1% in adolescents 12 to 17 years of age with 6.3% reporting one major depressive episode in the past year with severe impairment (National Institute of Mental Health [NIMH], 2012).
- Approximately 60 percent of adolescents with depression have recurrences throughout adulthood. Adults with a history of adolescent depression have a higher rate of suicide than those without such a history (Clark, Jansen, & Cloy, 2012).
- Complex factors contribute to adolescents experiencing depressive symptoms, including developmental stressors (e.g., peer relationships, school accomplishments, physical and emotional changes) and environmental and contextual stressors (e.g., poverty, crime, family separations, discrimination) (Garcia, 2010).
- Adolescent-onset depression has been associated with abuse and neglect; poor academic performance; substance use; early pregnancy; and disruptions in social, employment, and family settings into adulthood. Although the prevalence of adolescent depression is high, it is significantly underdiagnosed and undertreated (Clark et al., 2012).
- Adolescents, who lack adequate coping abilities and resilience, engage in risk behaviors such as smoking, substance abuse, reckless behavior, suicidal attempts, and high-risk sexual behavior (Hockenberry & Wilson, 2012).
- Attention deficit hyperactive disorder (ADHD) is one of the most common *neurodevelopmental* disorders of childhood. It is usually first diagnosed in childhood and often lasts into adulthood. Children with ADHD may have trouble paying attention, controlling impulsive behaviors (may act without thinking about what the result will be), or be overly active (CDC, 2015).
  - In the United States as of 2012, more than 1 in 10 (11%) US school-aged children had received an ADHD diagnosis by a health-care provider by 2011 (CDC, 2015).
  - Brain imaging studies have revealed that, in youth with ADHD, the brain matures in a normal pattern but is delayed, on average, by about 3 years. The delay is most pronounced in brain regions involved in thinking, paying attention, and planning. More recent studies have found that the outermost layer of the brain, the cortex, shows delayed maturation overall, and a brain structure important for proper communications between the two halves of the brain shows an abnormal growth pattern. These delays and abnormalities may underlie the hallmark symptoms of ADHD and help to explain how the disorder may develop (*The ADHD Molecular Genetics Network, 2002; CDC, 2015).
  - The symptoms of this developmental disorder change over time. The diagnosis is made when symptoms of inattention or hyperactivity–impulsivity persist for at least 6 months and are maladaptive and inconsistent with developmental level (American Psychiatric Association [APA], 2014).
  - Children and adolescents with ADHD may exhibit oppositional defiant behavior and conduct disorders and may use inappropriate ways to get their needs met (Halter, 2014; Varcarolis, 2011).

- This disruptive behavior creates conflict with parents and authority figures, interferes with making and keeping friends, and interferes with learning. "Intrapersonal and academic problems lead to high levels of anxiety, low self-esteem, and blaming others for one's trouble" (Halter, 2014; Varcarolis, 2011).

Geriatric Considerations

- Folkman, Lazarus, Pimley, and Novacek (*1987) found that younger subjects reported more stress related to finances and work, whereas older subjects reported stress related to health, home maintenance, and social and environmental issues.
- Successful aging is dependent upon the ability of the person, when confronted with for diminished sense of control, is to adjust their expectations. Realistic expectations can reduce the stress of the loss (Hayward & Strauss, 2013).
- Coping mechanisms related to successful aging is related to the capacity for adapting new strategies in place of those that are diminished in late life. "At the same time as declines were occurring in personal control, many older adults also exhibited significant increases in the sense of God-mediated control" (Hayward & Krause, 2013).
- No one life event has consistently negative effects on an older adult; rather, several events in a short period represent the greatest challenge (Miller, 2015).

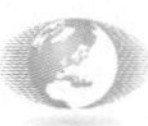

Transcultural Considerations

- Three major components of cultural systems influence responses to illness or chronic disease and a person's ability to make healthful changes in lifestyle: (1) family support systems, (2) coping behaviors, and (3) health beliefs and practices (Boyd, 2012).
- In certain cultures, the family plays a critical role in all aspects of the individual's life, including rejection or reinforcement of healthy lifestyle changes (Boyd, 2012).
- Asian cultures emphasize maintaining harmony and respect. It is not unusual for an Asian individual, who sees the nurse as an authority, to agree with all he or she suggests. Agreeing does not mean intended compliance, only good manners. This behavior opposes the assertive, questioning behavior emphasized in the dominant US culture (Boyd, 2012).
- Some symptoms that Western medicine would interpret as mental illness are considered normal in other cultures. Visions, hexes, and hearing voices are acceptable in some US subcultures: Appalachian, Asian, African American, Hispanic, and Native American (*Flaskerud, 1984).
- East Indian Hindu Americans believe in internal and external forces of control. Uncontrolled psychological factors, such as anger, shame, and envy, make a person more susceptible to disease. They also believe strong supernatural forces, external events or misfortune, such as the wrath of a disease goddess, malevolent spirits of dead ancestors, sins committed in previous lives, or jealous living relatives, cause illness. Hindus wear charms to ward off evil intentions. Exorcism is a treatment sought to expel evil spirits (Giger, 2013).
- The Chinese culture views mental illness as one's inability to control one's behavior and is shameful. Chinese families may wait until a relative's mental illness is unmanageable before seeking Western medicine, hospitalized Chinese psychiatric individuals will appear more symptomatic (Giger, 2013).

Focus Assessment Criteria

Ineffective coping can be manifested in various ways. An individual or family may respond with a disturbance in another functional pattern (e.g., spirituality, parenting). The nurse should be aware of this and use assessment data to ascertain the dimensions affected.

Subjective Data

Assess for Defining Characteristics

Physiologic Stress-Related Symptoms

Cardiovascular
Headache, Fainting (blackouts, spells), syncope
Chest pain, Increased pulse, Palpitations, Increased blood pressure

Respiratory
Shortness of breath; increased rate and depth of breathing
Chest discomfort (pain, tightness, ache)

Gastrointestinal
Nausea, Vomiting, Abdominal pain
Change in appetite
Unintentional change in weight

Musculoskeletal
Pain, Fatigue, Weakness

Genitourinary
Menstrual changes
Sexual difficulty
Urinary discomforts (pain, burning, urgency, hesitancy)

Dermatologic
Itching, Rash

Perception of Stressor
How have these stressors affected you?
How are you dealing with them? Has this help?

Obtain the History of Drinking Pattern From the Individual or Significant Other (*Kappas-Larson & Lathrop, 1993)
What was the date of the last drink?
How much was consumed on that day?
On how many days of the last 30 was alcohol consumed?
What was the average intake?
What was the most you drank?

Determine the Attitude Toward Drinking by Asking CAGE Questions (*Ewing, 1984)
Have you ever thought you should *C*ut down your drinking?
Have you ever been *A*nnoyed by criticism of your drinking?
Have you ever felt *G*uilty about your drinking?
Do you drink in the morning, as an Eye opener?

Symptoms of Depression (Mitchell et al., 2013)
Physiological concomitants of anxiety (i.e., effects of autonomic overactivity, "butterflies," indigestion, stomach cramps, belching, diarrhea, palpitations, hyperventilation, paresthesia, sweating, flushing, tremor, headache, urinary frequency).
Somatic Complaints (Heaviness in limbs, back, or head). Backaches, headaches, muscle aches. Loss of energy and fatigability
Reports of loss of libido, impaired sexual performance, menstrual disturbances
Depressed mood most of the day, nearly every day
Fatigue (loss of energy), markedly diminished interest or pleasure in almost all activities most of the day, nearly every day. Significant weight loss/gain
Insomnia/hypersomnia
Psychomotor agitation/retardation
Impaired concentration (indecisiveness)
Risk for suicide (refer to *Risk for Suicide* for assessment of critical warning signs and level of risk)
Refer to a valid test for a complete depression assessment (e.g., The Hamilton Rating Scale for Depression [HAM-D])

Assess for Related Factors

Current/recent stressors (number, type, duration)
Major life events and everyday stresses
Refer also to Related Factors above

Objective Data

Assess for Defining Characteristics

Appearance
Inappropriate altered affect
Inappropriate dress, grooming

Behavior
Calm
Hostile
Tearful
Sudden mood swings
Withdrawn

Cognitive Function
Impaired orientation to time, place, person
Impaired concentration
Altered ability to solve problems
Impaired memory
Impaired judgment

Risk-Prone/Abusive Behaviors

To self
Excessive smoking
Excessive alcohol intake
Excessive food intake
Drug abuse
Reckless driving
Suicide attempts
Unsafe sexual practices

To others
Does not care, is unwilling to listen, neglects needs of family members
Imposes physical harm on family members (bruises, burns, broken bones)

Assess for Attention Difficulties with parent and child (American Academy of Pediatrics [AAP], 2015)

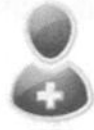

CLINICAL ALERT Hyperactivity may be or may not be ADHD, which is defined as persistent pattern of inattention and/or hyperactivity–impulsiveness present before the age of 7 years (AAP, 2015)

Persistent pattern of inattention and/or hyperactivity

Clear evidence that behavior interferes with developmentally appropriate social, academic, or occupational functioning

Cannot be accounted for by another mental disorder
A child with ADHD might (CDC, 2015)

- daydream a lot
- forget or lose things a lot
- squirm or fidget
- talk too much
- make careless mistakes or take unnecessary risks
- have a hard time resisting temptation
- have trouble taking turns
- have difficulty getting along with others

Goals

NOC
Coping, Stress level. Self-Esteem, Social Interaction Skills, Abusive Behavior Self=Restraint, Social Support, Sleep, Decision-Making, Behavior Modification,

The person will make decisions and follow through with appropriate actions to change provocative situations in the personal environment as evidenced by the following indicators:

- Verbalizes feelings related to emotional state
- Focuses on the present
- Identifies personal strengths
- Identifies response patterns and if their responses are helpful or not
- Identifies resources in community for individual and family

The child/adolescent will comply "with requests and limits on behavior in absence of arguments, tantrums, or other acting-out behaviors" as evidenced by the following indicators (Varcarolis, 2011):

- Demonstrates increased impulse control within (specify time)
- Demonstrates the ability to tolerate frustration and delay gratification within (specify time)
- Demonstrates an absence of tantrums, rage reactions, or other acting-out behaviors within (specify time)
- Describes the behavior limits and rationale to an authority figure
- Acknowledges the responsibility for misbehaviors, increased impulse control within (specify time)

Interventions

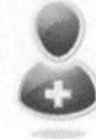

CLINICAL ALERT Proctor et al. (2014, p. 93) wrote "When we listen to understand, we are present and available and are only listening to what the person is saying, not thinking about other things." It requires self-discipline rather than launching into our own agenda.

NIC

Coping Enhancement, Counseling, Emotional Support, Active Listening, Assertiveness Training, Behavior Modification, Anger Control, Crisis Intervention, Self-responsibility Facilitation, Support System Enhancement.

Assess Causative and Contributing Factors

- Refer to Related Factors.

Establish Rapport

- Spend time with the individual. Provide supportive companionship.
- Consider how you would feel in this situation.
- Avoid being overly cheerful and cliché such as "Things will get better."
- Convey honesty and empathy.
- Offer support. Encourage expression of feelings. Let the person know you understand his or her feelings. Do not argue with expressions of worthlessness by saying things such as "How can you say that? Look at all you accomplished in life."
- Allow extra time for the individual to respond.

R: *The person with a chronic mental illness "must be helped to give up the role of being sick for that of being different" (*Finkelman, 2000).*

Assess Present Coping Status

- Determine the onset of feelings and symptoms and their correlation with events and life changes.
- Assess the ability to relate facts.
- Listen carefully as the individual speaks to collect facts; observe facial expressions, gestures, eye contact, body positioning, and tone and intensity of voice.

R: *Behavior is disrupted when both needs and goals are threatened.*

- Determine the risk of self-harm; intervene appropriately.
- Assess for signs of potential suicide:
  - History of previous attempts or threats (overt and covert)
  - Changes in personality, behavior, sex life, appetite, and sleep habits
  - Preparations for death (putting things in order, making a will, giving away personal possessions, acquiring a weapon)
  - Sudden elevation in mood
- See *Risk for Suicide* for additional information on suicide prevention.

Assess the Effects of Depression on Function

- Preform a Functional Health Assessment to determine the effects of their depression on functioning. Refer to appropriate nursing diagnoses for interventions.

R: *Depression can affect all aspects of a person's life, relationships and work (Halter, 2014).*

Assist in Developing Appropriate Problem-Solving Strategies

- Ask to describe previous encounters with conflict and how he or she resolved them.
- Evaluate whether his or her stress response is "fight or flight" or "tend and befriend."

- Encourage the individual to evaluate his or her behavior.
- "Did that work for you?" "How did it help?" "What did you learn from that experience?"
- Discuss possible alternatives (i.e., talk over the problem with those involved, try to change the situation, or do nothing and accept the consequences).
- Assist the individual in identifying problems that he or she cannot control directly; help the individual to practice stress-reducing activities for control (e.g., exercise, yoga).
- Be supportive of functional coping behaviors.
- "The way you handled this situation 2 years ago worked well then. Can you do it now?"
- Give options; however, leave the decision making to the person.

R: *Cognitive interventions help the person regain control over his or her life. They include identifying automatic thoughts and replacing them with positive thoughts (*Finkelman, 2000).*

Assist to Gradually Increase Activity

- Identify activities that were previously gratifying but have been neglected: personal grooming or dress habits, shopping, hobbies, exercise, and arts and crafts.
- Encourage these activities in the daily routine for a set time span, for example:
  - I will walk 20 minutes every day.
  - I will plant a small garden.
  - I will walk down steps rather than using an elevator.
  - I will park my car farther from my destination and walk.
  - I will volunteer, for example, in a literacy program or reading to children.
  - I will play the piano for 30 minutes every afternoon.

R: *Depression is immobilizing and immobilization increases depression. The person needs to make a conscious effort to fight inactivity to improve.*

Explore Outlets That Foster Feelings of Personal Achievement and Self-Esteem

- Make time for relaxing activities (e.g., dancing, exercising, sewing, woodworking).
- Find a helper to take over responsibilities occasionally (e.g., sitter).
- Learn to compartmentalize (do not carry problems around with you always; enjoy free time).
- Encourage longer vacations (not just a few days here and there).
- Provide opportunities to learn and use stress management techniques (e.g., jogging, yoga, thought-stopping).

R: *People with chronic mental illness experience low self-esteem and a lack of confidence, competence, and sense of efficacy. Altered perceptions, attention deficits, cognitive confusion, and labile emotions interfere with decision making, problem-solving, and interpersonal relationships (*Finkelman, 2000).*

Facilitate Emotional Support From Others

- During conversations try not to focus on your problems. Balance the conversation with some positives.
- Seek out people who share a common challenge: establish telephone contact, initiate friendships within the clinical setting, develop and institute educational and support groups.
- Establish a network of people who understand your situation.
- Decide who can best act as a support system (do not expect empathy from people who themselves are overwhelmed with their own problems).
- Maintain a sense of humor.
- Allow tears.

R: *Coping effectively requires successful maintenance of many tasks: self-concept, satisfying relationships with others, emotional balance, and stress.*

- Teach self-monitoring tools (*Finkelman, 2000):
  - Develop a daily schedule to monitor for signs of improvement or worsening.
  - Discuss reasonable goals for present relationships.
  - Write down what is done when in control, depressed, confused, angry, and happy.
  - Identify activities tried, would like to try, or should do more.
  - Create a warning sign checklist that indicates worsening and how to access help.

R: *Self-monitoring can help the individual learn how to observe symptoms and recognize when he or she needs more intensive help (*Finkelman, 2000).*

Teach Problem-Solving Techniques

- *Goal setting* is consciously setting time limits on behaviors, which is useful when goals are attainable and manageable. It may become stress-inducing if unrealistic or short sighted.
- *Information seeking* is learning about all aspects of a problem, which provides perspective and, in some cases, reinforces self-control.
- *Mastery* is learning new procedures or skills, which facilitates self-esteem and self-control (e.g., self-care of colostomies, insulin injection, or catheter care).

R: *Goals should be realistic and attainable to promote self-esteem and reduce stress.*

Initiate Health Teaching and Referrals, as Indicated

- Prepare for problems that may occur after transition:
  - Medications—schedule, cost, misuse, side effects
  - Increased anxiety
  - Sleep problems
  - Eating problems—access, decreased appetite
  - Inability to structure time
  - Family/significant other conflicts
  - Follow-up—forgetting, access, difficulty organizing time

R: *For depression-related problems beyond the scope of nurse generalists, referrals to an appropriate professional (marriage counselor, psychiatric nurse therapist, nurse practitioner, psychologist, and psychiatrist) will be needed.*

- Instruct the individual in relaxation techniques; emphasize the importance of setting 15 to 20 minutes aside each day to practice relaxation:
  - Find a comfortable position in a chair or on the floor.
  - Close the eyes.
  - Keep noise to a minimum (only very soft music, if desired).
  - Concentrate on breathing slowly and deeply.
  - Feel the heaviness of all extremities.
  - If muscles are tense, tighten, then relax each one from toes to scalp.
- Teach assertiveness skills.
- Teach the use of cognitive therapy techniques.

R: *The techniques can effectively reduce stress, which negatively affects functioning.*

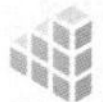

Pediatric Interventions

- If attention disorders are present, explain their etiology and behavioral manifestations to the child and caregivers.
- Help the child to understand he or she is not "bad" or "dumb."

R: *"Brain imaging studies have revealed that, in youth with ADHD, the brain matures in a normal pattern but is delayed, on average, by about 3 years. The delay is most pronounced in brain regions involved in thinking, paying attention, and planning." (The ADHD Molecular Genetics Network, 2002; CDC, 2015).*

- Establish target behaviors with the child and caregivers.
- Avoid repetitive lecturing.

R: *Interventions focus on helping the child develop self-control and self-respect. Children with attention disorders are often very intelligent and do not need repetitive lectures.*

- Work with parents and teachers to learn more effective behavioral strategies to support success:
  - Establish eye contact before giving instructions.
  - Set firm, responsible limits.
  - Avoid lectures; simply state rules.
- Maintain routines as much as possible.
- Attempt to keep a calm and simple environment.
- Reinforce appropriate behavior with a positive reinforcer (e.g., praise, hug).

R: *Routine helps to reduce stress for caregivers and child.*

R: *Children with attention disorders cannot filter extraneous stimuli and therefore respond to everything, thus losing focus.*

- Monitor for rising levels of frustration. Intervene early to calm child.

R: *This can prevent a potential outburst (Halter, 2014; Varcarolis, 2011).*

- Avoid power struggles and no-win situation. Look for a compromise.

R: *"Therapeutic goals are lost in power struggles" (Halter, 2014; Varcarolis, 2011).*

Allow the Child to Discuss the Requests Within Reason. Provide Simple Explanation. Provide Periodic Rewards for Positive Behaviors

R: *Discussions allow the child to maintain a sense of control and power (Varcarolis, 2011).*

Assist the child in improving play with peers

- Start with short play periods.
- Use simple, concrete games.
- Begin with sympathetic siblings or family members.
- Initially, select a quieter and less demanding peer as playmate.
- Provide immediate and instant feedback (e.g., "I see you are being distracted"; "You are playing nicely").

R: *Success with peers in play is critical for positive reinforcement and self-esteem.*

- Initiate health teaching and referrals as needed.
- Teach parents/caregivers of hyperactive children to (CDC, 2015):
  - **Create a routine**. Try to follow the same schedule every day, from wake-up time to bedtime.
  - **Get organized.** Put schoolbags, clothing, and toys in the same place every day, so your child will be less likely to lose them.
  - **Avoid distractions.** Turn off the TV, radio, and computer, especially when your child is doing homework.
  - **Limit choices.** Offer a choice between two things (this outfit, meal, toy, etc., or that one) so that your child isn't overwhelmed and overstimulated.
  - **Change your interactions with your child.** Instead of long-winded explanations and cajoling, use clear, brief directions to remind your child of responsibilities.
  - **Use goals and rewards.** Use a chart to list goals and track positive behaviors, then reward your child's efforts. Be sure the goals are realistic—baby steps are important!
  - **Discipline effectively.** Instead of yelling or spanking, use timeouts or removal of privileges as consequences for inappropriate behavior.
  - **Help your child discover a talent.** All kids need to experience success to feel good about themselves. Finding out what your child does well—whether it's sports, art, or music—can boost social skills and self-esteem.
- Provide information about medication therapy if indicated.
- Refer to specialists as needed (e.g., psychological, learning specialists).

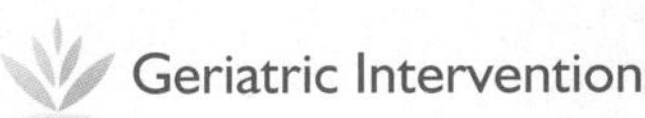

Geriatric Interventions

- Assess for risk factors for ineffective coping in older adults (Miller, 2015):
  - Inadequate economic resources
  - Several daily hassles at the same time
  - Several major events in short period
  - Unrealistic goals

R: *Miller (2015) identifies the following as risk factors for increased stress and poor coping in older adults: diminished economic resources, immature developmental level, unanticipated events, several daily hassles at the same time, several major life events in a short period, high social status, and high feelings of self-efficacy in situations that cannot change.*

Evaluate Coping Resources Available (Miller, 2015)

- Social supports especially religious support
- Instrumental support (meals, transportation, personal care)

- Emotional support that he or she is valued, loved, respected
- Information support regarding resources available

R: *Researchers have reported that stressful life events as predisposing factors and social connectedness as a buffer that serves to promote successful coping and reduce suicide risk.in older adults (Conwell, Van Orden, & Caine, 2011).*

- Specifically address daily stressors (food preparation, medication schedule, self-care, and housekeeping). Review possible options to reduce daily stress, for example, weekly pill boxes, frozen complete meals.

R: *Older adults who experience daily stressors more frequently reported their memory to be significantly worse and affects overall psychological functioning (Stawski, Mogle, & Sliwinski, 2013).*

Defensive Coping

NANDA-I Definition

Repeated projection of falsely positive self-evaluation based on a self-protective pattern that defends against underlying perceived threats to positive self-regard.

Defining Characteristics

Delay in seeking health care
Denies fear of death
Denies fear of invalidism
Displaces fear of impact of the condition
Displaces sources of symptoms
Does not admit impact of disease on life
Does not perceive relevance of danger
Does not perceive relevance of symptoms
Inappropriate affect
Minimizes symptoms
Refusal of health care
Use of dismissive gestures when speaking of distressing events
Use of treatment not advised by health-care professional

Related Factors*

Related to:

Threat of unpleasant reality
Conflict between self-perception and value system
Deficient support system
Fear of failure
Fear of humiliation
Fear of repercussions
Low level of confidence in others
Low level of self-confidence
Uncertainty
Unrealistic expectations of self

Author's Note

In selecting this diagnosis, it is important to consider the potentially related diagnoses of *Chronic Low Self-Esteem*, *Powerlessness*, and *Impaired Social Interaction*. They may express how the person established, or why he or she maintains, this defensive pattern.

Defensive Coping is the "repeated projection of falsely-positive self-evaluation based on a self-protection pattern that defends against perceived threats to positive self-regard" (Halter, 2014; Varcarolis, 2011). When a defensive pattern is a barrier to effective relationships, *Defensive Coping* is a useful diagnosis.

Key Concepts

General Considerations

- "Defenses are efficient mechanisms that help dealing with threatening and at times traumatic stressors. Pathology probably does not originate from the actual use of defense mechanisms; it is caused by a continuous reliance on defenses, instead of actually attempting to solve the core problems that cause their necessity in the first place" (Galor, 2012).
- Over time defense mechanisms do contribute to the development of severe pathology, yet the fact that they seem to help the individual to cope in a short-term should not be ignored nor dismissed.
- Defensive functioning is the ability to use defense mechanisms to protect the ego from overwhelming anxiety. If defensive mechanisms are overused, they become ineffective or ego-defeating (Varcarolis, 2011).
  - Some individuals with psychotic disorders of paranoia use defensive coping when they are suspicious, threatened, and vulnerable (Halter, 2014; Varcarolis, 2011).

Goals

NOC

Acceptance: Health Status, Coping, Self-Esteem, Social Interaction Skills, Information Processing

The individual will demonstrate appropriate interactions with others and report that they feel safe and are more in control as evidenced by the following indicators:

- Adheres to treatment, for example, medications, therapy, and goals
- Uses newly learned constructive methods to deal with stress and promote feelings of control
- Removes self from situations that increase their anxiety

Interventions

NIC

Coping Enhancement, Emotional Support, Self-Awareness Enhancement, Environment Management, Presence, Active Listening

Reduce Demands on the Individual If Stress Levels Increase

- Modify the level of or remove environmental stimuli (e.g., noise, activity).

R: *"Noisy environments can be perceived as threatening" (Halter, 2014; Varcarolis, 2011).*

- Decrease (or limit) contacts with others (e.g., visitors, other individuals, staff) as required.
- Clearly articulate minimal expectations for activities. Decrease or increase as tolerated.
- Identify stressors placing demands on the individual's coping resources; develop plans to deal with them.

R: *Increased stress increases defensive coping (Mohr, 2010).*

Establish a Therapeutic Relationship

- Maintain a neutral, matter-of-fact tone with a consistent positive regard. Ensure that all staff relate in a consistent fashion, with consistent expectations.
- Focus on simple, here-and-now, goal-directed topics when encountering the individual's defenses.
- Do not react to, defend, or dwell on negative projections or displacements; also do not challenge distortions or unrealistic/grandiose self-expressions. Try instead to shift to more neutral, positive, or goal-directed topics.
- Avoid control issues; attempt to present positive options to the individual, which allows a measure of choice.
- To promote learning from the individual's own actions (i.e., "natural consequences"), identify those actions that have interfered with the achievement of established goals.
- Reinforce more adaptive coping patterns (e.g., formal problem-solving, rationalization) that assist the person in achieving established goals.
- Evaluate interactions, progress, and approach with other team members to ensure consistency within the treatment milieu.

R: *Calm and consistent approaches can help to decrease anger and aggression (Halter, 2014; Varcarolis, 2011).*

Promote Dialogue to Decrease Paranoia and Permit a More Direct Addressing of Underlying Related Factors (see also *Chronic Low Self-Esteem*)

- Validate the individual's reluctance to trust in the beginning. Over time, reinforce the consistency of your statements, responses, and actions. Give special attention to your meeting of (reasonable) requests or your following through with plans and agreements.
- Use clear, simple language. Explain activities before you do them.
- Be honest, nonjudgmental, and nondefensive; take a neutral approach.
- Do not whisper, laugh, or engage in behavior that can be misinterpreted.

R: *A suspicious person can detect dishonesty. Neutrality and consistency discourages the person from misinterpreting the communication (Halter, 2014; Varcarolis, 2011).*

- Engage the individual in diversional, nongoal-directed, noncompetitive activities (e.g., relaxation therapy, games, and outings).
- Initially, provide solitary, noncompetitive activities (Halter, 2014; Varcarolis, 2011).

R: *Diversional, supportive interactions that do not encourage suspiciousness should be balanced with goal-directed/problem-focused interactions according to the individual's tolerance.*

- Encourage self-expression of neutral themes, positive reminiscences, and so forth.
- Encourage other means for self-expression (e.g., writing, art) if verbal interaction is difficult or if this is an area of personal strength.
- Listen passively to *some* grandiose or negative self-expression to reinforce your positive regard. If this does not lead to more positive self-expression or activity, then such listening may prove counterproductive.

Ineffective Impulse Control

NANDA-I Definition

A pattern of performing rapid, unplanned reactions to internal or external stimuli without regard to negative consequences of these reactions to the impulsive individual or to others

Defining Characteristics*

Acting without thinking
Irritability
Gambling addiction
Asking personal questions
Sensation seeking
Bulimia
Sexual promiscuity
Inability to save money or regulate finances
Inappropriate sharing personal details
Temper outbursts
Overly familiar with strangers
Violent Behavior

Related Factors

Alcohol dependence
Disorder of cognition*
Anger*
Disorder of development*
Codependency*
Disorder of mood*
Compunction*
Disorder of personality*
Delusion*
Disorder of body image
Denial*

Substance abuse (drugs)
Disorder of brain function
Environment that might cause irritation or frustration*
Fatigue*
Hopelessness*
Ineffective coping*
Insomnia*
Low self-esteem
Poor
Smoker*
Social isolation*
Stress vulnerability*
Suicidal feelings*
Unpleasant physical symptoms*

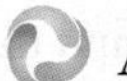

Author's Note

Ineffective Impulse Control is a new NANDA-I nursing diagnosis that represents a behavior that can cause a variety of problems in the individual or to others such as substance abuse, violence, sexual promiscuity, etc.

It is a component of the *DSM-5* diagnoses *Personality Disorders, Oppositional Defiant Disorder. Intermittent Explosive disorder, Conduct Disorder*.

It may be more clinically useful to view *Ineffective Impulse Control* as behavior that contributes to a nursing diagnosis and/or a manifestation rather than as the response or nursing diagnosis. For example, *Risk for Suicide, Risk for Other-Directed Violence, Dysfunctional Family Processes, Defensive Coping, Self-Mutilation, Impaired Social Interactions, Loneliness, Noncompliance, Ineffective Self Health Management, Impaired Parenting,* and *Stress Overload* all can have a component of poor impulse control that contributes to the diagnosis.

The clinician can choose to use *Ineffective Impulse Control* as a nursing diagnosis or can use a more specific nursing diagnosis as discussed in this Author's Note. The following interventions can also be used with the aforementioned diagnoses or as additional interventions for another nursing diagnosis, in which the individual has problems with impulse control.

Key Concepts

Refer also to *Ineffective Coping.*

- Impulse control disorders are often found in families. It may reflect a learned behavior and of neurobiological origins (Halter, 2014). Fahimm et al. (2012) reported that the gray matter is less dense and reduced in young in adolescents. Gray matter is associated with impulse control and self-regulation (Halter, 2014).

Focus Assessment Criteria

Refer to *Ineffective Coping.*

Goals

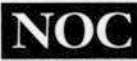

NOC

Impulse Self-Control, Suicide-self restraint

The individual will consistently demonstrate the use of effective coping responses as evidenced by the following indicators:

- Identifies consequences of impulsive behavior
- Identifies feelings that precede impulsive behavior
- Controls impulsive behavior

Interventions

"In a Respectful, Neutral Manner, Explain the Expected Individual's Behaviors, Limits, and Responsibilities" (Varcarolis, 2011)

NIC

Self-Awareness Enhancement, Presence, Counseling, Behavioral Modification, Anger Control, Coping Enhancement, Milieu Therapy, Limit Setting

R: *Individuals need to have explicit guidelines and boundaries and to be informed that they will be held responsible for their behavior (Varcarolis, 2011).*

Assist the Individual to Identify Problematic Situations

- Explore possible responses/actions and their benefits and consequences.
- Role-play acceptable social skills.

R: *Emphasizing alternative ways of responding to problematic situations can produce positive responses from others.*

Explain a Behavioral Contract and Its Components

R: *Instead of focusing on problem areas, a behavioral contract builds positive relationships and supports appropriate behavior.*

- The individual identifies their problematic behavior and how it affects others.
- Identifies an alternative to the problematic behavior.
- Identifies a reward (the reward may be that communication focuses on making a positive choice and the feeling of success).
- Identifies the consequences of a poor choice, which results in a negative response from others.
- If written, sign and date (both individual and clinician).
- When a positive choice is observed or related, specifically address how the individual feels.
- When a problematic choice is observed or related, specifically address the how the individual feels about the situational response. Focus on to continue the process of trying.

Engage in Role-Playing (Halter, 2014)

R: *This provides individuals or groups to learn and practice new behaviors or skills.*

- Start with low stress situations.
- If the response is problematic, ask the individual why they think it could be problematic.

Approach the Individual in a Consistent Manner in All Interactions (Halter, 2014)

- Initially avoid touch and physical closeness.
- If behavior is inappropriate or undesirable, redirect to appropriate dialogue and/or another activity.
- When indicated, if an individual has misbehaved, expect an apology and/or correcting a result of an outburst, for example, picking up thrown object.
- Prior to a previous problematic situation, provide direction and state expectation calmly.
- Ensure all staff are consistent.

R: *Consistency enhances feelings of security and clarifies expectations, while exceptions encourage manipulative behaviors (Halter, 2014).*

Teach Strategies to Help Reduce Tension and Negative Feelings (e.g., Assertiveness, Quieting Oneself)

- Be realistic. Begin in small steps.

R: *Ingrained maladaptive behaviors can be changed a little at a time (Varcarolis, 2011).*

Encourage Participation in Group Therapy

R: *The individual may be able to experiment with social relations within the safety of a group therapy setting (Mohr, 2010).*

- Avoid:
  - Giving attention to inappropriate behaviors.
  - Showing own frustration.
  - Accepting gift giving, flattery, seductive behaviors, and instilling guilt by individuals (Varcarolis, 2011).

R: *These behaviors are attempts are manipulative and serve to undermine the effectiveness of therapy.*

Provide and Encourage the Use of Other Services (e.g., Social Services, Vocational Rehabilitation, Legal Services)

R: *The consequences of impulsive behavior can be multiple social problems, for example, incarceration, divorce, truancy, addiction (Varcarolis, 2011).*

Ineffective Denial

NANDA-I Definition

Conscious or unconscious attempt to disavow the knowledge or meaning of an event to reduce anxiety and/or fear, leading to the detriment of health

Defining Characteristics[12]

Major* (Must Be Present)

Delays seeking or refuses health-care attention
Does not perceive personal relevance of symptoms or danger

Minor (May Be Present)

Uses home remedies (self-treatment) to relieve symptoms
Does not admit fear of death or invalidism*
Minimizes symptoms*
Displaces the source of symptoms to other areas of the body
Cannot admit the effects of the disease (substance abuse††) on life pattern
Makes dismissive gestures when speaking of distressing events*
Displaces the fear of effects of the condition
Displays inappropriate affect*

Related Factors

Pathophysiologic

Related to inability to tolerate consciously the consequences (of any chronic or terminal illness) secondary to:

AIDS
Cancer
HIV infection
Progressive debilitating disorders (e.g., multiple sclerosis, myasthenia gravis)

Treatment Related

Related to preferences to continue treatment with no positive results, for example, chemotherapy, radiation

Psychological

Related to inability to tolerate consciously the consequences of:
Loss of a job
Financial crisis
Negative self-concept, inadequacy, guilt, loneliness, despair, sense of failure
Smoking
Loss of spouse/significant other
Obesity
Domestic abuse

---

[12]*Source*: Lynch, C. S., & Phillips, M. W. (1989). Nursing diagnosis: Ineffective denial. In R. M. Carroll-Johnson (Ed.), *Classification of nursing diagnosis: Proceedings of the eighth conference*. Philadelphia, PA: J. B. Lippincott.

Related to inability to tolerate consciously physical and/or emotional dependence on (Halter, 2014; Varcarolis, 2011):

Alcohol
Stimulants
Cannabis
Hallucinogens
Cocaine, crack
Opiates
Barbiturates/sedatives

Related to long-term self-destructive patterns of behavior and lifestyle (Varcarolis, 2011)

Related to feelings of increased anxiety/stress, need to escape personal problems, anger, and frustration

Related to feelings of omnipotence

Related to genetic origins of alcoholism

Author's Note

Ineffective Denial differs from denial in response to loss. Denial in response to illness or loss is necessary and beneficial to maintain psychological equilibrium. *Ineffective Denial* is not beneficial when the person will not participate in regimens to improve health or the situation (e.g., denies substance abuse). If the cause is not known, *Ineffective Denial related to unknown etiology* can be used, such as *Ineffective Denial related to unknown etiology as evidenced by repetitive refusal to admit barbiturate use is a problem.*

Errors in Diagnostic Statements

See *Ineffective Coping.*

Key Concepts

- Denial is a set of dynamic processes that protects the person from threats to self-esteem. It is common in the grieving process.
- When action is essential to change a threatening or damaging situation, denial is maladaptive; however, when no action is needed or when the outcome cannot be changed, denial can be positive and can help reduce stress (*Lazarus, 1985).
- Denial can take several forms:
  - Denial of relevance to the person
  - Denial of immediacy of the threat
  - Denial of responsibility
  - Denial that threat is anxiety-provoking
  - Denial of threatening information
  - Denial of any information

Addictions (Substance, Behavioral)

- Denial is a major response in people with addictions. It is the inability to accept one's loss of control over the addictive behavior or severity of the associated consequences (Boyd, 2012).
- Addiction is defined as a chronic, relapsing brain disease that is characterized by compulsive drug seeking and use, despite harmful consequences (National Institute on Drug Abuse [NIDA], 2010).
- "The initial decision to take drugs is mostly voluntary. However, when drug abuse takes over, a person's ability to exert self-control can become seriously impaired. Brain imaging studies from drug-addicted individuals show physical changes in areas of the brain that are critical to judgment, decision-making, learning and memory, and behavior control" (NIDA, 2010).
- Behavioral addictions activate the release of higher levels of endogenous opioids cortisol, adrenaline, dopamine, glutamate and activate the limbic systems in the reward and pleasure neural pathways, for example, of the brain's limbic system the same as substance do (Grant, 2011).

- Behavioral addictions include pathological gambling, kleptomania, pyromania, compulsive buying, and compulsive sexual behavior (Grant, 2011). Potenza reported neuroimaging studies of impulse control disorders which showed similarities between behavioral and substance addictions, which was indicated by abnormal function (i.e., decreased activation) of the ventromedial prefrontal cortex of the brain, which is located in the frontal lobe and is implicated as a critical component in neuroimaging studies of impulse control disorders suggest similarities between behavioral and substance addictions in processing of risk and decision making (*Potenza, 2006)

Focus Assessment Criteria

See *Ineffective Coping* for general assessment.

Subjective Data

Assess for Defining Characteristics

Denies or minimizes the existence or severity of a problem, for example, health, family
Denies or minimizes that alcohol/drug/gambling use is problematic
Justifies the use of alcohol/drugs
Blames others for the use of alcohol/drugs

Objective Data

Assess for:

Missed appointments
Failure to schedule tests, consults
Reports not taking medication

Assess for effects of substance abuse on:

Work-Related Problems

Absenteeism
Frequent unexplained brief absences
Elaborate excuses
Daytime fatigue
Failed assignments
Loss of job

Social Problems

Mood swings
Arguments with mate/friends
Isolation (avoidance of others)

Legal Difficulties

Traffic accidents/citations
Violence while intoxicated

Physical Effects of Alcohol Abuse

Blackout
Memory impairment
Lower extremity paresthesias
Malnutrition
Pancreatitis
Withdrawal symptoms (e.g., tremors, nausea, vomiting, increased blood pressure and pulse, sleep disturbances, disorientation, hallucinations, agitation, seizures)
Liver dysfunction
Gout symptoms
Anemia
Gastritis/gastric ulcers
Cardiomyopathy

Physical Effects of Opioid Abuse

Drowsiness
Slurred speech
Pupillary constriction
Withdrawal symptoms (e.g., tearing, runny nose, gooseflesh, yawning, dilated pupils, mild hypertension, tachycardia, nausea, vomiting, restlessness, abdominal cramps, joint pain)
Malnutrition
Respiratory depression
Constipation
Respiratory infections
Decreased response to pain
Increased risk for HIV, Hepatitis C cellulitis (skin popping, IV route)

Impaired memory
Slowed motor movements

Physical Effects of Amphetamine and Cocaine Abuse

Hyperactivity
Paranoia
Skin infections
Cerebrovascular accident
Hallucinations
Cardiac dysrhythmias
Seizures
Respiratory depression
Left ventricular hypertrophy
Decreased appetite/weight loss
Increased heart rate
Dilated pupils
Chills
Nausea and vomiting
Hepatitis, HIV, cellulitis (IV route)
Increased alertness

Physical Effects of Hallucinogen Abuse

Increased heart rate
Sweating
Hallucinations
Flashbacks
Tremors
Incoordination
Blurred vision

Physical Effects of Cannabis Abuse

Dry mouth
Increased heart rate
Conjunctival infection
Increased appetite
Impaired lung structure
Sinusitis

Physical Effects of Barbiturate/Sedative—Hypnotic Abuse

Drowsiness
Impaired memory
Cellulitis (IV route)
Hepatitis, HIV (IV route)
Endocarditis
Pneumonia
Respiratory depression
Signs of intoxication and withdrawal

Goals

NOC

Acceptance: Health Status, Anxiety Self-Control, Fear Self-Control, Health Beliefs: Perceived Threat

The individual will use alternative coping mechanism in response to stressor instead of denial as evidenced by the following indicators:

- Acknowledges the source of anxiety or stress
- Uses problem-focused coping skills

Interventions

NIC

Teaching: Disease Process, Anxiety Reduction, Counseling, Active Listening

Initiate a Therapeutic Relationship

- Assess effectiveness of denial.
- Avoid confronting the individual that he or she is using denial.
- Approach the individual directly, matter-of-factly, and nonjudgmentally.

R: *Denial may be valuable in the early stages of coping, when resources are insufficient to manage more problem-focused approaches (*Lazarus, 1985).*

Encourage the Individual to Share Perceptions of the Situation (e.g., Fears, Anxieties)

- Focus on the feelings shared.
- Use reflection to encourage more sharing.

R: *As denial is reduced, interventions must focus on emerging strong feelings of anxiety and fear.*

When Appropriate, Help the Individual with Problem-Solving

- Attempt to elicit from the individual a description of the problem.

R: *Partial, tentative, or minimal denial allows the individual to use problem-focused coping skills while reducing distress (an emotion-focused coping skill) (*Lazarus, 1985).*

Ineffective Denial • Related to Impaired Ability to Accept Consequences of Own Behavior as Evidenced by Lack of Acknowledgment of an Addiction (Substance Abuse/Dependency: Pathological Gambling, Kleptomania, Pyromania, Compulsive Buying, Compulsive Sexual Behavior)

Goals

NOC

Anxiety Self-Control, Coping, Social Support, Addiction Consequences, Knowledge: Substance Use Control, Knowledge: Disease Process

The individual will maintain abstinence from alcohol/drug use and state recognition of the need for continued treatment as evidenced by the following indicators:

- Acknowledges an addiction problem and responsibility for own behavior
  - Identifies three areas of one's life that drugs have negatively affected*
  - Acknowledges when using denial rationalization and projection in relation to their addiction
  - Participates in a support group at least three times a week by (specify)*
  - Agrees to contact a support person when feeling the need to abuse*
- Abstain from substance or behavior addiction.
- State recognition of the need for continued treatment.
- Express a sense of hope.
- Identify three alternative strategies to cope with stressors.*
- Have a plan for high-risk situations for relapse (Halter, 2014; Varcarolis, 2011).

Interventions

NIC

Coping Enhancement, Anxiety Reduction, Counseling, Mutual Goal Setting, Substance Use Treatment, Support System Enhancement, Support Group

Assist the Individual in Understanding Addiction

- Be nonjudgmental. Explain addiction is a disorder with choices.

R: *Historically, individuals with addictions have been viewed as immoral and degenerate. Acknowledgment of their addiction as a disorder can increase the individual's sense of trust.*

- Assist the individual to gain an intellectual understanding that this is an illness, not a moral problem.
- Explain that addiction "does not cure itself" and that it requires abstinence and treatment of the underlying issues (Halter, 2014; Varcarolis, 2011).
- Have the individual identify triggers for their addiction. Discuss how to avoid.
- Provide opportunities to perform successfully; gradually increase responsibility.
- Provide educational information about the progressive nature of substance abuse and its effects on the body and interpersonal relationships.
- Refer to *Disturbed Self-Esteem* for further interventions.

R: *The individual most likely has been reprimanded by many and is distrustful.*

Provide Interventions Appropriate With the Phase of Addictive Behavior Change (*Prochasaska, DiClemente, & Norcross, 1982)

Precontemplation Phase (Unaware of Problems Related to Addictive Behaviors)

- Attempt to raise awareness of the problem and its consequences (e.g., relationships, job, finances).
- Discuss the possibility of change.
- Explore feelings about making changes.

R: *If the person does not think the behavior change is important to improved health, he or she is unlikely to initiate the change (*Bodenheimer, MacGregor, & Shariffi, 2005).*

Contemplation Phase (Aware of Addiction-Related Problems and Considering Change, But Ambivalent)

- Allow the individual to express past successful attempts.
- List the advantages and disadvantages for changing and continuing to use.

R: *If the importance and/or the confidence are low, an action plan with specific behavior changes would not reflect true collaboration.*

Preparation Phase (Intending to Take Action Within the Next Month or Unsuccessful in the Past Year)

- Initiate referrals to the next most acceptable, appropriate, and effective resource for the individual.
- Assist the individual in making a specific, detailed plan for change and identify barriers.

R: *The person's level of confidence will increase with success. Goals that are not easily achievable set the individual up for failure (*Bodenheimer et al., 2005).*

Action Phase (Overtly Involved in Behavioral Changes for at Least One Day)

- Reaffirm the decision to change.
- Emphasize successful actions.
- Help the individual anticipate and prepare for situations that may challenge decisions.

R: *The person's level of confidence will increase with success. Goals that are not easily achievable set the person up for failure (*Bodenheimer et al., 2005).*

Maintenance Phase (Free of Addictive Behavior for More Than 6 Months)

- Help the individual identify strategies to prevent relapse.
- Review reasons why change was made.
- Review the benefits gained from change.

R: *Compliance is increased with targeted interventions depending on the level of motivation present.*

Openly Discuss the Reality of Relapse; Emphasize That Relapse Does Not Mean Failure

- After the relapse, help to identify triggers.
- Plan an alternative action if triggers are present (e.g., call sponsor, take a walk).
- Encourage discussions of relapse with others recovering from similar addictions.
- Emphasize a "one day at a time" philosophy.

R: *Relapse must be addressed to increase motivation and to reduce abandoning all attempts to change behavior.*

Assist the Individual to Identify and Alter Patterns of Substance Abuse

- Explore situations in which the individual is expected to use a substance (e.g., after work with friends).
- Encourage avoidance of situations in which alcohol/drugs are being used.
- Assist in replacing drinking/smoking buddies with nonusers. (Alcoholics Anonymous and Narcotics Anonymous (AA/NA) are helpful. Each AA/NA group is unique; encourage the individual to find a comfortable group for him or her.)
- Assist the individual in organizing and adhering to a daily routine.
- Have the individual chart (amount, time, situation) alcohol/drug use (useful with early stage substance abusers resistant to treatment).

R: *Alcohol and drug abuse is reinforced by the drug itself (e.g., feelings of being high, increased congeniality, gaining attention) or avoiding unpleasant situations. Treatment approaches must aim at removing identified reinforcers (Halter, 2014).*

Discuss Alternative Coping Strategies

- Teach relaxation techniques and meditation. Encourage use when the individual recognizes anxiety.
- Teach thought-stopping techniques to use during thoughts about drinking/substance/gambling use. Instruct to say vocally or subvocally, "STOP, STOP," and to replace that thought with a positive one. The individual must practice the technique and may need assistance in identifying replacements.
- Assist to anticipate stressful events (e.g., job, family, social situations) in which alcohol/drug use/gambling is expected; role-play alternative strategies and teach assertiveness skills.
- Teach how to handle anger constructively.

R: *An addictive person sees engaging in their addiction as a solution to every problem. He or she needs new problem-solving techniques (*Smith-DiJulio, 2009).*

Assist the Individual in Achieving Abstinence from their Addiction

- Assist to set short-term goals (e.g., stopping one day at a time).
- Assist in structured planning:
  - Discard supplies.

- Break contact with dealers/users.
- Avoid high-risk places.
- Structure free time.
- Avoid large blocks of time without activities.
- Plan leisure activities not associated with alcohol/drug use.

- Assist the individual in recognizing stressors that lead to substance abuse (e.g., boredom, interpersonal situations).
- Assist the individual in evaluating the negative consequences of the behavior. Visualization may be helpful.
- When the individual denies alcohol/drug use, look for nonverbal clues to substantiate facts (e.g., deteriorating appearance, job performance, social skills).
- After you have established a trusting relationship, confront the individual's denial.
- Discourage the individual from trying to correct other problems (e.g., obesity, smoking) during this time.
- Do not attempt to probe past history in early abstinence.

R: *The purpose of the interventions is to assist the individual in recognizing and affirming the negative relationship between denial and resulting adverse consequences (health or social) (*Smith-DiJulio, 2009).*

Initiate Health Teaching and Referral, as Indicated

- "Expect sobriety. Reinforce for individuals to view their commitment to one day at a time" (Halter, 2014; Varcarolis, 2011).

R: *Individuals may be overwhelmed thinking they can never drink, use that drug or gamble again (Halter, 2014; Varcarolis, 2011).*

- Advise the individual to consult with primary care provider regarding pharmaceutical treatment if indicated. For example, opioid antagonists, (naltrexone, nalmefene), selective serotonin reuptake inhibitors (SSRIs).

R: *Opioid antagonists, such as naltrexone and nalmefene, which decrease dopamine release in the brain, have been found to reduce reward sensitivity and therefore may be effective in battling the urges that pathological gamblers experience neurotransmitter glutamate have also been effective in reducing gambling behavior in pathological gamblers. SSRIs, most commonly referred to antidepressants, have shown mixed results in impulse control disorders (SSRIs).*

- Refer to AA, Alanon, AlaTeen, or Gamblers Anonymous
- Refer for therapy and/or treatment facility.

R: *In controlled studies, several therapist-driven techniques such as cognitive-behavioral therapy, motivational interviewing and relapse prevention have demonstrated efficacy with substance and behavioral addictions (Grant, 2011),*

- Reinforce healthy living choices, for example, balanced diet, exercise, recreation, rest.

R: *Individuals who abuse drugs and/or alcohol do not engage in healthy lifestyles.*

Explain the Probability of Genetic Predisposition the Addiction and the Importance of Prevention

- Encourage a discussion of addictions, substances and behavioral with family.
- Monitor for early signs in children, for example, impulsivity, unable to delay gratification.
- Seek out appropriate assistance. Primary care provider, pediatrician, support groups.

R: *Family studies have reported that pathological gamblers have increased rates of first degree relatives—parents, children or siblings—with substance use disorders, suggesting a possible shared genetic vulnerability between pathological gambling and other addictions (Grant, 2011; *Shah et al., 2004).*

Labile Emotional Control

NANDA-I Definition

Uncontrollable outbursts of exaggerated and involuntary emotional expression.

Defining Characteristics

Absence of eye contact
Difficulty in use of facial expressions
Embarrassment regarding emotional expression
Excessive crying without feeling sadness
Excessive laughing without feeling happiness
Expression of emotional incongruent with triggering factor
Involuntary crying
Involuntary laughing
Tearfulness
Uncontrollable crying
Uncontrollable laughing
Withdrawal from occupational situation
Withdrawal from social situation
Mood swings[13]
Angry outbursts[13]
Behavior outbursts, threats, throwing objects[13]

Related Factors

Alternation in self-esteem
Brain injury,[13] for example, traumatic, stroke, tumors
Emotional disturbance
Fatigue
Functional impairment
Insufficient knowledge about symptom control
Insufficient knowledge of disease
Insufficient muscle strength
Mood disorder
Musculoskeletal impairment
Pharmaceutical agent
Physical disability
Psychiatric disorder
Social distress
Stressors
Substance abuse
Neurological Disorders, for example, Parkinson's disease, amyotrophic lateral sclerosis, extrapyramidal and cerebellar disorders, multiple sclerosis, Alzheimer's disease[13]

Author's Note

Labile Emotional Control as approved by NANDA-I represents two different responses, with two distinct origins. One is represented in a neurological disorder (affect [PBA]) "of emotional expression characterized clinically by frequent, involuntary, and uncontrollable outbursts of laughing and/or crying that are incongruous with or disproportionate to the patient's emotional state" (Ahmed & Simmons, 2013).

The other is "**emotional dysregulation,** a term used in the mental health community referring to an emotional response that is poorly modulated, and does not fall within the conventionally accepted range of emotive response. ED may be referred to as **labile mood** (marked fluctuation of mood) or **mood swings**" (Beauchaine, Gatzke-Kopp, & Mead, 2007).

Labile emotional responses that are mood swings, disrupt relationships. Smoking, self-harm, eating disorders, and addiction have all been associated with emotional dysregulation. A functional health assessment would be indicated to validate how these mood swings are negatively affecting the individual/family lives. Thus labile emotions would then be related factors or sign/symptoms of a nursing diagnosis. For example, *Risk for Violence*, *Disabled Family Coping*, *Fear*.

Labile Emotional Control as defined as "uncontrollable outbursts of exaggerated and involuntary emotional expression" would represent involuntary crying and/or laughing related to neurological etiology.

---

[13]Added by Lynda Juall Carpenito for clarity and usefulness

Key Concepts

- Estimated prevalence rates of pseudobulbar affect (PBA) in neurological disorders vary considerably, with one review showing rates ranging from 2% to 49% in amyotrophic lateral sclerosis and from 7% to as high as 95% in multiple sclerosis (Olney, Goodkind, & Lomen-Hoerth, 2011).
- PBA occurs secondary to multiple neurological diseases or injury, including stroke, amyotrophic lateral sclerosis (ALS), multiple sclerosis (MS), traumatic brain injury (TBI), Alzheimer's disease (AD), and Parkinson's disease (PD), among others (Olney et al., 2011).
- "The pathological laughing and crying is a disorder of voluntary emotion regulation rather than a state of generalized emotional hyperactivity" (Olney et al., 2011).
- PBA is associated with considerable burden incremental to that of the underlying neurological conditions, affecting QOL, QOR, health status, and social and occupational functioning (Colamonico, Formella, & Bradley, 2012).
- "Following brain injury an individual may also lose emotional awareness and sensitivity to their own and other's emotions, and therefore their capacity to control their emotional behaviour may also be reduced. They may overreact to people or events around them – conversations about particular topics, sad or funny movies or stories. Weaker emotional control and lower frustration tolerance, particularly with fatigue and stress can also result in more extreme changes in emotional responses" (Colamonico et al., 2012).
- Emotional reactions may be appropriate in the situation, but the behavior or expression may be (Colamonico et al., 2012).

Focus Assessment Criteria

Assess emotional responses of laughing and/or crying:

Appropriate for situation, voluntary
Frequency
Involuntary, and uncontrollable outbursts of laughing and/or crying
Disproportionate to the person's emotional state or the situation, for example, stronger, louder or last longer than would be usual for that person.

Assess for associated neurological diseases or injury:

Stroke, amyotrophic lateral sclerosis (ALS), multiple sclerosis (MS), traumatic brain injury (TBI), Alzheimer's disease (AD), and Parkinson's disease (PD)

Assess for associated psychiatric disorders:

Borderline Personality Disorder
ADHD
Bipolar disorder
Complex post-traumatic stress disorder

Goals

NOC
Coping: Self-Esteem, Knowledge: Stress Management

The person will report improved satisfaction with the response of others to their behavior as evidence by the following indicators:

- Describes responses of others as respectful
- Reports privacy is maintained

Interventions

NIC
Family Integrity Promotion, Coping Enhancement, Emotional Support, Caregiver Support

Explain the Cause of Labile Emotions

- The frontal lobe of our brain normally keeps our emotions under control. The cerebellum and brain stem are where our reflexes are mediated. In PBA, there is a disconnect between the frontal lobe of the brain and the cerebellum and brain stem.
- The response is often a normal reaction in standard contexts but is combined with evidence of impaired ability to regulate an excessive or prolonged emotional response. For example, laughs at a joke (Wilson, 1924; Wortzel et al., 2008).

R: *"Contrary to many clinical descriptions, episodes were often induced by contextually appropriate stimuli and associated with strong experiences of emotion that were consistent with the display" (Olney et al., 2011).*

Explain the possibility that Emotional Lability is Often Worse Soon After the Stroke Happens, but Usually Lessens or Goes Away With Time as the Person Recovers (Olney, et al., 2011)

R: *This is valid and may be helpful with the initial shock.*

Gently Explain the Effects on Home Life, Work, and Relationships

R: *The psychological consequences and the impact on social interactions may be substantial (Ahmed & Simmons, 2013). It may have socially and occupationally disabling consequences, which are superimposed on the burden of the primary neurological disorder (Olney et al., 2011)*

If Appropriate, Ask the Person Affected How They Would Like to be Treated When They Have an Episode of Crying

R: *This may provide insight into the person's experience*

- Observe for triggers (Acquired Brain Injury Outreach Service, 2011):
  - Fatigue
  - Increased stress
  - Excessive stimuli, for example, loud music, multiple conversations
  - Discussions of sensitive topics, for example, finances, work, speaking in a group.

Provide Rest Period Before an Activity, for Example, Physical Therapy, Mealtime, Visiting Time

R: *This may help the person adapt with the stress of the activity.*

In Response to Uncontrolled Crying or Laughing, It May be Helpful to (Acquired Brain Injury Outreach Service, 2011)

- Try and change the subject.
- Redirect the person to a different activity. For example, short walk.
- Instruct to take deep breaths.
- Avoid telling the person to control themselves.
- Be matter of fact.
- Touch their arm if appropriate.
- Ask if they want you to stay or leave.

R: *Interventions that communicate empathy and do not emphasize the emotional outburst can be comforting and reduce embarrassment.*

Provide Information and Education to Those Who Witness the Uncontrolled Outburst, Advise Them Not to Laugh

R: *The uncontrolled crying or laughing can be disturbing to others if they do not understand*

Explain the Benefits of

- Relaxation and breathing exercises to reduce tension and stress
- Using distractions—thinking of something else, imagining a peaceful image or picture, counting
- Doing an activity (going for a walk)
- Cognitive and behavioral strategies such as thought-stopping
- Counseling and support, for example, individual, family

R: *There are many sudden losses and changes with after a brain injury—loss of work, ability to drive, independence, changes in relationships or finances, changes in the quality of their life. There are feelings of sadness, grief, anger, frustration, disappointment, jealousy, or depression (Olney et al., 2011)*

Discuss the Possible Use of Medications for Labile Emotions With Their Primary Prescriber (Colamonico et al., 2012)

- Tricyclic antidepressants and selective serotonin reuptake inhibitors
- Dextromethorphan/quinidine combination (Nuedexta)

R: *A labile emotional response is caused by a disinhibition syndrome in which pathways involving serotonin and glutamate are disrupted. Dextromethorphan/quinidine combination has been FDA approved in 2011 also for treatment (Colamonico et al., 2012).*

Initiate Health Teaching and Referral as Needed

- Advise to pursue strategies to reduce stress, for example, exercise, relaxation breathing.
- Refer to community agencies if indicated, for example, home health care, social services.

Impaired Mood Regulation

Definition

A mental state characterized by shifts in mood or affect and which is comprised of a constellation of affective, cognitive, somatic, and/or psychological manifestations varying from mild to severe.

Defining Characteristics

Changes in verbal behavior
Disinhibition
Dysphoria
Excessive guilt
Excessive self-awareness
Excessive self-blame
Flight of thoughts
Hopelessness
Impaired concentration
Influenced self-esteem
Irritability
Psychomotor agitation
Psychomotor retardation
Sad effect
Withdrawal

Related Factors

Alteration in sleep pattern
Anxiety
Appetite change
Chronic illness
Functional impairment
Hypervigilance
Impaired social functioning
Loneliness
Pain
Psychosis
Recurrent thoughts of death
Recurrent thoughts of suicide
Social isolation
Substance misuse
Weight change

Author's Notes

The top five mental illness listed as the primary diagnosis for hospitalization are mood disorders, substance-related disorders, delirium/dementia, anxiety disorders, and schizophrenia (Halter, 2014). Mood disorders include bipolar disorders and major depressive disorders (APA, 2010). *Impaired Mood Regulation* as approved by NANDA-I above represents manifestations of individuals with bipolar or major depressive disorders. Some of related factors represent signs and symptoms of mood disorders, for example, alteration in sleep pattern, appetite changes, hypervigilance: some are individual's responses to *Impaired Mood Regulation* as social isolation, weight change, loneliness substance abuse, recurrent thoughts of death, recurrent thoughts of suicide, impaired social functioning, anxiety. The principle treatment for bipolar or major depressive disorders are medications, which can stabilize the individual's mood fluctuations.

Impaired Mood Regulation is not the focus of nursing interventions. Using a Functional Health Assessment, the nurse, the individual, and family will determine which patterns are disrupted by the individual's mood disorder. Some related nursing diagnoses are *Risk for Self-Harm, Insomnia, Ineffective Coping, Compromised Family Coping,* and *Defensive Coping Impaired Social Interactions, Risk for Violence to Others,* and *Ineffective Denial.* Refer to the specific nursing diagnoses throughout this book.

DECISIONAL CONFLICT

Decisional Conflict

Impaired Emancipated Decision Making
Risk for Emancipated Decision Making
Readiness for Emancipated Decision Making

NANDA-I Definition

Uncertainty about course of action to be taken when choice among competing actions involves risk, loss, or challenge to values and beliefs

Defining Characteristics*

Verbalized uncertainty about choices
Verbalizes undesired consequences of alternatives being considered
Vacillation among alternative choices
Delayed decision making
Self-focusing
Verbalizes feeling of distress while attempting a decision
Physical signs of distress or tension (e.g., increased heart rate, increased muscle tension, restlessness)
Questioning of personal values and/or beliefs while attempting to make a decision
Questioning moral values while attempting a decision
Questioning moral rules while attempting a decision
Questioning moral principles while attempting a decision

Related Factors

Many situations can contribute to decisional conflict, particularly those that involve complex medical interventions of great risk. Any decisional situation can precipitate conflict for an individual; thus, the examples listed below are not exhaustive, but reflect situations that may be problematic and possess factors that increase the difficulty.

Treatment Related

Related to lack of relevant information

Related to risks versus the benefits of (specify test, treatment):

Surgery

Tumor removal
Cosmetic surgery
Amputation
Transplant
Orchiectomy
Prostatectomy
Hysterectomy
Laminectomy
Mastectomy
Joint replacement
Cataract removal
Cesarean section

Diagnostics

Amniocentesis
Magnetic Resonance Assay

Treatments

Chemotherapy
Radiation

Dialysis
Mechanical ventilation
Enteral feedings
Intravenous hydration
Use of preterm labor medications
Participation in treatment study trials
HIV antiviral therapy

Situational (Personal, Environmental)

Related to perceived threat to value system

Related to risks versus the benefits of:

Personal

Marriage
Breast versus bottle feeding
Parenthood
Circumcision
Divorce
Abortion
Institutionalization (child, parent)
Contraception
Nursing home placement
Sterilization
In vitro fertilization
Transport from rural facilities
Artificial insemination
Adoption
Foster home placement
Separation

Work/Task

Career change
Professional ethics
Business investments
Relocation

Related to:

Lack of relevant information*
Confusing information

Related to:

Disagreement within support systems
Inexperience with decision making
Unclear personal values/beliefs[a]
Conflict with personal values/beliefs
Family history of poor prognosis
Hospital paternalism—loss of control
Ethical or moral dilemmas of:

- Quality of life, Palliative Care
- Cessation of life-support systems
- "Do not resuscitate" orders
- Termination of pregnancy
- Organ transplant
- Selective termination with multiple-gestation pregnancies

Maturational

Related to risks versus benefits of:

Adolescent

Peer pressure
Alcohol/drug use
Career choice
Use of birth control

Adult

College
Whether to continue a relationship
Career change
Relocation
Retirement
Sexual activity
Illegal/dangerous situations

Older adult

Retirement
Relocation
Out of home (relative's home, assisted living, skilled care)

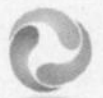

Author's Note

The nurse has an important role in assisting individuals and families with making decisions. Because nurses usually do not benefit financially from decisions made regarding treatments and transfers, they are in an ideal position to assist with decisions. Although, according to Danis et al. (*1991), "Nursing or medical expertise does not enable health care professionals to know the values of individuals or what individuals think is best for themselves," nursing expertise enables nurses to facilitate systematic decision making that considers all possible alternatives and possible outcomes, as well as individual beliefs and values. The focus is on assisting with logical decision making, not on promoting a certain decision.

When people are making a treatment decision of considerable risk, they do not necessarily experience conflict. In situations where the treatment option is "choosing life," individual perception may be one of submitting to fate and be relatively unconflicted. Because of this, nurses must be cautious in labeling patients with the nursing diagnosis of "Decisional Conflict" without sufficient validating cues (*Soholt, 1990).

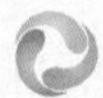

Errors in Diagnostic Statements

***Decisional Conflict* related to failure of physician to gain permission for mechanical ventilation from family**

In such a situation, this statement represents an unprofessional and legally problematic approach. Failure of the physician to gain permission for mechanical ventilation would be a practice dilemma necessitating formal reporting to the appropriate parties. Should the family have evidence that the individual did not desire this treatment (i.e., a living will), this situation would not be described as *Decisional Conflict*, because there is certainty about a course of action. The nurse should further assess the family for responses fitting other nursing diagnoses, such as *Grieving*.

***Decisional Conflict* related to uncertainty about choices**

Uncertainty about choices validates *Decisional Conflict;* it is not a causative or contributing factor. If the individual needed more information, the diagnosis would be *Decisional Conflict related to insufficient knowledge about choices and effects*.

Key Concepts

General Considerations

- "Nurses' judgments and decisions have the potential to help healthcare systems allocate resources efficiently, promote health gain and patient benefit and prevent harm." (Thompson, Aitken, Doran, & Dowding, 2013, p. 1721)
- The logical steps of decision making are well identified in clinical practice. They can be summarized in the following steps:
  - Define the problem.
  - List the possible alternatives or options.
  - Identify the probable outcomes of the various alternatives.
  - Evaluate the alternatives based on actual or potential threats to beliefs/values.
  - Make a decision.
- Policy makers perceive SDM as desirable because of its potential to (Légaré et al., 2010):
  - Reduce overuse of options not clearly associated with benefits for all (e.g., prostate cancer screening);
  - Enhance the use of options clearly associated with benefits for the vast majority (e.g., cardiovascular risk factor management);
  - Reduce unwarranted health-care practice variations;
  - Foster the sustainability of the health-care system;
  - Promote the right of individual to be involved in decisions concerning their health. Despite this potential, SDM has not yet been widely adopted in clinical practice.
- An National health service (NHS) patient survey found 48% of inpatients and 30% of outpatients want to be more involved in decisions about their care (NHS, 2010).
- Soholt (*1990) identified that the following factors may influence an individual when making a health-care treatment decision:
  - Reliance on the truth of medical advice
  - Submission to fate when the treatment option is "choosing life"
  - Consideration of values

- The decision-making process is complicated when there is a need for a rapid decision. Making an informed decision during acute stress is difficult, if not impossible. The stress can be enormous if a sense of urgency compounds the decision.
- Jezewski (*1993) reported that both intrapersonal and interpersonal conflicts occur when do-not-resuscitate decisions are being made. Intrapersonal conflict results from discord with individual values and life events. The most common interpersonal conflict arises between staff and family members, and among family members.
- The most important right that an individual possesses is the right of self-determination, or the right to make the ultimate decision concerning what will or will not be done to his or her body.
- Not all individuals desire the same degree of control over treatment decision making. The need to play an active, collaborative, or passive role is very individualized and must be assessed carefully.
- Perception of the effect of a treatment on an individual's life may be more important in his or her decision than considerations of the medical effectiveness.
- Value conflicts often lead to confusion, indecision, and inconsistency. Decision making is more complicated when an individual's goals conflict with those of significant others. People may decide against their values if the need to please others is greater than the need to please themselves.
- One study found that older adults' end-of-life decisions were strongly related to their religiosity and values regarding preservation of life and quality of life (*Cicirelli, MacLean, & Cox, 2000). Those who preferred "to hasten death were less religious and placed a higher value on quality of life" (*Cicirelli & MacLean, 2000). Most of the study group favored hastening death if terminally ill, regardless of religious beliefs (*Cicirelli & MacLean, 2000).

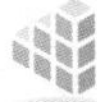

Pediatric Considerations

- In most cases, children do not make major decisions for themselves. A parent (or surrogate) must make the decision on the child's behalf.
- A child's ability to understand a situation and make a decision depends on age, developmental level, and past experience. Understanding, however, should not be confused with legal competence.
- As adolescents mature, their ability to analyze problems and make decisions increases.
- Researchers working with children should seek assent from children with a mental age of 7 years or older. Parents must give written, informed consent for the child to participate in the study (Hockenberry & Wilson, 2015).

Geriatric Considerations

- Decisions are often made for, not with, older adults.
- Barriers to decision making for older adults include dementia, depression, long-term passivity, and hearing or other communication problems (Miller, 2015).
- Reasons why decision makers exclude older adults from involvement in decisions that profoundly affect their lives include the desire to avoid discussion of sensitive topics (e.g., finances, relocation) and beliefs that older adults are incompetent, not qualified, or not interested (Miller, 2015).
- Family members making a decision to place an older family member in a long-term facility found information from health-care professionals inadequate. Friends who validated the situation were most helpful.

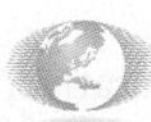

Transcultural Considerations

- Fatalism is a belief that little can be done to change life events and the best response is submission and acceptance. Americans of Latin, Irish, Appalachian, Filipino, Puerto Rican, and Russian Orthodox origins often believe in this external focus of control (Giger, 2013).
- Northern European and African Americans have been found to have both internal and external foci of control (Giger, 2012).

Focus Assessment Criteria

Decisional conflict is a subjective state that the nurse must validate with the individual. The nurse should assess each individual to determine his or her level of decision making within the conflict situation. Some of the same cues may be seen in people with *Hopelessness*, *Powerlessness*, and *Spiritual Distress*.

Decision-Making Patterns
"Tell me about the decision you need to make."
"How would you describe your usual method of making decisions?"
"How involved would you like to be in making the decision?"

Perception of the Conflict
"How do you feel when you think about the decision you have to make?"
"Has there been a change in your sleep patterns, appetite, or activity level?"

Assess for Related Factors

"Why is this a stressful decision for you?"
"What things make you uncomfortable about deciding?"
"In the past, how did you arrive at decisions that had a positive outcome?"
"What decisions have you made that you felt confident about?"
"When you make a decision, do you do it alone or do you like to involve other people? If so, whom do you consult for advice?"

Goals

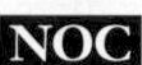

NOC
Decision-Making, Information Processing, Participation: Health Care Decisions

The individual/group will make an informed choice as evidenced by the following indicators:

- Relates the advantages and disadvantages of choices
- Shares fears and concerns regarding choices and responses of others
- Defines what would be most helpful to support the decision-making process

Interventions

Carp's Cues

Andrew Lansley wrote, "No decision about me without me" (Department of Health, 2010), which emphasizes that shared decision making (SDM) must be the norm rather than the exception (Lilley et al., 2010).

NIC
Decision-Making Support, Mutual Goal Setting, Learning Facilitation, Health System Guidance, Anticipatory Guidance, Patient Right Protection, Values Clarification, Anxiety Reduction

Assess Causative/Contributing Factors
Refer to Related Factors.

Address each element to ensure SDM (Lilley et al., 2010)

- Clarify the decision to be made.
- Explore what is important to the individual.
- Clarify options available.
- Communicate risks and benefits of the treatment options.

R: *With informed choice, individual make their own decisions and professionals act as sources of expert clinical information, but with no further active role in decision-making (Lilley et al., 2010).*

Clarify the Decision to be Made

- Encourage significant others to be involved in the entire decision-making process.
- Suggest the individual use significant others as a sounding board when considering alternatives.
- Respect and support the role that the individual desires in the decision, whether it is active, collaborative, or passive.
- Facilitate refocusing on the needed decision when the individual experiences fragmented thinking during high anxiety.
- Encourage the individual to take time in deciding.
- With adolescents, focus on the present—what will happen versus what will not. Help identify the important things because they do not have extensive past experiences on which to base decisions.

R: *People who are strongly self-directed and have taken past responsibility for health practice are more likely to assume an active role in decision making.*

Explore What is Important to the Individual (Lilley et al., 2010)

- Use values clarification techniques to assist the individual in reviewing the parts of his or her life that reflect his or her beliefs.

- Help the individual to identify his or her most prized and cherished activities.
- Ask reflective statements that lead to further clarification.
- Review past decisions in which the individual needed to publicly affirm opinions and beliefs.
- Evaluate the positions the individual has taken on controversial subjects. Does he or she view them in black-and-white terms, or various shades of gray?
- Identify the values the individual is proud of. Rank them in order of importance.

R: *Every decision is based on consciously or unconsciously held beliefs, attitudes, and values. Determining out what matters to individuals/families allows health professionals to explore how this may affect the decisions they make (Lilley et al., 2011).*

- Decisional conflict is greater when none of the alternatives is good. Assist the individual in exploring personal values and relationships that may affect the decision. Explore obtaining a referral with the individual's spiritual leader.

R: *People are the experts about their life goals and values; therefore, health-care professionals need to use a participatory decision-making model.*

- Support the decision—even if the decision conflicts with your own values.

R: *Difficult decisions create stress and conflict because values and actions are not congruent. Conflict may lead to fear and anxiety that negatively affect decision making. External resources become very important for the individual in decisional conflict with a low level of self-confidence in making autonomous decisions.*

Fear of Outcome/Response of Others

- Provide clarification regarding potential outcomes and correct misconceptions.
- Explore with the individual what the risks of not deciding would be.
- Encourage expression of feelings.
- Promote self-worth.
- Encourage the individual to face fears.
- Encourage the individual to share fears with significant others.
- Actively reassure the individual that the decision is his or hers to make and that he or she has the right to do so.
- Assist the individual in recognizing that it is his or her life; if he or she is comfortable with the decision, others should respect the conviction.

R: *The roles of individual values greatly influence the resolution of ethical decision-making dilemmas. Decisional conflict becomes more intense when it involves a threat to status and self-esteem.*

Clarify Options Available in Accordance With Individual Values

Communicate Risks and Benefits of the Treatment options

- Provide information comprehensively and sensitively.
- Correct misinformation.
- Give concise information that covers the major points when the decision must be made quickly.
- Enable the individual to determine the amount of information that he or she desires.
- Encourage verbalization to determine the individual's perception of choices.
- Ensure that the individual clearly understands what is involved in the decision and the various alternatives (i.e., informed choice).

R: *Information that is valid, relevant, and understandable is required for informed decisions (Lilley et al., 2010).*

- Encourage the individual to seek second professional opinions regarding health.

R: *Mastering content for effective decision making requires time. Time allows an individual to choose the option that provides the most benefit with the least risk.*

Controversy With Support System

- Reassure the individual that he or she does not have to give in to pressure from others, whether family, friends, or health professionals.
- Advocate for the individual's wishes if others attempt to undermine his or her ability to make the decision personally or are excluding him or her from decision making.
- Identify leaders within the support system and provide information.

R: *Sims, Boland, and O'Neill (*1992) interviewed families involved in caregiving and concluded that the process by which an individual "frames" a problem is key to understanding decision making. Values, feelings, and previous experiences significantly influenced caregivers' decision making.*

Impaired Emancipated Decision Making

NANDA-I Definition

A process of choosing a health-care decision that does not include personal knowledge and/or considerations of social norms, or does not occur in a flexible environment, resulting is decisional dissatisfaction.

Defining Characteristics

Verbalizes excessively fearing what others will think of the decision
Verbalizes feeling constraint in describing own opinion
Expresses inability in choosing the health-care option that best fits current lifestyle
Verbalizes not being able to describe how the option will fit in current lifestyle
Verbalizes being overly concerned about what everyone else thinks is best
Shows signs of distress when listening to other's opinions
Delays enactment of the chosen health-care option
Limits verbalization about health-care options in the presence of others

Related Factors

Impaired emancipated decision making in women's health care occurs because the traditional health-care structure in most societies has been built on patriarchal–hierarchical values systems that deem empirical findings as the best for all. When making health-care decision women must consider many variables and a significant factor is her own personal knowledge related to how the health-care option she chooses fits her value system and lifestyle (Scaffidi, Posmontier, Bloch, & Wittmann-Price, 2014).

Treatment Related

Related to barriers to understanding options, limited decision-making experience, and confidence in her ability to make decisions associated with:

Hormone replacement therapy
Lumpectomy versus mastectomy
Chemotherapy versus radiation
Repeat cesarean birth versus vaginal birth after cesarean
Circumcision of male newborn
Family planning method
Fetal genetic testing
Induction of labor
Uterine ablation versus dilation and curettage
Medical or surgical abortion
Medication continuance

Situational (Personal, Environmental)

Related to:

Lack of understanding of all health-care options available*
Inability to adequately verbalize perceptions about health-care options*
Lack of adequate time to discuss health-care options*
Limited decision-making experience*
Lack of privacy and confidence to discuss health-care options openly*
Traditional hierarchical family and health-care systems*

Related to barriers to understanding options and confidence in her ability to make decisions and fears associated with restrictions from her traditional hierarchical family.

Related to barriers to understanding options, fears, and confidence in her ability to make decisions associated with:

Breast or bottle feeding
Conception
Abortion
Abusive relationship
Nursing home placement

Related to barriers to understanding options and confidence in her ability to make decisions associated with work place (specify):

Well-lit building, parking and walking area
Appropriate, private, clean facilities

Maturational

Related to barriers to understanding options and confidence in her or his ability to make decisions and fears associated with restrictions from her traditional hierarchical family

Adolescent
Alcohol/drug use
Birth control
Sexual expression

Adult
Physical activity
Nutritional habits
Sexual expression
Healthy or unhealthy relationships

Older Adult
Nursing home placement

Key Concepts

General Considerations

- An antecedent to making an emancipated decision is recognition that existing oppression exists for many health-care decisions that women make (*Wittmann-Price, 2004).
- Paternalism still exists in the health-care decision-making processes (Goldberg & Shorten, 2014).
- To make an emancipated decision, women need to experience three elements:
  - Being aware of social norms about the options
  - Being able to make the decision in a flexible environment
  - Being able to use her personal knowledge (Whitmann-Price & Price, 2014).
- An emancipated decision is congruent with the current paradigm of SDM (Whitmann-Price & Fisher, 2009).
- Nurses have a distinct role in the SDM process and identified themes in the role include:
  - Knowledge as a basis for SDM
  - Sharing power in the nurse–client relationship
  - Utilization of decisional support strategies
  - Communication (Lewis, Starzomski, & Young, 2014)
- Women are often influenced in their decision-making process by those people they consider as close friends in their lives (Silva, de Jesus, Merighi, Domingos, & Oliveria, 2014).
- Nurses are in a prime position to assist women in the decision-making process but at times are counterproductive because of interprofessional conflicts related to communication and priorities. These nurse–primary care provider conflicts adversely affect individuals' decision-making process (Jacobson, Zlatnik, Kennedy, & Lyndon, 2013).

- Influences of social relationships and power affect women's decision-making processes (Lessa, Tyrrell, Alves, & Rodrigues, 2014).
- Appropriate information needs to be provided to women in order for them to make an informed decision (Hatfield & Pearce, 2014).
- Women who experience severe oppression, intimate partner violence (IPV), still make decisions based on their personal knowledge knowing that oppression exists (James, Taft, Amir, & Agius, 2014).
- Personal knowledge or knowledge about what works for them is a key component of emancipated decision making (*Wittmann-Price, 2006; Wittmann-Price & Bhattacharya, 2008; Wittmann-Price, Fliszar, & Bhattacharya, 2011).
- Personal knowledge is influenced by culture (Harris, 2014).
- Women can overcome oppressive forces by using an emancipated decision-making process (Stepanuk, Fisher, Wittmann-Price, Posmontier, & Bhattacharya, 2013).
- The decisional process for women can be described in the following steps:
  - Identify.
  - Contemplate—during this phase consideration is given to personal knowledge.
  - Resolve.
  - Engage (Hershberger, Finnegan, Pierce, & Scoccia, 2013).
- Women who make emancipated decisions will be more satisfied with their decision (Stepanuk, et al., 2013; *Wittmann-Price, 2006; Wittmann-Price & Bhattacharya, 2008; Wittmann-Price et al. 2011).
- Being satisfied with a decision will increase the likelihood of individuals carrying through with their chosen option (*Clark, O'Connor, Graham, & Wells, 2003).

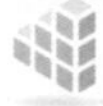

Pediatric Considerations

- Consideration of the ethical issues in pediatric decision making by using ethically-based questions assists parents to clarify the issues and move toward a shared decision (Delany & Galvin, 2014). This approach supports integrating parental personal knowledge into the SDM process.
- Children with complex health issues who require parental decisions in a time of crises are best served by parents and providers move through a decision-making process. Additional studies are needed to better understand what variables parents use to make decisions in crises (Allen, 2014).
- Decisional support tools for pediatric discharge planning are useful to match the parental preferences with the appropriate services for the child (Holland et al., 2014).
- SDM, which involves parents in management decisions about a child's care, supports satisfaction with the decision and treatment adherence leading to better individual outcomes (Rivera-Spoljaric, Halley, & Wilson, 2014).

Geriatric Considerations

- Registered dietitians (RD) assisting families to make decisions for the elderly about feeding tubes includes establishing a relationship, explaining options, and identifying the individuals' needs for family members (Szetok, O'Sullivan, Body, & Parrott, 2014).
- Sensory deficits such as hearing and communication must be considered within the realm of geriatric decision making (Hardin, 2012).
- Oncology treatment decisions for elderly individuals are best done after an evaluation of their personal needs, studies support that in 39% of the time treatment decisions are changed after a thorough evaluation is completed (Hamaker, Schiphorst, Aten Bokkel Huinink, Schaar, & van Munster, 2014).

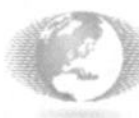

Transcultural Considerations

- Nurses are in a prime position to assess elderly individuals' ability to participate effectively in the decision-making process. Assessing and understanding the decisional ability of the individual can lead to better individual outcomes (Mahon, 2010).
- South Asian families' health-care decision making include issues of language, family values, and faith, all of which need to be considered by nurses working with this population (Brown, Patel, Kaur, & Coad, 2013).
- A large nursing cross-cultural study of inpatient orthopedic nursing units found that decision making was most often based on individualized care as the significant factor throughout seven counties studied (Suhonen et al., 2011).
- This study demonstrated that Muslim women living outside their original country who experience chronic pain benefited when making decisions from elements of a flexible environment which included time, dialogue, honesty, and understanding (Müllersdorf, Zander, & Eriksson, 2011).

Focus Assessment Criteria

Assisting female individuals to arrive at an emancipated decision includes dialogue between the nurse and the individual that specifically addressed the social norms placed on individual options. This will produce awareness of underlying oppressions that are present. In addition, discussion must include the individuals' personal knowledge about herself, what works for her and her lifestyle and what does not. All of the decision-making process must be conducted in a flexible environment that includes open discussion, SDM, and availability of information.

Subjective Data

Assess for Defining Characteristics

"What are you available options?"
"What have you heard about the available options?"
"What types of health-care options have worked for you in the past?"

Assess Perception of Oppression

"What do other people in your life feel that you should do?"
"Do you feel pressured by other people to pick a specific option?"

Assess for Related Factors

"Who do you rely on for assistance with health-care issues?"
"Do you feel as if the person or persons that you identified as being involved in your health-care decisions is/are supportive of your preferences?"
"What are the main concerns about your health-care choices?"
"Do you feel as if you have enough information about the options?"

Objective Data

Assess for Defining Characteristics

Cognitive Cues
Inability to discuss openly with family members or others in the room
Inability to list assets and deficits for each available option

Affective Cues
Choosing words carefully
Remaining noncommittal during the discussion about options

Psychomotor Cues
Continuously glancing or looking at others before answering
Tense facial expression
Glancing at watch or clock

Goals

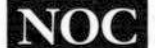

NOC
Coping, Decision-Making, Family Functioning, Capacity of the family system to meet the needs of its members during developmental transitions, Family Integrity

The individual/group will make an informed choice as evidenced by the following indicators:

- Relates the advantages and disadvantages of choices
- Shares fears and concerns regarding choices and responses of others
- Defines what would be most helpful to support the decision-making process

Interventions/Rationale

Assess Causative factors

- Refer to Related Factors.

NIC

Abuse Protection Support, Anticipatory Guidance, Anxiety Reduction, Assertiveness Training, Behavior Modification, Complex Relationship Building, Conflict Mediation, Coping Enhancement, Crisis Intervention, Culture Brokerage, Decision-Making Support, Family Integrity Promotion, Family Support

Reduce or Eliminate Causative or Contributing Factors

- Provide privacy and confidence to discuss health-care options openly to
  - Ensure that the individual has comfortable space to have an in-depth discussion about health-care options.
  - Suggest that all electronics be turned off and the door to the room closed to limit distractions.
  - Ensure that environmental issues (heat and light) are appropriate.
  - Ensure that the conversation will not be interrupted (place sign on the door that states "Conference in Progress").
  - Have nonjudgmental SDM tools available for the individual in order to assist her.
  - Be ready to make an "Advantages/Disadvantages" list for each health-care option.
  - Encourage the individual to reflect on what each decisional outcome will "look like" in relation to her current lifestyle.
  - Assure the individual that she is not pressured to make her final decision at the current time.

R: *Hain and Sandy (2014) found that a component of effective SDM is trust. In order to build trust nurses must demonstrate honesty, respect, and confidentiality so patients are not embarrassed to reveal concerns.*

Initiate the SDM process (Wittmann-Price & Fisher, 2009)

- Knowledge as a basis for SDM
- Review all the options presented to the individual as well as others that are available.
- Discuss specific timelines associated with each option.
- Dialogue about advantages and disadvantages of each option.
- Encourage the individual to verbalize how each option would affect their life and lifestyle.
- Ascertain the focus of the individual's value system (family, longevity, spirituality, peacefulness, etc.).

R: *Légaré and colleagues (2013) have identified two specific competencies to assist individuals in the SDM process and these include relational competencies or establishing a nurse–client relationship that is open and honest, and risk communication competencies or dialoguing about issues that may be difficult.*

R: *Wittmann-Price and Fisher (2009) discuss the utilization of SDM tools that originate at the Ottawa Hospital Research Institute (https://decisionaid.ohri.ca/decguide.html). The tools are interactive and there are tools for almost any health care of social decision that an individual is faced with. If there is not a tool for a specific issue, a generic tool is available.*

- Sharing power in the nurse–client relationship
- Sit with the individual to discuss options when adequate time is available
- Use therapeutic communication skills
- Encourage the individual to reflect
- Do not provide the individual with an opinion
- Refrain from stating "if it was me, I would…"

R: *Carling-Rowland, Black, McDonald, and Kagan (2014) demonstrated that in servicing health professionals about communication increased their effectiveness with vulnerable populations.*

- Utilization of decisional support strategies
- Discuss the relationship of others in individual's decision-making process.
- Ascertain if the individual has been the one making health-care decisions for herself and her family.
- Ask the individual her timeline for arriving at a decision.
- Assess what information the individual has available to her on the issue.
- Provide the individual with SDM tools if needed.

R: *Ernst and colleagues (2013) qualitatively studied individuals with complex care issues and found that individual decision-making participation decreased as the complications of illness increased.*

Effective Communication (Lewis, Starzomski, & Young, 2014)

- Provide time for individual to assimilate information.
- Remain nonjudgmental.
- Clarify information.
- Focus fully on the individual.
- Demonstrate interest.
- Refrain from interrupting.
- Use open-ended sentences or questions.
- Use positive body language.

R: *Boykins (2014) describes communication as a process that includes competencies for nurses. One of the most important competency is to understand one's own communication pattern and how it affects patient-centered care.*

Refer to Other Nursing Diagnoses for Treatment of Problematic Situations and to Provide More Specific Interventions as

- *Risk for or Disabled Family Coping* with clinical data to support or suspect abuse
- *Dysfunctional Family Processes*
- *Powerlessness*

Initiate health teaching and referral as indicated

- Counseling (individual, partner, family)
- Community services (Woman Against Violence, crisis hot line)
- Career planning services

Risk for Emancipated Decision Making

NANDA-I Definition

Vulnerable to a process of choosing a health-care decision that does not include personal knowledge and/or consideration of social norms, or does not occur in a flexible environment resulting in decisional dissatisfaction.

Risk Factors

Refer to Related Factors in *Impaired Emancipated Decision Making.*

Focus Assessment Criteria

Refer to *Impaired Emancipated Decision Making.*

Goals

Refer to *Impaired Emancipated Decision Making.*

Interventions

Refer to *Impaired Emancipated Decision Making.*

Readiness for Emancipated Decision-Making

NANDA-I Definition

Decisional satisfaction that can be strengthened by supporting the process of choosing a health-care decision to include personal knowledge and consideration of social norms in a flexible environment.

Defining Characteristics

Verbalizes there is no over-concern about what everyone else thinks is best
Verbalizes own opinion without constraint
Acknowledges that the chosen health-care option best fits current lifestyle
Describes how the option will fit current lifestyle
Verbalizes there is no over concerned about what everyone else thinks is best
Can listen to other's opinions without showing signs of distress
Does not delay enactment of the chosen health-care option
Does not limit verbalization about health-care options in the presence of others

Verbalizes understanding of all health-care options available
Verbalize perceptions about health-care options
Reports having adequate time to discuss health-care options
Reports having decision-making experience

Key Concepts

An individual is ready to make an emancipated decision making when she recognizes the social norms placed on health-care options and uses her personal knowledge in a flexible environment to arrive at a health-care option.

Focus Assessment Criteria

Refer to *Impaired Emancipated Decision Making.*

Goals

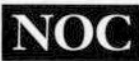

Refer to *Impaired Emancipated Decision Making.*

The individual will report making an emancipated decision about a health-care issue, as evidenced by the following indicators:

- The individual is satisfied with the decision.
- The individual used her personal knowledge to assist her to arrive at the decision.
- The individual was able to arrive at the decision in a flexible environment without oppressive forces from others.
- The option chosen fits in best with the individual's lifestyle.
- The individual is uninhibited when telling others about the option she chose.
- The individual is satisfied with the chosen option.
- The individual carries through with the option that was chosen.

Interventions

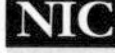

Refer to *Impaired Emancipated Decision-Making.*

Refer to *Impaired Emancipated Decision Making.*

DIARRHEA

NANDA-I Definition

Passage of loose, unformed stools

Defining Characteristics*

At least three loose, liquid stools per day
Urgency
Cramping/abdominal pain
Hyperactive bowel sounds

Related Factors

Pathophysiologic

Related to malabsorption* or inflammation* secondary to:

Colon cancer
Diverticulitis
Celiac disease (sprue)
Gastritis

Irritable bowel
Crohn's disease
Peptic ulcer
Spastic colon
Ulcerative colitis

Related to lactose deficiency, dumping syndrome

Related to increased peristalsis secondary to increased metabolic rate (hyperthyroidism)

Related to infectious processes* secondary to:

Food poisoning
Trichinosis
Typhoid fever
Malaria
Shigellosis
Cholera
Microsporidia
Dysentery
Infectious hepatitis
Cryptosporidium

Related to excessive secretion of fats in stool secondary to liver dysfunction

Related to inflammation and ulceration of gastrointestinal mucosa secondary to high levels of nitrogenous wastes (renal failure)

Treatment Related

Related to malabsorption or inflammation secondary to surgical intervention of the bowel

Related to adverse effects of pharmaceutical agents* of (specify):

Thyroid agents
Analgesics
Stool softeners
Chemotherapy
Antibiotics
Laxatives
Iron sulfate
Antacids
Cimetidine

Related to tube feedings

Situational (Personal, Environmental)

Related to stress or anxiety*

Related to irritating foods (fruits, bran cereals) or increase in caffeine consumption

Related to changes in water and food secondary to travel*

Related to change in bacteria in water

Related to bacteria, virus, or parasite to which no immunity is present

Author's Note

Noninfectious (infrequent), for example, congenital, inflammatory bowel disease; infectious (predominant), for example, bacterial, viral, parasitic

Errors in Diagnostic Statements

Diarrhea related to opportunistic enteric pathogens secondary to AIDS

Diarrhea, sometimes chronic, occurs in 60% to 90% of people with AIDS. Prolonged diarrhea represents a collaborative problem: *Risk for Complications of Fluid/Electrolyte/Nutritional Imbalances secondary to diarrhea.* Besides cotreating with a physician, the nurse treats other responses to chronic diarrhea (e.g., *Risk for Impaired Skin Integrity, Risk for Social Isolation*).

Key Concepts

General Considerations

- Acute infectious diarrhea is a yearly occurrence for most Americans and is associated with 1 million hospitalizations and about 600 deaths in the United States annually. Accurate numbers are difficult to acquire since most individuals do not seek medical treatment (*Goodgame, 2006; Wanke, 2016a).
- Noninfectious diarrhea (four loose or watery stools per day) is reported to be up to 28% of individual with HIV/AIDS (Clay & Crutchley, 2014). The etiology of noninfectious diarrhea in people infected with HIV is multifactorial and may include HIV-related enteropathy; cART; and, less commonly, autonomic neuropathy, chronic pancreatitis, and exocrine insufficiency (MacArthur, 2014). Siegal, Schrimshaw, Brown-Bradley, and Lekas (2010) reported that individuals with HIV/AIDS report diarrhea to cause "significant emotional distress and neatively affects patients' social lives by impacting their daily schedules and causing feelings of shame" (MacArthur, 2014). Diarrhea is an independent predictor of reduced quality of life (*Tramarin et al., 2004).
- Diarrhea can be acute or chronic. Causes of acute diarrhea include infection, medication side effects, heavy-metal poisoning, fecal impaction, and food. Causes of chronic diarrhea include irritable bowel syndrome, lactose deficiency, colon cancer, inflammatory bowel disease, malabsorption disorders, alcohol, medication side effects, and laxatives.
- For drugs that can induce diarrhea refer to Related Factors discussed earlier.
- Diarrhea may occur in 20% of individuals receiving broad spectrum antibiotics. Most resolve after finishing the antibiotic treatment (Arcangelo & Peterson, 2016). One study reported that in hospitalized patients receiving antibiotics, an antibiotic-associated diarrhea (AAD) period prevalence of 9.6% in individuals on antibiotics was found (Elseviers, 2015).
- Hyperperistalsis is the motor response to intestinal irritants. Rapid transit of feces through the large intestine results in decreased water absorption and unformed, liquid stool. Ongoing diarrhea leads to dehydration and electrolyte imbalance.
- Diarrhea may be related to an inflammatory process in which the intestinal mucosal wall becomes irritated, resulting in increased moisture content in the fecal masses.
- Up to 28% of individuals live with >4 loose or watery stools per day related to antiretroviral therapies (noninfectious diarrhea) (Clay & Crutchley, 2014).

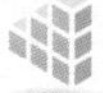

Pediatric Considerations

- Diarrhea in infants is always serious because of their small extracellular fluid reserve. Sudden losses result in circulatory collapse, renal failure, and irreversible acidosis and death (Pillitteri, 2014).
- Oral rehydration therapy is indicated for children with mild diarrhea and normal urine output.
- Signs of severe dehydration are sunken eyes; sunken fontanelles; loss of skin turgor; dry mucous membranes; rapid, thready pulse; cyanosis; rapid breathing; delayed capillary refill; and lethargy.
- Children who live in warm environments with poor sanitation and refrigeration or in crowded, substandard environments are at risk for eating contaminated food.

Geriatric Considerations

- The elderly are at high risk for dehydration from diarrhea.
- Elderly dehydration is related to (Miller, 2015)
  - Medications (e.g., diuretics)
  - Decreased thirst as one ages
  - Decreased ability of the kidney to concentrate urine
  - Vomiting and/or diarrhea can cause dehydration rapidly.
- Refer to the Key Concepts of *Deficient Fluid Volume* related to diarrhea.

Focus Assessment Criteria

Refer to *Constipation*.

Goals

NOC

Bowel Elimination, Electrolyte & Acid–Base Balance, Fluid Balance, Hydration, Symptom Control, Knowledge::prescribed diet, Self-management: Acute disease

The individual/parent will report less diarrhea as evidenced by the following indicators:

- Describes contributing factors when known
- Explains rationale for interventions
- Explains what foods and fluids to avoid

Interventions

NIC

Bowel Management, Diarrhea Management, Fluid/Electrolyte Management, Nutrition Management, Enteral Tube Feeding, Infection Control

Assess Causative Contributing Factors

- Tube feedings
- Dietetic foods
- Foreign travel
- Contaminated foods
- Food allergies
- Medications

Eliminate or Reduce Contributing Factors

Side Effects of Tube Feeding (Lutz & Przytulski, 2011)

- Control the infusion rate (depending on delivery set).
- Administer smaller, more frequent feedings.
- Change to continuous-drip tube feedings.
- Administer more slowly if signs of gastrointestinal intolerance occur.
- Control temperature.
- If formula has been refrigerated, warm it in hot water to room temperature.
- Dilute the strength of feeding temporarily.
- Follow the standard procedure for administration of tube feeding.
- Follow tube feeding with the specified amount of water to ensure hydration.
- Be careful of contamination/spoilage (unused but opened formula should not be used after 24 hours; keep unused portion refrigerated).

R: *High-solute tube feedings may cause diarrhea if not followed by sufficient water.*

Contaminated Foods (possible sources)

- Raw seafood
- Raw milk
- Shellfish
- Restaurants
- Excess milk consumption
- Improperly cooked/stored food

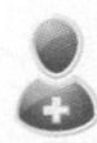

Clinical Alert When there is a high suspicion of diarrhea caused by food contamination, inform the board of health. This should not be punitive but instead a method to identify the cause of the contamination and the prevention measures needed. Food poisoning can be a minor event for some and extremely hazardous for the immunocompromised.

- Eliminate foods containing large amounts of the hexitol, sorbitol, and mannitol that are used as sugar substitutes in dietetic foods, candy, and chewing gum.

R: *The hexitols, a group of sugar alcohols that are slowly acted on by bacteria in the oral cavity and are slowly absorbed from the gastrointestinal tract, are capable of inducing osmotic diarrhea (e.g., sorbitol and mannitol) (*Ravry, 1980).*

Teach the Importance of Proper Hand Washing

- Wet hands and use plain or antibacterial soap.
- Rub together for 15 to 30 seconds.
- Wash the fingernails, between the fingers, and the wrists.
- Rinse the hands thoroughly and dry with a single use towel.

R: *Hand washing is an effective way to prevent the spread of infection.*

Reduce Diarrhea

- For short-term diarrhea, drink only clear liquids for 24 hours, for example, broth, water, noncaffeinated drinks. Avoid cold or hot drinks.
- Avoid milk (lactose) products, high-fat fiber foods, greasy, fried, and spicy foods, and fresh fruits and vegetables.
- Start with crackers, pretzels, yogurt, rice, bananas, and applesauce.
- If tolerated, gradually add potatoes, boiled eggs, white bread, cottage cheese, canned, peeled fruits, chicken without skin, and add salt.
- Eat small, frequent meals.
- Avoid caffeine and alcohol.

R: *Foods with complex carbohydrates (e.g., rice, toast, cereal) and salt facilitate fluid absorption into the intestinal mucosa (Lutz & Przytulski, 2011).*

- Instruct the individual to seek medical care if blood and mucous are in stool and fever greater than 101° F.

R: *Acute bloody diarrhea (dysentery) has certain causative pathogens (e.g., Campylobacter jejuni,* Shigella, Salmonella*) that require antibiotic therapy (Spies, 2009).*

Replace Fluids and Electrolytes

- Increase oral intake to maintain a normal urine specific gravity (light yellow in color).
- Encourage liquids (tea, water, apple juice, flat ginger ale).
- When diarrhea is severe, use an over-the-counter oral rehydration solution.
- Teach to monitor the color of urine to determine hydration needs. Increase fluids if urine color is amber or dark yellow.
- Caution against the use of very hot or cold liquids.
- Teach to gently clean the anal area after bowel movements; lubricants (e.g., petroleum jelly) can protect skin.

R: *The acidity of diarrheal stools can irritate the anal membranes.*

- See *Deficient Fluid Volume* for additional interventions.

Monitor Elderly Individuals for Signs of Dehydration (Miller, 2015)

- Confusion
- Dizziness or headaches
- Dry mouth
- Rapid heart rate
- Low blood pressure
- Low urine output
- Constipation

Conduct Health Teaching as Indicated

- Instruct person/family member to seek an evaluation if one or more of the following occurs (Wanke, 2016b):
  - Profuse watery diarrhea with signs of dehydration. Early features of dehydration include sluggishness, becoming tired easily, dry mouth and tongue, thirst, muscle cramps, dark-colored urine, urinating infrequently, and dizziness or lightheadedness after standing or sitting up. More severe features include abdominal pain, chest pain, confusion, or difficulty remaining alert.
  - Many small stools containing blood and mucus
  - Bloody or black diarrhea

- Temperature ≥38.5° C (101.3° F)
- Passage of ≥6 unformed stools per 24 hours, or illness that lasts more than 48 hours
- Severe abdominal pain or painful passage of stool

- Explain the interventions required to prevent future episodes and effects of diarrhea on hydration (e.g., probiotics, food safety, avoidance of ill persons).
- Advise not to treat traveler's diarrhea with antimobility agents (e.g., Lomotil (dipenoxylate/atropine), Imodium (loperamide)) for the first 24 hours.

R: *Antimobility agents can delay the clearance of organisms and thus can increase the severity of traveler's diarrhea with complications (e.g., sepsis, toxic megacolon).*

R: *Bismuth subsalicylate (Pepto-Bismol) has been found safe in a variety of diarrheal illnesses and to have antibacterial activity as well. It is also effective in controlling symptoms of traveler's diarrhea.*

Teach Precautions to Take When Traveling to Foreign Lands (Weller, 2015)

- Do not drink or brush the teeth with unboiled tap water.
- Do not drink beverages that contain ice made from unboiled tap water.
- Drink only boiled tap water, drinks made from boiled tap water, carbonated beverages, beer, and wine.
- Be wary of locally bottled water, because safety and bottling conditions might not be adequate. Other drinks are probably safer.
- Food can also contain infection-causing organisms. Reduce the risk of infection by following several food precautions:
  - Do not eat unpeeled fruit. Peel any fruit yourself before eating it.
  - Do not eat raw vegetables.
  - Do not eat or drink unpasteurized ("raw") dairy products.
  - Do not eat raw or rare meat, fish, or shellfish (including ceviche).
  - Refer a potential traveler to *Patient information: General travel advice (Beyond the Basics).*

R: *Microorganisms can multiply in foods not stored properly and/or washed with contaminated water. Ice can be contaminated.*

Reduce Food-Borne Infections by Properly Handling Foods (Weller, 2015)

- Do not drink raw (unpasteurized) milk or foods that contain unpasteurized milk.
- Wash raw fruits and vegetables thoroughly before eating. Try washing with baking soda, which dissolves well when rinsed off.
- Keep the refrigerator temperature at 40° F (4.4° C) or lower; the freezer at 0° F (−17.8° C) or lower.
- Use precooked, perishable, or ready-to-eat food as soon as possible.
- Keep raw meat, fish, and poultry separate from other food.
- Wash hands, knives, and cutting boards after handling uncooked food, including produce and raw meat, fish, or poultry.

R: *Failure to clean equipment used with raw foods can transfer microorganisms to cooked foods.*

- Thoroughly cook raw food from animal sources to a safe internal temperature: ground beef 160° F (71° C); chicken 170° F (77° C); turkey 180° F (82° C); pork 145° F (63° C) with a three minute rest time.
- Seafood should be cooked thoroughly to minimize the risk of food poisoning. Eating raw fish (e.g., sushi) poses a risk for a variety of parasitic worms (in addition to the risks associated with organisms carried by food handlers). Freezing kills some, although not all, harmful microorganisms. Raw fish that is labeled "sushi grade" or "sashimi grade" has been frozen.
- Cook chicken eggs thoroughly, until the yolk is firm.
- Never leave cooked foods at room temperature for more than 2 hours (1 hour if the room temperature is above 90° F/32° C).
- Keep cold foods cold and hot foods hot in the summer.

R: *Improper storage can cause microorganisms to multiply.*

In Addition, Pregnant Women or Those With a Weakened Immune System Should

- Not eat hot dogs, pâtés, luncheon meats, bologna, or other delicatessen meats unless they are reheated until steaming hot; avoid the use of microwave ovens since uneven cooking may occur.

- Avoid spilling fluids from raw meat and hot dog packages on other foods, utensils, and food preparation surfaces. In addition, wash hands after handling hot dogs, luncheon meats, delicatessen meats, and raw meat, chicken, turkey, or seafood or their juices.
- Not eat preprepared salads, such as ham salad, chicken salad, egg salad, tuna salad, or seafood salad.
- Not eat soft cheeses, such as feta, Brie, and Camembert, blue-veined cheeses, or Mexican-style cheeses, such as queso blanco, queso fresco, or Panela, unless they have a label that clearly states that the cheese is made from pasteurized milk.
- Not eat refrigerated pates or meat spreads. Canned or shelf-stable products may be eaten.
- Not eat refrigerated smoked seafood unless it has been cooked. Refrigerated smoked seafood, such as salmon, trout, whitefish, cod, tuna, or mackerel, is most often labeled as "nova-style," "lox," "kippered," "smoked," or "jerky." The fish is found in the refrigerator section or sold at deli counters of grocery stores and delicatessens. Canned or shelf-stable smoked seafood may be eaten.

R: *Some bacteria, although harmless to the pregnant woman, result in premature delivery, serious infection of the newborn, or even stillbirth (Food and Drug Administration, 2014).*

- Explain that a diet primarily made up of dietetic foods containing sugar substitutes (hexitol, sorbitol, and mannitol) can cause diarrhea.

R: *The hexitols, a group of sugar alcohols that are slowly acted on by bacteria in the oral cavity and are slowly absorbed from the gastrointestinal tract, are capable of inducing osmotic diarrhea (e.g., sorbitol and mannitol) (*Ravry, 1980).*

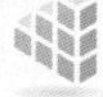

Pediatric Interventions

Monitor Fluid and Electrolyte Losses

- Fluid volume lost
- Urine color and output
- Skin color
- Mucous membranes
- Capillary refill time

Consult With Primary Care Provider If

- Diarrhea persists.
- Blood or mucus is in stools.
- Child is lethargic.
- Urine output is scanty.
- Stools suddenly increase.
- Child is vomiting.

R: *Children with signs of moderate or severe dehydration should be referred for possible parenteral therapy (Hockenberry & Wilson, 2012).*

Reduce Diarrhea

- Refer to the General Intervention for this nursing diagnosis.

Provide Oral Rehydration

- Use oral rehydration solutions (e.g., Pedialyte, Lytren, Ricelyte, Resol).
- Determine fluid loss by body weight loss. If less than 5% of total weight is lost, 50 mL/kg of fluid will be needed during the next 3 to 6 hours (Pillitteri, 2014).
- For more than a 5% weight loss, consult with the primary care provider for fluid replacement.
- Fluids must be given to replace losses and continuing losses until diarrhea improves (Pillitteri, 2014).

R: *Fluid replacement should be aggressive in infants and very young children.*

Reintroduce Food

- Begin with bananas, rice, cereal, pretzels, and crackers in small quantities.
- Gradually return to regular diet (except milk products) after 36 to 48 hours; after 3 to 5 days, gradually add milk products (half-strength skim milk to skim milk to half-strength milk (whole or 1%).
- Gradually introduce formula (half-strength formula to full-strength formula).

R: *Small quantities of nonirritating foods will decrease stimulation of the bowel.*

R: *Lactose-containing fluids or foods can worsen diarrhea in some children.*

For Breast-Fed Infants

- Continue breast-feeding.
- Use oral rehydration therapy if needed.

R: *Breast-feeding should be continued with fluid replacement therapy. Reduced severity and duration of the illness is attributed to breast milk's low osmolality and antimicrobial effects (Pillitteri, 2014).*

Protect Skin From Irritation With Nonwater-Soluble Cream (e.g., Petroleum Jelly)

R: *Diarrheal stools are acidic and irritating.*

Initiate Health Teaching as Needed

Teach Parents Signs That Indicate Medical Care is Needed

- Sunken eyes
- Dry mucous membranes
- Rapid, thready pulse
- Rapid breathing
- Lethargy
- Diarrhea increases

R: *Diarrhea in infants and small children can be serious because of their small extracellular fluid reserve. Early signs of hypovolemia need to be reported to prevent circulatory collapse, renal failure, and irreversible acidosis and death (Pillitteri, 2014).*

RISK FOR DISUSE SYNDROME

NANDA-I Definition

At risk for deterioration of body systems as the result of prescribed or unavoidable musculoskeletal inactivity

Defining Characteristics

Presence of a cluster of actual or risk nursing diagnoses related to inactivity:

Risk for Pressure Ulcer
Risk for Constipation
Risk for Altered Respiratory Function
Risk for Ineffective Peripheral Tissue Perfusion
Risk for Infection
Risk for Activity Intolerance
Risk for Impaired Physical Mobility
Risk for Injury
Powerlessness
Disturbed Body Image

Related Factors

(Optional) Refer to Author's Note.

Pathophysiologic

Related to:
Decreased sensorium
Unconsciousness

Neuromuscular impairment secondary to:

Multiple sclerosis
Muscular dystrophy
Parkinsonism
Partial/total paralysis
Guillain–Barré syndrome
Spinal cord injury

Musculoskeletal impairment secondary to:

Fractures
Rheumatic diseases

End-Stage Disease

AIDS
Cardiac
Renal Cancer

Psychiatric/Mental Health Disorders

Major depression
Catatonic state
Severe phobias

Treatment Related

Related to:

Surgery (amputation, skeletal)
Mechanical ventilation
Traction/casts/splints
Invasive vascular lines
Prescribed immobility

Situational (Personal, Environmental)

Related to:

Depression
Debilitated state
Fatigue
Pain

Maturational

Newborn/Infant/Child/Adolescent

Related to:

Down syndrome
Risser-Turnbuckle jacket
Legg–Calvé–Perthes disease
Juvenile arthritis
Cerebral palsy
Osteogenesis imperfecta
Mental/physical disability
Autism
Spina bifida

Older Adult

Related to:

Decreased motor agility
Muscle weakness
Presenile dementia

Author's Note

Risk for Disuse Syndrome describes an individual at risk for the adverse effects of immobility. *Risk for Disuse Syndrome* identifies vulnerability to certain complications and also altered functioning in a health pattern. As a syndrome diagnosis, its etiology or contributing factor is within the diagnostic label (*Disuse*); a "related to" statement is not necessary. As discussed in Chapter 2, a syndrome diagnosis comprises a cluster of predicted, actual, or risk nursing diagnoses because of the situation. Eleven risk or actual nursing diagnoses are clustered under *Disuse Syndrome* (see Defining Characteristics).

The nurse no longer needs to use separate diagnoses, such as *Risk for Ineffective Respiratory Function* or *Risk for Impaired Skin Integrity*, because they are incorporated into the syndrome category. If an immobile individual manifests signs or symptoms of pressure ulcer or another diagnosis, however, the nurse should use the specific diagnosis. He or she should continue to use *Risk for Disuse Syndrome*, so other body systems do not deteriorate.

Errors in Diagnostic Statements

***Risk for Disuse Syndrome* related to reddened sacral area (3 cm)**

A reddened sacral area is evidence of pressure ulcer. Thus, the nurse should use two diagnoses: *pressure ulcer* related to effects of immobility, as evidenced by reddened sacral area (3 cm) and continue also to use *Risk for Disuse Syndrome*.

Key Concepts

General Considerations

- "Observation of 45 hospitalised medical patients indicated that, on average, 83% of the hospital stay was spent lying in bed. The amount of time spent standing or walked ranged from 0.2–21%" (Kalisch, Lee, & Dabney, 2013).
- "Immobility is inconsistent with human life." Mobility provides control over the environment; without mobility, the individual is at the mercy of the environment (*Christian, 1982).
- Prolonged immobility decreases motivation to learn and ability to retain new material. Affective changes are anxiety, fear, hostility, rapid mood shifts, and disrupted sleep patterns (Halter, 2014).
- Bed rest reduces the hydrostatic pressure gradient within the cardiovascular system, reduces muscle force production, virtually eliminates compression on the bones, and lowers total energy expenditure (Stuempfle & Drury, 2007).
- Immobility restricts the ability to seek out sensory stimulation. Conversely, immobile people may be unable to remove themselves from a stressful or noisy environment (*Christian, 1982).
- Musculoskeletal inactivity or immobility adversely affects all body systems (Table II.5).
- Disuse of the muscles leads to atrophy and a loss of muscle strength at a rate of around 12% a week. Almost half the normal strength of a muscle is lost after 3 to 5 weeks of bed rest (Jiricka, 2008).
- Bed rest can cause an average vertical bone loss of 1% per week (*Nigam, Knight, & Jones, 2009).
- Prolonged immobility adversely affects psychological health, learning, socialization, and ability to cope. Table II.6 illustrates these effects.
- Probable long-term complications in individuals with traumatic spinal cord injury are pneumonia, atelectasis, autonomic dysreflexia, deep vein thrombosis, pulmonary embolism, pressure ulcers, fractures, and renal calculi.

Intensive Care Units

- "While the mean length of stay is currently 3.86 days in an ICU environment, critical care patients who are at risk for immobility often require prolonged hospital stays. These patients are often mechanically ventilated, confined to the bed, and sedated, which, in addition to their acute illness, contributes to the deconditioning of multiple organ systems. This deconditioning can occur in a few days of inactivity with some reports indicating that critically ill patients can lose up to 25% peripheral muscle weakness within 4 days when mechanically ventilated and 18% in body weight by the time of discharge. Loss of muscle mass particularly skeletal muscle is higher in the first 2–3 weeks of immobilization during an intensive care unit stay" (Zomorodi, Topley, & McAnaw, 2012).
- After transition to home, up to 60% of critically ill individuals exhibit long-term complications preventing them from complete functional recovery (*Timmerman, 2007).

Pediatric Considerations

- Mobility is essential for physical growth and development and mastery of developmental tasks (Hockenberry & Wilson, 2015). Restricted movement can thwart achievement of developmental tasks. Refer to Table II.7 in the diagnostic category *Delayed Growth and Development*.

Table 11.5 ADVERSE EFFECTS OF IMMOBILITY ON BODY SYSTEMS

System	Effect
Cardiac	Decreased myocardial performance
	Decreased aerobic capacity
	Decreased stroke volume
	Increased heart rate at rest and with increased activity
	Decreased oxygen uptake
	Reduction in plasma volume reduces cardiac preload, stroke volume, cardiac output
Circulatory	Reduction in plasma volume reduces cardiac preload, stroke volume, cardiac output
	Venous stasis
	Orthostatic intolerance
	Dependent edema
	Decreased resting heart rate
	Reduced venous return
Respiratory	Increased intravascular pressure
	Stasis of secretions
	Impaired cilia
	Drying of sections of mucous membranes
	Decreased chest expansion
	Slower, more shallow respirations
Musculoskeletal	Muscle atrophy
	Decreased skeletal muscle volume, most pronounced in the antigravity muscles
	Shortening of muscle fiber (contracture)
	Decreased strength/tone (e.g., back)
	Decreased bone density
	Joint degeneration
	Fibrosis of collagen fibers (joints)
Metabolic/hemopoietic	Increased bone resorption leads to a negative calcium balance (hypercalcemia) and eventually decreased bone mass
	Decreased nitrogen excretion
	Decreased tissue heat conduction
	Decreased glucose tolerance
	Insulin resistance
	Decreased red blood cells
	Decreased phagocytosis
	Change in circadian release of hormones (e.g., insulin, epinephrine)
	Anorexia
	Decreased metabolic rate
	Elevated creatine levels
Gastrointestinal	Constipation
	Anorexia
Genitourinary	Urinary stasis
	Urinary calculi
	Urinary retention
	Inadequate gravitational force

(continued)

Table 11.5 ADVERSE EFFECTS OF IMMOBILITY ON BODY SYSTEMS (*CONTINUED*)

System	Effect
Integumentary	Decreased capillary flow
	Tissue acidosis to necrosis
Neurosensory	Reduced innervation of nerves
	Decreased near vision
	Increased auditory sensitivity
	Increased sensitivity to thermal stimuli
	Altered circadian rhythm

Source: Hockenberry, M. J., & Wilson, D. (2015). *Wong's essentials of pediatric nursing* (10th ed.). New York: Elsevier; Grossman, S., & Porth, C. A. (2014). *Porth's pathophysiology: Concepts of altered health states* (9th ed.). Philadelphia: Wolters Kluwer; *Stuempfle, K., & Drury, D. (2007). The Physiological Consequences of Bed Rest. *Journal of Exercise Physiology Online, 10*(3), 32–41.

Table 11.6 PSYCHOSOCIAL EFFECTS OF IMMOBILITY

Psychological	Increased tension
	Negative change in self-concept
	Fear, anger
	Rapid mood changes
	Depression
	Hostility
Learning	Decreased motivation
	Decreased ability to retain, transfer learning
	Decreased attention span
Socialization	Change in roles
	Social isolation
Growth and development	Dependency

Source: Grossman, S., & Porth, C. A. (2014). *Porth's pathophysiology: Concepts of altered health states* (9th ed.). Philadelphia: Wolters Kluwer; Miller, C. (2015). *Nursing for wellness in older adults* (7th ed.). Philadelphia: Lippincott Williams & Wilkins; *Stuempfle, K., & Drury, D. (2007). The Physiological Consequences of Bed Rest. *Journal of Exercise Physiology Online, 10*(3), 32–41.

- Physical activity serves as a means of communication and expression for children. Major psychological consequences of immobility include the following:
  - Sensory deprivation, leading to alterations in self-perception and environmental awareness
  - Isolation from peers
  - Feelings of helplessness, frustration, anxiety, and boredom (Hockenberry & Wilson, 2012)
- Children who are restrained by casts, splints, or straps during the first 3 years of life have more difficulty with language than children with unrestricted activities (Hockenberry & Wilson, 2012).
- Children's responses to immobility may range from active protest to withdrawal or regression (Hockenberry & Wilson, 2012).

Geriatric Considerations

- "Beginning at about 40 years, muscle strength declines gradually, resulting in an overall decrease of 30% to 50% by age 80" (Miller, 2015, p. 468). The lower extremities have a great decline over the upper extremities. Muscle endurance and coordination decrease as a result of age-related changes in muscles and the central nervous system (Miller, 2015).
- Age-related changes in joint and connective tissues as degeneration of collagen and cartilage, calcifications in joint capsules, and decreased viscosity of synovial fluid result in impaired flexion and extension movements, decreased flexibility, and reduced cushioning protection for joints (Miller, 2015).

- Aging slows the response of the central nervous system to maintain balance, thus increasing the risk of falls (Miller, 2015).

Focus Assessment Criteria

This may be assessed by physical therapy.

Subjective Data

Assess for Factors Which Contribute to Immobility

Neurologic
Musculoskeletal
Debilitating diseases
History of symptoms (complaints) of pain, muscle weakness, fatigue
Cardiovascular
Respiratory
History of recent trauma or surgery
Severe mental illness (e.g., depression, catatonia, paranoia)

Objective Data

Assess for

Ability to Use Right Arm, Left Arm, Right Leg, and Left Leg

Assess for Ability or if Assistance is Needed to
Turn self
Sit
Stand
Transfer
Ambulate

Weight-Bearing (Assess Both Right and Left Sides)
Full
Partial
As tolerated
Nonweight-bearing

Gait
Stable
Unstable

Range of Motion of Shoulders, Elbows, Arms, Hips, and Legs

Assess for:

Assistive Devices

Crutches	Wheelchair	Cane
Prosthesis	Braces	Other
Walker		

Restrictive Devices

Cast or splint	Foley	Traction
Intravenous line	Braces	Monitor
Ventilator	Dialysis	Drain

Motivation (as Perceived by Nurse, Reported by the Individual, or Both)

Goals

NOC

Endurance, Immobility Consequences: Physiologic, Immobility Consequences: Psycho-Cognitive, Mobility Level Joint Movement, Ambulation, Joint Movements

The individual will not experience preventable complications of immobility as evidenced by the following indicators:

- Intact skin/tissue integrity
- Maximum pulmonary function
- Maximum peripheral blood flow
- Full range of motion
- Bowel, bladder, and renal functioning *within normal limits*
- Regular social contacts and activities when possible

The individual will be repositioned or mobilized dependent if hemodynamically stable at rest (Zomorodi et al., 2012)

- Position upright as soon as possible
- Implement ongoing extreme position changes every hour or as indicated
- Implement kinetic/rotating beds if indicated
  The individual will when possible
- Explain rationale for treatments
- Make decisions regarding care
- Share feelings regarding immobile state

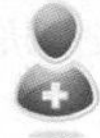

Clinical Alert "In several studies of missed nursing care, defined as required nursing care that is omitted or significantly delayed, ambulation of patients was identified as the most frequently missed element of inpatient nursing care, missed 76.1–88.7% of the time" (Kalisch et al., 2013).

Interventions

NIC

Activity Therapy, Energy Management, Mutual Goal Settings, Exercise Therapy, Fall Prevention, Pressure Ulcer Prevention, Body Mechanics Correction, Skin Surveillance, Positioning, Coping Enhancement, Decision-Making, Support Therapeutic Play

Identify Causative and Contributing Factors

- Pain; refer also to *Impaired Comfort*
- Fatigue; refer also to *Fatigue*
- Decreased motivation; refer also to *Activity Intolerance*
- Depression; refer also to *Ineffective Coping*
- Barriers to bed mobility and/or ambulation

Initiate a Mobility Ambulation Protocol for Hemodynamically Stable Individual (Refer to *Impaired Physical Mobility*)

For Individuals Unable to Ambulate, Aggressively Reposition, (Hourly if Possible) as (Zomorodi et al., 2012)

- Position upright as soon as possible

R: *This therapeutic goal is distinct from ambulation or mobilization.*

- Turning frequently from side to side, partial side to side
- Raising and lowering head of bed
- Bed in chair position

R: *"Early mobility has been linked to decreased morbidity and mortality as inactivity has a profound adverse effect on the brain, skin, skeletal muscle, pulmonary, and cardiovascular systems" (Zomorodi et al., 2012).*

Promote Optimal Respiratory Function

- Encourage deep breathing and controlled coughing exercises five times every hour.
- Teach to use a blow bottle or incentive spirometer every hour when awake (with severe neuromuscular impairment, the individual also may have to be awakened at night).
- For a child, use colored water in the blow bottle; have him or her blow up balloons, soap bubbles, or cotton balls with straw.
- Auscultate lung fields every 8 hours; increase frequency if breath sounds are altered.

- Encourage small, frequent feedings to prevent abdominal distention.

R: *Bed rest decreases chest expansion and cilia activity and increases mucus retention, increasing risks of pneumonia (Grossman & Porth, 2014).*

Maintain Usual Pattern of Bowel Elimination

- Refer to *Constipation* for specific interventions.

Prevent Pressure Ulcers

- Refer to *Risk for Pressure Ulcer.*

Promote Factors That Improve Venous Blood Flow

- Elevate extremity above the level of the heart (may be contraindicated if the individual is hemodynamically unstable).
- Teach to avoid standing or sitting with legs dependent for long periods.
- Reduce or remove external venous compression, which impedes venous flow.
- Avoid pillows behind the knees or suggest a bed that is elevated at the knees.
- Tell to avoid crossing the legs.
- Remind to change positions, move extremities, or wiggle fingers and toes every hour.
- Monitor legs for edema, tissue warmth, and redness daily.

R: *Increased serum calcium resulting from bone destruction caused by lack of motion and weight-bearing increases blood coagulability. This, in addition to circulatory stasis, makes the individual vulnerable to thrombosis formation (Grossman & Porth, 2014).*

Maintain Limb Mobility and Prevent Contractures (*Maher, Salmond, & Pellino, 2006)

Increase Limb Mobility

- Perform range-of-motion exercises (frequency to be determined by the individual's condition).
- Support extremity with pillows to prevent or reduce swelling.
- Encourage the individual to perform exercise regimens for specific joints as prescribed by physician or physical therapist.

Position in Alignment to Prevent Complications

- Point toes and knees toward ceiling when the individual is supine. Keep them flat when in a chair.
- Use footboard.
- Instruct to wiggle toes, point them up and downward, rotate their ankles inward and outward every hour.

R: *These strategies prevent footdrop, a serious complication of immobility and deep vein thrombosis.*

- Avoid placing pillows under the knee; support calf instead.
- Avoid prolonged periods of hip flexion (i.e., sitting position).
- To position hips, place rolled towel lateral to the hip to prevent external rotation.
- Keep arms abducted from the body with pillows.
- Keep elbows in slight flexion.
- Keep wrist neutral, with fingers slightly flexed and thumb abducted and slightly flexed.
- Change position of shoulder joints during the day (e.g., abduction, adduction, range of circular motion).

R: *Compression of nerves by casts, restraints, or improper positions can cause ischemia and nerve degeneration. Compression of the peroneal nerve results in footdrop; compression of the radial nerve results in wristdrop and possible permanent nerve damage after 6 to 8 hours (Hockenberry & Wilson, 2012).*

Provide or Assist in Range-of-Motion Exercises at Interval That are Appropriate for the Individual Condition

R: *Joints without range of motion develop contractures in 3 to 7 days, because flexor muscles are stronger than extensor muscles.*

Prevent Urinary Stasis and Calculi Formation

- Provide a daily fluid intake of 3,000 mL (unless contraindicated); see *Deficient Fluid Volume* for specific interventions.

R: *The peristaltic contractions of the ureters are insufficient when in a reclining position; thus, there is stasis of urine in the renal pelvis. Concentrated urine provides a medium for crystals to combine and precipitate into kidney stones (Lutz & Przytulski, 2011).*

Reduce and Monitor Bone Demineralization

R: *Prolonged immobility causes increased bone resorption resulting in hypercalcemia. Individuals with preexistent renal dysfunction are at increased risk (Lim et al., 2011).*

- Monitor serum levels of calcium.
- Monitor for signs of hypercalcemia, nausea/vomiting, polydipsia, polyuria, lethargy.
- Promote weight-bearing when possible (tilt-table).

R: *The upright position improves bone strength, increases circulation, and prevents postural hypotension (Grossman & Porth, 2014).*

Promote Sharing and a Sense of Well-Being

- Encourage to share feelings and fears regarding restricted movement.
- Encourage to wear own clothes, rather than pajamas, and unique adornments (e.g., baseball caps, colorful socks) to express individuality.

Reduce the Monotony of Immobility

- Vary daily routine when possible (e.g., give a bath in the afternoon so the person can watch a special show or talk with a visitor during the morning).

Include the Individual/family in Planning Daily Schedule

- Allow to make as many decisions as possible.
- Make daily routine as normal as possible (e.g., have the individual wear street clothes during the day, if feasible).
- Encourage the individual to make a schedule for visitors so everyone does not come at once or at inconvenient times.
- Spend time with the person just listening (i.e., not time that is task-oriented; rather, sit down and talk).

Be Creative; Vary the Physical Environment and Daily Routine When Possible

- Update bulletin boards, change pictures on the walls, and move furniture within the room.
- Maintain a pleasant, cheerful environment (e.g., plenty of light, flowers).
- Place the individual near a window, if possible.
- Provide reading material (print or audio), radio, and television.
- Discourage the use of television as the primary source of recreation unless it is highly desired.
- Consider using a volunteer to spend time reading to the individual or helping with an activity.
- Encourage suggestions and new ideas (e.g., "Can you think of things you might like to do?").

R: *Decreased activity reduces social contacts, reduces problem-solving ability, and decreases coping ability and orientation to time. Strategies are focused on increasing visual and auditory stimuli, engaging in decision making and activities to reduce monotony.*

Pediatric Interventions

Explain Types of Play in the Health-Care Setting

- Exercise/energy-releasing play: promotes use of large upper/lower extremities (e.g., throwing a ball, playing in water)
- Diversional/recreational play: provides enjoyable activities to combat boredom
- Developmentally supportive play: selected age-appropriated activities to challenge the infant/child
- Therapeutic play: provides the child with activities that with interactions with a health-care professional, facilitates expression of feeling and fears about the health-care experience. This dialogue clarifies misunderstandings and reasons for certain treatments.

Explain to Parents/Caregiver That Play Can[14]

- Relieve the stress caused by immobility.
- Allow for continued growth and development physically, mentally, and emotionally.

[14]*Source*: Arkansas Children's Hospital, A Parent's Guide... Play and Your Immobilized Child. Accessed at www.archildrens.org/documents/child_life/PlayImmoblizedChild.pdf

- Allow the parent and child to dialogue about concerns or misunderstandings about their care, procedures etc.
- Encourage sharing of feelings.
- Provide choices for the child, to increase his feeling of control.
- Provide "well role," as child sees he can still succeed.
- Provide for family support and involvement.
- Provide an escape from pain, boredom, and sadness.
- Help to minimize any possible physical side effects due to decreased activity.

Plan Appropriate Activities for Children

- Provide an environment with accessible toys that suit the child's developmental age; ensure they are well within reach.
- Encourage the family to bring in the child's favorite toys, including items from nature that will keep the "real world" alive (e.g., goldfish, leaves in fall).
- Limit TV watching to a few favorite programs.

R: *Watching TV can overstimulate a child and interfere with socialization (Pillitteri, 2014).*

Use Play Therapy (Pillitteri, 2014)

- As an energy release:
  - Pound pegs
  - Cut wood with pretend saw
  - Pound clay
  - Punch a balloon

R: *Play that releases energy substitutes for the usual hitting, running, and shouting of children.*

- As dramatic play:
  - Provide health-care equipment as dolls, doll beds, play stethoscopes, IV equipment, syringes, masks, and gowns.
  - Allow the child to choose the objects.
  - Allow the child opportunities to play and express their feelings.
  - Use opportunities to ask the child questions.
  - Reflect only what the child expresses.
  - Do not criticize.

R: *Dramatic play allows children to express feelings about illness and treatments.*

- As creative play:
  - Provide opportunities to draw pictures.
  - Ask the child to describe the picture.

R: *Picture drawing may express emotions that the child cannot verbally.*

- Vary the environment
- Transport child outside the room as much as possible

R: *Changes in the environment provide varied stimuli and increased social contact (Hockenberry & Wilson, 2015).*

- Access information for managing prolonged immobility. www.archildrens.org/documents/child_life/PlayImmobizedChild.pdf; www.chop.edu/health-resources/play-and-recreation-during-hospitalization#.VVdzYPlVhBc

DEFICIENT DIVERSIONAL ACTIVITY

NANDA-I Definition

Decreased stimulation from (or interest or engagement in) recreational or leisure activities

Defining Characteristics

Observed and/or statements of boredom due to inactivity

Related Factors

Pathophysiologic

Related to difficulty accessing or participating in usual activities secondary to:

Communicable disease
Pain

Situational (Personal, Environmental)

Related to unsatisfactory social behaviors

Related to no peers or friends

Related to monotonous environment

Related to long-term hospitalization or confinement

Related to lack of motivation

Related to difficulty accessing or participating in usual activities secondary to:

Excessive stressful work
No time for leisure activities
Career changes (e.g., new job, retirement)
Children leaving home (empty nest)
Immobility
Decreased sensory perception
Multiple role responsibilities

Maturational

Infant/Child

Related to lack of appropriate stimulation toys/peers

Older Adult

Related to difficulty accessing or participating in usual activities secondary to:

Sensory/motor deficits
Lack of transportation
Fear of crime
Lack of peer group
Limited finances
Confusion

Author's Note

The individual is the best person to express a deficit in diversional activities based on his or her determination, which types and amounts of activity are desired. Miller (2015) writes that activities associated with various roles affirm an individual's self-concept.

To validate *Deficient Diversional Activity*, explore the etiology of factors amenable to nursing interventions, keeping your main focus on improving the quality of leisure activities. For an individual with personality problems that hinder relationships and decrease social activities, *Impaired Social Interactions* is more valid. In this case, focus on helping the individual identify behavior that imposes barriers to socialization.

Errors in Diagnostic Statements

***Deficient Diversional Activity* related to boredom and reports of no leisure activities**

Boredom and reports of no leisure activities are manifestations, not contributing factors, of the diagnosis. Thus, write the diagnosis as *Deficient Diversional Activity related to unknown etiology*, as evidenced by reports of boredom and no leisure activities.

***Deficient Diversional Activity* related to inability to sustain meaningful relationships, as evidenced by "no one calls me to go out."**

In this situation, delay making a formal diagnosis and collect more data to explore more, specifically the meaning of "no one calls me to go out." Other diagnoses may be more applicable, such as *Impaired Social Interactions, Risk for Loneliness,* and *Ineffective Coping*.

Key Concepts

General Considerations

- All human beings need stimulation. In adults, lack of stimulation leads to boredom and depression. In infants and children, it causes "failure to thrive" and may stunt growth severely.
- The relationship between informal activity and life satisfaction is significant. The quality or type of activity is more important than the quantity (*Rantz, 1991).
- Boredom paralyzes an individual's productivity and causes a feeling of stagnation. It can be a major contributing factor to addictive behaviors (e.g., overeating, drug abuse, alcoholism, smoking).
- The bored individual has introspective feelings of being oppressed and trapped, which give rise to conscious or unconscious anger or hostility.
- In recent years, pet therapy has been appreciated increasingly for ill and older individuals.

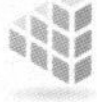

Pediatric Considerations

- Children who are at special risk for deficient diversional activity include those who are
  - Bored or immobilized
  - Hospitalized for long periods
  - Isolated to protect themselves or others
  - In diminished contact with family, friends, or both
- Age-appropriate activities should be provided to promote mental health and human development. Child-life specialists—experts who are certified in early childhood, creative arts, or recreation therapies—provide psychosocial assessment and therapeutic activities in group contexts (they give advice on individual clients, playroom design, and activities). They work with the multidisciplinary team to provide developmentally appropriate therapy and education to children and aiming to reduce the psychological trauma of illness. Refer to the table in the *Delayed Growth and Development* section.
- See also Key Concepts, Pediatric Considerations for *Anxiety*, *Risk for Disuse Syndrome*, and *Delayed Growth and Development*.

Geriatric Considerations

- Cultural background strongly influences the older individual's use of diversional activities because of the value placed on work versus leisure. Older, less educated, rural people tend to place less value on leisure activities.
- In Western society, retirement usually occurs between 62 and 70 years of age. About 80% of men and 90% of women older than 65 years are identified as retired. The lost work role can lead to depression, particularly if the individual has engaged in no preretirement planning (Miller, 2015).
- Cultivating varied interests and activities throughout life enhances aging (Miller, 2015).
- A change in living arrangements or environment might subject the older adult to a diversional activity deficit. For example, an organic gardener with her own private yard moves to a senior high-rise apartment with no land for a garden. Or an older man who plays the drums moves in with his adult children who have neither the space for his drum set nor the inclination to listen to his drum solos.
- Social isolation resulting from the death of a spouse, lack of transportation, hearing impairment, limited finances, fear of crime, or other physical or psychological disabilities places the older individual at risk for diversional activity deficit (*Rantz, 1991).
- Volunteer activities provide diversion for 21% of people 55 to 64 years of age and 14% of those 65 years and older. Those 65 years and older volunteered an average of 8 hours per week. Reasons cited for not volunteering included transportation difficulties, financial concerns, and age discrimination by some community organizations (Miller, 2015).

Focus Assessment Criteria

Subjective Data

Assess for Defining Characteristics

Perception of their current activity level: Ask to rate on a scale of 1 to 10 his or her satisfaction with current diversional activity level (1 = not at all satisfied and 10 = very satisfied).

Past activity patterns (type, frequency): work, leisure

Activities that he or she desires

Objective Data

Assess for Related Factors

Motivation

Interested	Withdrawn
Uninterested	Hostile

Any barriers to recreational activities

Physical Status

Immobility	Pain
Altered level of consciousness	Sensory deficits (visual, auditory)
Fatigue	Equipment (traction, intravenous [IV] lines)
Altered hand mobility	Communicable disease/isolation

Psychological/Cognitive Status

Depression	Language barrier
Embarrassment	Lack of knowledge
Socioeconomic status	Fear
Lack of support system	Financial limitations
Previous patterns of inactivity	Transportation difficulties

Goals

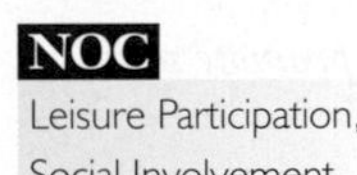

NOC
Leisure Participation, Social Involvement

The individual will rate that he or she is more satisfied with current activity level as evidenced by the following indicators:

- Relates methods of coping with anger or depression resulting from boredom
- Reports participation in one enjoyable activity each day

Interventions

NIC
Recreation Therapy, Socialization Enhancement, Self-Esteem Enhancement, Therapeutic Play

Assess Causative Factors

- Refer to Related Factors.

Reduce or Eliminate Causative Factors

Monotony

- Refer to Interventions, "Reduce the monotony of immobility," under *Disuse Syndrome*.
- Provide opportunities for reminiscence individually or in groups (e.g., past trips, hobbies).
- Provide music therapy with audiocassette players with lightweight headphones. For group music therapy (*Rantz, 1991), the following is recommended:
  - Introduce a topic.
  - Play related music.
  - Develop the topic with discussion.
  - Discuss responses.

R: *Music therapy can be valuable in relieving boredom, sparking interest, and assisting individuals to cope with social problems (*Rantz, 1991).*

- Consider using holistic and complementary therapies (e.g., aromatherapy, pet therapy, therapeutic touch). For pet therapy (*Rantz, 1991), the following is recommended:
  - Animals must be well groomed, healthy, and clean.
  - Animals should be relaxed with strangers.
  - Animals should eliminate before entering the facility.
  - Sponsors always should ask the individual if he or she likes the type of animal before approaching the individual.

R: *Complementary therapies serve to reduce stress, enhance coping, and foster well-being.*

Lack of Motivation

- Stimulate motivation by showing interest and encouraging sharing of feelings and experiences.
- Explore fears and concerns about participating in activities.

- Discuss likes and dislikes.
- Encourage sharing of feelings of present and past experiences.
- Spend time with the individual purposefully talking about other topics (e.g., "I just got back from the shore. Have you ever gone there?").
- Point out the need to "get going" and try something new.
- Help the individual work through feelings of anger and grief:
  - Allow him or her to express feelings.
  - Take the time to be a good listener.
  - See *Anxiety* for additional interventions.

R: *Reminiscing, or spending time focusing on significant memories, can be satisfying and stimulating for the bored, ill, confined, or elderly individual (*Rantz, 1991).*

- Encourage the individual to join a group of possible interest or help. (He or she may have to participate by way of intercom or special arrangement.)
- Consider the use of music therapy or reminiscence therapy.

R: *Membership in a group or a support group can boost self-esteem and self-worth, provide a sense of belonging and encourage activities that the individual otherwise may have avoided. Support groups can often assist those with stressful, costly, or time-consuming problems.*

Inability to Concentrate

- Plan a simple daily routine with concrete activities (e.g., walking, drawing, folding linens).
- If the individual is anxious, suggest solitary, noncompetitive activities (e.g., puzzles, photography).

R: *Tasks that match the individual's concentration and interest can increase contact with reality, promote socialization, and improve self-esteem (Varcarolis, 2011).*

Identify Factors That Promote Activity and Socialization

Encourage Socialization With Peers and All Age Groups (Frequently Very Young and Very Old Individuals Mutually Benefit From Interactions)

Acquire Assistance to Increase the Individual's Ability to Travel

- Arrange transportation to activities, if necessary.
- Acquire aids for safety (e.g., wheelchair for shopping, walker for ambulating in hallways).

Increase the Individual's Feelings of Productivity and Self-Worth

- Encourage the individual to use strengths to help others and self (e.g., assign him or her tasks to perform in a general project). Acknowledge these efforts (e.g., "Thank you for helping Mr. Jones with his dinner").
- Encourage open communication; value the individual's opinion ("Mr. Jones, what do you think about _____?").
- Encourage the individual to challenge him or herself to learn a new skill or pursue a new interest.
- Provide opportunities to interact with nature and animals.

R: *Exposure to various stimuli can increase social interactions and decrease boredom (*Barba, Tesh, & Courts, 2002).*

Refer to Social Isolation for Additional Interventions

 Pediatric Interventions

- Provide an environment with accessible toys that suit the child's developmental age; ensure that they are well within reach.
- Keep toys in all waiting areas.
- Encourage the family to bring in the child's favorite toys, including items from nature that will help to keep the "real world" alive (e.g., goldfish, leaves in fall).
- Consult a child-life specialist as indicated.
- Refer to Pediatric Interventions in the nursing diagnosis *Disuse Syndrome* for specifics on how to engage in therapeutic play.
- Refer to online sources for activities as favorite therapeutic activities for children, adolescents, and families: Practitioners share their most effective interventions (www.lianalowenstein.com/e-booklet.pdf).

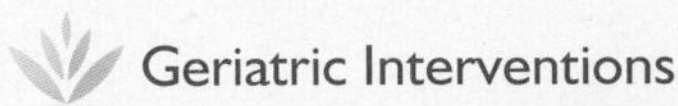

Geriatric Interventions

- Explore interests and the feasibility of trying a new activity (e.g., mobility).
- Use creative activities that produce a satisfying outcome. Avoid activities that only keep the person busy.
- Taylor activities to the person's capabilities.
- Arrange for someone to accompany or orient the individual during initial encounters.

R: *Change, although a welcome relief from boredom, increases anxiety initially.*

- Explore possible volunteer opportunities (e.g., Red Cross, hospitals).
- Initiate referrals, if indicated.
  - Suggest joining the American Association of Retired Persons (AARP).
  - Write local health and welfare council or agencies.
  - Provide a list of associations/clubs with senior citizen activities (i.e., YMCA) such as Sixty Plus Club, Churches, XYZ Group (Extra Years of Zest), Golden Age Club, Young at Heart Club, SOS (Senior Outreach Services), Encore Club, Leisure Hour Group, MORA (Men of Retirement Age), Gray Panthers.

R: *Cognitive impairment, musculoskeletal impairment, pain, metabolic abnormality, or sensory deficit may force an older adult to consider modifying long-time leisure activities or developing new activities. For example, an individual who likes to cook but has poor eyesight might obtain large-print cookbooks, have a friend write favorite recipes in bold print, or tape-record recipes (*Rantz, 1991).*

R: *Change, although a welcome relief from boredom, increases anxiety initially.*

AUTONOMIC DYSREFLEXIA

Autonomic Dysreflexia

Risk for Autonomic Dysreflexia

NANDA-I Definition

Life-threatening, uninhibited sympathetic response of the nervous system to a noxious stimulus after a spinal cord injury at T7 or above

Defining Characteristics

Major (Must Be Present)

The individual with spinal cord injury (T6 or above) with

Paroxysmal hypertension* (sudden periodic elevated blood pressure in which systolic pressure is above 140 mm Hg and diastolic is above 90 mm Hg)
Bradycardia or tachycardia* (pulse rate less than 60 or more than 100 beats/min)
Diaphoresis (above the injury)*
Red splotches on skin (above the injury)*
Pallor (below the injury)*
Headache (a diffuse pain in different portions of the head and not confined to any nerve distribution area)*
Apprehension
Dilated pupils

Minor (May Be Present)

Chilling*
Conjunctival congestion*
Horner's syndrome* (pupillary contraction; partial ptosis of the eyelid; enophthalmos; sometimes, loss of sweating over the affected side of the face)
Paresthesia*

Pilomotor reflex* (gooseflesh)
Blurred vision*
Chest pain*
Metallic taste in mouth*
Nasal congestion*
Penile erection and semen emission

Related Factors

Pathophysiologic (Stephenson, 2014)

Related to visceral stretching and irritation secondary to:

Gastrointestinal

Gallstones
Gastric ulcers
Hemorrhoids
Gastrocolic irritation
Anal fissure
Gastric distention
Constipation
Fecal impaction
Hemorrhoids
Acute abdominal condition, infection, trauma

Urologic

Bladder distension*
Urinary calculi
Urinary tract infection
Epididymitis or scrotal compression

Skin Irritation*

Pressure ulcers
Insect bites
Burns
Ingrown toenails
Sunburn
Blister
Insect bites
Contact with hard or sharp objects

Reproductive

Menstruation
Epididymitis
Ejaculation
Sexual intercourse
Pregnancy or delivery
Uterine contraction
Vaginal infection
Vaginal dilation

Related to fracture

Related to stimulation of skin (abdominal, thigh)

Related to spastic sphincter

Related to deep vein thrombosis

Related to pulmonary embolism

Related to pain

Related to fractures or other skeletal trauma

Related to surgical or diagnostic procedures

Treatment Related

Related to visceral stretching secondary to:

Removal of fecal impaction
Clogged or nonpatent catheter
Visceral stretching and irritation secondary to surgical incision, enemas
Catheterization, enema
Bowel instrumentation/colonoscopy
Cystoscopy/instrumentation
Urodynamic study

Situational (Personal, Environmental)

Related to deficient individual knowledge* of prevention or treatment

Related to visceral stretching secondary to:

"Boosting" (binding legs and distending bladder to boost norepinephrine production for competitive wheel-chair sports; *McClain, Shields, & Sixsmith, 1999)

Sexual activity

Related to neural stimulation secondary to immersion in cold water

Related to temperature fluctuations

Related to constrictive clothing, shoes, or appliances

Author's Note

Autonomic Dysreflexia represents a life-threatening situation that nurse-prescribed interventions can prevent or treat. Prevention involves teaching the individual to reduce sympathetic nervous system stimulation and not using interventions that can cause such stimulation. Treatment focuses on reducing or eliminating noxious stimuli (e.g., fecal impaction, urinary retention). If nursing actions do not resolve symptoms, initiation of medical intervention is critical. When an individual requires medical treatment for all or most episodes of dysreflexia, the situation can be labeled a collaborative problem: *Risk for Complications of Autonomic Dysreflexia*.

Errors in Diagnostic Statements

Autonomic Dysreflexia related to paroxysmal hypertension

Paroxysmal hypertension is a sign of dysreflexia, not a causative or contributing stimulus. The diagnosis should be restated: *Risk for Autonomic Dysreflexia related to possible reflex stimulation by visceral or cutaneous irritation, as evidenced by (specify)*.

Clinically, *Risk for Autonomic Dysreflexia* is more descriptive than *Autonomic Dysreflexia*. The individual usually is in a potential state, with associated nursing responsibilities of prevention, teaching, and early removal of stimulus.

Key Concepts

- The autonomic nervous system (sympathetic and parasympathetic) is located in the cerebrum, hypothalamus, medulla, brain stem, and spinal cord. With spinal cord injury, activity below the injury is deprived of the controlling effects from the higher centers. The result is poorly controlled responses (Stephenson, 2014).
- Stimulation of sensory receptors below a spinal lesion results in sympathetic discharge, mediated by the spinothalamic tract and posterior columns. This reflex stimulation of the sympathetic nervous system causes spasms of the pelvic viscera and arterioles. These spasms cause vasoconstriction below the level of injury. Baroreceptors in the aortic arch and carotid sinus respond to the hypertensive state with superficial vasodilation, flushing, diaphoresis, and piloerection (gooseflesh) above the level of the spinal lesion (Stephenson, 2014).
- Vagal stimulation slows the heart rate, but, because the cord is severed, vagal impulses to dilate vessels are prohibited (Grossman & Porth, 2014; *Teasell, Arnold, & Delaney, 1996).
- Failure to reverse dysreflexia can result in status epilepticus, stroke, and death. However, avoidance of noxious triggers can "prevent the episode entirely" (Somali, 2009).
- "Due to spinal cord injury, the upper brain centers are unable to modulate this sympathetic discharge, resulting in increased blood pressure. Autonomic dysreflexia is characterized by an increase in the baseline blood pressure, most often from 20 to 40 mmHg. However, the systolic pressure may vary from 250 to 300 mmHg and the diastolic from 200 to 220 mmHg. AD-associated hypertension may lead to retinal detachment, stroke, convulsion, myocardial infarction and death" (Andrade et al., 2013).
- Three types of stimuli can initiate dysreflexia: visceral distention (e.g., full bladder or rectum), stimulation of pain receptors (e.g., diagnostic procedure, pressure, injuries), and visceral contractions (e.g., ejaculation, bladder spasms, uterine contractions).
- The onset of autonomic dysreflexia occurred between 1 and 6 months after injury (Stephenson, 2014).

Focus Assessment Criteria

Subjective Data

Assess for Defining Characteristics

Initial Symptoms

Headache (severe, sudden)	Nasal congestion	Cold extremities
Sweating (where?)	Numbness	Pilomotor skin erections (goose bumps)
Chills	Pallor	Blurred vision
Metallic taste in mouth	Dyspnea	Other

Assess for Related Factors

History of Dysreflexia, Triggered by:

Anxiety	Skin lesion	Diagnostic study
Bladder distention	Pain	Pressure
Bowel distention	Sexual activity	
Tactile stimulation	Menstruation	

Knowledge of Dysreflexia

Cause	Medical treatment
Self-treatment	Prevention

Goals

NOC

Neurologic Status, Neurologic Status: Autonomic, Vital Signs Status

The individual/family will respond to early signs/symptoms. The individual/family will take action to prevent dysreflexia as evidenced by the following indicators:

- States factors that cause dysreflexia
- Describes the treatment for dysreflexia
- Relates indications for emergency treatment

Interventions

NIC

Dysreflexia Management, Vital Signs Monitoring, Emergency Care, Medication Administration

Assess for Causative or Contributing Factors

- See Related Factors.

Proceed as Follows if Signs of Dysreflexia Occur

- Stand or sit the individual up.
- Lower the individual's legs.
- Loosen all the individual's constrictive clothing or appliances.

R: *An upright position and removal of hose increase venous pooling, reduce venous return, and decrease blood pressure (Stephenson, 2014).*

Check for Distended Bladder

R: *Andrade et al. (2013) reported that bladder distention causes 89% of autonomic dysreflexia in the population studied.*

If the Individual Is Catheterized

- Check the catheter for kinks or compression.
- Irrigate the catheter with only 30 mL of saline, very slowly.
- Replace the catheter if it will not drain.

If the Individual Is Not Catheterized

- Insert the catheter using dibucaine hydrochloride ointment (Nupercainal).
- Remove 500 mL, then clamp for 15 minutes.
- Repeat the cycle until the bladder is drained.

R: *Bladder distension is the most common cause of dysreflexia. Bladder distention can trigger dysreflexia by stimulation of sensory receptors. Nupercainal ointment reduces tissue stimulation. Too rapid removal of urine can* *result in compensatory hypotension. These interventions aim to reduce cerebral hypertension and induce orthostatic hypotension (Stephenson, 2014).*

Check for Fecal Impaction

- First apply Nupercainal to the anus and into the rectum for 1 in (2.54 cm).
- Gently check the rectum with a well-lubricated glove using your index finger.
- Insert rectal suppository or gently remove impaction.

R: *Spasms of pelvic viscera and arterioles cause vasoconstriction below the level of injury, producing hypertension and pallor. Afferent impulses triggered by high blood pressure cause vagal stimulation, resulting in bradycardia. Baroreceptors in the aortic arch and carotid sinus respond to the hypertension, triggering superficial vasodilation, flushing, diaphoresis, and headache above the level of cord injury (Stephenson, 2014).*

Check for Skin Irritation

- Spray the skin lesion that is triggering the dysreflexia with a topical anesthetic agent.
- Remove support hose.

R: *Dysreflexia can be triggered by stimulation (e.g., of the glans penis or skin lesions).*

Continue to Monitor Blood Pressure Every 3 to 5 Minutes

R: *Failure to reverse severe hypertension can result in status epilepticus, retinal or intracerebral hemorrhage, and death.*

Immediately Consult Physician/PA/NP for Pharmacologic Treatment If Hypertension Is Double Baseline or Noxious Stimuli Are Unable to Be Eliminated

R: *Use an antihypertensive agent with rapid onset and short duration while the causes of autonomic dysreflexia (AD) are investigated. Nifedipine and nitrates are the most commonly used agents. Nifedipine used should be in the immediate-release form; sublingual nifedipine may lead to erratic absorption. Other drugs to treat AD with severe symptoms include hydralazine mecamylamine, diazoxide, and phenoxybenzamine. If 2% nitroglycerine ointment (or nitropaste) is used, it may be applied to the skin above the level of the spinal cord injury (SCI). For monitored settings, an IV drip of sodium nitroprusside can be used. Blood pressure is monitored (Stephenson, 2014).*

Initiate Health Teaching and Referrals as Indicated

- Teach the signs, symptoms, and treatment of dysreflexia to the individual and family. Advise to carry a wallet-sized card explaining symptoms and treatment for autonomic dysreflexia.
- Teach the indications that warrant immediate medical intervention.
- Explain situations that trigger dysreflexia (menstrual cycle, sexual activity, elimination).
- Teach to watch for early signs and to intervene immediately.
- Teach to observe for early signs of bladder infections and skin lesions (pressure ulcers, ingrown toenails).
- Document the frequency of episodes and precipitating factor(s).
- Provide printed instructions to guide actions during the crisis or to show to other health-care personnel (e.g., dentists, gynecologists).
- Advise athletes with high spinal cord injury about the danger of boosting.

R: *Researchers have reported responses of athletes with spinal cord injuries and in wheelchairs if "boosting" is dangerous. The responses were not dangerous (64.3%), somewhat dangerous (48.9%), dangerous (21.3%), and very dangerous (25.5%) to health.*

Risk for Autonomic Dysreflexia

NANDA-I Definition

Refer to *Autonomic Dysreflexia*.

Risk Factors

Refer to *Autonomic Dysreflexia*—Related Factors.

Key Concepts

Refer to *Autonomic Dysreflexia*.

Focus Assessment Criteria

Refer to *Autonomic Dysreflexia*—Focus Assessment Criteria.

Goal

Refer to *Autonomic Dysreflexia*.

Interventions

Refer to *Autonomic Dysreflexia*.

FRAIL ELDERLY SYNDROME

Frail Elderly Syndrome

Risk for Frail Elderly Syndrome

NANDA-I Definition

Dynamic state of unstable equilibrium that affects the older individual experiencing deterioration in one or more domain of health (physical, functional, psychological, or social) and leads to increased susceptibility to adverse health effects, in particular disability

Defining Characteristics

Presence of a cluster of nursing diagnoses (minimum of two) occurring simultaneously:

Activity Intolerance
Bathing self-care deficit
Decreased cardiac output
Dressing self-care deficit
Fatigue
Feeding self-care deficit
Hopelessness
Imbalanced nutrition: less than body requirements
Impaired memory
Impaired physical mobility
Impaired walking
Social isolation
Toileting self-care deficit

Related Factors

Abnormal function in inflammatory systems
Abnormal function in neuroendocrine systems
Alteration in cognitive functioning
Chronic illness
Depression
History of falls
Living alone
Malnutrition
Poor energy regulation
Prolonged hospitalization
Psychiatric disorder
Sarcopenia
Sarcopenic obesity
Sedentary lifestyle
Stress

Author's Note

Frail Elderly Syndrome and *Risk for Frail Elderly Syndrome* are newly accepted NANDA–I nursing diagnoses. According to the NANDA-I definition, syndrome nursing diagnoses are comprised of a cluster of nursing diagnoses. The etiology of all the nursing diagnoses in the cluster is the effects of the frail elderly condition. Thus *Frail Elderly Syndrome* does not have related factors. The interventions for *Frail Elderly Syndrome* are focused on reducing or preventing nursing diagnoses in the cluster.

Risk for Frail Elderly Syndrome represents a significant clinical condition, which nurses can address to prevent or reduce. In addition, physical therapists, nutritionists, occupational therapists, and social workers participate in prevention. Lifestyle choices, for example, exercise, socialization, nutrition, can impact its onset and its profound negative effects of functioning.

Key Concepts

Frailty can be Described as a Continuum (Ahmed, Mandel, & Fain, 2007; deVries et al., 2011)

Robust

- No long-term diagnostic characteristics of frailty.

Prefail

- Fewer than three diagnostic characteristics of frailty
- Increased risk of falls, institutionalization, and mortality
- At this stage, frailty syndrome may be reversed.

Fail

- Decline in the measurement of frailty markers over a 3-year period
- Higher risk of falls, institutionalization, and mortality
- Progressive course

Failure to Thrive

- Progressive apathy
- Decreased appetite
- Irreversible functional decline
- Last stage resulting in death
- Lifestyle factors over the lifespan, such as physical inactivity, inadequate nutrition, alcohol intake, and obesity, may impact the development of frail elderly syndrome.
- "Obesity is associated with the frailty syndrome in older women in cross-sectional data. This association remains significant even when multiple conditions associated with frailty are considered" (*Blaum, Xue, Michelon, Semba, Fried, 2005).
- Other health conditions, such as cardiovascular risk factors, diabetes, infections, subclinical vascular disease, cholesterol, and high blood pressure, may contribute to the development of frail elderly syndrome.
- Screening is most helpful early when interventions are most effective (Pijpers, Ferreira, Stehouwer, Nieuwenhuijzen, & Kruseman, 2012).
- There are eight factors that place an elder at risk. Physical factors include nutritional status, physical activity, mobility, strength, and energy. Psychological factors include cognition and mood, and social factors include lack of social contacts and social support (deVries et al., 2011).
- Frailty syndrome is characterized by a reduced functional reserve and impaired adaptive capacity resulting from cumulative decline of multiple subsystems, and causes increased vulnerability leading to adverse outcomes (Xue, 2011).
- Dysregulation in multiple physiologic systems, especially stress response systems, is a key feature of frailty. The basis of this dysregulation is likely related to age-related molecular changes (DNA damage, cell senescence, and mitochondrial dysfunction), genetics, and specific inflammatory disease states. This results in anorexia, osteopenia, decreased immune function, cognition, glucose metabolism, and increased clotting (Walston, 2013; *Walston et al., 2006).
- The risk factors of frailty are multidimensional. Physiologic factors, psychological and emotional state, coping, and social and environmental factors and their interaction contribute to unstable equilibrium.
- Fried et al. (*2001) reported "the overall prevalence of frailty in this community-dwelling population was 6.9%; it increased with age and was greater in women than men. Four-year incidence was 7.2%. Frailty was associated with being African American, having lower education and income, poorer health, and having higher rates of comorbid chronic diseases and disability.
- There is an overlap between frailty, chronic disease, and disability; each is separate clinical condition.
- Heart failure, renal impairment, stroke, osteoarthritis of hip and knee, and depression are conditions most highly associated with frailty (Pijpers et al., 2012).
- The presence of cognitive impairment increases the potential for poor outcomes.

Vitamin D Deficiencies

- The incidence of vitamin D deficiencies has been reported as (Kennel, Drake, & Hurley, 2010)
  - Nursing home/housebound individuals mean age 81 (25% to 50%)
    - Elderly ambulatory women, aged >80 years (0% to 25%)
    - Women with osteoporosis, aged 70 to 79 years (30%)
    - Individuals with hip fractures; mean age, 77 years (23%)
  - Adult hospitalized patients; mean age, 62 years (57%)
    - African American women, aged 15 to 49 years (42%)
- Vitamin D supplementation is effective for fall prevention and improving balance. In one report, lower serum levels of 25-hydroxyvitamin D (<20.0 ng/mL) were associated with a higher prevalence of frailty

at baseline in a group of 1,600 men over age 65, but did not predict greater risk for developing frailty at 4.6 years (Walston, 2013).

Obesity and Frailty

- "Although obesity is well known to be associated with disability, its association with the frailty syndrome is less obvious, particularly because frailty is considered a wasting disorder and weight loss is a possible but not necessary component of the syndrome of frailty" (*Blaum et al., 2005, p. 927).
- Blaum et al. (*2001) reported that several researchers have described a distinct syndrome of "sarcopenic obesity" 10–13% in obese people with a mismatch between fat and muscle. This syndrome is known to be strongly associated with decreased strength and increased mobility disability. Biochemical markers associated with frailty are higher in overweight people, particularly inflammatory markers such as C-reactive protein (CRP) and IL-6.14

Focus Assessment Criteria

Frailty phenotype or observable properties are defined as three or more of the following five criteria. Prefrailty is defined as one or two of these characteristics, and not frail has none of the five criteria below (Fried et al., 2001; Walston, 2013).

- Weight loss (≥5% of body weight in last year)
- Exhaustion (positive response to questions regarding effort required for activity)
- Weakness (decreased grip strength)
- Slow walking speed (gait speed) (>6 to 7 seconds to walk 15 feet)
- Decreased physical activity (kcals spent per week: males expending <383 kcal and females <270 kcal)

Refer to diagnosis *Risk for Frail Elderly Syndrome.*

Goals

The individual and/or significant other will engage in comfort care as evidenced by the following indicators:

Reports a reduction in specified symptoms
Describes his or her personal wishes/decisions
Reports an increase in social interactions with significant others
Plans for care transition to new health-care setting, if anticipated

Interventions

Identify Causative and Contributing Factors

- Refer to *Risk for Frail Elderly Syndrome.*
- Refer to *Adult Failure to Thrive.*

Weigh Benefits and Risks of Health-Care Interventions With Individual/Significant Others

- Once frail elderly syndrome has been diagnosed, counsel the individual and care provider on the benefits and risks of health interventions.
- Provide information on health interventions and allow opportunity for informed choices about their care.

R: *Since frailty is a vulnerable state, all invasive procedures or harmful medications should be evaluated in relation to risk versus benefits (Clegg, Young, Lliffe, Rickert, & Rockwood, 2013).*

Palliative Care

- Arrange for communication with physician/NP/PA with the individual/family to discuss available treatment options.
- Explore the individual's and significant others' understanding of the individual's relevant medical condition and each one's expectations, hopes, and concerns as related to the medical condition.
- Advocate for individual's expectations with physician/NP/PA and other health-care providers.
- Plan for care transitions by insuring that individual expectations for care are communicated to receiving care facility/health-care provider.

- Encourage open communication between individual and significant others regarding individual's expectations for care.
- Ensure that end-of-life discussions have occurred and relevant documents prepared. For example, living will, power of attorney.
- Assess for sources of discomfort and treat accordingly.

R: *Emergencies in palliative care, when death is expected, are different from those in other medical situations, which, if left untreated, will immediately threaten life. In palliative care, if the condition left untreated seriously threatens the quality of remaining life, interventions may be indicated (Carpenito, 2014). Frailty is an ongoing process. Movement to a level of worse frailty more commonly occurs than improvement in frailty. Frailty often leads to decline and increased frailty and places an individual at a higher risk for worsening disability, falls, admissions to hospitals and long-term care facilities, and death (Clegg et al., 2013).*

Initiate Health Teaching and Referrals as Needed

- Refer to Home Health Agency for an in-home nursing assessment.
- Refer to Social Service for occupational therapy and/or physical therapy.

R: The home environment should be assessed to evaluate safety and adequacy/availability of self-care aids, for example, bathing, toileting, meals (access, quality), support systems (availability, effectiveness).

Risk for Frail Elderly Syndrome

NANDA-I Definition

Vulnerable to a dynamic state of unstable equilibrium that affects the older individual experiencing deterioration in one or more domain of health (physical, functional, psychological, or social) and leads to increased susceptibility to adverse health effects, in particular disability.

Risk Factors

Activity intolerance*
Age >70 years
Alteration in cognitive functioning
Altered clotting processes (e.g. Factor VII, D-dimers)*
Anorexia*
Anxiety
Average daily physical activity is less than recommended for gender and age*
Chronic illness
Constricted life space
Decrease in energy*
Decrease in muscle strength*
Decrease in serum 25-hydroxyvitamin D concentration
Depression
Economically disadvantaged
Endocrine regulatory dysfunction (e.g., glucose intolerance, increase in IGF-1, androgen, DHEA, and cortisol)
Ethnicity other than Caucasian
Exhaustion*
Fear of falling
Female gender
History of falls*
Immobility
Impaired balance*
Impaired mobility*
Insufficient social support*
Living alone
Low educational level
Malnutrition*
Muscle weakness*
Obesity
Prolonged hospitalization
Sadness*
Sarcopenia (age-related loss of skeletal muscle and muscle strength), sarcopenic obesity
Sedentary lifestyle
Sensory deficit (e.g., visual, hearing)
Social isolation*
Social vulnerability (e.g., disempowerment, decreased life control)
Suppressed inflammatory response (e.g., IL-6, CRP)*
Unintentional loss of 25% of body weight over one year*
Unintentional weight loss > 10 pounds (>4.5 kg) in one year*
Walking 15 feet requires > 6 seconds (4 m > 5 seconds)*
Weakness in grip strength (related to BMI, gender) in lowest 20% of population*

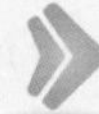

Carp's Cues

Asterisks (*) in the above list indicate that they are defining characteristics or signs/symptoms of frail elderly syndrome, not risk factors (determined in collaboration with this diagnosis, contributor—Collen Galambos).

Key Concepts

Refer to *Frail Elderly Syndrome.*

Focus Assessment Criteria

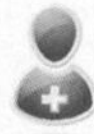

CLINICAL ALERT Frailty phenotype or observable properties are defined as meeting three or more of the following five criteria. Prefrailty is defined as one or two of the following characteristics, and not frail has none.

- Weight loss (≥5% of body weight in last year)
- Exhaustion (positive response to questions regarding effort required for activity)
- Weakness (decreased grip strength)
- Slow walking speed (gait speed) (>6 to 7 seconds to walk 15 feet)
- Decreased physical activity (kcals spent per week: males expending <383 kcal and females <270 kcal) Cognitive impairment was also associated with chronic disability.

Laboratory Findings (Walston, 2013; *Walston et al., 2006; Lab Test Online, 2015)

- Increased C-reactive protein (a protein made by the liver and released into the blood within a few hours after tissue injury, the start of an infection, or other cause of inflammation)
- Increased IL-6 (a protein produced by immune cells that acts on other cells to help regulate and/or promote an immune response)
- Decreased insulin-like growth factor-1 (helps promote normal bone and tissue growth and development)
- Decreased DHEA-S (to evaluate adrenal gland function to help diagnose tumors, adrenal cancers, congenital adrenal hyperplasia, and adult-onset adrenal hyperplasia)
- Increased cortisol (Cortisol is a hormone that plays a role in the metabolism of proteins, lipids, and carbohydrates.)
- 25-hydroxyvitamin D (<20.0 ng/mL) has been associated with muscle weakness and frailty in older adults) (Ensrud et al., 2011).

Assess for Related Factors

Refer to Related Factors.

Assessment Models

The Five Phenotype Model (Fried Ferrucci, Darer, Williamson, & Anderson, 2004)

Weight loss: self-reported, more than 4.5 kg or weight loss of greater than or equal to 5% per year

Self-reported exhaustion: Using the US Center for Epidemiological Studies Depression Scale (3 to 4 days/week or most of the time)

Low energy expenditure: <383 kcal/week (men) or <270 kcal/week (women)

Slow gait speed: standardized cutoff times to walk 4.57 m, stratified by sex and height

Weak grip strength: grip strength stratified by sex and body mass index

Objective Data and Physical Assessment

Use Five Phenotype Model criteria listed above. Add a cognitive assessment tool.

Obtain history of weight loss, exhaustion, energy level.

Measure walking time using a 15-foot walk test.

Obtain grip strength using a dynamometer.

Sarcopenia, or age-related loss of skeletal muscle and muscle strength, is a key physiologic component of frailty.

The Cumulative Deficit Model (*Rockwood, 2005)

Frailty is defined by the presence of symptoms, signs, abnormal laboratory values, disease states, and disabilities.

The Frailty Index is used which calculates the cumulative effect of individual deficits.

Additional Assessment Options

A standardized frailty instrument tool.
A standard cognitive assessment tool.
A standard depression scale.
Balance and gait performance (Get-up-and-Go test)
Fatigue scale
Depression assessment
Home assessment
Social supports (availability)
Medical history including diagnosis and prognosis for each diagnosis or health problem

Goals

The individual will contribute to an increase in functional ability as evidenced by the following indicators:

- Manages all illnesses contributing to functional weakness
- Participates in muscle strengthening exercises
- Improves nutritional intake
- Enhances social support system
- Demonstrates optimism with choices

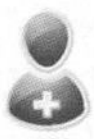

Clinical Alert "Although many different strategies may be used in treating vitamin D deficiency, a common oversight in management is to stop treatment or provide inadequate vitamin D maintenance dosing once the 25-(OH)D level reaches the optimal range. Regardless of initial vitamin D therapy, and assuming no change in lifestyle or diet, a maintenance/prevention daily dose of 800 to 2000 IU or more will be needed to avoid recurrent deficiency". "Others may appear robust but tolerate medical stress poorly, and never regain full function following illness or hospitalization." "Still others are noted to have gradual but unrelenting functional decline in the absence of apparent stress factors" (Walston, 2013).

Interventions

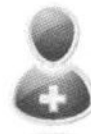

Clinical Alert Frailty and disability are two different but related health conditions. Frailty can be present without disability. There is an overlap between frailty and comorbidity with comorbidity defined as two or more of the following nine diseases: myocardial infarction, angina, congestive heart failure, claudication, arthritis, cancer, diabetes, hypertension, and chronic obstructive pulmonary disease (Clegg et al., 2013).

Identify Causative and Contributing Factors

- Refer to Related Factors.

Encourage a Positive Attitude to Promote Engagement (Refer to Appendix D for Practical Strategies to Increase Engagement in Self Health Management)

- Interact in a friendly, approachable, nonjudgmental style.
- Role model positive interaction.
- Encourage positive interaction between individual and family members/care providers.

Engage the Individual to Assess Their Life Style and Acceptable Alternatives

R: *Some factors that contribute to frailty in older adults can be prevented.*

Sedentary Life Style

- Explore activities daily and weekly. Elicit from individual options to increase motion.
- Emphasize walking as little as a mile in a one-week period was associated with a slower progression of functional limitations.
- Develop home-based exercise program to increase muscle functioning
  - Plan exercises based on strength and capabilities.
  - Encourage an exercise regime working up to 30 minutes a day three times/week.
  - Exercises should focus on strength and balance for optimal effect.
- Refer to *Sedentary Lifestyle* if the person has no physical barriers to increasing mobility or to *Impaired Physical Mobility* if a progressive ambulation program is indicated.

R: *Exercise is believed to be the most effective of all interventions proposed to improve quality of life and functionality in older adults. The demonstrated benefits of exercise in older adults include increased mobility, enhanced performance of activities of daily living (ADL), improved gait, decreased falls, improved bone mineral density, and increased general well-being. Exercise also reduces sarcopenia, or age-related loss of skeletal muscle and muscle strength, which is a key physiologic component of frailty (Clegg et al., 2013; Walston, 2013).*

Inadequate Nutrition

R: *In general, older adults need the same kind of balanced diet as any other group, but fewer calories. Diets of older individuals, however, tend to be insufficient in iron, calcium, and vitamins. The combination of long-established eating patterns, income, transportation, housing, social interaction, and the effects of chronic or acute disease influence nutritional intake and health (Miller, 2015).*

Encourage Nutritional Intake and Good Eating Habits

- Counsel individual and care provider on the importance of good nutrition.
- Identify any barriers that prevent nutritional intake and resolve barriers.
- Identify ways to promote appetite.
- Arrange for a nutritional consultation.

R: *The term nutritional frailty has been used to describe inadequate nutrition in the frail elderly associated with a variety of physical and social health problems (Byard, 2015).*

- Refer also to *Imbalanced Nutrition* for specific interventions.

Obesity (BMI >30)

R: *Obesity is associated with the frailty syndrome in older women in cross-sectional data. This association remains significant even when multiple conditions associated with frailty are considered (*Blaum et al., 2005).*

- Refer to *Obesity* or *Overweight* for specific interventions.

Impaired Mobility

- Refer to *Impaired Physical Mobility* if a progressive ambulation program is indicated.

Compromised Cognition

- Refer also to *Chronic Confusion*, *Acute Confusion*, or *Impaired Memory*.

Inadequate Socialization

Increase Social Support Network

- Explore barriers to connecting with social contacts and offer suggestions on how to resolve barriers.
- Explore with individual available personal and community resources to increase social support.
- Develop a plan to make contact with one or two identified resources. Increase connections according to individual's capabilities.
- Check on progress toward increasing connections.
- Refer to *Risk for Loneliness*, *Social Isolation*, *Compromised Family Coping*, or *Disabled Family Related to Multiple Stressors Associated with Elder Care*.

Impaired Self Care

- Refer to *Self-Care Deficits*.

Arrange for a Comprehensive Interdisciplinary Geriatric Assessment

- Involve a geriatrician or primary care physician with interdisciplinary team of geriatric nurse, social worker, occupational therapist, and physiotherapists.
- Obtain assessment covering health, physical, psychiatric, psychosocial, and restorative/rehabilitation capability.
- Based on this assessment, develop a plan of treatment.

R: *"Comprehensive geriatric assessment has become the internationally accepted method to assess elderly people in clinical practice. Comprehensive geriatric assessment is sensitive to the reliable detection of degrees of frailty" (Clegg et al., 2013).*

Arrange for a Medication Review and Develop a Self-Medication Program

- Consult with geriatrician, APRN, or NP with geriatric expertise, and pharmacist, and conduct a review of all medications and over-the-counter supplements taken by the individual.
- Assess individual's ability to manage medications independently.
- Arrange for a care provider to administer medications to individuals who are not independent in this skill.
- Provide education and training to individual and care provider on prescribed medications and proper ways to administer them.

R: *"Unrecognized drug side effects as well as drug-drug interactions can cause unexpected adverse effects that can predispose patients to weakness, slowness (both physical and mental) and falls"* (Palace & Flood-Sukhdeo, 2014).

Explain the Effects of Vitamin D Deficiency If Indicated and the Importance of Lifelong Replacement With Periodic Laboratory Monitoring (Kennel et al., 2010)

R: *"Even if regularly exposed to sunlight, elderly people produce 75% less cutaneous D3 than young adults"* (Kennel et al., 2010). *"Muscle weakness due to vitamin D deficiency is predominantly of the proximal muscle groups and is manifested by a feeling of heaviness in the legs, tiring easily, and difficulty in mounting stairs and rising from a chair; the deficiency is reversible with supplementation"* (Janssen, Samson, & Verhaar, 2002).

Initiate Health Teaching and Referrals as Needed

- If family members/care providers are stressed, refer to community resources such as support groups, online resources, or hot lines for care providers.

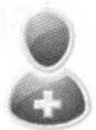

CLINICAL ALERT "A common oversight in management is to stop treatment or provide inadequate vitamin D maintenance dosing once the 25(OH)D level reaches the optimal range. Regardless of initial vitamin D therapy, and assuming no change in lifestyle or diet, a maintenance/prevention daily dose of 800 to 2000 IU or more will be needed to avoid recurrent deficiency" (Kennel et al., 2010).

RISK FOR ELECTROLYTE IMBALANCE

See also *Risk for Complications of Electrolyte Imbalance* in Section 3.

NANDA-I Definition

At risk for a change in serum electrolyte levels that may compromise health

Risk Factors*

Endocrine dysfunction
Diarrhea
Fluid imbalance (e.g., dehydration, water intoxication)
Impaired regulatory mechanisms (e.g., diabetes insipidus, syndrome of inappropriate secretion of antidiuretic hormones)
Renal dysfunction
Treatment-related side effects (e.g., medications, drains)
Vomiting

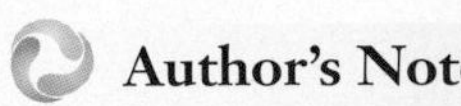

Author's Note

This NANDA-I diagnosis is a collaborative problem. Refer to Section 3 for *Risk for Complications of Electrolyte Imbalances*.

DISTURBED ENERGY FIELD

NANDA-I Definition

Disruption of the flow of energy surrounding a person's being that results in disharmony of the body, mind, and/or spirit.

Defining Characteristics*

Perception of changes in patterns of the energy flow, such as

- Temperature change (warmth, coolness)
- Visual changes (image, color)
- Disruption of the field (vacant, hole, spike, bulge, obstruction, congestion, diminished flow in energy field)
- Movement (wave, spike, tingling, dense, flowing)
- Sounds (tone, word)

Related Factors

Pathophysiologic

Related to slowing or blocking of energy flows secondary to:*

Illness (specify)
Pregnancy
Injury

Treatment Related

Related to slowing or blocking of energy flow secondary to:

Immobility*
Perioperative experience*
Labor and delivery*
Chemotherapy

Situational (Personal, Environmental)

Related to slowing or blocking of energy flow secondary to:

Pain*
Grieving*
Fear*
Anxiety*

Maturational

Related to age-related developmental difficulties or crises* (specify)

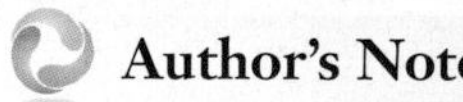

Author's Note

This diagnosis is unique for two reasons: (1) It represents a specific theory (human energy field theory) and (2) its interventions require specialized instruction and supervised practice. Meehan (*1991) recommends the following preparation:

- At least 6 months of professional practice in an acute care setting
- Guided learning by a nurse with at least 2 years of experience
- Conformance with practice guidelines
- Thirty hours of instruction in the theory and practice
- Thirty hours of supervised practice with relatively healthy people
- Successful completion of written and practice evaluations

Some may consider this diagnosis unconventional. Nurses may need to be reminded that there are many theories, philosophies, and frameworks of nursing practice, just as there are many definitions of clients and practice settings. Some nurses practice on street corners with homeless people, whereas others practice in offices attached to their homes. Nursing diagnosis should not represent only mainstream nursing (acute care, long-term care, home health). Nurses should celebrate diversity despite opinions that this diagnosis has little applicability. Fundamentally, nurses are all connected through the quest to improve the condition of individuals, families, groups, and communities.

Key Concepts

- Janet Mentgen, the founder of HEALING TOUCH, identified seven principles of self-care for healers as (Mentgen, 2007) follows:
  - Physical Clearing takes care of your physical body, your physical existence.
  - Emotional Clearing expresses your hurts, your pains.
  - Mental Clearing changes your cognitive thought process.
  - Sacred Space your sacred space at home, your sacred space when you are away.
  - Silence the silence of meditation, Holy silence.
  - Holy Leisure brings balance into your life, restores.
  - Holy Relationships being committed to your relationships.

  Note: Accessed the complete article at www.creativepathwaysinc.com/wp-content/uploads/2014/10/july2007.pdf
- Therapeutic touch is rooted in Eastern philosophy. The cultural orientation of Western medicine is to conduct research to explain a modality's effects. In the Eastern culture, if something works, research is unnecessary for proof. Western researchers have validated positive effects with no noted adverse effects.
- Weymouth (2002) explained that one of the theories on which healing touch is based "is that the human body has an energy field that interpenetrates and extends several feet from it in all directions" (p. 49). She said that some healers can feel the human energy field, and others may see it. "The healing practitioner uses her or his hands to influence the energy field in such a way as to bring harmony and balance to it" (p. 50).
- Therapeutic touch is derived from the basic premise that universal life energy sustains all living organisms. Health is defined as the state in which all of a client's energies are in harmony or dynamic balance. Health is compromised when there is disequilibrium, blockage, or deficits in energy flow (*Macrae, 1988).
- In nursing, the Rogerian conceptual system has provided the foundation for therapeutic touch. This model affirms that energy fields are fundamental units of human beings and their environment (*Meehan, 1991).
- "Therapeutic touch is a knowledgeable and purposive patterning of the patient–environmental energy field process" (*Meehan, 1991). It requires specialized instruction and supervised practice. See the Author's Note for recommended preparation.
- Life-giving, healing energy flows within the universal flow of energy. Such energy, present in all living systems, is composed of intelligence, order, and compassion (*Bradley, 1987).
- Rogers states that therapeutic touch is an example of how a nurse "seeks to strengthen the coherence and integrity of human and environmental fields and to knowingly participate in the patterning of human and environmental fields for the realization of optimum well-being" (*Meehan, 1991).
- *Wardell and Weymouth (2004) reported on a review of the literature on touch, through June 2003. Significant findings were reported after therapeutic touch sessions.
  - Individuals with cancer reported improvement in intrapersonal relations and a reduction in pain (seven out of nine studies).
  - Elderly individuals reported enhanced appetite and sleep quality, decrease pain, angry outbursts, and restlessness.
  - Individuals post hysterectomy reported decreased BP, pulse, and use of narcotics for pain.
- In a pilot study, Quinn and Strelkauskas (*1993) found that all the recipients of therapeutic touch experienced dramatic increases in all dimensions of positive effect (joy, vigor, contentment, and affection) and dramatic decreases in all dimensions of negative effect (anxiety, guilt, hostility, and depression). They also identified a shift in consciousness during therapeutic touch, which was measured by perception of time. The practitioner and the recipients reported the same time distortions, indicating a shift in consciousness.
- The use of healing touch with critically ill people resulted in no physiologic change before, during, or after therapy; however, recipients experienced significant improvements in relaxation and sleep (*Umbreit, 2000).
- An intrinsic relationship may exist between therapeutic touch and the placebo effect. Therapeutic touch may enhance the placebo effect and reduce discomfort and distress (*Meehan, 1998).
- Denison (*2004) reported that clients with fibromyalgia syndrome reported a decrease in pain with therapeutic touch. Using thermography, there was also an increase in cutaneous skin temperature.

Focus Assessment Criteria

Because assessment of the energy field is quickly followed by the intervention, and reassessment continues throughout, refer to Interventions for assessment.

Goals

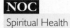

NOC
Spiritual Health

The individual will report relief of symptoms after therapeutic touch as evidenced by the following indicators:

- Reports increased sense of relaxation
- Reports decreased pain, using a scale of 0 to 10 before and after therapies
- Have slower, deeper respirations

Interventions

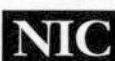

NIC
Therapeutic Touch, Spiritual Support, Presence

Note: The following phases of therapeutic touch are learned separately but rendered concurrently. Presentation of these interventions is to describe the process for nurses who do not practice therapeutic touch. This discussion may help them to support colleagues who practice therapeutic touch and also to initiate referrals. As discussed before, preparation for therapeutic touch requires specialized instruction, which is beyond the scope of this book. Refer to the reference Nurse Healers Professional Associates International for Standards.

Prepare the Individual and Environment for Therapeutic Touch (TT) (Bulbrook & Mentgen, 2009)

- Provide as much privacy as possible.
- Explain therapeutic touch and obtain verbal permission to perform it.
- Give the individual permission to stop the therapy at any time.
- Allow the individual to assume a comfortable position (e.g., lying on a bed, sitting on a couch).

R: *Early beliefs regarding therapeutic touch attributed its effects to an energy transfer and exchange between practitioner and recipient (*Quinn, 1989). Current beliefs are that the practitioner shifts "consciousness into a state that may be thought of as a 'healing meditation,' facilitates repatterning of the recipient's energy field through the process of resonance, rather than 'energy exchange or transfer'" (*Quinn & Strelkauskas, 1993).*

R: *The practitioner of therapeutic touch facilitates the flow of healing energy (*Umbreit, 2000).*

Shift From a Direct Focus on the Environment to an Inner Focus

- Perceived as the center of life within the nurse (centering)

R: *Centering allows the entry of healing (*Krieger, 1997).*

Assess the Individual

- Scan the client's energy field for openness and symmetry (*Krieger, 1987).
- Move the palms of your hands toward the individual, at a distance of 2 to 4 inches over his or her body, from head to feet in a smooth, light movement.
- Use calm and rhythmic hand movements.
- Sense the cues to energy imbalance (e.g., warmth, coolness, tightness, heaviness, tingling, and emptiness).

R: *This TT practitioner recognizes what is known and what is felt.*

Facilitate a Rhythmic Flow of Energy

- Moving hands vigorously from head to toe (unruffling/clearing)

R: *Unruffling enhances the energy flows in the healer's system (*Krieger, 1997).*

Focus Intent on the Specific Repatterning of Areas of Imbalance and Impeded Flow

- Using your hands as focal points, move them gently, sweeping from head to feet one time.
- Note the energy flow over lower legs and feet.
- If the energy flow is not open in this area, continue to move your hands or hold the feet physically to facilitate energy flow.
- Briefly shake your hands to dispel congestion from the field if needed.

- When therapeutic touch is complete, place your hands over the solar plexus area (just above the waist) and focus on facilitating the flow of healing energy to the individual.
- Provide the individual with an opportunity to rest.

R: *This corrects energy imbalance (*Krieger, 1987).*

Encourage the Individual to Provide Feedback

- Assess if the individual exhibits a relaxation response. Signs include drops of several decibels in voice volume; slower, deeper respirations; audible sign of relaxation; and a peripheral flush perceived on face.

Document Both the Procedure and the Feedback

R: *"At the core of the therapeutic touch process is the intent of the practitioner to help the recipient" (*Quinn & Strelkauskas, 1993). The practitioner focuses entirely on the recipient with unconditional love and compassion. The healer is intentionally motivated to help the recipient, who is willing to accept the change.*

R: *TT can promote feelings of calm, peace, well-being, and comfort (*Kierman, 2002).*

- Provide therapeutic touch to
  - Reduce acute pain (Monroe, 2009), chronic pain (Hart, 2008).
  - Reduce agitation in individuals with dementia (Woods, Craven, & Whitney, 2005).
  - Promote sleep (*Heidt, 1990, *Wardell & Weymouth, 2004).
  - Promote physiologic defense mechanisms (e.g., fibroblast proliferation) (Gronowicz, McCarthy, & Jhaveri, 2006), increase hemoglobin (*Movaffaghi, Hasanpoor, Farsi, Hooshmand, & Abrishami, 2006), and increase CD4 cell concentration (*Turner et al., 1998).
  - Improve activities of daily living in older adults.

R: *The results of a randomized, control study reported that the "Healing Touch group showed a small but clinically relevant improvement in the Basic Activities of Daily Living (BADL) subscale (median 0.0, interquartile range 0.0, +1.0), while the placebo group showed a small but clinically relevant decline (median 0.0, interquartile range –1.0, 0.0)" (Wicking, 2012).*

  - Increase sense of consecutiveness with decreased depression (Van Aken & Taylor, 2010).
  - Effectively decrease pain and fatigue of the cancer patients undergoing chemotherapy (Aghabati, Mohammadi, & Esmaiel, 2010).

R: *The clinical efficacy of healing touch is supported as a supportive care modality for many medical conditions, discomforts overall functioning (Anderson & Taylor, 2011).*

COMPROMISED ENGAGEMENT

Behavior of person and/or caregiver that fails to coincide with a health-promoting or therapeutic plan because of barriers in the individual/family, with health-care providers and/or the health-care system, which fail to strengthen patient activation (Carpenito, 2015).

Risk for Compromised Engagement

Vulnerable to behavior of person and/or caregiver that fails to coincide with a health-promoting or therapeutic plan because of barriers between the individuals and the health-care providers and/or the health-care system, which fail to strengthen patient activation, which may compromise heath (Carpenito, 2015)

Readiness for Enhanced Engagement

A pattern of choosing a course of action that is sufficient for meeting short- and long-term health-related decisions and goals that can be strengthened

IMPAIRED ENVIRONMENTAL INTERPRETATION SYNDROME

NANDA-I Definition

Consistent lack of orientation to person, place, time, or circumstances over more than 3 to 6 months necessitating a protective environment

Defining Characteristics*

Major (Must Be Present, One or More)

Consistent disorientation
Chronic confusional states

Minor (May Be Present)

Loss of occupation
Inability to concentrate
Loss of social functioning
Inability to reason
Slow in responding to questions
Inability to follow simple directions

Related Factors

Dementia* (Alzheimer's disease, multi-infarct dementia, Pick's disease, AIDS dementia)
Parkinson's disease
Huntington's disease*
Depression*
Alcoholism

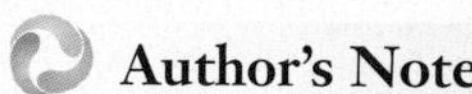

Author's Note

Environmental Interpretation Syndrome describes an individual who needs a protective environment because of consistent lack of orientation to person, place, time, or circumstances. This diagnosis is described under *Chronic Confusion, Wandering,* and *Risk for Injury.* Interventions focus on maintaining maximum level of independence and preventing injury. Until clinical research differentiates this diagnosis from the aforementioned diagnoses, use *Chronic Confusion, Wandering,* or *Risk for Injury* depending on the data presented.

FATIGUE

NANDA-I Definition

An overwhelming sustained sense of exhaustion and decreased capacity for physical and mental work at the usual level

Defining Characteristics*

Reports an unremitting and overwhelming lack of energy
Perceived need for additional energy to accomplish routine tasks
Reports inability to maintain usual routines
Reports feeling tired
Compromised concentration
Compromised libido
Increased physical complaints
Decreased performance

Disinterest in surroundings
Lethargic; drowsy
Reports inability to maintain usual level of physical activity
Increase in physical complaints
Increase in rest requirements
Reports guilt for not keeping up with responsibilities
Reports inability to restore energy even after sleep
Introspection
Listlessness

Related Factors

Many factors can cause fatigue; combining related factors may be useful (e.g., related to muscle weakness, accumulated waste products, inflammation, and infections secondary to hepatitis).

Bio-Pathophysiologic

Related to hypermetabolic state secondary to:

Viruses (e.g., Epstein–Barr)	Fever	Pregnancy*

Related to inadequate tissue oxygenation secondary to:

Chronic obstructive lung disease	Congestive heart failure	Anemia*
Peripheral vascular disease		

Related to biochemical changes secondary to:

Endocrine/Metabolic Disorders

Diabetes mellitus	Pituitary disorders	Acquired immunodeficiency syndrome (AIDS)
Hypothyroidism	Addison's disease	

Chronic Diseases

Renal failure	Cirrhosis	Lyme disease

Related to muscular weakness/wasting secondary to:

Myasthenia gravis	Parkinson's disease	Multiple sclerosis
AIDS	Amyotrophic lateral sclerosis	

Related to hypermetabolic state, competition between body and tumor for nutrients, anemia, and stressors associated with cancer

Related to malnutrition*

Related to nutritional deficits* or changes in nutrient metabolism secondary to:

Nausea	Side effects of medications	Vomiting
Gastric surgery	Diarrhea	Diabetes mellitus

Related to chronic inflammatory process secondary to:

AIDS	Cirrhosis	Arthritis
Inflammatory bowel disease	Lupus erythematosus	Renal failure
Hepatitis	Lyme disease	

Treatment Related

Biochemical changes secondary to:

Chemotherapy	Radiation therapy	Side effects of (specify)

Related to surgical damage to tissue and anesthesia

Related to increased energy expenditure secondary to:

Amputation	Gait disorder	Use of walker, crutches

Situational (Personal, Environmental)

Related to prolonged decreased activity and deconditioning secondary to:

Anxiety*
Nausea/vomiting
Pain
Social isolation
Diarrhea
Obesity
Fever
Depression

Related to excessive role demands

Related to overwhelming emotional demands

Related to extreme stress*

Related to sleep disturbance

Maturational

Child/Adolescent

Related to hypermetabolic state secondary to:

Mononucleosis
Fever

Related to chronic insufficient nutrients secondary to:

Obesity
Excessive dieting
Eating disorders

Related to effects of newborn care on sleep patterns and need for continuous attention

Related to hypermetabolic state during first trimester

Author's Note

Fatigue as a nursing diagnosis differs from acute tiredness. Tiredness is a transient, temporary state (*Rhoten, 1982) caused by lack of sleep, improper nutrition, increased stress, sedentary lifestyle, or temporarily increased work or social responsibilities. *Fatigue* is a pervasive, subjective, drained feeling that cannot be eliminated; however, the nurse can assist the person to adapt to it. Activity intolerance differs from fatigue in that the nurse will assist the person with activity intolerance to increase endurance and activity.

The focus for the person with fatigue is not on increasing endurance. If the cause resolves or abates (e.g., acute infection, chemotherapy, radiation), *Fatigue* as a diagnosis is discontinued and *Activity Intolerance* can be initiated to focus on improving the deconditioned state.

Individuals with peripheral vascular disease can serve as an example of the difference between *Fatigue* and *Activity Intolerance*. Early in the disease process, the individual is taught to walk as exercise and to walk into the pain (intermittent claudication), rest and to continue walking, this is *Activity Intolerance*. If the person does not exercise and/or continues to use tobacco, the condition will worsen and any walking is severely compromised. The person must plan activities and rest before and after, this is *Fatigue*.

Errors in Diagnostic Statements

***Fatigue* related to feelings of lack of energy for routine tasks**

When a person reports insufficient energy for routine tasks, the nurse performs a focus assessment and collects additional data to determine whether *Fatigue* is appropriate or actually a symptom of another diagnosis, such as *Activity Intolerance*, *Ineffective Coping*, *Interrupted Family Processes*, *Anxiety*, or *Ineffective Health Maintenance*. When acute or chronic conditions cause fatigue, the nurse must determine whether the person can increase endurance (which would call for *Activity Intolerance*) or needs energy conservation techniques to help accomplish desired activities. When fatigue results from ineffective stress management or poor health habits, *Fatigue* or *Activity Intolerance* is not indicated. During data collection to determine contributing factors, the nurse can record the diagnosis as *Possible Fatigue related to reports of lack of energy*. Using a "possible" diagnosis indicates the need for more data collection to rule out or confirm.

Key Concepts

General Considerations

- Fatigue is a subjective experience with physiologic, treatment-related, and psychological components. Fatigue in chronic diseases correlated strongly with abnormalities in mood, most typically depression and anxiety (Jong, Oudhoffc, & Epskamp, 2010).
- Acute tiredness is an expected response to increased physical exertion, change in daily activities, additional stress, or inadequate sleep. Acute physical fatigue occurs more rapidly in deconditioned muscles (Grossman & Porth, 2014).
- US society values energy, productivity, and vitality. It views those without energy as sluggish or lazy. Fatigue and tiredness are viewed negatively.
- Fatigue can be physical, mental, and motivational. Causes of fatigue are multifactorial. Careful assessment of the causes can indicate specific interventions to reduce them.
- "Fatigue in individuals with a chronic disease is divided into central and peripheral fatigue. Central fatigue results from alterations or abnormalities in neurotransmitter pathways within the central nervous system (CNS)" (Jong et al., 2010).
- Peripheral fatigue results from neuromuscular dysfunction outside the CNS and relates to impaired neurotransmission in peripheral nerves and/or defects in muscular contraction, due to energy depletion, inflammation, joint abnormalities, or muscle wasting. The contribution of peripheral and central fatigue to overall fatigue in individuals may vary significantly between different diseases (Jong et al., 2010).
- Individuals with chronic fatigue have increased sensitivity to serotonin-mediated hypothalamic activation, implying the existence of defective central serotonergic neurotransmission. This contributes to depression (Jong et al., 2010).
- The principal CNS components of the stress response include central corticotrophin-releasing hormone (CRH) and the sympathetic nervous system. Individuals with chronic fatigue have altered diurnal cortisol rhythm and blunted cortisol stress response, producing high stress levels causing fatigue (Jong et al., 2010).
- Self-reported fatigue has been associated with a worsening or altering of all of the following (Gambert, 2013):
    - *Physical function*: reduced activities, prolonged periods of rest, uncoordinated movements, increased risk of falling, and increased need for assistance to meet basic activities of daily living and instrumental activities of daily living
    - *Cognition*: reduced alertness, decreased concentration, reduced clarity of thoughts, and increased forgetfulness
    - *Emotional state*: increased anger, emotional lability, and depression
    - *Social isolation*: complete or near-complete lack of contact with other persons
- In addition, fatigue is an independent predictor of mortality and has been associated with a significant reduction in overall functional status (Gambert, 2013).
- Cancer-related fatigue has been reported in 35% to 100% of cases and is reported to be the most distressing side effect. Stressors contributing to fatigue in individuals with cancer are illustrated in Box II.1.
- The fatigue related to radiation is unexplained but may be related to increased metabolic effort by the body to repair damage caused by the radiotherapy to healthy cells.
- Women receiving localized radiation to the breast reported that fatigue decreased in the second week but increased and reached a plateau after week 4 until 3 weeks after treatment ceased. Fatigue levels did not change significantly on weekends between treatments (*Greenberg, Sawicka, Eisenthal, & Ross, 1992; Haas, 2011).
- When fatigue is a side effect of treatment, it does not resolve when the treatment ends, but gradually lessens over months (*Nail & Winningham, 1997; Bardwell & Ancoli-Israel, 2008).

Pediatric Considerations

- Infants and small children cannot express fatigue. The nurse can elicit this information by interviewing the parents and carefully assessing key functional health patterns (e.g., sleep–rest, activity–exercise [which may reveal respiratory difficulties or activity intolerance], and nutrition–metabolic [which may reveal feeding difficulties]).
- Children at risk for fatigue include those with acute or chronic illness, congenital heart disease, exposure to toxins, prolonged stress, or anemia.
- Children depend on parents/caregivers to modify the environment to mitigate effects of fatigue.

Box II.1 CONTRIBUTING FACTORS TO FATIGUE IN CLIENTS WITH CANCER

Pathophysiologic

Hypermetabolic state associated with active tumor growth
Competition between the body and the tumor for nutrients
Chronic pain
Organ dysfunction (e.g., hepatic, respiratory, gastrointestinal)

Treatment Related

Accumulation of toxic waste products secondary to radiation, chemotherapy
Inadequate nutritional intake secondary to nausea, vomiting
Anemia
Analgesics, antiemetics
Diagnostic tests
Surgery

Situational (Personal, Environmental)

Uncertainty about future
Fear of death, disfigurement
Social isolation
Losses (role responsibilities, occupational, body parts, function, appearance, economic)
Separation for treatments

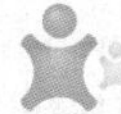

Maternal Considerations

- Fatigue is common in early pregnancy due to increased metabolic requirements (Pillitteri, 2014).
- Gardner reported that levels of fatigue in postpartum women increased at 2 weeks but decreased by 6 weeks. Factors associated with high postpartum fatigue were sleep alterations, additional children, child care problems, less household help, less education, low family income, and young age of mother (*Gardner, 1991; Pillitteri, 2014).
- "Postpartum fatigue is particularly challenging, because the new mother has demanding life tasks to accomplish during this period of time. Postpartum fatigue may impact postpartum maternal role attainment and may place a woman at increased risk for postpartum depression" (Corwin & Arbour, 2007).

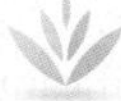

Geriatric Considerations

- "Although fatigue is common among older people, it is frequently underreported and often not even evaluated because, much like pain, it is often identified by both the older individual and his or her family or caregiver(s) as a natural part of the aging process" (Gambert, 2013).
- The normal effects of aging do not in themselves increase the risk of or cause fatigue. Fatigue in older adults has basically the same etiologies as in younger adults. The difference is that older adults tend to experience more chronic diseases than younger adults. Thus, fatigue in older adults is not the result of age-related factors, but related to such risk factors as chronic diseases and medications (Miller, 2015).
- The causes of fatigue in the older adults can be described under the following categories (Gambert, 2013):
  - Organic (infectious, immunologic/rheumatologic), chronic fatigue syndrome, physiologic, neoplastic-related, toxin-related, cardiovascular- and pulmonary disease-related fatigue
  - Medication-related fatigue, for example, nonsteroidal anti-inflammatory drugs, tetracycline, antipsychotics, antidepressants, sleep medications, and pain medications
  - Illicit drug- and alcohol-related fatigue
  - Physiological fatigue, for example, inadequate sleep, insufficient rest, overactivity, poor physical conditioning, stress, and changes in diet
  - Frailty related to weight loss and sarcopenia (degenerative loss of skeletal muscle mass [0.5% to 1% loss per year after the age of 50], quality, and strength associated with aging)
  - Psychogenic fatigue: Psychiatric problems commonly cause fatigue. Depression is the most commonly associated disease entity. Features suggesting that fatigue is psychogenic include fatigue being

present throughout the day, fatigue being present upon awakening, fatigue that improves later in the day, and fluctuations in mood.
- Nutrition lacking sufficient quantities of calories, protein, and/or the essential vitamins and minerals may lead to symptoms of fatigue.
    - Vitamin D-deficient state can cause nonspecific symptoms, such as fatigue, loss of muscle strength, bone and muscle pain, arthralgia, fibromyalgia-like syndromes, poor balance, and low mood.
    - Subclinical vitamin B_{12} deficiency is common in the elderly and can result from absorption problems, proton-pump inhibitor overuse, excessive alcohol intake, or "tea and toast" diets. It can result in fatigue, weight loss, neuropathy, memory impairment, and depression.
- Organic fatigue, the most common causes of which are infectious and immunologic/rheumatologic
- Chronic fatigue syndrome
- Disease-related fatigue, for example, cancer, cardiac, respiratory endocrine
- Toxin-related fatigue, for example, exposure to toxins, such as carbon monoxide and heavy metals. Wood-burning stoves, kerosene heaters, automobile exhaust, and coal-burning plants produce carbon monoxide. Acute exposure to high carbon monoxide levels can cause headaches, dizziness, and flu-like symptoms. When chronic, low-level exposure occurs; however, more subtle symptoms may develop, such as depression, fatigue, confusion, and memory loss (Gambert, 2013).

- According to Miller (2015), "the activity theory proposed that older adults would remain psychologically and socially fit if they remained active." Participation in activities affirms a person's self-concept.
- Chronic fatigue, reported by approximately 70% of older adults, can result in diminished motor activity and muscle tone. Note that anemia, very common in this population, is another possible contributor to complaints of chronic fatigue (Miller, 2015).

Focus Assessment Criteria

Subjective Data

Assess for Defining Characteristics

Description of Fatigue
Onset
Pattern: morning, evening, transient, unfading/all day
Precipitated by what?
Relieved by rest?

Effects of Fatigue on

Activities of daily living	Libido	Concentration
Mood	Leisure activities	Motivation

Assess for Related Factors

Medical Condition (Acute, Chronic; Refer to Key Concepts)

Nutritional Imbalances

Treatments

Chemotherapy	Radiation therapy
Medication side effects	Stressors (e.g., excessive role demands, career, financial, family)

Goals

NOC

Fatigue: Disruptive Effects, Fatigue Level, Self-Management: Chronic Disease, Energy Conservation, Nutritional Status, Depression Level

The person will participate in activities that stimulate and balance physical, cognitive, affective, and social domains as evidenced by the following indicators:

- Discusses the causes of fatigue
- Shares feelings regarding the effects of fatigue on life
- Establishes priorities for daily and weekly activities

Interventions

NIC
Energy Management, Environmental Management, Mutual Goal Setting, Socialization Enhancement, Coping Enhancement, Exercise Therapy

Nursing interventions for this diagnosis are for people with fatigue regardless of etiology that cannot be eliminated. The focus is to assist the individual and family to adapt to the fatigue state.

Assess Causative or Contributing Factors

- If fatigue has related factors that can be treated, refer to the specific nursing diagnosis as
  - Lack of sleep; refer to *Disturbed Sleep Pattern*
  - Poor nutrition; refer to *Imbalanced Nutrition*
  - Sedentary lifestyle; refer to *Sedentary Lifestyle*
  - Inadequate stress management; refer to *Stress Overload*
  - Chronic excessive role or social demands; refer to *Ineffective Coping*

Explain the Causes of Fatigue (See Key Concepts)

R: *In many chronic diseases, fatigue is the most common, disruptive, and distressing symptom, because it interferes with self-care activities (Gambert, 2013).*

Allow Expression of Feelings Regarding the Effects of Fatigue on Life

- Identify difficult activities.
- Help the individual verbalize how fatigue interferes with role responsibilities.
- Encourage the individual to convey how fatigue causes frustration.

Assist to Identify Strengths, Abilities, and Interests

- Identify values and interests.
- Identify areas of success and usefulness; emphasize past accomplishments.
- Use information to develop goals with the individual.
- Assist in identifying sources of hope (e.g., relationships, faith, things to accomplish).
- Assist in developing realistic short- and long-term goals (progress from simple to more complex; use a "goals poster" to indicate type and time for achieving specific goals).

R: *Focusing on strengths and abilities may provide insight into positive events and lessen the tendency to overgeneralize the severity of disease, which can lead to depression.*

Assist the Individual to Identify Energy Patterns

Instruct the Individual to Record Fatigue Levels Every Hour Over 24 Hours; Select a Usual Day

- Ask the individual to rate fatigue using the Rhoten fatigue scale (0 = not tired, peppy; 10 = total exhaustion).
- Record the activities during each rating.

Analyze Together the 24-Hour Fatigue Levels

- Times of peak energy
- Times of exhaustion
- Activities associated with increasing fatigue

Explain Benefits of Exercise and Discuss What Is Realistic

R: *Identifying times of peak energy and exhaustion can aid in planning activities to maximize energy conservation and productivity.*

Explain the Purpose of Pacing and Prioritization

- Explore what activities the individual views as important to maintain self-esteem.
- Attempt to divide vital activities or tasks into components (e.g., preparing menu, shopping, storing, cooking, serving, cleaning up); the individual can delegate some parts and retain others.
- Plan important tasks during periods of high energy (e.g., prepare all meals in the morning).
- Assist the individual in identifying priorities and to eliminate nonessential activities.
- Plan each day to avoid energy- and time-consuming, nonessential decision making.
- Distribute difficult tasks throughout the week.
- Rest before difficult tasks, and stop before fatigue ensues.

R: *The individual requires rest periods before or after some activities. Planning can provide for adequate rest and reduce unnecessary energy expenditure. Such strategies can enable continuation of most desired activities, contributing to positive self-esteem.*

Teach Energy Conservation Techniques

- Modify the environment.
  - Replace steps with ramps.
  - Install grab rails.
  - Elevate chairs from 3 to 4 inches.
  - Organize kitchen or work areas.
  - Reduce trips up and down stairs (e.g., put a commode on the first floor).
  - Use a taxi instead of driving self.
  - Delegate housework (e.g., employ a high school student for a few hours after school).

R: *Strategies can be utilized to decrease energy used in activities of daily living.*

- Discuss with individual some type of appropriate exercise component that could be integrated into their life, for example, strengthening, stretching, chair exercises.

R: *Predictors of healthy longevity are high intake of plant-based foods (fruits, vegetables, nuts), high levels of physical activity, and strong social networks (Hutnik, Smith, & Koch, 2012; Miller, 2015).*

Promote Socialization With Family and Friends (Miller, 2015)

- Encourage to participate in one social activity, weekly.
- Explain that feelings of connectedness decrease fatigue and stress.

R: *Quality or type of activity reportedly is more important than quantity. Informal activities promoted well-being the most, followed by formal structured activities, and last by solitary activities, which were found to have little or no effect on life satisfaction (*Longino & Kart, 1982).*

Explain the Effects of Conflict and Stress on Energy Levels

- Teach the importance of mutuality in sharing concerns.
- Explain the benefits of distraction from negative events.
- Teach and assist with relaxation techniques before anticipated stressful events. Encourage mental imagery to promote positive thought processes.
- Allow the individual time to reminisce to gain insight into past experiences.
- Teach to maximize aesthetic experiences (e.g., smell of coffee, feeling warmth of the sun).
- Teach to anticipate experiences he or she takes delight in each day (e.g., walking, reading favorite book, writing a letter).

R: *Focusing on strengths and abilities may provide insight into positive events and lessen the tendency to overgeneralize the severity of the disease, which can lead to depression.*

- Help to identify how he or she can help others. Listening to others' problems, using the computer to access information and making phone calls

R: *Reciprocity or returning support to one's support system is vital for balanced and healthy relationships (*Tilden & Weinert, 1987). Individuals with fatigue have difficulty with reciprocity.*

Provide Significant Others Opportunities to Discuss Feelings in Private Regarding

- Changes in person with fatigue
- Caretaking responsibilities
- Financial issues
- Changes in lifestyle, role responsibilities, and relationships
- See *Caregiver Role Strain* for additional strategies for caregivers.

Initiate Health Teaching and Referrals, as Indicated

- Counseling
- Community services (Meals On Wheels, housekeeper)
- Financial assistance

Maternal Interventions

- Explain the reasons for fatigue in first and third trimesters:
  - Increased basal metabolic rate
  - Changes in hormonal levels

- Anemia
- Increased cardiac output (third trimester)

- Emphasize the need for naps and 8 hours of sleep each night.

R: *Fatigue in the first and third trimesters is normal.*

- Discuss the importance of exercise (e.g., walking).

R: *Exercise provides emotional and physical benefits.*

- For postpartum women, discuss factors that increase fatigue:
  - Labor more than 30 hours
  - Preexisting chronic disease
  - Hemoglobin less than 10 g/dL or postpartum hemorrhage
  - Episiotomy, tear, or cesarean section
  - Sleeping difficulties
  - Ill newborn or a congenital anomaly
  - Dependent children at home
  - Child care problems
  - Unrealistic expectations
  - No daytime rest periods

R: *Explaining the reasons for fatigue can allay fears. Strategies can be discussed to reduce fatigue at home.*

FEAR

NANDA-I Definition

Response to perceived threat that is consciously recognized as a danger

Defining Characteristics

Verbal Reports of Panic*

Alarm*
Aggression
Apprehension*
Avoidance behaviors*
Being scared*
Decreased self-assurance*
Dread*
Excitement*
Impulsiveness*
Increased alertness*/tension
Narrowed focus on source of the fear*
Panic
Terror*

Visceral–Somatic Activity

Musculoskeletal

Shortness of breath
Fatigue*/limb weakness
Muscle tightness*

Respiratory

Increased rate*
Trembling

Cardiovascular

Palpitations
Rapid pulse*
Increased systolic blood pressure*

Skin

Flush/pallor*
Increased perspiration*
Paresthesia

Gastrointestinal

Anorexia*
Nausea/vomiting
Diarrhea*/urge to defecate
Dry mouth*/throat

Central Nervous System (CNS)/Perceptual

Syncope
Irritability
Insomnia
Absentmindedness
Lack of concentration
Nightmares
Pupil dilation*
Diminished problem-solving ability*

Genitourinary

Urinary frequency/urgency

Related Factors

Fear can be a response to various health problems, situations, or conflicts. Some common sources are indicated next.

Pathophysiologic

Related to perceived immediate and long-term effects of:

Cognitive impairment
Disabling illness
Long-term disability
Loss of body function or part
Sensory impairment
Terminal disease

Treatment Related

Related to loss of control and unpredictable outcome secondary to:

Hospitalization
Invasive procedures
Surgery and its outcome
Radiation
Anesthesia

Situational (Personal, Environmental)

Related to loss of control and unpredictable outcome secondary to:

Change or loss of significant other
Pain
New environment
New people
Success
Divorce
Lack of knowledge
Failure
Related to potential loss of income

Maturational

Preschool (2 to 5 years)

Related to:

Age-related fears
Animals
Being alone
Bodily harm
Dark, strangers, ghosts
Not being liked
Separation from parents, peers
Strangers

School-Age (6 to 12 years)

Related to:

Being lost
Being in trouble
Thunder, lightning
Bad dreams
Weapons

Adolescent (13 to 18 years)

Related to uncertainty of:

Appearance
Scholastic success
Peer support

Adult

Related to uncertainty of:

Marriage
Job security
Pregnancy
Effects of aging
Parenthood

Older Adult

Related to anticipated dependence:

Prolonged suffering
Financial insecurity
Vulnerability to crime
Abandonment

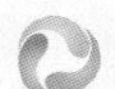

Author's Note

See *Anxiety*.

Key Concepts

General Considerations

- Psychological defense mechanisms are distinctly individual and can be adaptive or maladaptive.
- Fear differs from anxiety in that fear is aroused by an identified threat (specific object); anxiety is aroused by a threat that cannot be easily identified (nonspecific or unknown).
- Both fear and anxiety lead to disequilibrium.
- Anger may be a response to certain fears.
- A sense of adequacy in confronting danger reduces fear. Fear disguises itself. The expressed fear may be a substitute for other fears that are not socially acceptable. Awareness of factors that intensify fears enhances control and prevents heightened feelings. Confronting the safe reality of a situation reduces fear.
- Fear can become anxiety if it becomes internalized and serves to disorganize instead of becoming adaptive.
- Chronic physical reactions to stressors lead to susceptibility and chronic disease.
- Physiologic responses are manifested throughout the body primarily from the hypothalamus' stimulation of the autonomic and endocrine systems.
- People interpret the degree of danger from a threatening stimulus. The physiologic and psychological systems react with equal intensity (elevations in blood pressure and heart and respiratory rates).
- Fear is adaptive and a healthy response to danger.
- Fear differs from *phobia*, an irrational, persistent fear of a circumscribed stimulus (object or situation) other than having a panic attack (panic disorder) or of humiliation or embarrassment in certain social situations (social phobia) (American Psychiatric Association, 2014).

Pediatric Considerations

- Fear is a part of normal development in children. Fear can be a positive adaptive force when it teaches children an awareness of potential danger.
- Infants and small children experience fear but cannot identify the threat verbally. Verbal (crying, protesting) and nonverbal (kicking, biting, holding back) responses are important indicators of children's fear (*Broome, Bates, Lillis, & McGahee, 1990; Hockenberry & Wilson, 2015).
- Fear behaviors are *consistent* and *immediate* on exposure to or mention of a specific stressor; if the response is erratic, the diagnosis more accurately might be anxiety. Refer to the table in the *Delayed Growth and Development* section or the Key Concepts—Pediatric Considerations in the *Anxiety* section.
- Fears throughout childhood follow a developmental sequence and are influenced by culture, environment, and parental fears (Hockenberry & Wilson, 2012).
- Fears are most frequent in 8- to 10-year-old children (*Nicastro & Whetsell, 1999).
- Main fears of different age groups are as follows (Hockenberry & Wilson, 2012; *Nicastro & Whetsell, 1999):
  - *Infants and toddlers (birth to 2 years)*: Fears evolve from physical stimuli (e.g., loud noises, separation from parents/caregivers, strangers, sudden movements, animals, certain situations [i.e., doctor's office]).
  - *Preschoolers (3 to 5 years)*: Fears evolve from real or imagined situations (e.g., injury or mutilation, ghosts, devils, monsters, the dark, bathtub and toilet drains, being alone, dreams, robbers, wild animals, snakes).

- *School-aged children (6 to 8 years)*: Common fears are ghosts, monsters, dark, being alone, thunder, lightning, being lost, kidnapping, guns, and weapons.
- *School-aged children (9 to 12 years)*: Common fears are the dark, being lost or alone, bodily harm, strangers, bad dreams, punishment, grades and tests, and being in trouble.
- *Adolescents:* Fears may be verbalized and include loss of self-control, disturbance to body image, death, separation from peers, inept social performance, sexuality gossip, AIDS, being alone, and war.

- Fear is a momentary reaction to danger related to a low estimate of one's own power over the situation (Hockenberry & Wilson, 2012).

Maternal Considerations

The fears and concerns of pregnancy differ for each trimester.

First Trimester

- Uncertainty about timing of pregnancy
- Uncertainty about her own or her partner's adequacy as parent
- Concerns about material issues (e.g., finances)

Second Trimester

- Fears diminish as the fetus moves
- Decrease in physical symptoms

Third Trimester

- Fears for her own well-being and how she will tolerate labor
- Fears for the well-being of the fetus
- Obsessed with labor and delivery

Geriatric Considerations

- Cesarone (*1991) clustered the sources of fear in the elderly into five categories:
  - Disease, suffering, and falls
  - Dependence and abandonment
  - Dying
  - Illness or death of loved ones
  - Miscellaneous reasons (crime, financial insecurity, diagnostic tests)
- Fear of falling leads to activity avoidance and decline in functioning in up to 76% of older adults living in the community and between 40% and 75% living in long-term facilities (Kim & So, 2013; Lach & Parsons, 2013).

Focus Assessment Criteria

Subjective/Objective Data

Assess for Defining Characteristics

Onset
Have the individual tell you a "story" about his or her fearfulness.

Thought Process and Content
Are thoughts clear, coherent, logical, confused, or forgetful?
Can the individual concentrate or is he or she preoccupied?

Perception and Judgment
Does fear remain after the stressor is eliminated?
Is the fear a response to a present stimulus or distorted by past influences?

Visceral—Somatic Activity
Refer to Defining Characteristics.

Goals

Anxiety Self-Control, Fear Self-Control

The adult will relate increased psychological and physiologic comfort as evidenced by the following indicators:

- Shows decreased visceral response (pulse, respirations)
- Differentiates real from imagined situations
- Describes effective and ineffective coping patterns
- Identifies own coping responses

The child will exhibit or relate increased psychological and physiologic comfort, as evidenced by the following indicators:

- Discusses fears
- Exhibits less crying

Interventions

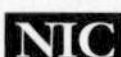

Anxiety Reduction, Coping Enhancement; Presence, Counseling, Relaxation Therapy

Nursing interventions for *Fear* represent interventions for any individual with fear regardless of the etiologic or contributing factors.

Assess Possible Contributing Factors

- Refer to Related Factors.

Reduce or Eliminate Contributing Factors

Unfamiliar Environment

- Orient to environment using simple explanations.
- Speak slowly and calmly.
- Avoid surprises and painful stimuli.
- Use soft lights and music.
- Remove threatening stimulus.
- Plan one-day-at-a-time, familiar routine.
- Encourage gradual mastery of a situation.
- Provide a transitional object with symbolic safeness (security blanket, religious medal).

R: *A quiet, calm professional can communicate calm to the individual (Varcarolis, 2011).*

Intrusion on Personal Space

- Allow personal space.
- Move the individual away from the stimulus.
- Remain with the individual until fear subsides (listen, use silence).
- Later, establish frequent and consistent contacts; use family members and significant others to stay with the individual.
- Use touch as tolerated (sometimes holding the individual firmly helps him or her maintain control).

R: *Minimizing environmental stimuli can help reduce escalation of fear (Varcarolis, 2011).*

Threat to Self-Esteem

- Support preferred coping style when individual uses adaptive mechanisms.
- Initially, decrease the individual's number of choices.
- Use simple, direct statements (avoid detail).
- Give direct suggestions to manage everyday events (some prefer details; others like general explanations).
- Encourage expression of feelings (helplessness, anger).
- Give feedback about expressed feelings (support realistic assessments).
- Refocus interaction on areas of capability rather than dysfunction.
- Encourage normal coping mechanisms.
- Encourage sharing common problems with others.
- Give feedback of effect the individual's behavior has on others.
- Encourage the individual to face the fear.

R: *Open, honest dialogue may help initiate constructive problem solving and can instill hope.*

When Intensity of Feelings Has Decreased, Assist With Insight and Controlling Response

- Bring behavioral cues into the individual's awareness.

R: *Severe fear or panic can interfere with concentrating and information processing (Varcarolis, 2011).*

- Ask to write their fears in narrative form.

R: *Writing down one's fears can give insight and control (*Crossley, 2003).*

- Teach how to solve problems.
  - What is the problem?
  - Who or what is responsible?
  - What are the options?
  - What are the advantages and disadvantages of each option?

R: *Open, honest dialogue may help initiate constructive problem solving and can instill hope.*

Initiate Health Teaching and Referrals, as Indicated

- Progressive relaxation technique
- Reading, music, breathing exercises
- Desensitization, self-coaching
- Thought stopping, guided fantasy
- Yoga, hypnosis, assertiveness training

R: *These methods can increase control and increase comfort or relaxation.*

Pediatric Interventions

Participate in Community Functions to Teach Parents Age-Related Fears and Constructive Interventions (e.g., Parent–School Organizations, Newsletters, Civic Groups)

- Provide child opportunities to talk and write about fears and to learn healthy outlets for anger or sadness, such as play therapy.
- Acknowledge illness, death, and pain as real; refrain from protecting children from the reality of existence; encourage open, honest sharing that is age-appropriate.
- Never make fun of the child. Share with child that these fears are okay.
- Fear of imaginary animals and intruders (e.g., "I don't see a lion in your room, but I will leave the light on for you, and, if you need me again, please call.")
- Fear of parent being late (establish a contingency plan [e.g., "If you come home from school and Mommy is not here, go to Mrs. S next door."]).
- Fear of vanishing down a toilet or bathtub drain:
  - Wait until child is out of the tub before releasing the drain.
  - Wait until child is off the toilet before flushing.
  - Leave toys in bathtub and demonstrate how they do not go down the drain.
- Fear of dogs and cats:
  - Allow child to watch a child and a dog playing from a distance.
  - Do not force child to touch the animal.
- Fear of death (See Key Concepts for *Grieving*.)
- Fear of pain (See Pediatric Interventions for *Pain*.)
- Refusal to go to sleep:
  - Establish a realistic hour for retiring.
  - Contract for a reward if the child is successful.
  - Do not sleep with the child or take the child to the parent's room.
- Discuss with parents the normality of fears in children; explain the necessity of acceptance and the negative outcomes of punishment, shaming, or forcing the child to overcome the fear.
- Provide the child with the opportunity to observe other children cope successfully with the feared object.
- Demonstrate strength and self-confidence.
- Take child's hand and gently guide into shallow water.
- Allow child to watch you pet a dog.

R: *Strategies focus on accepting the child's fear, providing an explanation, if possible, or some form of control. The more successfully a child handles a fearful situation, the more confidence and less vulnerability the child feels (*Nicastro & Whetsell, 1999).*

R: *Desensitization by gradually facing a fearsome object or situation is effective with most children (Hockenberry & Wilson, 2012).*

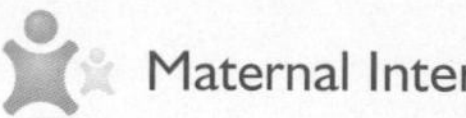
Maternal Interventions

- Provide opportunities to express fears during each trimester.

R: *Fears and concerns change with each trimester.*

- Refer to Key Concepts—Maternal Considerations for specifics.
- Provide opportunities for expectant father to share his concerns and fears.

R: *Expectant fathers are concerned about changes in the relationship with their partner, their competence as a provider/father, and meeting the newly evolving expectations of the mother (Pilitteri, 2014).*

DEFICIENT FLUID VOLUME

Definition

Decreased intravascular, interstitial, and/or intracellular fluid. This refers to dehydration, water loss alone without change in sodium (NANDA-I).

State in which a person who can take fluids (not NPO) experiences or is at risk of experiencing dehydration.[15]

Defining Characteristics

Major (Must Be Present, One or More)

Insufficient oral fluid intake
Dry skin*/mucous membranes*
Negative balance of intake and output
Weight loss

Minor (May Be Present)

Increased serum sodium
Thirst*/nausea/anorexia
Concentrated urine
Urivnary frequency
Decreased* or excessive urine output

Related Factors

Pathophysiologic

Related to excessive urinary output:
Uncontrolled diabetes
Diabetes insipidus (inadequate antidiuretic hormone)

Related to increased capillary permeability and evaporative loss from burn wound (nonacute)

Related to losses secondary to:
Abnormal drainage
Diarrhea
Excessive menses
Fever or increased metabolic rate
Peritonitis
Wound

[15]Added by Lynda Juall Carpenito for clarity and clinical usefulness.

Situational (Personal, Environmental)

Related to vomiting/nausea

Related to decreased motivation to drink liquids secondary to:

Depression
Fatigue

Related to fad diets/fasting

Related to high-solute tube feedings

Related to difficulty swallowing or feeding self secondary to:

Oral or throat pain
Fatigue

Related to extreme heat/sun/dryness

Related to excessive loss through:

Indwelling catheters
Drains

Related to insufficient fluids for exercise effort or weather conditions

Related to excessive use of:

Laxatives or enemas
Diuretics, alcohol, or caffeine

Maturational

Infant/Child

Related to increased vulnerability secondary to:

Decreased fluid reserve and decreased ability to concentrate urine

Older Adult

Related to increased vulnerability secondary to:

Decreased fluid reserve and decreased sensation of thirst

Author's Note

Deficient Fluid Volume is used frequently to describe individuals who are NPO, in hypovolemic shock, or experiencing bleeding. This author recommends its use only when an individual can drink but has an insufficient intake for metabolic needs or excessive losses. If the person cannot drink or needs intravenous therapy, refer to the collaborative problems in Section 3, *Risk for Complications of Hypovolemia* and *Risk for Complications of Electrolyte Imbalances*.

Should *Deficient Fluid Volume* be used to represent such clinical situations as shock, renal failure, or thermal injury? Most nurses would agree that these are collaborative problems that require nursing and medical interventions for treatment.

Errors in Diagnostic Statements

Risk for Deficient Fluid Volume related to increased capillary permeability, protein shifts, inflammatory process, and evaporation secondary to burn injuries

This diagnosis does not represent a situation for which nurses could prescribe interventions with achievable outcomes (e.g., "Client will have stable vital signs and adequate urine output [0.5 mL/kg/hr]"). Because both nurse- and physician-prescribed interventions are needed to accomplish this outcome, this situation is actually the collaborative problem *RC of Fluid/Electrolyte Imbalance* with the nursing goal of "The nurse will monitor to detect fluid and electrolyte imbalances."

Deficient Fluid Volume **related to effects of NPO status**

Managing fluid balance in an NPO individual is a nursing responsibility involving both nurse- and physician-prescribed interventions. Thus, this situation is best described as *RC of Fluid/Electrolyte Imbalance*. If the nurse wants to specify etiology, he or she can write *RC of Fluid/Electrolyte Imbalance related to NPO state*. This usually is not necessary, however.

When an individual can drink but is not drinking sufficient amounts, *Deficient Fluid Volume related to decreased desire to drink fluids secondary to fatigue and pain* may apply.

Key Concepts

General Considerations

- The two main causes of deficient fluid volume are inadequate fluid intake and increased fluid and electrolyte losses (e.g., gastrointestinal, urinary, skin, third-space [edema]).
- Vomiting or gastric suctioning results in fluid, potassium, and hydrogen losses.
- The thirst sensation primarily regulates fluid intake. The kidneys' ability to concentrate urine primarily regulates fluid output.
- Urine-specific gravity reflects the kidneys' ability to concentrate urine; the range of urine-specific gravity varies with the state of hydration and the solids to be excreted. (Specific gravity is elevated with dehydration, signifying concentrated urine.) Normal values are 1.010 to 1.025. Diluted values are less than 1.010. Concentrated values are greater than 1.025 (ranges of normal can vary from lab to lab).
- People at high risk for fluid imbalance include the following:
  - Those taking medication for fluid retention, high blood pressure, seizures, or "anxiety" (tranquilizers)
  - Those with diabetes, cardiac disease, excessive alcohol intake, malnourishment, or gastrointestinal distress
  - Adults older than 60 years and children younger than 6 years of age (decreased sensation of thirst)
  - Those who are confused, depressed, comatose, or lethargic (no sensation of thirst)
  - Athletes unaware of the need to replace electrolytes as well as fluids
- Excessive fluid and electrolyte loss can be expected during
  - Fever or increased metabolic rate
  - Climate extremes (heat/dryness, humidity)
  - Extreme exercise or diaphoresis
  - Excessive vomiting or diarrhea
  - Burns, tissue insult, fistulas
- Fluid balance maintenance is a major concern for all athletes competing in hot climates. The following is true for both men and women (*Maughan, Leiper, & Shirreffs, 1997):
  - Drinking large volumes of plain water will inhibit thirst and promote a diuretic response.
  - To maintain hydration during extreme exercise, high levels of sodium (as much as 50 to 60 mmol) and possibly some potassium to replace losses in sweat are needed.
  - Palatability of drinks is important to stimulate intake and ensure adequate volume replacement.
  - Because adequate hydration greatly affects athletic performance, the goal should be to be hydrated *at the beginning* of exercise and to maintain hydration as well as possible thereafter, focusing on replacing salt loss as well as water.

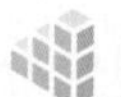

Pediatric Considerations

- Infants are vulnerable to fluid loss because of the following:
  - They can lose more water rapidly because their bodies have a higher proportion of water.
  - More fluid is in the extracellular space, from where it is lost more easily.
  - They have a greater metabolic turnover of water.
  - Homeostatic regulation (i.e., renal function) is immature.
  - They have a greater surface area relative to body mass.
- Recent research has proven that children and adolescents "do not have less effective thermoregulatory ability, insufficient cardiovascular capacity or lower physical exertion tolerance compared to adults during exercise in the heat when adequate hydration is maintained" (American Academy of Pediatrics, 2011, p. 1).
- Poor hydration status (before, during, after) in addition to one or more of the following can cause reduced performance and risk for exertional heat-illness risk as (American Academy of Pediatrics, 2011)
  - Undue physical exertion
  - Insufficient recovery between repeated exercise bouts or training

- Closely scheduled same-day training or sports competition
- Inappropriate wearing of clothing, uniforms, and protective equipment

- "Severe exertional heat injury or heat stroke is associated with significant morbidity and mortality, especially if diagnosis is delayed and appropriate medical management is not initiated promptly" (American Academy of Pediatrics, 2011, p. 1).
- Differentiation of heat stress, heat exhaustion, exertional heat stroke, and heat injury (American Academy of Pediatrics, 2011, p. 5):
  - *Heat stress*: High air temperature, humidity, and solar radiation that lead to perceived discomfort and physiologic strain when children and adolescents are exposed to such environmental conditions, especially during vigorous exercise and other physical activity.
  - *Exertional heat illness*: A spectrum of clinical conditions that range from muscle (heat) cramps, heat syncope, and heat exhaustion to life-threatening heat stroke incurred as a result of exercise or other physical activity.
  - *Heat exhaustion*: Moderate heat illness, characterized by the inability to maintain blood pressure and sustain adequate cardiac output, that results from strenuous exercise or other physical activity, environmental heat stress, acute dehydration, and energy depletion. Signs and symptoms include weakness, dizziness, nausea, syncope, and headache; core body temperature is 104° F (40° C).
  - *Exertional heat stroke*: Severe multisystem heat illness, characterized by central nervous system abnormalities such as delirium, convulsions, or coma, endotoxemia, circulatory failure, temperature-control dysregulation, and, potentially, organ and tissue damage, that results from an elevated core body temperature (104° F [40° C]) that is induced by strenuous exercise or other physical activity and typically (not always) high environmental heat stress.
  - *Heat injury*: Profound damage and dysfunction to the brain, heart, liver, kidneys, intestine, spleen, or muscle induced by excessive sustained core body temperature associated with incurring exertional heat stroke, especially for those victims in whom signs and/or symptoms are not promptly recognized and are not treated effectively (rapidly cooled) in a timely manner.

Geriatric Considerations

- A general decrease in thirst with aging puts older adults at risk for not drinking sufficient fluids to maintain adequate hydration.
- Older adults are more susceptible to fluid loss and dehydration because of the following (Miller, 2015):
  - Decreased percentage of total body water
  - Decreased renal blood flow and glomerular filtration
  - Impaired ability to regulate temperature
  - Decreased ability to concentrate urine
  - Increased physical disabilities (decrease access to fluids)
  - Self-limiting of fluids for fear of incontinence
  - Diminished thirst sensation
- About 75% of fluid intake in older adults occurs between 6 AM and 6 PM (Miller, 2015).
- Cognitive impairments can interfere with recognition of cues of thirst.
- Dehydration, defined as diminished total body-water content, is the most common fluid and electrolyte disturbance among older adults. Because it is associated with morbidity and mortality rates, careful screening and prevention in primary care settings are essential.
- Dehydration in nursing home residents is a complex problem that requires a comprehensive approach, including facility-wide involvement and use of checklists to ensure adequate hydration (Zembruski, 1997).

Focus Assessment Criteria

Subjective Data

Assess for Defining Characteristics

Decreased thirst

Assess for Related Factors

Refer to Related Factors.

Objective Data

Assess for Defining Characteristics

Present Weight/Usual Weight
Weight loss (How much? Since when?)
Fluid intake (amounts, type, *last 2 to 48 hours*)
Mucosa (lips, gums) (dry)
Skin moisture (dry or diaphoretic)
Color (pale or flushed)
Tongue (furrowed/dry)
Fontanelles of infants (depressed)
Eyeballs (sunken)
Tachycardia

Urine Output
Amount (varied; very large or minimal amount)
Color (amber; very dark or very light; clear? cloudy?)
Specific gravity (increased or decreased)
Odor

Assess for Related Factors

Abnormal or Excessive Fluid Loss
Liquid stools
Vomiting or gastric suction (e.g., fistulas, drains)
Diuresis or polyuria
Abnormal or excessive drainage
Diaphoresis
Fever
Loss of skin surfaces (e.g., healing burns)

Decreased Fluid Intake Related to
Fatigue
Decreased level of consciousness
Depression/disorientation
Nausea or anorexia
Physical limitations (e.g., cannot hold glass)

Goals

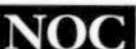
NOC

Electrolyte and Acid/Base Balance, Fluid Balance, Hydration

The individual will maintain urine-specific gravity within normal range as evidenced by the following indicators:

- Increases fluid intake to a specified amount according to age and metabolic needs
- Identifies risk factors for fluid deficit and relate need for increased fluid intake as indicated
- Demonstrates no signs and symptoms of dehydration

Interventions

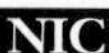
NIC

Fluid/Electrolyte Management, Fluid Monitoring

Assess Causative Factors

Prevent Dehydration in High-Risk Individuals (See Key Concepts)

- Monitor individual intake; ensure at least 2,000 mL of oral fluids every 24 hours unless contraindicated. Offer fluids that are desired hourly.
- Teach the individual to avoid coffee, tea, grapefruit juice, sugared drinks, and alcohol.

R: *Large amounts of sugar, alcohol, and caffeine act as diuretics that increase urine production and may cause dehydration.*

- Monitor output; ensure at least 5 mg/kg/hour.

R: *Monitoring of output will help to evaluate hydration status early.*

- Weigh the individual daily in the same clothes, at the same time. A 2% to 4% weight loss indicates mild dehydration; 5% to 9% weight loss indicates moderate dehydration.

R: *To monitor weight effectively, weights should be measured at the same time on the same scale with the same clothes.*

- Monitor urine and serum electrolytes, blood urea nitrogen, osmolality, creatinine, hematocrit, and hemoglobin.

R: *These laboratory studies will reflect hydration status.*

- For older people scheduled to fast before diagnostic studies, advise them to increase fluid intake 8 hours before fasting.

R: *This will reduce the risks of dehydration.*

- Review the individual's medications. Do they contribute to dehydration (e.g., diuretics)? Do they require increased fluid intake (e.g., lithium)?

R: *Certain medications can contribute to dehydration.*

R: *Output may exceed intake, which already may be inadequate to compensate for insensible losses.*

Initiate Health Teaching, as Indicated

- Give verbal and written directions for desired fluids and amounts.
- Include the individual/family in keeping a written record of fluid intake, output, and daily weight.
- Provide a list of alternative fluids (e.g., ice cream, pudding).
- Explain the need to increase fluids during exercise, fever, infection, and hot weather.
- Teach the individual/family how to observe for dehydration (especially in infants, elderly) and to intervene by increasing fluid intake (see Subjective and Objective Data for signs of dehydration).

R: *Careful monitoring after discharge will be needed for at-risk individuals.*

- For athletes, stress the need to hydrate before and during exercise, preferably with a high-sodium-content beverage. (Refer to *Hyperthermia* for additional interventions.)

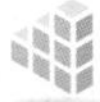 Pediatric Interventions

To Increase Fluid Intake, Offer

- Appealing fluids (popsicles, frozen juice bars, snow cones, water, milk, Jell-O); let the child help make them.
- Unusual containers (colorful cups, straws)
- A game or activity
  - On a chart, have the child cross out the number of cups he or she drank each day.
  - Read a book to the child and have him or her drink a sip when turning a page, or have a tea party.
  - Have child take a drink when it is his or her turn in a game.
  - Set a schedule for supplementary liquids to promote the habit of in-between-meal fluids (e.g., juice or Kool-Aid at 10 AM and 2 PM each day).
  - Decorate straws.
  - Let the child fill small cups with a syringe.
  - Make a progress poster; use stickers or stars to indicate fluid goals met.

R: *A variety of age-appropriate strategies can be used to increase fluid intake.*

- Older children usually respond to the challenge of meeting a specific intake goal.
- Rewards and contracts are also effective (e.g., a sticker for drinking a certain amount).
- Young children usually respond to games that integrate drinking fluids.

Take Measures for Fever in Children Younger Than 5 Years

- Work to attain a temperature below 101° F (38.4° C) with medication (acetaminophen or ibuprofen) only. Instruct parents to closely follow instructions for age.

R: *Aspirin is not to be used in children with fevers due to its association with Reye's syndrome.*

- Overdose of these medications can cause liver toxicity.
- Dress children in lightweight pajamas and infant in diapers only.

R: *Overdressing increases the child's temperature and does not prevent trembling (Pillitteri, 2014).*

- Should a seizure occur; instruct the parents to
  - Not give oral medications
  - Place cool washcloths on forehead, axillary, and groin areas
  - Transport the child to the emergency room

R: *Seizures can occur with high fevers (102° F to 104° F); immediate medical evaluation is needed.*

For Fluid Replacement, Refer to Pediatric Interventions Under Diarrhea

Prevention of Exertional Heat Illness (American Academy of Pediatrics, 2011)

- Teach risk factors to children and parents:
  - Hot and/or humid weather
  - Poor preparation
  - Not heat-acclimatized
  - Inadequate prehydration
  - Little sleep/rest
  - Poor fitness
  - Excessive physical exertion
  - Insufficient rest/recovery time between repeat bouts of high-intensity exercise (e.g., repeat sprints)
  - Insufficient access to fluids and opportunities to rehydrate
  - Multiple same-day sessions
  - Insufficient rest/recovery time between practices, games, or matches
  - Overweight/obese (BMI 85th percentile for age)
  - Clinical conditions (e.g., diabetes) or medications (e.g., attention-deficit/hyperactivity disorder medications)
  - Current or recent illness (especially if it involves/involved gastrointestinal distress or fever)
  - Clothing, uniforms, or protective equipment that contribute to excessive heat retention

R: *"Likewise, as the number of risk factors for exertional heat illness increases, the maximum environmental heat and humidity level for safe exercise, sports participation, or other physical activities will decrease" (American Academy of Pediatrics, 2011, p. 3).*

Preventive Interventions

- Provide and promote consumption of readily accessible fluids at regular intervals before, during, and after activity.

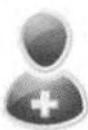

Clinical Alert Generally, 100 to 250 mL (approximately 3 to 8 oz) every 20 minutes for 9- to 12-year-olds and up to 1.0 to 1.5 L (approximately 34 to 50 oz) per hour for adolescent boys and girls is enough to sufficiently minimize sweating-induced body-water deficits during exercise and other physical activity as long as their preactivity hydration status is good. Electrolyte-supplemented beverages that emphasize sodium may justified in warm- to hot-weather conditions, when sweat loss is extensive so as to more effectively optimize rehydration (American Academy of Pediatrics, 2011).

- Allow gradual introduction and adaptation to the climate, intensity, and duration of activities and uniform/protective gear.
- Physical activity should be modified.
- Decrease duration and/or intensity.
- Increase frequency and duration of breaks (preferably in the shade).
- Cancel or reschedule to cooler time.
- Provide longer rest/recovery time between same-day sessions, games, or matches.
- Avoid/limit participation if child or adolescent is currently or was recently ill.
- Closely monitor participants for signs and symptoms of developing heat illness.
- Ensure that personnel and facilities for effectively treating heat illness are readily available on site.
- In response to an affected (moderate or severe heat stress) child or adolescent, promptly activate emergency medical services and rapidly cool the victim.

R: *"Each child and adolescent should be given the opportunity to gradually and safely adapt to preseason practice and conditioning, sport participation, or other physical activity in the heat by appropriate and progressive acclimatization. This process includes graduated exposure (typically over a 10- to 14-day period) to the environment, intensity, duration, and volume of physical activity and to the insulating and metabolic effects of wearing various uniform and protective-equipment configurations" (American Academy of Pediatrics, 2011 pp. 3, 4).*

Teach to Closely Monitor all Children and Adolescents at all Times During Sports and Other Physical Activity in the Heat for Signs and Symptoms of Developing Heat Illness

- Any significant deterioration in performance with notable signs of struggling
- Negative changes in personality or mental status
- Other concerning clinical markers of well-being, including pallor, bright-red flushing, dizziness, headache, excessive fatigue, vomiting
- Complaints of feeling cold or extremely hot

R: *First aid for evolving heat illness should not be delayed. Anyone experiencing exertional heat illness should not return to practice or competition, recreational play, or other physical activity for the remainder of the current session, game/match, or play/activity period (American Academy of Pediatrics, 2011).*

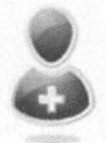

Clinical Alert An emergency medical services (EMS) communication should be activated immediately for any child or adolescent who collapses or exhibits moderate or severe central nervous system dysfunction or encephalopathy during or after practice, competition, or other physical activity in the heat, especially if the child or adolescent is wearing a uniform and/or protective equipment that is potentially contributing to additional heat storage.

Advise to Initiate Immediate Treatment

- When feasible, rectal temperature should be promptly checked by trained personnel and, if indicated (rectal temperature 40° C [104° F]), on-site whole-body rapid cooling using proven techniques should be initiated without delay. Move the victim to the shade, immediately removing protective equipment and clothing.
- Initiate cooling by cold- or ice-water immersion (preferred, most effective method) or by applying ice packs to the neck, axillae, and groin and rotating ice-water-soaked towels to all other areas of the body until rectal temperature reaches just under 39° C (approximately 102° F) or the victim shows clinical improvement.
- If rectal temperature cannot be assessed in a child or adolescent with clinical signs or symptoms suggestive of moderate or severe heat stress, appropriate treatment should not be delayed.
- Prompt rapid cooling for 10 to 15 minutes, and if the child or adolescent is alert enough to ingest fluid, hydration should be initiated by attending staff while awaiting the arrival of medical assistance.

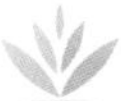

Geriatric Interventions

- Monitor for signs of dehydration, dizziness, and weakness; mucous membrane; and intake versus output.

R: *The elderly are at high risk for dehydration due to decreased thirst sensation, decreased fluid volume, and decreased ability to concentrate urine (Miller, 2015).*

- Avoid caffeine, alcohol, and high-sugar foods and drinks.

R: *Large amounts of sugar, alcohol, and caffeine act as diuretics that increase urine production and may cause dehydration.*

- Explain the need to drink fluids and to use a system for reminding himself or herself not to rely on thirst.
- Incorporate strategies to prompt fluid intake:
  - Fill a large pitcher of water in the morning to monitor intake.
  - Drink an extra glass of water with medications.
  - In care facilities, structure a schedule with a beverage cart with choices.

R: *Strategies that include verbal prompting and choices of fluids will increase fluid intake. Elderly individuals who live alone need help to design prompts that will remind them to drink.*

EXCESS FLUID VOLUME

NANDA-I Definition

Increased isotonic fluid retention

Defining Characteristics

Edema (peripheral, sacral)

Taut, shiny skin
Intake greater than output
Weight gain

Related Factors

Pathophysiologic

Related to compromised regulatory mechanisms secondary to:

Renal failure (acute or chronic)
Systemic and metabolic abnormalities
Endocrine dysfunction
Lipedema

Related to portal hypertension, lower plasma colloidal osmotic pressure, and sodium retention secondary to:

Liver disease
Cirrhosis
Ascites
Cancer

Related to venous and arterial abnormalities secondary to:

Varicose veins
Phlebitis
Infection
Peripheral vascular disease
Immobility
Trauma
Thrombus
Lymphedema
Neoplasms

Treatment Related

Related to sodium and water retention secondary to corticosteroid therapy

Related to inadequate lymphatic drainage secondary to mastectomy

Situational (Personal, Environmental)

Related to excessive sodium intake/fluid intake

Related to low protein intake:

Fad diets
Malnutrition

Related to dependent venous pooling/venostasis secondary to:

Standing or sitting for long periods
Immobility
Tight cast or bandage

Related to venous compression from pregnant uterus

Maturational

Older Adult

Related to impaired venous return secondary to increased peripheral resistance and decreased efficiency of valves

Author's Note

Excess Fluid Volume is frequently used to describe pulmonary edema, ascites, or renal failure. These are all collaborative problems that should not be renamed as *Excess Fluid Volume.* Refer to Section 3 for collaborative problems as *Risk for Complications of renal failure*, *Risk for Complications of Pulmonary Edema*, *Risk for Complications of Hepatic Dysfunction*. This diagnosis represents a situation for which nurses can prescribe if the focus is on peripheral edema. Nursing interventions center on teaching the individual or family how to minimize edema and protect tissue from injury.

Errors in Diagnostic Statements

Risk for Excess Fluid Volume related to left-sided mastectomy

For this diagnosis, the nurse would institute strategies to reduce edema and teach the individual how to manage it. Thus, the nurse would write the diagnosis as *Risk for Excess Fluid Volume related to lack of knowledge of techniques to reduce edema secondary to compromised lymphatic function*. If edema were present, the nurse might use *Risk for Impaired Physical Mobility related to effects of lymphedema on motion*.

***Excess Fluid Volume* related to portal hypertension and decreased colloid osmotic pressure secondary to cirrhosis**

This diagnosis requires frequent monitoring, electrolyte replacement, diuretic therapy, dietary restrictions, and plasma expander therapy. These interventions call for three collaborative problems: *Risk for Complications of Hepatic Dysfunction*. Because edema predisposes skin to injury and breakdown, the nurse could also use *Risk for Impaired Skin Integrity related to vulnerability of skin secondary to edema*.

Key Concepts

General Considerations

- See *Deficient Fluid Volume*.
- Edema results from the accumulation of fluid in the interstitial compartment of the extravascular space. Without intervention, edema can progress to further tissue damage and permanent swelling (Cooper, 2011).
- Determining the underlying cause is essential to identifying specific interventions.
- Peripheral edema should be classified as unilateral or bilateral. *Unilateral* usually results from venous and arterial abnormalities, lymphedema, infection, trauma, and neoplasms. *Bilateral* usually results from congestive heart failure, systemic and metabolic abnormalities, endocrine dysfunction, lipedema, and pregnancy.
- People with cardiac pump failure are at high risk for excesses in both vascular and tissue fluids (i.e., pulmonary and peripheral edema). Pulmonary edema is a medical emergency.

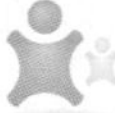

Maternal Considerations

- Increased estrogen levels during pregnancy cause water retention of 6 to 8 L to supply tissue needs for water and electrolytes.

Geriatric Considerations

- Older adults are prone to stasis edema of the feet and ankles as a result of increased vein tortuosity and dilatation and decreased valve efficiency (Miller, 2015).

Focus Assessment Criteria

Subjective Data

Assess for Defining Characteristics

History of Symptoms

Complaints of:

Weight gain
Edema

Onset/duration

Assess for Related Factors

See Related Factors.

Objective Data

Assess for Defining Characteristics

Signs of Fluid Overload
Pulse (bounding or dysrhythmic)
Respirations
Blood pressure (elevated)
Edema
Press thumb for at least 5 seconds into the skin, and note any remaining indentations.

Rate edema according to the following scale:
None = 0
Trace = +1
Moderate = +2
Deep = +3
Very deep = +4
Note degree and location (feet, ankles, legs, arms, sacral, generalized).
Weight gain (Weigh daily on the same scale, at the same time.)
Neck vein distention (Distended neck veins at 45° elevation of head may indicate fluid overload or decreased cardiac output.)

Goals

NOC
Electrolyte Balance, Fluid Balance, Hydration, Tissue Perfusion

The individual will exhibit decreased edema (specify site), as evidenced by the following indicators:

- Relates causative factors
- Relates methods of preventing edema

Interventions

NIC
Electrolyte Management, Fluid Management, Fluid Monitoring, Skin Surveillance

Identify Contributing and Causative Factors

- Refer to Related Factors.

Reduce or Eliminate Causative and Contributing Factors

Improper Diet

- Assess dietary intake and habits that may contribute to fluid retention.
- Be specific; record daily and weekly intake of food and fluids.
- Assess weekly diet for inadequate protein or excessive sodium intake.
  - Discuss likes and dislikes of foods that provide protein.
  - Teach the individual to plan a weekly menu that provides protein at an affordable price.
  - Teach the individual to decrease salt intake.
  - Read labels for sodium content.
  - Avoid convenience and canned and frozen foods.
  - Cook without salt; use spices (lemon, basil, tarragon, mint) to add flavor.
  - Use vinegar in place of salt to flavor soups, stews, etc. (e.g., 2 to 3 teaspoons of vinegar per 4 to 6 quarts, according to taste).

R: *High sodium intake leads to increased water retention. High-sodium foods include salted snacks, bacon, cheddar cheese, pickles, soy sauce, processed lunchmeats, monosodium glutamate (MSG), canned vegetables, ketchup, and mustard. Some over-the-counter drugs, such as antacids, are also high in sodium.*

Dependent Venous Pooling

- Assess for evidence of dependent venous pooling or venous stasis.
- Encourage alternating periods of horizontal rest (legs elevated) with vertical activity (standing); this may be contraindicated in congestive heart failure.
  - Keep the edematous extremity elevated above the level of the heart whenever possible (unless contraindicated by heart failure).
  - Keep the edematous arms elevated on two pillows or with IV pole sling.
  - Elevate the legs whenever possible, using pillows under them (avoid pressure points, especially behind the knees).
  - Discourage leg and ankle crossing.

R: *These strategies reduce venous stasis.*

- Reduce constriction of vessels.
  - Assess clothing for proper fit and constrictive areas.
  - Instruct the individual to avoid panty girdles/garters, knee-high stockings, and leg crossing and to practice elevating the legs when possible.

R: *Edema inhibits blood flow to the tissue, resulting in poor cellular nutrition and increased susceptibility to injury.*

Venous Pressure Points

- Assess for venous pressure points associated with casts, bandages, and tight stockings.
  - Observe circulation at edges of casts, bandages, and stockings.
  - For casts, insert soft material to cushion pressure points at the edges.
- Check circulation frequently.
- Shift body weight in the cast to redistribute weight within (unless contraindicated).
  - Encourage to do this every 15 to 30 minutes while awake to prevent venostasis.
  - Encourage wiggling of fingers or toes and isometric exercise of unaffected muscles within the cast.
  - If the individual cannot do this alone, assist him or her at least hourly to shift body weight.

R: *These strategies increase circulation and venous return.*

- See *Impaired Physical Mobility*.

Inadequate Lymphatic Drainage

- Keep the extremity elevated on pillows.
  - If the edema is marked, the arm should be elevated *but not in adduction* (this position may constrict the axilla).
  - The elbow should be higher than the shoulder.
  - The hand should be higher than the elbow.
- Measure blood pressure in the unaffected arm.
- Do not give injections or start IV fluids in the affected arm.
- Protect the affected limb from injury.
- Teach to avoid using strong detergents, carrying heavy bags, holding cigarettes, injuring cuticles or hangnails, reaching into hot ovens, wearing jewelry or a wristwatch, or using Ace bandages.
- Advise to apply lanolin or a similar cream, often daily, to prevent dry, flaky skin.
- Encourage to wear a Medic-Alert tag engraved with *Caution: lymphedema arm—no tests/no needle injections*.
- Caution the individual to visit a physician if the arm becomes red, swollen, or unusually hard.
- After a mastectomy, encourage range-of-motion exercises and use of the affected arm to facilitate development of a collateral lymphatic drainage system (explain that lymphedema often decreases within 1 month, but that the individual should continue massaging, exercising, and elevating the arm for 3 to 4 months after surgery).

R: *Compromised lymph drainage compromises the body defenses against infection. Trauma to tissue can increase lymphedema.*

Immobility/Neurologic Deficit

- Plan passive or active range-of-motion exercises for all extremities every 4 hours, including dorsiflexion of the foot.
- Change the individual's position at least every 2 hours, using the four positions (left side, right side, back, abdomen) if not contraindicated (see *Impaired Skin Integrity*).
- If the individual must remain in high Fowler's position, assess for edema of buttocks and sacral area; help the individual shift body weight every 2 hours to prevent pressure on edematous tissue.

R: *Contracting skeletal muscles increases lymph flow. Exercise increases muscle efficiency and can prevents thrombus.*

Protect Edematous Skin From Injury

- Inspect skin for redness and blanching.
- Reduce pressure on skin areas; pad chairs; and footstools.
- Prevent dry skin.
- Use soap sparingly.
- Rinse off soap completely.
- Use a lotion to moisten skin.
- Consider low air therapy with mattress overlays.

R: *Low air loss therapy with mattress overlays or mattress replacement products may help reduce skin moisture by constant motion of air across the mattress surface (Cooper, 2011).*

- See *Impaired Skin Integrity* for additional information about preventing injury.

R: *Edema inhibits blood flow to the tissues, resulting in poor cellular nutrition and increased susceptibility to injury. Skin tears over bony prominences and pressure ulcers, especially on the heels, are common with edema of a lower extremity (Cooper, 2011).*

Initiate Health Teaching and Referrals, as Indicated

- Give clear verbal and written instructions for all medications: what, when, how often, why, side effects; pay special attention to drugs that directly influence fluid balance (e.g., diuretics, steroids). Identify if any previous medications have been discontinued.
- Write down instructions for diet, activity, and use of Ace bandages.
- Have the individual demonstrate the instructions.
- With severe fluctuations in edema, have the individual weigh himself or herself every morning and before bedtime daily; instruct to keep a written record of weights. For less severe illness, the individual may need to weigh himself or herself only once daily and record the weight.
- Advised to call primary care provider for excessive edema/weight gain (greater than 2 lb/day) or increased shortness of breath at night or upon exertion. Explain that these signs may indicate early heart problems and may require medication to prevent them from worsening.
- Consider home care or visiting nurses referral to follow at home.
- Provide literature concerning low-salt diets; consult with a dietitian if necessary.

R: *Home management of edema will require specific instructions and monitoring.*

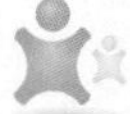

Maternal Interventions

- Explain the cause of edema of ankles and fingers.

R: *Increased estrogen levels cause fluid retention.*

- Advise the individual to limit salt intake moderately (e.g., eliminate processed meats, chips) and to maintain water intake of 8 to 10 glasses daily unless contraindicated.

R: *Sodium is important to maintain adequate circulatory blood volume. A health-care professional should supervise restrictions.*

- Consult with an advanced practice nurse or physician if individual has elevated blood pressure, proteinuria, facial puffiness, sacral or pitting edema, or weight gain of more than 2 lb in 1 week.

R: *A medical evaluation is needed.*

R: *During pregnancy, possible causes of edema are peripheral arterial vasodilation, sodium and water retention, decreased thirst threshold, the enlarging uterus increasing capillary pressure on the lower extremities, and changes in the renin–angiotensin–aldosterone system (Pillitteri, 2014).*

- Advise the individual to avoid reclining on her back, sitting for prolonged periods without elevating feet, or standing for prolonged periods (Davis, 1996).
- Instruct the individual to lie on the left side for short periods several times a day and to take a warm tub bath daily.

R: *Lying on the left side removes weight of the gravid uterus from the vessels, increases venous return to the heart, and improves renal function. Research findings have suggested that rest periods in water (i.e., baths) instead of bed rest may better reduce edema during pregnancy.*

RISK FOR IMBALANCED FLUID VOLUME

NANDA-I Definition

At risk for a decrease, increase, or rapid shift from one to the other of intravascular, interstitial, and/or intracellular fluid that may compromise health. This refers to body fluid loss, gain, or both.

Risk Factors*

Abdominal surgery	Pancreatitis
Ascites	Receiving apheresis
Burns	Sepsis
Intestinal obstruction	Traumatic injury (e.g., fractured hip)

Author's Note

This diagnosis can represent several clinical conditions, such as edema, hemorrhage, dehydration, and compartmental syndrome. If the nurse is monitoring a individual for imbalanced fluid volume, labeling the specific imbalance as a collaborative problem, such as hypovolemia, compartment syndrome, increased intracranial pressure, gastrointestinal bleeding, or postpartum hemorrhage, would be more useful clinically. For example, most intraoperative individuals would be monitored for hypovolemia. If the procedure was neurosurgery, then cranial pressure would also be monitored. If the procedure were orthopedic, compartment syndrome would be addressed. Refer to Section 3 for specific collaborative problems and interventions.

DYSFUNCTIONAL GASTROINTESTINAL MOTILITY

Dysfunctional Gastrointestinal Motility

Risk for Dysfunctional Gastrointestinal Motility

See also *Risk for Complications of Paralytic Ileus.*

NANDA-I Definition

Increased, decreased, ineffective, or lack of peristaltic activity within the gastrointestinal system

Defining Characteristics*

Absence of flatus
Abdominal cramping or pain
Abdominal distention
Accelerated gastric emptying
Bile-colored gastric residual
Change in bowel sounds (e.g., absent, hypoactive, hyperactive)
Diarrhea
Dry stool difficulty passing stools
Hard stools
Increased gastric residual
Nausea
Regurgitation, vomiting

Related Factors*

Aging
Anxiety
Enteral feedings
Food intolerance (e.g., gluten lactose)
Immobility
Ingestion of contaminates (e.g., food, water)
Malnutrition
Pharmaceutical agents (e.g., narcotics/opiates, antibiotics, laxatives, anesthesia)
Prematurity, sedentary lifestyle
Surgery

Author's Note

This NANDA-I diagnosis is too broad for clinical usefulness. It represents collaborative problems and some nursing diagnoses such as *Diarrhea*, *Constipation*. Refer to Section 3 for more specific collaborative problems as *Risk for Complications of Gastrointestinal Dysfunction*, *Risk for Complications of Paralytic Ileus*, and *Risk for Complications for GI Bleeding*.

Risk for Dysfunctional Gastrointestinal Motility

See also *Risk for Complications of Gastrointestinal Dysfunction*

NANDA-I Definition

At risk for increased, decreased, ineffective, or lack of peristaltic activity within the gastrointestinal system

Risk Factors*

Abdominal surgery
Aging
Anxiety
Change in food or water
Decreased gastrointestinal circulation
Diabetes mellitus
Food intolerance (gluten, lactose)
Gastroesophageal reflux disease (GERD)
Immobility
Infection (e.g., bacteria parasitic, viral)
Pharmaceutical agents (e.g., antibiotics, laxatives, narcotics/opiates, proton-pump inhibitors)
Prematurity
Sedentary lifestyle
Stress
Unsanitary food preparation

Author's Note

This NANDA-I diagnosis is too broad for clinical use. This diagnosis represents some collaborative problems such as *Risk for Complications of Gastrointestinal Dysfunction*, *Risk for Complications of GI Bleeding*, *Risk for Complications of Paralytic Ileus* and nursing diagnoses such as *Risk for Diarrhea*, *Risk for Constipation*, and *Risk for Infection*. Refer to Section 3.

Examine the risk factors in the individual and determine if the focus of nursing interventions is prevention; if yes, use *Risk for Infection*, *Risk for Diarrhea*, or *Risk for Constipationt*. If the focus is to monitor gastrointestinal function for complications that require medical and nursing interventions, use a collaborative problem as *Risk for Complications of (specify)*.

GRIEVING

Grieving

Anticipatory Grieving[16]
Complicated Grieving
Risk for Complicated Grieving

NANDA-I Definition

A normal complex process that includes emotional, physical, spiritual, social, and intellectual responses and behaviors by which individuals, families, and communities, incorporate an actual, anticipated, or perceived loss into their daily lives

Defining Characteristics

Major (Must Be Present)

[16]Added by Lynda Juall Carpenito for usefulness and clarity.

The individual reports an actual or perceived loss (person, pet, object, function, status, or relationship) with varied responses such as the following:

Denial
Suicidal thoughts
Guilt
Crying
Anger*
Sorrow
Despair*
Longing/searching behaviors
Inability to concentrate
In sleep patterns*
Blame*
Detachment*
Anergia
Disorganization*
Feelings of worthlessness
Numbness
Disbelief
Anxiety
Helplessness

Related Factors

Many situations can contribute to feelings of loss. Some common situations are as follows.

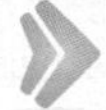

Carp's Cues

An example of a *Grieving* nursing diagnosis statement is *Grieving* related to loss of function or independence secondary to congestive heart failure as manifested by unable to drive anymore, dyspnea preventing usual hobbies (gardening, yard work), and interfering with activities of daily living.

Pathophysiologic

Related to loss of function or independence secondary to: (Insert disease, disorder, injury)

Neurologic
Digestive
Cardiovascular
Respiratory
Sensory
Renal
Musculoskeletal
Trauma

Treatment Related

Related to negative effects losses associated with:

Long-term dialysis
Surgery (e.g., mastectomy)

Situational (Personal, Environmental)

Related to loss of health

Related to losing a job

Related to loss of financial stability

Related to death of a pet

Related to loss of a cherished dream

Related to a loved one's serious illness

Related to loss of a friendship

Related to loss of home

Related to the negative effects and losses secondary to:

Chronic pain
Death
Terminal illness

Related to perceived negative effects and losses associated with:

Childbirth
Child leaving home
Marriage
Divorce
Separation
Role function

Maturational

Older Adult

Related to losses and/or changes attributed to aging:

Independence (loss of driving license, own home, meal preparation)
Friends
Function
Occupation
Sexual performance

Related to loss of hope, dreams

Author's Note

Grieving, Anticipatory, and *Complicated Grieving* represent three types of responses of individuals or families experiencing a loss. *Grieving* describes normal grieving after a loss and participation in grief work. *Anticipatory Grieving* (not a NANDA-I nursing diagnosis) describes engaging in grief work before an expected loss, for example, a family with a terminally ill child.

Complicated Grieving represents a maladaptive process in which grief work is suppressed or absent, or an individual exhibits prolonged exaggerated responses. For all three diagnoses, the goal of nursing is to promote grief work. In addition, for *Complicated Grieving*, the nurse directs interventions to reduce excessive, prolonged, problematic responses.

In many clinical situations, the nurse expects a grief response (e.g., loss of body part, death of significant other). Other situations that evoke strong grief responses are sometimes ignored or minimized (e.g., abortion, newborn death, death of one twin or triplet, death of secret lover, suicide, loss of children to foster homes, or adoption).

Errors in Diagnostic Statements

Complicated Grieving related to excessive emotional reactions (crying, anger) to recent death of son

Response to loss is highly individualized. Regardless of severity, no response to acute loss should be labeled "dysfunctional." *Complicated Grieving* is characterized by a sustained or prolonged detrimental response; this diagnosis cannot be validated until 18 to 24 months after the loss. The nurse should reword this diagnosis as *Grieving related to recent death of son,* as evidenced by emotional responses of anger and profound sadness.

Anticipatory Grieving related to perceived effects of spinal cord injury on life goals

Using *Anticipatory Grieving* here focuses on anticipated, not actual, losses. Because this individual is grieving for both actual and anticipated losses, the nurse should rewrite this as *Grieving related to actual or anticipated losses associated with recent spinal cord injury*.

Key Concepts

General Considerations

- "The grieving process takes time. Healing happens gradually; it can't be forced or hurried—and there is no 'normal' timetable for grieving" (Smith & Segal, 2016).
- US culture is devoted to youth and life. Even though death surrounds each person, society views it as pertaining to someone else. Society today has been called "death denying," failing to recognize and confront the realities of death and grief.
- Caregivers must recognize that their attitudes and beliefs about death, dying, and grief significantly influence their care of people experiencing loss.
- Loss can occur without death; when a person experiences any loss (object, relationship), grief and mourning ensue.
- Bereavement is the grieving response to events: loss, death, divorce, health, or body part.
- Grief is the emotional feeling: anger, frustration, loneliness, sadness, guilt, and regret related to the perception of the loss of health or body part.
- Mourning is the public display of grief and is influenced by one's beliefs, religious practices, and cultural context.

- The following tasks of *Grieving* have been identified by Worden (*2009) and can assist the nurse in identifying the individual's current progression in the grief process:
  - *Task 1*: To accept the reality of loss
  - *Task 2*: To feel the pain of grief
  - *Task 3*: To adjust to an environment in which the deceased is missing
  - *Task 4*: To emotionally relocate the deceased and move on with life
- The normal grief process may include the following (*Worden, 2009):
  - Feelings: numbness, shock, anger, frustration, irritation, misdirected hostility, sadness, fear, loneliness, relief, guilt, yearning, helplessness, out of control
  - Physical sensations:
    - Depersonalization—"Nothing seems real."
    - Shakiness, edginess
    - Lack of energy, weakness
    - Dry mouth, increased perspiration
    - Stomach hollowness, "butterflies"
    - Headache
    - Chest or throat pain or tightness, breathlessness
    - Same physical symptoms as the deceased
  - Thoughts:
    - Disbelief—"This isn't really happening."
    - Anger—"Why did it happen? It's not fair."
    - Forgetfulness, confusion
    - Guilt—"If only ______." "I wish ______."
    - Preoccupation or obsessive thinking about the deceased
    - Forging ahead—"I have to make changes/decisions now."
    - Suicide—"Life has no meaning."
    - Dread—fear of one's own or another's death
    - Extranormal experiences—sense of "presence" of the deceased, dreams, etc.
    - Finality—"Things will never be the same."
  - Behaviors:
    - Sleeping and appetite disturbances
    - Yelling, crying, sighing
    - Increased alcohol/nicotine intake
    - Absent-minded behavior
    - Activities regarding the deceased—calling out, visiting or avoiding places or objects that remind the survivor of the deceased, talking to the deceased (pictures/ashes)
    - Searching behavior—expecting the deceased
    - Social withdrawal
    - Change in work performance—tardiness, leaving early or working late, etc.
    - Shock and disbelief
- Divorce poses many losses for the partners and their families: roles, relationships, homes, possessions, finances, control, routines, and patterns.

Losses Associated with AIDS/HIV

- AIDS-related bereavement seems to differ from traditional grieving models in four ways (Kain, 2016):
  - Many individuals with AIDS die young, which is not expected in the 2015.
  - The stigma associated with AIDS prevents loved ones from openly grieving or acknowledging the cause of death.
  - Caregivers may respond to the end of caregiving responsibilities with guilty relief. In gay community, survivors may feel guilty about being HIV-negative in light of the suffering of their peers.
  - When survivors are HIV-positive, they suffer guilt about their status and worry about their own health status all of which confound bereavement.
- Disenfranchised grief occurs when social stigma is associated with a death or illness (e.g., suicide, AIDS); the individual may be alone, emotionally isolated, or fearful of public expressions of grief (*Bateman, 1999; *Leming & Dickinson, 2010).
- Complex social issues of morality, sexuality, contagion, and shame associated with AIDS-related losses interfere with the process of bereavement and healing (*Cotton et al., 2006; *Mallinson, 1999).
- Gay men who have experienced multiple AIDS-related losses (e.g., loss of friends and community, disintegrating family structures and social networks) may receive little understanding from heterosexuals (*Cotton et al., 2006; *Mallinson, 1999).

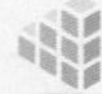

Pediatric Considerations (Hockenberry & Wilson, 2015)

Parental Grief

- Can be more complicated than others going through the bereavement process
  - Not only experience the primary loss of the child but then feel the secondary losses. These can include the parents' lost identity of being a parent, their hopes and dreams for their child's future that will now go unmet, and the void that is created in the family unit by the loss.
  - It is common for the parents of a child to suffer grief differently. It may cause strain in the marriage, and the family, as the parents work through their grief but also attempt to carry out their household/familiar responsibilities.
  - In dealing with their own grief, parents may have difficulty responding to surviving children's grieving needs.
- Use therapeutic statements when communicating with the bereaved parent.
  - Be nonjudgmental in any questions you may need to ask.
  - Show empathy, not sympathy.
  - It is okay to sit in silence. Knowing someone is there can be comforting. Let them know you are there to listen if they want to talk.
  - Assess the coping strategies of the parent and evaluate need for assistance.
  - It is okay to show emotion. It shows the parent that you, as their nurse, care about the child and will also mourn their loss. If the nurse has frequently taken care of the child, the family may recognize the nurse as a shared caregiver and find comfort in their presence.
  - In cases with chronically ill children, the nurse may have been on the journey with the family almost as long as the family has and can feel the loss profoundly.
    - Do not, however, become so emotional in front of the grieving family that your emotions take precedence over theirs. You need to be there for them, not them there for you.

Sibling Grief

- Each child grieves in their own way and that is different from adults. Their age and developmental status, as well as personality and already in-place coping techniques, influence the child's reaction to the death of their sibling.
- Infants and Toddlers:
  - May act as though person is still alive
  - Become upset and anxious about changes in their daily routine that occur with the loss
  - Respond and react to parental anxiety and sadness even if they do not understand it
- Preschool Children:
  - May feel guilt or responsible for death of their sibling, like they are being punished
  - May have unexpected responses or behaviors, such as regression to earlier stage of development, engage in attention seeking behavior, or engage in strange activities that are new for them
  - Fear separation from their parents
- School-Age Children:
  - With a better understanding of death, the school-aged child may have different fears such as what was the cause of the death and could it happen to them, the dying process itself, and overall fear of the unknown.
  - Show increased interest in post death rituals
  - May be inquisitive about what happens to the body after death
- Adolescents:
  - Have the most difficulty with processing and coping with death
  - Become overly concerned with living-in-the-now
  - Prone to feeling alone in their grief because they have a tendency to feel like they can't talk to anyone or that anyone would understand what they are going through

Nurse's Grief and Roles in Care for the Grieving Family

- A nurse may experience loss and grief as they come to understand the fatal prognosis of their patients. This can lead to burnout for the nurse who undergoes this process frequently, depending on the area of nursing they work in.
  - The nurse may experience anger or depression at the inability to change the patient's prognosis.
  - It is emotionally stressful to routinely care for the dying child and grieve with their families over and over. The nurse may find themselves caring for the child and family that has just died and then have to move on to their next patient assignment once postmortem care is complete with little or no downtime in between.
  - Self-awareness and having coping strategies are essential for the nurse.

- Debriefing can be beneficial after such an event in helping the nurse process and stay resilient. Seek professional help as needed. Practice a healthy lifestyle.
- Often, another hospital staff member (e.g., chaplain, social worker, grief counselor) may be on hand to assist with the immediate needs of the grieving parents. In some cases, however, it would fall to the nurse.
  - Help the parents to understand the reactions to death that their surviving children may be exhibiting.
  - Assist the parents in striving to find a balance that allows them to grieve over their profound loss but also keep an emotional reserve to allow them to still console and care for surviving children.
  - Attempt to maintain a normal environment and routine.
  - Encourage parents to answer questions the surviving children may have honestly.
  - Encourage the surviving sibling to talk openly and allow outlets for their grief.

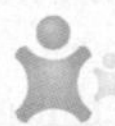

Maternal Considerations

- Unfortunately "miscarriage or death of a newborn are often not recognized as major losses but can precipitate prolonged grief" (Block, 2013).
- Jiong, Vestergaard, and Obel (2011) reported in a large cohort study that, "children born to mothers who lost a close relative (a child, a parent, or a sibling) during pregnancy, and those children are categorized as exposed children due to bereavement during fetal life." Maternal bereavement during pregnancy was associated with an increased risk of several adverse birth outcomes, such as low birth weight, preterm birth, low Apgar score at 1 minute and low Apgar score at 5 minutes.
- Jonas-Simpson, McMahon, Watson, and Andrews (2013) completed research-based documentary that explores nurses' experiences of grieving while caring for a family whose newborn died. The following represents the theme that evolved:
  - "Over the years, comfort with death grew and an ability to be with those who were bereaved developed, not only in the nurses' practices but also in their personal lives, as one nurse described."
  - "Another nurse connected her growth with her ability to mentor novice nurses and her growing comfort with perinatal death and bereavement."
  - Appreciating and cherishing their family even more; thinking about what would it be like to lose a child; not being able to fully enjoy pregnancy
  - Knowing the possibility of loss; and appreciating the significance of loss even more after becoming a mother
  - "Support from colleagues was very significant in helping them to find their way through grief."
  - "Providing authentic compassion and high quality care in the event of perinatal loss helped them to feel better about their own grief."

Geriatric Considerations

- Older adults can experience multiple losses in a short period of time, as death of spouse, partner, relative child, loss if income, loss of home, relocation, physical health, sensory losses. The multitude of losses in a short period of time can be overwhelming and a barrier to grieving (*Worden, 2009).
- Suicide in later life is a major public health concern in the United States, where more than 6,000 older adults take their own lives every year. Suicide prevention in this age group is made challenging by the high lethality of older adults' suicidal behavior; few survive their first attempt to harm themselves. Research has revealed that factors in each of five domains place older adults at increased risk for suicide—psychiatric illness, personality traits and coping styles, medical illness, life stressors and social disconnectedness, and functional impairment (Conwell, 2014).
- There seems to be some support for extending traditional bereavement periods to at least 24 months for older adults who have lost a spouse. Of greater influence than the loss of a significant other is the loss of a crucial relationship that provides meaning to the individual's life. Even in young widows, the estimate of adjustment period has been extended, based on research showing movement at the 24-month mark from high distress to low distress (as measured on the Goldberg General Health Questionnaire; (*Caserta, Lund, & Dimond, 1985).
- Bereavement is a risk factor for suicide. Older adults commit about 25% of all suicides. Suicide attempts are less frequent in older adults; however, the rate of attempted to successful suicide increases to 4:1 after 60 years of age, compared with 20:1 in those younger than 40 years. Men older than 65 years have the highest incidence of suicide; men 65 to 74 years of age have 30.4 suicides per 100,000; men 75 to 84 years of age have 42.3 suicides per 100,000; and men older than 85 years have the highest suicide rate, 50.6 suicides per 100,000 (Miller, 2015).

- Death of a pet can be a significant loss for many persons. Some are more vulnerable, such as an isolated older individual, and can result in a grieving process.
- Social supports, strong religious beliefs, and good prior mental health are resources that decrease psychosocial and physical dysfunction (*Hooyman & Kramer, 2006; Miller, 2015).

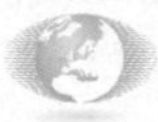

Transcultural Considerations

- Mourning, a behavioral response to death or loss, is culturally determined. There is a need to advocate for vulnerable populations to lessen the impact of death by understanding the cultural responses and rituals around death and dying (Purnell, 2013).
- Bereavement is a universal stressor but the magnitude of stress and its meaning vary cross-culturally. The dominant US culture assumes that the death of a child is more stressful than that of an older relative.
- Puerto Ricans believe that a person's spirit is not free to enter the next life if he or she has left something unsaid before death. Heightened grieving may occur if closure has not been achieved, such as through sudden death (Giger, 2013).
- Hispanics sometimes express grief with seizure-like behavior, hyperkinetic episodes, aggression, or stupor. This syndrome is called *elliptic* (Giger, 2013).
- The degree of mourning in the Chinese culture depends on the mourner's closeness to and the importance of the deceased person (Giger, 2013). Grief work for Haitians frequently includes taking on symptoms of the deceased person's last illness (Giger, 2013).

Focus Assessment Criteria

Subjective Data

Assess for Defining Characteristics

Present Interactions Between or Among Family Members
Adults
Children
Maturational level
Understanding of crisis
Degree of participation
Preexisting family tensions
Knowledge of expected grief reactions
History of relationship to ill or deceased person, for example, conflicted, overly dependent, abusive, hostile

Expressions of
Ambivalence
Anger
Denial
Depression
Fear
Guilt

Report of
Gastrointestinal disturbances
Insomnia
Preoccupation with sleep
Fatigue (decreased or increased)
Inability to carry out work, self-care, social responsibility

Assess for Related Factors

Family
Previous coping patterns for crisis
Quality of the relationship of the ill or deceased individual with each family member
Position or role responsibilities of the ill or deceased individual
Sociocultural expectations for bereavement
Religious expectations for bereavement

Individual Family Members

Previous experiences with loss or death (as child, adolescent, or adult)

Did family share their grief?

Did they practice any particular religious or cultural rituals associated with bereavement?

Objective Data

Assess for Defining Characteristics

Normative

Anger

Crying

Disbelief, denial

Hopelessness

Preoccupation

Sadness

Shock

Sorrow

Withdrawal

Problematic Pattern (Profound; Progressively Worsened Responses or no evidence of) (Subjective, Objective)

Lasting loss of normal patterns of social behavior

Progressively deeper regression and depression

Progressively deeper isolation

Somatic manifestations (prolonged)

Obsessions and phobias

Delusions and hallucinations

Attempted suicide

Substance abuse (e.g., prescription sedatives/opioids, alcohol, illicit drugs)

Goals

NOC

Coping, Family Coping, Community Grief Response, Grief Resolution, Psychosocial Adjustment, Life Change, Family Resiliency, Guilt resolution

The individual will express his or her grief, and grief will be freely expressed, as evidenced by the following indicators:

- Describe the meaning of the death or loss to him or her
- Share his or her grief with significant others

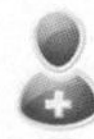

CLINICAL ALERT When a person has died in a health care facility, the nurse should contact family members not present. Offer them the option to see the body. If desired, a letter or card of condolence and/or attending the funeral is usually most appreciated.

Interventions

NIC

Active Listening, Family Support, Grief Work Facilitation, Coping Enhancement, Anticipatory Guidance, Emotional Support, Reminiscence Therapy

Assess for Factors That May Delay Grief Work

- Unavailable or no support system
- Dependency
- Previous emotional illness
- Uncertain loss (e.g., missing child)
- Inability to grieve
- Early object loss
- Failure to grieve for past loss
- Personality structure
- Nature of relationship
- Multiple losses

Reduce or Eliminate Factors, If Possible

Promote a Trust Relationship

- Establish a safe, secure, and private environment.
- Promote feelings of self-worth through one-on-one or group sessions.
- Allow for established time to meet and discuss feelings.
- Communicate clearly, simply, and to the point.
- Never try to lessen the loss (e.g., "She didn't suffer long"; or "You can have another baby.").
- Create a therapeutic milieu (convey that you care).
- Demonstrate respect for the individual's culture, religion, race, and values.
- Provide a presence of simply "being" with the bereaved.

R: *Grief work cannot begin until the individual acknowledges the loss. Nurses can encourage this acknowledgment by engaging in open, honest dialogue, providing the family an opportunity to view the dead person and recognizing and validating the grief (*Leming & Dickinson, 2010; Vanezis & McGee, 1999).*

Support Grief Reactions

- Explain that each person will grieve differently and at a different pace.

R: *Research findings have refuted the notion that grief is neat, orderly, linear, and completed at an arbitrary point (Wright & Hogan, 2008).*

- Explain grief reactions: shock and disbelief, developing awareness, and resolution.
  - Assure loved ones that the memory of your loved one will continue, but the pain will lessen in time and will not disappear.
  - Support the person on the realization (intellectually and emotionally) that the person is dead and will not return.
  - Allow the widowed person to share their fears of having to develop new skills and to take on roles that were formerly performed by the deceased.
- Describe varied acceptable expressions:
  - Elated or manic behavior as a defense against depression
  - Elation and hyperactivity as a reaction of love and protection from depression
  - Various states of depression
  - Various somatic manifestations (weight loss or gain, indigestion, dizziness)

Determine Whether Family Has Special Requests Regarding Viewing the Deceased (*Vanezis & McGee, 1999)

- Prepare them for possible body changes.
- Remove all equipment; change soiled linen.
- Ask them if they want to engage in a ritual or any other comforting activity (e.g. holding, washing, touching, kissing).
- Leave arms outside of sheets to encourage touching if desired.

Promote Family Cohesiveness

- Support the family at its level of functioning.
- Encourage self-exploration of feelings with family members.

R: *Each family member has his or her own perception of making sense of a loved one's death (*O'Mallon, 2009).*

- Recognize and reinforce the strengths of each family member.

R: *Understanding and strengthening families at the end of life and during bereavement are essential for health maintenance or restoration (*O'Mallon, 2009).*

- Encourage family members to share their feelings and support one another.

R: *Acknowledging that grief responses are expected and normal can support an anxious grieving individual (*Hooyman & Kramer, 2006).*

- Specifically, dialogue with the "strong" family members about their feelings.

R: *Mourners who were busy with the practical and necessary caregiving tasks of the dying person may not address the impending loss and, therefore, are at risk for delayed grieving response.*

Promote Grief Work With Each Response

Denial

- Recognize that response is useful and necessary.
- Explain the use of denial by one family member to the other members.
- Do not push the individual to move past denial without emotional readiness.

Isolation

- Convey acceptance by acknowledging grief.
- Create open, honest communication to promote sharing.
- Encourage family to increase supportive activities (e.g., support groups, church groups) gradually.
- Encourage client/family to let significant others know their needs (e.g., support, privacy, permission to share their experience).

Depression

- Identify the level of depression and develop the approach accordingly.
- Use empathic sharing; acknowledge grief ("It must be very difficult.").
- Identify any indications of suicidal behavior (frequent statements of intent, revealed plan).
- See *Risk for Self-Harm* for additional information.

Anger

- Acknowledge anger as a coping mechanism.
- Explain to the family that anger serves to try to control one's environment more closely because of an inability to control loss.

R: *Acknowledging that grief responses are expected and normal can support an anxious grieving individual (*O'Mallon, 2009).*

Identify Individuals at High Risk for Complicated Grieving Reactions

- Identify those at high risk for complicated grief reactions:
    - *Length of relationship*: more than 55 years, less than 5 years; consider significance and quality of relationship to the survivor
    - *Medical issues*: pending treatments or surgeries; history of acute or chronic illness
    - *Mental health history or treatment*: outpatient counseling/follow-up; psychiatric medications (depression, anxiety, sleep, etc.); psychiatric hospitalizations; suicide attempts; suicidal ideations
    - *Substance abuse*: alcohol or drug abuse treatment
    - *Suicidality*: in family history, suicidal ideation or potential for it
    - *Children*: 17 years or younger, either in home or with significant relationship to deceased (e.g., grandparent who lived in the same home)
    - *Multiple losses*: deaths, moves, retirement, divorce car accident
    - *Traumatic death*: circumstances of death, sudden or unexpected, as perceived by bereaved

R: *Sudden death or suicide is catastrophic. Interventions focus on helping survivors with valid perceptions of the event, and, in suicide, shame and embarrassment. Those left behind experience guilt, rejection, and disillusionment (*Gibson, 2003).*

Promote Physical Well-Being: Nutrition, Sleep/Rest, Exercise for Survivors of Suicide

- Encourage them to make an appointment with their primary care professional.
- Elicit their interpretation of the event. Clarify distortions.
- Discuss plans for the funeral and notification of friends and relatives.
- Discuss the hazards of secrecy.
- Allow for expression of guilt, rage, and blame (e.g., of professionals).
- Follow up with telephone contacts to family.
- Refer all survivors to counseling, especially those at high risk (surviving children; those with inadequate support; those who respond with blaming, scapegoating, or secrecy).

R: *Providing a caring environment of support, comfort, openness, and family involvement can facilitate positive family bereavement outcomes (*O'Mallon, 2009).*

Provide Health Teaching and Referrals, as Indicated

Teach the Individual and Family Signs of Resolution

- Grieving individual no longer lives in the past but is future oriented and establishes new goals.
- Grieving individual redefines relationship with the lost object/person.
- Grieving individual begins to resocialize.

- Suggest if comfortable to organize a gathering to recall these memories and share these rich stories and experiences.

R: *Reminiscence therapy gives people the opportunity to meet as a group.*

- Identify agencies that may be helpful (e.g., community agencies, religious groups).

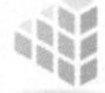

Pediatric Interventions

Explain What Caused the Death

- Clarify child's perceptions.
- Openly clarify that the child did not cause the death.

R: *Children need to feel the joys and sorrows of life to begin to incorporate both in their lives appropriately (*Hooyman & Kramer, 2006; Kübler-Ross, 1975).*

R: *Children of parents who commit suicide are at increased risk for future psychopathology and depression and for suicide as a coping measure (Boyd, 2012; *Hooyman & Kramer, 2006).*

Openly Discuss Possible Responses (*Hooyman & Kramer, 2006)

- "Sometimes when someone dies we feel bad if we said or did something bad to them."
- "Sometimes we feel glad we didn't die and then feel bad because ________ did."
- "When someone dies, we can become afraid that we may die also."
- "I remember when ________ said or did ________. What do you remember?"

Explain Rituals (e.g., Read Children's Book About Death)

R: *Children can be encouraged to communicate symbolically through writing, telling stories, or drawing pictures.*

Assist Family With the Decision About the Child Attending the Funeral and Determine If the Following Are Present (Boyd, 2012; *Hooyman & Kramer, 2006)

- Child has a basic understanding of death and good coping skills.
- Child is not afraid of adults' emotional responses.
- The ethnic group approaches death openly (e.g., children commonly attend funerals).
- A familiar adult who is coping well with his or her own grief is available to monitor the child's needs.
- Child expresses a desire to attend and has a basic understanding of what will happen.

Explore the Child's Modified Involvement in Funeral Activities (e.g., Visit Funeral Home Before Guests Come, Attend After-Service Gathering)

R: *Children need to be included in grief rituals based on their developmental level or "they may feel abandoned and left to face their fear alone" (Boyd, 2005).*

Allow Child to Grieve at Own Pace. Give Adolescents Permission to Grieve Openly. Consider a Sibling Support Group, If Indicated

R: *Children can feel rejected or unloved if parents or significant others fail to offer emotional support and nurturing because of their own grief (Hockenberry & Wilson, 2015).*

R: *Siblings of deceased children may experience guilt, anger, jealousy, and fear (Hockenberry & Wilson, 2015).*

The Child Who is Dying (Ball, Bindler, & Cowen, 2015)

- Cultural differences should be observed and respected as this aspect can be pivotal in the dying process for the family as well as the child who is about to die.
- Some examples of traditions involving the dying process based on religion:
  - *Catholicism*: commonly buried; sacrament of the sick performed
  - *Judaism*: seven-day mourning period; body to ritually washed; buried as soon as possible
  - *Islam*: deathbed should be turned to face Mecca; autopsy only for medical or legal reasons; body is washed only by Muslim of the same gender
  - *Jehovah's Witness*: organ donation is forbidden; autopsy only for legal reasons
- Sometimes the child is aware they are dying before being formally told. If the parents decide to keep the prognosis from the child for fear of causing child to lose hope, they can actually be causing child to feel isolated. This child may feel they can't talk about death or the fears they associate with it as they don't want to add to their parent's grief.

- Consult a bereavement specialist or counselor for suggestions and as a resource for the child as well as the parents/family.
- Listen to the child. Each child will cope differently. Allow the child to speak openly and answer their questions honestly. They may experience mood swings and the nurse should help facilitate outlets for their emotion such as play, drawing, or other activities. Allow the children to develop friendships with other children with similar interests or problems.

There's no tragedy in life like the death of a child. Things never get back to the way they were.

—President Dwight Eisenhower

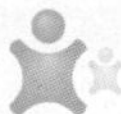

Maternal Interventions

Assist Parents of a Deceased Infant, Newborn, or Fetus With Grief Work (Hockenberry & Wilson, 2015; *Mina, 1985)

Promote Grieving

- Use baby's name when discussing the loss.
- Allow parents to share the hopes and dreams they had for the child.
- Provide parents with access to a hospital chaplain or religious leader of their choice.
- Encourage parents to see and to hold their infant to validate the reality of the loss.
- Design a method to communicate to auxiliary departments that the parents are in mourning (e.g., rose sticker on door, chart).
- Prepare a memory packet wrapped in a clean baby blanket (photograph [Polaroid], ID bracelet, footprints with birth certificate, lock of hair, crib card, fetal monitor strip, infant's blanket). Encourage them to take the memory packet home. If they prefer not to, keep the packet on file in case they change their minds later.
- Encourage parents to share the experience with their other children at home (refer to pertinent literature for consumers).
- Provide for follow-up support and referral services (e.g., support group) after discharge.

R: *Researchers have found that 100% of parents who held their deceased babies reported positive experiences. Parents who did not hold their infants reported problems with resolution of the grief process (*Ransohoff-Adler & Berger, 1989).*

R: *In a study, 80% of the parents who did not hold their deceased infants reported it was the decision of a health care professional (*Ransohoff-Adler & Berger, 1989).*

Assist Others to Comfort Grieving Parents

- Stress the importance of openly acknowledging the death.
- If the baby or fetus was named, use the name in discussions.
- Never try to lessen the loss with discussions of future pregnancies or other healthy siblings.
- Send sympathy cards. Create a remembrance (e.g., plant a tree).
- Be sensitive to the gravity of the loss for both the mother and father.

*R: Providing a caring environment of support, comfort, openness, and family involvement can facilitate positive family bereavement outcomes (*O'Mallon, 2009).*

Anticipatory Grieving[17]

Definition

State in which an individual/group experiences reactions in response to an expected significant loss

Defining Characteristics

Major (Must Be Present)

Expressed distress at potential loss

[17]This diagnosis is not presently on the NANDA-I list but has been added for clarity and usefulness.

Minor (May Be Present)

Anger
Change in communication patterns, eating habits, sleep patterns, and/or social patterns
Decreased libido
Denial
Guilt
Sorrow
Withdrawal

Related Factors

See *Grieving*.

Author's Note

"Anticipatory Grieving is thought to begin when an individual is forewarned of an impending death. Anticipatory grieving may take the form of sadness, anxiety, attempts to reconcile unresolved relationship issues, and efforts to reconstitute or strengthen family bonds. Caretaking behavior may be a form of anticipatory grieving, as the caretaker expresses affection, respect, and attachment through the physical acts of providing care. Anticipation and an opportunity to prepare psychologically for death is thought to ease the adaptation of the grieving individual after death" (Black, 2013).

Goals

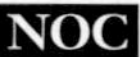

NOC
See also *Grieving*.

Individual will identify expected loss, and grief reactions will be freely expressed, as evidenced by the following indicators:

- Participates in decision making for the future
- Shares concerns with significant others

Interventions

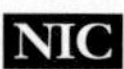

NIC
See also *Grieving*.

Assess for Causative and Contributing Factors of Anticipated or Potential Loss

- Frail elderly
- Body image, self-esteem, or role changes
- Impending retirement
- Terminal illness
- Separation (divorce, hospitalization, marriage, relocation, job)
- Socioeconomic status

Encourage to Share Concerns

- Use open-ended questions and reflection ("What are your thoughts today?" "How do you feel?").
- Acknowledge the value of the individual and his or her grief by using touch, sitting with him or her, and verbalizing your concern ("This must be very difficult," "What is most important to you now?").
- Recognize that some people may choose not to share their concerns, but convey that you are available if they desire to do so later ("What do you hope for?").

Assist the Individual and Family to Identify Strengths

- "What do you do well?"
- "What are you willing to do to address this issue?"
- "Is religion/spirituality a source of strength for you?"
- "Do you have close friends?"
- "Whom do you turn to in times of need?"
- "What does this person do for you?"
- "What sources of strength have you called upon successfully in the past?"

Promote Integrity of the Family by Acknowledging Strengths

- "Your brother looks forward to your visit."
- "Your family is so concerned for you."

Support With Grief Reactions

- Prepare them for possible grief reactions.
- Explain possible grief reactions.
- Focus on the current situation until the individual or family indicates the desire to discuss the future.

Promote Family Cohesiveness

Identify Availability of a Support System

- Meet consistently with family members.
- Identify family member roles, strengths, and weaknesses.

Identify Communication Patterns Within the Family Unit

- Assess positive and negative feedback, verbal and nonverbal communication, and body language.
- Listen and clarify messages being sent.

Provide for the Concept of Hope

- Supply accurate information.
- Resist the temptation to give false hope.
- Discuss concerns willingly.
- Help the family reframe hope (i.e., for a peaceful death).

Promote Group Decision Making to Enhance Group Autonomy

- Establish consistent times to meet with the individual and the family.
- Encourage members to talk directly with and to listen to one another.

Promote Grief Work With Each Response

Isolation

- Listen and spend designated time consistently with individual and family.
- Offer the opportunities to explore their emotions.
- Reflect on past losses and acknowledge loss behavior (past and present).

Depression

- Begin with simple problem-solving and move toward acceptance.
- Enhance self-worth through positive reinforcement.
- Identify level of depression and indications of suicidal behavior or ideas.
- Be consistent and establish times daily to speak with individual and family.

Anger

- Support crying as a release of this energy.
- Listen to and communicate concern.
- Encourage concerned support from significant others as well as professionals.

Guilt

- Listen and communicate concern.
- Promote more direct expression of feelings.
- Explore methods to resolve guilt, such as ritual forgiveness.

Fear

- Help the individual and family to recognize the feeling.
- Explain that fear is a normal aspect of grieving.
- Explore attitudes about loss, death, etc.
- Explore methods of coping.

Rejection

- Allow for verbal expression of this feeling to diminish the emotional strain.
- Recognize that expression of anger may cause rejection by significant others.

Provide for Expression of Grief

- Encourage emotional expressions of grieving.
- Caution about use of sedatives and tranquilizers, which may prevent or delay expressions.
- Encourage verbalization by all age groups.
  - Support family cohesiveness.
  - Promote and verbalize strengths of the family group.

- Encourage the individual and family to engage in life review.
  - Focus and support the social network relationships.
  - Reevaluate past life experiences and integrate them into a new meaning.
  - Convey empathic understanding.
  - Explore unfinished business.

Provide Health Teaching and Referrals, as Indicated

Refer the Individual With Potential for Dysfunctional Grieving Responses for Counseling (Psychiatrist, Nurse Therapist, Counselor, Psychologist)

Explain What to Expect
- Anger
- Fear
- Feelings of aloneness
- Feeling of "going crazy"
- Guilt
- Labile emotions
- Sadness
- Rejection

Teach the Signs of Resolution
- Grieving individual no longer lives in the past but establishes new goals for life.
- Grieving individual redefines relationship with the lost object/person.
- Grieving individual begins to resocialize.

Teach Signs of Complicated Responses and Referrals Needed
- Defenses used in uncomplicated grief work that become exaggerated or maladaptive responses
- Persistent absence of any emotion
- Prolonged intense reactions of anxiety, anger, fear, guilt, and helplessness

Identify Agencies That May Enhance Grief Work
- Self-help groups
- Widow-to-widow groups
- Parents of deceased children
- Single-parent groups

R: *Research validates that professional interventions and professionally supported voluntary and self-help services are capable of reducing the risk of psychiatric and psychoanalytic disorders resulting from bereavement (*Bonanno & Lilienfeld, 2008; Boyd, 2012).*

R: *Home care of a dying relative can provide the family with choice and control, reduce feelings of helplessness, and promote effective grieving after death (Wright & Hogan, 2008).*

Complicated Grieving

NANDA-I Definition

A disorder that occurs after the death of a significant person, of which the experience of distress accompanying bereavement fails to follow normative expectations and manifests in functional impairment

Defining Characteristics

Major (Must Be Present, One or More)

Unsuccessful adaptation to loss
Prolonged denial, depression
Delayed emotional reaction
Inability to assume normal patterns of living
Grief avoidance*
Yearning*

Minor (May Be Present)

Social isolation or withdrawal
Inability to develop new relationships/interests
Inability to restructure life after loss
Rumination*
Self-blame*
Verbalizes persistent painful memories*

Related Factors

See *Grieving*.

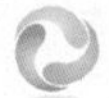

Author's Note

Complicated Grieving represents a maladaptive process in which grief work is suppressed or absent or an individual exhibits prolonged exaggerated responses. In the above definition, "fails to follow normative expectations" can be problematic. Who judges what a normal response to loss is. After a young mother loses her son to a tragic accident, she goes to the grave every day and leaves him a sandwich. Is this pathological? The question is what is she doing when she is not visiting the grave? How is she responding to her other children? Is this grave side activity preventing her from living her life? Is she slowly getting back to living her life again? If not then the Grieving is complicated but not because she leaves a sandwich for her child. It is because she is not engaged in grief work or resuming her previous life.

Key Concepts

General Considerations

- Unresolved grief may be difficult to determine because the grief experience has no clearly defined end point, nor is there a "right way" to grieve (Varcarolis, 2011). Some people do experience factors that interfere with the natural progress of grief work and, therefore, its resolution. *Rando (1984) outlines eight variations of unresolved grief:
  - *Absent grief:* as if the death never occurred
  - *Inhibited grief:* can mourn only certain aspects of the loss
  - *Delayed grief:* cannot experience grief at the time of loss (e.g., "I must be strong for my children now.")
  - *Conflicted grief:* often associated with a previous dependent or ambivalent relationship
  - *Chronic grief:* ongoing intense grief reaction, sometimes serves to keep the deceased "alive" through grief
  - *Unanticipated grief:* cannot grasp the full implications of loss; extreme bewilderment, anxiety, self-reproach, and depression
  - *Abbreviated grief:* often confused with unresolved grief, this shortened but normal form of grief might occur when significant grief work has been done before the loss
  - *Disenfranchised grief:* usually associated with a socially unacceptable or negated loss (e.g., suicide, AIDS)
- Unresolved grief is a pathologic response of prolonged denial of the loss or a profound psychotic response. Examples include the following:
  - Refusal to remove possessions of deceased after a reasonable time
  - Lasting loss of normal patterns of social behavior
  - Progressively deeper regression and depression
  - Progressively deeper isolation
  - Somatic manifestations (prolonged)
  - Obsessions and phobias
  - Delusions and hallucinations
  - Attempted suicide
  - Substance, alcohol, prescribed opioids/sedative abuse
- Predisposing factors attributed to *Complicated Grieving* are as follows (*Worden, 2009):
  - A socially unspeakable or negated loss (e.g., suicide, AIDS-related death)
  - New feelings of dependency and neediness associated with the loss
  - History of depressive illness or previous complicated grief reactions
  - Sudden, uncertain, or overcomplicated circumstances surrounding the loss
  - A highly ambivalent, narcissistic, or dependent relationship with the deceased

R: *Grief work cannot begin until the individual acknowledges the loss. Nurses can encourage this acknowledgment by engaging in open, honest dialogue, providing the family an opportunity to view the dead person and recognizing and validating the grief (*Leming & Dickinson, 2010; Vanezis & McGee, 1999).*

Focus Assessment Criteria

See *Grieving*.

Goals

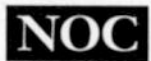

See also *Grieving*.

The individual will verbalize intent to seek professional assistance, as evidenced by the following indicators:

- Acknowledges the loss
- Acknowledges an unresolved grief process

Interventions

Carp's Cues

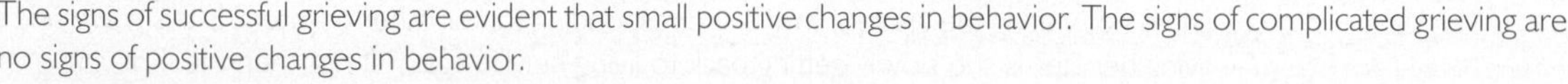

The signs of successful grieving are evident that small positive changes in behavior. The signs of complicated grieving are no signs of positive changes in behavior.

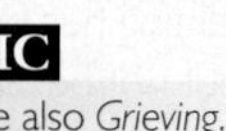

See also *Grieving*.

Assess for Causative and Contributing Factors

- Unavailable (or lack of) support system
- History of dependency on deceased
- History of a difficult relationship with the lost person or object
- Multiple past losses
- Ineffective coping strategies
- Unexpected or traumatic death
- Expectations to "be strong"

R: *The more dependent the individual was on the deceased person, the more difficult the resolution (Varcarolis, 2011).*

R: *Unresolved conflicts disrupt successful grief work (Varcarolis, 2011).*

Promote a Trust Relationship

- Implement the General Interventions under *Grieving*.

Support the Individual's and the Family's Grief Reactions

- Implement the General Interventions under *Grieving*.

Promote Family Cohesiveness

- Implement the General Interventions under *Grieving*.
- Slowly and carefully identify the reality of the situation (e.g., "After your husband died, who helped you most?").

R: *People with few supportive relationships have more difficulty grieving (*Leming & Dickinson, 2010; Varcarolis, 2011).*

Explore with loved ones for factors that can hinder grieving (*Worden, 2009)

- History of an ambivalent, hostile, overly dependent relationship
- Uncertainty of death, for example, missing inaction
- Multiple losses at the same time. For example, 9/11, entire family killed in accident
- History of complicated or delayed grieving
- Family member designated as the "strong one" is not allowed to grieve.

Promote Grief Work With Each Response

- Explain the use of denial by one family member to the other members.
- Do not force the individual to move past denial without emotional readiness.

Isolation

- Convey a feeling of acceptance by allowing grief.
- Create open, honest communication to promote sharing.
- Reinforce the individual's self-worth by allowing privacy.
- Encourage the individual/family gradually to increase social activities (e.g., support or church groups).

Depression

- Implement the General Interventions under *Grieving*.

Anger

- Understand that this feeling usually replaces denial.
- Explain to the family that anger serves to try to control one's environment more closely because of inability to control loss.
- Encourage verbalization of the anger.
- See *Anxiety* for additional information for anger.

Guilt/Ambivalence

- Acknowledge the individual's expressed self-view.
- Role play to allow the individual to "express" to dead person what he or she wants to say or how he or she feels.
- Encourage the individual to identify positive contributions/aspects of the relationship.
- Avoid arguing and participating in the individual's system of shoulds and should nots.
- Discuss the individual's preoccupation with dead person and attempt to move verbally beyond the present.

Fear

- Focus on the present and maintain a safe and secure environment.
- Help the individual to explore reasons for a meaning of the behavior.
- Consider alternative ways of expressing his or her feelings.

R: *Unresolved conflicts disrupt successful grief work (*Leming & Dickinson, 2010; Varcarolis, 2011).*

Provide Health Teaching and Referrals, as Indicated

Teach the Individual and the Family Signs of Resolution

- Grieving individual no longer lives in the past, but is future oriented and is establishing new goals.
- Grieving individual redefines the relationship with the lost object/person.
- Grieving individual begins to resocialize; seeks new relationships, experiences.

R: *The final task is to initiate the beginning of withdrawing from the paralyzing pain of the loss and to begin with baby steps to return to a productive life. It is represented by reengaging activities and relationships. Many have guilt that others will judge them badly. Taking these steps indicated integrating the loss into one's life. It does not diminish the love you had for the deceased person.*

Identify Agencies That May Be Helpful

- Support groups
- Mental health agencies
- Psychotherapists
- Grief specialists
- Faith communities

R: *Risk of death is greater in men than in women during the first 6 months of conjugal bereavement. Changes in health behavior patterns, such as nutrition, alcohol use, smoking, and decreased physical activity levels, may contribute to this increased mortality rate (*Leming & Dickinson, 2010).*

R: *People with few supportive relationships have more difficulty grieving (*Leming & Dickinson, 2010; Varcarolis, 2011).*

Risk for Complicated Grieving

NANDA-I Definition

Vulnerable to a disorder that occurs after the death of a significant other, in which the experience of distress accompanying bereavement fails to follow normative expectations and manifests in functional impairment, which may compromise health.

Risk Factors

Death of significant other
Insufficient social support
Emotional disturbance

Key Concepts

See *Grieving*.

Focus Assessment Criteria

See *Grieving*.

Goals

See *Grieving*.

Interventions/Rationales

See *Grieving*.

DELAYED GROWTH AND DEVELOPMENT

Delayed Growth and Development

Risk for Delayed Development
Adult Failure to Thrive

NANDA-I Definition

Deviations from age-group norms

Defining Characteristics

Inability or difficulty performing skills or behaviors typical of his or her age group
Altered physical growth in weight and/or height outside the expected percentile
Flat affect
Listlessness
Decreased response time
Slow or inappropriate social responses
Limited signs of satisfaction to caregiver
Difficulty feeding
Decreased appetite
Limited eye contact
Lethargy
Irritability
Negative mood
Regression or delay in self-toileting
Regression or delay in self-feeding

Related Factors

Pathophysiologic Causes

Disability related to trauma

Mental/Behavior disabilities
Child abuse or neglect
Cardiovascular defects or disease
Central nervous system dysfunction
Congenital anomalies of the extremities
Genetic disorders (e.g., cystic fibrosis)
GI dysfunction
Inadequate nutritional intake (e.g., failure to thrive)
Malabsorption syndrome
Prolonged pain
Muscular dystrophy
Repeated acute or chronic illness resulting in disability

Delays from Treatment Modalities

Confinement for ongoing treatment
Isolation secondary to their disease process
Prolonged bed rest
Prolonged, painful treatments
Traction, casts, splints, etc.
Repeated and/or prolonged hospitalizations

Situational Causes

Parent's insufficient knowledge of child care, development, and growth
Change in environment
Separation from significant persons in child's life (e.g., parents, friends, other caregivers)
School-related conflicts (e.g., bullying)
Death of significant persons in child's life (e.g., parents, friends, other caregivers)
Loss or lack of control over environment (e.g., established routines, rituals, or traditions)
Inadequate parental support, as in cases of neglect or abuse
Inadequate sensory stimulation, as in cases of neglect or isolation
Cultural beliefs or practices

Maturational Causes

Infant–Toddler (Birth to 3 Years)

Separation from parents/significant caregivers
Inadequate parental support and its resulting impact on child
Inability to communicate related to preexisting condition (e.g., hearing or vision dysfunction or loss)
Restriction of daily activities secondary to illness or defect
Inability to trust significant caregivers or parents in their life
Multiple caregivers
Excessive painful experiences (e.g., ongoing medical treatments or abuse)

Preschool (4 to 6 Years)

Inability or loss to communicate through preexisting condition or trauma
Lack of stimulation (e.g., neglect)
Instability in parent/caregiver's lives (e.g., divorce, domestic violence)
Death of parent/caregiver
Additional children being added to the family unit
Removal of child from home environment
Negative social interactions with peers

School-Aged Children (6 to 11 Years)

Negative social interactions with peers
Bullying
Self-consciousness about preexisting condition (mental disability or physical deformity)
Death or loss of parent/caregiver or significant friend

Adolescent (12 to 18 Years)
Negative social interactions with peers
  Bullying
  Self-consciousness about preexisting condition (mental disability or physical deformity)
Impact on body image (e.g., physical deformities from trauma or congenital malformation)
Loss of parent/caregiver or significant friend/loved one
Loss of independence of autonomy secondary to preexisting condition or trauma

Author's Note

Specific developmental tasks are associated with various age groups (e.g., to gain autonomy and self-control [e.g., toileting] from 1 to 3 years of age and to establish lasting relationships from 18 to 30 years of age). An adult's failure to accomplish a developmental task may cause or contribute to a change in functioning in a functional health pattern (e.g., *Impaired Social Interactions*, *Powerlessness*). Because nursing interventions focus on altered functioning rather than achievement of past developmental tasks, the diagnosis *Delayed Growth and Development* has limited use for adults. It is most useful for a child or an adolescent experiencing difficulty achieving a developmental task.

Errors in Diagnostic Statements

Delayed Growth and Development related to inability to perform toileting self-control appropriate for age (4 years)

Inability to perform toileting self-control is not a contributing factor but a diagnostic cue. The nurse should rewrite the diagnosis as *Delayed Growth and Development related to unknown etiology*, as evidenced by inability to perform toileting self-control appropriate for age (4 years). The use of "unknown etiology" directs nurses to collect more data on reasons for the problem.

Delayed Growth and Development related to mental retardation secondary to Down syndrome

When *Delayed Growth and Development* is used to describe an individual with mental or physical impairment, what is the nursing focus? What goals would nursing interventions achieve? If physical impairments represent barriers to achieve developmental tasks, the nurse can write the diagnosis as *Risk for Delayed Growth and Development related to impaired ability to achieve developmental tasks (specify—e.g., socialization) secondary to disability*. For a child with mental impairment, the nurse should determine what functional health patterns are altered or at high risk for alteration and amenable to nursing interventions and address the specific problem (e.g., *Toileting Self-Care Deficit*).

Key Concepts

- A developmental disorder can be defined as "an abnormal, slower rate of development in which a child demonstrates a functioning level below that observed in normal children of the same age" (Hockenberry & Wilson, 2015).
- Normal development follows a definable, predictable, and sequential pattern. Interruptions in this process due to congenital or environmental causes can result in disability or delay.
- Growth and development are most rapidly developing early in life. Disruptions that occur at these ages can have more significant impacts in the child's life.
- Growth and development are not always regimented processes. They can occur in spurts but are always continuous on some level. Every child develops at their own rate.
- Development occurs from simple to complex and occurs in all aspects of a child's life (motor, intellectual, personal, social, and language/sensory) (Table II.7).

Focus Assessment Criteria

Current Nutritional Patterns
Parental/child's knowledge of nutrition
Diet history
Height/weight at birth
Intake patterns
Child's habits/reactions related to eating/drinking or feeds
Diet recall (what and how much does child eat on a daily basis)

Table II.7 DEVELOPMENTAL GOALS BY AGE AND THE IMPACT OF ILLNESS OR DISABILITY

Developmental Goal	Impact of Illness or Disability	Interventions
Infant–Toddler		
Development of trust in the caregiver	• Multiple caregivers • Frequent separation or removal from parent/caregiver secondary to hospitalization for condition	• Encourage frequent, consistent visitation between child and parent/caregivers.
Formation of bonding attachment to parent/caregiver	• Separation of child from their parent/caregivers secondary to frequent hospitalizations or isolation (e.g., neonate in an Isolette and parent's limited ability to hold them) • Parent/caregiver's inability to accept patient's condition, disability, or deformity • Parent/caregiver's grief over loss of idea of the perfect child	• Emphasize the healthy aspects of the child and educate the parent/caregivers about how to manage and care for the child's illness/disability.
Learning through sensory stimulation	• Increased exposure to painful experiences/procedures and lack of pleasurable ones that encourage healthy learning and development • Sensory deprivation secondary to confinement or isolation related to disease process	• Encourage age-appropriate stimulation whenever possible and encourage family/caregivers to do the same. Encourage parent/caregivers to participate in child's care when possible.
Preschool-Age		
Mastering self-care skills	• Limited opportunities for learning these skills	• Encourage and offer opportunities for learning. • Provide assistance or devices that would help facilitate learning when appropriate.
Developing peer relationships	• Limited opportunities for interaction related to hospitalization or isolation	• Encourage relationships with others. • Provide opportunities for age-appropriate play. • Encourage socialization.
Developing body image	• Developing awareness of their disability and its possible impact on their appearance • Associates pain, failure, and anxiety when it comes to their physical existence	• Help the child learn to cope with criticism or social awkwardness.
School Age		
Developing sense of accomplishments	• Limited opportunities for achievements and competitions in peer-related activities	• Encourage school attendance and school activities. Whenever possible, schedule medical treatments around these social activities.
Forming peer relationships and bonds	• Limited opportunities for social interaction secondary to hospitalization or isolation	• Encourage and provide information about clubs and activities that child could safely participate in.
Adolescence		
Developing sexual and personal identity	• Increased realization of limitations from illness/disability on their appearance or the way they relate to others	• Encourage and provide education about coping skills.
Developing sense of independence from parent/caregiver	• Inability to be self-reliant and the impact that they may never be full independent	• Encourage socialization with peers of similar age and special needs.
Emergence of sexual behavior and relationships	• Doubt about whether they will have normal relationship as an adult or have children	• Encourage socialization in mixed-sex settings, especially those with similar limitations. • Encourage emphasis of child's perceived positive attributes such as make up, haircuts, and stylish clothes. • Provide information about reproductive options as appropriate.

Source: Hockenberry, M. J., & Wilson, D. (2015). *Wong's essentials of pediatric nursing* (10th ed.). New York: Elsevier

Physiologic Alterations
Nausea
Vomiting
Diarrhea
Food intolerances/allergies
Dysphagia

Fatigue

Parental Attitudes

What are the child's expectations of the child?
What are their feelings about being a parent?
What is the parent's approach to care and discipline of the child?
How do the parents feel about the home situation?
How do the parents feel about the child's illness or disability?
Assess the family's functioning level and identify areas that need attention.
Identify cultural beliefs or traditions that need to be observed and considered.

Stressors

Child's behavior and level of success in school
Child's peer and sibling relationships
Family living arrangements
Who does the child live with? Is it more than one person at more than one location?
Are parents/caregivers separated? Are they on good terms or is there tension?
Is there extended family or nonfamily members living in the home?
Is there any history of domestic violence in any of the child's environments?
Other illnesses or disabilities in the home

General Appearance

Cleanliness and grooming
Response to stimulation
Eye contact
Mood (e.g., flat, anxious)
Facial reactions

Responses/Interactions with Parent

Receptive to comfort from parent
Response to strangers or unpleasant stimuli
Reaction when separated from parent/caregiver

Nutritional/Elimination Status

Height/weight and compare to norms for age group
Head circumference
Bowel and bladder control

Personal/Social

Language
Cognition
Motor ability/activity

Goals

NOC
Child Development: specify age

The child will demonstrate increasing age-appropriate behaviors as evidenced by the following indicators:

- Socialization
- Language
- Motor skills
- Self-care
- Cognitive skills

Interventions

NIC
Anticipatory Guidance
Health Screening
Development Enchantment
Counseling

Assess for Causative or Contributing Factors to the Child's Developmental Stage and Carefully Evaluate the Child's Level of Functioning

Infant–Toddler

- Encourage the parent/caregiver's involvement in child's care/treatments.
- Demonstrate methods that parents can use when managing child's care at home.
- Use age-appropriate communication when preparing child for procedure.
- Consider cultural practices and beliefs.

- Encourage sensory stimulation as appropriate.
- Encourage tactile interactions between parent/caregiver and child.
- Provide frequent periods of rest/cluster care.
- Observe parent/caregiver's interactions with child and evaluate for potential risk factors.
- Respond to crying promptly and consistently.
- When possible, be consistent with staffing to limit number of people caring for and interacting with child.
- When possible and as tolerated, allow child's hands and feet to free.
- Encourage self-care as age appropriate.
- Provide periods of play and sensory stimulation as age appropriate.
- Perform unpleasant procedures in separate room from where child sleeps and plays whenever possible.

Preschool-Age

- Encourage and support parent/caregiver's presence and assistance with child's care.
- Provide child with age-appropriate play opportunities.
- Encourage social interactions with peers when possible.
- Consider cultural practices and beliefs.
- Encourage self-care as age appropriate.
- Use age-appropriate communication when preparing child for procedure.
- Provide periods of play and sensory stimulation as age appropriate.
- Use familiar routines to help child understand time.
- Verbalize frequently (e.g., saying words of equipment, reading/telling stories).
- Offer choices (e.g., which medicine do you want to take first?).
- Allow child to wear their own clothes when possible.

School Age-Adolescent

- Encourage and support parent/caregiver's presence and assistance with child's care.
- Use age-appropriate communication.
- Encourage and provide opportunities for completing schoolwork.
- Provide opportunities for play and interactions with peers when possible.
- Encourage visits from family and friends when possible.
- Allow child to wear their own clothes when possible.
- Consider cultural practices and beliefs.
- Talk frequently with the child about their feelings and thoughts and evaluate for need for possible further interventions.
- Identify child's interests/hobbies and encourage them as appropriate.
- Facilitate health care being tailored to child's developmental needs (e.g., making appointments for treatments during after-school hours).
- Provide opportunities for child to have new experiences to discover interests as appropriate (e.g., group outings or activities).

R: *Minimizing the impact of the child's illness/disability while maximizing the potential for the child's healthy development is at the heart of family-centered care (Hockenberry & Wilson, 2015).*

R: *The age of onset of child's illness/disability can determine the impact on the child but through promoting normal development, the detrimental outcomes may be minimized (Hockenberry & Wilson, 2015).*

Risk for Delayed Development

NANDA-I Definition

Vulnerable for delay of 25% or more in one or more of the areas of social or self-regulatory behavior, or cognitive, language, gorss of fine motor skills, which may be compromised.

Risk Factors

Refer to *Delayed Growth and Development.*

Goals

The child will continue to demonstrate appropriate behavior, as evidenced by the following indicators, allowing for age:

- Self-Care
- Social skills
- Language
- Cognitive skills
- Motor skills

Interventions

Refer to *Delayed Growth and Development*.

Adult Failure to Thrive

Definition

State in which the individual experiences insidious and progressive physical and psychosocial deterioration characterized by limited coping and diminished resilience in response to deteriorations in health (Carpenito, 1999).[18]

Defining Characteristics

Major (Must Be Present, One or More)

Altered mood state*
Anorexia*
Apathy*
Cognitive decline*
Consumption of minimal to no food at most meals*
Decreased social skills*
Denial of symptom(s)
Depression
Expresses loss of interest in pleasurable outlets*
Giving up
Loneliness
Neglect of home environment
Physical decline* (e.g., fatigue, dehydration, incontinence of bowel and bladder)
Social withdrawal*
Self-care deficit*
Unintentional weight loss* (e.g., 5% in 1 month, 10% in 6 months)

Related Factors

The cause of failure to thrive in adults (usually older adults) is unknown (*Kimball & Williams-Burgess, 1995; *Murray, Zentnrer, & Yakimo, 2009). Researchers have identified some possible contributing factors, listed below.

Situational (Personal, Environmental)

Related to diminished coping abilities

Related to limited ability to adapt to effects of aging

Related to loss of social skills and resultant social isolation

---

[18]This definition has been added by Lynda Juall Carpenito, the author, for clarity and usefulness.

Related to loss of social relatedness

Related to increasing dependency and feelings of helplessness

Author's Note

Adult Failure to Thrive was removed from the NANDA-I list in 2015 because it was replaced by *Frail Elderly Syndrome* (Herdman & Kamitsuru, 2014, p. 13). "Some elderly patients, including those who do not have acute illness or severe chronic disease, eventually undergo a process of functional decline, progressive apathy, and a loss of willingness to eat and drink that culminates in death" (*Robertson & Montagnini, 2004). "Failure to thrive should not be considered a normal consequence of aging, a synonym for dementia, the inevitable result of a chronic disease, or a descriptor of the later stages of a terminal disease" (*Robertson & Montagnini, 2004).

Errors in Diagnostic Statements

Adult Failure to Thrive related to dementia

Dementia does not cause *Adult Failure to Thrive*, but actually represents a cause of the condition. Because the cause is uncertain, the nurse may find *Adult Failure to Thrive related to unknown etiology* clinically useful. If dementia is also present, refer to *Chronic Confusion*.

Key Concepts

- Failure to thrive is a "complex presentation of symptoms causing gradual decline in physical and cognitive function that occurs without immediate explanation" (*Murray et al., 2009).
- The United States National Institute of Aging described FTT as a "syndrome of weight loss, decreased appetite and poor nutrition, and inactivity, often accompanied by dehydration, depressive symptoms, impaired immune function, and low cholesterol" (*Sarkisian & Lachs, 1996).
- The condition affects 5% to 35% of community-dwelling older adults, 25% to 40% of nursing home residents, and 50% to 60% of hospitalized veterans (Agarwal, 2014).
- In elderly individuals, failure to thrive is associated with increased infection rates, diminished cell-mediated immunity, hip fractures, decubitus ulcers, and increased surgical mortality rates (Agarwal, 2014).
- People who are not include are those who (*Haight, 2002; *Wagnil & Young, 1990) have pride; help others; have family supports in place; are perseverant and self-reliant; have experienced hardships; have cultural, spiritual, and religious values; and who regularly enhance their self-care activities.
- Older adults who cannot cope with changes after a stressful life event will feel unprotected, empty, and lonely (*Newbern & Krowchuk, 1994).
- "Interaction with the environment is as critical to thriving as a human being at the end of life as at the beginning" (*Newbern & Krowchuk, 1994).
- Older adults overwhelmed by a sense of helplessness and hopelessness give up.
- Failure to thrive implies that the older adult *should* thrive despite chronic illness and age-related changes. It is not a normal part of aging (*Kimball & Williams-Burgess, 1995).
- Resilience is a combination of abilities and characteristics that allow an individual to bounce back and/or cope successfully in spite of significant stress or adverse events (*Tusaie & Dyer, 2004).

Focus Assessment Criteria

Assessing and diagnosing *Adult Failure to Thrive* requires evaluation for new pathology or, if a condition is under treatment, a thorough functional assessment (physical, cognitive) and evaluation of the individual's strengths and coping patterns.

Determine If the Following Laboratory/Diagnostic Tests Have Been Assessed (*Robertson & Montagnini, 2004)

- Growth hormone, testosterone (men), serum albumin, and cholesterol levels
- Blood culture, HIV, RPR test, complete blood count, serum glucose level, thyroid-stimulating hormone level, urinalysis
- Serum BUN and creatinine levels, serum electrolyte levels
- Vitamin B_{12} and folate levels, vitamin D levels

- QuantiFERON-TB
- Chest radiography, EKG

Ensure the Following Are Evaluated (*Robertson & Montagnini, 2004)

- Medication review (side effects, necessary, alternatives)

R: *Several medications can cause cognition changes, anorexia, depression, dehydration, electrolyte abnormalities; for example, more than four prescription medications, beta blockers, tricyclic antidepressants, anticholinergic drugs, diuretics (high-potency combinations, benzodiazepines (*Robertson & Montagnini, 2004).*

- A standardized scale for assessing ADL activities and Up + Go test (by physical therapy
- Geriatric depression scale

R: *Depression in older adults has been identified in from 10% to 25% in community settings and 50% of nursing home residents (*Miller, 2015).*

- Ensure a nutritional reconciliation is performed, for example, daily caloric intake, the availability of food, oral pathology, ill-fitting dentures, problems with speech or swallowing, medication use that might cause anorexia, financial and social problems that may negatively impact nutrition.

R: *"Nutrition reconciliation is defined as the process of maximizing health by helping align an individual's current diet to the diet prescribed for him or her by the health care team" (Tuso & Beattle, 2015).*

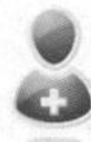

Clinical Alert An estimated 14.3% of American households were food insecure, and those with very low food security were 5.6% (Gregory & Singh, 2014). A high number of individuals admitted to the hospital suffer from protein energy malnutrition and obesity. These conditions are associated with unhealthy eating habits and food insecurity related to finances (Tuso & Beattle, 2015). Unfortunately, obesity is often not seen as state of malnutrition (Ibid).

- Presence of chronic diseases

R: *All medical conditions present in an individual with failure to thrive should be evaluated to determine if the treatment plan is optimal) (*Robertson & Montagnini, 2004)*

- Environmental Assessment (support system safety, socialization)

R: *Some of these contributors are unmodifiable, some are easily modifiable, and some are potentially modifiable but only with the use of resource-intensive strategies. Initial interventions should be directed at easily remediable contributors in the hope of improving overall functional status, because a single contributor may simultaneously influence several other syndromes that conspire to create the phenotype of failure to thrive (*Robertson & Montagnini, 2004).*

If indicated, refer to other nursing diagnoses such as:

- Self-care ability—refer to *Self-Care Deficit Syndrome*
- Cognition—refer to *Confusion*
- Coping—refer to *Ineffective Coping*
- Socialization—refer to *Risk for Loneliness*
- Nutrition—refer to *Imbalanced Nutrition*

Goals

NOC

Physical Aging, Psychological Adjustment, Self-Management, Will to Live, Personal Resiliency, Social Involvement, Leisure Participation

The individual will participate to increase functioning, as evidenced by the following indicators:

- Increases social relatedness
- Maintains or increase present weight

Interventions

NIC

Caregiver support, Nutrition management, Coping enhancement, Hope inspiration, Cognitive Stimulation

Keep an Open Mind Regarding the Possibility of Identifying and Correcting Causative Factors with a Correspondent Improvement in Functioning

R: *Often, the cause or causes of the deterioration are not identifiable or are irreversible (*Robertson & Montagnini, 2004).The most disturbing of these barriers is the reinforcement of a fatalistic expectation of aging "that events are fixed in advance so that human beings are powerless to change them" (Merriam-Webster, 2015)*

Ensure a Thorough Assessment and Diagnostic Work-Up Has Been Prescribed or Completed

- Refer to Focus Assessment Criteria.

Assure a Promote Socialization (Refer to *Risk for Loneliness*)

R: *Older adults who are more adaptive, report "that their social lives are determined through an ongoing struggle for identity and social relevance despite numerous later-life challenges?"(*Cornwell, Laumann, & Schumm, 2008)*

- Speak as one adult to another. Use average volume, appropriate eye contact, and slow rate of speech.
- Attempt to identify one activity that provides enjoyment.
- Engage in useful and meaningful conversations about likes, dislikes, interests, hobbies, and work history.
- Attempt to identify activities that the person can participate in without relying on family members.
- Encourage the individual to be as independent as possible.
- Stress the importance to increase exercise, for example, walking, chair exercises.
- Identify community resources for socialization and activities (*Gosline, 2003).
- Join a club or group with a shared interest, such as walking, knitting, sports, dancing, chess, or bridge.
- Join a senior center or church senior group.

R: *A constant effort must be made to maintain social roles and activity in the face of difficult later-life transitions. Since this effort is crucial in maintaining older adults' mental and physical well-being, social gerontologists view social integration as a key component of "successful aging" (*Cornwell et al., 2008).*

Institute Health Teaching and Referrals, as Indicated

RISK-PRONE HEALTH BEHAVIOR

Definition

Impaired ability to modify lifestyle/behaviors in a manner that improves health status (NANDA-I)

State in which a person has an inability to modify lifestyle/behavior in a manner consistent with a change in health status.[19]

Defining Characteristics*

Demonstrates nonacceptance of health status change
Failure to achieve optimal sense of control
Minimizes health status change
Failure to take action that prevents health problems

Related Factors

Situational (Personal, Environmental)

Related to:

Low self-efficacy*
Negative attitude toward health care*
Multiple stressors
Inadequate social support*
Inadequate resources
Inadequate finances
Multiple responsibilities

[19]This definition has been added by Lynda Juall Carpenito, the author, for clarity and usefulness.

Related to unhealthy lifestyle choices (e.g., tobacco use, excessive alcohol use, overweight)

Related to impaired ability to understand secondary to:

Low literacy
Language barriers

Author's Note

This nursing diagnosis replaces the NANDA diagnosis *Impaired Adjustment. Risk-Prone Health Behavior* has some commonalities with *Ineffective Health Maintenance* and *Noncompliance.* This author recommends that *Ineffective Health Maintenance* be used to describe a person with an unhealthy lifestyle that puts him or her at risk for a chronic health problem or disease. *Noncompliance* applies to a person who wants to comply, but factors are present that deter adherence.

Risk-Prone Health Behavior describes a person with a health problem who is not participating in management of the health problem because of lack of motivation, comprehension, or personal barriers.

Errors in Diagnostic Statements

***Risk-Prone Health Behavior* related to high-fat diet and sedentary lifestyle**

This diagnosis represents an unhealthy lifestyle. The related factors are actually signs and symptoms, not related factors; thus, the diagnosis would be *Ineffective Health Maintenance related to unknown etiology as evidenced by high-fat diet and sedentary lifestyle.* It is necessary for the nurse to assess what factors fall under "related to," such as lack of knowledge, inadequate time, or access barriers.

***Noncompliance* related to unknown etiology as evidenced by reports it is not necessary to monitor blood glucose levels daily**

Because the individual with diabetes does not desire to monitor blood glucose levels, the focus is on helping him or her understand the importance through motivation, attitude, and behavior changes. *Risk-Prone Health Behavior related to unknown etiology as evidenced by reports it is not necessary to monitor blood glucose levels daily* would be more appropriate because it would focus on behavior changes. *Noncompliance* should focus on barriers that do not relate to motivation.

Key Concepts

General Considerations

- "Self-management support is the assistance caregivers give individuals with chronic diseases to encourage daily decisions that improve health-related behaviors and clinical outcomes" (*Bodenheimer, MacGregor, & Sharifi, 2005).
- Help individuals to choose health behaviors in a collaborative partnership with the caregivers (*Bodenheimer et al., 2005).
- Refer to *Ineffective Health Maintenance Management* for key concepts on health education, self-efficacy, and barriers to learning.
- Motivational interviewing is a readiness to change the model in which readiness = importance × confidence. Techniques are used to assess readiness to change (importance and confidence) and to encourage individuals to increase their readiness (*Rollnick, Mason, & Butler, 2000).

Literacy

- Health literacy is "the degree to which individuals have that capacity to obtain, process, and understand basic health information and services needed to make appropriate health decisions" (*Cutilli, 2005).
- Those with the highest incidence of low literacy:
  - Are poor
  - Live in the South and West
  - Have less than a high school diploma
  - Are members of an ethnic/cultural minority older than 65 years of age
  - Have physical/mental disabilities
  - Are homeless or inmates

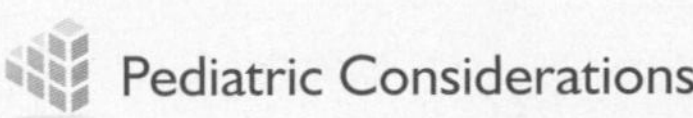

Pediatric Considerations

The Youth Risk Behavior Surveillance System

- The Youth Risk Behavior Surveillance System (YRBSS) monitors six categories of priority health-risk behaviors among youth and young adults: (1) behaviors that contribute to unintentional injuries and violence; (2) tobacco use; (3) alcohol and other drug use; (4) sexual behaviors that contribute to unintended pregnancy and sexually transmitted infections (STIs), including human immunodeficiency virus (HIV) infection; (5) unhealthy dietary behaviors; and (6) physical inactivity. In addition, YRBSS monitors the prevalence of obesity and asthma. YRBSS includes a national school-based Youth Risk Behavior Survey (YRBS) conducted by Centers for Disease Control and Prevention [CDC] and state and large urban school district school-based YRBSs conducted by state and local education and health agencies. This report summarizes results for 104 health-risk behaviors plus obesity, overweight, and asthma from the 2013 national survey, 42 state surveys, and 21 large urban school district surveys conducted among students in grades 9 to 12 (CDC, 2014).
- The findings reported:

Bicycle/Car Safety

- Of the 67.0% of students nationwide who had ridden a bicycle during the 12 months before the survey, 87.9% had never or rarely worn a bicycle helmet.
- Of the 64.3% students nationwide who drove a car or other vehicle during the 30 days before the survey, 10.0% had driven a car or other vehicle one or more times when they had been drinking alcohol during the 30 days before the survey.
- 21.9% of students nationwide had ridden one or more times in a car or other vehicle driven by someone who had been drinking alcohol during the 30 days before the survey.
- Of the 64.7% of students nationwide who drove a car or other vehicle during the 30 days before the survey, 41.4% had texted or e-mailed while driving a car or other vehicle on at least one day during the 30 days before the survey.

Weapons/Violence/Bulling

- 17.9% of students had carried a weapon (e.g., gun, knife, or club) on at least 1 day during the 30 days before the survey.
- 6.9% of students had been threatened or injured with a weapon (e.g., a gun, knife, or club) on school property one or more times during the 12 months before the survey.
- 8.1% of students had been in a physical fight on school property one or more times during the 12 months before the survey.
- 7.1% of students had not gone to school on at least 1 day during the 30 days before the survey because they felt they would be unsafe at school or on their way to or from school (i.e., did not go to school because of safety concerns).
- 14.8% of students had been electronically bullied, including being bullied through e-mail, chat rooms, instant messaging, websites, or texting, during the 12 months before the survey.

Sexual Violence

- 7.3% of students had been physically forced to have sexual intercourse when they did not want to.
- Of 73.9% of students nationwide who dated or went out with someone during the 12 months before the survey, 10.3% had been hit, slammed into something, or injured with an object or weapon on purpose by someone they were dating or going out with one or more times during the 12 months before the survey.
- Of 73.9% of students nationwide who dated or went out with someone during the 12 months before the survey, 10.4% of students had been kissed, touched, or physically forced to have sexual intercourse when they did not want to by someone they were dating.
- 29.9% of students nationwide had felt so sad or hopeless almost every day for 2 or more weeks in a row that they stopped doing some usual activities.

Suicide

- 17.0% of students had seriously considered attempting suicide during the 12 months before the survey.
- 13.6% of students nationwide had made a plan about how they would attempt suicide during the 12 months before the survey.
- 8.0% of students had attempted suicide one or more times during the 12 months before the survey.
- 2.7% of students nationwide had made a suicide attempt that resulted in an injury, poisoning, or overdose that had to be treated by a doctor or nurse during the 12 months before the survey.

Tobacco Use

- 9.3% of students had smoked a whole cigarette for the first time before age 13 years.
- 15.7% of students had smoked cigarettes on at least 1 day during the 30 days before the survey (i.e., current cigarette use).
- 8.8% of students had used smokeless tobacco (e.g., chewing tobacco, snuff, or dip) on at least 1 day during the 30 days before the survey.

Alcohol/Drug Use

- 18.6% of students had drunk alcohol (other than a few sips) for the first time before age 13 years.
- 20.8% of students had had five or more drinks of alcohol in a row (i.e., within a couple of hours) on at least 1 day during the 30 days before the survey.
- 40.7% of students had used marijuana one or more times during their life (i.e., ever used marijuana).
- 8.6% of students had tried marijuana for the first time before age 13 years.
- 23.4% of students had used marijuana one or more times during the 30 days before the survey.
- 5.5% of students had used any form of cocaine (e.g., powder, crack, or freebase) one or more times during their life.
- 7.1% of students had used hallucinogenic drugs (e.g., LSD, acid, PCP, angel dust, mescaline, or mushrooms).
- 8.9% of students had sniffed glue, breathed the contents of aerosol spray cans, or inhaled any paints or sprays to get high one or more times during their life.
- 6.6% of students had used ecstasy (also called MDMA) one or more times during their life.
- 2.2% of students had used heroin (also called "smack," "junk," or "China White") one or more times during their life.
- 3.2% of students had used methamphetamines (also called "speed," "crystal," "crank," or "ice") one or more times during their life.
- 17.8% of students had taken prescription drugs (e.g., OxyContin, Percocet, Vicodin, codeine, Adderall, Ritalin, or Xanax) without a doctor's prescription one or more times during their life (i.e., ever took prescription drugs without a doctor's prescription). The prevalence of having ever taken prescription drugs without a doctor's prescription was 17.8 %.

Sexual Behavior/Birth Control

- 46.8% of students had ever had sexual intercourse.
- 5.6% of students had had sexual intercourse for the first time before age 13 years.
- 15.0% of students had had sexual intercourse with four or more persons during their life.
- 34.0% of students had had sexual intercourse with at least one person during the 3 months before the survey.
- Of 34.0% of currently sexually active students nationwide, 59.1% reported that either they or their partner had used a condom during last sexual intercourse.
- Of 34.0% of currently sexually active students nationwide, 19.0% reported that either they or their partner had used birth control pills to prevent pregnancy before last sexual intercourse.
- Of 34.0% of currently sexually active students nationwide, 25.3% reported that either they or their partner had used birth control pills; an IUD (such as Mirena or Para Gard) or implant (such as Implanon or Nexplanon); or a shot (such as Depo-Provera), patch (such as OrthoEvra), or birth control ring (such as NuvaRing) to prevent pregnancy before last sexual intercourse.
- Of 34.0% of currently sexually active students nationwide, 13.7% reported that neither they nor their partner had used any method to prevent pregnancy during last sexual intercourse.
- Of 34.0% of currently sexually active students nationwide, 22.4% had drunk alcohol or used drugs before last sexual intercourse.

Dietary Behavior

- 5.0% of students had not eaten fruit or drunk 100% fruit juices during the 7 days before the survey.
- 62.6% of students had eaten fruit or drunk 100% fruit juices one or more times per day during the 7 days before the survey.
- 21.9% of students had eaten fruit or drunk 100% fruit juices three or more times per day during the 7 days before the survey.
- 6.6% of students had not eaten vegetables during the 7 days before the survey.
- 61.5% of students had eaten vegetables 1 or more, 28.8% had eaten 2 or more, 15.8 had eaten 3 or more vegetables per day during the 7 days before the survey.

- 19.4% of students had not drunk milk during the 7 days before the survey.
- Of 40.3% of students who had drunk one or more, 25.9% of students had drunk two or more and 12.5% of students had drunk 3 or more glasses of milk per day during the 7 days before the survey.
- 22.3% of students had not drunk soda or pop (not including diet soda or diet pop) during the 7 days before the survey.
- Of 27.0% of students who had one or more times, 19.4% of students had two or more times and 11.2% of students three or more times drank a can, bottle, or glass of soda or pop (not counting diet soda or diet pop) during the 7 days before the survey.
- 13.7% of students had not eaten breakfast during the 7 days before the survey.
- 38.1% of students had eaten breakfast on all 7 days before the survey.

Exercise

- 15.2% of students had not participated in at least 60 minutes of any kind of physical activity that increased their heart rate and made them breathe hard some of the time on at least 1 day during the 7 days before the survey.
- 27.1% of students had been physically active doing any kind of physical activity that increased their heart rate and made them breathe hard some of the time.

TV, Computer, Electronic Device Use

- 41.3% of students played video or computer games or used a computer for something that was not school work for 3 or more hours per day on an average school day (i.e., used computers 3 or more hours per day).
- 32.5% of students watched television 3 or more hours per day on an average school day.

Overweight/Obesity

- 13.7% of students were obese.
- 16.6% of students were overweight.
- 31.1% of students described themselves as slightly or very overweight.
- 47.7% of students were trying to lose weight.

Miscellaneous

- 10.1% of students most of the time or always wore sunscreen with an SPF of 15 or higher when outside for more than 1 hour on a sunny day.

Focus Assessment Criteria

Subjective/Objective Data

Assess Literacy Level (*Murphy, Davis, Long, Jackson, & Decker, 1993)

Have Individual Read the Following Words:

Fat	Pill	Jaundice
Fatigue	Colitis	Osteoporosis
Flu	Allergic	Anemia
Directed	Constipation	

Note: Fat, flu, and pill are not scored. A score of 6 or fewer correct can indicate an individual at risk for poor literacy.

Assess Knowledge of Condition

Examples:

Do you know what diabetes is?

What would you like to know about hypertension?

Do you know what to do to prevent complications of diabetes?

Assess for Barriers

What do you think is causing your blood pressure (blood sugar or weight) to remain high?

What could you do to decrease your blood pressure (weight, blood sugar)?

Would you like to stop smoking (or drinking alcohol)?

What is preventing you?

Goals

NOC

Adherence Behavior, Symptom Control, Health Beliefs, Treatment Behavior, Illness/Injury

The individual will verbalize the intent to modify one behavior to manage health problem, as evidenced by the following indicators:

- Describes the health problem
- Describes the relationship of present practices/behavior to decreased health
- Engages in goal setting

Interventions

NIC

Health Education, Mutual Goal Setting, Self-responsibility, Teaching: Disease Process, Decision-Making Process

Does your practice "give patients a fish" or "teach patients to fish?"

If Low Literacy Is Suspected, Start With What the Individual Is Most Stressed About (Refer to Index for Interventions in This Book)

R: *Persons who are identified as having reading problems will have difficulty with most verbal instructions and client education material (Kalichman et al., 2005).*

- For more on health literacy read, "Health Literacy: Challenges and Strategies," found at the website for the Online Journal of Issues in Nursing (Egbert & Nanna, 2009).

Engage in Collaborative Negotiation (Tyler & Horner, 2008)

- Ask the individual: "How can you be healthier?" Focus on the area they choose.
- Do not provide unsolicited advice.
- Accept that only the individual can make the change.
- Accept resistance.

For Example: Diabetes

- Exercise
- Healthy eating
- Medication
- Blood glucose monitoring
- Individual-defined choice

R: *Motivational interviewing involves helping the individual identify the discrepancy between present behaviors and future health goals (Tyler & Horner, 2008).*

Individuals Are Responsible for Day-to-Day Decisions (*Bodenheimer et al., 2005)

- Provide information as directed by the individual:
  - Ask: What do you want to know about __________?
  - Provide information the individual wants to know.
  - Ask the individual if he or she understood.
  - Ask if there are other questions.

R: *Individuals often receive too much or too little information. When the learner chooses what to learn, health-related outcomes are improved (*Bodenheimer et al., 2005).*

Ask the Individual to Repeat the Goal, Behavior, or Activity

R: *Assessing understanding can positively improve comprehension and outcomes.*

Assess Readiness to Change

- Determine how important the individual thinks the behavior change is. For example:
  - How important is it to you to increase your activity? Rate from 0 to 10 (0 = not important, 10 = important).

R: *If the individual does not think the behavior change is important to improved health, he or she is unlikely to initiate the change (*Bodenheimer et al., 2005).*

Determine How Confident the Individual Is to Make the Change

- For example:
  - How confident are you that you can get more exercise? Rate from 0 to 10.
  - Determine if the individual is ready for change.
  - If the importance level is 7 or above, assess confidence level. If the importance level is low, provide more information regarding the risks of not changing behavior.
  - If the level of confidence is 4 or less, ask the individual why it is not 1.
  - Ask individual what is needed to change the low score to 8.

R: *If the importance and/or the confidence is low, an action plan with specific behavior changes would not reflect true collaboration.*

Collaboratively, Set a Realistic Goal and Action Plan

- For example: How often each week could you walk around the block two times?

R: *The individual's level of confidence will increase with success. Advising that it is not easily achievable sets the individual up for failure (*Bodenheimer et al., 2005).*

Establish a Follow-Up Plan. Ask the Individual If You Can Call Him or Her in 2 Weeks to See How He or She Is Doing. Gradually Extend the Time to Monthly Calls

R: *Telephone support has been found to benefit persons with limited health literacy, those with multiple chronic health problems, and those with gaps in care (*Piette, 2005).*

Pediatric Interventions

- "Results from the 2013 national YRBS indicated that many high school students are engaged in priority health-risk behaviors associated with the leading causes of death among persons aged 10–24 years in the United States" (Kann et al., 2014).

INEFFECTIVE HEALTH MAINTENANCE

Ineffective Health Maintenance

Related to Insufficient Knowledge of Effects of Tobacco Use and Self-Help Resources Available
Ineffective Health Management

Definition

Inability to identify, manage, and/or seek out help to maintain health (NANDA-I)

The state in which a person experiences or is at risk of experiencing a disruption in health because of lack of knowledge to manage a condition or basic health requirements.[20]

Defining Characteristics*

Demonstrated lack of adaptive behaviors to environmental changes
Demonstrated lack of knowledge about basic health practices
Lack of expressed interest in improving health behaviors
History of lack of health-seeking behaviors
Inability to take responsibility for meeting basic health practices
Impairment of personal support systems

Related Factors

Various factors can produce ineffective health maintenance. Common causes are listed next.

[20]This definition has been added by Lynda Juall Carpenito, the author, for clarity and usefulness.

Situational (Personal, Environmental)

Related to:
Misinterpretation of information
Insufficient resources*
Lack of motivation
Lack of education or readiness
Deficient communication skills*
Lack of access to adequate health-care services
Cognitive impairments*
Perceptual impairment*

Maturational

Related to insufficient knowledge of age-related risk factors. Examples include the following:

Child
Sexuality and sexual development
Inactivity
Substance abuse
Poor nutrition
Safety hazards

Adolescent
Same as children practices
Vehicle safety

Adult
Parenthood
Safety practices
Sexual function

Older Adult
Effects of aging
Sensory deficits
Safety issues
Exercise

Author's Note

The nursing diagnosis *Ineffective Health Maintenance* applies to both well and ill populations. Health is a dynamic, ever-changing state defined by the individual based on his or her perception of highest level of functioning (e.g., a marathon runner's definition of health will differ from that of a paraplegic). Because individuals are responsible for their own health, an important associated nursing responsibility involves raising individual consciousness that better health is possible.

As focus shifts from an illness/treatment-oriented to a health-oriented health-care system, *Ineffective Health Maintenance* and *The Readiness for Enhanced Diagnoses* are becoming increasingly significant. The increasingly high acuity and shortened lengths of stay in hospitals require nurses to be creative in addressing health promotion (e.g., by using printed materials, Internet, community-based programs).

Errors in Diagnostic Statements

***Ineffective Health Maintenance* related to insufficient financial resources and knowledge for self-management of diabetes**

Ineffective Health Maintenance related to insufficient financial resources and knowledge for self-management of diabetes as evidenced by Hgb A1c 9.5, excessive CHO intake, and inconsistent use of daily insulin. *Ineffective Health Maintenance* represents difficulty or inability to engage in wellness practices. In contrast *Ineffective Health Management* represents difficulty managing their illness, for example, treatments, follow-up visits, because of barriers as knowledge, importance, finances, and no or unresponsive support system. Thus, this diagnosis should be *Ineffective Health*

Management related to insufficient financial resources and knowledge for self-management of diabetes as evidenced by Hgb A1c 9.5, excessive CHO intake, and inconsistent use of daily insulin.

***Ineffective Health Maintenance* related to increased alcohol and tobacco use in response to marital breakup and heavy family demands**

This diagnosis is inappropriate for the person who wants to alter personal habits but is not in good or excellent health. A more appropriate focus would be to promote constructive stress management without tobacco or alcohol through the nursing diagnosis *Ineffective Coping* related to inability to constructively manage the stressors associated with marital breakup and family demands.

Key Concepts

General Considerations

- Healthy people (U.S. Department of Health and Human Services [USDHHS], 2012):
  - Attain high-quality, longer lives free of preventable disease, disability, injury, and premature death.
  - Achieve health equity, eliminate disparities, and improve the health of all groups.
  - Create social and physical environments that promote good health for all.
  - Promote quality of life, healthy development, and healthy behaviors across life stages.
- Healthy People 2020 leading health indicators (Progress Update, 2014):
  - Target met
    - Air quality index (AQI) exceeding 100 (number of billion person days, weighted by population and AQI value)
    - Children exposed to secondhand smoke (percent; nonsmokers, 3 to 11 years)—target less than 47%
    - Homicides (age adjusted, per 100,000 population)—target lower than 5.5%
    - Adults meeting aerobic physical activity and muscle strengthening federal guidelines (age adjusted, percent, 18+ years)—target 20.5%
  - Improvements in
    - Adults receiving colorectal cancer screening based on most recent guidelines (age adjusted, percent, 50 to 75 years)
    - Adults with hypertension whose blood pressure is under control (age adjusted, percent, 18+ years)
    - Children receiving the recommended doses of DTaP, polio, MMR, Hib, hepatitis B, varicella, and PCV vaccines (percent, aged 19 to 35 months)
    - Infant deaths (per 1,000 live births):
      - Injury deaths (age adjusted, per 100,000 population)
      - Total preterm live births (percent, <37% gestation period)
  - Little or no detectable change
    - Adolescent cigarette smoking in past 30 days (percent, grades 9 to 12)
    - Binge drinking in past 30 days—adults (percent, 18+ years)
    - Obesity among adults (age adjusted, percent, 20+ years)
    - Obesity among children and adolescents (percent, 2 to 19 years)
    - Mean daily intake of total vegetables (age adjusted, cup equivalents per 1,000 calories, 2+ years)
    - Persons with diagnosed diabetes whose A1c value is >9% (age adjusted, percent, 18+ years)
      - Persons with a usual primary care provider (percent)
      - Persons with medical insurance (percent)
  - Getting worse
    - Persons who visited the dentist in the past year (age adjusted, percent, 2+ years)
    - Adolescents with major depressive episodes (percent, 12 to 17 years)
    - Suicide (age adjusted, per 100,000 population)

Carp's Cues

It is useful to review the online report that includes target percentages, with noted percentage at baseline (2005 to 2008) and reported percentage at year 2012. Some of the target percentages appear rather low as:

- Children exposed to secondhand smoke (percent; nonsmokers, 3 to 11 years)—52.2% (2005 to 2008), 41.3% (2009 to 2012), and 47.0% target
- Adults meeting aerobic physical activity and muscle strengthening federal guidelines (age adjusted, percent, 18+ years)—18.2% (2008), 20.6% (2012), and 20.1%
- Homicides (age adjusted, per 100,000 population)—6.1 (2007), 5.3 (2010), and 5.5

- Many people view health as the absence of disease. Rather, health can be viewed as a return (or recovery) to a previous state or to a heightened awareness of full potential and life meaning.
- Control of major health problems in the United States depends directly on modification of individual behavior and habits of living.
- The US poverty line is $22,350 for a family of four (U.S. Bureau of Census, 2011). The overall poverty rate is 14.3%, which is about 42.9 million people, 20% of whom are children younger than 6 (HHS Poverty Guidelines, 2011).
- In addition to addressing lifestyles to promote wellness, total health depends on the following (*Edelman & Mandle, 2009):
  - Eradication of poverty and ignorance
  - Availability of jobs
  - Adequate housing, transportation, and recreation
  - Public safety
  - Aesthetically pleasing and beneficial environment
- The goals of prevention are as follows:
  - Avoidance of disease through healthy lifestyles
  - Decreased mortality from disease through early detection and intervention
  - Improved quality of life
- The three levels of prevention are (1) primary, (2) secondary, and (3) tertiary.
  - Primary prevention involves actions that prevent disease and accidents and promote well-being. Key Concepts are as follows:
    - *Concept*: Wellness; *Example*: Diet low in salt, sugar, carbohydrates, and fat
    - *Concept*: A lifestyle that incorporates the principles of health promotion and is directed by self; *Example*: Regular exercise and stress management; elimination of smoking; minimal alcohol intake; responsibility
    - *Concept*: Mutual sharing with others who have similar needs; *Example*: La Leche League childbirth education; assertiveness training; specific written resources (books, pamphlets, magazines); public media
    - *Concept*: Safety; *Example*: Adherence to speed limits; use of seat belts and car seats; proper storage of household poisons
    - *Concept*: Immunizations; *Example*: Children: hepatitis B series; nonpregnant women of childbearing age: rubella if antibody titer is negative; elderly: influenza, pneumonia
  - Secondary prevention concerns actions that promote early detection of disease and subsequent intervention by examination by a health professional, self-examination, and screening tests. Types of screening include the following:
    - Physical findings (periodic examinations by health-care professionals and self-examinations of breasts, testicles, and skin)
    - Survey of risk factors (smoking, alcohol abuse)
    - Laboratory tests (serum—e.g., sickle cell in African Americans, phenylketonuria in newborns; urine—e.g., renal disease in older adults; X-ray—e.g., dental caries, PPD for tuberculosis, fasting blood glucose for diabetes mellitus)
  - Tertiary prevention involves actions that restore and rehabilitate and prevent complications in cases of illness. Examples for a person with coronary artery disease would be as follows:
    - Restorative (surgery, such as coronary artery bypass, angioplasty, and medications)
    - Rehabilitative (stress management, exercise program, stop smoking)

Health Promotion Behaviors

- A person is motivated to pursue health promotion behaviors if (Pender, Murdaugh, & Parsons, 2011)
  - The change is desired and has value.
  - The change will produce positive results.
  - It is likely that they will be successful.
- Several factors influence motivation (*Pender et al., 2006):
  - Previous experiences
  - Past as a predictor for future behavior
  - Perceived benefits of action
  - Perceived barriers, for example, discomfort, expense, time, dexterity
  - Perceived health status
  - Cognitive impairments
  - Problems with mobility, dexterity, strength, agility

- "Self-management support is the assistance caregivers give individuals with chronic diseases in order to encourage daily decisions that improve health related behaviors and clinical outcomes" (*Bodenheimer, MacGregor, & Sharifi, 2005).
- Individuals are helped to choose health behaviors in a collaborative partnership with the caregivers (*Bodenheimer et al., 2005). Researchers have validated that "members of the public had a significantly higher confidence in the ability of normal weight nurses to provide education about diet and exercise compared with overweight nurses" (Hisks et al., 2008).
- Refer to *Ineffective Health Management* for key concepts on health education, self-efficacy, and barriers to learning.
- Motivational interviewing is a readiness to change model. Techniques are used to assess readiness to change (importance and confidence) and to encourage individuals to increase their readiness (*Rollnick, Mason, & Butler, 2000).

Literacy/Health Literacy

- Refer to Key Concepts under *Ineffective Health Management*.

Stress

- Refer to *Anxiety* and *Ineffective Coping* for specific information on anxiety and ineffective coping.
- Stress is the physical, psychological, social, or spiritual effect of life's pressures and events and is present in all people (*Edelman & Mandle, 2009).
- Stress is an interactive process in response to the loss or threat of loss of homeostasis or well-being (Cahill, Gorski, & Le, 2003).
- Stress is a psychological, emotional state experienced by an individual in response to a specific stressor or demand that results in harm, either temporary or permanent, to the individuals (*Ridner, 2004).
- Excessive stress requires recognition, perception, and adaptation (Cahill, Gorski, & Le, 2003).
- A chronic state of stress or repeated episodes of psychological stress (depression, anger, hostility, anxiety) can lead to cardiovascular disease, arteriosclerosis, headaches, and gastrointestinal disorders (Edelman & Mandle, 2010).
- In response to stress, individuals initiate or increase unhealthy behaviors such as overeating, sedentary lifestyle, excessive use of drugs or alcohol, smoking, and social isolation (*USDHHS, 2000).

Nutrition

- See Key Concepts for *Imbalanced Nutrition*.

Exercise

- Regular exercise can increase the following:
  - Cardiovascular–respiratory endurance
  - Delivery of nutrients to tissue
  - Muscle strength
  - Tolerance for psychological stress
  - Muscle endurance
  - Ability to reduce body fat content
  - Flexibility
- Vigorous exercise sessions should include a warm-up phase (10 minutes at a slow pace), endurance exercises, and a cool-down phase (5 to 10 minutes of a slow pace and stretching).
- Current beliefs regarding optimal exercise are as follows:
  - Emphasize physical activity over "exercise."
  - Moderate physical activity is very beneficial.
  - Intermittent physical activity that accumulates to 30 or more minutes is beneficial.
- To enhance long-term exercise, the individual should (*Moore & Charvat, 2002):
  - Respond to relapses with a plan to prevent recurrences.
  - Set realistic goals.
  - Keep an exercise log.
  - Exercise with a friend.

Tobacco Use

- The percentage of US adults who smoke cigarettes was 17.8% in 2013, a drop from 20.9% in 2005, and the lowest rate of smoking since researchers began tracking this figure in 1965 (Centers for Disease Control and Prevention [CDC], 2015).
- Smoking remains particularly high among people who live below the poverty level, those who have less education, and those who have a disability or a limitation.

- Among US regions, people in the Midwest had the highest smoking rate, of 20.5%. The smoking rate was 19.2% among people in the South, and 16.9% among people in the Northeast. People who live in the West had the lowest smoking rate, of 13.6%, according to the report.
- "However there hasn't been a significant change in cigarette smoking or smokeless tobacco use across many states, the combined use of cigarettes and smokeless tobacco increased in five states—Delaware, Idaho, Nevada, New Mexico and West Virginia" (Nguyen, Marshall, Hu, & Neff, 2015).
- "Despite states collecting about $25 billion in 2015, they're spending less than $500 million—about 2 percent—on tobacco control" (Nguyen et al., 2015).
- "Tobacco use is the leading preventable cause of disease and premature death in the US" (MMWR, 2016). It has been proven that tobacco use causes the following cancers: lung, bronchial, laryngeal, oral cavity, pharyngeal, esophageal, stomach, pancreatic, kidney, urinary bladder, uterine, cervical, and acute myelogenous leukemia. It also causes abdominal aortic aneurysms, peripheral vascular disease, stroke, and chronic obstructive lung disease and contributes to osteoporosis (CDC, 2010).
- More deaths are caused by cigarette smoking than by all deaths from HIV, illegal drug use, alcohol use, motor vehicle accidents, suicide, and murders combined (CDC, 2011; Mokdad et al., 2011).
- Cigarette smoke contributes more than 4,000 chemicals, 250 of which are toxic, to be absorbed in the blood and swallowed into the gastrointestinal (GI) tract to act directly in the oral cavity and respiratory system (Andrews & Boyle, 2012; Mayo Foundation for Medical Education and Research, 2009).
- Nearly 18 of every 100 US adults aged 18 years or older (17.8%) currently smoke cigarettes. This means an estimated 42.1 million adults in the United States currently smoke cigarettes.
  - More than 20 of every 100 adult men (20.5%)
  - About 15 of every 100 adult women (15.3%)
- In the United States, 20.5% of men and 15.3% of women smoke
- Current cigarette smoking was highest among people of multiple races and non-Hispanic American Indians/Alaska Natives (26.1%) and lowest among Asians
- Smoking one to four cigarettes per day doubles an individual's risk of death from ischemic heart disease. Studies also report there is a steady increase in consumption over 10 to 20 years (Bjartveit & Tverdal, 2005).
- Women smoking during reproductive age are at risk for difficulty conceiving, infertility, spontaneous abortion, premature rupture of membranes, low birth weight, neonatal mortality, stillbirth, preterm delivery, and sudden infant death syndrome (SIDS) (CDC, 2011).
- On average, women metabolize nicotine more quickly than men, which may contribute to their increased susceptibility to nicotine addiction and may help to explain why, among smokers, it is more difficult for women to quit (CDC, 2010).
- Smoking has immediate and long-term effects on the cardiovascular system. Immediate effects are vasoconstriction and decreased oxygenation of the blood, elevated blood pressure, increased heart rate and possible dysrhythmias, and increased work by the heart. Long-term effects are an increased risk for coronary artery disease, stroke, hyperlipidemia, and myocardial infarction. Smoking also contributes to hypertension, peripheral vascular disease (e.g., leg ulcers), and chronically abnormal arterial blood gases (low oxygen, or PO_2, and high carbon dioxide, or PCO_2) (Halter, 2014).
- Smoking decreases pancreatic secretion of bicarbonate; this increases duodenal acidity. Tobacco delays the healing of gastric duodenal ulcers and increases their frequency (Katz, 2003).
- Use of smokeless tobacco (snuff, chewing tobacco) is associated with yellow teeth, gum recession, cavities, oral leukoplakia (premalignant lesions), oral cancer, pancreatic cancer, stroke and cardiovascular disease, higher cholesterol levels, gastric ulcers, heart disease, and nicotine addiction. At least 12 million Americans are at risk, mostly male teens and male adults (National Cancer Institute, 2009).
- Nicotine is the primary addicting substance in tobacco smoke and juice. Individuals with tobacco addiction need special assistance with short-term withdrawal and long-term maintenance of a tobacco-free life.
- Secondhand smoke (SHS) is also known as *environmental tobacco smoke* (ETS). SHS is a mixture of two forms of smoke that come from burning tobacco:
  - *Sidestream smoke*: Smoke from the lighted end of a cigarette, pipe, or cigar
  - *Mainstream smoke*: The smoke exhaled by a smoker
- SHS is the inhalation of tobacco smoke by nonsmokers. SHS contains formaldehyde, arsenic, cadmium, benzene, ammonia, carbon monoxide, methanol, hydrogen cyanide, and polonium. SHS has been shown to have negative health effects (Andrews, 1998; Mayo Clinic, 2009; Pletsch, 2002).
- Exposure to SHS increases the risk of coronary heart disease by 25% to 30% (Institute of Medicine, 2009). People with angina experience more discomfort in a smoke-filled room.
- Bronchospasm increases when a person with asthma is exposed to tobacco smoke.
- Children living with smoking parents have more upper respiratory and ear infections and dental caries than those living with nonsmokers.

- Passive smoking causes lung cancer, asthma, and bronchitis in nonsmokers.
- Pregnant women exposed to SHS have lower-birth-weight infants.
- Sudden infant death syndrome is two to four times more common in infants whose mothers smoked during pregnancy.

Osteoporosis

- Osteoporosis is classified as primary (associated with age- and menopause-related changes) or secondary (caused by medications or diseases) (Miller, 2015).
- Age-related changes beginning around age 40 years decrease cortical bone by 3% per decade in men and women. Lifetime cortical bone loss is 35% (women) and 23% (men), and lifetime trabecular bone loss is 50% (women) and 33% (men) (Miller, 2015).
- Woman older than age 50 and men older than age 70 are at higher risk for osteoporosis (NIH, 2014).
- Smoking contributes to osteoporosis by (Shahab, 2012)
  - Causing decrease in parathyroid hormone, which reduces calcium absorption
  - Reducing body mass, which is postulated to provide an osteogenic stimulus and is linked to higher BMD14
  - Reducing the level of vitamin D in the body, which is required for good bone health
  - Increasing free radicals and oxidative stress, which affects bone resorption
  - Causing peripheral vascular disease, reducing blood supply to the bones
  - The chemicals in tobacco smoke have a direct toxic effects on bone cells.

Vitamin D Deficiency

- Vitamin D promotes calcium absorption in the gut and maintains adequate serum calcium and phosphate concentrations to enable normal mineralization of bone and to prevent hypocalcemic tetany. It is also needed for bone growth and bone remodeling by osteoblasts and osteoclasts. Without sufficient vitamin D, bones can become thin, brittle, or misshapen. Vitamin D sufficiency prevents rickets in children and osteomalacia in adults. Together with calcium, vitamin D also helps protect older adults from osteoporosis (Institute of Medicine, 2010; NIH, 2014).
- Those at risk for vitamin D deficiency are older adults, breastfed infants, people with dark skin, people with limited sun exposure, people with inflammatory bowel disease and other conditions causing fat malabsorption, and people who are obese or who have undergone gastric bypass surgery (Institute of Medicine, 2010; NIH, 2014).
- Infants, children, and elderly adults are at risk for low vitamin D levels because of inadequate vitamin D intake. Human breast milk contains low levels of vitamin D, and most infant formulas do not contain adequate vitamin D. Elderly adults may avoid sunlight and often do not consume enough vitamin D-rich foods, and even when they do, absorption may be limited (Drezner, 2013).
- As many as half of older adults in the United States with hip fractures could have serum 25(OH)D levels <30 nmol/L (<12 ng/mL) (Institute of Medicine, 2010; NIH, 2014).
- Contributing factors to osteoporosis include loss of female hormones after menopause, hypogonadism, low calcium or vitamin D intake in adolescent and adult women, insufficient exercise, small stature, fair skin, family history, cigarette smoking, excessive consumption of alcohol or caffeine, use of corticosteroids daily for 3 months or longer, and use of antiseizure medications (NIH, 2010).
- Deficiencies in dietary calcium and vitamin D in young women can lead to osteoporosis in later years (Bohaty, Rocole, Wehling, & Waltman, 2008).

Pediatric Considerations

- Anticipatory health promotion, or *anticipatory guidance*, is essential to comprehensive health care. It encompasses focusing an individual or family on what could be expected in a specific situation such as pregnancy, relocation, retirement, or menopause. Anticipatory guidance varies in content with a child's age and involves teaching families what is likely in upcoming weeks, months, or years.
- Health maintenance begins with the prenatal visit and continues with comprehensive health supervision during the child's development.
- The child depends on a parent/adult caregiver to provide a safe environment and promote health (e.g., immunizations, well checkups, and chronic disease management).
- Risk of ineffective health maintenance varies with a child's age and health status. For example, the toddler is at risk for accidental poisoning, whereas the adolescent is more likely to engage in high-risk behavior such as unprotected sex.
- Many factors can influence a child's nutritional needs, including periods of rapid growth, stress, illness, metabolic errors, medications, and socioeconomic factors (e.g., inadequate income, poor housing, lack of food).

- By conservative estimates, more than one million youths run away from home each year. Alienated youth are frequently outside the health-care system and tend to remain there unless efforts are made to identify and develop acceptable health services for them. The adoption of destructive lifestyles by many of these youths contributes heavily to physical and psychological morbidity and to alarmingly high mortality.

Tobacco Use

- Almost 70% of adult smokers began smoking before they turned 18. Most smokers try their first cigarette around the age of 11, and many are addicted by the time they turn 14. So why do kids start smoking in the first place? (American Lung Association, 2015)
    - Their parents are smokers.
    - Peer pressure—their friends encourage them to try cigarettes, and to keep smoking.
    - They see smoking as a way of rebelling and showing independence.
    - They think that everyone else is smoking, and that they should, too.
    - Tobacco advertising targets teenagers.
- The Family Smoking Prevention and Tobacco Control Act in 2009 mandates (American Lung Association, 2015):
    - Ban all outdoor tobacco advertising within 1,000 feet of schools and playgrounds.
    - Ban all remaining tobacco-brand sponsorships of sports and entertainment events.
    - Ban free giveaways of any nontobacco items with the purchase of a tobacco product or in exchange for coupons or proof of purchase.
    - Limit advertising in publications with significant teen readership as well as outdoor and point-of-sale advertising, except in adult-only facilities, to black-and-white text only.
    - Restrict vending machines and self-service displays to adult-only facilities.
    - Require retailers to verify age for all over-the-counter sales and provide for federal enforcement and penalties against retailers who sell to minors.
    - Require bigger, stronger health warning.
    - Prohibit the use of descriptors, such as "light," "mild," and "low," to characterize a product.
    - Require detailed disclosure of ingredients, nicotine and harmful smoke constituents.
    - Grant FDA authority to restrict tobacco marketing.

Maternal Considerations

- Smoking in pregnancy (USDHHS, 2015):
    - Lowers the amount of oxygen available to you and your growing baby
    - Increases the following:
        - The baby's heart rate
        - The risk that the baby will be born prematurely
        - The risk that the baby will be born with low birth weight
        - The baby's risk of developing respiratory problems
        - The chances of stillbirth
        - The risk for certain birth defects like a cleft lip or cleft palate
        - The risk for sudden infant death syndrome (SIDS)
- Children whose mothers smoked during pregnancy are at greater risk of (USDHHS, 2015):
    - Behavioral problems, including Attention Deficit Hyperactivity Disorder (ADHD)
    - Learning disorders
    - Becoming smokers
- Women smoking during reproductive age are at risk for difficulty conceiving, infertility, spontaneous abortion, premature rupture of membranes, low birth weight, neonatal mortality, stillbirth, preterm delivery, and SIDS (CDC, 2014).

Geriatric Considerations

- It can be observed that while goals to extend life expectancy were coming to fruition, older adults were not typically valued in our society. The pursuit of wellness in older adults, he argued, would move our society toward supporting not only longevity, but also vitality" (McMahon & Fleury, 2011).

- According to Miller (2015), health is the ability of older adults to function at their highest capacity, despite age-related changes and risk factors. Of all age-related changes, osteoporosis is most likely to have serious negative functional consequences, even without additional risk factors.
- The Federal Interagency Forum on Aging-Related Statistics reported (AgingStats.org; Federal Interagency Forum on Age-Related Statistics, 2012):
  - 76% of people aged 65 and overrated their health as good, very good, or excellent.
  - 79% of those aged 65 to 74 reported good or better health.
  - At age 85 and over, 67% of people reported good or better health. This pattern was also evident within racial and ethnic groups.
- Differentiating between age-related changes and risk factors that affect the functioning of older people is important. Risk factors such as inadequate nutrition, fluid intake, exercise, and socialization can have more influence on functioning than can most age-related changes.
- Older adults have decreased sweating, shivering, peripheral circulation, subcutaneous tissue, and inefficient vasoconstriction. These age-related changes diminish the ability to adapt to adverse temperatures and increase their risk of hypothermia and hyperthermia. This can also affect thermoregulation during and tolerance of physical activity (Miller, 2015).
- Regular exercise has been shown to correlate positively with increased self-esteem, longevity, and decreased falls (Miller, 2015).

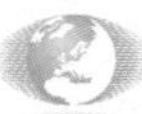

Transcultural Considerations

- All cultures have systems of health beliefs to explain what causes illness, how it can be cured or treated, and who should be involved in the process. The extent to which patients perceive patient education as having cultural relevance for them can have a profound effect on their reception to information provided and their willingness to use it. Western industrialized societies such as the United States, which see disease as a result of natural scientific phenomena, advocate medical treatments that combat microorganisms or use sophisticated technology to diagnose and treat disease. Other societies believe that illness is the result of supernatural phenomena and promote prayer or other spiritual interventions that counter the presumed disfavor of powerful forces. Cultural issues play a major role in patient compliance. One study showed that a group of Cambodian adults with minimal formal education made considerable efforts to comply with therapy but did so in a manner consistent with their underlying understanding of how medicines and the body work (*McLaughlin & Braun, 1998).
- Health and illness are culturally prescribed. One culture may view an obese person as strong and healthy, whereas another culture views that same person as weak and unhealthy. Nurses must remember that treatment strategies consistent with an individual's cultural beliefs may have a better chance of success (Andrews & Boyle, 2012).
- A future orientation to illness, disease, and health care is necessary for prevention. The dominant US culture is oriented to the future, whereas other cultures have a present-oriented perception (e.g., African American, Hispanic, Southern Appalachian, traditional Chinese) (Andrews & Boyle, 2012). Some members of these cultures, however, are future oriented.
- Some cultures believe that fate depends on God or other supernatural forces. Humans are at the mercy of these forces despite their behavior (Andrews & Boyle, 2012).
- Some Asian cultures believe in balance and harmony for health. They emphasize moderation and avoid excesses. In the *yin/yang theory*, the yin force in the universe represents female aspects of nature: cold and darkness. The yang force represents male aspects of nature: fullness, light, and warmth. An imbalance of yin and yang creates illness (Andrews & Boyle, 2012).
- In Hispanic and African American cultures, health is maintained by the hot/cold humoral theory. This ancient Greek concept describes four body humors: yellow bile, black bile, phlegm, and blood. When these humors are balanced, health is present. Treatment of illness consists of restoring humoral balance by adding or deleting substances (e.g., foods, beverages, herbs, drugs) that are either hot or cold. For example, an earache is classified as cold and thus needs hot substances for treatment (Andrews & Boyle, 2012).
- Because the family is usually the individual's most important social unit, the nurse can promote their help to support lifestyle changes (Andrews & Boyle, 2012).
- Cigarette smoking remains particularly high among certain groups, including adults who are male, younger, multiracial or American Indian/Alaska Native, have less education, live below the federal poverty level, live in the South or Midwest, have a disability/limitation, or who are LGB (CDC, 2015).
- Despite a myriad of concomitant health concerns, excessive fatness continues to be embraced by many countries as a sign of health, wealth, happiness, and does not have AIDS, especially for woman in certain countries.

Focus Assessment Criteria

Subjective Data

Assess for Defining Characteristics

Health Status

Individual's description of health

Immediate health concerns

Frequency of:

- Bowel irregularity
- Headaches
- Influenza
- Fatigue
- Feeling overwhelmed
- Mouth lesions
- Urinary tract infections
- Respiratory infections
- Skin rashes

Assess for Related Factors

Influencing Factors: Health Management and Adherence Behavior

What factors make it difficult to follow health advice?

What daily health management activities are practiced?

How much control does the individual believe he or she has?

Risk Factors

Family incidence of:

- Abuse or violence
- Cancer
- Cardiovascular disease
- Depression
- Diabetes mellitus
- Drug, tobacco, or alcohol abuse
- Hypertension
- Overweight/obesity
- Other (specify)

Exposure to tobacco smoke

Health habits

Define Tobacco Use Behavior

Type and Quantity

Cigarettes, pipe, cigars, smokeless (chewing) tobacco

Pack-years

Number of smokers in household

Smoke in car, home, in presence of others, for example, children

Alcohol use (daily, weekly, seldom number of drinks). Refer to *Ineffective Denial* if indicated.

Drug use (prescribed, over-the-counter, street)

Dietary consumption of fat/salt/sugar, carbohydrates, protein; frequency; and amount of portions (Refer to *Imbalanced Nutrition* for assessment criteria.)

Exercise program (Refer to *Sedentary Lifestyle* for assessment criteria.)

Environmental Risk Factors

Do you use seat belts or child restraints?

Is home child-proofed? (If appropriate, determine measures taken.)

Could any factors in the home or at work cause falls or accidents?

Could any other factors potentially threaten your health or cause injury?

Preventive Health Activities

Refer to Table II.8 for Primary and Secondary Prevention for Age-Related Conditions.

Table II.8 PRIMARY AND SECONDARY PREVENTION FOR AGE-RELATED CONDITIONS (1,4,5)

Developmental Level	Primary Prevention	Secondary Prevention
Infancy (0–1 year)	Parent education Infant safety Nutrition Breast feeding Sensory stimulation Infant massage and touch Visual stimulation Activity Colors Auditory stimulation Verbal Music Immunizations DPT or DTaP IPV, Hib Hepatitis B (three-dose series) Hepatitis A (2) Rotavirus (RV) Pneumococcal (PCV) Meningococcal Influenza (yearly) Oral hygiene Teething biscuits Fluoride (if needed >6 months) Avoid sugared food and drink	Complete physical examination every 2–3 months Screening at birth Congenital hip dysplasia PKU G-6-PD deficiency in blacks, Mediterranean, and far Eastern origin children Sickle cell Hemoglobin or hematocrit (for anemia) Cystic fibrosis Vision (startle reflex) Hearing (response to and localization of sounds) TB test at 12 months Developmental assessments Screen and intervene for high risk Low birth weight Maternal substance abuse during pregnancy Alcohol: fetal alcohol syndrome Cigarettes: SIDS Drugs: addicted neonate, AIDS Maternal infections during pregnancy
Preschool (1–5 years)	Parent education Teething Discipline Nutrition Accident prevention Normal growth and development Child education Dental self-care Dressing Bathing with assistance Feeding self-care Immunizations DTaP IPV MMR HIB *H. Influenzae* (yearly) Varicella Hepatitis A (2) (two-dose series) Pneumococcal Hepatitis B (3 dose series) Dental/oral hygiene Fluoride treatments Fluoridated water	Complete physical examination between 2 and 3 years and preschool (UA, CBC) TB test at 3 years Development assessments (annual) Speech development Hearing Vision Screen and intervene Lead poisoning Developmental lag Neglect or abuse Strong family history of arteriosclerotic diseases (e.g., MI, CVA, peripheral vascular disease), diabetes, hypertension, gout, or hyperlipidemia—fasting serum cholesterol at age 2 years, then every 3–5 years if normal Strabismus Hearing deficit Vision deficit Autism
School age (6–11 years)	Health education of child "Basic 4" nutrition Accident prevention Outdoor safety Substance abuse counsel Anticipatory guidance for physical changes at puberty Immunizations DTaP age 11–12 MMR (two lifetime doses) OPV/IPV (four lifetime doses) Hepatitis B three-dose series if needed Hepatitis A (2) Pneumococcal (3)	Complete physical examination TB test every 3 years (at ages 6 and 9) Developmental assessments Language Vision: Snellen charts at school 6–8 years, use "E" chart Older than 8 years, use alphabet chart Hearing: audiogram Cholesterol profile, if high risk, every 3–5 years Serum cholesterol one time (not high risk)

(continued)

Table II.8 PRIMARY AND SECONDARY PREVENTION FOR AGE-RELATED CONDITIONS (1,4,5) *(continued)*

Developmental Level	Primary Prevention	Secondary Prevention
	Varicella (at age 11–12 if no history of infection) Gardisil (HPV) series of three for girls, 9–26 years, for boys age 9–18 years Dental hygiene every 6–12 months Continue fluoridation Complete physical examination	
Adolescence (12–19 years)	Health education Proper nutrition and healthful diets Calcium 100 mg and vitamin D 400 units daily Sex education Choices Risks Precautions Sexually transmitted diseases Safe driving skills Adult challenges Seeking employment and career choices Dating and marriage Confrontation with substance abuse Safety in athletics, water Skin care Dental hygiene every 6–12 months Immunizations Tdap if not received then Td every 10 years thereafter Hepatitis B three-dose series if needed Hepatitis A series (2) two-dose series TOPV (if needed to complete four-dose series) Gardisil (HPV) (series of three for girls ages 11–26, for boys aged 9–18) Pneumococcal (3)	Complete physical examination yearly Blood pressure Cholesterol profile PPD test at 12 years and yearly if high risk RPR, CBC, U/A Female: Breast self-examination (BSE) Male: Testicular self-examination (TSE) Female, Pap and pelvic exam yearly after 3 years of onset of sexual activity or at age 21 Urine gonorrhea and chlamydia tests with yearly PE's screening Depression Suicide Tobacco use Eating disorders Substance abuse Pregnancy Family history of alcoholism or domestic violence Sexually transmitted infections
Young adult (20–39 years)	Health education Weight management with good nutrition as BMR changes Low-cholesterol diet Calcium 100 mg daily (females) Vitamin D 400 units daily (females) Lifestyle counseling Stress management skills Safe driving Family planning Divorce Sexual practices Parenting skills Regular exercise Environmental health choices Alcohol, drug use Use of hearing protection devices Dental hygiene every 6–12 months Immunizations If needed one time dose of Tdap, then Td every 10 years thereafter Influenza yearly Pneumovax (3) Varicella (two-dose series for those with no evidence of immunity) Female: rubella, if serum negative for antibodies Hepatitis B three-dose series Hepatitis A (2) Gardisal (three-dose series for females from age 11 to 26) MMR (If born in 1957 or later, one or more doses) Pneumococcal Diabetes mellitus	Complete physical examination at about 20 years, then every 5–6 years Female: BSE monthly, Pap 1–2 years unless high risk Male: TSE monthly Parents to be: high-risk screening for Down syndrome, Tay-Sachs Female pregnant: RPR, rubella titer, Rh factor, amniocentesis for women 35 years or older (if desired) All females: baseline mammography between ages 35 and 40 If high risk, female with previous breast cancer: annual mammography at 35 years and yearly after, a female with mother or sister who has had breast cancer, same as above Family history colorectal cancer or high risk: annual stool guaiac, digital rectal, and colonoscopy at intervals determined after baseline colonoscopy. PPD if high risk Glaucoma screening at 35 years and along with routine physical examinations Cholesterol profile every 5 years, if normal Cholesterol profile every year if borderline Screening (Refer to *Adolescent* section)

(continued)

Table II.8 PRIMARY AND SECONDARY PREVENTION FOR AGE-RELATED CONDITIONS (1,4,5) (*continued*)

Developmental Level	Primary Prevention	Secondary Prevention
Middle-aged adult (40–59 years)	Health education: continue with young adult Calcium 1,000–1,500 mg daily Vitamin D 400 units daily Midlife changes, male and female counseling (see also Young adult) "Empty nest syndrome" Anticipatory guidance for retirement Menopause Grandparenting Dental hygiene every 6–12 months Immunizations Hepatitis B three-dosed series Hepatitis A (2) If needed one time dose of Tdap, then Td every 10 years thereafter Influenza—yearly Pneumococca (3) at age 65 for all those who were not high risk for vaccine prior	Complete physical examination every 5–6 years with complete laboratory evaluation (serum/urine tests, X-ray, ECG) DEXA scan (screening for high-risk men and women for osteoporosis) once then as needed Female: BSE monthly Male: TSE monthly PSA yearly after age 40 for African Americans and Hispanics and after age 50 for others All females: mammogram every 1–2 years (40–49 years) then annual mammography 50 years and older Screening (Refer to *Adolescent* section) Schiotz's tonometry (glaucoma) every 3–5 years Colonoscopy at 50 and 51, then at intervals determined after baseline colonoscopy. Stool guaiac annually at 50 and yearly after
Older adult (60–74 years)	Health education: continue with previous counseling Home safety Retirement Loss of spouse, relatives, friends Special health needs Calcium 1,000–1,500 mg daily Vitamin D 400 units daily Changes in hearing or vision Dental/oral hygiene every 6–12 months Immunizations Tdap one dose then Td every 10 years Influenza—annual Hepatitis B 3 dose series Hepatitis A (2) Pneumococcal (3) Herpes zoster 60 years or older unless a live vaccine is contraindicated	Complete physical examination every 2 years with laboratory assessments Blood pressure annually Female: BSE monthly, Pap every 1–3 years, annual mammogram Male: TSE monthly, PSA yearly Annual stool guaiac Colonoscopy (interval determined by baseline results) Complete eye examination yearly DEXA scan once and as needed Screen for high risk Depression Suicide Alcohol/drug abuse "Elder abuse"
Old-age adult (75 years and older)	Dental/oral hygiene every 6–12 months Immunizations Tetanus every 10 years Influenza—annual Pneumococcal—if not already received	

Objective Data

Assess for Defining Characteristics

General appearance
Weight
Height
Body Mass Index (BMI)
Lack of knowledge of age-related preventive health measures, for example, immunizations, avoiding sun exposure, safe driving skills, water safety, sport safety, and home safety
Dental self-care, professional dental care

Goal

NOC

Health Promoting Behavior, Health Seeking Behaviors, Knowledge: Health Promotion, Knowledge: Health Resources, Participation: Health-Care Decisions, Risk Detection

The individual or caregiver will verbalize intent to engage in health maintenance behaviors, as evidenced by the following indicators:

- Identifies barriers to health maintenance

Interventions

NIC

Health Education, Self-Responsibility Facilitation, Health Screening, Risk Identification, Family Involvement Promotion, Nutrition Counseling, Weight Reduction Assistance

Assess for Barriers to Health Maintenance

- Refer to Related Factors.

Explain Primary and Secondary Prevention Measures for Age-Related Conditions (see Table II.8).

R: *Many injuries, physical or mental disorders, or health-threatening situations can be prevented or decreased by immunizations, health education, safety programs, and healthy lifestyles or detected early with screening and treated promptly (*Murray, Zentner, & Yakimo, 2009).*

Identify Strategies to Improve Access for the Vulnerable Populations (e.g., Uninsured, Displaced, Homeless, Poor)

- Community centers, school-based clinics, planned parenthood, faith-based clinics
- Pharmaceutical companies' assistance programs, generic alternative medications

R: *Low-income families usually focus on meeting basic needs (food, shelter, and safety) and seek help with curing illness, not preventing it. The cost of medications and office visits, hours of operation, and transportation are barriers for the poor.*

Assist Individual and Family to Identify Behaviors That Are Detrimental to Their Health

- Tobacco use (Refer to *Ineffective Health Maintenance*)
- High-fat, high-carbohydrate, high-calorie diets (Refer to *Imbalanced Nutrition*)
- Sedentary life styles (Refer to *Sedentary Lifestyle*)
- Inadequate immunizations (Refer to *Ineffective Health Maintenance*)
- Excessive stress (Refer to *Stress Overload*)

R: *Providing information and resources can help foster a sense that change is possible.*

Older Adults Interventions

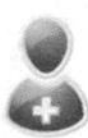

CLINICAL ALERT Try to clear your mind of negative bias regarding aging. Be determined to identify areas where the person can be healthier. Be creative, for example, cannot walk around the block but can do chair exercises. Determine with the individual what they can do.

R: *Focusing on problems and deficits alone limits the exploration of individual strengths, thereby compounding the risk for vulnerability to diminished health and well-being (McMahon & Fleury, 2012).*

Discuss their Feelings About Their Life.

- What do they like about their life?
- What gives meaning to their life?
- Discuss what they would like to do but don't.
- Discuss if realistic modifiable.
- Is there another option that is acceptable?
- Explore if assistance is needed, who or what is the source.

R: *Kiefer (2008) reported a component of wellness is subjective well-being, which is defined by the person as how they feel and think about their life.*

Ineffective Health Maintenance • Related to Insufficient Knowledge of Effects of Tobacco Use and Self-Help Resources Available

Goals

NOC

Health Seeking Behaviors, Knowledge: Health Promotion, Knowledge: Health Resources, Participation: Health-Care Decisions, Risk Detection

- Identify benefits of abstinence from tobacco use.
- Verbalize commitment to personal health and desire to eliminate tobacco use.[21]
- Devise strategies to assist in smoking/chewing cessation.[21]

Carp's Cues

Smokers know that smoking is harming their health. Everyone tells them to quit. This implies quitting is in fact easy. Addiction to tobacco is stronger than addiction to heroin. About 70% of smokers say they want to quit and about half try to quit each year, but only 4% to 7% succeed without help. This is because smokers not only become physically dependent on nicotine, but also have a strong psychological dependence (CDC, 2010).

Nicotine reaches the brain within seconds after taking a puff. Nicotine alters the balance of chemicals in your brain. It mainly affects chemicals called dopamine and noradrenaline. Nicotine induces pleasure and reduces stress and anxiety. Smokers use it to modulate levels of arousal and to control mood (CDC, 2010).

Interventions

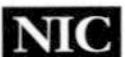

NIC

See *Ineffective Health Maintenance*

Advise All Tobacco Users to Quit

During hospitalization, focus on the individual's readiness to quit, and clarify misinformation. Ask the individual:

- How smoking has affected their health?
- Have they ever tried to quit?
- How long did they stop?
- Do they want to quit?
- What is your reason to quit smoking?

R: *Focusing the discussion on the person's experiences and perceptions may provide insight into assisting the person to quit. Quitting tobacco is the most important thing a person can do to protect his or her health (CDC, 2010).*

Explain That There Is No Such Thing as "a Few Cigarettes a Day"

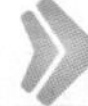

Carp's Cues

More deaths are caused by cigarette smoking than by all deaths from HIV, illegal drug use, alcohol use, motor vehicle accidents, suicide, and murders combined (CDC, 2011; Mokdad et al., 2008).

R: *Smoking one to four cigarettes per day increases one's risk of death from ischemic heart disease and from all other causes. Studies also report there is a steady increase in consumption over 10 to 20 years.*

Explain the Hazards of SHS for Smokers and Nonsmokers

- SHS is a mixture of two forms of smoke that come from burning tobacco:
  - *Sidestream smoke*: Smoke from the lighted end of a cigarette, pipe, or cigar
  - *Mainstream smoke*: The smoke exhaled by a smoker

---

[21] These outcome criteria are established only *if* the individual desires to quit tobacco use. For the individual who does not wish to change tobacco use behaviors, provide information regarding health risks and benefits so he or she makes an *informed* choice. Avoid being judgmental. Always "keep the door open" should the individual later change his or her mind.

- Sidestream smoke has higher concentrations of cancer-causing agents (carcinogens) and is more toxic than mainstream smoke.

R: *It has smaller particles than mainstream smoke. These smaller particles make their way into the lungs and the body's cells more easily.*

- Nonsmokers who breathe in SHS take in nicotine and toxic chemicals by the same route smokers do. The more SHS you breathe, the higher the level of these harmful chemicals in your body.
- Smokers take in the toxins of tobacco when they smoke and when they breathe in their exhaled smoke.
- When more than one person smoke together, they increase their inhalation of the toxins in tobacco smokes.

Assess Readiness to Quit (CDC, 2010)

- Ask if ready to quit now, if yes (Healthy People, 2010)
  - Set a quit date within 2 weeks.
  - Reduce caffeine intake.
  - Throw away all tobacco, lighters, and ashtrays.
  - Clean car, clothes, and house of smell of smoke.
  - Have teeth cleaned.
  - Avoid tempting situations (e.g., alcohol use).
  - Total abstinence is necessary.
  - Put money saved from not smoking in a fund for your use only. Treat yourself with it.
  - Tell their family, friends, coworkers of the plan.
- Others smoking in the household hinders successful quitting.
- Review past attempts: what helped, what causes relapse?
- Prepare for challenges, for example, nicotine withdrawal (Perea, 2008).
  - Craving for tobacco
  - Irritability
  - Tension
  - Difficulty concentrating
  - Restlessness
  - Headaches
  - Drowsiness
  - Increased appetite
  - Trouble sleeping
- Advise to choose a time to quit of relatively low stress.
- The severity of symptoms is related to duration of smoking and how many cigarettes smoked.

R: *These symptoms occur whether the individual stops suddenly or cuts back.*

- Nicotine withdrawal usually takes 2 to 4 weeks.
- Review of options available can enhance autonomy and decision making.

Assess Associated Activities, Motivation, Previous Quitting Attempts (Leon, 2002)

- When do you smoke first cigarette of the day?
- When do you want a cigarette (e.g., after a meal, with coffee)?
- What happens if you can't smoke for a few hours?
- When you are sick, do you still smoke?
- When did you last try to stop smoking, and what motivated you?
- Have you had any successes, and for how long?
- What were your three toughest obstacles to quitting, and what could we do about them?
- What made you start smoking again?
- What is your present motivation for quitting?
- What method(s) do you think would be best for you to try now?
- Who or what has helped you when you tried to stop in the past?

R: *Exploration of personal smoking habits provides information that can increase confidence in success. This may precipitate a decision to cease smoking (Andrews & Boyle, 2012; Health People 2020, 2010).*

Explain Early Withdrawal Symptoms

- Intense cravings
- Anxiety, tension, or frustration

- Drowsiness or trouble sleeping
- Increased appetite

Explain the Grieving Process Related to Giving up Smoking

- For some people, allowing for a grieving process helps let go of the habit. Smoking is like a companion, and it's probably been there for you for celebrations and disappointments alike. Allow yourself to say goodbye by really enjoying your last cigarette. When you're facing cravings later, dial up a friend before you run out to buy a pack, whip out your "reasons to quit" list, and remember that you've already let it go; you don't need to smoke anymore.

Explain the Effects of Smoking on One's Body and a Timeline of the Body Recovery from the Effects of Smoking. After Quitting for

- Less than 20 minutes, your heart rate will already start to drop back toward normal levels (CDC, 2004).
- 2 hours, your heart rate and blood pressure will have decreased to near normal levels and you may feel the tips of your fingers and toes may start to feel warm.
- Before 8 hours, your sense of smell and taste will improve (Cleveland Clinic, 2014) and the nicotine in the bloodstream has reduced by 93.75%.
- 12 hours, the carbon monoxide in your body decreases to lower levels, and your blood oxygen levels increase to normal (CDC, 2004).
- 24 hours, your anxiety level is the highest and within 2 weeks should return to near precessation levels.
- 24 hours, your **risk for heart attack** will already have begun to drop (The heart attack rate for smokers is 70% higher than for nonsmokers; but, believe or not, just one full day after quitting smoking.).
- 72 hours, the nicotine level in your body is zero.
- 2 weeks to 3 months, your heart attack risk has started to drop. Your lung function is beginning to improve. Your circulation has substantially improved. Walking has become easier. Your chronic cough, if any, has likely disappeared.
- 8 weeks, insulin resistance in smokers has normalized despite average weight gain of 6 lb.
- 1 year, your increased risk of coronary heart disease, heart attack, and stroke has dropped to less than half that of a smoker.
- 5 to 15 years, your risk of stroke has declined to that of a nonsmoker.
- 10 years, your risk of being diagnosed with lung cancer is between 30% and 50% of that for a continuing smoker.
- 13 years, your risk of smoking-induced tooth loss has declined to that of a never-smoker. The average smoker who is able to live to age 75 has 5.8 fewer teeth than a nonsmoker.
- 15 years, your risk of coronary heart disease and pancreatic cancer is now the same as a person who has never smoked.
- 20 years, in women the risk of death from all smoking-related causes, including lung disease and cancer, has now reduced to that of a never-smoker.

Explore Strategies Available to Quit

- Discuss various available methods to quit smoking. Explain that most individuals take several attempts at quitting before success.
- Individual/group counseling
- Self-help materials (written, audio, video)
- Nicotine replacement therapy (transdermal patch, gum, spray)

R: *Each of these modalities has varying degrees of effectiveness. Individuals should be encouraged to continue trying different therapies until they succeed (*Sheahan & Latimer, 1995). Comprehensive smoking cessation guidelines are available at http://www.surgeongeneral.gov/tobacco.*

- Provide information about or initiate referrals to community resources such as the American Lung Association, self-help groups, Meals on Wheels, and home health agencies.

R: *These resources can provide the Individuals needed assistance with home management and self-care.*

- Individual methods: self-help books and tapes, "cold turkey"
- Group methods: contact local chapters of American Cancer Society, American Lung Association, and state-funded hotlines
- Hypnosis, acupuncture
- Over-the-counter products: filters, tablet regimens, nontobacco cigarettes, nicotine-containing chewing gum
- Prescription medications varenicline (Chantix), bupropion (Wellbutrin, Zyban), antidepressants

- Transdermal nicotine patch: stress the hazards of smoking with patch

R: *The best quit-smoking programs are those that combine multiple strategies (Stead, Lancaster, & Perera, 2006).*

Avoid Urges to Smoke

- Spend more time with nonsmokers.
- Engage in activities that cannot include smoking (e.g., exercising).
- Keep low-calorie oral substitutes handy (e.g., gum, fruit).
- Use a relaxation technique such as deep breathing.

Engage in the Following If Relapse Occurs

- Stop smoking immediately.
- Get rid of cigarettes.
- Realize that relapse is common before successful quitting.
- Learn from mistakes.
- Set a new date.

R: *Assessment of previous attempts to quit provides insight, which can increase motivation and success. Specific strategies can increase motivation.*

Discuss Strategies to Minimize Weight Gain and to Increase Exercise

- Refer to *Sedentary Lifestyle.*

If Unwilling to Quit at This Time, Help Motivate the Individual. Identify Reasons to Quit

Explore Negative Aspects of Tobacco Use With the Individual

- *Physical*: exercise intolerance, cough, sputum, frequent respiratory infections, dental disease, increased risk of diseases, premature facial wrinkling, bad breath
- *Environmental*: burned clothing/furniture, discolored interiors of home/workplace, malodorous clothing/furniture, dirty ashtrays, house and occupational fires
- *Social*: inability to smoke in public places; offensive nature of tobacco use behaviors to family members, friends, coworkers
- *Financial*: help the individual calculate monetary cost of habit
- *Psychological*: unpleasant withdrawal symptoms when tobacco is not available (e.g., midnight "nicotine fits"), decreased self-esteem from dependency

Identify Positive Aspects of Tobacco Use With the Individual (Use the Individual's Own Words). Have Person List All Reasons Why He or She Wants to Quit

R: *To assist an individual to initiate a health behavior change, the nurse provides information to increase perceptions of the seriousness of the behavior and susceptibility to disease if behavior continues (Andrews, 1998; *Murray et al., 2009).*

Provide Information on Health Risks

- Address health risks of tobacco use to self—Refer to Key Concepts
- Address health risks of tobacco use to others—Refer to Key Concepts
- Discuss the benefits of quitting
  - Decreased pulse and blood pressure
  - Improved taste/smell
  - Lower risk of cancer, stroke, chronic obstructive pulmonary disease, myocardial infarction
  - Decreased sputum production
  - Pulmonary mucosa regenerates
  - Improved dental hygiene
  - Improved circulation
  - Increased social acceptance
  - Fewer respiratory infections

R: *To assist an individual to initiate a health behavior change, the nurse provides information to increase perceptions of the seriousness of the behavior and susceptibility to disease if behavior continues (Andrews, 1998; *Murray et al., 2009). Discuss with the individual who is not ready to quit now the strategies for quitting at a later date.*

Help the Person Prepare to Stop

- List all reasons for wanting to quit.
- Determine when smoking is most desirable (e.g., upon awaking, after a meal). Continue to smoke but delay smoking, when desired, for half to 1 hour.

- Choose a quit date after 4 weeks of changing smoking patterns.
- Refer to Getting Started to Quit Smoking on thePoint at http://thePoint.lww.com/Carpenito6e. Print it to share with a smoker.

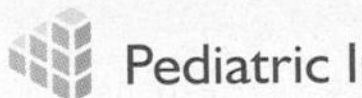

Pediatric Interventions

Assess If Adolescent Knows Someone Who Smokes (Peers, Relatives)

- Use an open-ended, nonjudgmental approach (e.g., "What do you think about smoking?").

Relate Short-Term Rather Than Long-Term Consequences of Smoking (e.g., Early Wrinkling of Skin, Yellow Stains on Teeth and Fingers, Tobacco Odor on Breath and Clothing, Gum Disease, Tooth Staining)

Emphasize Ostracization of Smokers (e.g., Standing Outside Buildings in the Cold to Smoke)

R: *Teenagers are preoccupied with appearance and peer acceptance. The incidence of use of smokeless tobacco has increased among school-aged children, many of whom see it as less of a health hazard than smoking cigarettes.*

Discuss Hazards of Smokeless Tobacco (Cancer of Mouth and Tongue, Tooth Erosion and Loss, Foul Breath, Gum Disease, Tooth Staining, Heart Disease)

Advise that Smokeless Tobacco in Your Mouth for 30 Minutes Is the Same as Smoking Three Cigarettes

R: *Smokeless tobacco is not harmless and can cause serious health problems (Stead et al., 2006).*

Assist Adolescent Not to Start Smoking (DuRant & Smith, 1999)

- Counteract advertising images.
- Practice assertive behavior.
- Discuss smoking myths.
- Address health consequences of tobacco use.
- Most smokers would like to quit. Advise adolescent to ask smokers if they would like to quit.

R: *Helping teens to appreciate that most smokers would like to quit may deter them from starting (Hockenberry & Wilson, 2009).*

Maternal Interventions

Explain the Adverse Effects of Smoking (CDC, 2006; Mitchell et al., 1999)

During Pregnancy

- Crosses the placenta
- Reduces oxygen to the fetus
- Reduces transport of nutrients, calcium, glucose, hormones
- Causes low birth weight
- Causes stillbirths, congenital deformities

In Infants and Children

- Contributes to allergies, otitis media, bronchitis, asthma, and SIDS

If Desired, Establish a Plan to Decrease the Number of Cigarettes Smoked per Day and, If Possible, Set a Date for Total Cessation

Approach Relapses as Temporary Setbacks

Identify Situations That Lead to Smoking

R: *Adverse effects are proportional to daily cigarettes smoked; thus, any decrease is beneficial.*

Sources:

- American Heart Association Smoke-free. (2015). Living: Benefits & Milestones. Retrieved from http://www.heart.org/HEARTORG/GettingHealthy/QuitSmoking/QuittingSmoking/Smoke-free-Living-Benefits-Milestones_UCM_322711_Article.jsp
- Stop Smoking Recovery Timetable (2015). Retrieved from http://whyquit.com/whyquit/A_Benefits_Time_Table.html
- Heathline. (2015). What Happens When You Quit Smoking? Retrieved from http://www.healthline.com/health/quit-smoking

Ineffective Health Management

NANDA-I Definition

Pattern of regulation and integrating into daily living a therapeutic regimen for the treatment of illness and its sequelae that is unsatisfactory for meeting specific health goals

Defining Characteristics

Difficulty with prescribed regimen
Failure to include treatment regimen in daily living
Failure to take action to reduce risk factor (s)
Ineffective choices in daily living for meeting health goal(s)

Related Factors

Treatment-related

Related to the
Complexity treatment regimen
Complexity of health-care system
Insufficient knowledge of therapeutic regimen

Situational (Personal, Environmental)

Related to
Insufficient social support
Perceived barrier(s)
Perceived benefit(s)
Perceived seriousness of condition
Perceived susceptibility
Powerlessness

Related to Barriers to comprehension secondary to:
Cognitive deficits
Fatigue
Hearing impairments
Low literacy
Motivations
Anxiety
Memory problems

Author's Note

In 2010 the costs of health care in the United States exceeded $2.7 trillion and accounted for 17.9% of the gross domestic product. Projections indicate health care will account for 20% of the US gross domestic product by 2020. Twenty to thirty percent of dollars spent in the US health-care system have been identified as wasteful. Providers and administrators have been challenged to contain costs by reducing waste and by improving the effectiveness of care delivered. Patient nonadherence to prescribed medications is associated with poor therapeutic outcomes, progression of disease, and an estimated burden of billions per year in avoidable direct health-care costs (Iuga & McGuire, 2014).

Some reasons for nonadherence are low health literacy, financial, and lack of or unsatisfactory teaching strategies. *Ineffective Self-Help Management* is a very useful diagnosis for nurses in most settings. Individuals and families experiencing various health problems, acute or chronic, usually face treatment programs that require changes in previous functioning or lifestyle. Medication nonadherence is a significant contributor to poor outcomes and health-care costs associated with use of emergency rooms and hospital admissions.

Ineffective Health Management focuses on assisting the person and family to identify barriers in management of the condition and to prevention complications at home.

The nursing diagnosis *Risk for Ineffective Health Maintenance* is useful to describe a person who needs teaching or referrals before discharge from an acute care center to prevent problems with health maintenance at home or in community settings.

Risk-Prone Health Behavior, approved in 2006, is different. This diagnosis focuses on habits or lifestyles that are unhealthy and can aggravate an existing condition or contribute to developing a disease.

Errors in Diagnostic Statements

Ineffective Health Management related to reports that he does not believe he has diabetes mellitus as manifested by reports he did not fill medications and a fasting blood sugar of 200.

The man's denial of a diabetic mellitus diagnosis is the primary barrier to managing his condition. Ineffective denial related inability to accept consciously the consequences the chronic disease of diabetes mellitus and its implications. The focus will be on addressing his denial and its hazards to his health. An initial question can be "I am concerned that you doubt this diagnosis, what do you think is causing your blood sugar to remain high?"

Key Concepts

Transition from Acute Care Setting (Carpenito-Moyet, 2014)

- Barriers that effectively transition from acute care setting are as follows:
  - Personal
  - Support system
  - Home environment

Personal Barriers

- Determine if any of these barriers to self-care are responsible for this admission. Access the appropriate resource in the institution as early as possible to initiate resolving or reducing barriers (e.g., social service, home care).
- Individuals are assessed for disabilities and compromised functioning at admission. Assess if the individual:
  - Is homeless
  - Has no medical insurance
  - Is unable to live alone
  - Is physically impaired
  - Is mentally compromised
  - Can read, level of comprehension
  - Understands English
  - Is abusing drugs, alcohol

Support System Barriers

- Preparing family members/support persons for home care is addressed in each care plan in Section 3. If a support system is not present, nonexistent, or incapable to providing home care, refer to the appropriate resource in the institution as early as possible (e.g., social service, home care agency).
- Determine the present status of a support system. Assess:
  - What kind of assistance is needed for home care 24/7 (e.g., daily visits, phone calls, etc.)?
  - Is there a support system? Who?
  - Are they willing/available to provide assistance?
  - Will they arrange for assistance from others?
  - Are they capable of providing needed care at home (e.g., elderly spouse)?

Home Environment

- If there are barriers to home care due to the environment, refer to the appropriate resource in the institution as early as possible (e.g., social service, home health agency).
- Determine the status of the home environment. Assess:
  - Where does the person live? Home alone? Shelter? Homeless? With others?
  - Can equipment for home care be accessed? Insurance coverage? Home barriers?
  - Is the person capable accessing home/apartment? Stairs?
  - Is there access to a bathroom without using stairs?
  - Is there a temporary alternative (e.g., family member's home)?
- The Centers for Medicare and Medicaid Services (CMS) in 2008 published "Roadmap for Implementing Value Driven Healthcare in the Traditional Medicare Fee-for-Service-Program."
- The CMS objective is "to improve the accuracy of Medicare's payment under the acute care hospital inpatient prospective payment system . . . while providing additional incentives for hospitals to engage

in quality improvement efforts" (CMS, 2008). Of equal importance is that additional payments will be denied for the treatment of the following 14 hospital-acquired conditions (CMS, 2008):

- Stage II and IV pressure ulcers
- Falls and trauma such as fractures, dislocations, intracranial injuries, crushing injuries, burns, and other injuries
- Manifestations of poor glycemic control (e.g., ketoacidosis, hyperosmolar coma, hypoglycemic coma, secondary diabetes with ketoacidosis, or hyperosmolarity)
- Catheter-associated UTIs
- Vascular catheter-associated infections
- Surgical-site infection, mediastinitis, following coronary artery bypass graft (CABG)
- Surgical-site infection following bariatric surgery for obesity (laparoscopic gastric bypass, gastroenterostomy, laparoscopic gastric restrictive surgery)
- Surgical-site infection following certain orthopedic procedures (spine, neck, shoulder, elbow)
- Surgical-site infection following cardiac implantable electronic device (CIED)
- Foreign objects retained after surgery
- Deep vein thrombosis (DVT) pulmonary embolism (PE) following certain orthopedic procedures (total knee replacement, hip replacement)
- Iatrogenic pneumothorax with venous catheterization
- Air embolism
- Blood incompatibility

- In addition to adequate nursing staffing, the following were noted to enhance quality (Di Leonardi, Faller, & Siroky, 2011, p. 15):
  - Understanding that there will be unfinished or incomplete care to handover to next shift.
  - Use of standardized technique, such as hand washing, skin preparation, wound dressings
  - Prudent monitoring of invasive medical devices, such as catheters, chest tubes, IVs
  - Systematic skin inspection, cleaning, and positioning
  - Adherence to care pathways/protocols
  - Ensure medication reconciliation is complete on admission and transition.
  - Refer to interventions under *Ineffective Health Maintenance*.

Literacy, Health Literacy

- Health literacy is "the degree to which individuals have that capacity to obtain, process, and understand basic health information and services needed to make appropriate health decisions" (*Cutilli, 2005).
- Parker and Ratzan (2010) wrote, "Recognizing health literacy is foundational to reforming health and healthcare in America". Those with the highest incidence of low literacy are often:
  - Poor
  - Live in the South and West
  - Do not have a high school diploma
  - Are members of an ethnic/cultural minority older than age 65
  - Have physical/mental disabilities
  - Are homeless or inmates

Functional Illiteracy/Health Literacy

Functional Illiteracy

- When someone who has minimal reading and writing skills
- And does not have the capacity for literacy to manage ordinary everyday needs and requirements of most employments
- Individuals who are illiterate (who cannot read or write) are easier to identify than someone who is functionally illiterate.

Health Literacy

- Health literacy is the capacity to obtain, process, and understand basic health information and services needed to make appropriate health decisions (Parker & Ratzan, 2010) and to follow instructions for treatment.
- Health literacy can be defined as "the knowledge, motivation and competences to access. Understand, appraise and apply health information in order to make judgments and take decisions in everyday life concerning health care, disease prevention and health promotion to maintain or improve quality of life throughout the course of life" (Sørensen et al. 2012; cited in Pelikan et al., 2015).

- In 2003, the National Assessment of Adult Literacy (NAAL) reported that 9 out of 10 English-speaking adults in the United States do not have health literacy (*Kutner, Greenberg, Jiny, & Paulsen, 2006).
- A large study on the scope of health literacy at two public hospitals found the following (*Williams et al., 1995):
  - Half of English-speaking patients could not read and understand basic health education material.
  - 60% could not understand a routine consent form.
  - 26% could not understand the appointment card.
  - 42% failed to understand directions for taking their medications.
- The European Health Literacy Project investigated health literacy in nine countries in the European Union (Austria, Bulgaria, Germany, Greece, Ireland, and Netherlands) in 2011. Using four levels health literacy as insufficient, problematic, sufficient, and excellent. The following findings reported are (Pelikan et al., 2015) given below:
  - None of the countries' studied had a health literacy score of excellent. The Netherlands had the highest score under sufficient health literacy category; Bulgaria the lowest. Non-EU citizens were not included in the study.
  - Forty-seven percent (47%) of the populations studied had limited health literacy.
  - Those with the reported worst health and high use of health-care services reported lowest levels of health literacy.
  - Health literacy worsened with age.
  - Financial deprivation was the highest predictor of low health literacy.
  - For a comprehensive, practical tool for of improving health literacy, refer to DeWalt et al. (2010).

Older Adults

- "A variety of physical and/or psychological factors may interfere with the older adult's ability to process information, demonstrate learning, or adopt the target behavior. Some of these factors include depression, fatigue, stress, functional limitations from physical aging and chronic illnesses, and lack of motivation to learn" (Speros, 2009).
- Risk of chronic illness, functional decline, and geriatric syndromes threaten the well-being of older adults. Forty-three percent of Medicare beneficiaries have three or more chronic conditions such as arthritis, cancer, and heart disease (Federal Interagency Forum on Age Related Statistics, 2010).
- Survey research also reveals that at least 42% of persons over the age of 65 have a functional limitation. One study reported that 25% of older persons with one or more chronic condition also have one or more coexisting geriatric syndrome (Lee, Cigolle, & Blaum, 2009).
- "In addition to changing physical and health circumstances, older adults tend to spend less of their leisure time socializing and communicating as they grow older" (Federal Interagency Forum on Age Related Statistics, 2010).

Goals

NOC

Adherence Behavior, Symptom Control, Health Beliefs Treatment Behavior Illness/Injury

The person will verbalize intent to modify one behavior to manage health problem as evidenced by the following indicators:

- Describes the relationship of present lifestyle to his or her health problems
- Identifies two resources to access after discharge
- Sets a date to initiate change

Interventions

NIC

Heath Education, Mutual Goal Setting, Self-Responsibility, Teaching: Disease Process, Decision-Making Process

On Admission Complete a Medication Reconciliation

- Develop a list of current medications.
- Develop a list of medications to be prescribed.
- Compare the medications on the two lists.
- Make clinical decisions based on the comparison.
- Communicate the new list to the individual and/or appropriate caregivers.
- Table II.9 outlines a comprehensive list of medications to review during medication reconciliations

R: *Medication errors occur 46% of the time during transitions, admission, transfer, or discharge from a clinical unit/hospital. Almost 60% of individuals have at least one discrepancy in their medication history completed on*

Table II.9 SOURCES OF MEDICATION HISTORY

The medication history can be obtained from a variety of sources:

- The client
- A list the patient may have
- The medications themselves, if brought in from home
- A friend or family member
- A medical record
- The individual's pharmacy

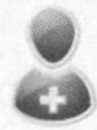

Clinical Alert According to the Joint Commission (2010, p. 1), Medication reconciliation is the process of comparing an individual's medication orders to all of the medications that the patient has been taking. This reconciliation is done to avoid medication errors such as omissions, duplications, dosing errors, or drug interactions. It should be done at every transition of care in which new medications are ordered or existing orders are rewritten. Transitions in care include changes in setting, service, practitioner, or level of care.

admission (Cornish et al., 2005). "The most common error (46.4%) was omission of a regularly used medication. Most (61.4%) of the discrepancies were judged to have no potential to cause serious harm. However, 38.6% of the discrepancies had the potential to cause moderate to severe discomfort or clinical deterioration" (p. 424).

Ask the Individual/Family Member, for Each Medication, the Following:

- What is the reason you are taking each medication?
- Are you taking the medication as prescribed? Specify once a day, twice a day, etc.
- Are you skipping any doses? Do you sometimes run out of medications?
- How often are you taking the medication prescribed "if needed as a pain medication?"
- Have you stopped taking any of these medications?
- How much does it cost you to take your medications?
- Are you taking anybody else's medication?

R: *After acquiring a list of medications, additional assessment questions are critical, which are the defining elements for medication reconciliation: The list alone is not medication reconciliation.*

Engage in Collaborative Negotiation

- Ask: How can you be healthier? Focus on the area the he or she chooses.

R: *Motivational interviewing involves helping the person identify the discrepancy between present behaviors and future health goals. Asking someone to identify an unhealthy lifestyle versus telling him or her that he or she needs to lose weight, stop smoking, exercise, eat better, etc., starts a mutual conversation versus a one-direction dictum.*

Evaluate the Following:

- Primary language, ability to read and write in primary language
- English as a second language
- English as primary language, ability to read, write

Carp's Cues

For successful outcomes for self-heath management at home. Specific teaching techniques have proven to be effective. Refer to Appendix C: Strategies to Promote Engagement of Individual/Families for Healthier Outcomes.

Identify Red Flags for Low Literacy (DeWalt et al., 2010)

- Frequently missed appointments
- Incomplete registration forms
- Noncompliance with medication
- Unable to name medications, explain purpose, or dosing
- Identifies pills by looking at them, not reading label
- Unable to give coherent, sequential history
- Asks fewer questions
- Lack of follow-through on tests or referrals

R: *Persons who are identified as having reading problems will have difficulty with most verbal instructions and individual education material (*Kalichman et al., 2005).*

For Comprehension to Occur, the Nurse Must Accept That There Is Limited Time and That the Use of This Time Is Enhanced by (DeWalt et al., 2010)

Using Every Contact Time to Teach Something

- Creating a relaxed encounter
- Using eye contact
- Slowing down—break it down into short statements
- Limited content—focus on two or three concepts
- Using plain language (refer to Box II.2)
- Engaging individual/family in discussion
- Using graphics
- Explaining what you are doing to the individual/family and why
- Asking them to tell you about what you taught. Tell them to use their own words.

R: *Research shows that individuals remember and understand less than half of what clinicians explain to them (*Roter, Rune, & Comings, 1998; *Williams et al., 1995).*

Box II.2 REPLACING MEDICAL JARGON/WORDS WITH PLAIN WORDS

Medical Jargon/Words	Plain Words
Hepatic	Livers
Pulmonary Function	Lungs
Medications	Pills
Nutrition	Food
Beverages	Drinks
Dermatologist	Skin doctor
Ophthalmology	Eye doctor
Dermatitis	Rash
Conjunctivitis	Eye infection
Gastrointestinal Specialist	Stomach doctor
Antihypertensive Medicine	Blood pressure medications
Anticoagulant	Blood thinner
Enlarge	Bigger infection
Lesion	Sore
Lipids	Fats
Menses	Period
Osteoporosis	Decrease in the inside of the bone
Depression	Feeling sad
Normal range	Good
Toxic	High levels
Anti-inflammatory	Helps swelling and irritation go away
Dose	How much medicine you should take
Contraception	Helps you not get pregnant
Generic	General name for a type of medication
Oral	By mouth
Monitor	Keeps track of
Referral	See another doctor/nurse practitioner

- Avoid information overload with older adults and those with low literacy. Consider a home health nurse assessment visit to evaluate competencies at home.

R: *"Rushing an older adult to demonstrate a new skill can lead to incapacitating anxiety, frustration, and unwillingness to perform for fear of failure and shame" (Speros, 2009).*

Carp's Cues

For a comprehensive resource on how to reduce the barriers to learning and comprehension in older adults, refer to Speros (2009).

Use the Teach-Back Method (Refer to Figure II.4)

- Explain/Demonstrate.
  - Explain one concept (e.g., medication, condition, when to call PCP).
  - Demonstrate one procedure (e.g., dressing charge, use of inhaler).
- Assess.
  - I want to make sure, I explained ______ clearly, can you tell me ______.
  - Tell me what I told you.
  - Show me how to ______.
  - Avoid asking, Do you understand?
- Clarify.
  - Add more explanation if you are not satisfied the person understands or can perform the activity.
  - If the person cannot report the information, don't repeat the same explanation; rephrase it.

R: *Low health literacy is not only linked to worse health outcomes and greater mortality risk, but to unnecessary health-care services use and costs (Parker & Ratzan, 2010).*

Carp's Cues

Be careful the person/family does not think you are testing him or her. Assure them it is important that you help them to understand that the teaching method can help you teach and also diagnose educational needs.

Teach-Back Questions (Examples)

- When should you call your PCP?
- How do you know your incision is healing?
- What foods should you avoid?
- How often should you test your blood sugar?
- What should you do for low blood sugar?
- What weight gain should you report to your PCP?

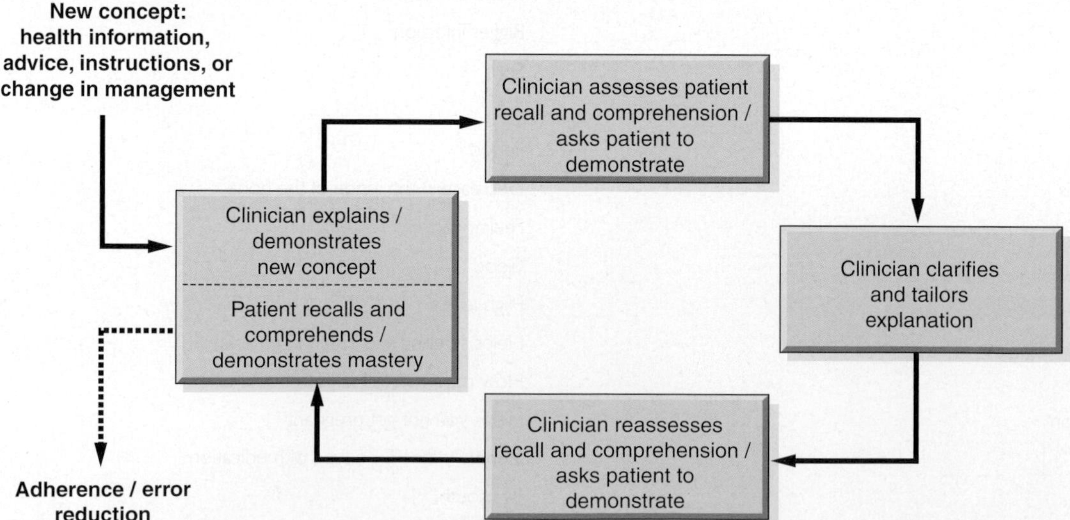

FIGURE II.4 The Teach-Back Process. (From Berkman, N. D., DeWalt, D. A., Pignone, M. P., Sheridan, S. L., Lohr, K. N., Lux, L., Sutton, S. F., Swinson, T., & Bonito, A. J. (2004). *Literacy and health outcomes*. Evidence Report/Technology Assessment No. 87 (Prepared by RTI International—University of North Carolina Evidence-based Practice Center under Contract No. 290-02-0016). AIIRQ Publication No. 04/Æ007-2. Rockville, MD: Agency for Healthcare Research and Quality.)

Box II.3 TEACH-BACK METHOD: REMINDER CARD

- Who—*me*
- What—*anything important I want them to understand*
- When—*every time*
- Why—*I need to know they understand*
- How—Focus on "need to know" and "need to do"
- Practice with and improve one's teach-back skills

- Which inhaler is your rescue inhaler?
- Is there something you have been told to do that you do not understand?
- What should you bring to your PCP office?
- Is there something you have a question about?

Carp's Cues

Use every opportunity to explain a treatment, a medication, the condition, and/or restrictions (see Box II.3). For example, as you change a dressing:

- Explain and ask the individual/family member to redress the wound.
- Point out how the wound is healing and what would indicate signs of infection.

R: *Based on the person's response or demonstration, the nurse can evaluate if the person/family can apply the teaching to safe self-care at home.*

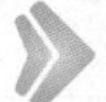

Carp's Cues

When individual/family does not understand what was said or demonstrated, the teach-back needs to be revised in a manner that will improve understanding. Teach-back has the potential to improve health outcomes because if done correctly, it forces the nurse to limit the information to need to know. The likelihood of success is increased when the individual is not overwhelmed. If needs, recommend a home health nurse assessment.

Teach Self-Care or Care at Home by Addressing the Following:

The Condition

Medical Conditions

- What do you know about your condition?
- How do you think this condition will affect you after you leave the hospital?
- What do you want to know about your condition?

Surgical Procedure

- What do you know about the surgery you had?
- Do you have any questions about your surgery?
- How will surgery affect you after you leave the hospital?

Medications

- Renew all the medications that the individual will continue to take at home.
- Explain what OTC not to take.
- Finish all the meds like antibiotics.
- Do not to take any medications that are at home unless approved by PCP.
- Ask to bring all his or her medications to next visit to PCP (e.g., prescribed, OTC, vitamins, herbal medicines).
- Depending on the literacy level of the individual/family, provide the following:
  - A list of each medication, what used for, times to take, with food or without food
  - Create a pill card with columns.
    - Pictures of pill
    - Simple terms for used for
    - Time using symbols with pictures of pills in spaces
- Figure II.5 illustrates a pill card. For a printable pill card to use with individuals, refer to thePoint at http://thePoint.lww.com/Carpenito6e.
- Explain the following:
  - If a pill looks different, check with pharmacy.
  - Do not take any other medications except those on list unless approved by PCP.

FIGURE II.5 Example of a Pill Card. (From DeWalt, D. A., Callahan, L. F., Hawk, V. H., Broucksou, K. A., Hink, A, Rudd, R., & Brach, C. (2010). *Health literacy universal precautions tool kit*. Retrieved from http://www.ahrq.gov/professionals/quality-patient-safety/quality-resources/tools/literacy-toolkit/index.html.)

Name: Sarah Smith **Pharmacy phone number: 123-456-7890**						**Date Created: 12/15/07**
Name	**Used For**	**Instructions**	**Morning**	**Afternoon**	**Evening**	**Night**
Simvastatin 20mg	Cholesterol	Take 1 pill at night				
Furosemide 20mg	Fluid	Take 2 pills in the morning and 2 pills in the evening				
Insulin 70/30	Diabetes (Sugar)	Inject 24 units before breakfast and 12 units before dinner	24 units		12 units	

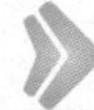

Carp's Cues

In the author's primary care practice, hospitalized individuals may be given a different medication in the same class due to formulary restrictions. When the individual has a follow-up used in the office, during medication reconciliation, it is discovered he or she is taking two β-blockers, one prescribed in the hospital and the one previously taken.

Evaluate the Financial Implications of Prescribed Medication

- Does the person have insured medication coverage? If yes, does it cover the medication ordered? If yes, what is the copay? Can the person afford this?
- If there is no insurance or no medication coverage, how will the person access these medications?
- Is there an inexpensive generic available?
- Which medications are critical and need immediately?
- Explain that most pharmaceutical companies provide free branded medications (not generic) through patient assisted programs. Applications can be accessed via the pharmaceutical website. Social service departments can also assist with this process.
- Some medications (e.g., oral diabetic medications, antibiotics) can be acquired free in supermarkets (e.g., Pathmark, ShopRite) or at low cost (e.g., Target).
- Advise individual/family to call PCP office if they do not want to continue a medication.

Dietary recommendations

- Ask individual/family to report if there are any dietary limitations.
- Ensure there are written directions.
- Explain why some foods/beverages are to be avoided (e.g., avoid olives, pickles on a low-salt diet).

Activities

- Provide instructions on activities permitted and restrictions.
- When they can drive.
- Return to work; what kind of job do they have?

Treatments

- Explain each treatment to be continued at home.
- Equipment needed, frequency of treatment.
- Write down what signs and symptoms should be reported (e.g., decrease in output for catheter).

Competence

- Can this treatment be provided safely by the individual or caregiver?
- If not, consult with the transition specialist in the health-care agency.

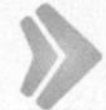

Carp's Cues

If a home health agency is referred to, validate that their arrival will be timely in order to begin the treatment on time.

Provide Specific Teaching for Management of a Medical Disorder and/or Postoperative Care and/or Postpartum Care, Signs of Complications, Activity Restrictions, Dietary Recommendations Medications Prescribed, and Follow-up Care.

- Refer to medical surgical textbooks, specialty textbooks for specific information to teach associated with the individual's condition.
- Refer to Carpenito-Moyet (2014) *Nursing Care Plans: Transitional Patient and Family Centered Care* for specific content to teach the individual/family self-care at home for 68 medical and surgical conditions.

For Individual Living With a Chronic Condition With Unsatisfactory Outcomes, for Example, Hgb A1c > 8, B/P > 130/85, a Smoker with Frequent Upper Respiratory Infections, a 10-lb Weight Gain With a BMI of 31 in 3 months:

Assess for Barriers

- What do you think is causing your BP (blood sugar or weight) to remain high?
- What could you do to decrease your BP (weight, blood sugar)?
- Would you like to stop smoking (or drinking alcohol)?
- What is preventing you?

If Low Literacy Is Suspected, Start with What the Person Is Most Stressed About

- What do you want to know about __________?
- Speak simply.
- Repeat and ask person to repeat.
- Use appropriate examples, for example, affordable sources of protein.
- Identify with the person one to three changes they can make as:
  - Do not skip meals, eat breakfast as cereal, boiled egg.
  - Substitute sugar drinks, for example, soda, juices with water or a noncalorie drink.
  - Walk when you can, park car farther away in parking lot, walk down stairs. Plan to walk with a friend, for example, mall in hot weather, safer place for some (avoid food or shopping).

R: *Individuals often receive too much or too little information. When the learner chooses what to learn, health-related outcomes are improved (*Bodenheimer et al., 2005).*

- For example: What did you have for dinner last night?
- Response: fried chicken.
- What else?
- Response: that is all.
- How could you prepare the chicken to have less fat?
- What could you add to that dinner that is healthy?

R: *The person's level of confidence will increase with success. Advice that is not easily achievable sets the person up for failure (*Bodenheimer et al., 2005).*

- Refer to thePoint at http://thePoint.lww.com/Carpenito6e for printed material Getting Started to provide the person with strategies to improve health, for example, smoking cessation, exercise, better food choices, weight loss, stress management.

HOPELESSNESS

NANDA-I Definition

Subjective state in which an individual sees limited or no alternatives or personal choices available and is unable to mobilize energy on own behalf

Defining Characteristics

Expresses profound, overwhelming, sustained apathy in response to a situation perceived as impossible

Physiologic

Increased sleep
Lack of energy
Decreased response to stimuli*

Emotional

Person Feels

As though they do not receive any breaks and there is no reason to believe they will in the future
Empty or drained
Demoralized
Helpless
Lack of meaning or purpose in life

Person Exhibits

Passivity* and lack of involvement in care
Decreased affect*
Giving up–given up complex
Isolating behaviors
Decreased verbalization*
Lack of ambition, initiative*, and interest
Fatigue
Risk-taking behaviors such as failure to wear seat belt, helmet, or driving while intoxicated

Cognitive

Rigidity (e.g., all-or-none thinking)
Lack of imagination and wishing capabilities
Inability to identify or accomplish desired objectives and goals
Inability to plan, organize, make decisions, or problem-solve
Inability to recognize sources of hope
Suicidal thoughts

Related Factors

Pathophysiologic

Any chronic or terminal illness (e.g., heart disease, diabetes, kidney disease, cancer, acquired immunodeficiency syndrome [AIDS]) can cause or contribute to hopelessness.

Related to impaired ability to cope secondary to:

Failing or deteriorating physiologic condition
New and unexpected signs or symptoms of previously diagnosed disease process (i.e., recurrence of cancer; Robinson, Hoover, Venetis, Kearney, & Street, 2012).
Prolonged pain, discomfort, and weakness
Impaired functional abilities (walking, elimination, eating, dressing, bathing, speaking, writing)

Treatment Related

Related to:

Prolonged treatments (e.g., chemotherapy, radiation) that cause pain, nausea, and discomfort
Treatments that alter body image (e.g., surgery, chemotherapy)
Prolonged diagnostic studies
Prolonged dependence on equipment for life support (e.g., dialysis, respirator)
Prolonged dependence on equipment for monitoring bodily functions (e.g., telemetry)

Situational (Personal, Environmental)

Related to:

Prolonged activity restriction (e.g., fractures, spinal cord injury, imprisonment)
Prolonged isolation (e.g., infectious diseases, reverse isolation for suppressed immune system)
Abandonment by, separation from, or isolation from significant others (Mair, Kaplan, & Everson-Rose, 2012)
Inability to achieve valued goals in life (marriage, education, children)
Inability to participate in desired activities (walking, sports, work)
Loss of something or someone valued (spouse, children, friend, financial resources)
Prolonged caretaking responsibilities (spouse, child, parent)
Exposure to long-term physiologic or psychological stress
Recurrence of breast cancer (Robinson et al., 2012)
Loss of belief in transcendent values/God
Ongoing, repetitive losses in community related to AIDS
Repetitive natural disasters (hurricanes, tornadoes, flooding, fires)
Prolonged exposure to violence and war

Maturational

Child

Loss of autonomy related to illness (e.g., fracture)
Loss of bodily functions
Loss of caregiver
Loss of trust in significant other
Inability to achieve developmental tasks (trust, autonomy, initiative, industry)
Rejection, abuse, or abandonment by caregivers

Adolescent

Change in body image
Inability to achieve developmental task (role identity)
Loss of bodily functions
Loss of significant other (peer, family)
Rejection by family

Adult

Abortion
Impaired bodily functions, loss of body part
Impaired relationships (separation, divorce)
Inability to achieve developmental tasks (intimacy, commitment, productivity)
Loss of job, career
Loss of significant others (death of spouse, child)
Miscarriage

Older Adult

Cognitive deficits
Dementia
Inability to achieve developmental tasks
Loss of independence
Loss of significant others, things (in general)
Motor deficits
Sensory deficits

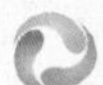

Author's Note

Hopelessness describes a person who sees no possibility that his or her life will improve and maintains that no one can do anything to help. *Hopelessness* differs from *Powerlessness* in that a hopeless person sees no solution or no way to achieve what is desired, even if he or she feels in control. In contrast, a powerless person may see an alternative or answer, yet be unable to do anything about it because of lack of control or resources. Sustained feelings of powerlessness may lead to hopelessness. Hopelessness is commonly related to grief, depression, and suicide. For a person at risk for suicide, the nurse also should use the diagnosis *Risk for Suicide*. Hopelessness is a distinct concept and not merely a symptom of depression.

Errors in Diagnostic Statements

Hopelessness related to AIDS

This diagnostic statement does not describe a situation the nurse can treat. The statement should include specific factors the person has identified as overwhelming, as in the following diagnostic statement: *Hopelessness related to recent diagnosis of AIDS and rejection by parents.*

Key Concepts

General Considerations

Hope

- Hope is an unconscious cognitive behavior that energizes and allows a person to act, achieve, and use crisis as an opportunity for growth. It activates motivation and defends against despair (*Korner, 1970). It has been defined as any expectation greater than zero for achieving a given goal (*Stotland, 1969). Hope is a "common human experience in that it is a way of propelling self towards envisioned possibilities in everyday encounters with the world" (*Parse, 1990).
- Early childhood experiences influence a person's ability to hope. A trusting environment promotes hope.
- Mihaljević, Aukst-Margetić, Vuksan-Ćusa, Koić, and Milošević (2012) found high indices of hope in people who have a relationship with a higher being, participate in religious services, and can control their immediate environment. Spiritual practices provide a source of hope.
- Watson (*1979) has identified hope as both a curative and a "carative" factor in nursing. Hope, with faith and trust, provides psychic energy to draw on to aid the curative process.
- Researchers have observed that hope prolongs life in critical survival conditions, whereas loss of hope often results in death (*Korner, 1970).
- Kübler-Ross (*1975) observed that those who expressed hope coped more effectively during their difficult dying periods. She also noted that death occurred soon after these people stopped expressing hope.
- Notewotney (*1989) identified six dimensions of hope: confidence in outcome, possibility of a future, relating to others, spiritual beliefs, emergence from within, and active involvement.
- Miller (*1989) studied 60 critically ill individuals to determine hope-inspiring strategies:
  - Thinking to buffer threatening perceptions
  - Using positive thinking
  - Feeling that life has meaning and growth results from crises
  - Engaging in beliefs and practices that enable transcendence of suffering
  - Receiving from caregivers a constructive view, expectations of individual's ability to manage difficulty, and confidence in therapy
  - Sustaining relationships with loved ones
  - Perceiving that knowledge and actions can affect outcomes
  - Having desired activities and outcomes to attain
  - Other specific behaviors that thwart despair, including distraction and humor

Hopelessness

- Hopelessness is an emotional state in which a person feels that life is too much or impossible. A person without hope sees no possibility that life will improve and that there are no solutions. He or she believes that no one can do anything to help. Hopelessness is related to despair, helplessness, doubt, grief, apathy, sadness, depression, and suicide. It is present- and past-oriented and a de-energizing state.
- Hopelessness results in three basic categories of feeling:
  - *Sense of the impossible*: what a person feels compelled to do, he or she cannot; thus, he or she feels trapped
  - *Overwhelmed*: the person perceives tasks and others as too big and difficult to handle and self as small
  - *Apathy*: the person has no goals or sense of purpose
- Hopeless people lack internal resources and strengths (e.g., autonomy, self-esteem, integrity). Regardless of age, they reach outside for help because their internal resources are depleted.
- Engel (*1989) identified the "giving up–given up" complex as having five characteristics:
  - Experiencing the feeling of giving up as helplessness or hopelessness

  - Having a depreciated image of self
  - Experiencing a sense of loss of gratification from relationships or roles
  - Feeling disruption
  - Reactivating memories of earlier periods of giving up
- Often, when internal and external resources are exhausted, a person relies on his or her relationship with God for hope. The person may feel more secure placing hope in God than in others or self. Hoping in God may not mean an abrupt end to the crisis, but it may give a sense of God's control of circumstances and ability to provide support during this time. Meaning and purpose for life and suffering may be found in an individual's relationship with God and the knowledge of His control. Hope for an individual's future may depend on his or her perception of a promise of eternal fellowship with God that continues after life on earth ends. With this eternal relationship comes the belief in God's promise to end all suffering and restore harmonious relationships—with God, self, and others (*Jennings, 1997).
- Hopelessness can be found in the gay community in response to multiple AIDS-related losses, such as loss of friends and community and disintegrating family structures and social networks. These losses are unending and repetitive and receive little understanding from many heterosexuals (Liu & Mustanski, 2012).

Pediatric Considerations

- Ninety-four percent of parents who have children with cancer were found to have feelings of hopelessness based on the follow-up results at a university center (Bayat, Erdem, & Kuzucu, 2008).
- Consistent nurturing, trustworthiness, and achievement of hoped-for things and events nurture hope in children.
- Families of children with life-threatening diseases may feel hopeless and become dysfunctional. The nurse may need to identify dysfunctional family interactions, use strategies from family therapy, or make appropriate referrals.
- To become an adult, the adolescent must first achieve hopefulness. Hinds, Martin, and Vogel (*1987) found that adolescents with cancer progress through four sequential, self-sustaining phases to cope and achieve hopefulness:
  - Cognitive discomfort
  - Distraction
  - Cognitive comfort
  - Personal competence
- Nursing interventions that have been found to influence hopefulness in adolescents include truthful explanations, doing things with them, nursing knowledge of survivors, caring behaviors, focusing on the future, competency, and conversing about less-sensitive areas. In addition, humor has been identified as promoting cognitive distraction and facilitating hope. Nursing interventions that inhibit cognitive distraction (e.g., focusing on nursing tasks and on negative adolescent behaviors) promote hopelessness (*Hinds et al., 1987).

Geriatric Considerations

- Older adults are at risk for hopelessness because of the many psychosocial and physiologic changes that accompany normal aging, which often are perceived as losses. Older adults also have decreased energy, and energy is necessary for hopefulness (Miller, 2015).
- Healthy coping in older adults is related to acquiring developmental resources in later adulthood. Older adults must learn to give up less useful operations and acquire more effective resources to deal with age-related life changes (Sirey, Bruce, & Alexopoulos, 2014).
- Stressors for older adults are unique and differ from those of other age groups. They include changes in personal care, longing for absent children or grandchildren, fear of being a victim of crime, and fear of being taken advantage of by the "system." The nurse may be able to assist older individuals to identify stressors and locate resources to prevent hopelessness.

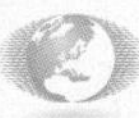

Transcultural Considerations

- Nurses who subscribe to the dominant US culture may misinterpret cultural differences related to values, expectations, and loci of control (*Leininger, 1978).
- Hopelessness focuses on an inability to achieve goals, which is future oriented. The concept of hopelessness may not be relevant to cultures that are not future oriented.

- Interventions for hopelessness vary among cultures (Polanco-Roman & Miranda, 2013).
- Disease (as in cancer) perceived as hopelessness in certain cultures may be taboo to discuss and delay early detection and treatment.

Focus Assessment Criteria

Hopelessness is a subjective emotional state in which the nurse must validate with the individual. The nurse must assess emotional and cognitive areas carefully to infer that the individual is experiencing hopelessness. Some of these same cues may be seen in people with diagnoses of *Social Isolation*, *Powerlessness*, *Disturbed Self-Concept*, *Spiritual Distress*, or *Ineffective Coping*.

Subjective Data

Assess for Defining Characteristics

Activities of Daily Living
Change(s) is usual activities of daily living, sleep, appetite, eating patterns, exercise, and recreation.

Energy and Motivation
Is the individual exhausted, tired?
Does he or she have any goals or desires?
Does the individual feel overwhelmed?
Does he or she express an interest in any activities?
Can the individual solve day-to-day typical problems?

Meaning and Purpose in Life
What does this individual value most in life? Why?
What does this individual describe as his or her purpose or role in life?
Is this purpose or role fulfilled?
Are perceptions of his or her meaning and purpose realistic or achievable?
What kind of relationship does he or she have with God or a higher being?
Does this relationship give meaning or purpose to his or her life?
What does this illness mean to the person?

Choice or Control in Situations
What does the individual perceive to be his or her most difficult problem? Why?
What does he or she believe is the solution? Is this solution realistic?
Is his or her perception of the problem distorted? If so, how?
Has the individual considered or tried other alternatives?
Does this individual believe he or she has any control in the situation?
How flexible or rigid are this individual's thought processes?

Future Options
What does the individual believe the future will bring? Negative or positive things?
What does he or she see as worth living for?
How does the future look to this individual?
How does this individual perceive his or her present illness? Its effect on his or her life? Its effect on his or her relationships?
How does this person perceive current treatments for his or her illness? Promising, or stressful and useless?
Can this individual describe something to which he/she is looking forward to happening?
Does this individual recognize any sources of hope?
What does he or she want most in life?
Does this individual have suicidal thoughts? If so, refer to *Risk for Suicide*.

Assess for Related Factors

Presence of Illness or Treatment
Chronic, prolonged, deteriorating, and exhausting.

Significant Relationships
Whom does this individual perceive as the most significant other?
What is this individual's current relationship with this significant other?

Has divorce or death of a spouse, child, sibling, friend, or pet occurred recently?
Has this individual moved away from or been rejected by significant others?

Objective Data

Assess for Defining Characteristics

General appearance (grooming, eye contact, posture)
Speed of activities
Interaction with others
Involvement in self-care activities

Goals

NOC

Decision-Making, Depression Control, Hope, Quality of Life, Mood Equilibrium, Personal Resiliency

- Demonstrate increased energy, as evidenced by an increase in activities (e.g., self-care, hobbies).
- Express desirable expectations for the near future. Describe one's own meaning and purpose in life.
- Demonstrate initiative, self-direction, and autonomy in decision making. Demonstrate effective problem-solving strategies.
- Redefine the future, setting realistic goals with expectation to meet these goals.

Interventions

NIC

Hope Instillation, Values Classification, Decision-Making Support, Spiritual Support, Support System Enhancement

Assist Individual to Identify and Express Feelings

- Listen actively, treat the individual as an individual, and accept his or her feelings. Convey empathy to promote verbalization of doubts, fears, and concerns.
- Validate and reflect impressions with the person. It is important to realize that individuals with cancer often have their own reality, which may differ from the nurse's.
- Assist the individual in recognizing that hopelessness is part of everyone's life and demands recognition. The individual can use it as a source of energy, imagination, and freedom to consider alternatives.

R: *Hopelessness can lead to self-discovery.*

- Assist the individual to understand that he or she can deal with the hopeless aspects of life by separating them from the hopeful aspects. Help the individual to distinguish between the possible and impossible.
- The nurse mobilizes an individual's internal and external resources to promote and instill hope. Assist the individuals to identify their personal reasons for living that provide meaning and purpose to their lives.

R: *This gives the individual permission to talk and explore his or her life, which is a hopeful intervention (Robinson et al., 2012).*

Assess and Mobilize the Individual's Internal Resources (Autonomy, Independence, Rationality, Cognitive Thinking, Flexibility, Spirituality)

- Emphasize strengths, not weaknesses.
- Compliment the individual on appearance or efforts as appropriate.
- Identify areas of success and usefulness; emphasize past accomplishments. Use this information to develop goals with the individual.
- Assist the individual in identifying things he or she has fun doing and perceives as humorous. Such activities can serve as distractions to discomfort and allow the individual to progress to cognitive comfort (Sar & Sayar, 2013).
- Assist the individual in adjusting and developing realistic short- and long-term goals (progress from simple to more complex; may use a "goals poster" to indicate type and time for achieving specific goals). Attainable expectations promote hope.
- Encourage "means–end" thinking in positive terms (i.e., "If I do this, then I'll be able to.").

R: *It is important to recognize constructive possibilities in adults living with HIV/AIDS to promote a life worth living and to recognize a glimmer of hope. Otherwise, one becomes stuck and sinks to a narrowing existence, focusing on the impossible, and loses a future perspective (Govender & Schlebusch, 2012).*

Assist the Individual With Problem Solving and Decision Making

- Respect the individual as a competent decision-maker; treat his or her decisions and desires with respect.
- Encourage verbalization to determine the individual's perception of choices.

- Clarify the individual's values to determine what is important.
- Correct misinformation.
- Assist the individual in identifying those problems he or she cannot resolve to advance to problems he or she can. In other words, assist the individual to move away from dwelling on the impossible and hopeless and to begin to deal with realistic and hopeful matters.
- Assess the individual's perceptions of self and others in relation to size. (People with hopelessness often perceive others as large and difficult to deal with and themselves as small.) If perceptions are unrealistic, assist the individual to reassess them to restore proper scale.
- Promote flexibility. Encourage the individual to try alternatives and take risks.

R: *If a person recognizes and deals with hopelessness imaginatively, movement, growth, and resourcefulness can result. Rigidity never overcomes hopelessness.*

R: *Motivation is essential to recovering from hopelessness. The individual must determine a goal even if he or she has low expectation of achieving it. The nurse is the catalyst to encourage the individual to take the first step to identify a goal. Then, the individual must create another goal.*

- Explain the benefits of distraction from negative events.
- Teach and assist with relaxation techniques before anticipated stressful events.
- Encourage mental imagery to promote positive thought processes.
- Teach to maximize aesthetic experiences (e.g., smell of coffee, back rub, feeling warmth of the sun, or a breeze) that can inspire hope.
- Teach to anticipate experiences he or she delights in daily (e.g., walking, reading favorite book, writing a letter).
- Teach ways to conserve and generate energy through moderate physical exercise.
- Encourage music therapy, aromatherapy, and message with essential oils to improve the individual's physical and mental status.

R: *Music therapy, aromatherapy, and massage with essential oils were found to help learn to release stress and express feelings to adapt to current life and face the impact of illness with a positive attitude (Ye & Yeh, 2007).*

R: *People can cope with a part of life they view as hopeless if they realize that other factors in life are hopeful. For example, a person may realize that he or she may never walk again but will be able to go home, be with grandchildren, and move around. Therefore, hopelessness can lead to the discovery of alternatives that provide meaning and purpose in life. It is essential to keep hopelessness out of the way of hope.*

Assess and Mobilize the Individual's External Resources

Family or Significant Others

- Involve the family and significant others in plan of care.
- Encourage the individual to spend increased time or thoughts with loved ones in healthy relationships.
- Teach the family members their role in sustaining hope through supportive, positive relationships.

R: *Maintaining family role responsibilities is essential for hope and coping. In addition, hope is essential for families of the critically ill to facilitate coping and adjustment.*

- Empower the individuals who have chronic disease by instilling hope through the bolstering of support systems.

R: *Individuals who live alone with no family support were found to have more symptoms of hopelessness. Brothers and Anderson (2007) found that women who reported feelings of hopelessness and were alone (without a partner) were more inclined to develop depressive symptoms than those with a partner.*

- Convey hope, information, and confidence to the family because they will convey their feelings to the individual.
- Use touch and closeness with the individual to demonstrate to the family its acceptability (provide privacy).
- Herth (*1993) found the following strategies to foster hope in caregivers of terminally ill people:
  - Cognitive reframing—positive self-talk, praying/meditating, and envisioning hopeful images (this may involve letting go of expectations for things to be different)
  - Time refocusing—focusing less on the future and more on living one day at a time
  - Belief in a power greater than self—empowering the caregiver's hope
  - Balancing available energy—listening to music or other favorite activities to empower the caregiver's hope through uplifting energy

R: *Hope is related to help from others, in that an individual believes external resources may be supportive when his or her internal resources and strengths seem insufficient to cope (i.e., a family or significant other is often a source of hope) (*Benzein & Berg, 2005).*

R: *Hope maintained by family members has a contagious effect on individuals.*

Health-Care Team

- Develop a positive, trusting nurse–client relationship by:
  - Answering questions
  - Respecting individual's feelings
  - Providing consistent care
  - Following through on requests
  - Providing comfort
  - Being honest
  - Conveying positive attitude
  - Keeping communication patient-centered
  - Recommending cognitive-behavioral therapy
- Convey attitude of "We care too much about you to let you just give up," or "I can help you."

R: *The health-care team must be hopeful if the individual is to be hopeful; otherwise, the individual views efforts of the team as a waste of time.*

- Keep communication patient-centered. Patient-centered communication (PCC) was found to significantly decrease the hopelessness of cancer patients.

Support Groups

- Encourage the individual to share concerns with others who have had a similar problem or disease and positive experiences from coping effectively with it.
- Provide information on self-help groups (e.g., "Make today count"—40 chapters in the United States and Canada; "I can cope"—series for individuals with cancer; "We Can Weekend"—for families of individuals with cancer).

R: *Isolation, concurrent losses, and poorly controlled symptom management hinder hope (Öztunj, Yeşil, Paydaş, & Erdoğan, 2013).*

R: *Hopelessness was found to be a predictor of suicide.*

God or Higher Powers

- Assess the individual's belief support system (value, past experiences, religious activities, relationship with God, meaning and purpose of prayer; refer to *Spiritual Distress*).
- Create an environment in which the individual feels free to express spirituality.
- Allow the individual time and opportunities to reflect on the meaning of suffering, death, and dying.
- Accept, respect, and support the individual's hope in God.

R: *Individuals with enhanced psycho-spiritual well-being were found to cope more effectively by finding meaning and purpose in the lived experience (*Jennings, 1997; *Lin & Bauer-Wu, 2003). Hope was found to be positively correlated with spiritual well-being in women with breast cancer.*

RISK FOR COMPROMISED HUMAN DIGNITY

NANDA-I Definition

Vulnerable for perceived loss of respect and honor, which may compromise health

Risk Factors

End-of-Life Decisions*

Related to providing treatments that were perceived as futile for terminally ill client (e.g., blood transfusions, chemotherapy, organ transplants, mechanical ventilation)

Related to conflicting attitudes toward advanced directives

Related to participation of life-saving actions when they only prolong dying

Treatment Decisions

Related to disagreement among health-care professions, family members, and/or the individual regarding

Treatments
Transition to home, relative's home, or community nursing care facility
The individual's living will
End-of-life care

Related to the client's/family's refusal of treatments deemed appropriate by the health-care team

Related to inability of the family to make the decision to stop ventilator treatment of terminally ill client

Related to a family's wishes to continue life support, even though it is not in the best interest of the client

Related to performing a procedure that increases the client's suffering

Related to providing care that does not relieve the client's suffering

Related to conflicts between wanting to disclose poor medical practice and wanting to maintain trust in the physician

Cultural Conflicts

Related to decisions made for women by male family members

Related to cultural conflicts with the American health-care system

Related to individual's compromised ability to comprehend and//or to communicate preferences, decisions

Author's Note

Risk for Compromised Human Dignity was accepted by NANDA-I in 2006.

This nursing diagnosis presents a new application for nursing practice. All individuals are at risk for this diagnosis. Providing respect, honor, and protection to all individuals, families, and communities is a critical core element of professional nursing. Prevention of compromised human dignity must be a focus of all nursing interventions. It is the central concept of a caring profession.

This diagnosis can also apply to prisoners, who as part of their penalty will be deprived of some rights, for example, privacy and movement. Prisoners, however, should always be treated with respect and not be tortured or humiliated. Nurses have the obligation to honor and "do no harm" in all settings in which they practice.

This author recommends that this diagnosis be developed and integrated into a Standard Care of the Nursing Department for all individuals and families in their health-care facility. The outcomes and interventions apply to all individuals, families, and groups. This Department of Nursing Standards of Practice could also include *Risk for Infection, Risk for Infection Transmission, Risk for Falls,* and *Risk for Compromised Family Coping*.

Errors in Diagnostic Statements

Risk for Compromised Human Dignity related to perceived dehumanizing treatments

This diagnosis represents actual compromised human dignity, not an at-risk diagnosis. This situation should be reported and investigated, and reported to the appropriate authority in the agency for immediate action.

Key Concepts

- "Dignity is a slippery concept, most easily understood when it has been lost" (*Reed, Smith, Fletcher, & Bradding, 2003). Nurses have a responsibility and commitment to protect and preserve client dignity (*Walsh & Kownako, 2002).
- Dignity exists when an individual is "capable of exerting control or choice over his or her behavior, surroundings, and the way he or she is treated by others. He or she should be capable of understanding information and making decisions. He or she should feel comfortable with his or her physical and psychosocial status quo" (*Mairis, 1994).

- The ability to maintain dignity is dependent on one's ability in the presence of the threat to keep intact one's beliefs about oneself (*Haddock, 1994).
- "Dignity is the ability to feel important and valuable in relation to others, in contexts which are perceived as threatening. Dignity is a dynamitic subjective belief but also has a shared meaning among humanity. Dignity is striven for and its maintenance depends on one's ability to keep intact the boundary containing beliefs about oneself and the extent of the threat. Context and possession of dignity within oneself affects one's ability to maintain or promote the dignity of another" (*Haddock, 1996).
- To have dignity is to have control over oneself. The effects of loss of dignity are emotional distress, humiliation, and embarrassment (*Mairis, 1994; *Walsh & Kowanko, 2002).
- The Principles of Medical Ethics (*American Medical Association [AMA], 2001) has nine elements, three apply to dignity and truth-telling as follows:
  - A physician shall be dedicated to providing competent medical care, with compassion and respect for human dignity and rights.
  - A physician shall uphold the standards of professionalism, be honest in all professional interactions, and strive to report physicians deficient in character or competence, or engaging in fraud or deception, to appropriate entities.
  - A physician shall, while caring for a patient, regard responsibility to the patient as paramount.
- The American Nursing Association (ANA) published in 2012, Nursing Care and Do Not Resuscitate (DNR) and Allow Natural Death (AND) Decisions, which included the following:
  - Nursing care is directed toward meeting the comprehensive needs of patients and their families across the continuum of care. This is particularly vital in the care of patients and families at the end of life to prevent and relieve the cascade of symptoms and suffering that are commonly associated with dying. Nurses are leaders and vigilant advocates for the delivery of dignified and humane care. Nurses actively participate in assessing and assuring the responsible and appropriate use of interventions in order to minimize unwarranted or unwanted treatment and patient suffering.

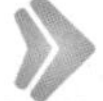

Carp's Cues

Please refer to the ANA website for access to all of the ANA position statements. The nurse's roles in ethics and human rights: protecting and promoting individual worth, dignity, and human rights in practice settings, nursing care and do not resuscitate (DNR) and allow natural death (and) decisions.

- In the United States, fewer than one in five deaths involve hospitalization with the use of the intensive care unit (*Angus et al., 2004). Twenty percent of all hospital deaths occur in intensive care units (*Halcomb, Daly, Jackson, & Davidson, 2004). The distinction between critical illness and terminal illness is not clear (*Elpern, Covert, & Kleinpell, 2005). Dying while receiving aggressive interventions to extend life produces confusion, conflicts, and distress in caregivers, clients, and families (*Elpern et al., 2005; *Zomorodi & Lynn, 2010).
- Elpern et al. (*2005), using the moral distress scale, reported the following factors with the highest levels of moral distress to be related to the following:
  - Continue to participate in care for the terminally ill client who is being sustained on a ventilator when no one will make a decision to "pull the plug."
  - Follow a family's wishes to continue life support, even though it is not the best interest of the client.
  - Initiate extensive life-saving actions when I think it only prolongs death.
  - Follow the family's wishes for the client's care when I do not agree with them but do so because the hospital administration fears a lawsuit.
  - Carry out the physician's orders for unnecessary tests and treatments for terminally ill clients.
  - Provide care that does not relieve the client's suffering because the physician fears increasing doses of pain medication will cause death.
- Zuzelo (*2007) used Corley's moral distress scale with a Likert scale of 0 to 6 (0 = no moral distress; 6 = extreme moral distress). The most distressing events were given below:
  - Working with unsafe nurses
  - Working with physicians (nurse practitioners [NPs], physician assistants [PA]) not competent in providing the care a client needs
  - Ineffective prescribed pain medication regimens
  - Family wishes to continue life support measures when it is not in the best interest of the client.
  - Implement a physician's (NP's, PA's) order for unnecessary tests or treatments.
  - When clients were used by students, interns, residents to practice a painful procedure

Focus Assessment Criteria

A focus assessment is not needed for this nursing diagnosis. Any client or group who is in any health-care facility—for example, hospitals, ambulatory settings, private office, and long-term facility or certain facilities such as residential homes, group homes, jails, and prisons—is at risk for compromised human dignity. *Risk for Compromised Human Dignity* is related to multiple negative factors associated with the procedures and environment of a health-care facility.

Goals

NOC
Abuse Protection, Comfort Level, Dignified Dying, Information Processing, Knowledge: Illness Care, Self-Esteem, Spiritual Well-Being

The individual/family will report respectful and considerate care as evidenced by the following indicators:

- Respect for privacy
- Consideration of emotions
- Anticipation of feelings
- Given options and control
- Asked for permission
- Given accurate explanations
- Minimization of body part exposure
- No unnecessary procedure, treatments

Interventions

NIC
Client Satisfaction: Protection of Rights, Client Satisfaction: Caring, Client Satisfaction: Cultural Needs Fulfillment, Client Satisfaction: Physical Care, Client Satisfaction: Psychological Care, Client Satisfaction: Communication, Dignified Life Closure, Comfortable Death, Neglect Recovery. Anticipatory Guidance, Family Support, Mutual Goal Setting, and Teaching: Procedure/Treatment, Touch

Determine and Accept Your Own Moral Responsibility

- Can a nurse maintain and defend the dignity of an individual or a group if she or he cannot maintain and defend her or his own dignity?

R: *Nurses have reported feelings of powerlessness within the work environment because of not addressing unacceptable care conditions and their own moral distress (*Hamric, Borchers, & Epstein, 2012).*

Determine if the Agency Has a Policy for Prevention of Compromised Human Dignity (Note: This Type of Policy or Standard May Be Titled Differently)

R: *Agency policies can assist the nurse when problematic situations occur; however, the moral obligation to protect and defend the dignity of clients or groups does not depend on the existence of a policy.*

Review the Policy (*Walsh & Kowanko, 2002)

- Does it include the following:
  - Protection of privacy and private space
  - Acquiring permission continuously
  - Providing time for decision-making
  - Advocating for the individual

Ensure That There Are Clear Guidelines Regarding the Number of Personnel (e.g., Students, Nurses, Physicians [Residents, Interns]) That Can Be Present When Confidential and/or Stressful Information Is Discussed, or When Procedures That Leave a Client Exposed Need to Be Done

R: *This type of policy can project the philosophy and culture of moral and respectful care of the institution among its personnel. "Practice expecting that honoring and protecting the dignity of individual/groups is not a value but a way of being" (*Söderberg, Lundman, & Norberg, 1999).*

When Appropriate, Request the Client or Family Members to Provide the Following Information

- Person to contact in the event of emergency
- Person whom the client trusts with personal decisions, power of attorney
- Signed living will/desire to sign a living will
- Decision on organ donation

R: *Clients and families should be encouraged to discuss their directions to be used to guide future clinical decisions, and their decisions should be documented. One copy should be given to the person designated as the decision-maker in the event the client becomes incapacitated or incompetent, with another copy retained in a safe deposit box and one copy on the chart.*

When Providing Care

- Provide care to each individual and family as you would expect or demand for your family, partner, child, friend, or colleague.
- Provide opportunities to participate as fully as they can in self-care.

R: *Setting this personal standard can spur you to defend the client/group, especially when they do not belong to the same socioeconomic group as you.*

- Make a priority to provide the individual with choices and control in their care and life in accordance with their ability.

R: *Choice and control are key defining aspects of dignity. Withdrawal of respect inhibits choice and control (European Commission, 2016).*

Reduce Exposure of the Individual's Body with the Use of Drapes and Limit the Gaze of Others Who Are Not Needed

R: *Clients have reported being exposed as their central concern of humiliation, along with high levels of indignity (*Walsh & Kowanko, 2002).*

When Performing a Procedure, Engage in a Conversation, Act as If the Situation Is Matter of Fact for You in Order to Reduce Embarrassment, Use Humor If Appropriate, and Talk to the Client Even If He or She Is Unresponsive

R: *Individuals reported that when in embarrassing situations that were unavoidable (e.g., a bowel or bladder accident), a nurse who was matter of fact made them feel at ease with small talk or humor (*Walsh & Kowanko, 2002).*

Explain the Procedure to the Client during Painful or Embarrassing Procedures and Explain What He or She Will Feel

R: *Clients reported that they did not like being rushed and needed time to understand the upcoming procedure.*

Determine if Unnecessary Personnel Are Present Before a Vulnerable or Stressful Event Is Initiated (e.g., Code or a Painful or Embarrassing Procedure); Advise Them That They Are Not Needed

R: *Protecting the dignity and privacy of individual also includes unconscious or deceased clients (*Mairis, 1994).*

- Allow an opportunity to share his or her feelings after a difficult situation and maintain privacy for the client's information and emotional responses.

R: *Allowing the client to share his or her feelings can help him or her maintain or regain dignity. Recognition of the client as a living, thinking, and experiencing human being enhances dignity (*Walsh & Kowanko, 2002).*

Role-Model and Advocate to Maintain Dignity When Living and After Death

R: *Role-modeling considerate and respectful care can assist others to a heightened awareness and encourage them to perform this care themselves.*

Engage in Dialog With the Individual and Family Regarding Their Understanding of the Individual's Condition, Prognosis, and Present Plan of Care and Decisions That May Need to Be Explained. If Experienced Consult an Experienced Nurse

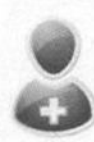

CLINICAL ALERT It is imperative for the individuals and families that they are provided with current, accurate information about the person's condition, prognosis, and treatment options. The expected sequela or the after effects of the disease, condition, or injury should be explained. Treatment options are outlined addressing purpose (cure, palliative hospice), risks, and advantages. If the person is terminally ill what are their end-of-life decisions?

Decisions that protect an individual from unnecessary pain and suffering and protect dignity come from informed individuals and/or families. This information should be provided by the physician, nurse practitioner, or physician assistant, who is primarily responsible for the care. The nurse's responsibility is to assess understanding, to encourage dialogue and questioning, and to ensure truth-telling.

- How do you think you are doing? How do you think he/she is doing?
- What have you been told about your condition? Your _____condition?
- To family, how well do you think your _______will be in 1 month?
- If the person is terminally ill what are his/her end-of-life decisions?
- Does the family agree with the decision?
- Explain the present situation, for example, renal function, metastasis, and congestive heart failure

R: *Providing directions in questions may help to uncover misunderstandings, denial, secrets, and the need for clarifications and/or other interventions.*

Contact the Physician, Nurse Practitioner, or Physician Assistant Who is Primarily Responsible for the Care of the Patient to Clarify Misunderstandings and/or Deliberate Isolation of the Individual From Prognosis Information

Gently Explore the Client/Family End-of-Life Decisions

- Explain the options (e.g., "If you or your loved one dies. . .").
  - Give medications, oxygen
  - Cardio defibrillation (shock)
  - Cardiopulmonary resuscitation
  - Intubation and use of respirator

R: *When someone is dying avoid using terms like, "If you or your loved one stops breathing or their heart stops…" This may imply to the individual or family that the event is unexpected and therefore CPR should be initiated. Successful resuscitation will be painful and temporary, and thus, the person will die again.*

- Advise the individual/family that they can choose all, some, or none of the above. The family, however, needs to support the individual's decisions.
- If family members disagree, the individual can be advised to name the family member that supports their decisions as their legal delegate/power of attorney.
- Differentiate between prolonging life versus prolonging dying.
- Document the discussion and decisions according to institute on policy.

R: *Direct but gentle inquiries and discussions can assist the individual//family to examine the situation clearly and the implications of treatment options and decisions.*

If Indicated, Explain "No Code" Status and Explain the Focus of Palliative Care That Replaces Aggressive and Futile Care (e.g., Pain Management, Symptom Management, Less or No Intrusive/Painful Procedures)

R: *Often, families think that "no code" status means no care. Palliative care focuses on comfort during the dying process.*

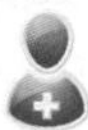

Clinical Alert The choices and values of the competent patient should always be given highest priority, even when these wishes conflict with those of the health-care team and family. An exception to this is when one or more physicians determine that CPR attempts would be medically ineffective or if the decision of the patient/surrogate is in conflict with the informed opinion of the agency/provider as to what constitutes beneficent care of the patient. In this situation, requests from a patient or surrogate will not be honored (ANA, 2012; *Ditillo, 2002).

Seek to Transfer the Individual from Intensive Care Unit, If Possible

R: *Intensive care unit (ICU) environments have many barriers to a palliative care environment (e.g., noise, frequent interruptions, close quarters).*

When Extreme Measures That Are Futile Are Planned or Are Being Provided for a Client, Discuss the Situation with the Physician/NP/PA

- "Use the chain of command to share and discuss issues that have escalated beyond the problem-solving ability and/or scope of those immediately involved" (LaSala & Bjarnason, 2010, p. 6).
- The urgency of the situation requires immediate attention.

SBAR

Situation: (To physician/NP) I have just assessed Mr. Black. Pulse ox is 90, with labored breathing.

Background: As you know, he is end-stage congestive heart failure. He is lethargic and not eating or drinking. The family are questioning if he should have a feeding tube.

Assessment: I cared for him yesterday. His condition is deteriorating.

Recommendation: I would like a consult for the palliative care specialist to speak to the family regarding his changing condition and comfort measures that can be implemented to prevent prolonging his suffering with enteral nutritional therapy.

R: *Protecting dignity is the acknowledgment of humanity in people, alive or dead, rather than treating them as inanimate objects (*Haddock, 1996). When people are helpless or unconscious, preserving their dignity is of the utmost priority (*Mairis, 1994).*

- "Extreme measures, when futile, are an infringement of the basic respect for the dignity innate in being a person" (*Walsh & Kowanko, 2002, p. 146).

When There is Disagreement on the Care Proposed or Is Being Provided, Consider the Following

- A multidisciplinary care conferences
- Consulting with a respected nurse
- Contact the ethics expert in the institution'

R: *"The purpose is to add clarity from other viewpoints. However, these committees may deal with the ethical issue, but not address the moral distress associated with it,"* says Hamric.

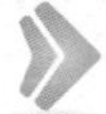

Carp's Cues

Some disturbing clinical situations are ethical dilemmas, in that both sides are sincere in their beliefs but disagree.

Discuss With Involved Personnel an Incident That Was Disrespectful to an Individual Client or Family and Report Any Incident That May Be a Violation of a Client's Dignity to the Appropriate Person

R: *Professionals have a responsibility to practice ethically and morally and to address situations and personnel that compromise human dignity.*

Discuss With Involved Personnel Any Incident That Was Disrespectful to the Client or His or Her Family

- Professionals have a responsibility to practice ethical and moral care and to address situations and personnel that compromise human dignity.
- A zero tolerance for abuse or neglect should be the institution's model.
- Report repetitive incidents or any egregious incident that is a violation of client's dignity to the appropriate personnel.

STAR

Stop	Did you witness or have reported to you an unsatisfactory treatment of client and/or family?
Think	Can I discuss this with the involved personnel or is it serious enough to report it to nurse manager?
Act	If desired, discuss the situation with a trusted colleague. Report the incident to nurse manager. Complete an incident report. Do not document the incident in the client's record, unless instructed to by manager.
Review	Are you satisfied with the actions taken in response to your report? If not, discuss your options with a trusted colleague.

If You Decide to Speak to the Involved Coworker, Use SBAR

SBAR

Situation: I overheard you talking to Mr. White's family. You told them to "stop ringing the call bell" and that they were being too demanding.

Background: Mr. White is critically ill with a poor prognosis.

Assessment: Do you know how much his family knows about his condition? Do they understand the concept of palliative care?

Recommendation: I would suggest you assess for their understanding of the situation. Ask them "How do you think your father is doing?" Engage in dialogue with individual and family regarding their thoughts on the present plan of care and decisions that may need explanation. If more information is needed, contact the appropriate person (e.g., physician/NP, nurse manager).

If You Are Dissatisfied With the Response of the Nurse to Your Discussion, Discuss this With the Nurse Manager

- Practice expecting that honoring and protecting the dignity of a client/group is not a value, but a way of being.

DISORGANIZED INFANT BEHAVIOR

Disorganized Infant Behavior

Risk for Disorganized Infant Behavior

NANDA-I Definition

Disintegrated physiologic and neurobehavioral responses of infant to the environment

Defining Characteristics (Hockenberry & Wilson, 2015; *Vandenberg, 1990)

Autonomic System

Cardiac
Arrhythmia
Decreased heart rate (bradycardia)
Increased heart rate (tachycardia)

Respiration
Pauses (apnea)
Decreased respirations (tachypnea)
Gasping

Skin Color Changes*
Paling around nostrils
Perioral duskiness
Mottling
Cyanosis
Grayness
Flushing/ruddiness

Visceral
Hiccuping*
Straining as if producing a bowel movement
Spitting up
Gagging
Grunting

Motor
Seizures
Sneezing*
Tremors/startles*
Yawning
Twitches*
Sighing*
Coughing*

Motor System

Fluctuating Tone

Flaccidity of the following:

Trunk
Face
Extremities

Hypertonicity
Extending legs
Arching
Saluting
Splaying fingers*
Airplaning
Extending tongue
Sitting on air
Fisting*

Hyperflexions
Trunk

Fetal tuck
Extremities

Frantic Diffuse Activity

Uncoordinated Movements

State System (Range)

Difficulty maintaining state control
Difficulty in transitions from one state to another

Sleep

Twitches*	Grimaces	Fusses in sleep
Whimpers	Makes jerky movements	Has irregular respirations
Makes sounds		

Awake

Eyes floating	Weak cry	Staring*
Panicky, worried*, dull look	Strain, fussiness	Abrupt state changes
Glassy eyes	Irritability*	Gaze aversion*

Attention–Interaction System

Impaired response to sensory stimuli (Herdman & Kamitsuru, 2015)
Difficulty consoling

Related Factors (Askin & Wilson, 2007)

Pathophysiologic

Related to immature or altered central nervous system (CNS) secondary to:

Prematurity*	Infection	Prenatal exposure to drugs/alcohol
Perinatal factors	Intraventricular hemorrhage	Decreased oxygen saturation
Hyperbilirubinemia	Congenital anomalies	Respiratory distress
Hypoglycemia		

Related to nutritional deficits secondary to:

Reflux	Swallowing problems	Colic
Feeding intolerance*	Emesis	Poor suck/swallow coordination

Related to excess stimulation secondary to:

Oral hypersensitivity
Frequent handling and position changes

Treatment Related

Related to excess stimulation secondary to:

Invasive procedures*	Medication administration	Chest physical therapy
Movement	Restraints	Feeding
Lights	Noise (e.g., prolonged alarm, voices, environment)	Tubes, tape

Related to inability to see caregivers secondary to eye patches

Situational (Personal, Environmental)

Related to unpredictable interactions secondary to multiple caregivers

Related to imbalance of task touch and consoling touch

Related to decreased ability to self-regulate secondary to (Holditch-Davis & Blackburn, 2007):

Sudden movement
Noise
Prematurity*
Disrupted sleep–wake cycles
Fatigue
Stimulation that exceeds the infant's tolerance threshold
Environmental demands

Author's Note

Disorganized Infant Behavior describes an infant who has difficulty regulating and adapting to external stimuli due to immature neurobehavioral development and increased environmental stimuli associated with neonatal units. When an infant is overstimulated or stressed, he or she uses energy to adapt; this depletes the supply of energy available for physiologic growth. The goal of nursing care is to assist the infant to conserve energy by reducing environmental stimuli, allowing the infant sufficient time to adapt to handling, and providing sensory input appropriate to the infant's physiologic and neurobehavioral status.

Key Concepts

- Als (*1986) explained that an infant's primary route of communication of competency and efforts at self-regulation is through behavioral indices.
- Infant behavior is a continual interaction with the environment by means of five subsystems (Blackburn, 2007; Kenner & McGrath, 2010; *Merenstein & Gardner, 2002; *Yecco, 1993):
  - *Autonomic/physiologic*: regulation of respiration, color, and visceral functions (e.g., gastrointestinal, swallowing)
  - *Motor*: regulation of tone, posture, activity level, and specific movement patterns of the extremities, head, trunk, and face
  - *State/organizational*: the range, transition between, and quality of states of consciousness (e.g., sleep to arousal, awake to alert, crying)
  - *Attention–interactive*: ability to orient and to focus on sensory stimuli (e.g., faces, sounds, objects) and to take in cognitive, social, and emotional information
  - *Self-regulatory*: maintenance of the integrity and balance of the other subsystems, smooth transitions between states, and relaxation among subsystems
- In full-term infants, these systems function smoothly and are synchronized and regulated with ease (Blackburn, 2007).
- Premature infants have immature subsystems, so with this "maturation process" they may have a temporary vulnerability to being physiologically instable (*Merenstein & Gardner, 2002).
- Premature infants must adapt to the extrauterine environment with underdeveloped body systems, usually in a neonatal intensive care unit (NICU) (Kenner & McGrath, 2010; *Merenstein & Gardner, 2002).
- Although mortality and morbidity rates have been reduced greatly in high-risk infants, these infants experience various neurobehavioral problems. These problems have been labeled as *the new morbidities of low-birth-weight infants* and include hyperexcitability, language problems, attention-deficit disorders, higher-order cognitive problems, and schooling problems (Blackburn, 2007).
- The six stages of CNS development are dorsal induction, ventral induction, proliferation and neurogenesis, neuron migration, organization, and myelinization. The first three occur completely before the fourth month of gestation. The last three stages continue until development is complete. The *migration stage* involves the movement of millions of cells from their point of origin in the periventricular region to their terminal location within the cerebral cortex and cerebellum. The *organization stage* peaks from 6 months gestation and can extend several years after birth (Blackburn, 2007). The *myelinization stage* peaks from 8 months gestation to 1 year after birth. Myelinization insulates individual nerve fibers to facilitate specificity of connections, increases the number of alternative pathways, and increases the speed of transmission (Blackburn & Ditzenberger, 2007).
- Neurologic dysfunctions resulting from neurologic underdevelopment (e.g., weak transmission, slow nerve conduction, decreased inhibitory potential; *Blackburn, 1993; Kenner & McGrath, 2010):
  - For too long, researchers believed that newborns could not perceive, respond to, or remember pain. Findings have validated, however, that newborns do feel and express pain much like adults. Williamson and Williamson (*1983) found that infants who received local anesthesia for circumcision cried less and had less variation in heart rate and higher oxygen saturation compared with infants who did not have a local anesthetic.

- Loudness of sound is measured in decibels (db). Adult speech is recorded at about 45 to 50 db. Sound levels in infant incubators have been reported to be 50 to 80 db. Hearing loss in adults has been associated with levels above 80 to 85 db (*Blackburn, 1993, Kenner & McGrath, 2010)
- A noise level >45 dB in the NICU is of concern. NICU personnel should develop ways to reduce noise (*American Academy of Pediatrics [AAP], 1997).
- Incidence of sensorineural hearing impairment is 4% in low-birth-weight infants and 13% in very-low-birth-weight infants (*Thomas, 1989).
- Padron et al. (2014) reported that "disorganized infants who do not display direct fear in the presence of the caregiver may have started out with compromised emotional regulation abilities at birth."

Focus Assessment Criteria

Experts recommend three assessment tools for neurobehavioral function: (1) the Brazelton Neonatal Behavioral Assessment Scale (NBAS) for healthy, full-term newborns; (2) Assessment of Preterm Infant Behavior (APIB) for preterm newborns; and (3) Newborn Individualized Developmental Care and Assessment Program (NIDCAP). All tools require training to use.

Objective Data

Assess for Defining Characteristics

Autonomic System
Note: See Defining Characteristics for all listed.
Respirations
Color changes
Visceral
Motor

Motor System (Fluctuating Tone)
Flaccid trunk, extremities, face
Hypertonic
Hyperflexions
Frantic, diffuse activity

State System (Range)
Sleep (see Defining Characteristics)
Awake

Attention–Interaction System
Imbalance of withdrawal versus engaging behaviors (see Defining Characteristics)

Goals

NOC

Newborn Adaptation, Neurologic Status, Preterm Infant Organization, Sleep, Comfort Level, Parent–Infant Attachment

The infant will demonstrate increased signs of stability as evidenced by the following indicators:

- Exhibits smooth, stable respirations; pink, stable color; consistent tone; improve posture; calm, focused alertness; well-modulated sleep; responsive to visual and social stimuli
- Demonstrates self-regulatory skills as sucking, hand to mouth, grasping, hand holding, hand and foot clasping, tucking

The parent(s)/caregiver(s) will describe techniques to reduce environmental stress in agency, at home, or both.

- Describe situations that stress the infant.
- Describe signs/symptoms of stress in the infant.
- Describe ways to support infant's efforts to self-calm (Vandenberg, 2007).

Interventions

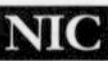

Environmental Management: Comfort Neurologic Monitoring, Sleep Enhancement, Newborn Care, Parent Education: Newborn Positioning, Pain Management

- See Related Factors.

Reduce or Eliminate Contributing Factors, If Possible

Pain

- Observe for responses that are different from baseline and have been associated with neonatal pain responses (*Bozzette, 1993; Kenner & McGrath, 2010):
  - Facial responses (open mouth, brow bulge, grimace, chin quiver, nasolabial furrow, taut tongue)
  - Motor responses (flinch, muscle rigidity, clenched hands, withdrawal) (*AAP, 2006)
  - Pain management requires routine assessment using a reliable pain-assessment tool which measures both physiologic and behavioral indicators of pain.
  - Develop strategies to minimize the number and frequency of painful or stressful procedures in the NICU.
  - Provide pharmacologic and/or nonpharmacologic pain relief for all painful procedures, such as gavage tube placement, tape removal, needle insertions, heel sticks, insertion and removal of chest tubes, intubation, prolonged mechanical ventilation, eye exams, circumcision, and surgery.
- Pharmacologic implications:
  - Doses of effective medications to reduce pain may be close to doses that cause toxicity in the neonate.
  - Early administration of pain medication may reduce the effective dose needed and thereby reduce toxicity.
  - Treatment of pain must be guided by ongoing pain assessments.
  - Pain relief for circumcisions should be provided.
  - Topical anesthetics can reduce pain for some procedures such as venipuncture, lumbar puncture, and IV insertion. Due to a risk of methemoglobinemia, in certain situations, use should be on intact skin only, no more than once a day, and not with other drugs known to cause methemoglobinemia.
- Nonpharmacologic interventions:
  - Developmental care that includes attention to behavioral cues and reducing environmental stimuli, has shown to be effective in reducing pain from minor procedures.
  - Facilitated tuck
  - Swaddling
  - Supportive bedding
  - Side-lying position kangaroo care
  - Nonnutritive suck
  - Oral sucrose solution combined with sucking has proved to be an effective distraction from pain.

R: *Repeated painful experiences can cause permanent behavioral abnormalities and altered pain sensitivity. There is concern that repeated pain in vulnerable infants may result in emotional, behavioral, and learning disabilities.*

Disrupted 24-Hour Diurnal Cycles

- Evaluate the need for and frequency of each intervention.
- Consider 24-hour caregiving assignment and primary caregiving to provide consistent caregiving throughout the day and night for the infant from the onset of admission. This is important in terms of responding to increasingly more mature sleep cycles, feeding ability, and especially emotional development.
- Consider supporting the infant's transition to and maintenance of sleep by avoiding peaks of frenzy and overexhaustion; continuously maintaining a calm, regular environment and schedule; and establishing a reliable, repeatable pattern of gradual transition into sleep in prone and side-lying positions in the isolette or crib.

R: *Intervention to facilitate motor–sleep–wake organization improves behavioral organization.*

Problematic Feeding Experiences

- Observe and record infant's readiness cues for participating with feedings (Kenner & McGrath, 2010).

Hunger Cues

- Transitioning to drowsy or alert state
- Mouthing, rooting, or sucking
- Bringing hands to mouth
- Crying that is not relieved with pacifier or nonnutritive sucking alone

Physiologic Stability

- Look for regulated breathing patterns, stable color, and stable digestion.
- Promote nurturing environment in support of a coregulatory feeding experience.

- Decrease environmental stimulation.
- Provide comfortable seating (be especially sensitive to the needs of postpartum mothers: e.g., soft cushions, small stool to elevate legs, supportive pillows for nursing).
- Encourage softly swaddling the infant to facilitate flexion and balanced tone during feeding.
- Explore feeding methods that meet the goals of both infant and family (e.g., breastfeeding, bottle-feeding, gavage).

R: *Preterm infants may have difficulty or demonstrate disorganization in the progression of their feeding behaviors (e.g., readiness, availability of hunger cues) and gastrointestinal motility (e.g., esophageal motility, intestinal motility, gastric emptying time (Kenner & McGrath, 2010).*

R: *Individualized developmental care can cause an earlier transition to full oral feedings (*Als et al., 2003).*

Support the Infant's Self-Regulatory Efforts

- When administering painful or stressful procedures, consider actions to enhance calmness.
- Support the flexed position with another caregiver.
- Provide opportunities to feed while shielding the infant from other stresses.
- Consider the efficient execution of necessary manipulations while supporting the infant's behavioral organization.
- Consider *unhurried* reorganization and stabilization of the infant's regulation (e.g., position prone, give opportunities to hold onto caregiver's finger and suck, encase trunk and back of head in caregiver's hand, provide inhibition to soles of feet).
- Consider removing extraneous stimulation (e.g., stroking, talking, shifting position) to institute restabilization. Consider spending 15 to 20 minutes after manipulation; over time, the infant's self-regulatory abilities will improve, making the caregiver's intervention less important.
- Consider supporting the infant's transition to and maintenance of sleep by avoiding peaks of frenzy and overexhaustion; by continuously maintaining a calm, regular environment and schedule; and by establishing a reliable, repeatable pattern of gradual transition into sleep in prone and side-lying positions in the isolette or crib.
- Consider initiating calming on the caregiver's body and then transferring the baby to the crib as necessary. For other infants, this may be too arousing, and transition is accomplished more easily in the isolette with the provision of steady boundaries and encasing without any stimulation.
- A nonstimulating sleep space with minimal exciting visual targets, social inputs, and so forth, may need to be made available to facilitate relaxation before sleep. A regular sleep routine helps many infants.

R: *When a premature newborn is ill, the combination of an immature CNS, exposure to inappropriate and unexpected patterned sensory input, and multiple caregivers leads to disorganization and imbalance of the behavioral indices to regulation.*

R: *Individualized interventions are implemented to increase organized behavior.*

Reduce Environmental Stimuli (Kenner & McGrath, 2010; *Merenstein & Gardner, 1998; *Thomas, 1989)

Noise

- Do not tap on incubator.
- Place a folded blanket on top of the incubator if it is the only work surface available.
- Slowly open and close porthole.
- Pad incubator doors to reduce banging.
- Use plastic instead of metal waste cans.
- Remove water from ventilator tubing.
- Speak softly at the bedside and only when necessary.
- Slowly drop the head of the mattress.
- Eliminate radios.
- Close doors slowly.
- Position the infant's bed away from sources of noise (e.g., telephone, intercom, unit equipment).
- Consider the following methods to reduce unnecessary noise in the NICU:
  - Perform rounds away from the bedsides.
  - Adapt large equipment to eliminate noise and clutter.
  - Alert staff when the decibel level in the unit exceeds 60 db (e.g., by a light attached to a sound meter). Institute quiet time for 10 min to lower noise.
  - Move more vulnerable infants out of unit traffic patterns.

R: *Noise levels in NICUs are hazardous because of potential damage to the cochlea with subsequent hearing loss and because of arousal effects on infants who cannot inhibit their responses. Noise interferes with sleep, increases heart rate, and leads to vasoconstriction (*Blackburn, 1993). The infant expends energy he or she needs to grow and to supply the brain with glucose and oxygen (*Thomas, 1989).*

R: *Thomas (*1989) found that NICUs have a loud, continuous pattern of background noise. In addition, peak noises over the continuous noise level can raise the decibel level 10-fold. Examples of peak noises are monitor alarms (67 db), NICU radios (62 db), opening of plastic sleeves (67 db), tappings of hoods (70 db), and sinks (66 db).*

Lights

- Use full-spectrum instead of white light at bedside. Avoid fluorescent lights.
- Cover cribs, incubators, and radiant warmers completely during sleep and partially during awake periods.
- Install dimmer switches, shades, and curtains. Avoid bright lights.
- Shade infants' eyes with a blanket tent.
- Avoid visual stimuli on cribs.
- Shield eyes from bright procedure lights. Avoid patches unless for phototherapy.

R: *When a premature newborn is ill, the combination of an immature CNS, exposure to inappropriate and unexpected patterned sensory input, and multiple caregivers leads to disorganization and imbalance of the behavioral indices to regulation.*

Position Infant in Postures That Permit Flexion and Minimize Flailing

- Consider gentle, *unhurried* reorganization and stabilization of infant's regulation by supporting the infant in softly tucked prone position, giving opportunities to hold onto caregiver's finger and suck, encasing trunk and back of head in caregiver's hand, and providing inhibition to soles of feet.
- To minimize infant flailing consider using boundaries (e.g. blanket rolls, snuggly).
- Use the prone/side-lying position.
- Swaddle baby, if possible, to maintain flexion.
- Create a nest using soft bedding (e.g., natural sheepskin, soft cotton, flannel).
- Avoid oversized diapers to allow you to perceive normal hip alignment.
- Avoid tension on lines or tubing.

R: *Developmentally correct handling and positioning can decrease stress, conserve energy, and enhance normal development (*Aita & Snider, 2003).*

Reduce the Stress Associated With Handling

- When moving or lifting the infant, contain him or her with your hands by swaddling or placing rolled blankets around the body.
- Maintain containment during procedures and caregiving activities.
- Handle slowly and gently. Avoid stroking.
- Initiate all interactions and treatments with one sense stimulus at a time (e.g., touch), then slowly progress to visual, auditory, and movement.
- Assess child for cues for readiness, impending disorganization, or stability; respond to cues.
- Support minimal disruption of the infant's own evolving 24-hour sleep–wake cycles.
- Use PRN instead of routine suctioning or postural drainage.
- Use minimal adhesive tape. Remove any carefully.

R: *Stress reduction will conserve energy, promote comfort, and enhance adaptation.*

R: *Stroking preterm infants who are unstable results in decreased levels of oxygen saturation (*Harrison et al., 1996).*

Reduce Disorganized Behavior during Active Interventions and Transport

- Have a plan for transport, with assigned roles for each team member.
- Establish behavior cues of stress on this infant with the primary nurse before transport.
- Minimize sensory input:
  - Use calm, quiet voices.
  - Shade the infant's eyes from light.
  - Protect infant from unnecessary touch.
- Support the infant's softly tucked postures with your hands and offer something to grasp (your finger or corner of a soft blanket or cloth).
- Swaddle the infant or place him or her in a nest made of blankets.

- Ensure that the transport equipment (e.g., ventilator) is ready. Warm mattress or use sheepskin.
- Carefully and smoothly move the infant. Avoid talking, if possible.
- Consider conducting caregiving routines while parent(s) or designated caregiver holds the infant, whenever possible.
- Reposition in 2 to 3 hours or sooner if infant behavior suggests discomfort.

R: *Interventions seek to reduce stimuli to prevent a disorganized response.*

Engage Parents in Planning Care

- Encourage them to share their feelings, fears, and expectations.
- Consider involving parents in creating the family's developmental plan:
  - My strengths are:
  - Time-out signals:
  - These things stress me:
  - How you can help me:
- Teach caregivers to continually observe the changing capabilities to determine the appropriate positioning and bedding options, for example, infant may fight containment (Hockenberry & Wilson, 2015).

R: *Anticipatory guidance and support can prevent overstimulation of their infant.*

Risk for Disorganized Infant Behavior

NANDA-I Definition

At risk for alteration in integrating and modulation of the physiological and behavioral systems of functioning (i.e., autonomic, motor, state-organization, self-regulatory, and attentional-interactional systems)

Risk Factors

Refer to Related Factors.

Related Factors

Refer to *Disorganized Infant Behavior.*

Focus Assessment Criteria

Refer to *Disorganized Infant Behavior.*

Interventions

Refer to *Disorganized Infant Behavior.*

RISK FOR INFECTION

NANDA-I Definition

Vulnerable to invasion and multiplication of pathogenic organisms, which may compromise health

Risk Factors

See Related Factors.

Related Factors

Various health problems and situations can create favorable conditions that would encourage the development of infections (see Key Concepts). Some common factors follow.

Pathophysiologic

Related to compromised host defenses secondary to:

Cancer
Altered or insufficient leukocytes
Arthritis
Respiratory disorders
Periodontal disease
Renal failure
Hematologic disorders
Hepatic disorders
Diabetes mellitus*
AIDS
Alcoholism
Immunosuppression*
Immunodeficiency secondary to (specify)

Related to compromised circulation secondary to:

Lymphedema
Obesity*
Peripheral vascular disease

Treatment Related

Related to a site for organism invasion secondary to:

Surgery
Invasive lines
Dialysis
Intubation
Total parenteral nutrition
Enteral feedings

Related to compromised host defenses secondary to:

Radiation therapy
Organ transplant
Medication therapy (specify; e.g., chemotherapy, immunosuppressants)

Situational (Personal, Environmental)

Related to widespread disease outbreak

Related to insufficient information on preventive measures

Related to compromised host defenses secondary to:

History of infections
Malnutrition*
Prolonged immobility
Stress
Increased hospital stay
Smoking

Related to a site for organism invasion secondary to:

Trauma (accidental, intentional)
Postpartum period
Bites (animal, insect, human)
Thermal injuries
Warm, moist, dark environment (skin folds, casts)

Related to contact with contagious agents (nosocomial or community acquired)

Maturational

Newborns

Related to increased vulnerability of infant secondary to:

HIV-positive mother
Lack of maternal antibodies (dependent on maternal exposures)
Lack of normal flora
Maternal substance addiction
Open wounds (umbilical, circumcision)
Immature immune system

Infant/Child/Adolescent

Related to increased vulnerability secondary to:

Lack of immunization
Multiple sex partners

Older Adult

Related to increased vulnerability secondary to:

Diminished immune response
Debilitated condition
Chronic diseases

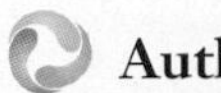

Author's Note

All people are at risk for infection and the risk is increased when in a health-care facility. Thus *Risk for Infection* represents the activation of a standard of care to prevent infection (e.g., hand washing, catheter-care protocols).

Secretion control, environmental control, and hand washing before and after contact can reduce the risk of transmission of organisms. Included in the population of those at risk for infection is a smaller group who are at high risk for infection. High risk for infection describes a person whose host defenses are compromised, thus increasing susceptibility to environmental pathogens or his or her own endogenous flora (e.g., a person with chronic liver dysfunction or with an invasive line). Nursing interventions for such a person focus on minimizing introduction of organisms and increasing resistance to infection (e.g., improving nutritional status). For a person with an infection, the situation is best described by the collaborative problem *Risk for Complications of Sepsis*.

Risk for Infection Transmission describes a person at high risk for transferring an infectious agent to others. Some people are at high risk both for acquiring opportunistic agents and for transmitting infecting organisms, warranting the use of both *Risk for Infection* and *Risk for Infection Transmission*.

Errors in Diagnostic Statements

Risk for Infection related to progression of sepsis secondary to failure to treat infection

Sepsis is a collaborative problem, not a nursing diagnosis. This person is not at risk for infection; rather, he or she requires medical and nursing interventions to treat the sepsis and prevent septic shock.

Risk for Infection related to direct access to bladder mucosa secondary to Foley catheter and lack of staff knowledge of aseptic technique

If the staff's lack of knowledge of aseptic technique is valid, the nurse should proceed with reporting the situation to nursing management in an incident report. Adding this to a nursing diagnosis statement would be legally and professionally inadvisable. Nurses should never use nursing diagnostic statements to criticize an individual, group, or member of the health team or to expose unsafe or unprofessional practices or behavior. Nurses must use other organizational channels of communication for these purposes.

Key Concepts

General Considerations

- The current report is based on 2014 data. On the national level, the report found increases and decreases as (Centers for Disease Control and Prevention [CDC], 2016; Magill et al., 2014):
  - A 46% decrease (NJ < 39%, PA < 51%) in central line–associated bloodstream infection (CLABSI) between 2008 and 2014
  - A 19% decrease (NJ < 17%, PA < 7%) in surgical site infections (SSIs) (hysterectomy) related to the 10 select procedures tracked in the report between 2008 and 2014
  - A 6% increase (NJ > 2%, PA > 2%) in catheter-associated urinary tract infections (CAUTI) between 2009 and 2013, although initial data from 2014 seem to indicate that these infections have started to decrease
  - An 8% decrease (NJ > 14%, PA > 8%) in hospital-onset methicillin-resistant *Staphylococcus aureus* (MRSA) bacteremia between 2011 and 2014
  - A 10% increase (NJ > 2%, PA > 8%) in hospital-onset *Clostridium difficile* infections between 2011 and 2014

Carp's Cues

There is significant variation from state to state on the status of the incidence of infections as listed earlier. (This author has inserted the preceding finding from New Jersey where she lives and Pennsylvania where she practices.) The reader is encouraged to refer to this website to access the data from their state.

The common pathogens, which are the specific causative agents of diseases, are (Grossman & Porth, 2014) as follows:

- Viruses
- Bacteria
- Fungi
- Protozoa
- Worms

Pathogens enter the body by (Grossman & Porth, 2014)

- Penetration of the skin/mucous membranes (e.g., abrasion, burn, surgery)
- Direct contact with mucous membranes/tissue—sexually transmitted infections, newborn exposure during birth through placenta (e.g., Herpes [HSV])
- Ingestion—parasites, food poisoning (e.g., hepatitis A)
- Inhalation—measles, meningitis, tuberculosis, pneumonia

Wounds/Surgical Wounds (2015d)

- Skin provides a first line of defense; the opening of the skin, either surgically or traumatically, potentiates infection.
- The type of procedure is also associated with different rates of SSIs (Owens et al. 2014, cited in Anderson & Sexton, 2015).
- The highest rates occur after abdominal surgery: small bowel surgery (5.3% to 10.6%), colon surgery (4.3% to 10.5%), gastric surgery (2.8% to 12.3%), liver/pancreas surgery (2.8% to 10.2%), exploratory laparotomy (1.9% to 6.9%), and appendectomy (1.3% to 3.1%).
- High-volume surgeries are associated with higher rates of SSI, and therefore, more common infections include coronary bypass surgery (3.3% to 3.7%), cesarean section (3.4% to 4.4%), vascular surgery (1.3% to 5.2%), joint prosthesis (0.7% to 1.7%), and spinal fusion (1.3% to 3.1%).
- Eye surgery is associated with an extremely low rate of SSI (0.14%).
- The rate of SSI following ambulatory surgery is relatively low (3 per 1,000 procedures at 14 days and 4.8 per 1,000 procedures at 30 days).
- The process of wound healing begins with a clot formed 1 to 6 hours after surgery or injury. Epithelialization is the basal cell proliferation and epithelial migration occurring inside a clot, beginning to form a scab in 48 hours and complete in 3 to 5 days. The superficial layer of epithelium creates a barrier to bacteria and other foreign bodies. This barrier is very thin, easily traumatized, and has little strength (Armstrong & Mayr, 2014).
- A wound essentially closes within 24 hours, eliminating the risk of direct inoculations of organisms.
- Wound infections rely on the capabilities of other host defenses to assist in healing.
- Risk factors associated with wound infections depend on (1) endogenous factors such as the presence of confounding factors, skin preparation, and the use of prophylactic antibiotics and (2) exogenous factors such as the preoperative scrub, barrier techniques, airborne contamination, environmental disinfection, wound care, and the condition of the wound at the time of closure.
- Wounds are at risk for infection due to the following factors:
  - Sutures and staples, unlike tape, create their own wounds, act like drains, and cause their own inflammatory response.
  - Drains provide a site for microorganism entry.
  - The incidence of infection in individuals who are not shaved or clipped is 0.9%. It increases to 1.4% with electric shaving, 1.7% with clipping, and 2.5% with razor shaving (*Kovach, 1990).
  - If it is necessary to remove hair prior to surgery, research has reported that both clipping and depilatory cream result in fewer SSIs than shaving with a razor (Grade A).
  - If removing hair is with a clipper, it is suggested that this is carried out on the day of surgery (The Joanna Briggs Institute, 2007; Tanner, Norrie, & Melen, 2011).

Sexually Transmitted Disease/Infections

- Since 2012, gonorrhea rates of infection have decreased 0.6%, chlamydia rates of infection have decreased 1.5%, congenital syphilis increased by 4%, and syphilis has increased by 10%. "This national rate increase was only among men, particularly gay and bisexual men" (CDC, 2015b).
- "While surveillance data show signs of potential progress in reducing chlamydia and gonorrhea among young people aged 15 to 24, both the numbers and rates of reported cases of these two diseases continue to be highest in this group compared to other age groups" (CDC, 2015a, 2015e).

- Both young men and young women are heavily affected by sexually transmitted diseases (STDs)—but for young women these infections can cause serious infections of the uterus (pelvic inflammatory disease) and infertility (CDC, 2015e).
- The Youth Risk Behavior Surveillance System reported risky sexual behavior among teenagers contributing to the high rates of sexually transmitted infections and pregnancy (CDC, 2015e).
  - 46.8% of students had ever had sexual intercourse.
  - 5.6% of students had sexual intercourse for the first time before age 13.
  - 34.0% of currently sexually active student nationwide, 59.1% reported that either they or their partner had used a condom during last sexual intercourse.
  - 34.0% of currently sexually active students nationwide, 19.0% reported that either they or their partner had used birth control pills to prevent pregnancy before last sexual intercourse.
  - 34.0% of currently sexually active students nationwide, 25.3% reported that either they or their partner had used birth control pills; an IUD (such as Mirena or ParaGard) or implant (such as Implanon or Nexplanon); or a shot (such as Depo-Provera), patch (such as Ortho Evra), or birth control ring (such as NuvaRing) to prevent pregnancy before last sexual intercourse.
  - 34.0% of currently sexually active students nationwide, 13.7% reported that neither they nor their partner had used any method to prevent pregnancy during last sexual intercourse.
  - 34.0% of currently sexually active students nationwide, 22.4% had drunk alcohol or used drugs before last sexual intercourse.
- The rate of sexually transmitted diseases (STDs) has more than doubled among middle-aged adults and the elderly over the last decade (CDC, 2013b), possibly related to
  - Medication treatments for erectile dysfunction
  - Culture of the "baby boomers" to stay sexually active as they age
  - The low rate of using condoms due to the belief there is no STD risk or risk for pregnancy.

Pediatric Considerations

- Infectious diseases are the leading cause of death in children (Pillitteri, 2014).
- Congenital infections, those acquired in utero, usually result from exposure to such viruses as cytomegalovirus, rubella, hepatitis B, herpes simplex, herpes zoster, varicella, and Epstein-Barr virus. Nonviral agents also may cause some infections, such as toxoplasmosis, syphilis, tuberculosis, trypanosomiasis, HIV, and malaria (Grossman & Porth, 2014).
- "About 62 percent of children in developed countries will have their first episode of OM by the age of one, more than 80 percent by their third birthday, and nearly 100 percent will have at least one episode by age five. In the U.S. alone, this illness accounts for 25 million office visits annually with direct costs for treatment estimated at $3 billion." (American Academy of Otolaryngology, 2014).
- Newborns are at increased risk for infections due to their inability to produce antibodies until age 2. By the time a child is a toddler, production of antibodies is well established. Phagocytosis is much more efficient in toddlers than in infants (Hockenberry and Wilson, 2015).

Geriatric Considerations

- The urinary tract is one of the most common sites of health-care–associated infections, accounting for 20% to 30% of infections reported by long-term care facilities (Center for Disease Control and Prevention, 2016).
- Infection is the primary cause of death in one-third of individuals aged 65 and older and is a contributor to death for many others.
- Infection also has a marked impact on morbidity in older adults, exacerbating underlying illnesses and initiating functional decline (High, 2015), therefore increasing the risk of infection.
- Factors contributing to increased risk for infection in older adults:
  - The supply of cutaneous nerves and blood vessels decreases with age. There is a decrease of 20% of dermis thickening. There is loss of collagen and decreased ability to produce more collagen, which decreases strength and elasticity. These physiologic changes associated with aging contribute to slowed or impaired wound healing in the elderly (Grossman & Porth, 2014).
  - Decreased antibody response to vaccines is caused by reductions in toll-like receptors, senescence of CD8+ T cells, reductions in naïve CD4+ T cells, and changes in B-cell biology.

- Immune function is also compromised by the increasing number of concomitant medical problems that occur with aging. Impaired immunity correlates more with an individual's disease burden than with chronologic age. Older adults who have chronic diseases (e.g., diabetes, chronic obstructive pulmonary disease, or heart failure) are more susceptible to common infections and exhibit poorer vaccine responses than those who do not have underlying health issue (High, 2015).
- Age-related changes in respiratory function do not significantly increase risk for infection. Rather, non–age-related risk factors, such as smoking and exposure to occupational toxins, increase risk.
- Studies have shown 5% to 20% of residents in long-term care facilities to have infections. The most frequent are those of the urinary tract, respiratory system, and skin and soft tissues (usually pressure ulcers; Miller, 2015).
- The increased susceptibility of older adults to infections is multifactorial (either host factors or environmental). Host factors include age-related changes in skin, underlying diseases, invasive treatment modalities, indiscriminate use of antibiotics, malnutrition, dehydration, impaired mobility, and incontinence. Environmental factors in institutions include limited surveillance for infection, crowded areas, cross-contamination, and delay in early detection.
- Skin and urinary tract colonization is a greater problem in older than in younger individuals. Changes in immune competence as decreased function of helper T cells with aging increase susceptibility to fungal, viral, and mycobacterial pathogens (Miller, 2015).
- The point prevalence of asymptomatic bacteriuria in long-term care residents can range from 25% to 50% (CDC, 2013b). Older adults do not exhibit the usual signs of infection (fever, chills, tachypnea, tachycardia, leukocytosis), but, instead, present with anorexia, weakness, change in mental status, normothermia, or hypothermia (Miller, 2015).
- "Fevers >38° C (100.4° F) indicate a potential for serious infection, while hypothermia relative to baseline body temperatures may signify severe infection or even sepsis" (High, 2015).

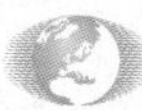

Transcultural Considerations

- The incidence of tuberculosis in American Indians is 7 to 15 times that of non-Indians. African Americans have an incidence three times that of white Americans. Urban American Jews are the most resistant to tuberculosis.
- Susceptibility to disease may also be environmental or a combination of genetic, psychosocial, and environmental factors (Giger, 2013).
- American Indians and Alaskan natives have twice the reported rate of gonorrhea and syphilis than other Americans (Giger, 2013).

Focus Assessment Criteria

Subjective Data

Assess for Signs/Symptoms of Infection

Does the Individual Complain of the Following?

Pain or swelling (generalized, localized)	Chills
Hemoptysis	Loss of appetite
Productive, prolonged cough	Night sweats
Chest pain associated with other criteria	Weight loss
Systemic symptoms	Older adult
Fever, continuous or intermittent	Anorexia, change in mental status
Easy fatigability	Normothermia, or hypothermia weakness

History of Recent Travel

Within United States

Outside United States

History of Exposure to Infectious Diseases

Airborne (most childhood infections result from communicable diseases [e.g., chickenpox, tuberculosis])

Vector-borne and other vector-associated infections (malaria, plague)

Vehicle-borne and other food- and water-borne infections (hepatitis A, salmonellas)

Contact spread (most common type of exposure)

Direct (person-to-person)

Indirect (e.g., by instruments, clothing, and so forth)

Contact droplet (e.g., pneumonias, colds)

Objective Data

Assess for the Following Risk Factors for SSIs

Record the number of risk factors in the ( ) as High Risk for Surgical Site Infection (1 to 10) or add the risk factors, for example, as High Risk for Surgical Site Infection related to obesity, diabetes mellitus, and tobacco use

R: *The Risk of Surgical Site Infection is influenced by the amount and virulence of the microorganism and the ability of the individual to resist it (Pear, 2007).*

Infection colonization of microorganisms (1)
Preexisting remote body site infection (1)
Preoperative contaminated or dirty wound (e.g., post trauma) (1)
Glucocorticoid steroids (2)
Tobacco use (3)
Malnutrition (4)
Obesity (5)
Perioperative hyperglycemia (6)
Diabetes mellitus (7)
Altered immune response (8)
Chronic alcohol use/acute alcohol intoxication (9)

1. Preoperative nares colonization with *Staphylococcus aureus* noted in 30% of most healthy populations, and especially methicillin-resistant *S. aureus* (MRSA) predisposes individuals to have higher risk of SSI (Price et al., 2008). Presence of invasive devices (indwelling catheters tracheostomy, intravenous [IV], drains) can be sources of colonization of microorganisms.
2. Systemic glucocorticoids (GC), which are frequently used as anti-inflammatory agents, are well-known to inhibit wound repair *via* global anti-inflammatory effects and suppression of cellular wound responses, including fibroblast proliferation and collagen synthesis. Systemic steroids cause wounds to heal with incomplete granulation tissue and reduced wound contraction (Franz et al., 2008).
3. "Smoking has a transient effect on the tissue microenvironment and a prolonged effect on inflammatory and reparative cell functions leading to delayed healing and complications". Quit smoking four weeks before surgery restores tissue oxygenation and metabolism rapidly (Sørensen, 2012).
4. Malnourished individuals have been found to have less competent immune response to infection and decreased nutritional stores, which will impair wound healing (Speaar, 2008).
5. An obese individual may experience a compromise in wound healing due to poor blood supply to adipose tissue. In addition, antibiotics are not absorbed well by adipose tissue. Despite excessive food intake, many obese individuals have protein malnutrition, which further impedes the healing (Guo & DiPietro, 2010).
6. There are two primary mechanisms that place individuals experiencing acute perioperative hyperglycemia at increased risk for SSI. The first mechanism is the decreased vascular circulation that occurs, reducing tissue perfusion and impairing cellular-level functions. A clinical study by Akbari, Fazle, & Onji (*1998) noted that when healthy, nondiabetic subjects ingested a glucose load, the endothelial-dependent vasodilatation in both the micro and macro circulations were impaired similar to that seen in diabetic patients. The second affected mechanism is the reduced activity of the cellular immunity functions of chemotaxis, phagocytosis, and killing of polymorphonuclear cells as well as monocytes/macrophages that have been shown to occur in the acute hyperglycemic state.
7. Postsurgical adverse outcomes related to diabetes mellitus are believed to be related to the preexisting complications of chronic hyperglycemia, which include vascular atherosclerotic disease and peripheral as well as autonomic neuropathies (Geerlings et al., 1999).
8. Suppression of the immune system by disease, medication, or age can delay wound healing (Guo & DiPietro, 2010).
9. Chronic alcohol exposure causes impaired wound healing and enhanced host susceptibility to infections. Wounds from trauma in the presence of acute alcohol exposure have a higher rate of postinjury infection due to decreased neutrophil recruitment and phagocytic function (Guo & DiPietro, 2010).

Goals

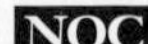

Infection Severity, Wound Healing: Primary Intention, Immune Status, Knowledge Infection Control

The person will report risk factors associated with infection and precautions needed as evidenced by the following indicators:

- Demonstrates meticulous hand washing technique by the time of discharge
- Describes the methods of transmission of infection
- Describes the influence of nutrition on prevention of infection

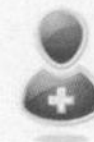

Clinical Alert Administer the preoperative antibiotic on time as prescribed. Investigation of antibiotics on inflammatory response to surgical incision yielded the current recommendation to administer antibiotic prophylaxis 1 hour before incision (Diaz & Newman, 2015).

Interventions

NIC

Infection Control, Wound Care, Incision Site Care, Health Education

Identify Individuals at High Risk for Nosocomial Infections

- Refer to Key Concepts.

Identify Individuals at High Risk for Health-Care Acquired Infections (HAI)

- Refer to Key Concepts.

R: *A recent prevalence study reported that SSIs account for 31% of all HAIs and are the most common health-care–associated infection (Magill et al., 2014).*

Use Appropriate Universal Precautions for Every Individual

R: *Assume everyone is potentially infected or colonized with an organism that could be transmitted in the health-care setting (Grossman & Porth, 2014).*

Antiseptic Hand Hygiene (Quoted From Diaz & Newman, 2015; CDC, 2015c)

- Wash with antiseptic soap and water for at least 15 seconds followed by alcohol-based hand rub.
- If hands were not in contact with anyone or thing in the room, use an alcohol-based hand rub and rub until dry (CDC, 2015c).
- Plain soap is good at reducing bacterial counts, but antimicrobial soap is better, and alcohol-based hand rubs are the best (CDC, 2015c).

Before Putting on Gloves and After Taking Them off

- Before and after touching a patient, before handling an invasive device (Foley catheter, peripheral vascular catheter) regardless of whether or not gloves are used
- After contact with body fluids or excretions, mucous membranes, nonintact skin, or wound dressings
- If moving from a contaminated body site to another body site during the care of the same patient
- After contact with inanimate surfaces and objects (including medical equipment) in the immediate vicinity of the patient
- And after removing sterile or nonsterile gloves
- Before handling medications or preparing food

R: *Numerous studies have proved that health-care workers' hands transmit microorganisms to patients (CDC, 2015). Evidence proves that effective hand washing is the cornerstone for preventing health-care–associated infections. It is also important in preventing specific site infections such as catheter-related bloodstream infections, catheter-related urinary tract infections, ventilator-associated pneumonia, and SSIs. Studies continue to demonstrate that hand hygiene practices among health-care workers is at an abysmally low rate (Diaz & Newman, 2015).*

Personal Protective Equipment (PPE) (2013a)

- Wear PPE when the individual interaction indicates that contact with blood/body fluids may occur.

R: *This will prevent contamination of clothing and skin during the process of care.*

- Before leaving room, remove and discard all PPE in the room or cubicle.

Gloves

- Wear gloves when providing direct individual care.

R: *Gloves provide a barrier from contact with infectious secretions and excretions.*

- Wear gloves for potential contact with nonintact skin, mucous membranes blood, and body fluids. Handle the blood of all individuals as potentially infectious.
- Remove gloves properly to prevent hand contamination. Deposit gloves in the proper container in the room.
- After removing gloves, wash hands with soap and water.
- Do not substitute alcohol-based hand rubs for physical action of washing and rinsing hands with antimicrobial soap and water upon any contact with individuals or any object in the room. Alcohol, chlorhexidine, and other antiseptic agents alone have poor activity against some organisms (e.g., spores *C. difficile*)

(*Siegel, Rhinehart, Jackson, Chiarello, & The Healthcare Infection Control Practices Advisory Committee, 2007, p. 78).

Masks

- Use PPE (masks, goggles, face shields) to protect the mucous membranes of your eyes, mouth, and nose during procedures and individual-care activities that may generate splashes or sprays of blood, body fluids, secretions, and excretions.

Gowns

- Wear a gown for direct contact with uncontained secretions or excretions.

R: *Gowns are needed to prevent soiling or contamination of clothing during procedures and individual-care activities.*

- Remove gown and perform hand hygiene before leaving the individual's room/cubicle.
- Do not reuse gowns even with the same individual.
- When suctioning oral secretion, wear gloves and mask/goggles or a face shield—sometimes gown (CDC, 2013a).

R: *These precautions prevent the transmission of pathogens to the caregiver and then to others (e.g., other individuals, visitors, other staff).*

Educate All Staff, Visitors, and Individuals on the Importance of Preventing Droplet Transmission From Themselves to Others

- Offer a surgical mask to persons who are coughing.

R: *Surgical masks decrease contamination of the surrounding environment.*

Instruct to

- Cover the mouth and nose during coughing and sneezing.
- Use tissues to contain respiratory secretions with prompt disposal into a no-touch receptacle. Wash hands with soap and water.
- Turn the head away from others and maintain spatial buffer, ideally >3 feet, when coughing.

R: *These measures are targeted to all individuals with symptoms of respiratory infection and their accompanying family members or friends beginning at the point of initial encounter with a health-care setting (e.g., reception/triage in emergency departments, ambulatory clinics, health-care-provider offices) (www.cdc.gov).*

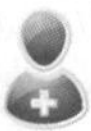

Clinical Alert If the ill individual or visitors refuse to comply with infection prevention requirements, report situation to manager or infection control officer.

Determine the ill Individual's Room Placement Based on (*Siegel et al., 2007, p. 81)

- Route of transmission of known or suspected infectious agent
- Risk factors for transmission in the infected individual
- Risk factors for adverse outcomes resulting from an HAI in other individuals in the area or room
- Availability of single-individual rooms
- Individual options for room-sharing (e.g., placing individuals with the same infection in the same room)
- Immediately report any situation that increases the risk of infection transmission to individuals, visitors, or staff.

Assess Individual-Care Equipment, Instruments, Devices, and Environment for Contamination From Blood or Body Fluids

- Follow policies and procedures for containing, transporting, handling, cleaning prior to confirmation of infectious agent.

Initiate Specific Precautions for the Suspected Agent

- Meningitis: droplet, airborne precautions
- Maculopapular rash with cough, fever
- Rubella: airborne precautions
- Abscess
- MRSA: contact, droplet precautions
- Cough/fever/pulmonary infiltrate in HIV infected or someone high risk of HIV infection

- Tuberculosis: airborne/contact (respirators)

R: *Prevention strategies are indicated when high-risk infections are suspected but not yet confirmed.*

Reduce Entry of Organisms

Surgical Site Infection (SSI) (2015d)

- Identify individuals at high risk for delayed wound healing (refer to Focus Assessment Criteria).

R: *Intervention can be implemented to control or influence the degree of risk associated with predictors and confounding factors.*

Maintain Normothermia

- Monitor temperature every 4 hours; notify physician/NP if temperature is greater than 100.8° F.

R: *Hypothermia also increases the risk of surgical wound infection. Hypothermia directly impairs immune function, including T-cell-mediated antibody production. Thermoregulatory vasoconstriction decreases subcutaneous oxygen tension and increases the risk of wound infection (Sessler, 2006).*

Monitor for Inadequate Tissue Oxygen in High-Risk Individuals (e.g., pulse oximetry)

R: *Deceased tissue oxygen impairs tissue repair (Grossman & Porth, 2014).*

Advise Smokers That the Risk of Wound Infection Is Tripled in Smokers (Armstrong & Mayr, 2014; Sessler, 2006)

Monitor for Hyperglycemia in Diabetic and Nondiabetic Individuals (Armstrong & Mayr, 2014)

R: *A large study found "Perioperative and postoperative hyperglycemia in general surgery patients with and without diabetes was associated with nearly 2-fold higher risk of infection, in-hospital mortality, and operative complications. Interestingly, the greatest risk of infection was among patients with no history of diabetes who experienced hyperglycemia" (Kwon, Thompson, & Dellinger, 2013).*

- Consult with physician/NP/PA for interventions to achieve rigorous postoperative glucose control.

R: *Surgical site infections have been found to double in both diabetic and nondiabetic postcardiac surgical individuals when blood glucose exceeds 200 mg/dL in the first 48 hours. Aggressive insulin infusion protocol has been shown to reduce wound infections, multiple organ failure, sepsis, and mortality in critical care individuals (Sessler, 2006).*

- Aggressively manage postoperative pain using prevention vs. PRN medication administration.

R: *Postoperative pain provokes an autonomic response that produces arteriolar vasoconstriction and reduces circulation needed for wound healing (Sessler, 2006). New data suggest that stress alters multiple physiologic pathways that are involved in wound repair processes (Gouin & Kiecolt-Glaser, 2010).*

- Prevent hypovolemia.

R: *Small volume deficits can substantially reduce peripheral circulation (Sessler, 2006).*

- Assess wound site every 24 hours and apply dressing if indicated; report any abnormal findings (e.g., increased redness, change in drainage, failure for edges to seal).

R: *Wound healing by primary intention requires a dressing to protect it from contamination until the edges seal (usually 24 hours). Wound healing by secondary intention requires a dressing to maintain adequate hydration; the dressing is not needed after wound edges seal.*

- Assess nutritional status to provide adequate protein and caloric intake for healing.

R: *To repair tissue, the body needs adequate stores of protein, carbohydrates, fats, vitamins A, B_{12}, C, K, and minerals, and adequate hydration for vascular transport of oxygen and wastes (Grossman & Porth, 2014).*

Catheter-Associated Urinary Tract Infection [CAUTI]

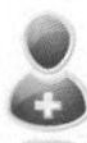

Clinical Alert Approximately 20% of hospital-acquired bacteremias arise from the urinary tract, and the mortality associated with this condition is about 10% (Fekete, 2015; Gould et al., 2009). When a catheter is in place, remind the prescriber every 2 days to reconsider whether catheter is still indicated (e.g., using reminder protocols or institute the nursing protocol which allows reassessment and determination if the catheter can be removed).

Insert Catheters Only for Appropriate Indications (Fekete, 2015; Gould et al., 2009)

R: *"The single most important factor for preventing urinary catheter-related complications is limiting their use to appropriate indications" (Schaeffer, 2015).*

- Presence of acute urinary retention or bladder outlet obstruction
- Need for accurate measurements of urinary output in critically ill individuals
- Perioperative use for selected surgical procedures:
  - Those undergoing urologic surgery or other surgery on contiguous structures of the genitourinary tract— colorectal
  - Management of hematuria associated with clots
  - Management of patients with neurogenic bladder
  - Anticipated prolonged duration of surgery (Catheters inserted for this reason should be removed in PACU.)
  - Individuals anticipated to receive large-volume infusions or diuretics during surgery
  - Need for intraoperative monitoring of urinary output
  - To assist in healing of open sacral or perineal wounds in incontinent individuals
  - Intravesical pharmacologic therapy (e.g., bladder cancer)
  - Prescribed prolonged immobilization (e.g., potentially unstable thoracic or lumbar spine, multiple traumatic injuries such as pelvic fractures)
  - To improve comfort for end-of-life care if needed

R: *A 6% increase in catheter-associated urinary tract infections (CAUTI) was reported between 2009 and 2013; although initial data from 2014 seem to indicate that these infections have started to decrease (CDC, 2015f).*

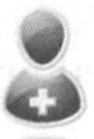

Clinical Alert Fekete (2015) cited, "Unwarranted urinary catheters are placed in 21 to 50 percent of hospitalized patients. The most common inappropriate indication for placing an indwelling urethral catheter is management of urinary incontinence. While catheter use in these patients may have a short-term benefit, the increased risk of complications associated with their use outweighs any benefit".

Consider Condom Catheters or Alternatives to Indwelling Catheter such as Intermittent Catheterization If Possible

Follow Evidence-Based Procedure for Catheter Insertion and Management

- Use a single-use packet of lubricant jelly on the catheter, and one should use clinical judgment when deciding whether or not to use anesthetic lubricant or plain lubricant.
- Use the smallest gauge catheter as possible.

R: *This is to reduce urethra trauma.*

- Maintain unobstructed urine flow; keep tubing free from kinks.
- Cleanse the patient's genitalia area with an aseptic cleanser prior to catheter insertion. Do not clean the periurethral area with antiseptics to prevent CAUTI while the catheter is in place. Routine hygiene (e.g., cleaning of the metal surface during daily bathing or showering) is appropriate.
- Secure to the thigh with a securement device.

R: *This will prevent movement and urethral traction, which can cause irritation and tissue breakdown and become an entry site for pathogens.*

- Keep the IUC drainage bag below the level of the bladder at all times.
- Empty the drainage bag every 8 hours and when the bag is two-thirds full or prior to all patient transfers. Empty using a separate, clean collecting container for each individual.

R: *A full drainage bag will cause traction on the catheter with pressure on the urethra, which can cause irritation and tissue breakdown and become an entry site for pathogens.*

- Consult with physician/nurse practitioner to discuss the inappropriate use of indwelling catheter in a particular individual.
  - Convenience of nursing staff
  - Individual with incontinence
  - Access for obtaining urine for culture or other diagnostic tests when the individual can voluntarily void
  - For prolonged postoperative duration without appropriate indications (e.g., structural repair of urethra or contiguous structures, prolonged effect of epidural anesthesia)

- If the IUC has been in place for more than 2 days, provide a daily reminder to the health-care provider to evaluate continued need for the device.
- Once an IUC is removed, if the patient does not void within 4 to 6 hours, use a bedside bladder scanner to determine urine volume. In and out catheterize the patient if the volume is greater than 500 mL; avoid replacing an IUC.
- Once an IUC is removed, offer the patient a bedside commode if they cannot ambulate safely to the bathroom.

R: *Every attempt to minimize urinary catheter use and duration of use in all individuals, especially with those at higher risk for CAUTI or mortality from catheterization such as women, the elderly, and those with impaired immunity.*

- Avoid use of urinary catheters for management of incontinence.
- For operative individuals who have an indication for an indwelling catheter, remove the catheter as soon as possible postoperatively, preferably within 24 hours.

R: *For urethral catheters avoid wiping the periurethral area with antiseptics to prevent CAUTI. Routine hygiene (e.g., cleansing of the metal surface during daily bathing or showering) is appropriate.*

R: *Antiseptic agents can cause tissue breakdown or the introduction of resistant bacteria at the meatus (Fekete, 2015).*

Obtain Urine Samples Aseptically

- For a sample of fresh urine (i.e., urinalysis or culture), aspirate the urine from the needleless sampling port with a sterile syringe/cannula adapter after cleansing the port with a disinfectant.
- For samples of large volumes of urine for special analyses (not culture), acquire aseptically from the drainage bag.
- After removal of indwelling urinary catheter, use bladder scan 4 hours after removal until the individual voids with a postvoid residual of less than 150 mL (Newman, 2015).

R: *To prevent the onset of urinary retention following indwelling catheter (Foley) removal and to assist with bladder retraining by determining the need to void is based on bladder volume. Bladder scanning can minimize instrumentation while preventing bladder distension and additional complications such as infection (Newman, 2015).*

- If intermittent cauterization is needed, bladder scan at the bedside can determine when catheterization is indicated.

R: *This noninvasive procedure has a high degree of accuracy and may enable unnecessary catheterization to avoid intermittent catheterization (Newman, 2015).*

Invasive Access Sites

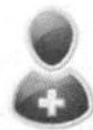

CLINICAL ALERT O'Grady et al. (2011) summarized research, "Reports spanning the past four decades have consistently demonstrated that risk for infection declines following standardization of aseptic care, and that insertion and maintenance of intravascular catheters by inexperienced staff might increase the risk for catheter colonization and CRBSI. Specialized 'IV teams' have shown unequivocal effectiveness in reducing the incidence of CRBSI, associated complications, and costs. Additionally, infection risk increases with nursing staff reductions below a critical level."

- Follow protocol for invasive access sites for insertion and maintenance. Some general interventions (O'Grady et al., 2011) are as follows:
  - Evaluate the catheter insertion site daily by palpation through the dressing to discern tenderness and by inspection if a transparent dressing is in use. If the patient is diaphoretic or if the site is bleeding or oozing, use gauze dressing until this is resolved. Gauze and opaque dressings should not be removed if the patient has no clinical signs of infection. If the patient has local tenderness or other signs of possible CRBSI, an opaque dressing should be removed and the site inspected visually (O'Grady et al., 2011).

R: *Transparent, semipermeable polyurethane dressings permit continuous visual inspection of the catheter site. Transparent dressings can be safely left on peripheral venous catheters for the duration of catheter insertion without increasing the risk for thrombophlebitis (O'Grady et al., 2011).*

  - Encourage the individual to report any changes in their catheter site or any new discomfort to their nurse.
  - Monitor temperature at least every 24 hours or more often as indicated; notify prescribing physician, NP, or PA if greater than 100.8° F.

- Remove peripheral venous catheters if the individual develops signs of phlebitis (warmth, tenderness, erythema, or palpable venous cord), infection, or a malfunctioning catheter.
- Maintain aseptic technique for all invasive devices, changing sites, dressings, tubing, and solutions per policy schedule.
- Use maximal sterile barrier precautions, including the use of a cap, mask, sterile gown, sterile gloves, and a sterile full body drape, for the insertion of CVCs, PICCs, or guidewire exchange.
- Use a 2% chlorhexidine wash instead of soap and water for daily skin cleansing.
- Daily cleansing of ICU patients with a 2% chlorhexidine impregnated washcloth may be a simple, effective strategy to decrease the rate of primary blood stream infections (O'Grady et al., 2011).
- Evaluate all abnormal laboratory findings, especially cultures/sensitivities and CBC.

R: *The CDC (2016) reported a 46% decrease in central line–associated bloodstream infection (CLABSI) was reported between 2008 and 2013, which is attributed to adhering to protocols.*

R: *Invasive lines provide a site for organism entry. Interventions focus on prevention and identification of early signs of infection.*

Respiratory Tract Infections

- Practice protective measures:
  - Practice respiratory hygiene (providing masks, tissues, hand hygiene products, designated handwashing sinks, and no-touch waste receptacles).
  - Assess the individual's personal hygiene habits. Correct any behavior that increases risk for infection.
  - If indicated, use airborne infection isolation rooms.
- Monitor temperature at least every 8 hours, and notify physician/NP/PA if greater than 100.8° F.
- Evaluate sputum characteristics for frequency, purulence, blood, and odor.
- Assess lung sounds every 8 hours or PRN.
- If prompt to cough, deep breathe hourly.
- If individual has had anesthesia, monitor for appropriate clearing of secretions in lung fields.
- Evaluate need for suctioning if individual cannot clear secretions adequately.
- Assess for risk of aspiration, keeping head of bed elevated at 30° unless otherwise contraindicated.
- Ensure optimal pain management to enhance effective coughing.

R: *Individuals with pain, postanesthesia, compromised ability to move, and those with ineffective cough are at risk for infection due to pooling of respiratory secretions.*

Protect the Individual With Immune Deficiency From Infection

- Place the individual in private room.
- Instruct the individual to ask all visitors and personnel to wash their hands before approaching.
- Limit visitors when appropriate.
- Screen all visitors for known infections or exposure to infections.
- Limit invasive devices to those that are necessary.
- Teach the signs and symptoms of infection that need reporting.
- Evaluate the individual's personal hygiene habits.

R: *Persons with compromised immune systems are more vulnerable to infection.*

RISK FOR INFECTION TRANSMISSION[22]

Risk for Infection Transmission

Related to Lack of Knowledge of Reducing the Risk of Transmitting HIV

Definition

Vulnerable to the risk for transferring an opportunistic or pathogenic agent to others

[22]This diagnosis is not on the NANDA-I list but has been included for clarity or usefulness by the author.

Risk Factors

Presence of risk factors (see Related Factors).

Related Factors

Pathophysiologic

Related to:
Colonization with highly antibiotic-resistant organism
Airborne transmission exposure (sneezing, coughing, spitting)
Contact transmission exposure (direct, indirect, contact droplet)
Vehicle transmission exposure (food, water, contaminated drugs or blood, contaminated sites [IV, catheter])
Vector-borne transmission exposure (animals, rodents, insects)

Treatment Related

Related to exposure to a contaminated wound

Related to devices with contaminated drainage:

Urinary, chest, endotracheal tubes
Suction equipment

Situational (Personal, Environmental)

Related to:
Unsanitary living conditions (sewage, personal hygiene)
Areas considered high risk for vector-borne diseases (malaria, rabies, bubonic plague)
Areas considered high risk for vehicle-borne disease (hepatitis A, *Shigella*, *Salmonella*)
Exposures to sources of infection as
- Intravenous/intranasal/intradermal drug use (sharing of needles, drug paraphernalia [straws])
- Contaminated sex paraphernalia
- Multiple sex partners
- Natural disaster (e.g., flood, hurricane)
- Disaster with hazardous infectious material

Maturational

Newborn

Related to birth outside hospital setting in uncontrolled environment

Related to exposure during prenatal or perinatal period to communicable disease through mother

Key Concepts

General Considerations

- To spread an infection, three elements are required (Fig. II.6):
  - A source of infecting organism
  - A susceptible host
  - A means of transmission for the organism
- Sources of infecting organisms include the following:
  - Individuals, personnel, and visitors with acute disease, incubating infection, or colonized organisms without apparent disease
  - Individual's own endogenous flora (autogenous infection)
  - Inanimate environment, including equipment and medications
- Susceptibility of the host varies according to
  - Immune status

FIGURE II.6 Breaking the chain of infection. (Adapted from the APIC Starter Kit with permission from the Association for Professionals in Infection Control and Epidemiology. Washington, DC, copyright APIC, 1978.)

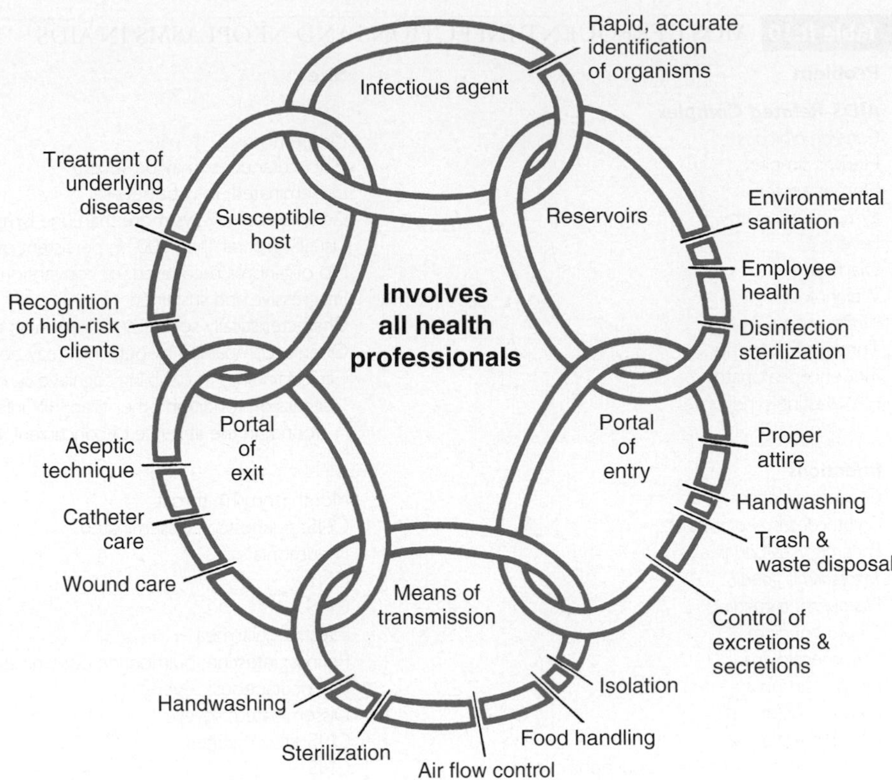

- Ability to develop a commensal relationship with the infecting organism and become an asymptomatic carrier
- Preexisting diseases

- Means of transmission for the organism include one or more of the following (Grossman & Porth, 2014):
  - Contact transmission, the most frequent method of transferring organisms, can be divided into four subgroups:
    - *Direct contact*—involves direct physical transfer between a susceptible person and an infected or colonized person: sexually transmitted infections (e.g., rubella, herpes simplex viruses, varicella [chickenpox], herpes zoster, HIV); vertical transmission (mother to newborn during birth) (e.g., Herpes simplex); congenital infection (transmission to infant during gestation) (e.g., HIV, cytomegalovirus, syphilis, varicella-zoster); infected blood in contact with another person's blood (e.g., HIV, hepatitis C, hepatitis B)
    - *Penetration*—disruption of the skin or mucous membranes (e.g., abrasion, burns, penetrating wound, bite, skin popping, or IV drug use)
    - *Ingestion*—entry of pathogenic microorganisms or toxins into oral cavity and gastrointestinal tract (e.g., parasites, contaminated foods, hepatitis A, dysentery)
    - *Inhalation/droplet*—involves an infected person transferring organisms into the conjunctivae, nose, or mouth of a susceptible host by coughing, sneezing, or talking. Droplets travel no more than 3 feet (e.g., tuberculosis, bacterial pneumonia, viral pneumonia, meningitis)
- Universal body substance precautions require precautions with all blood and body fluids. Those individuals with a suspected or confirmed medical diagnosis indicative of an infectious disease process, however, need documentation with a comprehensive plan of care for that infection or potential infection. The nursing diagnosis *Risk for Infection Transmission* can be used to document specific universal precaution practices.

Human Immunodeficiency Virus

- The cause of AIDS is a retrovirus labeled human immunodeficiency virus (HIV). Transmission is by exposure to contaminated blood, semen and preseminal fluid, vaginal and cervical secretions, and breast milk.
- HIV infection has a latency or incubation period of 18 months to 5 years. During this period, the person transmits disease through sexual activity or through contaminated blood or body fluids.
- HIV destroys the body's T and B lymphocytes, thus making the host susceptible to a select group of diseases (Table II.10).

Table II.10 MOST FREQUENT INFECTIONS AND NEOPLASMS IN AIDS

Problem	Site
AIDS-Related Complex	
Candida albicans	Mouth (thrush), throat
Herpes simplex	Mucocutaneous; may be severe
Herpes zoster	Disseminated; may be severe
Lymphadenopathy	Generalized (always more than one lymph node)
Fevers	Usually greater than 100° F; persistent over months
Diarrhea	No organisms recovered, or conventional organisms recovered
Weight loss	Progressive and sustained
Night sweats	Characteristically severe and drenching; persistent and sustained over months
Thrombocytopenia	Often accompanied by petechia; may be severe and life-threatening
HIV encephalopathy	Clinical findings of disabling cognitive or motor dysfunction in absence of concurrent illness or condition other than HIV infection
HIV wasting syndrome	Profound, in the absence of concurrent illness or condition other than HIV infection
Infections	
Candida albicans	Mouth (thrush); throat
Cryptococcus neoformans	CNS; pulmonary; disseminated
Pneumocystis carinii	Pneumonia
Toxoplasma gondii	CNS
Histoplasma gondii	CNS
Cryptosporidium	Intestine; diarrhea
Cytomegalovirus	Retinas; intestine; pulmonary; disseminated
Herpes simplex	Mucocutaneous; severe
Herpes zoster	Disseminated; severe
HIV dementia	CNS; disseminated
Progressive multifocal leukoencephalopathy	CNS
Mycobacterium avium-intracellulare	Disseminated
Mycobacterium tuberculosis	Pulmonary; tuberculosis
Neoplasms	
Kaposi's sarcoma	Skin; disseminated
Burkitt's lymphoma	Lymphatic system
Non-Hodgkin's lymphoma	Lymphatic system
Mycosis fungoides	Skin (dermal lymphoma)

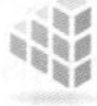

Pediatric Considerations

- Infections in newborns can be acquired transplacentally or transcervically. They can occur before, during, or after birth.
- Children are at greater risk for transmission of infections because of the following factors:
  - Close contact with other children
  - Frequency of infectious disease in children
  - Lack of hygienic habits (e.g., not washing hands after toileting or before eating)
  - Frequent hand-to-mouth activity, increasing risk for infection and reinfection (e.g., pinworms).

Focus Assessment Criteria

Refer to *Risk for Infection*.

Goals

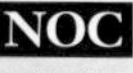

Infection Status, Risk Control, Risk Detection

The individual will describe the mode of transmission of disease by the time of discharge as evidenced by the following indicators:

- Relates the need to be isolated until noninfectious (e.g., TB)
- Relates factors that contribute to the transmission of the infection
- Relates methods to reduce or prevent infection transmission
- Demonstrates meticulous hand washing

Interventions

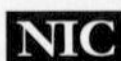

Teaching: Disease Process, Infection Control Infection Protection

Identify the Mode of Transmission Based on Infecting Agent

- Inhalation/Airborne
- Direct contact:
  - Infected blood
  - Ingestion
  - Penetration

R: *To prevent transmission of infection, the mode of transmission (i.e., airborne, contact, vehicle-borne, or vector-borne) must be known. For example, tuberculosis is spread airborne by coughing, sneezing, and spitting.*

Reduce the Transfer of Pathogens

- Isolate individuals with airborne communicable infections (Table II.11).

Table II.11 AIRBORNE COMMUNICABLE DISEASES

Disease	Apply Airborne Precautions for How Long	Comments
Anthrax, inhalation	Duration of illness	Promptly report to infection control office
Chickenpox (varicella)	Until all lesions are crusted	Immune person does not need to wear a mask. Exposed susceptible individuals should be placed in a private special airflow room on STOP SIGN alert status beginning 10 d after initial exposure until 21 d after last exposure. Report to epidemiology.
Diphtheria, pharyngeal	Until two cultures from both nose and throat taken at least 24 hr after cessation of antimicrobial therapy are negative for *Corynebacterium diphtheriae*.	Promptly report to epidemiology.
Epiglottis, due to *Haemophilus influenzae*	For 24 hr after cessation of antimicrobial therapy	Report to epidemiology.
Erythema infectiosum	For 7 d after onset	Report to epidemiology.
Hemorrhagic fevers	Duration of illness	Call epidemiology office immediately. May call the State Health Department and CDC for advice about management of a suspected case.
Herpes zoster (varicella-zoster), disseminated	Duration of illness	Localized; does not require STOP SIGN.
Lassa fever	Duration of illness	Call epidemiology office immediately.
Marburg virus disease		May call the State Health Department and CDC for advice about management of a suspected case.
Measles (rubeola)	For 4 d after start of rash, except in immunocompromised individuals for whom precautions should be maintained for duration of illness	Immune people do not need to wear a mask. Exposed susceptible individuals should be placed in a private special air flow room on STOP SIGN alert status beginning the fifth day after exposure until 21 d after last exposure.
Meningitis, *Haemophilus influenzae* known or suspected	For 24 hr after start of effective antibiotic therapy	Call epidemiology to report.
Neisseria meningitidis (meningococci) known or suspected	For 24 hr after start of effective antibiotic therapy	Promptly report to epidemiology.
Meningococcal pneumonia	For 24 hr after start of effective antibiotic therapy	Promptly report to epidemiology.
Meningococcemia	For 24 hr after start of effective antibiotic therapy	Consult with epidemiology.
Multiply resistant organisms	Until culture negative or as determined by epidemiology	Consult with epidemiology.
Mumps (infectious parotitis)	For 9 d after onset of swelling	People with history do not need to wear a mask. Call epidemiology office to report.
Pertussis (whooping cough)	For 7 d after start of effective therapy	Call epidemiology to report.

Table II.11 AIRBORNE COMMUNICABLE DISEASES (*continued*)

Disease	Apply Airborne Precautions for How Long	Comments
Plague, pneumonic	For 3 d after start of effective therapy	Promptly report to epidemiology.
Pneumonia, *Haemophilus* in infants and children any age	For 24 hr after start of effective therapy	Call epidemiology.
Pneumonia, meningococcal	For 24 hr after start of effective antibiotic therapy	Promptly report to epidemiology.
Rubella (German measles)	For 7 d after onset of rash	Immune people do not need to wear a mask. Promptly report to epidemiology.
Tuberculosis, bronchial, laryngeal, pulmonary, confirmed or suspect	Individuals are not considered infectious if they meet all these criteria: Adequate therapy received for 2–3 wk; Favorable clinical response to therapy; Three consecutive negative sputum smear results from sputum collected on different days	Call epidemiology to report; prompt use of effective antituberculosis drugs is the most effective means of limiting transmission.
Varicella (chickenpox)	Until all lesions crusted over	See chickenpox.

Source: Centers for Disease Control and Prevention, www.cdc.gov.

- Secure appropriate room assignment depending on the type of infection and hygienic practices of the infected individual.
- Use universal precautions to prevent transmission to self or other susceptible host.
- Refer to *Risk for Infection* for specific interventions.

R: *Nurses must use precautions with blood and body fluids from all individuals to protect themselves from exposure to HIV and hepatitis B and C.*

Initiate Health Education and Referrals as Indicated

- Discuss the mode of transmission of infection with the ill person, family, and significant others.

R: *Practices to prevent infection transmission must be continued after discharge.*

Risk for Infection Transmission • Related to Lack of Knowledge of Reducing the Risk of Transmitting HIV

Goals

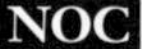

NOC
Infection Status, Risk Control, Risk Detection

The individual will relate practices that reduce the transmission of HIV as evidenced by the following indicators:

- Describes the causes of AIDS
- Identifies risk behaviors that contribute to its transmission
- Describes how to disinfect equipment

Interventions

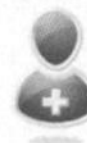

Clinical Alert Centers for Disease Control and Prevention (CDC) (2015) estimates that 1,201,100 persons aged 13 and older are living with HIV infection, including 168,300 (14%) who are unaware of their infection. There are about 50,000 new HIV infections per year. In 2010, the estimated number of new HIV infections among men who have sex with men (MSM) was 29,800 of the 50,000 new HIV infections. This was a significant 12% increase from the 26,700 new infections among MSM in 2008.

NIC

Teaching: Disease Process, Infection Control Infection Protection, Sexual Counseling, Behavior Management: Sexual Behavior

Identify Susceptible Individuals

- Homosexual practices
- Bisexual practices
- Intravenous/intranasal/intradermal drug users
- Blood transfusions before 1985
- Multiple sexual partners with sexually transmitted diseases
- High-risk behaviors
- Health-care workers
- Tattoo by unlicensed persons
- First responders (police, rescue workers, ambulance, firefighters)

Counsel Susceptible Individuals to Be Tested for HIV

- Emphasize early diagnosis can increase positive outcomes with treatment to prevent AIDS.
- Knowledge of HIV-positive status can decrease risk of transmission.

R: *Testing can provide baseline data and can help predict onset of infection, enabling the individual to receive treatment.*

Discuss the Mode of Transmission of the Virus

- Unprotected vaginal, anal, or oral sex with infected hosts or infected sex paraphernalia
- Sharing intravenous needles and syringes; intranasal drug paraphernalia
- Contact of infected fluids with broken skin or mucous membrane
- Breastfeeding, perinatal transmission

R: *HIV is transmitted by sexual contact, by contact with infected blood, body fluid, and blood products, and perinatally (from mother to fetus).*

Use Appropriate Universal Precautions for All Body Fluids

R: *Universal precautions reduce contact with contagious substances.*

- Wash hands before and after all contact with individual or specimen.

R: *Hand washing is one of the most important means to prevent the spread of infection.*

- Handle the blood of all individuals as potentially infectious.
- Wear gloves for potential contact with blood and body fluids.
- Handle all linen soiled with blood or body secretions as potentially infectious.
- Process all laboratory specimens as potentially infectious.

R: *Gloves provide a barrier from contact with infectious secretions and excretions.*

- Place used syringes immediately in a nearby impermeable container; do not recap or manipulate the needle in any way! Use retractable needle syringes when possible.

R: *Needle sticks can transmit infectious blood.*

- Wear protective eyewear and mask if splatter with blood or body fluids is possible

R: *Eye coverings protect the eyes from accidental exposure to infectious secretions present; gowns prevent soiling of clothes if contact with secretions/excretions is likely. Wear mask for tuberculosis and other respiratory organisms (HIV is not airborne).*

R: *Masks prevent transmission by aerosolization of infectious agents if oral mucosal lesions are present.*

Reduce the Risk of Transmission of HIV

- Explain low-risk sexual behaviors:
  - Mutual masturbation
  - Massage
- Vaginal intercourse with condom

R: *The risk of developing sexually transmitted infections is prevented with abstinence. Activities that do not include penile, vaginal, anal, or oral contact carry low or no risk. Transmission is reduced by condom use and avoiding multiple partners.*

- Explain other risks such as alcohol and drug use and having multiple partners.

R: *Alcohol and drug use reduce the individual's ability to make safe decisions regarding sexual activity. The risk of acquiring a sexually transmitted infection does increase as the number of partners increase.*

- Explain the effects of sexually transmitted infections on the risk of an HIV infection transmission.
- "STIs cause the mucous membrane in the mouth, penis, vagina, and rectum to become inflamed. When these tissues are inflamed, the immune system becomes activated to fight the infection with more immune cells, including CD4+ cells, being brought to the infected area. Activated immune cells, specifically CD4+ cells, are easier for HIV to infect. It is also easier for HIV to pass into the bloodstream when inflammation is present."
- Some STIs, such as herpes and syphilis, can cause open sores or lesions, which provide entry points into the body for HIV.
- Men with inflammation of the urethra (urethritis) had 10 times as much HIV in their semen compared to after they received treatment for their urethritis (Cohen et al., 1997).
- Explain the risk of ejaculate contact with broken skin or mucous membranes (oral, anal).

R: *These measures aim to prevent contact of body fluids with mucous membranes.*

Condom Use

- Teach the individual to use condoms of latex rubber, not "natural membrane"; teach appropriate storage to preserve latex. Avoid spermicides with nonoxynol-9.
- Explain the need for water-based lubricants to reduce prophylactic breaks. Avoid petroleum-based lubricants, which dissolve latex.
- Explain that a condom with a spermicide may provide additional protection by decreasing the number of viable HIV particles.

R: *Nonoxynol-9 spermicides may increase the risk of HIV transmission. Natural membrane condoms do not prevent transfer of infected fluids.*

Teach the Individual How to Disinfect Equipment at Home (e.g., Needles, Syringes, Drug Paraphernalia, Sex Aids)

- Wash under running water.
- Fill or wash with household bleach.
- Rinse well with water.

R: *Exposure to disinfecting agents rapidly inactivates HIV. Household bleach solution (dilute 1:10 with water) is an inexpensive choice.*

Provide Facts to Dispel Myths Regarding HIV Transmission

- The AIDS virus is not transmitted by mosquitoes, swimming pools, clothes, eating utensils, telephones, toilet seats, or close contact (e.g., at work, school).
- Saliva, sweat, tears, urine, and feces do not transmit HIV.
- AIDS cannot be contracted during blood donations.
- Blood for transfusions is tested to substantially reduce the risk of contracting the AIDS virus.

R: *Dispelling myths and correcting misinformation can reduce anxiety and allow others to interact more normally with the individual.*

Initiate Health Teaching and Referrals as Indicated

- Explain preexposure chemoprophylaxis for HIV prevention in high-risk individuals, (e.g., Truvada). Refer to primary care provider (Grant et al., 2010).
- Provide the community and the schools with facts regarding AIDS transmission, and dispel myths.
- In a case of acute exposure to HIV (e.g., sexual assault, needlestick, break in barrier with HIV-infected person), immediately refer to health-care facility/emergency room for immediate initiation of postexposure prophylaxis of antiviral therapy.

R: *Protocols for exposure to body fluids possibly contaminated with HIV are available in all health-care facilities.*

RISK FOR INJURY

NANDA-I Definition

Vulnerable to physical damage due to environmental conditions interacting with the individual's adaptive and defensive resources, which may compromise health

Risk Factors

Presence of risk factor (see Related Factors).

Related Factors

Pathophysiologic

Related to altered cerebral function secondary to hypoxia

Related to syncope

Related to vertigo or dizziness

Related to impaired mobility secondary to:
Postcerebrovascular accident
Arthritis
Parkinsonism
Artificial limb(s)

Related to impaired vision

Related to hearing impairment

Related to fatigue

Related to orthostatic hypotension

Related to vestibular disorders

Related to lack of awareness of environmental hazards secondary to:
Confusion
Unfamiliar setting

Related to tonic–clonic movements secondary to seizures

Treatment Related

Related to prolonged bed rest

Related to effects of (specify) or sensorium

Sedatives
Antihistamines
Antihypertensives
Antispasmodics
Vasodilators
Diabetic medications

Muscle relaxants
Diuretics
Psychotropics
Phenothiazine
Pain medications

Related to casts/crutches, canes, walkers

Situational (Personal, Environmental)

Related to decrease in or loss of short-term memory

Related to faulty judgment secondary to:

Stress
Depression
Drug abuse
Alcohol abuse
Dehydration

Related to household hazards (specify):

Unsafe walkways
Slippery floors
Bathrooms (tubs, toilets)
Stairs
Inadequate lighting
Improperly stored poisons
Unsafe toys
Faulty electric wires
Throw rugs

Related to automotive hazards:

Lack of use of seat belts or child seats
Mechanically unsafe vehicle

Related to fire hazards

Related to unfamiliar setting (hospital, nursing home)

Related to improper footwear

Related to inattentive caretaker

Related to improper use of aids (crutches, canes, walkers, wheelchairs)

Related to history of accidents

Related to unstable gait

Maturational

Infant/Child

Related to lack of awareness of hazards

Older Adult

Related to faulty judgments, secondary to cognitive deficits

Related to sedentary lifestyle and loss of muscle strength

Author's Note

This diagnosis has eight subcategories: *Risk for Aspiration, Poisoning, Suffocation, Risk for Falls, Risk for Perioperative Positioning Injury, Risk for Thermal Injury, Risk for Trauma,* and *Risk for Urinary Tract Trauma.* Interventions to prevent poisoning, suffocation, falls, and trauma are included under the general category *Risk for Injury.* Should the nurse choose to isolate interventions only for prevention of poisoning, suffocation, or trauma, then the diagnoses *Risk for Poisoning, Risk for Suffocation, Risk for Falls, Risk for Trauma,* or *Risk for Urinary Tract Trauma* would be useful.

Nursing interventions related to *Risk for Injury* focus on protecting an individual from injury and teaching precautions to reduce the risk of injury. When the nurse is teaching an individual or family safety measures to prevent injury but is not providing on-site protection (as in the community or outpatient department, or for discharge planning), the diagnosis *Risk for Injury related to insufficient knowledge of safety precautions* may be more appropriate.

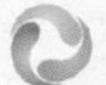

Errors in Diagnostic Statements

Risk for Injury: Hemorrhage related to abnormal blood profile secondary to cirrhosis

This diagnosis does not represent a situation that a nurse can prevent, but one that he or she monitors and comanages with physicians as the collaborative problem *Risk for Complications of Hemorrhage related to altered clotting factors*. Refer to Section 3, *Manual of Collaborative Problems*, for additional interventions.

Key Concepts

General Considerations

- Injury is the leading cause of death in ages 1 to 44 year and the fifth cause of death in all ages (Centers of Disease Prevention and Control [CDC], 2011).
- Health education activities that focus on fire safety, home safety, water safety, seat belt use, motor vehicle safety, cardiopulmonary resuscitation (CPR) training, poison control, and first aid can reduce the rate of accidents (*Clemen-Stone, Eigasti, & McGuire, 2002).
- Obesity appears to be associated with greater risk of falling in older adults, as well as a higher risk of greater ADL disability after a fall (Himes & Reynolds, 2012).
- Cell phone use is now estimated to be involved in 26% of all motor vehicle crashes—up from the previous year.
- Poisonings, including those from unintentional opioid prescription painkiller overdoses, were the leading cause of death in 18 states and Washington, DC (National Safety Council, 2014).
- Table II.12 lists the common sources of poisoning at home.
- Estimated rate of sports-related injuries among individuals above the age of 25 is:
  - Bicycling: 126.5 per 100,000 individuals
  - Basketball: 61.2 per 100,000 individuals
  - Baseball and softball: 41.3 per 100,000 individuals
  - Football: 25.2 per 100,000 individuals
  - Soccer: 23.8 per 100,000 individuals (Misra, 2014)

Table II.12 POISONOUS SUBSTANCES AROUND THE HOUSE

Drugs			
Aspirin	Cough medicines	Laxatives	Tranquilizers
Vitamins	Oral contraceptives	Barbiturates	Acetaminophen
Petroleum Products			
Cleaning Agents	Soaps and polishes	Disinfectants	Drain cleaners
Poisonous Plants			
Amaryllis	Iris	Philodendron	Azalea
Jack-in-the-pulpit	Poinsettia	Baneberry	Jerusalem cherry
Poison hemlock	Belladonna	Jimsonweed	Poison ivy
Bittersweet	Lily of the valley	Pokeweed	Bloodroot
Marijuana	Potato leaves	Castor-bean plant	Mistletoe
Rhododendron	Climbing nightshade	Morning glory	Rhubarb leaves
Daffodil	Mountain laurel	Schefflera	Devil's ivy
Mushrooms	Tomato leaves	Dieffenbachia	Oleander
Wisteria	Foxglove	Peace lily	Yew
Holly			
Miscellaneous			
Baby powder	Cosmetics	Lead paint	

Orthostatic Hypotension

- When autonomic reflexes are impaired or intravascular volume is markedly depleted, a significant reduction in blood pressure occurs upon standing, a phenomenon termed orthostatic hypotension. Orthostatic hypotension can cause dizziness, syncope, and even angina or stroke (Kaufman & Kaplan, 2015a).
- Postural (orthostatic) hypotension is diagnosed when, within 2 to 5 minutes of quiet standing (after a 5-minute period of supine rest), one or both of the following is present (Kaufman & Kaplan, 2015a).
  - At least a 20-mm Hg fall in systolic pressure
  - At least a 10-mm Hg fall in diastolic pressure
- Postural hypotension can affect the quality of life if it contributes to falls or fear of falling. It also can precipitate stroke and myocardial infarction (Miller, 2015).

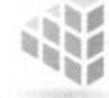 Pediatric Considerations

- Unintentional injuries—such as those caused by burns, drowning, falls, poisoning, and road traffic—are the leading cause of morbidity and mortality among children in the United States. Each year, among those 0 to 19 years of age, more than 12,000 people die from unintentional injuries and more than 9.2 million are treated in emergency departments for nonfatal injuries (CDC, 2012).
- The three leading causes of death for Americans in their 20s are tied to risky behavior and are largely preventable: accidents (unintentional injuries), homicide, and suicide.
- More than 9,000 children die each year (equivalent to 150 school busses all loaded with children each year).
- More than 225,000 children are hospitalized annually.
- Almost 9 million children are treated for their injuries in hospital emergency departments (EDs) each year.
- The CDC reports the following age-related causes of deaths from unintentional causes. Refer to Table II.13 (CDC, 2012).
  - Each year, car crashes injure and kill more children than do any disease. Used properly, safety seats and belts protect children and adults in crashes and help save lives (National Safety Council, 2014).
  - Children should be taught early (2 years of age) and reminded constantly about the rules for streets, playground equipment, fires, water (pools, bathtubs), animals, and strangers.
  - Swimming programs that use total submersion put infants at risk for water intoxication, hypothermia, and bacterial infections. In addition, infants may learn to fear the water.
  - Children 1 to 3 years of age are at greatest risk for being scalded by hot water. More than one-third of children 3 to 8 years of age are burned while playing with matches. When a fire strikes, young children need help to escape (Hockenberry & Wilson, 2015).
  - For children younger than 3 years, choking is the fourth leading cause of accidental death.
  - Toddlers are at highest risk for poisoning. Children are poisoned by medications as well as by common household items (e.g., plants, makeup, cleaning products).
  - For children 1 to 4 years of age, the leading cause of accidental death and serious injury is falls at home (Hockenberry & Wilson, 2015).

Table II.13 THE FIVE LEADING CAUSES AND NUMBER OF UNINTENTIONAL INJURY DEATHS AMONG CHILDREN, BY AGE GROUP, UNITED STATES, 2009

Age <1	Ages 1–4	Ages 5–9	Ages 10–14	Ages 15–19
Suffocation 907 (77%)	Drowning 450 (31%)	Motor Vehicle (MV) Traffic 378 (49%)	MV Traffic 491 (68%)	MV Traffic 3,242 (67%)
MV Traffic 91 (8%)	MV Traffic 363 (25%)	Drowning 119 (15%)	Transportation—Other 117 (15%)	Poisoning 715 (15%)
Drowning 45 (4%)	Fire/Burns 169 (12%)	Fire/Burns 88 (11%)	Drowning 90 (10%)	Drowning 279 (6%)
Fire/Burns 25 (2%)	Transportation—Other 147 (10%)	Transportation—Other 68 (9%)	Fire/Burns 53 (6%)	Transportation—Other 203 (4%)
Poisoning 22 (2%)	Suffocation 125 (9%)	Suffocation 26 (3%)	Suffocation 41 (5%)	Fall 58 (1%)

- Nearly 2 million people every year, many of whom are otherwise healthy, suffer sports-related injuries and receive treatment in EDs. Some sports-related injuries, such as sprained ankles, may be relatively minor, while others, such as head or neck injuries, can be quite serious.

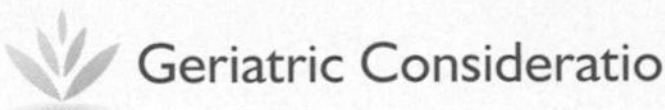

Geriatric Considerations

Falls

- The CDC (2015) reports:
    - One out of three older adults (those aged 65 or older) falls each year, but less than half talk to their health-care providers about it.
    - Among older adults, falls are the leading cause of both fatal and nonfatal injuries.
    - In 2013, 2.5 million nonfatal falls among older adults were treated in EDs and more than 734,000 of these patients were hospitalized.
    - Over 95% of hip fractures are caused by falls. Each year, there are over 258,000 hip fractures, and the rate for women is almost twice the rate for men.
    - One out of five hip fractures individuals (16.9%) dies within a year of their injury.
- Falls are more frequent in older adults; and the mortality, dysfunction, disability, and need for medical services that result are greater than in younger age groups. Unintentional injury, a category including falls, motor vehicle collisions, and burns, is the seventh leading cause of death in older adults, and the incidence of falls represents more than 60% of that category.
- Fear of falling affects 20% to 50% of older adults, which may be a rational psychological response to previous falls, but it is also reported by those who have not fallen. The response to fear of falling is to reduce activity, avoid exercising, and even less leaving their home. The result of decreasing activity leads to decreased muscle strength and less ability to prevent falling if they trip (Jefferis et al., 2014).
- A fall-free existence is not always possible for some people. Increased independence and mobility may be an important and valuable trade-off for increased risk of falling. Collaboration among individual, family, and team members helps arrive at the decision of a less-restricted environment.
- With age comes some loss of the postural control system. To not fall, an individual must be able to keep his or her center of gravity over an adequate base, as well as to rapidly process and respond to sensory information (*Baumann, 1999).
- Older adults frequently lack sufficient lower extremities and inability to produce muscle force to prevent falling muscle strength in lower extremities and have insufficient torque in their ankles, which results in lack of sufficient lower extremity strength and inability to rapidly produce muscle force in response to unexpected slip or trip (*Baumann, 1999; Miller, 2015). Enhancement of lower extremity strength contributed to improvements in balance stability demonstrated by greater ankle force production, in response to balance threats.
- Regular walking, as little as 60 minutes twice a week, can improve sensory function, balance, stability, hip flexion strength, hip extension, and dorsiflexion, all of which can reduce falls (Schoenfelder, 2000).

Focus Assessment Criteria

This entire assessment is indicated only when an individual is at high risk for injury because of personal deficits, alterations (e.g., mobility problems), or maturational age. In households without such a family member, the functional assessment of the individual can be deleted with the focus on the environment.

For assessment tools to evaluate risk for falls, refer to *Risk for Falls*.

Subjective Data

These consist of the individual's physical capabilities (as reported by individual or caretaker).

Assess for Risk Factors

Vision
Corrected (date of last prescription)
Complaints of
Blurriness | Difficulty focusing | Loss of side vision
Inability to adjust to darkness | Sensitivity to light

Hearing
Need to read lips, use of hearing aid, inadequate (condition, batteries)

Thermal/Tactile
Altered sense of hot/cold/pressure/sharp/dull

Mental Status
Drowsy
Confused
Oriented to time, place, events
Complaints of
Vertigo — Altered sense of balance
Orthostatic hypotension — Cognitive stage (immature reasoning/judgment)

Mobility
Reports of
Feeling light-headed, dizzy — Losing balance — Difficulty standing, sitting
Wandering — Falling or almost falling
Ability to ambulate:
Around room, house, up- and downstairs, and outside of the house
Ability to travel:
Drive car (date of last reevaluation)
Use public transportation
Motorized wheelchair/scooter
Assistive Devices:
Cane — Walker — Condition of devices
Wheelchair — Prosthesis — Competence in their use
Shoes/slippers
Communication ability:
Write — Use telephone — Make needs known
Contact emergency assistance
Support system/primary caregiver
Help available from relatives, friends, neighbors, club, and church contacts
History of "blackouts"
Urinary frequency or incontinence

Objective Data

Assess for Related Factors

Blood pressure (left, right, sitting/lying more than 5 minutes, 1 minute after standing)

Gait
Steady — Requires aids — Unsteady

Strength
Can stand on one leg — Can sit-stand-sit

Cognitive Processes
Can communicate needs
Can interact
History of wandering (witnessed and reported by others)
Can understand cause and effect

Presence of
Anger — Withdrawal — Depression
Faulty judgment

Ability for Self-Care Activities
Dress and undress — Bathe — Groom self
Feed self — Reach toilet

Assess for Risk Factors in the Home

Safety
Toilet facilities — Water supply — Heating
Sewage — Ventilation — Garbage disposal

Safety of Walkways (Inside and Outside)
Sidewalks (uneven, broken)
Stairs (inside and outside):
Broken steps
Lighting
No hand rails
Protection for children

Halls:
Cluttered
Poor lighting

Electrical Hazards
No outlet covers
Cords frayed and unanchored
Outlets overloaded; accessible to children; near water
Switches too far from bedside

Inadequate Lighting
At night
Outdoors
To bathroom at night

Unsafe Floors
Even or uneven
Highly polished
Rugs not anchored

Kitchen Hazards
Pot handles not turned inward
Stove (grease or flammable objects on stove)
Refrigerator (improperly stored food; inadequate temperatures)

Toxic Substances
Stored in food containers; not properly labeled; accessible to children
Medications kept beyond date of expiration
Poisonous household plants

Fire Hazards
Matches/lighters accessible to children
No fire extinguishers
Improper storage of corrosives, combustibles
Lack of furnace maintenance
No fire escape plan, no fire extinguishers
Emergency telephone numbers not accessible (fire, police)

Hazards for Children in Nursery
Cribs near drapery cords
Cribs with wide slat openings
Plastic bags
Pillows in crib
Unattended without crib rails up
Space between mattress and crib rails
Unattended on changing table
Pacifier hung around infant's neck
Propped bottle placed in infant's crib
Toys with pointed edges, removable parts

Hazards for Children in Household
Walkers
Accessible medications, lighters, matches, and cleaning products
Objects with lead paint
Poisonous plants (see Table II.12)
Open windows with loose or no screens
Plastic bags
Furniture with glass or sharp corners

Open doorways, stairways

Outdoor Hazards for Children
Porches without rails
Play area without fence
Backyard pools
Domestic/wild animals, pets as sources of bacteria (e.g., turtles) or dangerous (e.g., snakes)

Goals

NOC

Risk Control, Safe Home Environment, Falls Occurrence, Fall Prevention Behavior

The individual will relate fewer or no injuries as evidenced by the following indicators:

- Identifies the factors that increase the risk for injury
- Relates intent to use safety measures to prevent injury (e.g., remove or anchor throw rugs)
- Relates intent to practice selected prevention measures (e.g., wear sunglasses to reduce glare)
- Increases daily activity, if feasible

Interventions

NIC

Fall Prevention, Environmental Management: Safety, Health Education, Surveillance: Safety, Risk Identification

Refer to Related Factors

Reduce or Eliminate Causative or Contributing Factors, If Possible

Unfamiliar Surroundings

- Orient to surroundings on admission; explain the call system, and assess the individual's ability to use it.
- Closely supervise the individual during the first few nights to assess safety.
- Use a night light.
- Encourage to request assistance during the night.
- Teach about the side effects of certain drugs (e.g., dizziness, fatigue).
- Keep bed at lowest level during the night.
- Consider use of a movement detection monitor (bed-based alarm or personal alarm), if needed.

R: *An unfamiliar environment and problems with vision, orientation, mobility, and fatigue can increase the risk of falling.*

Impaired Vision

- Provide safe illumination and teach to
  - Ensure adequate lighting in all rooms, with soft light at night.
  - Have a light switch easily accessible next to the bed.
  - Provide background light that is soft.
- Teach how to reduce glare:
  - Avoid glossy surfaces (e.g., glass, highly polished floors).
  - Use diffuse rather than direct light; use shades that darken the room.
  - Turn the head away when switching on a bright light.
  - Wear sunglasses or hats with brims, or carry umbrellas, to reduce glare outside.
  - Avoid looking directly at bright lights (e.g., headlights).
- Teach to provide sufficient color contrast for visual discrimination and to avoid green and blue:
  - Color-code edges of steps (e.g., with colored tape).
  - Avoid white walls, dishes, and counters.
  - Avoid clear glasses (i.e., use smoked glass).
  - Choose objects colored black on white (e.g., black phone).
  - Avoid colors that merge (e.g., beige switches on beige walls).
  - Paint doorknobs with bright colors.

R: *Visual difficulty because of glare is often responsible for falls in older adults, who have increased susceptibility to glare. Incandescent (nonfluorescent) lighting produces less glare and therefore provides better illumination for older individuals.*

Decreased Tactile Sensitivity

- Teach preventive measures:
  - Assess the temperature of bathwater and heating pads before use.
  - Use bath thermometers.
  - Assess extremities daily for undetected injuries.
  - Keep the feet warm and dry and skin softened with emollient lotion (lanolin, mineral oil) (*Note*: Use socks with grips after just putting on lotion to prevent slips/falls).

R: *Loss of sensation in the limbs can increase the risk of burns and undetected injuries.*

- See *Ineffective Peripheral Tissue Perfusion* for additional interventions.

Orthostatic Hypotension

- See *Risk for Injury Related to Vertigo Secondary to Orthostatic Hypotension* for additional interventions.

Decreased Strength/Flexibility

- Perform strengthening exercises daily (Schoenfelder, 2000). The CDC (2015) outlines a safe beginning exercise program with warm-up and cooldown for older adults of: (search physical activity through the CDC website at www.cdc.gov/)
  - Squats
  - Wall push-ups
  - Toe stands
  - Finger marching
- Perform ankle-strengthening exercises daily (Schoenfelder, 2000)
  - The following is an example of toe stands (CDC, 2015).

R: *Toe stands are a good way to strengthen calves and ankles restore stability and balance, which can help prevent a fall if one slips or trips.*

  - Near a counter or sturdy chair, stand with feet shoulder-width apart. Use the chair or counter for balance.
  - To a count of four, slowly push up as far as you can, onto the balls of your feet and hold for 2 to 4 seconds.
  - Then, to a count of four, slowly lower your heels back to the floor.
  - Repeat 10 times for one set. Rest for 1 to 2 minutes. Then complete a second set of 10 repetitions.
- Walk at least two or three times a week.
  - Use ankle exercises as a warm-up before walking.
  - Begin walking with someone at side, if needed, for 10 minutes.
  - Increase time and speed according to capabilities.

R: *Ankle-strengthening and a walking program can improve balance, increase ankle strength, improve walking speed, decrease falls and fear of falling, and increase confidence in performing activities of daily living (CDC 2015; Schoenfelder, 2000).*

Hazardous Environmental Factors

- Teach to:
  - Eliminate throw rugs, litter, and highly polished floors.
  - Ensure nonslip surfaces in bathtub or shower by applying commercially available traction tapes.
  - Install handgrips in bathroom.
  - Install railings in hallways and on stairs.
  - Remove protruding objects (e.g., coat hooks, shelves, light fixtures) from stairway walls.
- Instruct staff to:
  - Keep side rails on bed in place and bed at the lowest position when the individual is left unattended.
  - Keep the bed at the lowest position with wheels locked when stationary.
  - Teach if in the wheelchair to lock and unlock the wheels.
  - Ensure that shoes or slippers have nonskid soles.

R: *Goals to prevent or manage falls focus on reducing their likelihood by minimizing environmental hazards and strengthening individual competence to resist falls and fall-related injuries.*

- If cognitively impaired, refer to *Wandering*.
- Teach lawn mower, snowblower safety (access www.aboutorthowest.com/data/fact/thr_771.htm)

Risk for Injury • Related to Lack of Awareness of Environmental Hazards

Goals

NOC

Safe Home Environment, Risk Control, Parenting: Infant/Toddler/Early Childhood/Middle Childhood, Adolescent Safety

The parent or family will identify and reduce environmental hazards as evidenced by the following indicators:

- Teach children safety habits
- Safely stores hazardous items
- Repairs hazards as needed
- Removes environmental hazards when possible
- Installs safety measures (e.g., locks, rails)

Interventions

NIC
Area Restriction, Surveillance: Safety, Environmental Management: Safety, Home Maintenance Assistance, Risk Identification, Teaching: Infant, Toddler Safety

Identify Situations That Contribute to Accidents

- Unfamiliar setting (homes of others, hotels)
- Peak activity periods (meal preparation, holidays)
- New equipment (bicycle, chain saw, lawn mower, snowblower)
- Lack of awareness of or disregard for environmental hazards (reckless driving)

R: *Injury is the fourth leading cause of death in the general population and the leading cause of death in children and young adults (*Clemen-Stone et al., 2002).*

Reduce or Eliminate Hazardous Situations

- Teach about safety with potentially dangerous equipment.
- Teach to read directions completely before using a new appliance or piece of equipment
- Teach children to stay away from all running lawn mowers.
- Children should not be allowed to play in or near where a lawn mower is being used.
- Never allow a child or another passenger to ride on a mower, even with parents. Doctors commonly see children with severe injuries to their feet caused by riding on the back of a rider mower with a parent or grandparent.
- Children should be at least 12 years of age before operating a push lawn mower, and age 16 to operate a riding lawn mower.
- Remove stones, toys, and other objects from the lawn before you start mowing.
- Unplug and turn off any appliance that is not functioning before examining it (e.g., lawn mower, snowblower, electric mixer).
- Most injuries happen when you try to clear the auger/collector or discharge chute with your hands.
- Do not remove safety devices, shields, or guards on switches, and keep hands and feet away from moving parts.
- Add fuel before starting the engine, not when it is running or hot.
- Use a stick or broom handle—not your hands or feet—to remove debris in lawn mowers or snowblowers.
- Do not leave a lawn mower or snowblower unattended when it is running. If you must walk away from the machine, shut off the engine (American Academy of Orthopedic Surgeons, 2012).

R: *Each year, many thousands of people suffer deep cuts, loss of fingers and toes, crushed and broken bones, joint injuries, burns, infections, other injuries, and even death due to improper or careless use of lawn mowers and snowblowers. Injuries happen to people from all age groups, mostly adults aged 25 to 64.*

Review Unsafe Practices

Automobiles

- Avoid driving
  - A mechanically unsafe vehicle
  - Without seat restraints on everyone
  - With unrestrained babies and children in the car
  - Excessive speeds
  - Without necessary visual aids
  - With unsafe road or road-crossing conditions
  - While medicated or buzzed/intoxicated (illegal drugs, prescription drugs, alcohol, etc.)
  - While tired
  - When distracted (cell phone use, texting, adjusting radio, etc.)
  - With children riding in the front seat of the car
- Avoid backing up without checking the location of small children
- Avoid warming a car in a closed garage

Flammables

- Igniting gas leaks
- Delayed lighting of gas burner or oven
- Experimenting with chemicals or gasoline
- Using unscreened fires, fireplaces, or heaters
- Inadequately storing combustibles, matches, or oily rags
- Smoking in bed or near oxygen
- Buying highly flammable children's toys or clothing

- Playing with fireworks or gunpowder
- Playing with matches, candles, cigarettes, or lighters
- Wearing plastic aprons or flowing clothing around an open flame

Kitchen

- Allowing grease waste to collect on stoves
- Wearing plastic aprons or flowing clothing around an open flame
- Using cracked glasses or dishware
- Using improper canning, freezing, or preserving methods
- Storing knives uncovered
- Keeping pot handles facing front of stove
- Using thin or worn pot holders or oven mitts
- Placing stove controls on front
- Using dishes that have lead in them

Bathroom

- Keeping the medicine cabinet unlocked
- Not having grab rails in the bathtub
- Not having nonskid mats or emery strips in the bathtub
- Maintaining poor lighting in the bathroom and hallways
- Improperly placing electrical outlets

Chemicals and Irritants

- Improperly labeling medication containers
- Keeping medications in containers other than the original ones
- Maintaining poor illumination at the medicine cabinet
- Improperly labeling containers of poisons and corrosive substances
- Keeping expired medications that dangerously decompose
- Storing toxic substances in accessible areas (e.g., under the sink)
- Storing corrosives (e.g., lye) inadequately
- Having contact with intense cold
- Being overexposed to sun, sunlamps, or heating pads

Lighting and Electrical

- Using uncovered outlets
- Using unanchored electrical wires
- Overloading electrical outlets
- Overloading fuse boxes
- Using faulty electrical plugs, frayed wires, or defective electrical appliances
- Maintaining inadequate lighting over landings and stairs
- Maintaining inaccessible light switches (e.g., bedside)
- Using machinery or appliances without prior instruction

R: *Specific instructions can reduce the rate of accidents and injury (Clemen-Stone et al., 2002).*

Initiate Health Teaching and Referral, as Indicated

Teach Measures to Prevent Car Accidents

- Frequently reevaluate the ability to drive.
- Wear good-quality sunglasses (gray or green) to reduce glare.
- Keep windshields clean and wipers in good condition.
- Place mirrors on both sides of the car.
- Stop periodically to stretch and to rest eyes.
- Know the effects of medications on driving ability.
- Do not smoke while driving or drive after drinking.
- Do not use a cellular phone while driving.

Teach Measures to Prevent Pedestrian Accidents

- Allow enough time to cross streets.
- Wear garments that reflect light (beige, white) or with reflective tape at night.
- Wait to cross on the sidewalk, not the street.
- Look both ways.

- Do not rely solely on green traffic lights to provide safe crossing (right turn on red light may be legal, or driver may disobey traffic regulations). Teach measures to prevent burns.
- Equip the home with a smoke alarm system and check its function each month.
- Have a handheld fire extinguisher.
- Set thermostats for water heater to provide warm, but not scalding, water.
- Use baking soda or a lid cover to smother a kitchen grease fire.
- Do not wear loose-fitting clothing (e.g., robes, nightgowns) when cooking.
- Do not smoke when sleepy.
- Ensure that portable heaters are safely used.
- Provide health teaching and referrals as indicated.

R: *Accidents occur more frequently*

- During the initial period of hospitalization and between 6:00 PM and 9:00 PM
- During peak activity periods (meals, playtime)
- In unfamiliar surroundings
- With adequate lighting
- At holidays
- On vacation
- During home repairs

R: *Injury prevention requires anticipation and recognition of where safety measures are applicable. Passive strategies provide automatic protection without choice (e.g., air bags, product design). Active strategies require persuasion through teaching or legislation to practice safety measures (Hockenberry & Wilson, 2009).*

Refer Individuals with Motor or Sensory Deficits for Assistance in Identifying Environmental Hazards

- Local fire company
- Community nursing agency
- Accident-prevention information (see Bibliography)

Refer to Physical Therapist for Evaluation of Gait

Pediatric Interventions

Teach Parents Basic Safety Measures and Assessments

- Instruct parents to expect frequent changes in infants' and children's abilities and to take precautions (e.g., an infant who suddenly rolls over for the first time might be on a changing table unattended).
- Discuss the necessity of constantly monitoring small children.
- Explain that walkers are dangerous and in addition walker use typically delays motor development and cognitive development. They allow the child to reach higher and walk faster which can cause them to roll down the stairs, to reach higher, for example, spill hot coffee, grab pot handles off the stove, touch radiators, fireplaces, or space heaters (American Academy of Pediatrics, 2015).

R: *"An estimated 197200 infant walker-related injuries occurred among children who were younger than 15 months and treated in US emergency departments from 1990 through 2001." (*Shields & Smith, 2015)*

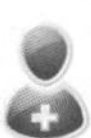

CLINICAL ALERT Sale of walkers is banned in Canada but not in the United States.

- Provide information to assist parents in selecting a babysitter:
  - Determine previous experiences and knowledge of emergency measures.
  - Observe interaction of sitter with child (e.g., have sitter arrive 30 minutes before you are ready to leave).
- Teach parents to expect children to mimic them and to teach what children can do with or without supervision.
  - Tell the child to ask you before attempting a new task.
- Explain and expect compliance with certain rules (depending on age) concerning:
  - Streets
  - Fire
  - Playground equipment

  - Animals
  - Water (pools, bathtubs)
  - Strangers
  - Bicycles
- Role-play with children to assess understanding of the problem.
  - "You're walking home. A strange man pulls up in a car near you. What do you do?"
  - "While walking past a barbecue, your dress catches on fire. What do you do?"

Identify Situations That Contribute to Accidents

Sports

Bicycles, Wagons, Skateboards, and Skates

- No reflectors or lights
- Not in single file
- Riding a too-large bicycle
- No training wheels
- Use of skateboards or skates in heavily traveled areas
- Lack of knowledge of the rules of the road
- Lack of helmet, protective pads
- Safe riding area for young children (not in street)

R: *Almost 50% of head injuries occur during sports such as recreational biking, skateboarding, and skating (American Academy of Orthopedic Surgeons, 2016).*

R: *Prevention strategies to decrease serious injuries resulting from skateboarding include warnings against skateboard use by children younger than 5 years of age, prohibition of skateboards on streets and highways, and the promotion of use of helmets and other protective gear (Hockenberry & Wilson, 2015).*

Water and Pools

- Discourage use of flotation or swim aids (water wings, tubs) with children who cannot swim.
- Teach safe water behavior:
  - No running, pushing
  - No jumping on others
  - No swimming alone
  - No playful screaming for help
  - No diving in water less than 8 feet deep
  - No swimming after meals
  - No excessive alcohol use
  - Keep sharp objects out of the pool.
  - No swimming during electrical storms
- Enclose the pool:
  - Use a 5- to 12-foot fence.
  - Use a fence that children cannot climb.
  - Use self-locking gates with an alarm system.
- Remove the pool cover completely.
- Avoid free-floating pool covers.
- Teach safe diving and sliding techniques:
  - Allow diving only from diving boards.
  - Discourage running dives.
  - Teach to steer upward with hands and head.
  - Descend pool slide sitting with feet first.
- Have lifesaving equipment at poolside (life preserver, rope, or hook).
- Learn CPR and how to respond to accidental submersion:
  - Remove the child from the water (bring child's head above water, supporting head/neck).
  - If spinal injury is suspected, immobilize on a board and apply a cervical collar.
  - Clear airway of debris (if visible only).
  - If the individual is unresponsive but has a pulse and is breathing, place on side if vomiting occurs.
  - Remove wet clothes, dry, and cover with blankets (including head).
  - If no pulse, begin CPR and continue until help arrives.

R: *Drowning is the second leading cause of death from injury during childhood. Children younger than 4 years of age are at especially high risk (National Safety Council, 2009).*

R: *Many near-drownings take place while a parent is supervising the child but has a momentary lapse of attention (Hockenberry & Wilson, 2015).*

R: *Effective swimming depends on intellectual as well as physical maturity. Organized swimming lessons may give parents a false sense of security that their child "can swim."*

Miscellaneous

- Unsupervised contact with animals and poisons in the environment (plants, pool chemicals, pills)
- Obstructed passageways
- Unsafe window protection in home with young children
- Guns or ammunition stored in unlocked fashion
- Large icicles hanging from roof
- Icy walkways
- Glass sliding doors that look open when closed
- Low-strung clothesline
- Discarded or unused refrigerators or freezers without removed doors

Infants and Toddlers

- Household
  - Pillows in crib
  - Staircases without stair gates
  - Crib mattresses that do not fit snugly
  - Cribs with slat openings that allow the child's body to fall through, catching the head
  - Glass or sharp-edged tables
  - Porches and decks without railings
  - Poisonous plants (see Table II.12)
  - Furniture painted with lead paint
  - Unsupervised bathing
  - Open windows
  - Propped bottle in crib
- Toys
  - Sharp edges
  - Balloons
  - Easily breakable parts
  - Lollipops
  - Removable small pieces
  - Pacifier around neck
- Miscellaneous
  - Child unattended in a shopping cart
  - Child unattended in a car
  - Cribs, walkers, or high chairs with movable parts that trap the child (e.g., springs)
  - Put the child in a car safety seat in the back seat only.

Assist Parents to Analyze an Accident

- What happened?
- How did it happen?
- Where, when did it happen?
- Why did the accident happen?

R: *Analysis of an accident may prevent recurrence.*

- Teach the Heimlich maneuver for choking on an object or piece of food.

R: *This procedure creates an artificial cough that forces air and the foreign object out of the child's airway.*

Teach Poison Prevention

- Instruct parents how to childproof the home.
- Instruct parents to keep poisons and corrosive substances in tightly closed, carefully marked containers in locked closets.
- Instruct parents to avoid taking medications in front of children.
- Parents should discard unused supplies of medications and keep needed medications in a locked, inaccessible medicine closet.

- Parents should be taught how to administer antidotes for specific toxic substances, if advised by the Poison Control Center.
- Parents should also have the phone number of the Poison Control Center in a convenient place.
- Refer individuals to the local poison control center for "Mr. Yuk" poison warning stickers and advice on emergency procedures; teach the child what the "Mr. Yuk" sticker means.
- Instruct parents to call the Poison Control Center. Post the telephone number in the kitchen: 1-800-222-1222.

R: *Poisoning is common in toddlers. They put everything into their mouths.*

Initiate Health Teaching and Referrals, as Indicated

- Assist the family in evaluating environmental hazards at home and when visiting others.
- Install specially designed locks to prevent children from opening closets where combustible, corrosive, or flammable materials or medications are stored.
- Instruct parents to use socket covers to prevent accidental electrical shocks to children.
- Teach parents about the hazards of lead paint ingestion and how to identify "pica" in a child.
- Refer parents to public health department if lead paint screening is necessary.
- Encourage the use of childproof caps.
- Advise parents to avoid storing dangerous substances in containers ordinarily used for foods.

R: *All environmental hazards cannot be removed. Strategies that include supervision and education of parents can reduce accidents (*Clemen-Stone et al., 2002).*

R: *Analysis of an accident may prevent recurrence.*

R: *Injury prevention requires anticipation and recognition of where safety measures are applicable. Passive strategies provide automatic protection without choice (e.g., air bags, product design). Active strategies require persuasion through teaching or legislation to practice safety measures.*

R: *Prevention strategies to decrease serious injuries resulting from skateboarding include warnings against skateboard use by children younger than 5 years of age, prohibition of skateboards on streets and highways, and the promotion of use of helmets and other protective gear.*

Risk for Injury • Related to Lack of Awareness of Environmental Hazards Secondary to Maturational Age

Goals

NOC

Risk Control, Fall Prevention Behavior

- The child/adolescent will be free from injury from potentially hazardous factors identified in the hospital environment.
- The family will reinforce and demonstrate safe practices in the hospital.

Interventions

NIC

Refer to *Risk for Infection.*

Protect the Infant/Child From Injury in the Hospital by Controlling Age-Related Hazards

Assess Each Unique Situation for Risk of Injury to the Infant, Young Child, School-Aged Child, or Adolescent. Inform Parents of the Risk for Injury

Infant (1 to 12 Months)

- Ensure that the infant can be identified by an identification band and a tag on his or her crib.
- Do not shake powder directly on an infant; rather, place powder in the hand and then on infant's skin.
- Keep powder out of an infant's reach.
- Keep unsafe toys out of reach (e.g., buttons, beads, balloons, broken toys, sharp-edged toys, other small toys).
- Use mitts to prevent an infant from removing catheters, eye patches, intravenous (IV) infusions, dressings, and feeding tubes, as needed.
- Keep side rails up in locked position when the child is in the crib.
- Pad side rails if an infant can move out of bed or is at risk for seizures.

- Use a cool-mist vaporizer.
- Do not use an infant walker.
- Ascertain identity of all visitors.
- Use a firm mattress that fits crib snugly.
- Do not feed honey to infants younger than 12 months because of the danger of botulism.
- Fasten safety straps on infant seats, swings, high chairs, and strollers.
- Do not allow bottles to be propped. The infant should be held with his or her head upright.
- Do not place pillows in the crib.
- Place one hand on the child while weighing, changing diapers, and so forth, to keep him or her from falling off the scale, changing table, etc.
- Do not allow an infant to wear pacifier on a string around the neck.
- Check bathwater to make sure the temperature is appropriate. Never leave an infant alone while bathing! Support the small infant's head out of the water.
- Check the temperature of formula, especially if you have heated it in the microwave. Shake the bottle before testing temperature.
- Position the crib away from the bedside stand, infusion pumps, and so forth to prevent the child from reaching unsafe objects (e.g., suction machine, electrical outlets, flowers, dials on infusion pump).
- Do not allow parents to smoke or drink hot beverages in an infant's room.
- Do not offer the child foods that must be chewed or are small enough to occlude the airway (e.g., nuts, popcorn, hard candy, whole hot dogs). Forks and knives are not appropriate utensils for infants.
- Discard syringes, needles, med packets, and plastic bags safely.
- Protect the feet of the infant who can walk with shoes or slippers.
- Transport the infant safely to other areas of the hospital (e.g., X-ray, laboratory).
- Remind parents to have an approved car seat in their automobile to transport the child home.

Early Childhood (13 Months to 5 Years)

- Ensure that the young child is identifiable by name band and name tag on the crib.
- Keep the side rails up in the locked position when the child is in the crib—top and bottom compartments; use side rails on youth beds.
- Monitor the child at all times when eating, bathing, playing, and toileting.
- Keep cleaning agents, sharp items, and plastic bags out of reach.
- Secure the thermometer while taking temperature (use rectal or axillary method with toddler, oral method when child is old enough not to bite down on thermometer) or use an infrared instant thermometer in the ear canal.
- Assess for loose teeth and document findings on records.
- Check the temperature of the bathwater before immersing the child.
- Use electric beds with extreme caution. For example, children may get their fingers caught or get under the bed and be at risk for a crushing injury.
- Position the crib/bed away from the bedside stand, infusion pumps, flowers, and so forth, to prevent child from reaching unsafe objects.
- Keep the child safe when mobile:
  - Protect the child's feet with shoes or slippers when ambulating.
  - Keep the bathroom and closet doors firmly shut.
  - Check any tubing attached to the child to prevent kinking or dislodgment.
  - Apply safety straps when the child is in the high chair or stroller or on a cart.
  - Transport the child safely to other areas of the hospital (e.g., X-ray).
  - Use mitts to prevent the child from removing catheters, eye patches, IV infusion, dressings, and feeding tubes, as needed.
  - Place one hand over the child when weighing, changing diapers, and so forth, to prevent falls.
- Do not call medications "candy."
- Do not permit the child to chew gum or eat hard candy, nuts, whole hot dogs, or fish with bones.
- Set limits. Enforce and repeat what the child can do and not do in the hospital and areas in which he or she can and cannot go.
- Provide age-appropriate, safe toys (see manufacturer's guidelines).
- Do not allow parents to smoke or drink hot beverages in the child's room.
- Feed the child in a quiet environment; ensure that he or she sits while eating to prevent choking.
- Remind parents to have an approved car seat in the automobile to transport the child home.
- Ascertain identity of all visitors.

School-Aged/Adolescent (6 to 12 Years/13 to 18 Years)

- Ensure that the child or adolescent can be identified by a name band and a tag on his or her bed. School-aged children may claim to be someone else as a joke, not realizing the danger of this.
- Assess for loose teeth; document findings on records.
- Assess for self-care deficits and activity intolerance, because the school-aged child or adolescent may not ask for help when ambulating, bathing, toileting, and so forth.
- Apply safety straps when transporting by cart or wheelchair.
- Set limits. Enforce and repeat what the child can and cannot do and areas in which he or she can and cannot go in the hospital.
- Provide age-appropriate activities. Supervise therapeutic play closely. Do not allow the child to use syringes as squirt guns.
- Do not allow parents to smoke or drink hot beverages in the child's room.
- Encourage the child or adolescent to wear a MedicAlert necklace or bracelet, if appropriate. Encourage the child to carry identification in a wallet or purse.
- Remind the child to wear his or her seat belt in the car when discharged.
- Discourage smoking and use of illicit drugs, including alcohol.

R: *The nurse should assess each child's unique risk of potential for injury. This includes the child with sensory or motor deficits and developmental delay. Environmental changes, such as hospitalization, visiting relatives' homes, and celebrating holidays, pose special hazards for children (Hockenberry & Wilson, 2015).*

R: *To protect children from injury, caretakers must be aware of the age-related behavioral characteristics that increase the child's vulnerability to injury (Hockenberry & Wilson, 2015).*

R: *Anatomically, children are more susceptible to head injuries because of their large head, to liver and spleen trauma because these organs are larger, and to being thrown more easily (in a car) because of their small, light bodies (Hockenberry & Wilson, 2015).*

R: *Infants explore the environment through taste and touch.*

Risk for Injury • Related to Vertigo Secondary to Orthostatic Hypotension

Goals

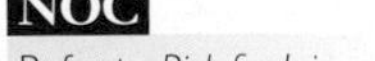

NOC

Refer to *Risk for Injury*.

The individual will relate fewer episodes of dizziness or vertigo as evidenced by the following indicators:

- Identifies situations that cause vertigo
- Relates methods of preventing sudden decreases in cerebral blood flow
- Demonstrates maneuvers to change position and avoid a sudden drop in cerebral pressure

Interventions

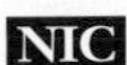

NIC

Refer to *Risk for Injury*.

Identify Contributing Factors (Kaufamn & Kaplan, 2015a)

- Recent medical history of potential volume loss (vomiting, diarrhea, fluid restriction, fever)
- Medical history of congestive heart failure, malignancy, diabetes, alcoholism
- Evidence on neurologic history and examination of parkinsonism, ataxia, peripheral neuropathy or dysautonomia (e.g., abnormal pupillary response, history of constipation, or erectile dysfunction)
- Cardiovascular disorders (systolic hypertension, heart failure cerebral infarct, anemia, dysrhythmias)
- Fluid or electrolyte imbalances
- Diabetes
- Certain medications (diuretics, antihypertensives, beta-blockers, alpha-blockers anticholinergics, biturates, vasodilators, antidepressants, antipsychotic drugs: olanzapine, risperidone, for example)
- Antihypertensive drugs, nitrates, monoamine oxidase inhibitors, phenothiazine, narcotics sedatives, muscle relaxants, vasodilators, antiseizure medications (Perlmuter, Sarda, Casavant, & Mosnaim, 2013)
- Alcohol use
- Age 75 years or older
- Prolonged bed rest
- Surgical sympathectomy
- Valsalva maneuver during voiding or defecating
- Arthritis (spurs on cervical vertebrae)

Assess for Orthostatic Hypotension

- Take bilateral brachial pressures with the individual supine.
- If the brachial pressures are different, use the arm with the higher reading and take the blood pressure immediately after the individual stands up quickly. Report differences to the physician/PA/NP.

R: *Postural (orthostatic) hypotension is diagnosed when, within 2 to 5 minutes of quiet standing (after a 5-minute period of supine rest), one or both of the following is present: at least a 20-mm Hg fall in systolic pressure and/or at least a 10-mm Hg fall in diastolic pressure (Kaufamn & Kaplan, 2015a).*

- Ask to describe sensations (e.g., light-headed, dizzy).
- Assess skin and vital signs.

R: *Use of the arm with the higher pressure gives a more accurate assessment of the blood pressure.*

Teach Techniques to Reduce Orthostatic Hypotension

- Change positions slowly especially in the morning, when orthostatic tolerance is lowest.
- Move from lying to an upright position in stages.
  - Sit up in bed.
  - Dangle first one leg, then the other, over the side of the bed.
  - Allow a few minutes before going on to each step.
  - Gradually pull oneself from a sitting to a standing position.
  - Place a chair, walker, cane, or other assistive device nearby to use to steady oneself when getting out of bed.
- Sleep with the head of the bed elevated 10° to 20°.

R: *This "decreases renal perfusion, thereby activating the renin-angiotensin-aldosterone system and decreasing nocturnal diuresis, which can be pronounced in these patients. These changes relieve orthostatic hypotension by expanding extracellular fluid volume and may reduce end organ damage by reducing supine hypertension" (Kaufamn & Kaplan, 2015b).*

- During day, rest in a recliner rather than in bed.

R: *Prolonged bed rest increases venous pooling which reduces circulation to the brain. Gradual position change allows the body to compensate for venous pooling (Grossman & Porth, 2014).*

- Avoid prolonged bed rest

R: *Prolonged bed rest promotes a reduction in plasma volume (after 3 to 4 days), decreased venous tone, peripheral vasoconstriction, and muscle weakness (after 2 weeks).*

- Avoid prolonged standing.
- Avoid stooping to pick something up from the floor; use an assistive device available from an orthotics department or a self-help store.
- Avoiding straining, coughing, and walking in hot weather; these activities reduce venous return and worsen orthostatic hypotension.
- Maintaining hydration and avoiding overheating. Drink water prior to exposure to hot weather.
- Refer to prescribing provider a discussion about the possible effectiveness of waist-high stockings.

R: *Compression waist-high stockings expand extracellular fluid volume and may reduce end organ damage by reducing supine hypertension (Kaufamn & Kaplan, 2015b).*

Encourage to Increase Daily Activity, If Permissible

- Discuss the value of daily exercise.
- Establish an exercise program.

R: *Exercise increases circulation and energy levels, decreases stress and the process of osteoporosis, and contributes to overall well-being.*

Teach to Avoid Dehydration and Vasodilation

- Replace fluids prior, during, and after periods of excess fluid loss (e.g., hot weather).
- Minimize diuretic fluids (e.g., coffee, tea, cola).
- Minimize alcohol consumption.
- Avoid sources of intense heat (e.g., direct sun, hot showers, baths, electric blankets).

- Avoid taking nitroglycerin while standing.

R: *Adequate hydration is necessary to prevent decreased circulating volume. Certain fluids are diuretics and reduce body fluids. Heat and alcohol can cause vasodilation.*

Teach to Reduce Postprandial Hypotension (Kaufamn & Kaplan, 2015b)

- Take antihypertensive medications after meals rather than before.
- Avoid large meals; plan instead five small meals.
- Ingest meals low in carbohydrate.
- Minimize alcohol intake.
- Drink water with meals.
- Avoid activities or sudden standing immediately after eating.
- Refer to prescribing professional to determine if an increase in dietary salt is indicated.

R: *This can increase central blood volume.*

R: *Studies have shown that in healthy older adults, blood pressure is reduced by 20 mm Hg within 1 hour of eating the morning or afternoon meal. This is thought to result from an impaired baroreflex compensatory response to splanchnic blood pooling during digestion (Kaufmann, Freeman & Kaplan, 2010).*

Institute Environmental Safety Measures

- Refer to *Risk for Injury—Related to Lack of Awareness of Environmental Hazards.*

Risk for Aspiration

NANDA-I Definition

Vulnerable to entry of gastrointestinal secretions, oropharyngeal secretions, solids, or fluids into the tracheobronchial passages, which may compromise health

Risk Factors

Pathophysiologic

Related to reduced level of consciousness secondary to:

Presenile dementia
Head injury
Cerebrovascular accident
Parkinson's disease
Alcohol- or drug-induced
Coma
Seizures
Anesthesia

Related to depressed cough/gag reflexes

Related to increased intragastric pressure secondary to:

Lithotomy position
Ascites
Obesity
Enlarged uterus

Related to impaired swallowing or decreased laryngeal and glottic reflexes secondary to:

Achalasia
Cerebrovascular accident
Myasthenia gravis
Catatonia
Muscular dystrophy
Esophageal strictures

Debilitating conditions
Multiple sclerosis
Scleroderma
Parkinson's disease
Guillain–Barré syndrome

Related to tracheoesophageal fistula

Related to impaired protective reflexes secondary to:

Facial/oral/neck surgery or trauma*
Paraplegia or hemiplegia

Treatment Related

Related to depressed laryngeal and glottic reflexes secondary to:

Tracheostomy/endotracheal tube*
Sedation
Tube feedings

Related to impaired ability to cough secondary to:

Wired jaw*
Imposed prone position

Situational (Personal, Environmental)

Related to inability/impaired ability to elevate upper body

Related to eating when intoxicated

Maturational

Premature

Related to impaired sucking/swallowing reflexes

Neonate

Related to decreased muscle tone of inferior esophageal sphincter

Older Adult

Related to poor dentition

Author's Note

Risk for Aspiration is a clinically useful diagnosis for people at high risk for aspiration because of reduced level of consciousness, structural deficits, mechanical devices, and neurologic and gastrointestinal disorders. People with swallowing difficulties often are at risk for aspiration; the nursing diagnosis *Impaired Swallowing* should be used to describe an individual with difficulty swallowing who also is at risk for aspiration. *Risk for Aspiration* should be used to describe people who require nursing interventions to prevent aspiration, but do not have a swallowing problem.

Errors in Diagnostic Statements

Risk for Aspiration related to bronchopneumonia

This diagnostic statement does not direct the nurse to the risk factors that could be reduced. If the nurse were monitoring and comanaging bronchopneumonia, the correct statement would be the collaborative problem *Risk for Complications of Bronchopneumonia*.

Risk for Aspiration related to difficulty swallowing

Difficulty swallowing is validation for *Impaired Swallowing*; thus, *Impaired Swallowing related to difficulty swallowing secondary to effects of Parkinson's disorder* would be more informative. Nursing measures would include prevention of aspiration.

Key Concepts

General Considerations

- Central nervous system (CNS) depression interferes with the protective mechanism of the sphincters.
- Nasogastric and endotracheal tubes cause incomplete closure of the esophageal sphincters and depress the gag and cough reflexes.
- Difficulty swallowing is a disturbing symptom that occurs in the vast majority of palliative care patients. In fact, swallowing disorders are part of the natural process of the end of life, irrespective of the etiology (Goldsmith & Cohen, 2014).
- The risk of aspiration is high with corresponding pneumonia.
- Food and eating is an important social event. Swallowing dysfunction can negatively impact social interaction, communication, intimacy, food consumption and nutrition (Goldsmith & Cohen, 2014).
- The volume and characteristics of the aspirated contents influence morbidity and mortality. Food particles can cause mechanical blockage. Gastric juice erodes alveoli, and capillaries and causes chemical pneumonitis.

Pediatric Considerations

- A proportionately oversized airway diameter in infants and small children increases the risk of aspiration of foreign objects (Hockenberry & Wilson, 2015).
- Children, especially toddlers, have a natural curiosity, seek attractive objects, and frequently put things in their mouth. Children cannot comprehend danger to self or others.
- Common household objects and food items that are aspirated include balloons (toy rubber balloons are the leading cause of choking deaths from children's products), baby powder, hot dogs, candy, nuts, grapes, and small batteries.
- Children with certain congenital anomalies (e.g., tracheoesophageal fistula, cleft palate, gastroesophageal reflux) are at greater risk for aspiration.

Focus Assessment Criteria

Subjective Data

Assess for Related Factors

History of a problem with swallowing or aspiration
Presence or history of (see Related Factors—Pathophysiologic)

Objective Data

Assess for Related Factors

Ability to swallow, chew, feed self
Neuromuscular impairment:
- Decreased/absent gag reflex
- Decreased strength on excursion of muscles involved in mastication
- Perceptual impairment
- Facial paralysis

Mechanical obstruction:
- Edema
- Tracheostomy tube
- Tumor

Perceptual patterns/awareness
Level of consciousness
Condition of oropharyngeal cavity
Nasal regurgitation
Hoarseness
Aspiration
Coughing 1 or 2 seconds after swallowing
Dehydration
Apraxia

Goals

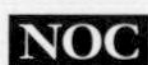
Aspiration Control

The individual will not experience aspiration as evidenced by the following indicators:

- Relates measures to prevent aspiration
- Names foods or fluids that are high risk for causing aspiration

The parent will reduce opportunities for aspirations as evidenced by the following indicators:

- Removes small objects from child's reach
- Inspects toys for removable small objects
- Discourages the child from putting objects in his or her mouth

Interventions

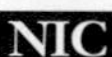
Aspiration Precautions, Airway Management, Positioning, Airway Suctioning

Assess Causative or Contributing Factors

- Refer to Related Factors

Ensure a Consult with Speech–Language Pathologist Is Initiated

R: *Speech–language pathologists (SLPs) are expert in assessment and management of oropharyngeal swallowing disorders.*

Reduce the Risk of Aspiration in

Individuals with Decreased Strength, Decreased Sensorium, or Autonomic Disorders

- Maintain head-of-bed elevation at an angle of 30° to 45°, unless contraindicated.

R: *There is evidence that a sustained supine position (zero-degree head-of-bed elevation) increases gastroesophageal reflux and the probability for aspiration (*American Association of Critical Care Nurses, 2011).*

- Use sedatives as sparingly as feasible.

R: *Sedation causes reduced cough and gag reflexes. It can impair the person's ability clear oropharyngeal secretions and refluxed gastric contents (American Association of Critical Care Nurses, 2011).*

- Maintain a side-lying position if not contraindicated by injury.
- If the individual cannot be positioned on the side, open the oropharyngeal airway by lifting the mandible up and forward and tilting the head backward. (For a small infant, hyperextension of the neck may not be effective.)
- Assess for position of the tongue, ensuring it has not dropped backward, occluding the airway.
- Keep the head of the bed elevated, if not contraindicated by hypotension or injury.
- Maintain good oral hygiene. Clean teeth and use mouthwash on cotton swab; apply petroleum jelly to lips, removing encrustations gently.
- Clear secretions from mouth and throat with a tissue or gentle suction.
- Reassess frequently for obstructive material in mouth and throat.
- Reevaluate frequently for good anatomic positioning.
- Maintain side-lying position after feedings.

R: *Regurgitation is often silent in people with decreased sensorium or depressed mental states.*

- Positions are maintained to reduce aspiration.

R: *Increased intragastric pressure can contribute to regurgitation and aspiration. Causes include bolus tube feedings, obstructions, obesity, pregnancy, and autonomic dysfunction.*

Individuals With Gastrointestinal Tubes and Feedings

- Confirm that tube placement has been verified by radiography or aspiration of greenish fluid (check hospital/organizational policy for preferred method).

R: *Verifying correct placement of feeding tubes is done most reliably by radiography. Aspiration of green-colored fluid or gastric aspirant with a pH of 6.5 or lower is also reliable.*

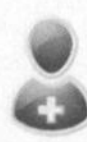

CLINICAL ALERT Verifying placement by instilling air and simultaneously auscultating or by aspirating nongreen fluid has proven inaccurate.

- Observe for a change in length of the external portion of the feeding tube, as determined by movement of the marked portion of the tube (American Association of Critical Care Nurses, 2011).
- If there is a doubt about the tube's position, request an X-ray.
- Maintain head-of-bed elevation at an angle of 30° to 45°, unless contraindicated.

R: *This helps to prevent reflux by use of reverse gravity.*

- Aspirate for residual contents before each feeding for tubes positioned gastrically.
- Measure gastric residual volumes (GRVs) every 4 hours in critically ill person. Delay tube feeding if GRV is greater than 150 mL.

R: *Gastric distention predisposes to regurgitation*

- Regulate gastric feedings using an intermittent schedule, allowing periods for stomach emptying between feeding intervals.
- Monitor for tolerance to enteral feedings by noting abdominal distention, complaints of abdominal pain, observing for passage of flatus and stool at 4-hour intervals (American Association of Critical Care Nurses, 2011).
- Avoid bolus feedings in those at high risk for aspiration.

R: *To administer an entire 4-hour volume of formula over a period of a few minutes is more likely to predispose to regurgitation of gastric contents than is the steady administration of the same volume over a period of 4 hours (American Association of Critical Care Nurses, 2011).*

For an Older Adult With Difficulties Chewing and Swallowing

- See *Impaired Swallowing*.

Initiate Health Teaching and Referrals, as Indicated

- Instruct on causes and prevention of aspiration.
- Maintain oral hygiene to prevent pneumonia related to oral bacteria aspiration.
- Have the family demonstrate tube-feeding technique.
- Refer to a community nursing agency for assistance at home.
- Teach the Heimlich or abdominal thrust maneuver to remove aspirated foreign bodies.

R: *The risk of aspiration increases after discharge due to less supervision.*

Risk for Falls

NANDA-I Definition

Vulnerable to increased susceptibility to falling that may cause physical harm and compromised health.

Risk Factors

Pathophysiologic

Related to altered cerebral function secondary to hypoxia

Related to syncope, vertigo, or dizziness

Related to impaired mobility secondary to (e.g., cerebrovascular accident, arthritis, parkinsonism)

Related to loss of limb

Related to impaired vision

Related to hearing impairment

Related to fatigue

Related to orthostatic hypotension

Treatment Related

Related to lack of awareness of environmental hazards secondary to (e.g., confusion)

Related to improper use of aids (e.g., crutches, canes, walkers, wheelchairs)

Related to tethering devices (e.g., IV, Foley, compression therapy, telemetry)

Related to prolonged bed rest

Related to side effects of medication(s)

Situational (Personal, Environmental)

Related to history of falls

Related to improper footwear

Related to unstable gait

Older Adult

Related to faulty judgments, secondary cognitive deficits

Related to sedentary lifestyle and loss of muscle strength

Related to fear of falling and the resulting physiologic deconditioning

Author's Note

This new nursing diagnosis can be used to specify an individual at risk for falls. If the individual is at risk for various types of injuries (e.g., a cognitively impaired individual), the broader diagnosis *Risk for Injury* is more useful.

Errors in Diagnostic Statements

Risk for Falls related to inadequate supervision

This diagnosis represents a legally inappropriate statement. Even if it is true, the diagnosis should be rewritten as *Risk for Falls related to inability to identify environmental hazards.*

Key Concepts

- Refer to *Risk for Injury.*

Focus Assessment Criteria

Fall Risk Assessment

Assess for the Following Risk Factors

Record the number of checks in the fall assessment scores in the brackets () as *High Risk for Falls* (score) or add the risk factors, for example, as *High Risk for Falls related to* instability, postural hypotension, and IV equipment.

Assess all individuals for risk factors for falls, using the assessment tool in the institution. The following represents one assessment tool:

Variables Score

History of falling

No (score as 0)
Yes (score as 25)

Secondary diagnosis

No (score as 0)
Yes (score as 15)

Ambulatory aid

Bed rest/nurse assist (score as 0)
Crutches/cane/walker (score as 15)
Furniture (score as 30)

IV or IV access

No (score as 0)
Yes (score as 20)

Gait

Normal/bed rest/immobile (score as 0)
Weak (score as 10)
Impaired (score as 20)

Mental status

Knows own limits (score as 0)
Overestimates or forgets limits (score as 15)

Total Score __________

Risk Level MFS Score Action

No risk

0 to 24 Good basic nursing care

Low to moderate risk

25 to 45 Implement standard fall prevention interventions.

High risk

46+ Implement high-risk fall prevention interventions.
Morse Fall Scale (*Morse, 1979). Used with permission.

Timed Up and Go (TUG) (*Podsiadlo & Richardson, 1991)

For individuals who are independent and ambulatory but frail, fatigued, and/or with possible compromised ambulation, assess the person's ability to TUG:

Have the person wear their usual footwear and use any assistive device they normally use.
Have the person sit in the chair with their back to the chair and their arms resting on the arm rests.
Ask the person to stand up from a standard chair and walk a distance of 10 feet (3 m).
Have the person turn around, walk back to the chair, and sit down again.
Timing begins when the person starts to rise from the chair and ends when he or she returns to the chair and sits down.

The person should be given one practice trial and then three actual trials if needed. The times from the three actual trials are averaged.

Predictive Results

Seconds	***Rating***
<10	Freely mobile
10 to 19	Mostly independent
20 to 29	Variable mobility
>29	Impaired mobility

Goals

NOC

Risk Control, Fall Occurrence, Fall Prevention Behavior, Personal Safety Behavior, Safe Home Environment

The individual will not injure himself or herself during hospital stay as evidenced by the following indicators:

- Identifies factors that increase risk of injury
- Describes appropriate safety measures
- Will agree to ask for help when needed

Interventions

NIC

Fall Prevention; Environmental Management: Safety, Health Education; Surveillance: Safety, Risk Identification; Technology Management; Medication Management; Family Involvement Promotion; Environmental Management: Home Preparation

Involve All Hospital Personnel on Every Shift in the Fall Prevention Program

R: *Approximately 14% of all falls in hospitals are accidental, another 8% are unanticipated physiologic falls, and 78% are anticipated physiologic falls.*

- Always glance into the room of a high-risk person when passing his or her room.
- Alert other departments of high-risk individuals when off unit for tests, procedures.
- Address fall prevention and risks with every hand-off and transfer.
- Seek to identify reversible risk factors in all individuals. Be aware of changing individual conditions and a change in risk status.
- Identify in a private conference room the number of falls on the unit monthly (e.g., poster).

R: *Intradisciplinary approach to fall prevention is effective when falls are viewed not as inevitable accidents but as preventable events.*

Identify the Individual's Risk for Falls

- Assess the person's ability to TUG (Podsiadlo & Richardson, 1991).
- Have the person wear his or her usual footwear and use any assistive device he or she uses.
- Refer to Focus Assessment criteria.

R: *Numerous researchers have reported that the TUG test is reliable (87% sensitivity and specificity) for community-dwelling older adults (Beling & Roller, 2009). Loss of strength in legs and ankles is a common cause of falls in older persons; however, it is not an outcome of aging but one of a sedentary lifestyle. It is not inevitable; it is preventable.*

- Initiate the institution's standard and protocol to prevent falls. One example is:
  - "Both Carondelet St. Joseph's Hospital (Tucson, Az) and Providence Health Center used the Ruby Slippers Program as part of their fall prevention programs. Patients at high risk of falling were provided with a pair of bright red double treaded slipper socks. Staff throughout both organizations were oriented to the fact that patients wearing these socks were at high risk of falling. Staff not involved in direct patient care (e.g., housekeepers) knew to summon help if they observed these patients trying to get out of bed or if they saw them unattended. At St. Joseph's, a picture of a ruby slipper on the door to patient rooms also alerted staff that the patient was at high risk of falling, whereas Providence used a red falling star on the doors and charts to identify these patients for staff" (Lancaster et al., 2007, p. 372).

R: *Standard interventions to prevent any individual from falling are instituted on admission. In addition, high-risk individuals are identified using the institution's protocol (e.g., red slippers, colored bracelet). Ensure that tables and chairs with side arms are stable. Persons with lower extremity weakness will benefit from sturdy chairs.*

Reduce or Eliminate Contributing Factors for Falls

Related to Unfamiliar Environment

- Orient to his or her environment (e.g., location of bathroom, bed controls, call bell). Leave a light on in the bathroom at night. Ensure that path to bathroom is clear.

R: *Orientation helps provide familiarity; a light at night helps the individual find the way safely.*

- Teach him or her to keep the bed in the low position with side rails up at night.

R: *The low position makes it easier for the individual to get in and out of bed.*

- Make sure that the telephone, eyeglasses, urinal, and frequently used personal belongings are within easy reach.

R: *Keeping objects at hand helps prevent falls due to overreaching and overextending.*

- Instruct to request assistance whenever needed.

R: *Getting needed help with ambulation and other activities reduces a individual's risk of injury.*

- For individuals with difficulty accessing toilet:
  - If urgency exists, evaluate for a urinary tract infection.

R: *New onset urinary urgency can be a sign of an infection.*

- Provide an opportunity to use bathroom/urinal/bedpan every 2 hours while awake, at bedtime, and upon awakening.

R: *Thirty percent of falls are related to attempting to access the bathroom and can be prevented by timed toileting schedule (Alcee, 2000).*

- Frequently scan floor for wet areas, objects on floor.
- Implement an elimination protocol, for example, toileting rounds every hour to offer bathroom assistance.

R: *Providing regular times for elimination can reduce getting out of bed to toilet or incontinence.*

Related to Gait Instability/Balance Problems

- Explain that gait and balance problems are due to underuse and deconditioning, *not aging.*
- Alert individuals that they may not be able to prevent a fall if they trip.

R: *Weak leg muscles and decreased range of motion (ROM) in ankles prevent a safe recovery from a slip or trip.*

- Explain that deficiencies in vitamin D interferes with one's postural balance, propulsion, and navigation and vitamin B_{12} deficiencies cause weakness, tiredness, or light-headedness

R: *Vitamin D supplements improve gait performance and prevent falls by more than 22% in older adults (Annweiler et al., 2010).*

- Seek to include a vitamin D and vitamin B_{12} level in next laboratory tests. Explain that the normal range is 30 to 100 nmol/L.

R: *Researchers have reported that the level should be at least 60 nmol/L to affect a reduction of falls (Annweiler et al., 2010).*

- Refer to Getting Started for strategies and exercises to improve gait and balance on thePoint at http://thePoint.lww.com/Carpenito6e.
- Instruct the individual to wear slippers with nonskid soles and to avoid shoes with thick, soft soles.

R: *These precautions can help prevent falls from slipping. Thick soles require adequate lifting of feet as one walks or the soles will catch and trip the person.*

- Ensure that mobility aids are available and reachable. Wheelchairs should always be locked. Remind that IV poles are on wheels and are not sturdy.

R: *Falls occur when an individual is reaching for a mobility aid or for a wheelchair not in the locked position.*

- Ensure that call bell, TV controls, and telephone are within reach.

R: *Stretching and reaching can contribute to rolling out of bed.*

Related to Tethering Devices (IVs, Foley, telemetry, compression devices)

- Evaluate if tethering devices can be discontinued at night.
- Can the IV be converted to a saline port?
- If the individual is competent, teach him or her how to safely ambulate with devices to bathroom or advise to call for assistance.

R: *Individuals can become entangled in lines and tubes and fall.*

- Creation of elimination protocol
- Pharmacy oversight of high-risk medications
- Use of low beds
- Prepackaging of components used for falls prevention tool kits
- Use of bed alarms
- Collaboration with physicians to reduce falls (e.g., medication orders such as sedatives)
- Diversion therapy (e.g., aprons, lacing boards)
- Staff scripting (e.g., what to say to patients when entering and leaving the room)

Related to Orthostatic Hypotension

- Refer to *Risk for Injury—Related to Vertigo Secondary to Orthostatic Hypotension.*

Related to Medication Side Effects

- Review the person's medication reconciliation completed on admission.

- Question regarding alcohol use.

R: *Alcohol can potentiate side effects of sombulence/dizziness.*

- Question if the person has side effects when taking certain meds.
- Question if, in the person's opinion, he or she is taking a medication for pain that is not working.

R: *Some medications might need to be discontinued because of side effects or ineffective therapeutic response.*

- Review with pharmacist/physicians/NP the present medications and evaluate those that can contribute to dizziness and if they should be discontinued, have dose reduced, or replaced with an alternative (Kaufamn & Kaplan, 2015a; *Riefkohl, Bieber, Burlingame, & Lowenthal, 2003).
  - Antidepressants (e.g., SSRIs)
  - Antipsychotics
  - Benzodiazepines
  - Antihistamines (e.g., Benadryl, hydroxyzine)
  - Anticonvulsants
  - Nonsteroidal anti-inflammatory drugs
  - Muscle relaxants
  - Narcotic analgesics
  - Antiarrhythmics (type 1A)
  - Digoxin

R: *The use of medications is one of the many different factors that can contribute to balance problems and the risk of falls. Published research suggests an association between the use of these drugs or drug class and an increased risk of falling (Riefkohl et al., 2003).*

Related to Confused/Uncooperative/Impaired Cognition

- Consider use of electronic devices in bed, chair, video surveillance.
- Follow institutional policy for side rails.
- Consider use of sitter.
- Move person to a more observable room.
- Plan to complete shift documentation in room of high-risk person.

R: *In some cases, extra measures are necessary to ensure an individual's s safety and prevent injury to him or her and others. The cost of extra surveillance will be less than the cost of injury and human suffering related to a fall.*

If a Person Falls or Reports a Fall

- Call out for help immediately and continue to attend to the individual.
- Implement the following:
  - Do not move initially.
  - If person hit head or if unknown, immobilize cervical spine.
  - Assess if loss of consciousness was experienced, complaints of pain, is confused.
  - Take baseline vital signs, blood glucose.
  - Determine baseline Glascow coma scale.
  - Assess risk for intracranial bleed (anticoagulants, thrombocytopenia, coagulopathy).
  - Assess for lacerations, fractures, contusions, decreased ROM.
  - Clean and dress any wounds.
  - Implement neuro checks q2 hours $\times$ 24 hours.
  - Contact the appropriate physician/NP to discuss findings and implications.

R: *Immediate assessment with notification of medical staff is indicated in order to determine the extent of injuries and the need for diagnostic tests and or treatments.*

R: *Postfall huddles can identify falls amenable to prevention interventions as individual education, staff heightened awareness, and reduction of risk factors (Gray-Miceli, Ratcliffe, & Johnson, 2010).*

SBAR

Situation: Ask individual and witnesses what happened, at what time, location, who witnessed.

Background: Prior fall risk score, history of falls

Assessment: Evaluate the following:

Side rails up/down	Fall risk alerts present (placards, wrist band)	
Position of bed	Call light reachable	Sitter present
Nonskid footwear	Use of assistive devices	Visitors present
Presence of clutter	Bed alarm on	Presence of IV, Foley
Staffing ratios		

Recommendation: Communicate identified factors that caused or contributed to the fall.

- Engage in a postfall huddle within 1 hour of fall. Involve all staff. Avoid all discussions of blaming. Refer institution's protocol for documentation guidelines of postfall huddles.

Teach strategies to decrease risk of falling at home.

- Ensure proper use of assistive devices. Consult with physical therapist.

R: *Expert instruction is needed to ensure proper equipment and use.*

- Perform ankle-strengthening exercises daily (*Schoenfelder, 2000):
  - Stand behind a straight chair, with feet slightly apart.
  - Slowly raise both heels until body weight is on the balls of the feet; hold for a count of three (e.g., 1 Mississippi, 2 Mississippi, 3 Mississippi).
  - Do 5 to 10 repetitions; increase repetitions as strength increases.
- Walk at least two or three times a week.
  - Use ankle exercises as a warm-up before walking.
  - Begin walking with someone at side, if needed, for 10 minutes.
  - Increase time and speed according to capabilities.

R: *Ankle-strengthening and a walking program can improve balance, increase ankle strength, improve walking speed, decrease falls and fear of falling, and increase confidence in performing activities of daily living (Schoenfelder, 2000).*

- Go to thePoint at http://thePoint.lww.com/Carpenito6e and access Getting Started for take-home guidelines to prevent falls at home and exercises to improve muscle strength and balance.

Older Adults

- Refer to *Risk for Injury*.

Risk for Poisoning

NANDA-I Definition

Vulnerable for accidental exposure to or ingestion of drugs or dangerous products in sufficient doses that may compromise health

Risk Factors

Presence of risk factors (see Risk Factors for *Risk for Injury*).

Risk for Suffocation

NANDA-I Definition

Vulnerable to inadequate air available for inhalation, which may compromise health

Risk Factors

External

Access to empty refrigerator/freezer
Eating large mouthfuls of food
Gas leak
Low-strung clothesline
Pacifier around infant's neck
Playing with plastic bags
Propped bottle in infant's mouth
Small object in airway
Smoking in bed
Soft items in crib
Unattended in water
Unvented fuel-burning heater
Vehicle running in closed garage

Other

Insufficient knowledge of safety precautions
Impaired cognitive, motor emotional, olfactory functioning

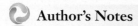

Author's Notes

The above risk factors can be taught to children/caretakers and adults to help prevent suffocation. Refer to *Risk for Injury* for additional focus topics.

Risk for Thermal Injury

NANDA-I Definition

Vulnerable to extreme temperature damage to skin and mucous membranes, which may compromise health

Risk Factors*

Cognitive impairment (e.g., dementia, psychoses)
Developmental level (infants, aged)
Exposure to extreme temperatures
Fatigue
Inadequate supervision
Inattentiveness
Intoxication (alcohol, drug)
Lack of knowledge (individual, caregiver)
Lack of protective clothing (e.g., flame-retardant sleepwear, gloves, ear covering)
Neuromuscular impairment (e.g., stroke, amyotrophic lateral sclerosis, multiple sclerosis)
Neuropathy
Smoking
Treatment-related side effects (e.g., pharmaceutical agents)
Unsafe environment

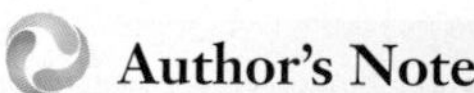

Author's Note

Risk for Thermal Injury is a new NANDA-I diagnosis that focuses on thermal injury only. The risk factors listed represent those related to most type of injuries. It is probably more useful to use *Risk for Injury*, to cover all the types of injury including thermal. Individuals who are at risk for thermal injury are also at risk for a multitude of injuries. *Risk for Thermal Injury* could be used in a standard of care to emphasize environmental hazards such as combustibles, fireworks, heaters, and fires.

Goals

Refer to *Risk for Injury* related to lack of awareness of environmental hazards.

Interventions

Refer to *Risk for Injury* related to lack of awareness of environmental hazards.

Risk for Trauma

NANDA-I Definition

Vulnerable to accidental tissue injury (e.g., wound, burns, fracture), which may compromise health

Risk Factors

Presence of risk factors (see Risk Factors for *Risk for Injury*).

Risk for Perioperative Positioning Injury

NANDA-I Definition

Vulnerable to inadvertent anatomical and physical changes as a result of posture or equipment used during an invasive/surgical procedure, which may compromise health

Risk Factors

Presence of risk factors (see Related Factors).

Related Factors

Hereditary Predisposition\Pathophysiologic

Related to increased vulnerability secondary to (Webster, 2012):

Preexisting generalized neuropathy
Structural anomaly/congenital abnormality (e.g., constriction at thoracic outlet or condylar groove, or arthritic narrowing of joint space)
Chronic disease
Cancer
Thin body frame
Radiation therapy
Osteoporosis
Compromised immune system
Renal, hepatic dysfunction
Infection

Related to compromised tissue perfusion secondary to:
Diabetes mellitus
Anemia
Ascites
Cardiovascular disease
Hypothermia
Dehydration
Hypovolemia
Peripheral vascular disease
History of thrombosis
Edema*
Coagulopathy or presence of hematoma near nerve
Infection/presence of abscess near nerve

Related to vulnerability of stoma during positioning

Related to preexisting contractures or physical impairments secondary to:
Rheumatoid arthritis
Polio

Treatment Related

Related to position requirements and loss of usual sensory protective responses secondary to anesthesia

Related to surgical procedures of 2 hours or longer

Related to vulnerability of implants or prostheses (e.g., pacemakers) during positioning

Situational (Personal, Environmental)

Related to compromised circulation secondary to:

Obesity*
Tobacco use
Pregnancy
Infant status
Cool operating suite
Elder status

Maturational

Related to increased vulnerability to tissue injury secondary to:

Author's Note

This diagnosis focuses on identifying the vulnerability for tissue, nerve, and joint injury resulting from required positions for surgery. The addition of *perioperative positioning* to *Risk for Injury* adds etiology to the label.

If an individual has no preexisting risk factors that make him or her more vulnerable to injury, this diagnosis could be used with no related factors because they are evident. If related factors are desired, the statement could read *Risk for Perioperative Positioning Injury related to position requirements for surgery and loss of usual sensory protective measures secondary to anesthesia*.

When an individual has preexisting risk factors, the statement should include these—for example, *Risk for Perioperative Positioning Injuries* related to compromised tissue perfusion secondary to peripheral arterial disease.

Errors in Diagnostic Statements

***Risk for Perioperative Positioning Injury* related to inadequate protective measures**

These related factors are legally problematic. Even if inadequate protective measures are a problem, they must not be included in the diagnostic statement. Instead, this problem should be referred to nursing management.

Key Concepts

General Considerations

- Perioperative peripheral nerve injuries (PPNI) are a common and potentially catastrophic complication of anesthesia and surgery. These injuries include a range of morbidity from transient and clinically minor injury to severe permanent injury (Webster, 2012).
- Retrospective studies have found that the incidence of permanent nerve damage after a surgical procedure and anesthesia is 0.03% to 1.4% (Webster, 2012).
- Commonly injured nerves include the ulnar nerve (28%), brachial plexus (20%), lumbosacral root (16%), and spinal cord (13%). Injury is less common for the sciatic, median, radial, and femoral nerves (Webster, 2012).
- Prolonged immobility diminishes the pulmonary capillary blood flow volume. Positional pressure on the ribs or the diaphragm's ability to force abdominal contents downward limits lung expansion.
- Anesthesia causes peripheral blood vessels to dilate, resulting in hypotension, and decreases blood return to heart and lungs. Prolonged immobility causes pooling in vascular beds.
- Hypothermia (there is a high incidence of nerve injury after induced hypothermia) (Webster, 2012)
- People with obesity are at increased risk for injury from surgical positions as a result of the following:
  - Lifting them into position is difficult.
  - Massive tissue and pressure areas need extra padding.
  - The mechanics of manipulating adipose tissue may prolong length of surgery.

- Recovery period may be prolonged because adipose tissue retains fat-soluble agents and slows elimination of agents.
- Venous stasis decreases circulation, and adipose tissue has a poor blood supply.
- Anesthesia causes the less normal defenses to protect against excessive manipulation.

Geriatric Considerations

- Osteoarthritis, loss of subcutaneous fat, decreased peripheral circulation, and wasted flaccid muscles can contribute to injury or trauma to bones, joints, nerves, and skin when on the operating table (*Martin, 2000).

Focus Assessment Criteria

Subjective Data

Assess for Preexisting Risk Factors

Refer to Related Factors.

Objective Data

Assess for Presurgical Risk Factors

Skin
- Temperature (cool, warm)
- Color (pale, dependent erythema, flushed, cyanotic, brown discolorations)
- Ulcerations (size, location, description of surrounding tissue)

Bilateral pulses (radial, posterior tibial, dorsalis pedis)
- Rate, rhythm
- Volume
- +0 = Absent, nonpalpable
- +1 = Thready, weak, fades in and out
- +2 = Present but diminished
- +3 = Normal, easily palpable
- +4 = Aneurysmal

Paresthesia (numbness, tingling, burning)
Edema (location, pitting)
Capillary refill (normal less than 3 seconds)
Range of motion (normal, compromised)
Current muscle or joint pain
- 0 = No pain; 10 = Worst pain

Goals

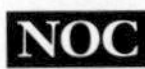

Circulation Status, Neurologic Status, Tissue Perfusion: Peripheral

The individual will have no neuromuscular damage or injury related to the surgical position as evidenced by the following indicators:

- Padding is used as indicated for procedure.
- Limbs are secured when at risk.
- Limbs are flexed when indicated.

Interventions

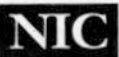

Positioning Intraoperative, Surveillance, Pressure Management

- Determine whether the individual has preexisting risk factors (refer to Risk Factors); communicate findings to surgical team.
- Before positioning, assess and document:
  - Range-of-motion ability
  - Physical abnormalities (skin, contractions)
  - External/internal prostheses or implants
  - Neurovascular status
  - Circulatory status
- Advise if any preexisting factors exist and determine if the position will be arranged before or after anesthesia.

R: *Documentation of all visible abnormalities is critical before surgery. Tissue and skin can be injured by excessive pressure or bruised by hitting a hard surface. People more vulnerable to pressure injuries are the very young; older adults; those who are dehydrated, very thin, or obese; and those undergoing more than 2 hours of immobility.*

- Discuss with the surgeon the surgical position desired.
- Move the individual from the transport stretcher to the operating room (OR) bed.
  - Have a minimum of two people with their hands free (e.g., not holding an IV bag).
  - Explain the transfer to the individual. Lock all wheels on the stretcher and bed.
  - Ask to move slowly to the OR bed. Assist during the move. Do not pull or drag the individual.
  - When the individual is on the OR bed, attach a safety belt a few inches above the knees with a space of three fingerbreadths.
  - Check that legs are not crossed and that feet are slightly separated and not over the edge.
  - Do not leave the person unattended.

R: *These strategies reduce injury from shearing and trauma.*

- Always ask the anesthesiologist or nurse anesthetist for permission before moving or repositioning an anesthetized. Move the person slowly and gently, watching all tubes, drains, lines, etc.

R: *If repositioning is necessary after induction, lifting, rather than rolling or pulling, the individual prevents shearing forces and friction. Shearing occurs when the dermal layers stay fixed because of the friction between linen and skin, and tissues attached to bony structures move with the weight of the torso. Tissue layers slide on each other, resulting in the kinking or stretching of subcutaneous blood vessels, thus obstructing blood flow to and from areas (Grossman & Porth, 2014).*

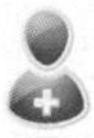

CLINICAL ALERT At no time should the individual's body be leaned on, pressed on, or impinged in any way by staff, equipment, or the devices used to secure safe positioning (Conner, 2006).

- Reduce vulnerability to injury (soft tissue, joint, nerves, blood vessels)
  - Align the neck and spine at all times.
  - Gently manipulate the joints. Do not abduct more than 90°.
  - Do not let limbs extend off the OR bed. Reposition slowly and gently.
  - Use a drawsheet above the elbows to tuck in arms at the side or abduct arm on an arm board with padding.
- Attempt to maintain natural positions without stretch to nerves/muscles/tendons/vessels

R: *Anesthetic agents interfere with normal vasodilation and constriction, thus reducing perfusion to bony prominences or compressed or dependent limbs.*

- Protect eyes and ears from injury.
  - Use padding or a special headrest to protect ears, superficial nerves, and blood vessels of the face if the head is on its side.
  - Ensure that the ear is not bent when positioned.
  - If needed, protect eyes from abrasions with an eye patch or shield.

R: *Excessive pressure of position, equipment, or surgery can injure the face and eyes. Excessive pressure to the eyes can cause thrombosis of the central renal artery. Eyes should be kept closed and lubricated to prevent drying and scratching.*

- Depending on the surgical position used, protect vulnerable areas; document position and protection measures used (*Rothrock, 2003).

Supine

- If the supine position is maintained for long periods of time, skin breakdown, lumbar strain, nerve injury, and circulatory compromise can occur, and respiratory compromise if the person is in the Trendelenburg position (Conner, 2006).
  - Pad the calcaneus, sacrum, coccyx, olecranon process, scapula, ischial tuberosity, and occiput.
  - Keep the arms at side, palms down or abducted on an arm board.
  - Protect the head and ears if the head is turned to the side.

Trendelenburg

- If the supine position is maintained for long periods of time, skin breakdown, lumbar strain, nerve injury, and circulatory compromise can occur, and respiratory compromise if the person is in the Trendelenburg position (Conner, 2006).
  - Use a well-padded shoulder brace over the acromion process, not soft tissue, and away from the neck.

Reverse Trendelenburg

- Use a padded footboard.

Jackknife (Modified Prone)

- The adverse effects of the jackknife position includes skin breakdown, nerve injury, and reduced respiration (Conner, 2006).
  - Use padded arm boards at correct heights to allow elbows to bend comfortably.
  - Place a soft pillow under the down ear.
  - Cushion hips and thighs with large pillows.
  - Cushion breasts.
  - Cushion male genitalia in natural position.
  - Use a large pillow under the lower legs and ankles to raise the toes off the bed.
  - Use additional padding on the shoulder girdle, olecranon, anterosuperior iliac spine, patella, and dorsum of the foot.
  - Apply a safety strap across the thighs.

Prone

- The prone position can cause skin breakdown, reduced respiration, circulation, nerve damage, eye or ear damage, damage to the breasts in women, or genitals in men (Conner, 2006).
  - Position two large body rolls longitudinally from the acromioclavicular joint to the iliac crest.
  - Refer to jackknife for additional information.

Laminectomy

- After induction of anesthesia, at least six people help roll the individual from the stretcher to the OR bed onto the laminectomy brace.
- Keep body aligned.
- Protect limbs from torsion.
- Place rolled towels in axillary regions.
- Follow precautions for jackknife.

Lithotomy

- The potential hazards lithotomy position are skin breakdown, nerve damage, musculoskeletal injury (improper raising and lowering of the legs), and circulatory compromise. The person may also experience hypotension if the legs are raised or lowered too quickly (Conner, 2006).
- Prepare stirrups with padding.
- Have two people simultaneously and slowly raise the individual's legs with slight rotation of the hips. Gently position the knees slightly flexed.
- Position the person's buttocks about 1 inch over the end of the table.
- Use a small lumbar pad and extra padding in the sacral area.
- Cover the legs with cotton boots.
- Position arms on arm boards or loosely over abdomen, supported with a sheet.

Fowler

- Position the neck in straight alignment.
- Use a padded footboard.
- Support the knees with a pillow.
- Cross the arms loosely over the abdomen and tape them on the pillow.

Sims (Lateral)

R: *Potential injury in the lateral position includes skin breakdown, nerve injury, and reduced respiration (Conner, 2006).*

- Position the individual on the side with arms extended on double-arm boards.
- Flex the lower leg.
- Use a small pillow under the head.
- Use a rolled towel in the axillary area of the downside arm.
- Elevate and pad the flank.
- Flex the lower leg and place a long pillow along the length of the leg to the groin.

- Use a 4-in strip of adhesive tape attached to one side of the table, over the iliac crest and to the other side.
- Protect ankles and feet from pressure.
- Protect male genitalia, female breasts, and ear as for jackknife position.

R: *Prolonged positioning can cause mechanical pressure on peripheral and superficial nerves. Hyperextension (greater than 90° angle) of a limb of an anesthetized person can cause nerve injuries (Conner, 2006; *Rothrock, 2003)*

- Hyperextension of the arm on an arm board can injure the brachial plexus (in the arm). Improper positioning of the brace also can injure the brachial plexus.
- Ulnar nerve injuries occur when an elbow slips off the mattress and is compressed between the table and the medial epicondyle.
- Position the forearm supine, which helps protect the ulnar nerve, as prolonged pronation of the forearm can compress the ulnar nerve in the cubital tunnel (Conner, 2006).
- Radial nerve injuries occur when the nerve is compressed between the individual and the table surface or from striking the table.
- Saphenous and peroneal nerve damage occurs with the use of stirrups with lithotomy—compression of the peroneal nerve against the stirrups or of the saphenous nerve between the metal popliteal knee support stirrup and the medial tibial condyle.

R: *Anesthesia and muscle relaxants cause the loss of the normal protective range-of-motion limitations (e.g., muscles stretch and strain, causing joint, tendon, or ligament injuries) (Conner, 2006).*

R: *Anesthetic agents interfere with normal vasodilation and constriction, thus reducing perfusion to bony prominences or compressed or dependent limbs. Padding protects bony prominences and limbs from injury.*

- If feasible, ask if he or she feels pain, burning, pressure, or any discomfort after positioning.

R: *This can direct the nurse to assess the area.*

- Continually, assess that team members are not leaning on the individual, especially limbs.
- Ensure that the head is lifted slightly every 30 minutes.
- Slowly reposition or return the person to supine position after certain surgical positions (e.g., Trendelenburg, lithotomy, reverse Trendelenburg, jackknife, lateral).

R: *Positions are changed slowly to prevent severe hypotension.*

- Assess skin condition when surgery is over; document findings; continue to assess and to relieve pressure to vulnerable areas postoperatively

R: *The OR nurse is continuously assessing and reporting abnormal data to the appropriate professionals to relieve pressure to vulnerable areas.*

Risk for Urinary Tract Injury

Definition

Vulnerable to damage of the urinary tract injury from use of catheters, which may compromise health

Risk Factors

Condition preventing ability to secure catheter (e.g., burn, trauma, amputation)
Long-term use of urinary catheter
Multiple catheterizations
Retention balloon inflated to ≥30 mL
Use of large caliber urinary catheter

Author's Note

This new NANDA-I nursing diagnosis represents prevention of trauma to the urethra during catheterization and/or with prolonged catheter use. Preventive strategies for reducing or eliminating urethra trauma are part of the protocols for preventing infection. The primary interventions are preventing unnecessary catheterizations, reducing the length of time and management of the catheter to prevent trauma/infection. Thus, this diagnosis is incorporated in *Risk for Infection*.

Goals

Refer to *Risk for Infection.*

Interventions

Note: These interventions are also found with *Risk for Infection.*

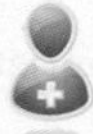

Clinical Alert Approximately 20% of hospital-acquired bacteremias arise from the urinary tract, and the mortality associated with this condition is about 10% (Fekete, 2015; Gould et al. 2009). When a catheter is in place, remind the prescriber every 2 days to reconsider if catheter is still indicated, for example, using reminder protocols or institute the nursing protocol which allows reassessment and determination if the catheter can be removed.

Insert Catheters Only for Appropriate Indications:

R: *"The single most important factor for preventing urinary catheter-related complications is limiting their use to appropriate indications (Fekete, 2015; Gould et al. 2009; Schaeffer, 2015).*

- Presence of acute urinary retention or bladder outlet obstruction
- Need for accurate measurements of urinary output in critically ill individuals
- Perioperative use for selected surgical procedures:
- Urologic surgery or other surgery on contiguous structures of the genitourinary tract or colon-rectal
- Management of hematuria associated with clots
- Management of neurogenic bladder
- Anticipated prolonged duration of surgery (catheters inserted for this reason should
- Need for intraoperative monitoring of urinary output
- Large-volume infusions or diuretics during surgery
- Assist in healing of open sacral or perineal wounds in incontinent individuals.
- Intravesical pharmacologic therapy (e.g., bladder cancer)
- Prescribed prolonged immobilization (e.g., potentially unstable thoracic or lumbar spine, multiple traumatic injuries such as pelvic fractures)
- Improve comfort for end-of-life care if needed

R: *A 6% increase in catheter-associated urinary tract infections (CAUTI) was reported between 2009 and 2013; although initial data from 2014 seem to indicate that these infections have started to decrease (CDC, 2013).*

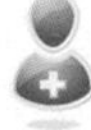

Clincal Alert Fekete cited "Unwarranted urinary catheters are placed in 21% to 50% of hospitalized patients The most common inappropriate indication for placing an indwelling urethral catheter is management of urinary incontinence. While catheter use in these patients may have a short-term benefit, the increased risk of complications associated with their use outweighs any benefit" (Fekete, 2015).

Consider Condom Catheters or Alternatives to Indwelling Catheter Such as Intermittent Catheterization If Possible

Follow Evidence-Based Procedure for Catheter Insertion and Management

- Using a single-use packet of lubricant jelly on the catheter is important in the placement of any catheter, and one should use clinical judgment when deciding whether or not to use anesthetic lubricant or plain lubricant.
- Use the smallest gauge catheter as possible.

R: *This is to reduce urethra trauma.*

- Maintain unobstructed urine flow, keep tubing free from kinks.
- Cleanse the patient's genitalia area with an aseptic cleanser prior to catheter insertion. Do not clean the periurethral area with antiseptics to prevent CAUTI while the catheter is in place. Routine hygiene (e.g., cleaning of the metal surface during daily bathing or showering) is appropriate.
- Secure the thigh with a securement device.

R: *This will prevent movement and urethral traction, which can cause irritation, tissue breakdown, and become an entry site for pathogens.*

- Keep the IUC drainage bag below the level of the bladder at all times.

R: *This prevents stagnant urine from backing into the person.*

- Empty the drainage bag every 8 hours and when the bag is two-thirds full or prior to all patient transfers. Empty using a separate, clean collecting container for each individual.

R: *A full drainage bag will cause traction on the catheter with pressure on the urethra, which can cause irritation, tissue breakdown, and become an entry site for pathogens.*

- Consult with physician/nurse practitioner/physician assistant to discuss the inappropriate use of indwelling catheter in a particular person.
  - Convenience of nursing staff
  - Person has incontinence.
  - Access for obtaining urine for culture or other diagnostic tests when the individual can voluntarily void.
  - For prolonged postoperative duration without appropriate indications (e.g., structural repair of urethra or contiguous structures, prolonged effect of epidural anesthesia)
  - If the IUC has been in place for more than 2 days, provide a daily reminder to the health-care provider to evaluate continued need for the device.
  - Once an IUC is removed, if the person does not void within 4 to 6 hours, use a bedside bladder scanner to determine urine volume. In and out catheterize the patient if the volume is greater than 500 mL; avoid replacing an IUC.
  - Once an IUC is removed, offer a bedside commode if they cannot ambulate safely to the bathroom.

DECREASED INTRACRANIAL ADAPTIVE CAPACITY

NANDA-I Definition

Intracranial fluid dynamic mechanisms that normally compensate for increases in intracranial volumes are compromised, resulting in repeated disproportionate increases in intracranial pressure (ICP) in response to a variety of noxious and nonnoxious stimuli

Defining Characteristics

Baseline intracranial pressure (ICP) ≥10 mm Hg 5 of
Disproportionate increase in ICP following stimuli
Elevated P2 ICP waveform*
Repeated increase in intracranial pressure (ICP) ≥10 mm Hg for more than 5 following external stimuli.
Volume–pressure response test variation (volume:pressure ratio 2, pressure–volume index ≥10 mm Hg*
Wide-amplitude ICP waveform*

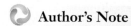

Author's Note

This diagnosis represents increased intracranial pressure. It is a collaborative problem because it requires physician/NP/PA to diagnose and two disciplines to treat—nursing and medicine. In addition, it requires invasive monitoring for diagnosis and assessments. The collaborative problem *Risk for Complications of Increased Intracranial Pressure* represents this clinical situation.

NEONATAL JAUNDICE

Neonatal Jaundice

Risk for Neonatal Jaundice

See also *Risk for Complications of Hyperbilirubinemia.*

NANDA-I Definition

The yellow-orange tint of the neonate's skin and mucous membranes that occurs after 24 hours of life as a result of unconjugated bilirubin in the circulation

Defining Characteristics*

Abnormal blood profile (hemolysis; total serum bilirubin greater than 2 mg/dL: inherited disorder; total serum bilirubin in high-risk range on age in hour-specific nomogram)
Abnormal skin bruising
Yellow-orange skin
Yellow sclera

Related Factors*

Abnormal weight loss (>7% to 8% in breastfeeding newborn; 15% in term infant)
Feeding pattern not well established
Infant experiences difficulty making transition to extrauterine life
Neonate aged 1 to 7 days
Stool (meconium) passage delayed

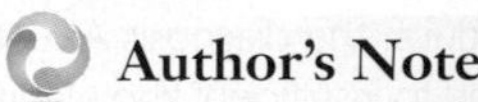

Author's Note

This NANDA-I diagnosis is a collaborative problem (the reader is referred to Section 3, *Risk for Complications of Hyperbilirubinemia*) that requires a laboratory test for diagnosis and treatment from medicine and nursing. Refer to Section 3 on *Risk for Complications of Hyperbilirubinemia* for neonates at risk for or experiencing hyperbilirubinemia.

Risk for Neonatal Jaundice

NANDA-I Definition

At risk for yellow-orange tint of the neonate's skin and mucous membranes that occurs after 24 hours of life as a result of unconjugated bilirubin in the circulation

Risk Factors*

Abnormal weight loss (>7% to 8% in breastfeeding newborn, 15% in term infant)
Feeding pattern not well established
Infant experiences difficulty making the transition to extrauterine life
Neonate aged 1 to 7 days
Prematurity
Stool (meconium) passage delayed

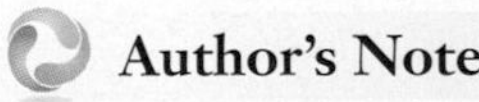

Author's Note

Refer to Author's Note under *Neonatal Jaundice*.

DEFICIENT KNOWLEDGE

NANDA-I Definition

Absence or deficiency of cognitive information related to a specific topic

NANDA-I Defining Characteristics

Accurate performance of test*
Inappropriate behaviors (e.g., hysterical, hostile, agitated, apathetic)*
Inaccurate follow-through of instruction*

Related Factors*

Alteration in cognitive functioning
Alteration in memory
Insufficient intolerance
Misinformation presented by others
Insufficient interest in learning
Insufficient knowledge of resources

Author's Note

Deficient Knowledge does not represent a human response, alteration, or pattern of dysfunction; rather, it is an etiologic or contributing factor (Jenny, 1987). Lack of knowledge can contribute to a variety of responses (e.g., anxiety, self-care deficits). All nursing diagnoses have related individual/family teaching as a part of nursing interventions (e.g., *Impaired Bowel Elimination, Impaired Verbal Communication*). When the teaching relates directly to a specific nursing diagnosis, incorporate the teaching into the plan. When specific teaching is indicated before a procedure, the diagnosis *Anxiety related to unfamiliar environment or procedure* or *Risk for Ineffective Health Management* related to insufficient knowledge of diabetic diet, risk of infection, signs/symptoms of high and low blood glucose levels and management, benefits of exercise, medication regimen can be used.

LATEX ALLERGY RESPONSE

Latex Allergy Response

Risk for Latex Allergy Response

NANDA-I Definition

A hypersensitive reaction to natural latex rubber products

Defining Characteristics

Major (Must be Present)

Positive skin or serum test to natural rubber latex (NRL) extract.

Minor (May be Present)

Allergic conjunctivitis
Asthma
Rhinitis
Urticaria

Related Factors

Biopathophysiologic

Related to hypersensitivity response to the protein component of NRL

Key Concepts

- NRL has been widely used in many products for more than 100 years. The first case of immediate hypersensitivity to latex was reported in 1979 (*Reddy, 1998).

- Use of latex gloves and condoms has increased dramatically since 1985. The increase in total exposure to latex has led to more people with latex sensitivity (Centers for Disease Control and Prevention [CDC], 2015).
- The current statistics for people sensitized to NRL are broken down by risk groups and are as follows (American Latex Allergy Association, 2010):
  - 8% to 17% of health-care workers
  - Up to 68% of children with spina bifida (related to frequent surgeries—anyone who has multiple surgeries is at risk)
  - Less than 1% of the general population in the United States (about 3 million people)
- Risk groups for latex allergy are health-care workers; rubber industry workers; people with spina bifida, history of barium enema, history of indwelling catheter, repeated catheterizations, urogenital abnormalities, or history of repeated or prolonged surgeries or mucous membrane exposure to latex; and people with atopic history or history of food allergy (banana, avocado, mango, kiwi, passion fruit, chestnut, melon, tomato, celery).
- Some reactions to latex products are delayed immunologic responses caused by chemical irritants used in the manufacture of latex gloves. This is a type IV allergic reaction, which is not a true latex allergy. A true latex allergy (type I reaction) occurs shortly after exposure to the proteins in NRL (CDC, 2015; *Kleinbeck, English, Sherley, & Howes, 1998).
- Irritant contact dermatitis is the most common reaction to latex products. Irritant contact dermatitis is not a true allergy. It is the development of dry, itchy, irritated areas on the skin, usually the hands. This reaction is caused by irritation from wearing gloves and by exposure to the powders added to them. Allergic contact dermatitis (sometimes called chemical sensitivity dermatitis) results from the chemicals added to latex during harvesting, processing, or manufacturing. These chemicals can cause a skin rash similar to that of poison ivy (CDC, 2015).

Focus Assessment Criteria

Subjective Data

Assess for Defining Characteristics

History of Swelling, Itching, Sneezing, Itchy Throat, Watery Eyes, or Redness of Skin or Mucous Membranes Upon Exposure to Any of the Following

Dental work	Condom use	Blowing up a balloon
Adhesive tape	Rubber cement	Elastic underwear
Rubber gloves	Shoes	Tennis racket
Golf grip	Garden hose	

Personal History of Any of the Following

Skin rash	Asthma	Eczema
Flushing	Urticaria	Anaphylactic reaction
Nasal, eye, or sinus symptoms		

Allergies to Any of the Following

Avocado	Passion fruit	Peach
Chestnut	Tomato	Banana
Mango	Raw potato	Kiwi
Papaya		

History of Adverse Reaction to or Complication of Surgery

Positive diagnostic testing (e.g., antilatex immunoglobulin E)

Assess for Risk Factors

Occupation with frequent contact with latex in the present or past

History of surgeries, urinary catheterizations, barium enema (before 1992)

Congenital abnormalities; spina bifida

Goals

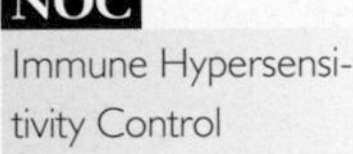

Immune Hypersensitivity Control

The individual will report no exposure to latex, as evidenced by the following indicators:

- Describes products of NRL
- Describes strategies to avoid exposure

Interventions

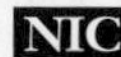

Allergy Management, Latex Precautions, Environmental Risk Protection

Assess for Causative and Contributing Factors

- Refer to Focus Assessment Criteria.

Eliminate Exposure to Latex Products

Use Nonlatex Alternative Supplies

- Clear disposable amber bags
- Silicone baby nipples
- 2 × 2 gauze pads with silk tape in place of adhesive bandages
- Clear plastic or Silastic catheters
- Vinyl or neoprene gloves
- Kling-like gauze

R: *Nonlatex items are sometimes available.*

Protect from Exposure to Latex

- Cover the skin with cloth before applying the blood pressure cuff.
- Do not allow rubber stethoscope tubing to touch the client.
- Do not inject through rubber parts (e.g., heparin locks); use syringe and stopcock.
- Change needles after each puncture of rubber stopper.
- Cover rubber parts with tape.

For Health-Care Workers and Others Who Regularly Wear gloves (CDC, 2015)

- Avoid hypoallergic latex gloves.

R: *Hypoallergic latex gloves do not contain the chemical additives that can cause contact dermatitis, but they still contain latex (CDC, 2015).*

Teach Which Products Are Commonly Made of Latex

Health-Care Equipment

- Natural latex rubber gloves, powdered or unpowdered, including those labeled "hypoallergenic"
- Blood pressure cuffs
- Stethoscopes
- Tourniquets
- Electrode pads
- Airways, endotracheal tubes
- Syringe plunges, bulb syringes
- Masks for anesthesia
- Rubber aprons
- Catheters, wound drains
- Injection ports
- Tops of multidose vials
- Adhesive tape
- Ostomy pouches
- Wheelchair cushions
- Briefs with elastic
- Pads for crutches
- Some prefilled syringes

Office/Household Products

- Erasers
- Rubber bands
- Dishwashing gloves
- Balloons
- Condoms, diaphragms
- Baby bottle nipples, pacifiers
- Rubber balls and toys
- Racket handles

- Cycle grips
- Tires
- Hot water bottles
- Carpeting
- Shoe soles
- Elastic in underwear
- Rubber cement

Initiate Health Teaching as Indicated

- Explain the importance of completely avoiding direct contact with all NRL products.
- Advise that an individual with a history of a mild skin reaction to latex is at risk for anaphylaxis.
- Instruct to wear a Medic-Alert bracelet stating "Latex Allergy" and to carry autoinjectable epinephrine.
- Instruct to warn all health-care providers (e.g., dental, medical, surgical) of the allergy.

R: *Any exposure (tactile, inhaled, ingested) can precipitate an anaphylactic reaction.*

- Refer interested individuals to Latex Allergy: A Prevention Guide at http://www.cdc.gov/niosh/docs/98-113/pdfs/98-113.pdf
- For a comprehensive list of products containing latex refer to American Latex Allergy Association website.

Risk for Latex Allergy Response

NANDA-I Definition

Risk of hypersensitivity to natural latex rubber products that may compromise health

Risk Factors

Biopathophysiologic

Related to history of atopic eczema

Related to history of allergic rhinitis

Related to history of asthma*

Treatment Related

Related to multiple surgical procedures, especially beginning in infancy*

Related to frequent urinary catheterizations

Related to frequent rectal impaction removal

Related to frequent surgical procedures

Related to barium enema (before 1992)

Situational (Personal, Environmental)

Related to history of allergies*

History of food allergy to banana, kiwi, avocado, chestnuts, tropical fruits (mango, papaya, passion fruit), poinsettia plants,* tomato, raw potato, peach, and so forth

History of allergy to gloves, condoms, and so forth

Frequent occupational exposure to NRL,* such as follows:

Workers making NRL products
Food handlers
Greenhouse workers
Health-care workers
Housekeepers

Author's Note

Frequent exposure to airborne latex has contributed to latex allergies. All individuals who do not have latex allergies should use nonpowder nonlatex gloves (DeJong et al., 2011).

Key Concepts

Refer to *Latex Allergy Response*.

Focus Assessment Criteria

While the general population has a low incidence of latex allergy, ranging from 1.0% to 6.7%, certain groups remain at high risk. These groups include health-care workers who frequently wear latex gloves (8% to 16%) and children with spina bifida, spinal cord trauma, and urogenital malformations who may have had repeated exposure to latex products because of multiple surgeries (24% to 64%). Other groups at risk for latex allergy include the following (American Association of Nurse Anesthetist, 2014):

Workers with occupational exposure to latex (e.g., hairdressers, latex glove manufacturers, housekeeping personnel)
Individuals with a history of asthma, dermatitis, or eczema
Individuals exposed to repeated bladder catheterization as a result of spinal cord trauma or neurogenic bladder
Individuals with food allergy, especially to bananas, avocados, kiwi, or chestnuts
Individuals with a history of anaphylaxis of uncertain etiology, especially during past surgeries, hospitalization, or dental visits
Individuals with a history of multiple surgeries or medical procedures during childhood
Female individuals facing greater exposure to latex-containing products due to obstetric procedures, gynecologic examinations, and contact with contraceptives

Goals

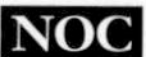

NOC

Immune Hypersensitivity Control

Refer to *Latex Allergy Response*.

Interventions

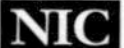

NIC

Allergy Management, Latex Precautions, Environmental Risk Protection

Refer to *Latex Allergy Response*.

SEDENTARY LIFESTYLE

NANDA-I Definition

Reports a habit of life that is characterized by a low physical activity level

Defining Characteristics[23]

Chooses a daily routine lacking physical exercise
Demonstrates physical deconditioning
Verbalizes preference for activities low in physical activity

[23]This definition has been added by Lynda Juall Carpenito, the author, for clarity and usefulness.

Related Factors*

Pathophysiologic

Related to decreased endurance secondary to obesity[1]

Situational (Personal, Environment)

Related to inadequate knowledge of health benefits of physical activity

Related to inadequate knowledge of exercise routines[1]

Related to insufficient resources (money, facilities)

Related to perceived lack of time

Related to lack of motivation

Related to lack of interest

Related to lack of training for accomplishment of physical exercise

Author's Note

This is the first nursing diagnosis submitted by a nurse from another country, accepted by NANDA in 2004. Congratulations to J. Adolf Guirao-Goris of Valencia, Spain.

Key Concepts

General Considerations

- Consensus Guidelines for Physical Activity and Public Health from the American Heart Association and American College of Sports Medicine call for at least 150 min/week of moderate exercise or, 75 min/week of vigorous exercise in the general adult population. Those guidelines also suggest that larger doses of ET may be necessary in some groups, such as those with or at risk for CHD (30 to 60 minutes daily), adults trying to prevent the transition to overweight or obesity (45 to 60 min/day), and formerly obese individuals trying to prevent weight regain (60 to 90 min/day) (Haskell, Lee, & Pate, 2007).
- Regular exercise can increase
  - Cardiorespiratory endurance
  - Delivery of nutrients to tissue
  - Muscle strength
  - Tolerance for psychological stress
  - Muscle endurance
  - Ability to reduce body fat content
  - Flexibility
- Vigorous exercise sessions should include a warm-up phase (10 minutes at a slow pace), endurance exercise, and a cool-down phase (5 to 10 minutes of a slow pace and stretching).
- Current beliefs regarding optimal exercise are as follows (*Allison & Keller, 1997):
  - Emphasize physical activity over "exercise."
  - Moderate physical activity that accumulates to 30 or more minutes is beneficial.
  - To enhance long-term exercise, the individual should (*Moore & Charvat, 2002)
    - Respond to relapse with a plan to prevent recurrences
    - Set realistic goals
    - Keep an exercise log
    - Exercise with a friend
- A regular pattern of moderate-intensity physical activity of 30 minutes or more, which can be accumulated throughout the day, four to five times a week, can be beneficial. Previously, vigorous exercise was recommended for a continuous 30 minutes or more.
- Forty percent of adults are completely sedentary in their leisure time (*Nies & Chruscial, 2002).
- At least 1 hour of walking per week can lower the risk of coronary heart disease in women (*Lee, 2001).

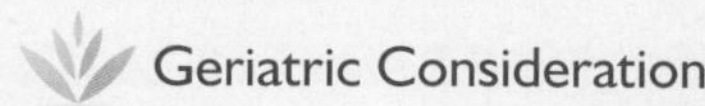

Geriatric Considerations

- The benefits of regular physical activity/exercise for older adults (Thompson, 2014):
  - Decreased anxiety and depression
  - Improved cognitive functioning
  - Enhanced physical functioning and independent functioning
  - Enhanced feelings of well-being
  - Enhanced performance of work, recreational and sport activities
  - Reduced risk of falls
  - Reduced injuries from falls
  - Effective therapy for many chronic diseases
- Additional benefits of exercise for older adults are (Edelman & Mandel, 2010)
  - Better sleep
  - Reduced constipations
  - Lower cholesterol
  - Lower blood pressure\better digestion
  - Weight loss socializing opportunities
- Only about 9% of American women older than 59 years get at least 150 minutes of physical activity each week (Lacharité-Lemieux, Brunelle, Dionne, 2015).
- Tai Chi improved balance, functional mobility, and fear of falling among older women (*Taggart, 2002).
- Falls among older women are a major health concern (*Young & Cochrane, 2004).

Focus Assessment Criteria

Subjective Data

Assess for Defining Characteristics

Regular exercise pattern (none, daily weekly)
Reports fatigue, shortness of breath with increased activity

Goals

NOC
Knowledge: Health Behaviors, Physical Fitness

The individual will verbalize intent to or engage in increased physical activity, as evidenced by the following indicators:

- Sets a goal for weekly exercise
- Identifies a desired activity or exercise

Interventions

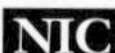

NIC
Exercise Promotion, Exercise Therapy

Discuss the Benefits of Exercise

- Reduces caloric absorption
- Improves body posture
- Increases metabolic rate
- Preserves lean muscle mass
- Suppresses appetite
- Improves self-esteem
- Reduces depression, anxiety, and stress
- Provides fun, recreation, diversion
- Increases oxygen uptake
- Increases caloric expenditure
- Maintains weight loss
- Increases restful sleep
- Increases resistance to age-related degeneration

R: *The process of seeking and attaining positive lifestyle change is known as "empowering potential." It occurs in three stages: appraising readiness, changing, and integrating change. As an individual strives to improve health, he or she moves through a process of introspection: planning new, healthier activities; coping with barriers and setbacks; and ultimately absorbing these new behaviors into everyday life.*

R: *The individual is responsible for choosing a healthy pattern of living. The nurse is responsible for explaining the choices.*

Assist the Individual to Identify Realistic Exercise Program

Consider

- Physical limitations (consult nurse or physician)
- Personal preferences
- Lifestyle
- Community resources (e.g., safe places to exercise)
- Individuals must learn to monitor pulse before, during, and after exercise to assist them to achieve target heart rate and not to exceed maximum advisable heart rate for age.

Age (years)	*Maximum Heart Rate (bpm)*	*Target Heart Rate (bpm)*
30	190	133 to 162
40	180	126 to 153
50	170	119 to 145
60	160	112 to 136

- A regular exercise program should
  - Be enjoyable
  - Use a minimum of 400 calories in each session
  - Sustain a heat rate of approximately 120 to 150 bpm
  - Involve rhythmic, alternating contracting and relaxing of muscles
  - Be integrated into the individual's lifestyle of 4 to 5 days/week for at least 30 to 60 minutes

Discuss the Aspects of Starting the Exercise Program

- Start slow and easy; obtain clearance from primary care provider
- Read, consult experts, and talk with friends/coworkers who exercise. Access the internet.
- Enlist another person to exercise with, include entire family.

R: *Any increase in activity also increases energy output and caloric deficits.*

- Plan a daily walking program:
  - Start at 5 to 10 blocks for 0.5 to 1 mile/day; increase 1 block or 0.1 mile/week.
  - Gradually increase the rate and length of walk; remember to progress slowly.
  - If you are breathing hard but you can talk comfortably, continue pace. If not, slow the pace. Remember: Increase only the rate or the distance of walking at one time.
- Avoid straining or pushing too hard and becoming overly fatigued.
- Stop immediately if any of the following occur:
  - Lightness or pain chest
  - Dizziness, lightheadedness
  - Severe breathlessness
  - Loss of muscle control
  - Nausea
- Add supplemental activity (e.g., parking far from destination, gardening, using stairs, spending weekends at activities that require walking).
- Work up to 1 hour of increased activity per day at least 4 days/week.

R: *The safest activities for the unconditioned obese person are walking, water aerobics, and swimming.*

Assist to Increase Interest and Motivation

- Develop a contract listing realistic short- and long-term goals.
- Keep intake/activity records.
- Increase knowledge by reading and talking with health-conscious friends and coworkers.
- Make new friends who are health conscious.
- Get a friend to follow the program or be a source of support.
- Be aware of rationalization (e.g., a lack of time may be a lack of prioritization).
- Keep a list of positive outcomes.

R: *Friends have the most positive influence to keep on an exercise program (*Resnick, Orwig, & Magaziner, 2002).*

Older Adults Interventions

Carp's Cues

Differentiating between age-related changes and risk factors that affect the functioning of older people is important. Risk factors such as inadequate nutrition, fluid intake, exercise, and socialization can have more influence on functioning than can most age-related changes (Miller, 2015).

- Explain the benefits of activity/exercise of 150 minutes a week. Explain the every 10 minutes count. Refer to Key Concepts.

R: *The total time can be 150 minutes a week or 25 minutes a day, However, you can increase your activity 10 minutes each session weekly.*

- Specifically ask primary provider what activities are safe prior to starting.
- Explain the difference between aerobic and muscle-strengthening activities:
  - Aerobic exercises cause one to breathe harder and heart to beat faster as, walking faster, climbing stairs, housekeeping.
  - Muscle-strengthening exercises build muscle strength and bone density, which can decrease with aging.
- Determine with the individual what they can do.

R: *"Focusing on problems and deficits alone limits the exploration of individual strengths, thereby compounding the risk for vulnerability to diminished health and well-being" (McMahon & Fleury, 2011). Some individuals may not be able to walk unassisted but they still can increase their activities.*

- Perform ankle-strengthening exercises daily (Liu & Latham, 2009; *Schoenfelder, 2000).
  - Stand behind a straight chair, with feet slightly apart.
  - Slowly raise both heels until body weight is on the balls of the feet; hold for a count of three (e.g., 1 Mississippi, 2 Mississippi, 3 Mississippi).
  - Do 5 to 10 repetitions; increase repetitions as strength increases.
- Walk at least two or three times a week.
  - Use ankle exercises as a warm-up before walking.
  - Begin walking with someone at side, if needed, for 10 minutes.
  - Increase time and speed according to capabilities.

R: *Ankle-strengthening and a walking program can improve balance, increase ankle strength, improve walking speed, decrease falls and fear of falling.*

RISK FOR IMPAIRED LIVER FUNCTION

See also *Risk for Complications of Hepatic Dysfunction.*

NANDA-I Definition

Vulnerable to a decrease in liver function which may compromise health

Risk Factors*

Hepatotoxic medications (e.g., acetaminophen, statins)
HIV coinfection
Substance abuse (e.g., alcohol, cocaine)
Viral infection (e.g., hepatitis A, hepatitis B, hepatitis C, Epstein–Barr virus)

Author's Note

This diagnosis represents a situation that requires collaborative intervention with medicine. Diagnostic studies, which cannot be ordered by nurses, are necessary to monitor for impaired liver function. This author recommends the collaborative problem *Risk for Complications of Hepatic Dysfunction* be used instead. Refer to Section 3 for interventions. Students should consult with their faculty for advice on the use of *Risk for Impaired Liver Function* or *Risk for Complications of Hepatic Dysfunction*.

RISK FOR LONELINESS

NANDA-I Definition

Vulnerable to experiencing discomfort associated with a desire or need for more contact with others, which may compromise health

Risk Factors

Pathophysiologic

Related to fear of rejection secondary to:

Obesity
Cancer (disfiguring surgery of head or neck, superstition from others)
Physical handicaps (paraplegia, amputation, arthritis, hemiplegia)
Emotional handicaps (extreme anxiety, depression, paranoia, phobias)
Incontinence (embarrassment, odor)
Communicable diseases (acquired immunodeficiency syndrome [AIDS], hepatitis)
Psychiatric illness (schizophrenia, bipolar affective disorder, personality disorders)

Related to difficulty accessing social events secondary to:

Debilitating diseases
Physical disabilities

Treatment Related

Related to therapeutic isolation

Situational (Personal, Environmental)

Related to affectional or cathectic deprivation*

Related to physical or social isolation*

Related to insufficient planning for retirement

Related to death of a significant other

Related to divorce

Related to visible physical disabilities

Related to fear of rejection secondary to:

Obesity
Hospitalization or terminal illness (dying process)
Extreme poverty
Unemployment

Related to moving to another culture (e.g., unfamiliar language)

Related to history of unsatisfactory social experiences secondary to:

Drug abuse
Unacceptable social behavior
Alcohol abuse
Delusional thinking
Immature behavior

Related to loss of usual means of transportation

Related to change in usual residence secondary to:

Long-term care
Relocation

Maturational

Child

Related to protective isolation or a communicable disease

Related to autism

Older Adult

Related to loss of usual social contacts secondary to:

Retirement
Relocation
Death of (specify)
Loss of driving ability

Author's Note

Risk for Loneliness was added to the NANDA list in 1994. Currently, *Social Isolation* is also on the NANDA list. *Social Isolation* is a conceptually incorrect diagnosis because it does not represent a response, rather a cause. ElSadr, Noureddine, and Kelley (2009), in a concept analysis of loneliness, found the literature that supports social isolation as a possible cause of loneliness. *Loneliness* and *Risk for Loneliness* better describe the negative state of aloneness.

Loneliness is a subjective state that exists whenever an individual says it does and perceives it as imposed by others. Social isolation is *not* the voluntary solitude necessary for personal renewal, nor is it the creative aloneness of the artist or the aloneness—and possible suffering—an individual may experience from seeking individualism and independence (e.g., moving to a new city, going away to college).

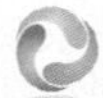

Errors in Diagnostic Statements

Loneliness related to inability to engage in satisfying personal relationships since death of wife 1 year ago

When an individual fails to resume activities or to renew or to initiate social relationships after the death of a spouse, the nurse should suspect *Complicated Grieving*. Prolonged social isolation after a death is a cue for unresolved grief. The nurse should conduct a focus assessment to identify other cues, such as prolonged denial, depression, or other evidence of unsuccessful adaptation to the loss. Until additional data are confirmed, the diagnosis *Possible Complicated Grieving* related to failure to resume or initiate relationships after wife's death 1 year ago would be appropriate.

Loneliness related to multiple sclerosis

Using multiple sclerosis as a related factor clusters all people with this condition as socially isolated and for the same reasons. This not only violates the uniqueness of each individual but also does not specify how a nurse can intervene. If mobility and incontinence problems are present but no data support social isolation, the nurse can record the diagnosis as *Risk for Loneliness* related to mobility and incontinence problems secondary to multiple sclerosis.

Key Concepts

General Considerations

- Being socially connected is not only influential for psychological and emotional well-being but it also has a significant and positive influence on physical well-being (Uchino, 2006) and overall longevity (Holt-Lunstad, Smith, & Layton, 2010; Holt-Lunstad, Smith, Baker, Harris, & Stephenson, 2015).
- A meta-analysis of 148 studies (308,849 participants) found "a 50% increased likelihood of survival for participants with stronger social relationships. This finding remained consistent across age, sex, initial health status, cause of death, and follow-up period of overall longevity (Holt-Lunstad et al., 2010, 2015).
- "Whereas social isolation can be an objectively quantifiable variable, loneliness is a subjective emotional state" (Holt-Lunstad et al., 2015). Loneliness is the perception of social isolation, or the subjective experience of being lonely, and thus involves necessarily subjective measurement. Loneliness has also been described as the dissatisfaction with the discrepancy between desired and actual social relationships (Holt-Lunstad et al., 2015).
- Loneliness differs from aloneness, solitude, and grief. *Aloneness* refers to being without company (not necessarily a negative state). *Solitude* involves being alone with a positive affective state. *Grief* is a response to traumatic loss (*Hillestad, 1984).

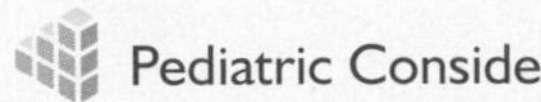

Pediatric Considerations

- Children at high risk for social isolation include the chronically ill or disabled, terminally ill, and disfigured and their siblings.
- A child in protective isolation or with a communicable disease may not understand the rationale for separation from others.
- Gay or lesbian teenagers often suffer emotional isolation and lack access to information specific to their needs (e.g., they are at increased medical risk for sexually transmitted diseases, substance use, and violence; *Bidwell & Deisher, 1991).

Geriatric Considerations

- Adjusting to the changes that accompany old age requires that an individual is flexible and develops new coping skills to adapt to the changes that are common to this time in their lives (*Warnick, 1995).
- "Aging research has demonstrated a positive correlation of someone's religious beliefs, social relationships, perceived health, self-efficacy, socioeconomic status and coping skills, among others, with their ability to age more successfully" (Singh & Misra, 2009).
- "Though the belief persists that depression is synonymous with aging and that depression is in fact inevitable, there has been recent research which dispels this faulty notion" (Singh & Misra, 2009).
- Society often devalues the elderly because of their decline (actual or perceived) in knowledge, skills, power, and importance. Some view elders as preoccupied in relaxation and freedom from certain worries and responsibilities or as slow and worthless. Both views label elders as having nothing to contribute to society (Elsen & Blegen, 1991).
- Family roles become altered and stressed when parents become dependent on their children and children begin to assume traditional parental tasks or decision making. To help older adults meet affiliative needs and increase satisfaction with social encounters, it is suggested that small groups (rather than large, noisy crowds) be formed to promote interaction and that one or two meaningful relationships (confidantes) be encouraged.
- Factors increasing social isolation in older adults include hearing impairment, limited mobility, fatigue, caregiving responsibilities, inability to drive, mental or psychosocial impairments, and separation from spouse, friends, and/or relatives by death, illness, or physical distance (Miller, 2015).
- Life changes, including widowhood and relocation, are associated with increased vulnerability to loneliness. Gender, social, and cultural factors influence the experience of loneliness in older women.
- Sensory deficits rate highest on the list of problems in the older adult with the potential to cause social isolation (Miller, 2015).

Depression

- "Depression or the occurrence of depressive symptomatology is a prominent condition amongst older people, with a significant impact on the well-being and quality of life. Though the belief persists that depression is synonymous with aging and that depression is in fact inevitable, there has been recent research which dispels this faulty notion" (Singh & Misra, 2009).
- Depression has a causal link to numerous social, physical, and psychological problems. These difficulties often emerge in older adulthood, increasing the likelihood of depression; yet depression is not a normal consequence of these problems (Singh & Misra, 2009).
- Studies have found that age isn't always significantly related to level of depression, and that the oldest of olds may even have better coping skills to deal with depression, making depressive symptoms more common but not as severe as in younger populations (Singh & Misra, 2009).

Focus Assessment Criteria

Social isolation can result in intense feelings of loneliness and suffering. Suffering associated with social isolation is not always visible. To diagnose this state, nurses must first be able to identify those at risk (Hawkley & Cacioppo, 2010; Holt-Lunstad et al., 2015).

Subjective Data

Assess for Related Factors

Self-Reports Feelings of
Being left out
Dissatisfaction with present quantity and/or quality of relationships
Lack of companionship
Being unable to increase the quantity and/or quality of relationships to the level the person desires

Social Resources (Support)

"Who lives with you?"

"Where does your family live?"

"About how many times did you talk to someone—friends, relatives, or others—on the telephone in the past week (either you called them or they called you)?" If subject has no telephone, ask, "How many times during the past week did you spend some time with someone who does not live with you; that is, you went to see them, or they came to visit you, or you went out to do things together?"

To whom does the individual turn in time of need?

Does the individual rely on friends or neighbors for such things as meals and transportation?

"Do you see your relatives and friends as often as you want to, or are you somewhat unhappy about how little you see them?"

If institutionalized, ask, "In the past year, about how often did you leave here to visit your family or friends for weekends or holidays or to go on shopping trips or outings, or are most of your friends here in the institution with you?"

Barriers to Social Contacts

Does the individual lack knowledge of resources available, where to meet others, how to initiate conversation with strangers?

Is individual housebound? (Illness or incapacity—lack of mobility on steps or curbs—and weather hazards can physically isolate older adults, as can loss of usual transportation, living in dangerous area, and lack of access to public transportation.)

Are there changes in the individual's sensory ability (tactile sense, hearing, visual acuity, ability to write letters)?

Change in Living Arrangement

Has the individual moved recently (to nursing home, child's home, apartment, strange location)?

Objective Data

Assess for Related Factors

Aesthetic Problems

Mutilating surgery

Odor (e.g., ulcerating tumor)

Extreme obesity

Incontinence

Personality Problems

Does this individual lack certain social skills or have personality features (e.g., aggression, egocentricity, racism, sexism, complaining, critical, problem drinker) that may discourage others from befriending him or her?

Goals

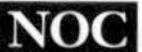

Loneliness, Social Involvement

The individual will report decreased feelings of loneliness, as evidenced by the following indicators:

- Identifies the reasons for his or her feelings of isolation
- Discusses the ways to increase meaningful relationships

Interventions

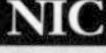

Socialization Enhancement, Spiritual Support, Behavior Modification: Social Skills, Presence, Anticipatory Guidance

The nursing interventions for various contributing factors that might be associated with *Risk for Loneliness* are similar.

Identify Causative and Contributing Factors

- Refer to Related Factors.

Reduce or Eliminate Causative and Contributing Factors

- Support the individual who has experienced a loss as he or she works through grief (refer to *Grieving*).
- Encourage to talk about the feelings of loneliness and their causes.

- Encourage the development of a support system or mobilize the individual's existing family, friends, and neighbors to form one.
- Discuss the importance of high-quality, rather than high-quantity, socialization.
- Refer to social skills teaching (see *Impaired Social Interaction*).
- Offer feedback on how the individual presents himself or herself to others (refer to *Impaired Social Interaction*).

R: *Longino and Kart (*1982) reported that type and quality of social interactions are more important than quantity. Informal activities promote well-being more so than formal, structured activities.*

Decrease the Barriers to Social Contact and That Will Promote Social Interactions

- Determine available transportation in the community (public, church-related, volunteer).
- Assist with the development of alternative means of communication for people with compromised sensory ability (e.g., amplifier on phone, taped instead of written letters; refer to *Impaired Communication*).
- Refer to *Impaired Urinary Elimination* for specific interventions to control incontinence.

Identify the Strategies to Expand the World of the Isolated. Dialogue With Individual to Determine What Activities They Are Interested in

- Senior centers and church groups
- Volunteer assignments (e.g., hospital, church)
- Foster grandparent programs
- Adult day care centers
- Retirement communities
- House sharing, group homes, community kitchens
- Adult education classes, special interest courses
- Pets
- Regular contact to diminish the need to obtain attention through a crisis (e.g., suicidal gesture)
- Psychiatric day hospital or activity program

R: *Older adults are at high risk for loneliness because they often have fewer natural opportunities to be among others. Retirement from work, difficulty securing transportation, health problems that restrict visiting, sensory deficits that make communication laborious or frustrating, or isolation from the mainstream in institutions (hospitals or nursing homes) can significantly limit natural interpersonal encounters (Osborne, 2012).*

Implement the Following for People With Ineffective Social Skills

- Refer to *Impaired Social Interactions*.

Older Adults Interventions

Discuss the Anticipatory Effects of Retirement

R: *The most important psychological challenge resulting from retirement is the loss of a work/life structure and the task of building a retirement/life structure to replace it.*

- Prepare for ambivalent feelings and short-term negative effects on self-esteem:
  - "Some losses may be missed (e.g., friendships in the workplace, various fringe benefits and perks, and the ways in which work provided a center point for a work/life structure)" (Osborne, 2012, p. 47).

R: *In our society, working people have a higher status than nonworking people. Retirement requires coping with a change in social status (Miller, 2015).*

Provide Anticipatory Guidance Related to Effects of Aging on the Individual and Life Style

- Explore some of the losses associated with aging: retirement, deaths of loved ones, friends, chronic illnesses, sensory changes, relocation, loss of driving licence.

R: *As one grows older, adults face numerous physical, psychological, and social role changes that challenge their sense of self and capacity to live happily.*

Discuss the Person's Activity and Exercise Patterns

- Refer to *Sedentary Life Style* for specifics on increasing activities for older adults.

R: *Research has reported that the level of daily physical and/or cognitive activities in working behaviors, volunteering, and/or home can help to maintain retirees' physical health. Perception of physical health is the major cause of depression in late life. An active older person in good physical health has a relatively low risk of depression.*

Emphasize the Need to Prevent Isolation, Which Can Lead to Loneliness and Depression

- Consider bridge employment (a limited hours job, post retirement to help to adjust to not working full time)
- Explore opportunities for making new friends, developing new interests, discovering opportunities for service/volunteering, spending more time in fellowship as clubs, faith-based organizations.

R: *Volunteering gives purpose to the day, requires getting dressed and groomed, and promotes feeling of engagement and achievement (*Edelman & Mandle, 2010).*

- Emphasize that it is not the number of activities one has but whether one is satisfied with their life style (Singh & Misra, 2009).

R: *"Adjusting to the changes that accompany old age requires that an individual is flexible and develops new coping skills to adapt to the changes that are common to this time in their lives" (*Warnick, 1995 quoted in Singh & Misra, 2009).*

Discuss Those Factors That Contribute to Successful Retirement

R: *"Retirement is a significant life event that requires preplanning and realistic expectation of life changes" (*Edelman & Mandle, 2010).*

- Stable health status
- Adequate income and health benefits
- Active in community, church, or professional organizations
- Higher education level and ability to pursue new goals/activities
- Extended social network, family friends, colleagues
- Satisfied with life before retirement
- Satisfied with living arrangements
- Plan to ensure adequate income.
- Decreased time at work for the last 2 to 3 years (e.g., shorter days, longer vacations)
- Cultivate friends outside work.
- Develop routines at home to replace work structure.
- Rely on others rather than spouse for leisure activities.
- Cultivate realistic leisure activities (energy, cost).
- Engage in community or church programs or professional organizations.

R: *"Among postretirement activities, research has unequivocally shown that retirees who engaged in bridge employment and voluntary work had fewer major diseases and functional limitations than retirees who chose full retirement" (Wang & Hesketh, 2012, p. 15).*

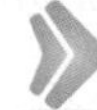

Carp's Cues

Singh and Misra (2009) write ". . .at the same time, old age can also be an opportunity. It can be happy and winsome or empty and sad — depending largely on the faith and grace of the person involved." Nurses can provide the guidance to dispel the myth that aging well can be enhanced by looking forward not backward. Embrace a new, different life. An older adult can celebrate that they will not die young!

Initiate Health Teaching/Referrals, as Indicated

- Volunteer (e.g., to tutor, read to children/elders, library work)
- Community-based groups that contact the socially isolated
- Self-help groups for those isolated because of specific medical problems (e.g., Reach to Recovery, United Ostomy Association)
- Wheelchair groups
- Psychiatric consumer rights associations

R: *Chronic illness can contribute to social isolation because of lack of energy, decreased mobility, discomforts, fear of exposure to pathogens, and distancing by previous friends who are uncomfortable with the ill individual's disabilities or the stigma associated with psychiatric problems (Miller, 2015).*

IMPAIRED MEMORY

NANDA-I Definition

Inability to remember or recall bits of information or behavioral skills

Defining Characteristics*

Major (Must Be Present, One or More)

Reports experiences of forgetting
Inability to recall if a behavior was performed
Inability to learn or retain new skills or information
Inability to perform a previously learned skill
Inability to recall factual information
Inability to recall events

Related Factors

Pathophysiologic

Related to neurologic disturbances* secondary to:

Degenerative brain disease (e.g. multiple sclerosis, Parkinson's disease)
Lesion
Head injury
Cerebrovascular accident

Related to reduced quantity and quality of information processed secondary to:

Visual deficits
Poor physical fitness
Learning habits
Educational level
Hearing deficits
Fatigue
Intellectual skills

Related to nutritional deficiencies (e.g., vitamins C and B_{12}, folate, niacin, thiamine)

Treatment Related

Related to effects of medication (specify) on memory storage

Situational (Personal, Environmental)

Related to self-fulfilling expectations

Related to excessive self-focus and worry secondary to:

Grieving
Anxiety
Depression

Related to alcohol consumption

Related to lack of motivation

Related to lack of stimulation

Related to difficulty concentrating secondary to:

Stress
Distractions

Sleep disturbances
Pain
Lack of intellectual stimulation

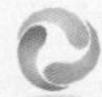

Author's Note

This diagnosis is useful when the individual can be helped to function better through strategies that improved memory. If the person's memory cannot be improved because of cerebral degeneration, this diagnosis is not appropriate. Instead, the nurse should evaluate the effects of impaired memory on functioning, such as *Self-Care Deficits* or *Risk for Injury.* The focus of interventions for these nursing diagnoses would be improving self-care or protection, not improving memory. *Chronic confusion* should also be considered.

Key Concepts

General Considerations

- Memory is a continuum of processing. First an information is perceived, then stored, and later retrieved when needed or desired (Miller, 2015). Memory problems associated with normal aging reflect a decrease in the efficiency with which the information is processed and retrieved (Grossman & Porth, 2014).
- Memory function worries people more than any other cognitive function. When an older person forgets, it is interpreted as a sign of disease; when a younger person forgets, it is attributed to many things on a person's mind.
- Short-term memory shows a slight decline with aging, this is attributed to belief that the longer the information is stored the longer it will last (Miller, 2015).

Focus Assessment Criteria

Acquire from the individual and significant others.

Subjective Data

Assess for Defining Characteristics

Remote events: "Where were you born?" "Where did you go to grade school?" "What was your first job?" "When were you married?"
Recent events: "Do you live with anyone?" "Do you have any grandchildren?" "What are the names of your grandchildren?" "When was the last time you went to the doctor?"
Immediate memory, retention: State three unrelated facts and ask the client to repeat the information immediately and again after 5 minutes.
Immediate memory, general grasp, and recall: Have the client read a short story and then summarize the information.
Immediate memory, recognition: Ask a multiple-choice question and ask the client to choose the correct answer.
Ability to remember:
Self-care activities
To shop for necessities
To take medications
Appointments
To pay bills

Goals

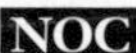

NOC
Cognitive Orientation, Memory

The individual will report increased satisfaction with memory, as evidenced by the following indicators:

- Identifies three techniques to improve memory
- Relates factors that deter memory

Interventions

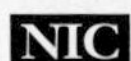

Reality Orientation, Memory Training, Environmental Management

Discuss Beliefs About Memory Deficits

- Correct misinformation.
- Explain that negative expectations can result in memory deficits.

R: *Many personal, such as level of education and expectations, and environmental factors, as multiple conversations at once, influence memory significantly.*

Assess for Factors That May Negatively Affect Memory (e.g., Pathophysiologic, Literacy, Stressors, Rushing)

R: *Memory problems can be related to many factors (e.g., CNS pathology, nutritional deficiencies, low literacy, sensory deficits, disinterest, stress, pain, or depression).*

If the Individual Has Difficulty Concentrating, Use Simpler Explanations and Reduce Environmental Distraction

Teach Two or Three of the Following Methods to Improve Memory Skills (*Maier-Lorentz, 2000; Miller, 2015)

- Write things down (e.g., use lists, calendars, notebooks).
- Use auditory cues (e.g., timers, alarm clocks) in conjunction with written cues.
- Use environmental cues (e.g., you might remove something from its usual place, then return it to its normal location after it has served its purpose as a reminder).
- Have specific places for specific items; keep items in their proper place (e.g., keep keys on a hook near the door).
- Put reminders in appropriate places (e.g., place shoes to be repaired near the door).
- Use visual images ("A picture is worth a thousand words"). Create a picture in your mind when you want to remember something; the more bizarre the picture, the more likely you will remember.
- Use active observation—pay attention to details around you and be alert to the environment.
- Make associations or mental connections (e.g., "Spring ahead and fall back" for changing clocks to and from daylight savings time).
- Make associations between names and mental images (e.g., Carol and Christmas carol).
- Rehearse items you want to remember by repeating them aloud or writing them on paper.
- Use self-instruction—say things aloud (e.g., "I'm putting my keys on the counter so I remember to turn off the stove before I leave").
- Divide information into small chunks that can be remembered easily (e.g., to remember an address or a zip code, divide it into groups ["seven hundred sixty, fifty-five"]).
- Organize information into logical categories (e.g., shampoo and hair spray, toothpaste and mouthwash, soap and deodorant).
- Use rhyming cues (e.g., "In 1492, Columbus sailed the ocean blue").
- Use first-letter cues and make associations (e.g., to remember to buy carrots, apples, radishes, pickles, eggs, and tea bags, remember the word *carpet*).
- Make word associations (e.g., to remember the letters of your license plate, make a word, such as "camel" for CML).
- Search the alphabet while focusing on what you are trying to remember (e.g., to remember that someone's name is Martin, start with names that begin with "A" and continue naming names through the alphabet until your memory is jogged for the correct one).
- Make up a story to connect things you want to remember (e.g., if you have to go to the cleaners and post office, create a story about mailing a pair of pants).

R: *If one wants to improve one's memory, both the intent to remember and the knowledge about techniques for remembering are needed (Miller, 2015).*

When Trying to Learn or Remember Something

- Minimize distractions.
- Do not rush.
- Maintain some form of organization of routine tasks.
- Carry a note pad or calendar or use written cues.

R: *Memory impairment can be improved when information is meaningful and logical rather than abstract.*

When Teaching (Miller, 2015)

- Determine if there are barriers to learning (e.g., stress, alcohol use/abuse, pain, depression, low literacy).
- Eliminate distractions.
- Present information as concretely as possible.
- Use practical examples.
- Allow learner to pace the learning.
- Use visual, auditory aids.
- Provide advance organizers: outlines, written cues.
- Encourage use of aids.
- Make sure glasses are clean and lights are soft white.
- Correct wrong answers immediately.
- Encourage verbal responses.
- Try to organize self-care activities in the same order and same time each day.

R: *Simple, direct teaching strategies with visual prompts can increase learning and retention.*

IMPAIRED PHYSICAL MOBILITY

Impaired Physical Mobility

Impaired Bed Mobility
Impaired Sitting
Impaired Standing
Impaired Walking
Impaired Wheelchair Mobility
Impaired Transfer Ability

NANDA-I Definition

Limitation in independent, purposeful physical movement of the body or of one or more extremities

Defining Characteristics

Compromised ability to move purposefully within the environment (e.g., sitting up, bed mobility, standing up, transfers, ambulation)
Range-of-motion (ROM) limitations
Altered gait
Physiologic instability with increased activity
Uncoordinated movements
Spastic movements
Postural instability
Movement-induced tremor

Related Factors

Pathophysiologic

Related to deconditioning secondary to physiologic instability

Related to decreased muscle strength and endurance secondary to:

Neuromuscular impairment
Autoimmune alterations (e.g., multiple sclerosis, arthritis)
Nervous system diseases (e.g., Parkinson's disease, myasthenia gravis)
Respiratory conditions (e.g., chronic obstructive pulmonary disease [COPD])
Muscular dystrophy
Partial paralysis (spinal cord injury, stroke)

Central nervous system (CNS) tumor
Trauma
Cancer
Increased intracranial pressure
Sensory deficits
Musculoskeletal impairment
Fractures
Connective tissue disease (systemic lupus erythematous)
Cardiac conditions

Related to joint stiffness* or contraction* secondary to:

Inflammatory joint disease
Post–joint-replacement or spinal surgery
Degenerative joint disease
Degenerative disc disease

Related to edema

Treatment Related

Related to equipment (e.g., ventilators, enteral therapy, dialysis, total parenteral nutrition)

Related to external devices (casts or splints, braces)

Related to insufficient strength and endurance for ambulation with (specify):

Prosthesis
Crutches
Walker

Situational (Personal, Environmental)

Related to compromised ability to move secondary to:

Fatigue
Decreased motivation
Pain*
Obesity (BMI over 30)
Cognitive impairment*
Depressive mood state*
Deconditioning*
Dyspnea

Maturational

Children

Related to abnormal gait secondary to:

Congenital skeletal deficiencies
Congenital hip dysplasia
Legg–Calvé–Perthes disease
Osteomyelitis

Older Adult

Related to decreased motor agility

Related to decreased muscle mass and strength*

Related to fear of falling

Author's Note

Impaired Physical Mobility describes an individual with deconditioning from immobility resulting from a medical or surgical condition. The literature is full of the effects of immobility on body system function. Early progressive mobility programs and progressive mobility activity protocol (PMAP) are designed to prevent these complications. These programs are appropriate for individuals in intensive care units, other hospital units, and skill nursing care facilities.

These programs necessitate continuous nursing attention. Several potential barriers for maintaining PMAP have been identified as lack of mobility education, safety concerns, and lack of interdisciplinary collaboration (King, 2012).

Gillis, MacDonald, and MacIssac (2008) reported that time constraints due to increased acuity and staffing issues have lowered the priority and time available for basic mobility.

Acuity levels on units must address the workload associated to PMAP and factor this into staffing. Several studies have shown the cost effectiveness of PMAP with decreased ICU stays, decreased ventilator use, and decreased hospital stays in addition to decreased complications of immobility such as decreased deep vein thrombosis, ventilator-associated pneumonia, and delirium.

Nursing interventions for *Impaired Physical Mobility* focus on early mobilization muscle strengthening and restoring function and preventing deterioration. *Impaired Physical Mobility* can also be utilized to describe someone with limited use of arm(s) or leg(s) or limited muscle strength.

Impaired Physical Mobility is one of the cluster of diagnoses in *Risk for Disuse Syndrome*. Limitation of physical movement of arms/legs also can be the etiology of other nursing diagnoses, such as *Self-Care Deficit* and *Risk for Injury*. If the individual can exercise but does not, refer to *Sedentary Lifestyle*. If the individual has no limitations in movement but is deconditioned and has reduced endurance, refer to *Activity Intolerance*.

Errors in Diagnostic Statements

***Impaired Physical Mobility* related to traumatic amputation of left arm**

Listing traumatic amputation of the left arm as a related factor does not describe the problem. Rather, the diagnostic statement should reflect how the loss has affected functioning. A more appropriate diagnosis might be *Self-Care Deficit: Feeding* related to insufficient knowledge of adaptations needed secondary to loss of left arm.

***Impaired Physical Mobility* related to limited motivation secondary to cerebrovascular accident (CVA)**

Limited motivation is a sign of *Impaired Physical Mobility*, not a related factor. Related factors should represent direction for nursing intervention, as reflected in the diagnosis *Impaired Physical Mobility related to decreased muscle strength and endurance secondary to CVA and decreased motivation.*

Key Concepts

General Considerations

- Winkelman and Peereboom (2010) studied the perceived barriers and facilitators of ICU nurses to increase in-bed and out-of-bed movement. They reported the factor that facilitated success with in-bed or out-of-bed mobilization as follows:
  - The presence of a protocol in the institution, which guided decisions about readiness for increased activity
  - Glasgow coma score greater than 10
  - Beds that provided a chair position
  - Prescriber's order
  - Expert mentor (nurse, physical therapist)
- Winkelman and Peereboom (2010) reported barriers as follows:
  - Absence of the above facilitators
  - Nurse's perception of the individual's nonreadiness for increased activity
  - Physical therapy is not consulted
- Inexperience ICU nurses may believe that increased mobility contributes to falls or disruption of equipment integrity, for example, ventilators, parenteral therapy. A shift is needed in the culture, that individuals in the ICU on complete bed rest is not acceptable routine.

Effects of Bed Rest

- In 12 healthy older adults after 10 days of bed rest. Deconditioning has a significant effect on the skeletal muscles used in standing and walking and has been linked to falls, functional decline, increased frailty, and immobility (Gillis et al., 2008).
- "Sarcopenia, a loss of muscle mass, can begin after only 2 days of bed rest, decreasing muscle strength by 1% to 3% per day. One week of bed rest can result in a 20% decrease in muscle strength and an additional 20% muscle strength loss for each week on bed rest" (De Jonghe et al., 2009 cited in King, 2012)
- "The act of lying down shifts 11% of the total blood volume away from the legs, with most going to the chest. Within the first 3 days of bed rest, an 8% to 10% reduction in plasma volume occurs, with the loss stabilizing to 15% to 20% by the fourth week. These changes result in increased cardiovascular workload, elevated resting heart rate, and a decrease in stroke volume with a reduction in cardiac output" (Vollman, 2012, p. 70).

- The four ROM categories are passive, active assistive, active, and active resistive (*Addams & Clough, 1998).
    - *Passive ROM* is the movement of the client's muscles by another person with the client's help.
    - *Active assistive ROM* is active contraction of a muscle with assistance by an external force such as a therapist, mechanical appliance, or the uninvolved extremity.
    - *Active ROM* is active contraction of a muscle against the force of gravity, such as straight leg lifts.
    - *Active resistive ROM* is active contraction of a muscle against resistance, such as weights.
- *Isometric exercises* are when muscles contract or tense without joint movement. They are contraindicated for people with cardiac conditions because they increase left ventricular function. When done, muscles should be tensed for 5 to 15 seconds (Grossman & Porth, 2014)
- *Ambulation* is a complex, three-dimensional activity involving the legs, pelvis, trunk, and upper extremities. *Gait* is a complex movement involving the musculoskeletal, neurologic, and cardiovascular systems. Cognitive factors such as mentation and orientation are critical for safe ambulation (*Addams & Clough, 1998).

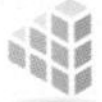

Pediatric Considerations

- Refer to *Disuse Syndrome*.

Geriatric Considerations

- Keller and Watt examined the effects of two extra walks per day on the mobility, independence, and exercise self-efficacy of a population of elderly persons on a medical unit in an acute regional public hospital. The walking program increased the older person's mobility and independence which gives support to the implementation of extra walking as a worthwhile nursing intervention in this group of elderly medical unit inpatients (*Killey & Watt, 2006).
- In particular among older people, immobility while being ill may result in critical mobility decline. Among older people, mobility may not spontaneously recover to its preillness level (Rantanen, 2013).
- Effects of immobility are particularly dangerous in older adults. Muscle weakness, atrophy, and decreased endurance occur quickly, and biochemical and physiologic effects such as nitrogen loss and hypercalciuria are important to consider (Grossman & Porth, 2014). Permanent functional loss is more likely with prolonged immobility, and older adults also are vulnerable to new morbidity such as pneumonia, pressure sores, falls and fracture, osteoporosis, incontinence, confusion, and depression. Every effort toward prevention and mobilization should be made (Miller, 2015).
- Age-related changes in joint and connective tissue impair flexion and extension movements, decrease flexibility, and reduce cushioning protection for joints (Miller, 2015).

Focus Assessment Criteria

Subjective Data

Assess for Defining Characteristics

History of Symptoms (Complaints of)
Pain
Muscle weakness
Dyspnea
Fatigue
Attributed to (specify) amount of time in bed
Attributed to (specify) amount of time sleeping or resting

Assess for Related Factors

History of Systemic Disorders that Compromise Movement, Strength
Neurologic, cardiovascular, respiratory, musculoskeletal, debilitating diseases (e.g., cancer, renal disease, autoimmune, endocrine)

Miscellaneous
Postsurgical status
Trauma

Objective Data

This assessment may be completed by physical therapy.

Assess for Defining Characteristics

Dominant Hand

Motor Function

Right arm	Strong	Weak	Absent	Spastic
Left arm	Strong	Weak	Absent	Spastic
Right leg	Strong	Weak	Absent	Spastic
Left leg	Strong	Weak	Absent	Spastic

Mobility

Ability to turn self	Yes	No	Assistance needed (specify)
Ability to sit	Yes	No	Assistance needed (specify)
Ability to stand	Yes	No	Assistance needed (specify)
Ability to get up	Yes	No	Assistance needed (specify)
Ability to transfer	Yes	No	Assistance needed (specify)
Ability to ambulate	Yes	No	Assistance needed (specify)

Weight-Bearing (Assess Both Right and Left Sides)

Full, partial weight-bearing   Gait (stable, unstable)   Non–weight-bearing

Assistive Devices

Crutches	Walker	Prosthesis
Braces	Cane	
Wheelchair	Other	

Restrictive Devices

Cast or splint	Monitor	Dialysis
Braces	Traction	Parenteral therapy
Drain	Ventilator	Enteral therapy
Foley	IV	

Range of Motion (Neck, Shoulders, Elbows, Arms, Spine, Hips, Legs)

Full   Limited (specify)   None

Assess for Related Factors

Endurance (Refer to *Activity Intolerance* for Additional Information)

Resting pulse, blood pressure, oxygen saturation, and respirations
Blood pressure, respirations, oxygen saturation, and pulse immediately after activity
Pulse every 2 minutes until pulse returns to within 10 beats of resting pulse
During and after activity, assess for indicators of hypoxia (showing intensity, frequency, or duration of activity must be decreased or discontinued) as follows:

Blood Pressure

Failure of systolic rate to increase
Increase in diastolic of 155 mm Hg

Respirations

Excessive rate increases
Decrease in rate
Dyspnea
Irregular rhythm

Cerebral and Other Changes

Confusion
Pallor
Weakness
Change in equilibrium
Incoordination

Goals

NOC

Ambulation, Joint Movement, Mobility, Fall Prevention Behavior, Adaption to Physical Disability, Transfer Performance, Immobility Consequences, Motivation, Knowledge: Prescribed Activity

The individual will report increased strength and endurance of limbs, as evidenced by the following indicators:

- Demonstrate the use of adaptive devices to increase mobility.
- Use safety measures to minimize potential for injury.
- Describe rationale for interventions.
- Demonstrate measures to increase mobility.
- Evaluate pain and quality of management.

Interventions

NIC

Progressive Mobility Protocol, [24]Body Mechanics Promotion, Bed Rest Care, Exercise Promotion, Positioning, Self-Care Assistance

Determine if individual is physiologically stable for progressive mobilization; e.g., cardiac stability, use of 2 or more vaopressors.

Consult With Physical Therapist for Evaluation and Development of a Mobility Plan

R: *Physical therapists are professional experts on mobility.*

Promote Optimal Mobility and Movement in All Health-Care Settings With Stable Individuals Regardless of Ability to Walk

R: *"As technology and medications have improved and increased, survival rates are also increasing in intensive care units (ICUs), so it is now important to focus on improving the individual outcomes and recovery. To do this, ICU individuals need to be assessed and started on an early mobility program, if stable" (Zomorodi, Topley, & McAnaw, 2012, p. 1).*

R: *Early mobility has been linked to decreased morbidity and mortality as inactivity has a profound adverse effect on the brain, skin, skeletal muscle, pulmonary, and cardiovascular systems.*

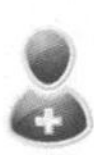

Clinical Alert "Critically ill individuals who are older, with comorbid conditions such as diabetes and preexisting cardiac disease and/or the presence of vasoactive agents, will be at greater risk for not tolerating in-bed mobilization. It is critical that the nurse assess the risk factors and plan when activity will occur to allow sufficient physiological rest to meet the oxygen demand that positioning will place on the body" (Vollman, 2012, p. 174).

Initiate an In-Bed Mobility Program Within Hours of Admission If Stable (Vollman, 2012)

- Maintain HOB 30°, including individual on ventilators unless contraindicated.

R: *This allows increased perfusion in all lung tissue.*

- Initiate a turning schedule within hours of admission if stable.

R: *This can prevent prolonged gravitational equilibrium. Prolonged periods in a stationary position result in greater hemodynamic instability when the individual turned (Vollman, 2012).*

- Assess tolerance to position change 5 to 10 minutes after apposition change.

R: *This time frame is needed to sufficiently assess response.*

- Initially turn slowly to right side.

R: *"The right lateral position should be used initially to prevent the hemodynamic challenges reported with use of the left lateral position" (Vollman, 2012, p. 174).*

R: *When the individual's positions are changed, their gravitational reference from one side to another, lying to sitting position, the body goes through a series of physiological adaptations to maintain cardiovascular homeostasis. With prolonged bed rest, a number of the normal compensatory mechanisms to posture change are disrupted (*Convertino et al., 1997).*

[24]Added by Lynda Juall Carpenito.

Initiate Early Progressive Mobility Protocol. Consult with Physical Therapy and Prescribing Provider (American Association of Critical Care Nurses [AACN] 2012; American Hospital Association, 2014; Timmerman, 2007; Zomorodi et al., 2012)

Prior to Initiating Step 2

- Evaluate need for analgesics versus risk of increased sedation prior to activity.
- Progress each step to 30 to 60 minutes duration as per individual's tolerance.
- Repeat each step until individual demonstrates hemodynamic and physical tolerance to stated activity/position for 60 minutes, then advance to next step at the next activity period.

Step 1: Safety Screening (AACN, 2012)

- M—Myocardial stability
  - No evidence of active myocardial ischemia × 24 hours
  - No dysrhythmia requiring new antidysrhythmic agent × 24 hours
- O—Oxygenation adequate on:
  - $FiO_2 < 0.6$
  - PEEP < 10 cmH_2O
- V—Vasopressor(s) minimal
  - No increase of any vasopressor × 2 hours
- E—Engages to voice
  - Individuals responds to verbal stimulation
- Reevaluate in 24 hours

Step 2: Progressive Mobility

- Level 1
  - Elevate head of bed (HOB) ≥30° TID, progress to 45° plus legs in dependent position (partial chair position).
  - Range of motion (ROM) TID
  - Turn Q 2 hours.
  - Passive ROM TID with RN, PCT, PT, OT, or family
  - Turn Q 2 hours.
  - Active resistance PT
  - Sitting on edge of bed
  - Sitting position: full-chair position 20 minutes TID
- Level 2
  - Passive ROM TID
  - Turn Q 2 hours.
  - Active resistance PT
  - Sitting position 20 minutes TID
  - Sitting on edge of bed
  - Active transfer to chair 20 min/day
- Level 3
  - Self- or assisted turning Q 2 hours
  - Passive ROM TID
  - Turn Q 2 hours with RN, PCT, PT, OT, or family
  - Active resistance with PT
  - Elevated HOB to 65° plus legs in full dependent position (full-chair position).
  - Consider lower HOB angle if individual's abdomen is large.
  - Sitting position 20 minutes TID
  - Sitting on edge of bed every 2 hours
  - Active transfer to chair 20 to 60 min/day
  - Ambulation (marching in place, walking in halls) (Patient must meet all criteria)
- Level 4
  - Passive ROM TID
  - Turn Q 2 hours.
  - Active resistance PT
  - Sitting position: 20 minutes TID
  - Sitting on edge of bed/stand at bedside with RN, PT, OT
  - Active transfer to chair 20 to 60 min/day (meal time) 3 × day
  - Ambulation (marching in place, walking in halls)
  - Encourage AAROM/AROM 3 × day with RN, PCT, PT, OT, or family

Assess for Clinical Signs and Symptoms Indicating Terminating a Mobilization Session (Adler & Malone, 2012)

Heart Rate

- >70% age-predicted maximum heart rate
- >20% decrease in resting HR
- <40 beats/min; >130 beats/min
- New onset dysrhythmia
- New antiarrhythmia medication
- New MI by ECG or cardiac enzymes

Pulse Oximetry/Saturation of Peripheral Oxygen (SpO_2)

- >4% decrease
- <88% to 90%

Blood Pressure

- Systolic BP >180 mm Hg
- >20% decrease in systolic/diastolic BP; orthostatic hypotension
- Mean arterial blood pressure <65 mm Hg; >110 mm Hg
- Presences of vasopressor medication; new vasopressor or escalating dose of vasopressor medication

Mechanical Ventilation

- Fraction of saturation of peripheral oxygen, (FiO_2) ≥0.60
- Positive end expiratory pressure (PEEP) ≥10
- Patient-ventilator asynchrony
- MV mode change to assist control
- Tenuous airway

Respiratory Rate

- <5 breaths/min; >40 breaths/min

Alertness/Agitation and Patient symptoms

- Patient sedation or coma—Richmond agitation sedation scale, ≤−3
- Patient agitation requiring addition or escalation of sedative medication; Richmond agitation sedation scale, >2
- Complaints of intolerable dyspnea on exertion

Initiate a Progressive Mobility Activity Protocol (PMAP) for Individuals in All Settings as Medical Stability Increases (e.g., Step-Down Unit, Medical, Surgical Units, Skilled Nursing Facilities)

R: *The PMAP is a nursing and interdisciplinary team approach to increase movement through a series of progressive steps from passive range of motion to ambulating independently as their medical stability increases (Hopkins & Spuhler, 2009).*

Explain to Individual and Family Why the Staff Are Frequently Moving the Individual

R: *An explanation of what the movement is preventing, for example, muscle wasting, blood clots, pneumonia may improve acceptability.*

Promote Motivation and Adherence (*Addams & Clough, 1998; Halstead & Stoten, 2010)

- Explain the effects of immobility.
- Explain the purpose of progressive mobility, passive and active ROM exercises.
- Establish short-term goals.
- Ensure that initial exercises are easy and require minimal strength and coordination.
- Progress only if the individual is successful at the present exercise.
- Provide written instructions for prescribed exercises after demonstrating and observing return demonstration.
- Document and discuss improvement specifically (e.g., can lift leg 2 in higher).

R: *Mobility is one of the most significant aspects of physiologic functioning because it greatly influences maintenance of independence (Miller, 2015). Motivation can be increased if short-term goals are accomplished.*

- Evaluate the level of motivation and depression. Refer to a specialist as needed.

R: *Effective management of pain and depression is sometimes necessary. Inadequate pain relief may be a primary factor leading to depression in some people, but depression should not be discounted as a secondary feature of pain. Depression may require aggressive management, including drugs and other therapies.*

Increase Limb Mobility and Determine Type of ROM Appropriate for the Client (Passive, Active Assistive, Active, Active Resistive)

- For passive ROM:
  - Begin exercises slowly, doing only a few movements at first.
  - Support the limb below the joint with one hand.
  - Move joint slowly and smoothly until you feel the stretch.
  - Move the joint to the point of resistance. Stop if the person complains of discomfort or you observe a facial grimace.
  - Do the exercise 10 times and old the position for a few seconds.
  - Do all exercises on one side and then repeat them on the opposite side if indicated.
  - If possible, teach the person or caregiver how to do the passive ROM.
  - Refer to ROM exercises at the website: alsworld.org for specific instructions and photos of passive ROM
- Perform active assistive ROM exercises (frequency determined by individual's condition):
  - If possible teach the individual/family to perform active ROM exercises on unaffected limbs at least four times a day, if possible.
  - Perform ROM on affected limbs. Do the exercises slowly to allow the muscles time to relax, and support the extremity above and below the joint to prevent strain on joints and tissues.
  - For ROM, the supine position is most effective. The individual/family member. who performs ROM himself or herself can use a supine or sitting position.
  - Do ROM daily with bed bath and three times daily if there are specific problem areas. Try to incorporate into activities of daily living.
- Support extremity with pillows to prevent or reduce swelling.
- Medicate for pain as needed, especially before activity.
- Apply heat or cold to reduce pain, inflammation, and hematoma per instructions.
- Encourage to perform exercise regimens for specific joints as prescribed by physical therapist (e.g., isometric, resistive).

R: *Active ROM increases muscle mass, tone, and strength and improves cardiac and respiratory functioning. Passive ROM improves joint mobility and circulation and decreases the likelihood of contractures.*

Position in Alignment to Prevent Complications

- Use a footboard.

R: *This measure prevents foot drop.*

- Avoid prolonged sitting or lying in the same position.

R: *This prevents hip flexion contractures.*

- Change the position of the shoulder joints every 2 to 4 hours.

R: *This helps to prevent shoulder contractures.*

- Use a small pillow or no pillow when in Fowler's position.

R: *This prevents flexion contracture of neck.*

- Support the hand and wrist in natural alignment.

R: *This prevents dependent edema and flexion contractures of the hand.*

- If it is supine or prone, place a rolled towel or small pillow under the lumbar curvature or under the end-of-the-rib cage.

R: *This prevents flexion or hyperflexion of lumbar curvature.*

- Place a trochanter roll alongside the hips and upper thighs.

R: *This presents external rotation of the femur and hips.*

- If in the lateral position, place pillow(s) to support the leg from groin to foot, and use a pillow to flex the shoulder and elbow slightly. If needed, support the lower foot in dorsal flexion with a towel roll or special boot.

R: *These measures prevent internal rotation and adduction of the femur and shoulder and prevent foot drop.*

- For upper extremities:
  - Arms abducted from the body with pillows
  - Elbows in slight flexion
  - Wrist in a neutral position, with fingers slightly flexed and thumb abducted and slightly flexed
  - Position of shoulder joints changed during the day (e.g., adduction, abduction, range of circular motion)

R: *These positions prevent contractures.*

Encourage Use of Affected Arm When Possible

- Encourage to use affected arm for self-care activities (e.g., feeding self, dressing, brushing hair).
- For post-CVA neglect of upper limb, see *Unilateral Neglect*.
- Instruct to use the unaffected arm to exercise the affected arm.
- Use appropriate adaptive equipment to enhance the use of arms.
  - Universal cuff for feeding in clients with poor control in both arms and hands
  - Large-handled or padded silverware to assist clients with poor fine-motor skills
  - Dishware with high edges to prevent food from slipping
  - Suction-cup aids to prevent sliding of plate.
- Use a warm bath to alleviate early morning stiffness and improve mobility.
- Encourage to practice handwriting skills, if able.
- Allow time to practice using affected limb.
- Determine if other factors are interfering with mobility.
  - If the pain is interfering with mobility, refer to *Acute* or *Chronic Pain*.
  - If depression is interfering with mobility, refer to *Ineffective Individual Coping*.
  - If fatigue is interfering with mobility, refer to *Fatigue*.

R: *Specific strategies are implemented to increase the use of affected arm and motivation.*

Consult with Physical Therapy to Teach Methods of Transfer From Bed to Chair or Commode and to Standing Position

Consult with PT for Instructions on Using Adaptive Equipment (e.g., Crutches, Walkers, and Canes)

Initiate Health Teaching and Referrals, as Indicated

- Home health nurse and physical therapist.

R: *This will ensure an assessment to determine if inpatient, outpatient, or home rehabilitation is indicated.*

Impaired Bed Mobility

NANDA-I Definition

Limitation of independent movement from one bed position to another

Defining Characteristics*

Impaired ability to turn from side to side
Impaired ability to move from supine to sitting to supine
Impaired ability to reposition self in bed
Impaired ability to move from supine to prone or prone to supine
Impaired ability to move from supine to long sitting or long sitting to supine

Related Factors

Refer to *Impaired Physical Mobility*.

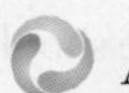 **Author's Note**

Impaired Bed Mobility may be a clinically useful diagnosis when an individual is a candidate for rehabilitation to improve strength, ROM, and movement. *Impaired Physical Mobility* addresses impaired bed mobility. This more specific diagnosis may be clinically useful with rehabilitative specialists such as nurses, physical therapists. More specialized interventions are beyond the scope of this book. The nurse can consult with a physical therapist for a specific plan. This diagnosis is inappropriate for an unconscious or terminally ill client.

Key Concepts

Refer to *Impaired Physical Mobility*.

Focus Assessment Criteria

Refer to *Impaired Physical Mobility*.

Goals

NOC

Bed Positioning: Self-limited

Refer to *Impaired Physical Mobility*.

Interventions

NIC

Exercise Therapy: Joint Mobility, Exercise Promotion: Strength Training, Exercise Therapy: Ambulation, Positioning, Teaching: Prescribed Activity/Exercise, Prosthesis Care

Refer to *Impaired Physical Mobility*.

Impaired Sitting

Definition

Limitation of ability to independently and purposefully attain and/or maintain a rest position that is supported by the buttocks and thighs, in which the torso is upright.

Defining Characteristics

Impaired ability to adjust position of one or both lower limbs on uneven surface
Impaired ability to attain a balanced position of the torso
Impaired ability to flex or move both hips
Impaired ability to flex or move both knees
Impaired ability to maintain the torso in balanced position
Impaired ability to stress torso with body weight
Insufficient muscle strength

Related Factors

Alteration in cognitive functioning
Insufficient endurance
Malnutrition
Impaired metabolic functioning
Insufficient energy
Neurological disorder

Orthopedic surgery
Prescribed posture
Sarcopenia
Pain
Psychological disorder
Self-imposed relief posture

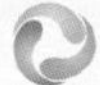

Author's Note

Impaired Sitting (a newly accepted NANDA-I nursing diagnosis) can be a clinically useful diagnosis when an individual is a candidate for rehabilitation to improve strength, ROM, and balance. *Impaired Physical Mobility* addresses impaired sitting. This more specific diagnosis may be clinically useful with rehabilitative specialists as nurses, physical therapists. More specialized interventions are beyond the scope of this book. The nurse can consult with a physical therapist for a specific plan.

Key Concepts

Refer to *Impaired Physical Mobility*.

Focus Assessment Criteria

Refer to *Impaired Physical Mobility*.

Impaired Standing

Definition

Limitation of ability to independently and purposefully attain and/or maintain the body in an upright position from feet to head.

Defining Characteristics

Impaired ability to adjust position of one or both lower limbs on uneven surface
Impaired ability to attain a balanced position of the torso
Impaired ability to extend one or both hips
Impaired ability to extend one or both knees
Impaired ability to flex one or both hips
Impaired ability to flex one or both knees
Impaired ability to maintain the torso in balanced position
Impaired ability to stress torso with body weight
Insufficient muscle strength

Related Factors

Circulatory perfusion disorder
Impaired metabolic functioning
Insufficient endurance
Malnutrition
Obesity
Prescribed posture
Self-imposed relief posture
Emotional disturbance
Injury to lower extremity
Insufficient energy
Neurologic disorder
Pain
Sarcopenia
Surgical procedure

Author's Note

Impaired Standing (a newly accepted NANDA-I Nursing diagnosis) can be a clinically useful diagnosis when an individual is a candidate for rehabilitation to improve strength, ROM, and balance. *Impaired Physical Mobility* addresses impaired standing. This more specific diagnosis may be clinically useful with rehabilitative specialists as nurses, physical therapists. More specialized interventions are beyond the scope of this book. The nurse can consult with a physical therapist for a specific plan.

Key Concepts

Refer to *Impaired Physical Mobility*.

Focus Assessment Criteria

Refer to *Impaired Physical Mobility*.

Impaired Walking

NANDA-I Definition

Limitation of independent movement within the environment on foot

Defining Characteristics*

Impaired ability to climb stairs
Impaired ability to walk required distances
Impaired ability to walk on an incline
Impaired ability to walk on uneven surfaces
Impaired ability to navigate curbs

Author's Note

Impaired Walking can be a clinically useful diagnosis when an individual is a candidate for rehabilitation to improve strength, ROM, and balance. *Impaired Physical Mobility* addresses *Impaired Walking*. This more specific diagnosis may be clinically useful with rehabilitative specialists as nurses, physical therapists. More specialized interventions are beyond the scope of this book. The nurse can consult with a physical therapist for a specific plan.

Related Factors

Refer to *Impaired Physical Mobility*.

Key Concepts

Refer to *Impaired Physical Mobility*.

Focus Assessment Criteria

Refer to *Impaired Physical Mobility*.

Goals

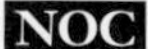

Refer to *Impaired Physical Mobility*.

The client will increase walking distances (specify distance goal) as evidenced by the following indicators:

- Demonstrates safe mobility
- Uses mobility aids correctly

Interventions

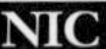

Refer to *Impaired Physical Mobility*.

Explain That Safe Ambulation Is a Complex Movement Involving the Musculoskeletal, Neurologic, and Cardiovascular Systems and Cognitive Factors Such as Mentation and Orientation

R: *A client who is deconditioned needs a progressive exercise program.*

Consult With a Physical Therapist for Evaluation and Planning Prior to Initiation

R: *Physical therapy consultation is imperative to prevent injury and to maintaining weight-bearing limitations.*

- Ascertain that the person is:
  - Using ambulatory aids (e.g., cane, walker, crutches) correctly and safely:
    - Wears well-fitting shoes
    - Can ambulate on inclines, uneven surfaces, and up and down stairs
    - Is aware of hazards (e.g., wet floors, throw rugs)

R: *Evaluation is needed to prevent injury to tissue structures and falls.*

- Refer to *Impaired Physical Mobility*.

Provide Progressive Mobilization, If Indicated

- Refer to *Impaired Physical Mobility*.

Impaired Wheelchair Mobility

NANDA-I Definition

Limitation of independent operation of wheelchair within the environment

Defining Characteristics*

Impaired ability to operate manual or power wheelchair on an even or uneven surface
Impaired ability to operate manual or power wheelchair on an incline
Impaired ability to operate manual or power wheelchair on a decline
Impaired ability to operate the wheelchair on curbs

Related Factors

Refer to *Impaired Physical Mobility*.

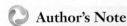

Author's Note

Impaired Wheelchair Mobility can be a clinically useful diagnosis when an individual is in need of instruction on using a wheelchair safely. This more specific diagnosis may be clinically useful with rehabilitative specialists as nurses, physical therapists. More specialized interventions are beyond the scope of this book.

Key Concepts

Refer to *Impaired Physical Mobility*.

Focus Assessment Criteria

Refer to *Impaired Physical Mobility*.

Goals

NOC

Body Mechanics Promotion, Exercise Therapy:: Positioning: Wheelchair, Fall Prevention Ambulation: Wheelchair

The individual will report satisfactory, safe wheelchair mobility as evidenced by the following indicators:

- Demonstrates safe use of the wheelchair
- Demonstrates safe transfer to/from the wheelchair
- Demonstrates pressure relief and safety principles

Interventions

NIC
Exercise Therapy: Balance, Exercise Promotion: Joint Mobility, Exercise Promotion: Strength Training, Positioning: Wheelchair, Fall Prevention, Body Mechanics Promotion, Exercise Therapy: Ambulation

Consult With Physical Therapist for a One–One Sessions to Teach and Assess Wheel Chair Use, Safety Issues

R: *The specialists should direct the plan with nursing reinforcing the teaching.*

Refer to a Physical Therapist for Instruction on Using the Wheelchair on Flat Surfaces, Curbs, in Elevators, and So Forth

R: *Specialists should be consulted to improve confidence and to prevent injuries.*

Refer to Home Health Nurse and Physical Therapist for Evaluation of Home Environment

R: *Wheelchair accessibility and other barriers to safe wheelchair use need to be assessed. Research has reported falls with sustained injuries and failure to make home modifications in a home with a individual in a wheelchair*

For More Specific Information Regarding Wheel Chair Use and Components

- Refer individual/family regarding the wheel chair sitting page at www.uab.edu.

Impaired Transfer Ability

NANDA-I Definition

Limitation of independent movement between two nearby surfaces

Defining Characteristics*

Impaired ability to transfer:
From bed to chair and chair to bed
On or off a toilet or commode
In and out of tub or shower
Between uneven levels
From chair to car or car to chair
From chair to floor or floor to chair
From standing to floor or floor to standing
From bed to standing or standing to bed
From chair to standing or standing to chair

Related Factors

Refer to *Impaired Physical Mobility*.

Author's Note

Impaired Transfer Ability can be a clinically useful diagnosis when an individual is in need of instruction on transferring from one surface to another. This more specific diagnosis may be clinically useful with rehabilitative specialists as nurses, physical therapists. More specialized interventions are beyond the scope of this book.

Key Concepts

Refer to *Impaired Physical Mobility*.

Focus Assessment Criteria

Refer to *Impaired Physical Mobility*.

Goals

NOC
Body Positioning: Self-Initiated Transfer Performance, Fall Prevention Behavior

The individual will demonstrate transfer to and from the wheelchair as evidenced by the following indicators:

- Identifies when assistance is needed
- Demonstrates ability to transfer in varied situations (e.g., toilet, bed, car, chair, uneven levels)

Interventions

NIC
Positioning: Wheelchair, Fall Prevention, Body Mechanic, Environmental Management: Safety

Consult With and Refer to a Physical Therapist to Evaluate the Person's Ability to Transfer

- Consider weight, strength, movement ability, tolerance to position changes, balance, motivation, and cognition.
- Use manual transfer or device-assisted lift.
- Consider ratio of staff to clients.

R: *A consultation with a physical therapist is needed to create a care plan for this client under Impaired Transfer Ability.*

Proceed With Established Plan to Transfer

- Before transferring, assess the number of personnel needed for assistance.
- The person should transfer toward the unaffected side.
- Position person on the side of the bed. His or her feet should be touching the floor, and he or she should be wearing stable shoes or slippers with nonskid soles.
- For getting in and out of bed, encourage weight-bearing on the uninvolved or stronger side.
- Lock the wheelchair before the transfer. If using a regular chair, be sure it will not move.
- Instruct to use the arm of the chair closer to him or her for support while standing.
- Use a gait belt (preferred) or place your arm around the client's rib cage and keep the back straight, with knees slightly bent.
- Tell to place his or her arms around your waist or rib cage, *not the neck*.
- Support legs by bracing his with yours. (While facing the client, lock his or her knees with your knees.)
- Instruct the person with hemiplegia to pivot on the uninvolved foot.

R: *Specific instructions and sufficient staff can prevent injury to the client and staff*

R: *Approximately 35% of fall-related injuries occur among the nonambulatory residents in skilled nursing facilities.*

Initiate Health Teaching and Referrals as Indicated

- Consult and refer the family to home health nurses/physical therapist for a home evaluation and to access resources for transition.

MORAL DISTRESS

Moral Distress

Risk for Moral Distress

Definition

Response to the inability to carry out one's chosen ethical/moral decision/action (NANDA-I)

The state in which a person experiences psychological disequilibrium, physical discomforts, anxiety, and/or anguish that results when a person makes a moral decision but does not follow through with the moral behavior.[25]

[25]This definition has been added by Lynda Juall Carpenito, the author, for clarity and clinical usefulness.

Defining Characteristics*

Expresses anguish (e.g., powerlessness, guilt, frustration, anxiety, self-doubt, fear) over difficulty acting on one's moral choice

Related Factors

When *Moral Distress* is used to describe a response in nurses, as explained in this section, related factors are not necessary or useful. These diagnoses are not documented in an individual's health/medical record, but rather represent a response that requires actions by the nurse, unit, and/or institution. The institution should have a standard of practice, which addresses moral and ethical conflict.

The related factors listed below represent the numerous sources of moral distress in nursing:

Situational (Personal, Environmental)

End-of-Life Decisions*

Related to providing treatments that were perceived as futile for terminally ill individual (e.g., blood transfusions, chemotherapy, organ transplants, mechanical ventilation)

Related to conflicting attitudes toward advanced directives

Related to participation of life-saving actions when they only prolong dying

Treatment Decisions

Related to the individual's/family's refusal of treatments deemed appropriate by the health-care team

Related to inability of the family to make the decision to stop ventilator treatment of terminally ill individual

Related to a family's wishes to continue life support even though it is not in the best interest of the individual

Related to performing a procedure that increases the individual's suffering

Related to providing care that does not relieve the individual's suffering

Related to conflicts between wanting to disclose poor medical practice and wanting to maintain trust in the physician

Professional Conflicts

Related to insufficient resources for care (e.g., time, staff)

Related to failure to be included in the decision-making process

Related to more emphasis on technical skills and tasks than on relationships and caring

Cultural Conflicts

Related to decisions made for women by male family members

Related to cultural conflicts with the American health-care system

Author's Note

There are over 180 NANDA-I-approved nursing diagnoses. None are more critical to professional nursing practice than *Moral Distress* and *Risk for Compromised Human Dignity*.

Moral Distress and *Risk for Compromised Human Dignity* diagnoses represent the core practice competencies that are mandated by the American Nurses Association in *Nursing scope and standards* and *Code of ethics for nurses with interpretive statements*. When a nurse practices without these competencies, they, the ill, and their loved ones will be destined to increased suffering, disrespect, and demoralization. Eighty-six percent of Americans polled reported nurses have very high or high ethical standards, ranking nurses at the top of all other professions (Gallup Poll, 2014).

To be successful in maintaining these high ethical standards, nurses must strive for moral competence to prevent *Moral Distress* and *Risk for Compromised Human Dignity* in those for whom you care and in yourself. Moral competence has eight attributes: loving kindness, compassion, sympathetic joy, equanimity, responsibility, discipline, honesty, and respect for human values, dignity and rights.

"Healthy work environments (HWEs) are important for the overall health of nurses, for successful nurse recruitment and retention, and for the quality and safety of patient care" (Kupperschmidt, Kientz, Ward, & Reinholz, 2010). "Healthy work environments are healing, empowering environments that have been correlated with employee engagement and organizational commitment" (Kupperschmidt et al., 2010).

". . .a healthy work environment must begin with each nurse being intentional and reflective about their experiences" (Kupperschmidt et al., 2010). This means one must avoid self-depiction, for example, "It is not that bad,*" " not my patient, acknowledging the reality, owning one's feelings, sharing thoughts on difficult or challenging concerns and listening to the views of others (Kupperschmidt et al., 2010). When nurses feel supported within a safe, ethical environment in which their clinical reasoning and judgment are valued, moral distress decreases and job satisfaction increases (Kupperschmidt et al., 2010).

If moral distress occurs in an individual patient or family, this author suggests a referral to a professional expert in this area; for example, a counselor, therapist, or spiritual advisor. Refer also to *Spiritual Distress*. Nurses should expect to experience moral distress as they struggle to make clinical decisions involving conflicting ethical principles (Zuzelo, 2007).

In the 14th edition of this book this author developed and included *Risk for Moral Distress*.

Risk for Moral Distress represents proactive strategies for individuals, groups, and institutions to prevent moral distress in themselves and other nurses. This diagnosis has not yet been submitted to NANDA-I.

"Most Americans fear how they will die more than death itself" (*Beckstrand, Callsiter, & Kirchkoff, 2006). Nurses should expect to experience moral distress as they struggle to make clinical decisions involving conflicting ethical principles (Zuzelo, 2007).

Key Concepts

- Hamric, Borchers, and Epstein (2012, p. 1) reported "The proportion of physicians and nurses who had left a previous position or who were considering leaving their current positions due to moral distress was high (16% and 31%, respectively)."
- Moral courage is the willingness of individuals, despite adversity, fear, and personal risk, to act on and fully support ethical responsibilities (*Gallagher, 2010; *Lachman, 2010; *Murray, 2010).
- "Moral competence is the individual's ability to live in a manner consistent with a personal code and role responsibilities. Society expects moral competence in nurses" (*Jormsri, Kunaviktikul, Ketefian, & Chaowalit, 2005, pp. 582–583).
- Baxter (2012) reported research on "the experience and meaning of becoming certain of the right course of action in the context of moral distress". "Participants 'recognized' or 'knew' the right action as they considered the situation within the context and their own personal context."… When resources were not available to provide alternative views, participants had to rely on only what they knew, thus creating moral certitude.
- Moral certitude (or certainty) is the term used to describe a very firm belief based on an inner conviction. Morally certain individuals believe that they are correct in their beliefs to the extent that they have no reservations whatsoever about the rightness of their beliefs (*Murray, 2010).
- "Moral arrogance involves truly believing that one's own moral stand or judgment is the only correct option regarding a controversial issue, even though others consider differing moral decisions or judgments to be morally acceptable" (*Gert, Culver & Clouser, 2006 in *Murray, 2010; *Jameton, 1984).
- Moral arrogance and moral certitude inhibit the thoughtful assessment needed in ethical practice. These attitudes bring with them the risk of suppressing open dialogue and forthright deliberation regarding ethical issues (*Murray, 2010).
- Gutierrez (*2005) reported "nurses' moral judgment and perceptions of appropriate moral actions [are] linked to strong moral values to ease suffering (nonmaleficence), respect individual wishes (autonomy), maintain truthfulness (veracity), and distribute scarce health care resources appropriately (justice)."
- Nurses are in a unique position to advocate for the individual and family and assist in decision making because they are closely integrated with them during caregiving and because they do not benefit financially from treatment decisions that are offered.
- Rodney et al. (*2002) reported that nurses were influenced by constraining and facilitating factors perceived as being beyond their control. Examples of constraining factors are privileges of physicians and corporate ethos. Examples of facilitating factors are supportive colleagues, professional guidelines, standards, and ethical educational forums (*Rodney et al., 2003;Zuzelo, 2007).

- Barriers to acting on one's moral distress are external and internal (*Wilkinson, 1988). These powerful constraints can prevent moral actions
  - External
    - Physicians
    - Fear of lawsuits
    - Unsupportive nursing administrators, agency administration policies
  - Internal
    - Fear of losing their job
    - Self-doubts
    - Futility of past actions
    - Socialization to follow orders
    - Lack of courage
- In 2010, 29% of Americans died in hospitals, down from 32% in 2000, possibly due to increased use of hospice care (Hall, Levant, & DeFrances, 2013).
- Aging Stats.gov (2012) reported
  - Both hospice and ICU/CCU use are common in the last month of life. In 2009, 43% of elderly decedents used hospice services in the last 30 days of life, and 27% used ICU/CCU services.
  - Use of hospice has increased substantially in recent years, from 19% of decedents in 1999 to 43% in 2009. Use of ICU/CCU services has grown more slowly, from 22% in 1999 to 27% in 2009.
- The distinction between critical illness and terminal illness is not clear (*Elpern, Covert, & Kleinpell, 2005). Dying while receiving aggressive interventions to extend life produces confusion, conflicts, and distress in caregivers, individuals, and families (*Elpern et al., 2005; Zomorodi, 2010).
- In *2001, Corley and coworkers reported that 15% of the nurses studied related that they have left a job because of moral distress. In 2005, the same investigators reported the percentage to be greater than 25.5%. An estimated 30% to 50% of all new RNs elect either to change positions or leave nursing completely within the first 3 years of clinical practice (American Association of Colleges of Nursing, 2010; *Cipriano, 2006).
- Researchers with a descriptive correlational study of new RNs ($n = 187$), found up to half had considered leaving nursing within the first year. By the third year, almost one-third of the new RNs had left nursing or decreased work hours to part-time (*Cowin & Hengstberger-Sims, 2006).
- Using a phenomenological research design, MacKusick & Minick (2010) interviewed nurses who were no longer working in nursing. Three themes emerged from the interviews:
  - "Unfriendly workplace was reported by all RNs in the study. Participants described being left alone or ignored as new RNs or being told to 'toughen up' under the auspices of making them 'better nurses'" (p. 337).
  - "Overly aggressive treatment, lack of collaboration between physicians and staff, and lack of respect for patient and family wishes caused recurrent emotional distress among the interviewees" (p. 338).
  - "Working in an unfriendly workplace and being exposed to emotionally distressing dilemmas on a frequent basis was followed typically by insurmountable fatigue and exhaustion" (p. 339).

Clinical Alert As one reviews the above conflicts that have and continue to demoralize new and seasoned nurses, it is soul breaking to note that we as nurses continue to fail to bond together to improve our collective lived experiences. Are we so damaged, that we cannot care for ourselves and each other? We and only we as nurses know how difficult nursing is. We get along by

- Offering a hand instead of criticism
- Praising and defending each other in public
- Discuss conflicts in private and only with each other
- Letting the gossip stop with you
- Stopping this dreadful rite of passage for our new nursing colleagues. We know they need our help
- Holding your criticism. Are our memories so short that we have forgotten how poorly we were treated as new graduates?
- And when a new nurse arrives on your unit, reaching out with a warm greeting, having a welcome cake or rose.

We spend more time with the people we work with than who we live with, so let us laugh together and cry together.

- Elpern et al. (*2005), using the Moral Distress Scale, reported the following factors with the highest levels of moral distress to be related to:
  - Continue to participate in care for the terminally ill individual who is being sustained on a ventilator when no one will make a decision to "pull the plug."
  - Follow a family's wishes to continue life support even though it is not the best interest of the individual.
  - Initiate extensive life-saving actions when I think it only prolongs death.
  - Follow the family's wishes for the individual's care when I do not agree with them but do so because the hospital administration fears a lawsuit.
  - Carry out the physician's orders for unnecessary tests and treatments for terminally ill individuals.
  - Provide care that does not relieve the individual's suffering because the physician fears increasing doses of pain medication will cause death (*Elpern et al., 2005).
- Zuzelo (2007) used Corley's Moral Distress Scale with a Likert scale of 0 to 6 (0 = no moral distress; 6 = extreme moral distress). The most distressing events were:
  - Working with unsafe nurses
  - Working with physicians (nurse practitioners [NPs], physician assistants [PAs]) not competent in providing the care the person needs.
  - Ineffective prescribed pain medication regimens
  - Family wishes to continue life support measures when it is not in the best interest of the individual.
  - Implement a physician's (NP's, PA's) order for unnecessary tests or treatments
  - When individuals were used by students, interns, residents to practice a painful procedure
- Edmonson (2015) has produced important work to strengthen the moral courage of nurse leaders, by identifying "factors that would increase their ability to act courageously in morally distressing situations." In phase one of the study, participants self-evaluated their current level of professional moral courage as baseline data. In phase two, the group was taught about ethics and moral courage. In phase three, 2 weeks after the course, participants completed a post course self-evaluation of their level of professional moral courage.
- Edmonson (2015) wrote, "Organizational leaders need to recognize the need for an environment conducive to moral acts through a balanced, safe, and open forum for discussion. Discussions may include internal/external influencing factors, participant/observer emotions, a learning environment, a strong ethics foundation, and an environment where courageous acts are encouraged, recognized, and rewarded."

Focus Assessment Criteria

Subjective Data

Assess for the Psychological and Physical Effects of Moral Distress and Caregiver Fatigue on Yourself or Colleagues (*American Association of Critical Care Nurses, 2004)

R: *Self-hatred, low self-esteem, burnout, hardening, or jading can develop in nurses who experience prolonged exposure to unrelieved moral distress.*

- Fatigue, exhaustion, headaches, lethargy, forgetfulness
- Gastrointestinal hyperactivity disturbances, weight gain/weight loss
- Impaired sleep, impaired mental susceptibility processes such as to illness, anger, sarcasm, guilt, emotional outbursts, emotional shutdown, cynical
- Apathy, indifference, avoidance, agitation, shaming others, victim behaviors
- Overinvolvement/underinvolvement/disengagement in care situations
- Spiritual distress, loss of meaning, loss of self-worth

R: *Moral stress is "commonly experienced by healthcare professionals as they struggle to make clinical decisions involving conflicting ethical principles" (Zuzelo, 2007). Nurses may also displace negative feelings or actions toward the offending source through horizontal violence, bullying, job dissatisfaction, lack of focus on primary work or disruptive behavior. This creates a toxic work environment (Edmonson, 2015).*

Goals

NOC

Not applicable

The nurse will relate the strategies to address moral distress as evidenced by the following indicators:

- Identifies the source(s) of moral distress
- Shares their distress with a colleague
- Identifies two strategies to enhance decision making with individual and family
- Identifies two strategies to enhance the discussion of the situation with the prescribing professional

Interventions

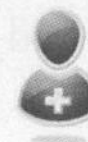

Clinical Alert "Most Americans fear how they will die more than death itself" (*Beckstrand et al., 2006). Eighty-six percent of Americans polled reported nurses have very high or high ethical standards, ranking nurses at the top of other professions (Gallup Poll, 2014).

NOC

Not applicable

Identify Sources of Moral Stress (*American Association of Critical Care Nurses, 2004)

- Inadequate Staffing
- Competency of team members (e.g., nurses, physicians, medical assistants, managers, technicians)
- Unsatisfactory response to requests
- Futile care
- Needless pain and suffering
- End-of-life challenges
- Deception/incomplete information
- Inadequate symptom management
- Disrespectful interactions
- Violence in the workplace

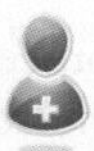

Clinical Alert Jameton (*1984) was the first to describe moral distress as a painful feeling that can cause psychological imbalance when nurses know what is the right thing to do but feel unable to do it. Jameton also described moral arrogance or certainty is when one believes their own moral judgment is the only correct option.

Consider the CODE Approach Prior to Responding to a Problematic Situation (*Lachman, 2010)

- Refer to Box II.4.

R: *Plato wrote that moral character is composed of courage, temperance, justice, and wisdom (*Lachman, 2010; Stanford Encyclopedia of Philosophy, 2007). "Moral courage is the ability to deal with the dilemmas inherent between these four virtues, along with an ability to endure distress, and the ability to overcome fear and stand up for one's values" (*Lachman, 2010).*

Box II.4 THE CODE APPROACH TO RESPONDING TO A PROBLEMATIC SITUATION (Lachman, 2010)

- **C**ourage to be moral requires:
- **O**bligations to honor (What is the right thing to do?)
  - The following documents serve to describe the ethical and moral obligations of all nurses.
    - ANA. (2010a). *Nursing social policy statement*/the essence of the profession. Silver Springs, MD: Author.
    - ANA. (2010b). *Nursing scope and standards*. Silver Springs, MD: Author.
    - ANA. (2015). *Code of ethics for nurses with interpretive statements*. Silver Springs, MD: Author.
    - ANA. (2012). *Nursing care and Do Not Resuscitate (DNR) and Allow Natural Death (AND) decisions*. Silver Springs, MD: Author.
  - For example in Standard 11 Communication in the ANA Scope of Practice (2010)
    - The registered nurse communicates effectively in all areas of practice with the following related competencies:
      - Seeks continuous improvement of communication and conflict resolution skills
      - Conveys information to health-care consumers, families, the interprofessional team, and others in communication formats that promote accuracy
      - Questions the rationale supporting care processes and decisions when they do not appear to be in the best interest of the patient
      - Discloses observations or concerns related to hazards and errors in care or the practice environment to the appropriate level
- **D**anger management (What do I need to handle my fear?)

R: *"One danger or hindrance to moral courage is that of ethical incompetence. Ethical competence requires cognitive strategies, including the ability to analyze and thoughtfully respond to a moral problem unrestrained by automatic responses and belief/emotional fixations" (*Lachman, 2010). Ethical competence demands emotional control which enhances insight into both the situation and one's reaction to the situation (*Lachman, 2010).*

  - Deliberate the risk analysis is important—"What is the worse outcome that could happen if I speak up?" "What is the worst outcome that could happen if I do not speak up?" Are you prepared for these possible outcomes if they occur?
- **E**xpression and action (What action do I need to take to maintain my integrity?)
  - "Strong communication skills, including assertiveness and negotiation, are necessary in situations demanding moral courage" (*Lachman, 2010). "These crucial skills help individuals deal with the hostility, defensiveness, and a variety of other tactics used by people to prevent one from acting in a morally courageous manner" (*Lachman, 2010).

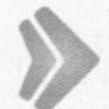

Carp's Cues

The reader is referred to the source, Lachman, V. D. (2010). Strategies necessary for moral courage. *The Online Journal of Issues in Nursing, 15*, 3. Accessed at www.nursingworld.org

Avoid Rationalization

R: *Rationalization is when nurses have justifications for their behaviors to protect themselves from grief and distress. This self-deception can over time transform the nurse from a caring to an uncaring professional (Coverston & Lassetter, 2010).*

"Use the Chain of Command to Share and Discuss Issues That Have Escalated Beyond the Problem-Solving Ability and/or Scope of Those Immediately Involved" (LaSala & Bjarnason, 2010)

R: *The urgency of the situation requires immediate attention.*

Explore Moral Work and Action

- Educate yourself about moral distress. Refer to articles on Bibliography.
- Share your stories of moral distress. Elicit stories from coworkers.
- Read stories of moral action. Refer to Gordon's *Life Support: Three Nurses on the Front Lines* and Kritek's *Reflections on Healing: A Central Construct* (see Bibliography).

R: *Stories can help nurses identify strengths, insights, shared distress, and options for moral actions (*Tiedje, 2000). Nurses responded positively when they were asked to discuss their feelings regarding moral issues (*Elpern et al., 2005).*

Investigate How Clinical Situations That Are Morally Problematic Are Managed in the Institution

R: *Organizational practices that support open discussions about individual care issues and problems with ethical and moral implications contribute to perceptions of an ethical climate for clinicians. "Organizational constraints included limited finances (resources), poor staffing patterns, and weak policies. These constraints result in organizational culpability for nurses who feel unrelieved distress because they could not advocate effectively for their own or their patients' well-being" (Edmonson, 2015).*

If an Ethics Committee Exists, Determine Its Mission and Procedures

Initiate Dialogue With the Individual, If Possible, and Family

- Explore what the perception of the situation is (e.g., How do you think your ___ is doing?)
- Pose questions (e.g., "What options do you have in this situation?"). Elicit feelings about the present situation. Does the family know that the individual is terminal? Is the individual improving?
- Access the physician to clarify misinformation. Stay in the room to promote sharing.
- Encourage the individual/family to write down questions for the physician.
- Be present during physician's round to ensure individual's/family's understanding.
- Avoid deception or supporting deception.

R: *Inadequate or poor communication is the primary cause of problematic situations that contribute to moral distress (*Gutierrez, 2005; LaSala & Bjarnason, 2010; Zuzelo, 2007).*

Gently Explore the Individual/Family End-of-Life Decisions

- Explain the options (e.g., "If you or your loved one's heart/breathing stops…"):
    - Medications, oxygen
    - Cardio defibrillation (shock)
    - Cardiopulmonary resuscitation
    - Intubation and use of respirator
- Advise the individual/family that they can choose all, some, or none of the above.
- Differentiate between prolonging life versus prolonging dying.
- Document the discussion and decisions according to institute on policy.

R: *Direct but gentle inquiries and discussions can assist the individual/family to examine the situation clearly and the implications of treatment options and decisions.*

If Indicated, Explain "No Code" Status and Explain the Focus of Palliative Care That Replaces Aggressive and Futile Care (e.g., Pain Management, Symptom Management, Less or No Intrusive/Painful Procedures)

R: *Often, families think that "no code" status means no care. Palliative care focuses on comfort during the dying process.*

Seek to Transfer the Individual From Intensive Care Unit, If Possible

R: *Intensive care unit (ICU) environments have many barriers to a palliative care environment (e.g., noise, frequent interruptions, close quarters)*

Dialogue With Unit Colleagues About the Situation That Causes Moral Distress

R: *Elpern et al. (*2005) found that nurses were relieved that their personal distress was shared and that they were not unique in their feelings. Sharing moral concerns may lead to less moral distress (Zuzelo, 2007).*

Seek Support and Information From Nurse Manager

R: *"Nurse managers may be an important first step in enhancing the ethical reasoning and moral assertiveness of nurses" (Zuzelo, 2007).*

Enlist a Colleague as a Coach or Engage as a Coach for a Coworker

- For advice, seek out colleagues who implement actions when they are distressed.

R: *A coach is a colleague who can listen, guide, and provide feedback throughout the process (*Tiedje, 2000). Gutierrez (*2005) reported 67% of nurses sought out support from other nurses. These nurses reported support for their negative feelings but did not receive help to initiate moral action.*

Engage in Open Communication With Involved Physicians or Nurse Manager; Start the Conversation With Your Concern, for Example, "I Am Not Comfortable With…," "The Family Is Asking/Questioning/Feeling…," "Mr. X Is Asking/Questioning/Feeling…"

R: *Each professional has rights and duties, and conflict may be resolved through open communication and sharing of feelings and values (*Caswell & Cryer, 1995; LaSala & Bjarnason, 2010). Nonthreatening language can reduce embarrassment and blame.*

Dialogue With Other Professionals: Chaplains, Social Workers, or Ethics Committee

R: *Nurses can be assisted in moral work with support from others in the organization.*

Advocate for End-of-Life Decision Dialogues With All Individuals and Their Families, Especially When the Situation is Not Critical; Direct the Individual to Create Written Documents of Their Decisions, and Advise the Family About the Document

R: *Exploring end-of-life decisions when there are no imminent threats to survival provide the most optimal setting for discussions. Decisions that are viewed as well thought out may assist the family with honoring their loved one's decision.*

Integrate Health Promotion and Stress Reduction in Your Lifestyle (e.g., Smoking Cessation, Weight Management, Regular Exercise, Meaningful Leisure Activities)

R: *Healthy lifestyles can reduce stress and increase energy levels for moral work.*

Risk for Moral Distress

Definition[26]

The state in which a person is at risk to experience psychological disequilibrium, physical discomforts, anxiety, and/or anguish that results when a person makes a moral decision but does not follow through with the moral behavior

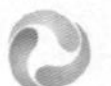

Author's Note

Refer to *Moral Distress*.

Risk Factors

Refer to *Moral Distress*—Related Factors.

[26]This definition has been added by Lynda Juall Carpenito, the author, for clarity and clinical usefulness.

Key Concepts

Refer to *Moral Distress*.

Focus Assessment Criteria

Refer to *Moral Distress*.

Goals

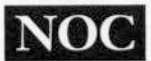

NOC
Nonapplicable

The nurse will relate the strategies to prevent moral distress, as evidenced by the following indicators:

- Identifies risk situations for moral distress
- Shares their distress with a colleague
- Identifies two strategies to enhance decision making with individuals and families
- Identifies two strategies to enhance communication patterns with proscribing professionals
- Engages institutional programs to prevent or decrease moral distress
- Engages in self-care strategies to enhance your health and prevent compassion fatigue

Interventions

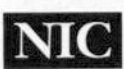

NIC
Nonapplicable

The following interventions are indicated for the institution and department of nursing:

Create a Just Culture That Fosters Moral Courage (American Nurses Association [ANA], 2010a)

- Commitment to organizational improvement
- Resilience
- Mission, vision, and values that support high-quality individual outcomes and increasing situational awareness
- Identifying at-risk behavior creates incentives for healthy behaviors.
- Address the problem of behaviors that threaten the performance of the health-care team.
- Make choices that align with organizational values.

R: *A just culture recognizes that individual care, safety, and quality are based on teamwork, communication, and a collaborative work environment (ANA, 2010a; LaSala & Bjarnason, 2010).*

Explore Moral Work and Action

- "Determining, assessing and exploring personal values, and then identifying the impact of these values on nursing practice are essential for dealing with day to day ethical issues" (*Scanlon & Fleming, 1989 in *Jormsri et al., 2005, p. 584).
  - Educate yourself about moral distress. Refer to articles on Bibliography.
  - Share your stories of moral distress. Elicit stories from coworkers.
  - Read stories of moral action. Refer to Gordon's *Life Support: Three Nurses on the Front Lines* and Kritek's *Reflections on Healing: A Central Construct* (see Bibliography).

R: *Stories can help nurses identify strengths, insights, shared distress, and options for moral actions (*Tiedje, 2000). Nurses respond (*Elpern et al., 2005).*

- Consider the words of Dr. Arthur Frank (2007), a sociologist, provisional resolutions for a recovering caregiver offered for dialogue and revision by professionals who feel a need to reflect on what care means in their lives and their conditions of work (6 of 13 from his paper provided here):
  - I will ask myself: By telling or not telling a truth at this moment, whom is that serving (or whom is that hurting)?
  - I am responsible for how I offer care, but I do not work in conditions of my own choosing.
  - I forgive myself for doing what my working conditions require, but forgiveness requires working to change whatever is detrimental to care.
  - My words and gestures, and the attitudes I project through my actions, affect the healing of my patients, the morale of my coworkers, and the moral self I become.
  - If I ever feel my work is out of my control, then I have ceased to be an effective professional and need either a day off, or to lead a protest, or both.
  - I will recognize who—patient, coworker, or myself—pays what price in which currency—money, time, physical risk, dignity—to keep the institution running.

Investigate How Clinical Situations That Are Morally Problematic Are Managed in the Institution; If an Ethics Committee Exists, Determine Its Mission, Procedures, and Accessibility

R: *Organizational practices that support open discussions about individual care issues and problems with ethical and moral implications contribute to perceptions of an ethical climate for clinicians. Barriers to reporting problematic situations (e.g., access, retaliation) have been reported.*

Ensure That There Are Clear Guidelines Regarding the Number of Personnel (e.g., Students, Nurses, Physicians [Residents, Interns]) That Can Be Present When Confidential and/or Stressful Information Is Discussed, or When Procedures That Leave an Individual Exposed Need to Be Done

R: *This type of policy can project the philosophy and culture of moral and respectful care of the institution among its personnel. "Practice expecting that honoring and protecting the dignity of individual/groups is not a value but a way of being" (*Söderberg, Gilje, & Norberg, 1997).*

Create or Reorganize the Ethics Committee With Membership of Multiple Disciplines (e.g., Medicine, Nursing, Ethics Expert, Administration)

R: *The ethics committee must be disciplined neutral and open to discussion of any situation that evokes moral distress.*

Ensure Accessibility by Health-Care Professionals With No Punitive Results for Reporting

R: *Gordan and Hamric (2006) reported that nurses who sought ethics consultation in their institution experienced physician anger, strained relationships with other team members, and threats of termination.*

The following interventions are indicated for the nursing units and nursing staff.

Clarify the Difference of Medical/Surgical Unit Care, ICUs, and Palliative/Hospice Care

Define and Promote "a Good Death" (Beckstrand et al., 2006). For Example:

- Not allowing the person to die alone
- Managing pain and discomforts
- Knowing the person wishes for end-of-life care
- Following their wishes
- Promoting cessation of intrusive treatments sooner rather than later
- Not initiating aggressive or distressing treatments at all
- Communicates effectively as a health-care team with the individual's choices priority

Advocate for the Individual Family With Their Primary Care Provider or Prescribing Specialist Before Conflicts Arise

- Explore the physician's/NP's/PA's understanding of the situation, prognosis.
- Elicit the individual's and/or family's perception of the situation.
- Explore individual's and family's expectations.
- Explore if the individual's and/or family's expectations are realistic.
- Ask: How will your ______ be in 1 month?
- Offer your observations of the individual's/family's understanding of the situation to involved health-care professionals (e.g., manager, nurse colleagues, specialists).

R: *Being less than truthful, unrealistic, or both is a barrier to providing appropriate care and eventually a "good death" (Beckstrand et al., 2006), and is a breach in the ANA Code of ethics for nurses.*

- Consult with palliative care nurse to dialogue regarding the transition from acute care to palliative care.

If Indicated, Explain "No Code" Status and Explain the Focus of Palliative Care That Replaces Aggressive and Futile Care (e.g., Pain Management, Symptom Management, Less or No Intrusive/Painful Procedures)

R: *Often, families think that "no code" status means no care. Palliative care focuses on comfort during the dying process.*

- If their code status has not been determined, ask if you (your ___) die, what do you want done or what does your ___ want if he or she dies? Do not ask, "If your heart stops or your ___ heart stops, what do you want done?"

R: *When someone is terminally ill, it is important that the person and their family understand that they are dying and will die. Attempts at resuscitation are futile and horrific. If resuscitation is "successful," then the person has to die again.*

- Gently focus the individual and family on what can be done to promote their comfort.
- Enlist the services of palliative or hospice nurses when indicated.

R: *Palliative/Hospice nurse has the expertise and resources to provide end-of-life care to the individual and those who love them.*

- Seek to transfer the individual from ICU, if possible.

R: *ICU environments have many barriers to palliative care (e.g., noise, frequent interruptions, close quarters, aggressive interventions).*

- If feasible, plan a transition of individual out of the hospital. Explore the "Going Home Initiative" at Baystate Medical Center, Springfield, Massachusetts (Lusardi et al., 2011).

Develop an On-Unit Process for Individual Nurses to Seek Assistance With Situations That May Precipitate Moral Stress

R: *Nurses need to know that conflicts regarding moral stress are expected and ever present in health care and that sharing of feelings to initiate constructive problem solving is expected.*

Establish Formal On-Unit Forums to Discuss Cases That Present Moral Stress or Have Caused Moral Distress; Record Discussions to Share With Other Staff

- Evaluate the causes of unsatisfactory outcomes.
- Discuss alternative approach measures.
- Discuss the interventions that resulted in optimal outcomes.

R: *Planned discussions of situations that can cause moral stress or distress communicate the importance of providing caring, respectful, individualized care.*

Advocate for End-of-Life Decision Dialogues With All Individuals and Their/Your Families, Especially When the Situation Is Not Critical

- Refer them to Aging with Dignity's (2013) Five Wishes that lets your family and doctors know
  - Who you want to make health-care decisions for you when you can't make them
  - The kind of medical treatment you want or don't want
  - How comfortable you want to be
  - How you want people to treat you
  - What you want your loved ones to know
- The Conversation Project is dedicated to helping people talk about their wishes for end-of-life care. The Conversation Starter Kit is accessed at theconversationproject.org/

Direct the Individual to Create Written Documents of Their Decisions and Advise the Family of the Document. If the Adult Children Disagree With Their Parent(s)' Decisions, Direct the Parent(s) to Select the Person Who Agrees With Them to Have Their Power of Attorney

R: *Exploring end-of-life decisions when there are no imminent threats to survival provides the most optimal setting for discussions. Decisions that are viewed as well thought out may assist the family with honoring their loved one's decision.*

Refer to Sources for Assistance for Advanced Care Planning as

- Centers for Disease Control and Prevention (2012). *Advance Care Planning: Ensuring Your Wishes Are Known and Honored If You Are Unable to Speak for Yourself.* Accessed at www.cdc.gov/
- "Making your healthcare wishes known," accessed at www.practicalbioethics.org

R: *Only 28% of home health care patients, 65% of nursing home residents, and 88% of hospice care patients have an advance directive on record (Jones, Moss, & Harris-Kojetin, 2011). Even among severely or terminally ill patients, fewer than 50% had an advance directive in their medical record. Between 65% and 76% of physicians whose patients had an advance directive were not aware that it existed (*Kass-Bartelmes, Hughes, & Rutherford, 2003).*

Integrate Health Promotion and Stress Reduction in Your Lifestyle (Barnsteiner, Disch, & Walton, 2014)

- Smoking cessation
- Weight management
- Regular exercise
- Meaningful leisure activities

Refer to *Altered Health Maintenance*

- Consider utilizing "The Compassion Fatigue Workbook" by Mathieu (2012) New York: Routledge.

R: *Healthy lifestyles can reduce stress and increase energy levels for moral work.*

SELF NEGLECT

NANDA-I Definition

A constellation of culturally framed behaviors involving one or more self-care activities in which there is a failure to maintain a socially accepted standard of health and well-being (Gibbons, Lauder, & Ludwick, 2006)

Defining Characteristics*

Inadequate personal hygiene
Inadequate environmental hygiene
Nonadherence to health activities

Related Factors*

Capgras syndrome
Cognitive impairment (e.g., dementia)
Depression
Learning disability
Fear of institutionalization
Frontal lobe dysfunction and executive processing ability
Functional impairment
Lifestyle choice
Maintaining control
Malingering
Obsessive-compulsive disorder
Schizotypal personal disorders
Substance abuse
Major life stressor

Author's Note

Self-Neglect is defined above as inadequate personal hygiene and/or inadequate environmental hygiene. If the person is unable cognitively to perform personal or environmental hygiene activities, then self-neglect does not represent a response but instead signs/symptoms of another problem as caregiver abuse, or ineffective coping. If they physically cannot perform these activities, then refer to *Self-Care Deficit* or *Home Management. Self-neglect* can also be the contributing factor for *Social Isolation* related to inadequate personal hygiene. Thus *Self-Neglect* can represent a variety of nursing diagnoses, depending on the assessment results. Refer to *Impaired Home Maintenance* for additional interventions.

UNILATERAL NEGLECT

NANDA-I Definition

Impairment in sensory and motor response, mental representation, and special attention of the body, and the corresponding environment characterized by inattention to one side and over-attention to the opposite side. Left-side neglect is more severe and persistent than right-side neglect.

Defining Characteristics

Alteration in safety behaviors on the neglected side
Disturbance in sound lateralization
Failure to
- Dress neglected side
- Eat food from portion on plate on neglected side
- Failure to groom the neglected side
- Move eyes in the neglected hemisphere
- Move head in the neglected hemisphere
- Move limbs in the neglected hemisphere
- Move trunk in the neglected hemisphere
- Notice people approaching from the neglected side

Hemianopsia
Impaired performance on line cancelation, line bisection, and target cancelation tests
Left hemiplegia from cerebrovascular accident
Marked deviation of the eyes to stimuli on the nonneglected side
Marked deviation of the trunk to stimuli on the nonneglected side
Omission of dressing on the neglected side
Perseveration
Representational neglect (e.g., distortion of drawing on the neglected side)
Substitution of letters to form alternative words when reading
Transfer of pain sensation to nonneglected side
Unaware of positioning of neglected side
Unilateral visuospatial neglect
Use of vertical hall of page only when writing
Positive Prevost's sign (with both eyes and the head fixed toward the right). This ipsilesional deviation of the head and eyes is specific to unilateral neglect (Becker & Karnath, 2010; *Berger, Pross, Ilg, & Karnath, 2006).

Related Factors

Pathophysiologic

Relaed to brain injury secondary to:

Cerebrovascular accident*
Cerebral aneurysms
Cerebrovascular problems*
Infection, for example, meningitis, encephalitis
Trauma*
Tumors

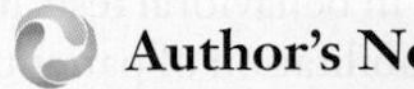

Author's Note

Unilateral Neglect represents a disturbance in the reciprocal loop that occurs most often in the right hemisphere of the brain. This diagnosis could also be viewed as a syndrome diagnosis, *Unilateral Neglect Syndrome*. As mentioned in Chapter 3, syndrome diagnoses encompass a cluster of nursing diagnoses related to the situation. The nursing interventions for *Unilateral Neglect Syndrome* would focus on *Self-Care Deficit*, *Anxiety*, and *Risk for Injury*.

Errors in Diagnostic Statements

Unilateral Neglect **related to lack of grooming and hygiene for right side of face, head, and right arm**

Lack of grooming on one side of the body can be an indicator of *Unilateral Neglect* if neurologic disease or damage is present; it is not a related factor. When writing the diagnostic statement, the nurse should ask, "How does the nurse treat unilateral neglect?" Because the nursing focus is on teaching adaptive techniques, phrasing the diagnosis *Unilateral Neglect related to lack of knowledge of adaptive techniques* would be appropriate. If *Unilateral Neglect* were viewed as a syndrome diagnosis, the appropriate diagnostic statement would be *Unilateral Neglect Syndrome*. No "related to" is needed with a syndrome diagnosis because the label includes the etiology. The interventions would have the same focus, reducing neglect by using adaptive techniques.

Key Concepts

General Considerations

- Unilateral neglect is a heterogeneous perceptual disorder that often follows stroke, especially after right-hemisphere lesion. Its most characteristic feature is inability to report or respond to stimuli presented from the contralateral space, including visual, somatosensory, auditory, and kinesthetic sources (Yang, Li-Tsang, Fong, 2013).
- Individual may not be able to visually track, orient, or reach to the neglected side (Grossman & Porth, 2014).
- Horizontal eye-in-head deviation on clinical brain scans appeared to be associated with spatial neglect rather than with brain damage (Becker & Karnath, 2010).
- Most individuals with neglect show early recovery, particularly within the first month, and marked improvement may be seen within 3 months. At least 10% of individuals with acute neglect will experience symptoms in the chronic phase (Barrett, 2014).
- The reported incidence following right-hemisphere stroke is 10% to 82% and from 15% to 65% following left-hemisphere stroke (*Plummer, Morris, & Dunai, 2003).
- Homonymous hemianopsia (loss of vision on the contralateral side) usually occurs with unilateral neglect. Unilateral neglect and hemianopsia are two separate phenomena, and either can be present without the other. When they occur together, the client has more difficulty compensating for the loss (Grossman & Porth, 2014).
- The client with a parietal lobe injury demonstrates problems with body schema, spatial judgment, and sensory interpretation.
- In addition, the individual with this type of brain injury may exhibit some or all of the following characteristics that complicate the neglect syndrome:
  - Impulsiveness
  - Short attention span
  - Lack of insight into the extent of the disability
  - Diminished learning skills
  - Inability to recognize faces
  - Decrease in concrete thinking
  - Confusion

Prism Adaption Therapy

- During prism adaptation therapy, an individual wears special prismatic goggles that are made of prism wedges that displace the visual field laterally or vertically. In most cases, the visual field is shifted laterally either in the rightward or in the leftward direction. While wearing the goggles, the individual engages in a perceptual motor task such as pointing to a visual target directly in front of him or her (Mizuno et al., 2011).
- "Prism Adaptation (PA) therapy can significantly improve ADL in individuals with subacute stroke. Moreover, PA also produced a generalized beneficial effect both in conventional and in behavioral tests in near as well as in far space, and it is therefore a good candidate treatment for the rehabilitation of patients with neglect" (Mizuno et al., 2011). "It has become clear that with respect to being used as a long-term rehabilitative tool, prism adaptation is only effective when it is repeated over many sessions and with sufficiently strong prism goggles" (Newport and Schenk, 2012).

Contralesional Limb Activation

- "Because the right arm is controlled by the intact left hemisphere, using this arm may exacerbate visual neglect, because activation of the left hemisphere (by right arm use) would tend to further inhibit the already damaged right hemisphere. Conversely, left limb activation would lead to increased activity in the right hemisphere" (*Bailey, Riddoch, & Crome, 2002).

- Hemispheric activation has been used to account for the reduction in visual neglect found in several studies. Even quite small active movements of the left upper limb have reduced visual neglect on the left side of the subject in single cases (*Bailey et al., 2002).

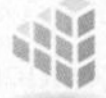

Pediatric Considerations

- Children at greatest risk for development of unilateral neglect are those with acquired hemiplegia (e.g., from stroke). Strokes may occur in children with congenital heart disease, sickle cell anemia, meningitis, or head trauma.
- These results add to the evidence in favor of an attentional deficit in developmental dyslexia, implicating a lesion in the neural structures subserving spatial attention (*Sireteanu, Goertz, Bachert, & Wander, 2006).

Geriatric Considerations

- Most people who experience unilateral neglect are older adults, simply because the incidence of stroke is greatest in this population.

Focus Assessment Criteria

This assessment may be completed by a physical therapist.

Subjective and Objective Data

Assess for Defining Characteristics

Client's Perception of the Problem

Effects on Activities of Daily Living (ADLs)

Bathing, grooming, and hygiene—Does the individual

- Wash the affected side of the body?
- Shave both sides of the face?
- Brush all the teeth?
- Put eyeglasses on straight?
- Put dentures in straight?
- Comb only part of the hair?
- Apply makeup to both sides of the face?

Feeding—Does the individual

- Pocket food on the affected side of the mouth?
- Eat only half of his or her food (i.e., eat food only on the unaffected side of the plate/tray)?

Dressing—Does the individual

- Dress the affected limbs?

Mobility/positioning:

- When sitting in a wheelchair, does the client lean or tilt toward the unaffected side?
- Does the affected arm dangle off the lapboard?
- Are the head and eyes turned toward the unaffected side?
- When propelling the wheelchair or when ambulating, does the client bump or run into objects on the affected side?

Safety—Does the individual

- Attempt to walk or transfer out of the chair or bed when unable to ambulate?
- Have sensation in the affected limbs?
- Frequently injure the affected arm or hand (cuts, bumps, bruises)?
- Feel pain when injured?
- Realize when injury occurs?
- Scan the entire visual field?
- Turn the head to the affected side to compensate?
- Respond to stimuli presented from the affected side?
- Does the affected arm dangle at the side and get caught in the wheelchair spokes, side rails, doorways, and so forth?

Goals

NOC
Heedfulness of Affected Side; Neurological Status: Peripheral; Sensory Function: Proprioception; Adaption to Physical Disability; Self-Care Status

The individual will demonstrate an ability to scan the visual field to compensate for loss of function/sensation in affected limbs as evidenced by the following indicators:

- Identifies safety hazards in the environment
- Describes the deficit and the rationale for treatment

Our systematic review indicates that there is modest evidence for the use of prism adaptation to reduce unilateral neglect in stroke, with immediate and long-lasting effects, and eye patching as shown by BIT-C scores for immediate effects. Other studies obtained positive effects from the use of visual scanning training (Ferreira, Leite Lopes, Luiz, Cardoso, & André, 2011).

Interventions

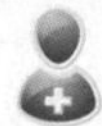

Clinical Alert Speech and language, memory, and other mental abilities may be unaffected in brain-injured individuals with spatial neglect. Nonetheless, the prognosis for recovery of independent function in those with persisting spatial neglect is significantly worse than in those with what appears to be more disabling deficits without spatial defects (Barrett, 2014; Jehkoneen et al., 2000).

NIC
Unilateral Neglect Management, Self-Care Assistance; Body Image Enhancement; Environmental Management: Safety, Exercise Therapy

Consult With a Neuropsychologist, Physical Therapist, Occupational Therapist, and a Nurse Rehabilitation Specialist to Create a Multidisciplinary Plan With and for the Individual/Family

- Ensure the individual/family understands unilateral neglect and the nursing and other treatment plans, for example, visual scanning training, limb activation treatment, prism adaptation.

R: *Priftis, Passarini, Pilosio, Meneghello, and Pitteri (2013) reported that all three treatments can lead to similar positive outcomes concerning left-sided neglect rehabilitation.*

R: *"It is therefore reasonable that individual should start a neglect intervention as soon as possible in the acute stage, in order to avoid non-use of the hemiplegic limbs, by increasing multisensory inputs or stimulation to the ipsilateral brain regions, and thus slowing down the secondary changes in the brain related to neglect" (Yang et al., 2013).*

Assist the Individual to Recognize the Perceptual Deficit

- Take every opportunity, large or small, to help them "tune in" to that side (Davis, 2013).
- Initially adapt the environment to the deficit:
  - Position the call light, bedside stand, television, telephone, and personal items on the unaffected side. Position the bed with the unaffected side toward the door.
  - Ensure the control for calling the nurse in on the strong side, where they can find it quickly.
- Approach and speak from the unaffected side.
- If you must approach from the affected side, announce your presence as soon as you enter the room to avoid startling him or her.
- When working with the affected extremity, position the unaffected side near a wall to minimize distractions.
- Take their hand in your hand and guide them to the task, for example, hold a fork (Davis, 2013).
- Teach and remind to scan from left to right frequently.
- Gradually change the environment as you teach him or her to compensate and to learn to recognize the forgotten field; move furniture and personal items out of the visual field. Speak to the individual from the affected side (after introducing yourself on the unaffected side).
- Provide a simplified, well-lit, uncluttered environment:
  - Provide a moment between activities.
  - Provide concrete cues: "You are on your side facing the wall."
- Provide a full-length mirror to help with vertical orientation and to diminish the distortion of the vertical and horizontal plane, which manifests itself in the client leaning toward the affected side.
- Use verbal instructions rather than mere demonstrations. Keep instructions simple.
- For an individual in a wheelchair, obtain a lapboard (preferably Plexiglas); position the affected arm on the lapboard with the fingertips at midline. Encourage the individual to look for and stroke the arm on the board.
- For an ambulatory individual, obtain an arm sling to prevent the arm from dangling and causing shoulder subluxation.

- When in bed, elevate the affected arm on a pillow to prevent dependent edema.
- Encourage to wear a watch, favorite ring, or bracelet on affected arm to draw attention to it.

R: *Strategies are provided to stimulate the individual to focus on the affected side.*

R: *The restorative approach attempts to reinstate preinjury capacity of injured brain-behavior systems via visual, tactile, or auditory stimulation cuing. This stimulation is gradually reduced and then eliminated when the goal activities are integrated and spontaneous (Riestra & Barrett, 2013).*

Assist with Adaptations Needed for Self-Care and Other ADLs

- Encourage to wear prescribed corrective lenses or hearing aids for bathing, dressing, and toileting.
- Instruct to attend to the affected extremity side first when performing ADLs.
- Instruct to always look for the affected extremity when performing ADLs, to know where it is at all times.
- Teach to dress and groom in front of a mirror.
- Suggest using color-coded markers sewn or placed inside shoes or clothes to help distinguish right from left.
- Encourage to integrate affected extremity during bathing and to feel extremity by rubbing and massaging it.
- Use adaptive equipment as appropriate.
- Refer to *Self-Care Deficit* for additional interventions.

R: *The restorative approach attempts to reinstate preinjury capacity of injured brain-behavior systems via visual, tactile, or auditory stimulation cuing. This stimulation is gradually reduced and then eliminated when the goal activities are integrated and spontaneous (Riestra & Barrett 2013).*

- For eating:
  - Set up meals with a minimum of dishes, food, and utensils.
  - Instruct the client to eat in small amounts and place food on unaffected side of mouth.
  - Instruct to use the tongue to sweep out "pockets" of food from the affected side after every bite.
  - After meals/medications, check oral cavity for pocketed food/medication.
  - Provide oral care TID and PRN.
  - Initially place food in their visual field; gradually move the food out of the field and teach the client to scan entire visual field.
  - Use adaptive feeding equipment as appropriate.
  - Refer to *Self-Care Deficit: Feeding* for additional interventions.
  - Refer to *Imbalanced Nutrition related to swallowing difficulties* if the individual has difficulty chewing and swallowing food.

R: *Adapting the environment minimizes sensory deprivation. Initially, however, attempts should be made to have the individual attend to both sides.*

R: *Reminders can help to adapt to the environment.*

Teach Scanning to Reduce Neglect Behavior and Prevent Injury

- Ensure a clutter-free, well-lit environment.
- Retrain to scan entire environment.
- Instruct to turn the head past midline to view the scene on the affected side.
- Perform activities that require turning the head.
- Remind the individual to scan when ambulating or propelling a wheelchair.

R: *Chan and Man (2013) found that a visual scanning training program was more effective treatment strategy for reducing neglect behavior. Scanning can help prevent injury and increase awareness of entire space.*

Use Tactile Sensation to Reintroduce Affected Arm/Extremity to the Individual

- Have the individual stroke the involved side with the uninvolved hand, and watch the arm or leg while stroking it.
- Rub different-textured materials to stimulate sensations (hot, cold, rough, soft).

R: *The restorative approach attempts to reinstate preinjury capacity of injured brain-behavior systems via visual, tactile, or auditory stimulation cuing. This stimulation is gradually reduced and then eliminated when the goal activities are integrated and spontaneous (Riestra & Barrett 2013).*

Instruct to Keep the Affected Arm and/or Leg in View

- Position the arm on the lapboard. (Plexiglas lapboards allow the client to view the affected leg, thereby helping to integrate the leg into the body schema.)
- Provide an arm sling for an ambulatory client.
- Instruct the client to take extra care around sources of heat or cold and moving machinery or parts to protect the affected side from injury.

R: *Decreased sensation or motor function increases the vulnerability to injury.*

Initiate Health Teaching and Referrals

- Ensure that follow-up appointments have been made, for example, neurologist, primary care provider, occupational therapy, physical therapy, home health nurse.
- Ensure that both the individual and the family understand the cause of unilateral neglect and the purpose of and rationale for all interventions.
- When performing relearning techniques (e.g., cueing, scanning visual field) demonstrate how and explain why to the individual/family. Request a return demonstration and questions.
- Teach use of adaptive equipment, if appropriate.
- Teach principles of maintaining a safe environment.

R: *These strategies can activate the individual/family to understanding their roles in the care process beyond the acute period by increasing their knowledge, skills, and confidence (Hibbard & Greene, 2013).*

NONCOMPLIANCE[27]

Definition

Behavior of person and/or caregiver that fails to coincide with a health-promoting or therapeutic plan agreed on by the person (and/or family and/or community) and health-care professional. In the presence of an agreed-upon, health-promoting, or therapeutic plan, the person's or caregiver's behavior is fully or partially nonadherent and may lead to clinically ineffective or partially ineffective outcomes.

Defining Characteristics

Development-related complication
Exacerbation of symptoms
Failure to meet outcomes
Missing appointments
Nonadherance behavior

Related Factors

Health System

Difficulty in client–provider relationship
Inadequate access to care
Inconvenience of care
Ineffective communication skills of provider
Insufficient follow-up with provider
Insufficient health insurance
Insufficient provider reimbursement
Insufficient teaching skill of provider
Low satisfaction with care
Perceived low credibility of provider
Provider discontinuity

Health-Care Plan

Complex treatment regimen
Financial barriers
High-cost regimen
Intensity of regimen
Lengthy duration of regimen

[27]This author has chosen retire this nursing diagnosis and replace it with *Compromised Engagement* and *Risk for Compromised Engagement*. Refer to the Table of Contents to access these diagnoses.

Individual

Cultural incongruence
Health beliefs incongruent with plan
Insufficient knowledge about regimen
Insufficient skills to perform regimen
Expectation incongruent with developmental phase
Insufficient motivation
Insufficient social support
Insufficient motivation
Values incongruent with plan

Network

Insufficient involvement of members in plan
Perception that beliefs of significant other differ from plan
Low social value attributed to plan

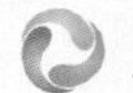

Author's Note

The nursing diagnosis *Noncompliance* was last revised in 1998. The label *Noncompliance* has never reflected a proactive approach to an individual/family who was not participating in recommended treatments or lifestyle changes. Criticism of the term noncompliant surfaced in the literature a decade ago. Recent health-care literature is full of alternative strategies for health-care professionals to improve health outcomes with individuals/families.

Merriam-Webster defines compliance as the act or process of complying to a desire, demand, proposal, or regimen, or to coercion. Compliance occurs when an individual obeys a directive from a health-care provider.

Gruman (2011) wrote, "Saying 'engagement' when meaning 'compliance' supports the belief that we are the only ones who must change our behavior. . . Doing so misrepresents the magnitude of shifts in attitude, expectations and effort that are required for all health care stakeholders to ensure that we have adequate knowledge and support to make well-informed decisions. . . And it fails to recognize that our behaviors are powerfully shaped by many contingencies, money, culture, time, illness status, and personal preference. . . Being engaged in our health and care does not mean following our clinician's instructions to the letter. . . Rather, it means being able to accurately weigh the benefits and risks of a new medication, of stopping smoking or getting a PSA test in the context of the many other demands and opportunities that influence our pursuit of lives that are free of suffering for ourselves and those we love."

Note: We = consumer/clients/family

IMBALANCED NUTRITION

Imbalanced Nutrition

Related to Anorexia Secondary to (Specify)
Related to Difficulty or Inability to Procure Food
Impaired Dentition
Impaired Swallowing
Ineffective Infant Feeding Pattern

NANDA-I Definition

Intake of nutrients insufficient to meet metabolic needs

Defining Characteristics

The individual who is not NPO reports or is found to have food intake less than the recommended daily allowance (RDA) with or without weight loss

and/or

Actual or potential metabolic needs in excess of intake with weight loss
Weight 10% to 20% or more below ideal for height and frame
Triceps skinfold, mid-arm circumference, and mid-arm muscle circumference less than 60% standard measurement
Muscle weakness and tenderness
Mental irritability or confusion
Decreased serum albumin
Decreased serum transferring or iron-binding capacity

Related Factors

Pathophysiologic

Related to increased caloric requirements and difficulty in ingesting sufficient calories secondary to:

Burns (postacute phase)
Cancer
Infection
Trauma
Chemical dependence (cocaine, crystal methamphetamine)
Preterm infants
Gastrointestinal (GI) complications/deformities
AIDS

Related to dysphagia secondary to:

Cerebrovascular accident (CVA)
Parkinson's disease
Möbius syndrome
Muscular dystrophy
Cerebral palsy
Cleft lip/palate
Amyotrophic lateral sclerosis
Neuromuscular disorders

Related to decreased absorption of nutrients secondary to:

Crohn's disease
Lactose intolerance
Necrotizing enterocolitis
Cystic fibrosis

Related to self-induced vomiting, physical exercise in excess of caloric intake, or refusal to eat secondary to anorexia nervosa

Related to reluctance to eat for fear of poisoning secondary to paranoid behavior

Related to anorexia, excessive physical agitation secondary to bipolar disorder

Related to anorexia and diarrhea secondary to protozoal infection

Related to vomiting, anorexia, and impaired digestion secondary to pancreatitis

Related to anorexia, impaired protein and fat metabolism, and impaired storage of vitamins secondary to cirrhosis

Related to anorexia, vomiting, and impaired digestion secondary to GI malformation or necrotizing enterocolitis

Related indigestion secondary to gastroesophageal reflux

Treatment Related

Related to increased protein and vitamin requirements secondary to inadequate absorption post bariatric surgery

Related to protein and vitamin requirements for wound healing and decreased intake secondary to:

Surgery
Surgical reconstruction of mouth
Radiation therapy
Medications (chemotherapy)
Wired jaw

Related to inadequate absorption as a medication side effect of (specify):

Example (Gröber & Kisters, 2007):
Colchicine
Neomycin
Pyrimethamine
Antacid
Antiepileptics
Antineoplastic drugs
Antibiotics (clotrimazole, rifampicin)
Dexamethasone
Antihypertensives (nifedipine, spironolactone)
Antiretroviral drugs (ritonavir, saquinavir)
Herbal medicines: Kava kava
St. John's wort (hyperforin)

Related to decreased oral intake, mouth discomfort, nausea, and vomiting secondary to:

Radiation therapy
Tonsillectomy
Chemotherapy
Oral trauma

Related to diarrhea* secondary to (specify)

Situational (Personal, Environmental)

Related to decreased desire to eat secondary to:

Social isolation
Depression
Nausea and vomiting
Stress

Related to inability to procure food (physical limitation or financial or transportation problems)

Related to inability to chew (damaged or missing teeth, ill-fitting dentures)

Maturational

Infant/Child

Related to inadequate intake secondary to:

Lack of emotional/sensory stimulation
Lack of knowledge of caregiver
Inadequate production of breast milk

Related to malabsorption, dietary restrictions, and anorexia secondary to:

Celiac disease
Lactose intolerance
Necrotizing enterocolitis
Cystic fibrosis
GI malformation
Gastroesophageal reflux

Related to sucking difficulties (infant) and dysphagia secondary to:

Cerebral palsy
Cleft lip and palate
Neurologic impairment

Related to inadequate sucking, fatigue, and dyspnea secondary to:

Congenital heart disease
Viral syndrome
Hyperbilirubinemia
Prematurity
Respiratory distress syndrome
Developmental delay

Author's Note

Because of their 24-hour presence, nurses are usually the primary professionals responsible for improving nutritional status. Although *Imbalanced Nutrition* is not a difficult diagnosis to validate, interventions for it can challenge the nurse. Secondary screening for individual determined to be at increased risk for nutritional deficits are performed by clinical nutritionists.

This nursing diagnosis will focus on nutritional deficits in individuals in health-care settings. In addition, assessments and interventions will be presented to assist the individual or family to improve nutrition and food security.

Many factors influence food habits and nutritional status: personal, family, cultural, financial, functional ability, nutritional knowledge, disease and injury, and treatment regimens. *Imbalanced Nutrition* describes people who can ingest food but eat an inadequate or imbalanced quality or quantity. For instance, the diet may have insufficient protein or excessive fat. Quantity may be insufficient because of increased metabolic requirements (e.g., cancer, pregnancy, trauma, or interference with nutrient use [e.g., impaired storage of vitamins in cirrhosis]).

Nurses should not use this diagnosis to describe individuals who are NPO or cannot ingest food. They should use the collaborative problems *Risk for Complications of Fluid/Electrolyte Imbalance* and *Risk for Complications of Negative Nitrogen Balance* to describe those situations.

Errors in Diagnostic Statements

Imbalanced Nutrition **related to insulin deficiency, altered consciousness, and hypermetabolic state**

This diagnosis represents individuals with diabetes experiencing diabetic ketoacidosis. In such a situation, nursing responsibility focuses on two major problems: managing the ketoacidosis with the prescribing provider and teaching the individual and family how to prevent future episodes. The first is described by the collaborative problem *Risk for Complications of Ketoacidosis*, for which the nurse would be responsible for monitoring for physiologic instability, initiating timely interventions, and evaluating the individual's response. The nurse would investigate the second problem, described by the nursing diagnosis *Possible Ineffective Health Management* related to adherence to diabetic diet and insufficient knowledge of adaptation needed when sick, after the individual is stable.

Imbalanced Nutrition **related to parenteral therapy and NPO status**

This diagnosis represents a situation with which nurses are intricately involved (parenteral therapy). From a nutritional perspective, however, what interventions do nurses prescribe to improve the nutritional status of an NPO individual? Parenteral nutrition in an individual who is NPO influences several actual or potential responses that nurses treat, representing both nursing diagnoses, such as *Impaired Comfort*, and the collaborative problems *Risk for Complications of Fluid/Electrolyte Imbalance* and *Risk for Complications of Negative Nitrogen Balance*.

Key Concepts

Food Security and Insecurity

- In 2013, 85.7% of US households were food secure throughout the year. The remaining 14.3% (17.5 million households) were food insecure (Coleman-Jensen, Gregory, & Singh, 2013).
- In 2013, 5.6% of US households (6.8 million households) had very low food security, essentially unchanged from 5.7% in 2011 and 2012 (Coleman-Jensen et al., 2013).
- Food security and insecurity are defined as follows:
  - Food secure: households with no or minimal indication of food insecurity
  - Food insecure with hunger: Households in which one or more members (mainly adults) have decreased the amount of food they consume to the extent that they have repeatedly experienced the physical sensation of hunger (Coleman-Jensen et al., 2013).

General Considerations

- Nutritional assessments are required within 24 hours of admission to a hospital and within 14 days of admission to a long-term facility (the Joint Commission).
- Dietary Guidelines for Americans recommends (U.S. Department of Agriculture and U.S. Department of Health and Human Services, 2010):
  - Balance calories to manage weight.
  - Prevent and/or reduce overweight and obesity through improved eating and physical activity behaviors.
  - Control total calorie intake to manage body weight. For people who are overweight or obese, this will mean consuming fewer calories from foods and beverages.
  - Increase physical activity and reduce time spent in sedentary behaviors.
  - Maintain appropriate calorie balance during each stage of life—childhood, adolescence, adulthood, pregnancy and breastfeeding, and older age.
- For proper metabolic functioning, the body requires adequate carbohydrates, protein, fat, vitamins, minerals, electrolytes, and trace elements. Figure II.7 depicts MyPlate, developed by the U.S. Department of Agriculture (2011). It recommends daily servings of five food groups. The sixth group—fats, oils, and sweets—should be eaten sparingly and should not exceed 30% of total calorie intake. Refer to www.choosemyplate.gov for extensive resources on healthy eating.
- More than one-third (34.9% or 78.6 million) of US adults are obese (Ogden,Carroll, Kit, & Flegal, 2014).
- Studies report that US women consume insufficient iron, calcium, and vitamins A and C (Dudek, 2014).
- Americans eat half of the fiber requirement and 20% more fat than needed (Dudek, 2014).
- The National Research Council (1989) compiled the dietary recommendations outlined in Box II.5.
- The body requires a minimum level of nutrients for health and growth. During the life span, nutritional needs vary, as indicated in Table II.14 (Dudek, 2014; Hockenberry & Wilson, 2015).
- Body mass index (BMI) is a score calculated from the height:weight ratio of an individual and used to determine the likeliness of health problems, as illustrated in Table II.15.
- Alcohol may directly alter the level of nutrient intake through its effect on appetite, displacement of food in the diet, or by virtue of its deleterious effects at almost every level of the GI tract. Deficiencies

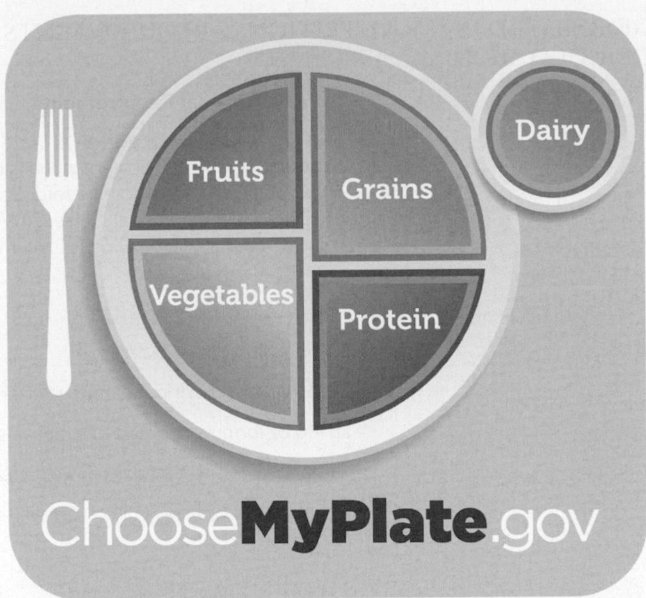

FIGURE II.7 MyPlate. Source: http://www.choosemyplate.gov/MyPlate

Box II.5 DIETARY RECOMMENDATIONS OF THE NATIONAL RESEARCH COUNCIL REPORT

Consume a variety of nutrient-dense foods and beverages within and among the basic food groups while choosing foods that limit the intake of saturated and trans fat, cholesterol, added sugars, salt and alcohol.

Reduce total fat intake to 20% to 35% or less of calories; saturated fatty acid intake to less than 10% of kilocalories; and cholesterol to less than 300 mg daily.*

Drink 8–10 glasses of water or noncaffeinated beverages.

Choose fiber-rich fruits, vegetables, and whole grains often.

Choose and prepare foods and beverages with little added sugars or caloric sweeteners.

Maintain protein intake at moderate levels.† Increase dry beans, fish.

Eat 3-ounce or more equivalents of whole-grain products daily.

Eat 2 to 4 servings of fruit daily.

Eat 3 to 5 servings of vegetables daily.

Limit total daily intake of salt (sodium chloride) to 1 teaspoon (2,300 mg) or less.‡

Consume 3 cups per day of fat-free or low-fat milk or equivalent milk products.

Avoid taking dietary supplements in excess of the recommended daily allowance (RDA) in any one day.

Balance food intake and physical activity to maintain appropriate body weight.

Engage in at least 30 minutes of moderate-intensity physical activity, not including usual activity at work/home on most days of the week.

For those who drink alcoholic beverages, limit consumption to one drink per day for women and up to two drinks per day for men.

---

* The intake of fat and cholesterol can be reduced by substituting fish, poultry without skin, lean meats, and low-fat or nonfat dairy products for fatty meats and whole-milk dairy products; by choosing more vegetables, fruits, cereals, and legumes; and by limiting oils, fats, egg yolks, and fried and other fatty foods.

† Meet at least the RDA for protein, do not exceed twice the RDA.

‡ Limit the use of salt in cooking, and avoid adding it to food at the table. Salty, highly processed salty, salt-preserved, and salt-pickled foods should be consumed sparingly.

§ The Committee does not recommend alcohol consumption.

National Research Council, Committee on Diet and Health of Food and Nutrition Board. (1989). Diet and health: Implications for reducing chronic disease risk. *Nutrition Reviews, 47*, 142–149; Food guide pyramid: A guide to daily food choices. Leaflet No. 572. Washington, DC: US Department of Agriculture; *Dietary guidelines for Americans*. (2005). Available from www.health.gov/dietaryguidelines/dga2005/document/html/executivesummary.htm. Accessed June 7, 2011.

Dudek, SG. (2009). *Nutrition essentials for nursing practice* (6th ed.) Philadelphia,PA: Lippincott Williams & Wilkins.

Table II.14 AGE-RELATED DAILY NUTRITIONAL REQUIREMENTS (U.S. DEPARTMENT OF AGRICULTURE, 2016)

Age	Daily Nutritional Requirements
Infants	100–120 kcal/kg/day for growth Breastfeeding is highly recommended and for at least 1 year (American College of Nursing-Midwives [ACNM], 2011; American Pediatric Association [APA], 2010; Association of Women's Health, Obstetrics, and Neonatal Nurses [AWHONN], 2007; WHO, 2012). For breastfed infants a daily supplement of vitamin D of 400 International Units/day beginning in the first few days of life... (APA, 2008)
Newborn	12–18 oz formula or breast milk
2–3 months	20–30 oz formula or breast milk
4–5 months	25–35 oz formula or breast milk; strained vegetables and fruits; egg yolks
6–7 months	28–40 oz formula or breast milk; above solids, plus meat, finger foods
8–11 months	24 oz formula or breast milk; three regular meals, chopped table food
1–2 years	24 oz formula or breast milk; 100 cal/kg same as for 8–11 months
Children	
Preschool (3–5 years)	90 cal/kg; 1.2 g/kg protein
	Basic food groups/servings; refer to Box II.2
	Calcium 800 mg
School (6–12 years)	80 cal/kg; 1.2 g/kg protein
	Basic food groups (as preschool)
	1.5–2 g calcium
	400 units vitamin D
	1.5–3 L water
Adolescent (13–17 years)	2,200–2,400 cal for girls
	3,000 cal for boys
	Basic food groups (as preschool)
	50–60 g protein
	1,200–1,500 mg calcium (to age 25)
	400 units vitamin D
Adults	1,600–3,000 cal range (based on physical activity, emotional state, body size, age, and individual metabolism)
	Basic food groups
	Refer to Box II.2
	Men need increased protein, ascorbic acid, riboflavin, and vitamins E and B_6. Vitamin D 800–2,000 International Units (from diet or supplements) : Serum levels of 25-hydroxyvitamin D are recommended.
Women	All of the above as well as increased iron, calcium, (calcium 19–50 years, 1,000 mg from diet or supplements) and vitamins A and B_{12}
Pregnant women (second and third trimesters)	Daily calorie requirement
	11–15 years: 2,500, calcium 1,300 mg
	16–22 years: 2,400, calcium 1,300 mg
	23–50 years: 2,300, calcium 1,300 mg
	Increase protein 10 g or 1 serving meat
	1.2–3.5 g calcium
	Increase vitamins A, B, and C

(continued)

Table II.14 AGE-RELATED DAILY NUTRITIONAL REQUIREMENTS (U.S. DEPARTMENT OF AGRICULTURE, 2013) *(continued)*

Age	Daily Nutritional Requirements
Lactating women	30–60 mg iron
	2,500–3,000 cal (500 more than regular diet)
	Basic food groups
	4 servings protein
	5 servings dairy
	4+ servings grain
	5+ servings vegetables
	2+ servings vitamin C-rich
	1+ green leafy
	2+ others
	Fluids 2–3 qt (1 qt milk)
	Increase in vitamins A and C, niacin
Older than 65 years	Basic food groups (same as adult)
	Caloric requirements decrease with age (1,600–1,800 for women; 2,000–2,400 for men), but dependent on activity, climate, and metabolic needs
	Ensure intake of essential amino acids, fatty acids, vitamins, elements, fiber, and water
	60 mg ascorbic acid
	40–60 mg protein
	Vitamin D 800–2,000 International Units (from diet or supplements) *Note*: Serum levels of 25-hydroxyvitamin D are recommended.
	1,000 mg calcium (from diet or supplements)
	10 mg iron

associated with alcoholism are vitamins A, D, riboflavin, and minerals; for example, magnesium, zinc, selenium (Lutz, Mazur, & Litch, 2015).

- Individuals with alcoholism consume almost 50% of their calories in alcohol, causing significant nutritional deficiencies (Beier, Landes, Mohammad, & McClain, 2014).

Cancer-Related Nutritional Disturbance

- Nutritional disturbances in individuals with cancer (*Cunningham & Huhmann, 2011) are as follows:
  - Cancer-induced alterations in nutrient intake:
    - Changes in appetite
    - Changes in taste and smell
    - Early satiety
    - Cancer cachexia
    - Changes in electrolyte balance
  - Cancer-induced changes in energy balance:
    - Changes in energy expenditure
    - Changes in nutrient metabolism
    - Changes in GI tract
    - Changes in body storage
  - Treatment-induced alterations in nutrient intake:
    - Changes in appetite
  - Treatment-induced changes in energy balance:
    - Changes in energy expenditure
    - Changes in the GI tract

Table II.15 BODY MASS INDEX[a]

BMI	19	20	21	22	23	24	25	26	27	28	29	30	31	32	33	34	35
Height	***Weight in Pounds***																
410″	91	96	100	105	110	115	119	124	129	134	138	143	148	153	158	162	167
4′11″	94	99	104	109	114	119	124	128	133	138	143	148	153	158	163	158	173
5′	97	102	107	112	118	123	128	133	138	143	148	153	158	163	158	174	179
5′1″	100	106	111	116	122	127	132	137	143	148	153	158	164	169	174	180	185
5′2″	104	109	115	120	126	131	136	142	147	153	158	164	169	175	180	186	191
5′3″	107	113	118	124	130	135	141	146	152	158	163	169	175	180	186	191	197
5′4″	110	116	122	128	134	140	145	151	157	163	169	174	180	186	192	197	204
5′5″	114	120	126	132	138	144	150	156	162	168	174	180	186	192	198	204	210
5′6″	118	124	130	136	142	148	155	161	167	173	179	186	192	198	204	210	216
5′7″	121	127	134	140	146	153	159	166	172	178	185	191	198	204	211	217	223
5′8″	125	131	138	144	151	158	164	171	177	184	190	197	203	210	216	223	230
5′9″	128	135	142	149	155	162	169	176	182	189	196	203	209	216	223	230	236
5′10″	132	139	146	153	160	167	174	181	188	195	202	209	216	222	229	236	243
5′11″	136	143	150	157	165	172	179	186	193	200	208	215	222	229	236	243	250
6′	140	147	154	162	169	177	184	191	199	206	213	221	228	235	242	250	258
6″	144	151	159	166	174	182	189	197	204	212	219	227	235	242	250	257	265
6′2″	148	155	163	171	179	186	194	202	210	218	225	233	241	249	256	264	272
6′3″	152	160	168	176	184	192	200	208	216	224	232	240	248	256	264	272	279
	Healthy Weight							Overweight						Obese			

[a]BMI of 19 to 24 = healthy weight; BMI of 25 to 29 = overweight; BMI of 30 and above = obese; 40 or above = extreme obesity.
Source: NHLBI Obesity Education Initiative Expert Panel on the Identification, Evaluation, and Treatment of Obesity in Adults (United States). (1998). *Evidence report of clinical guidelines on the identification, evaluation, and treatment of overweight and obesity in adults*. Bethesda, MD: NIH/National Heart, Lung, and Blood Institute (NHLBI).

- Researchers report that "increased caloric intake may neither reverse weight loss nor improve survival" (Tisdale, 2003, as cited in *Cunningham & Huhmann, 2011). Specialized nutritional interventions "are not recommended for individuals who are adequately nourished, who are not anticipated to be unable to eat for 10 to 14 days, or who have uncontrolled disease" (*MacFie et al., 2000, as cited in *Cunningham & Huhmann, 2011).
- Consideration of these criteria may assist with ethical concerns regarding providing or withholding nutritional supplements (*Cunningham & Huhmann, 2011).

Pediatric Considerations

- Changes in nutritional needs characterize each growth period (see Table II.14).
- Children at special risk for inadequate nutritional intake include those with
  - Congenital anomalies (e.g., tracheoesophageal fistula, GI malformation, cardiac, or neurologic anomalies)
  - Prematurity, developmental delay, and intrauterine growth retardation
  - Inborn errors of metabolism (e.g., phenylketonuria)
  - Gastroesophageal reflux
  - Malabsorption disorders
  - Developmental disorders (e.g., cerebral palsy)
  - Chronic illness (e.g., cystic fibrosis, chronic infections, diabetes)
  - Accelerated growth rates (e.g., prematurity, infancy, adolescence)
  - Parents who have inadequate attachment

- Parents should follow sound feeding practices to prevent nutritional deficits in their infants (Hockenberry & Wilson, 2015):
  - Infants who are breastfed can have semisolid foods introduced at 6 months. Solid foods can be introduced at 6 months for breastfed infants.
  - Bottle-fed infants should be fed iron-fortified formula for the first year. For bottle-fed infants, the infant should be able to control their head and trunk, usually 4 to 6 months (Lutz et al., 2015).

Fast Foods

- "The National Restaurant Association estimates that the average American eats out an average of four times a week. About 33 percent of children and adolescents in the United States consume fast food on a typical day, and intake increases with age" (Demory-Luce & Moti, 2014).
- "Socioeconomic trends, such as longer work hours, more women employed outside the home, and a high number of single-parent households have changed the way families obtain their meals. As parents experience busier lifestyles, they demand convenience for their family meals. The consumption of fast food is fostered because of the quick service, convenience, good taste, and inexpensive prices relative to more traditional home-style restaurants" (Demory-Luce & Moti, 2014).
- The findings from a national household survey among children highlight the nutritional effects of fast food consumption (*Bowman, Gortmaker, Ebbeling, Pereira, & Ludwig, 2004; Demory-Luce & Moti, 2014). Compared to children who did not eat fast food on a given day, children who did consumed
  - More total energy (2,236 vs. 2,049 kcal/day)
  - More total fat (84 vs. 75 g/day)
  - More total carbohydrates (303 vs. 277 g/day)
  - More added sugars (122 vs. 94 g/day)
  - More sugar-sweetened carbonated beverages (471 vs. 243 g/day)
  - Less milk (236 vs. 302 g/day)
  - Less fiber (13.2 vs. 14.3 g/day)
  - Fewer fruits and nonstarchy vegetables (103 vs. 148 g/day)
- The frequent eating of fast food (high in salt, sugar, and fat) and the increasing rate of obesity in children have created a problem that needs specific interventions (Hockenberry & Wilson, 2015). Refer to the nursing diagnosis *Overweight or Obesity*.

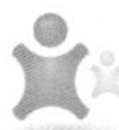

Maternal Considerations

- "A woman's nutritional status should be assessed preconceptionally with the goal of optimizing maternal, fetal, and infant health. Pregnancy-related dietary changes should begin prior to conception, with appropriate modifications across pregnancy and during lactation" (Goldstein, Roque, & Ruvel, 2015).
- For woman capable of becoming pregnant (U.S. Department of Agriculture & U.S. Department of Health and Human Services, 2010):
  - Choose foods that supply heme iron, which is more readily absorbed by the body, additional iron sources, and enhancers of iron absorption such as vitamin C-rich foods.
  - Consume 400 micrograms (mcg) per day of synthetic folic acid (from fortified foods and/or supplements) in addition to food forms of folate from a varied diet.
  - Consume 8 to 12 ounces of seafood per week from a variety of seafood types.
  - Due to their high methyl mercury content, limit white (albacore) tuna to 6 ounces/week and do not eat the following four types of fish: tilefish, shark, swordfish, and king mackerel.
  - If pregnant, take an iron supplement, as recommended by an obstetrician or other health-care provider.
- Nutritional needs change during pregnancy (refer to Table II.14).
- Recommendations for total weight gain during pregnancy vary. Women underweight before pregnancy should gain 28 to 40 lb; women at a desirable weight, 25 to 35 lb; women who are moderately overweight, 15 to 25 lb (Pillitteri, 2014).
- Overweight pregnant woman with a BMI of 25.0 to 29.9 are recommended to gain 5 to 25 0.6 (0.5 to 0.7). Obese pregnant woman (includes all classes) with a BMI ≥30.0 should gain 11 to 20 (*Institute of Medicine, 2009).
- "American women are now a more diverse group; they are having more twin and triplet pregnancies, and they tend to be older when they become pregnant. Women today are also heavier; a greater percentage of them are entering pregnancy overweight or obese, and many are gaining too much weight during pregnancy. Many of these changes carry the added burden of chronic disease, which can put the mother and her baby's health at risk" (*Institute of Medicine, 2009).
- The emphasis on nutrition and weight gain during pregnancy does not include dieting but instead healthy choices and portions.

- Dieting during pregnancy may result in insufficient maternal intake to provide the fetus with the necessary energy for growth. The fetus depends on the mother's dietary intake for growth and development, taking only iron and folate from maternal stores.

Geriatric Considerations

- Older people are prone to develop vitamin D deficiency because of various risk factors: decreased dietary intake, diminished sunlight exposure, reduced skin thickness, impaired intestinal absorption, and impaired hydroxylation in the liver and kidneys (Janssen, Samson, & Verhaar, 2002).
- In the United States, approximately 18% of older adults have complete tooth loss, which can challenge the ability to chew and swallow nutritious foods (Posthauer, Collins, Dorner, & Sloan, 2013).
- In general, older adults need the same kind of balanced diet as any other group, but fewer calories. Diets of older individuals, however, tend to be insufficient in iron, calcium, and vitamins. The combination of long-established eating patterns, income, transportation, housing, social interaction, and the effects of chronic or acute disease influence nutritional intake and health (Miller, 2015).
- People taking diuretics must be observed closely for adequate hydration (intake and output) and electrolyte balance, especially sodium and potassium. Potassium-rich foods should be included regularly in the diet or if necessary oral potassium should be prescribed.
- The recommendations for vitamin D and calcium change with aging:
  - 51 to 70 years old: Ca > 1,000/vitamin D > 600
  - 51- to 70-year-old females: Ca > 1,200/vitamin D > 600
  - 71+ years old: Ca > 1,200/vitamin D > 800
- Daily calcium requirements are recommended to achieve through dietary sources, not pills. If supplements are desired, consult with primary care provider prior to initiating OTC calcium.
- Iron-deficiency anemia usually occurs over time and may be related to chronic diseases and insufficient dietary iron. Increasing the intake of foods rich in vitamin C, folic acid, and dietary iron can improve the conditions necessary for optimal absorption of iron. Iron supplementation is often necessary.

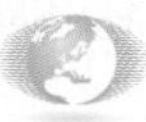

Transcultural Considerations

- Many cultures have used diet for centuries to treat specific diseases, promote health during pregnancy, foster growth and development in children, and prolong life (Andrews & Boyle, 2012).
- Some cultures view health as a state of balance among the body humors (blood, phlegm, black bile, and yellow bile). In this framework, a humoral imbalance that causes excessive dryness, cold, hot, or wetness leads to illness. For example, an upset stomach is believed to result from eating too many foods identified as cold. Foods, herbs, and medicines are classified as hot or cold or wet or dry. They are used to restore the body to its natural balance. For example, bananas are classified as a cold food, whereas cornmeal is a hot food (Andrews & Boyle, 2012).
- Weight gain is linked to the acculturation process experienced by foreign-born individuals migrating to the United States (*Park, Neckerman, Quinn, Weiss, & Rundle, 2008).
- The prevalence of primary lactose intolerance varies according to race. As many as 25% of the white population (prevalence in those with southern European roots) is estimated to have lactose intolerance, while among African American, Native American, and Asian American populations, the prevalence of lactose intolerance is estimated at 75% to 90% (*Roy, 2011).
- Nutritional practices can be categorized as beneficial, neutral, or harmful. Beneficial and neutral practices should be encouraged. Harmful practices should be approached with sensitivity and their detrimental effects explained (Andrews & Boyle, 2012).
- Group dining, which is encouraged in some settings (e.g., rehabilitation, long-term, mental health), may be in conflict with certain cultures (e.g., women eating with men) (Andrews & Boyle, 2012).
- Maintaining a kosher diet for a Jewish client is possible even if the agency does not have a kosher kitchen. Fish with fins or scales will meet dietary requirements. Dairy products are also possible. Paper plates with disposable utensils should be used so that meat and milk dishes are not mixed (Giger, 2013).

Focus Assessment Criteria (*Chima, 2004; Lutz et al., 2015)

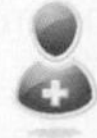

CLINICAL ALERT This assessment is designed to identify individuals who are malnourished and have an increased nutritional risk. Those identified should be referred to the registered dietician for a more detailed assessment (*Chima, 2004; Lutz et al., 2015).

Subjective Data

Recent weight loss of greater than 10 lb in the last 30 days?
Been on a weight reduction diet?
Recent change of appetite?
Problems with

Swallowing	Chewing	Sore mouth
Nausea	Diarrhea	Vomiting
Constipation	Indigestion	Bloating?

Special diet?
Supplements
Food allergies

Usual Intake

What is the usual for breakfast, lunch, and dinner?
Is intake of the basic five food groups sufficient?
Is fluid intake sufficient?

Appetite (Usual, Changes)

Food and Fluid Preferences

Food/fluid likes, dislikes, habits, and taboos
Religious/cultural dietary practices
Frequency of fast food consumption

Activity Level

Occupation, exercise (type, frequency)

Barriers to Food Procurement/Preparation (Who)

Functional ability, kitchen facilities, transportation, financial

Objective Data

General Appearance

Height
Weight
BMI
Mouth
Teeth

Laboratory Studies

For nutritional status and deficiencies (American Association for Clinical Chemistry, 2013):
- Iron tests such as serum iron, TIBC, and ferritin
- Vitamins and trace minerals such as B_{12} and folate, vitamins A, D, and K, B vitamins, calcium, and magnesium
- Prealbumin: although commonly used as a marker of malnutrition, levels of this protein may be affected by a number of conditions other than malnutrition.
- Albumin has been used in the past along with or instead of prealbumin to evaluate nutritional status, but now is more often used to screen for and help diagnose liver or kidney diseases.

Screen for risk inpatient infant–child–adolescents (*Chima, 2004; *Hammond, 2011):
- Recent weight loss
- On special diet and *needs education*
- Has feeding tube or on parenteral feedings
- Diabetic
- Receives high-calorie feeds/concentrated formula
- Food allergy
- Failure to thrive
- Feeding problems/intolerance
- Teen who is pregnant or lactating
- Child being breastfed

***Assess for Food Security** (Coleman-Jensen et al., 2013)*

Carp's Cues

This assessment tool is designed for determining if food insecurity exists and is appropriate in primary care or community settings. In the acute care setting, yes; answers to questions 1 and 2 indicate the individual/family should be referred to a social service professional.

1. "We worried whether our food would run out before we got money to buy more." Was that often, sometimes, or never true for you in the last 12 months?
2. "The food that we bought just didn't last and we didn't have money to get more." Was that often, sometimes, or never true for you in the last 12 months?
3. "We couldn't afford to eat balanced meals." Was that often, sometimes, or never true for you in the last 12 months?
4. In the last 12 months, did you or other adults in the household ever cut the size of your meals or skip meals because there wasn't enough money for food? (Yes/No)
5. (If yes to question 4) How often did this happen—almost every month, some months but not every month, or in only 1 or 2 months?
6. In the last 12 months, did you ever eat less than you felt you should because there wasn't enough money for food? (Yes/No)
7. In the last 12 months, were you ever hungry, but didn't eat, because there wasn't enough money for food? (Yes/No)
8. In the last 12 months, did you lose weight because there wasn't enough money for food? (Yes/No)
9. In the last 12 months, did you or other adults in your household ever not eat for a whole day, because there wasn't enough money for food? (Yes/No)
10. (If yes to question 9) How often did this happen—almost every month, some months but not every month, or in only 1 or 2 months?

(Questions 11 to 18 were asked only if the household included children age 0- to 17.)

11. "We relied on only a few kinds of low-cost food to feed our children, because we were running out of money to buy food." Was that often, sometimes, or never true for you in the last 12 months?
12. "We couldn't feed our children a balanced meal, because we couldn't afford that." Was that often, sometimes, or never true for you in the last 12 months?
13. "The children were not eating enough because we just couldn't afford enough food." Was that often, sometimes, or never true for you in the last 12 months?
14. In the last 12 months, did you ever cut the size of any of the children's meals because there wasn't enough money for food? (Yes/No)
15. In the last 12 months, were the children ever hungry but you just couldn't afford more food? (Yes/No)
16. In the last 12 months, did any of the children ever skip a meal because there wasn't enough money for food? (Yes/No)
17. (If yes to question 16) How often did this happen—almost every month, some months but not every month, or in only 1 or 2 months?
18. In the last 12 months, did any of the children ever not eat for a whole day because there wasn't enough money for food? (Yes/No)

Goals

NOC

Nutritional Status, Symptom Control. Nutritional Counseling, Nutritional Monitoring. Teaching: Individual

The individual will ingest daily nutritional requirements in accordance with activity level and metabolic needs, as evidenced by the following indicators:

- Relates importance of good nutrition
- Identifies age-related nutritional recommendations
- Will differentiate between nutritionally dense foods and foods that have low density

Interventions

NIC

Nutrition Management, Weight Gain Assistance, Nutritional Counseling

Refer to Appendix D: Practical Strategies to increase engagement in improving nutrition.

Assess for Food and Nutrient Intake Risk Factors (*Chima, 2004; *Hammond, 2011)

- Calorie or protein, vitamin, and mineral intake greater or less than required
- Swallowing difficulties

- GI disturbances, bowel irregularity
- Impaired cognitive function or depression
- Unusual food habits (pica)
- Misuse of supplements
- Restricted diet
- Inability or unwillingness to consume food
- Increase or decrease in activities of daily living

Psychological Social/Cultural Risk Factors

- Language barriers
- Low literacy
- Cultural or religious factors
- Emotional disturbances associated with feeding difficulties (e.g., depression)
- Limited resources for food preparation or obtaining food or supplies
- Alcohol or drug addiction
- Limited or low income
- Lack of ability to communicate needs
- Limited use or understanding of community resources

Physical Risk Factors

- Extreme age (adults >80 years, premature infants, very young children)
- Pregnancy: adolescent, closely spaced, or three or more pregnancies
- Alterations in anthropometric measurements, marked overweight/underweight for age, height, both; depressed somatic fat and muscle stores (*Note*: Recent unintentional weight loss is more predictive of morbidity/mortality than BMI).
- Chronic renal/cardiac disease, diabetes, pressure ulcers, cancer, AIDS, GI complications, hypermetabolic stress, immobility, osteoporosis, neurologic impairments, visual impairments

R: *Nutrients provide energy sources, build tissue, and regulate metabolic processes.*

Consult With a Nutritionist to Establish Appropriate Daily Caloric and Food Type Requirements for the Individual

R: *Consultation can help ensure a diet that provides optimal caloric and nutrient intake.*

Encourage to Rest Before Meals

R: *Fatigue further reduces an anorectic individual's desire and ability to eat.*

Offer Frequent, Small Meals Instead of a Few Large Ones; Offer Foods Served Cold

R: *Even distribution of total daily caloric intake helps prevent gastric distention, possibly increasing appetite.*

Encourage and Help the Individual to Maintain Good Oral Hygiene

R: *Poor oral hygiene leads to bad odor and taste, which can diminish appetite.*

Arrange to Have High-Calorie and High-Protein Foods Served at the Times That the Individual Usually Feels Most Like Eating

R: *Presenting high-calorie and high-protein food when the individual is most likely to eat increases the likelihood that he or she will consume adequate calories and protein.*

Take Steps to Promote Appetite

- Refer to *Imbalance Nutrition related to anorexia.*

Provide for Supplemental Dietary Needs Amplified by Acute Illness

R: *Metabolic demands are increased by the catabolic processes that occur through stages of acute illness, usually increasing nutritional demand.*

Initiate Health Teaching and Referrals as Needed

- Explain foods and nutrients to increase and foods and food components to reduce. Refer to Key Dietary Recommendations issued by the U.S. Department of Agriculture and U.S. Department of Health and Human Services (2010).

- Refer to thePoint for a printable handout on "Getting Started to Better Nutrition."
- Refer to Dietary Guidelines for Americans at the U.S. Department of Health and Human Services website www.health.gov.

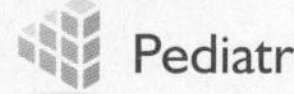

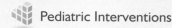

Pediatric Interventions

- Teach parents the following regarding infant nutrition:
  - Adequate infant feeding schedule and weight gain requirements for growth: 100 to 120 kcal/kg/day for growth
  - Proper preparation of infant formula
  - Proper storage of breast milk and infant formula
  - Proper elevation of infant's head during and immediately after feedings
  - Proper chin/cheek support techniques for orally compromised infants
  - The age-related nutritional needs of their children (Consult an appropriate textbook on pediatrics or nutrition for specific recommendations.)
- Discuss the importance of limiting snacks high in salt, sugar, or fat (e.g., soda, candy, chips) to limit risks for cardiac disorders, obesity, and diabetes mellitus. Advise families to substitute healthy snacks (e.g., fresh fruits, plain popcorn, frozen fruit juice bars, fresh vegetables).
- If eating "fast foods," teach healthier choices as follows:
  - Encourage portion control; educate children/adolescents that "large," "extra," "double," or "triple" will be higher in calories and fat.
  - Recommend smaller portions, since a regular serving is enough for most children, or sharing with a parent or sibling.
  - Look for whole grain foods, fruits, vegetables, and calcium-rich foods.
  - When planning a fast food meal, select an establishment that promotes healthier options at the point of purchase.
- Address strategies to improve nutrition when eating fast foods:
  - Drink skim milk.
  - Avoid French fries or share one order.
  - Choose grilled foods.
  - Eat salads and vegetables.
- Explore healthier fast foods at home (e.g., frozen dinners with three food groups).
- Suggest healthy snacks at home. Offer fresh fruits, vegetables, cheese and crackers, low-fat milk, calcium-fortified juices, and frozen yogurt as snacks.

R: *Making healthful food available and convenient and increasing healthy snacks reduces the pressure for the child to eat a certain amount at mealtime.*

- Avoid describing foods as bad or good. Explain nutrient density of foods (*Hunter & Cason, 2006).

R: *Nutrient dense foods give the most nutrients for the fewest amount of calories.*

- Foods that are nutrient dense:
  - Fruits and vegetables that are bright or deeply colored
  - Foods that are fortified
  - Lower fat versions of meats, milk, dairy products, and eggs
- Foods that are less nutrient dense:
  - Be lighter or whiter in color
  - Contain a lot of refined sugar
  - Be refined products (white bread as compared to whole grains)
  - Contain high amounts of fat for the amount of nutrients compared to similar products (fat-free milk vs. ice cream)
  - For example:
    - Apple is a better choice than a bag of pretzels with the same number of calories, but the apple provides fiber, vitamin C, and potassium.
    - An orange is better than orange juice because it has fiber.
- Allow the child to select one type of food he or she does not have to eat.
- Provide small servings (e.g., 1 tbs of each food for every year of age).
- Make snacks as nutritiously important as meals (e.g., hard-boiled eggs, raw vegetable sticks, peanut butter/crackers, fruit juices, cheese, and fresh fruit).
- Offer a variety of foods.

- Involve the child in monitoring healthy eating (e.g., create a chart where the child checks off intake of healthy foods daily).
- Replace passive television watching with a group activity (e.g., Frisbee tossing, biking, walking).
- Substitute quick, nutritious fast meals (e.g., frozen dinners).

R: *Nutritional requirements vary greatly for each age group. Periods of accelerated physical growth (e.g., infancy, puberty) may necessitate doubling iron, calcium, zinc, and protein intake (Hockenberry & Wilson, 2015).*

R: *Family nutritional patterns are the primary influence on the development of food habits (e.g., unhealthy snacks, excessive television watching, obesity (Dudek, 2014).*

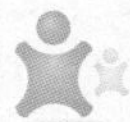

Maternal Interventions

- Pregnant or lactating mother admitted to unit other than antepartum or mother–baby (*Chima, 2004; *Hammond, 2011).
- Teach the importance of adequate calorie and fluid intake while breastfeeding in relation to breast milk production.
- Explain physiologic changes and nutritional needs during pregnancy (see Table II.14).
- Discuss the effects of alcohol, caffeine, and artificial sweeteners on the developing fetus.

R: *Studies have shown caffeine to have few effects on pregnancy outcome, but moderation is recommended. Consumption of artificial sweeteners during pregnancy has not been found to be contraindicated, but moderation is suggested (Dudek, 2014).*

- Discuss with pregnant adolescents that their nutritional needs are greater since they are still developing and now are pregnant (Pillitteri, 2014). Emphasize the growing fetus.

R: *Young adolescent mothers had smaller and thinner newborns than those born to older women who were aware of the need to adjust their nutrition during pregnancy and at delivery (Pillitteri, 2014).*

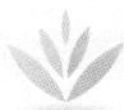

Geriatric Interventions

Consider a Consult With Registered Dietician for (*Chima, 2004; *Hammond, 2011)

- Individual with significant unintentional weight loss of 10 lb or more in past 1 to 2 months
- Individual desires education on a more nutritious diet
- Individual unable to take oral or other feedings ≥5 days prior to admission
- Individual on enteral or parenteral feedings
- Individual 80+ years admitted for surgical procedure
- Individual with skin breakdown (decubitus ulcer) consumes foods fortified with vitamin B_{12}, such as fortified cereals, or dietary supplement

Determine the Individual's Understanding of Nutritional Needs With

- Aging
- Medication use
- Illness
- Activity

R: *Certain medications or illnesses may require an adjustment in diet (e.g., potassium, sodium, fiber).*

Assess Whether Any Factors Interfere With Ingesting Foods (Lutz et al., 2015; Miller, 2015)

- Anorexia from medications, grief, depression, or illness
- Impaired mental status leading to inattention to hunger or selecting insufficient kinds/amounts of food
- Voluntary fluid restriction for fear of urinary incontinence
- Small frame or history of undernutrition
- New dentures or poor dentition
- Dislike of cooking and eating alone
- Regularly eats alone
- Has more than two alcoholic drinks daily

R: *Multiple factors can interfere with access or ingestion of food. Strategies to improve nutrition should address specific factors (Dudek, 2014).*

Assess Whether Any Factors Interfere With Preparing and/or Procuring Foods (Miller, 2015)

- Inadequate income to purchase food
- Lack of transportation to buy food
- Inadequate facility to cook
- Impaired mobility or manual dexterity (paresis, tremors, weakness, joint pain, or deformity)
- Safety issues (e.g. fires, spoiled foods)

Assess for Food Insecurity

- Refer to Focus Assessment Criteria.

Explain Decline in Sensitivity to Sweet and Salty Tastes; But Not Bitter and Sour (Lutz et al., 2015). **Caution on Oversalting Foods**

R: *Older adults can consume excessive salt and sugar to compensate for loss of sensitivity to these tastes (Miller, 2015).*

If Indicated, Consult With Home Health Nurse to Evaluate Home Environment (e.g., Safety Issues, Cooking Facilities, Food Supply, and Cleanliness)

Access Community Agencies as Indicated (e.g., Nutritional Programs, Community Centers, Home-Delivered Grocery Services)

R: *A home assessment may provide valid data in cases of suspected nutritional problems and/or food insecurity (Miller, 2015).*

Imbalanced Nutrition • Related to Anorexia Secondary to (Specify)

Goals

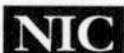

NOC Nutritional Status, Appetite

The individual will increase oral intake, as evidenced by the following indicators (specify):

- Describes causative factors when known
- Describes rationale and procedure for treatments

Interventions

NIC Nutrition Management, Nutrition Monitoring: Weight Gain Assistance, Nutritional Counseling

Assess Causative Factors

- Refer to Related Factors.

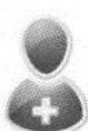

Clinical Alert "Investigators report that increased caloric intake may neither reverse weight loss nor improve survival" (Tisdale, 2003, as cited in *Cunningham & Huhmann, 2011). Sometimes methods to increase intake are taxing to the ill individual who is terminally ill. Discuss with individual/family members, primary care provider, specialists, and family regarding the benefits versus the distress of aggressive nutritional supplementation.

When Anorexia Is Present, Stress the Importance of Consuming Foods Higher in Nutrition (*Hunter & Cason, 2006)

- Avoid describing foods as bad or good. Explain nutrient density of foods.

R: *Nutrient dense foods give the most nutrients for the fewest amount of calories.*

- Foods that are nutrient dense:
  - Fruits and vegetables that are bright or deeply colored
  - Foods that are fortified

   - Lower fat versions of meats, milk, dairy products, and eggs
- Foods that are less nutrient dense:
   - Tend to be lighter or whiter in color
   - Contain a lot of refined sugar
   - Tend to be refined products (white bread as compared to whole grains)
   - Contain high amounts of fat for the amount of nutrients compared to similar products (fat-free milk vs. ice cream)
   - For example:
      - Apple is a better choice than a bag of pretzels with the same number of calories, but the apple provides fiber, vitamin C, and potassium.
      - An orange is better than orange juice because it has fiber.

Reduce or Eliminate Contributing Factors, If Possible

- Teach the effects of diminished sense of taste or smell on appetite (*Cunningham & Huhmann, 2011).
- Explain to the individual the importance of consuming adequate nutrients.
- Increase oral hygiene; alter food choices.
- Teach the individual to use spices (e.g., lemon juice, mint, cloves, basil, thyme, cinnamon, rosemary, bacon bits) to help improve the taste and aroma of food.
- Avoid sight, smell of food.
- Eat tart, sour, or cold foods.
- Teach low-fat protein sources that the individual may find more acceptable than red meat:
   - Eggs and dairy products
   - Poultry
   - Fish
   - Marinated meat (in wine, vinegar)
   - Soy products (tofu)
- Chopped- or ground-meat protein sources may be more acceptable.
- Mixing protein and vegetables may be more acceptable.
- Refer to meals as "snacks" to make them sound smaller.

R: *Strategies to stimulate appetite and increase the nutrition in food consumed are used.*

Social Isolation

- Encourage the individual to eat with others (meals served in the dining room or group area at the local meeting place such as the community center or by church groups).
- Provide daily contact through phone calls by the support system.
- See *Risk for Loneliness* for additional interventions.

R: *For most people, meals are social events. Loneliness at meals can reduce the incentive to prepare nutritious meals.*

- Assist individual in securing a safe environment.

R: *The fears associated with anorexia may influence food limitations (Soussignan, Jiang, Rigaud, Royet, & Schaal, 2010).*

Noxious Stimuli (Pain, Mucositis, Fatigue, Odors, Nausea, and Vomiting)

Pain

- Plan care so that unpleasant or painful procedures do not take place before meals.
- Schedule pain relief medications so that optimal relief without drowsiness is achieved at mealtime.
- Provide a pleasant, relaxed atmosphere for eating (no bedpans in sight; no rushing); try a "surprise" (e.g., flowers with meal).

R: *Arrange to decrease or eliminate pain and painful procedures near mealtimes.*

Mucositis

- Refer to *Impaired Oral Mucous Membrane* for interventions.

Fatigue

- Teach or assist the individual to rest before meals.
- Teach the individual to expend minimal energy in food preparation (cook large quantities and freeze several meals at a time; request assistance from others).

R: *Fatigue will decrease appetite and interfere with the effort needed to eat.*

Odor of Food

- Teach the individual to avoid cooking odors—frying foods, brewing coffee—if possible (take a walk; select foods that can be eaten cold).
- Suggest using foods that require little cooking during periods of anorexia.

R: *The smell of cooking foods can increase nausea and anorexia.*

Nausea and Vomiting

- Refer to *Nausea.*

See *Impaired Swallowing* for Additional Interventions

Promote Foods That Stimulate Eating and Increase Protein Consumption

- Maintain good oral hygiene (brush teeth, rinse mouth) before and after eating.

R: *Maintaining good oral hygiene before and after meals decreases microorganisms that can cause foul taste and odor, inhibiting appetite.*

- Offer frequent small feedings (six per day plus snacks). Restrict fluids with meals.

R: *Small feedings and fluid restriction with meals can help to prevent gastric distention, which can decrease appetite.*

- Practice relaxation techniques prior to meals.
- To stimulate appetite (*Cunningham & Huhmann, 2011):
  - Try a different food choice.
  - Avoid sight and smell of food prior to eating.
  - Eat sour foods.
  - Eat cold foods.
  - Use a straw.
  - Increase seasoning.
  - Use plastic utensils.

R: *Attempts to vary the taste and texture can improve appetite and prevent food aversion.*

- To increase intake:
  - Arrange to serve the highest protein/calorie nutrients when the individual feels most like eating (e.g., if chemotherapy is in the early morning, serve food in the late afternoon).
  - Eat dry foods (toast, crackers) on arising.
  - Try salty foods, if permissible.
  - Avoid overly sweet, rich, greasy, or fried foods.
  - Try clear, cool beverages. Sip slowly through a straw.
  - Try whatever the individual feels can be tolerated.
  - Eat small portions low in fat. Eat more frequently.
  - Review nutritionally dense foods versus low-calorie foods. Avoid empty-calorie foods (e.g., soda).
  - Encourage family to bring in favorite foods from home and to socialize during meals.
  - Try commercial supplements available in many forms (liquids, powder, pudding); keep switching brands until some are found that are acceptable to the individual in taste and consistency.

R: *Varied techniques should be attempted to increase intake of nutritious foods and beverages.*

- Teach techniques for home food preparation:
  - Add powdered milk to milkshakes, gravies, sauces, puddings, cereals, meatballs, or milk to increase protein and calorie content.
  - Add blended foods or baby foods to meat juices or soups.
  - Use fortified milk (i.e., 1 cup of instant nonfat milk to 1 quart of fresh milk).
  - Use milk or half-and-half cream instead of water when making soups and sauces; soy formulas can also be used.
  - Add cheese or diced meat.
  - Add cream cheese or peanut butter to toast, crackers, or celery sticks.
  - Add extra butter or margarine to soups, sauces, or vegetables.
  - Spread butter on toast while hot.
  - Use mayonnaise (100 cal/tbs) instead of salad dressing.

- Add sour cream or yogurt to vegetables or as dip.
- Use whipped cream (60 cal/tbs).
- Add raisins, dates, nuts, and brown sugar to hot or cold cereals.
- Have extra food (snacks) easily available.

R: *Certain measures can increase the nutritional content of foods even when intake is limited.*

Initiate Health Teaching and Referrals, as Indicated

- Dietitian for meal planning
- If anorexia is of psychiatric origins, refer to psychiatric therapy when indicated.
- Community meal centers

R: *Resources in the community can assist the individual and family.*

Imbalanced Nutrition • Related to Difficulty or Inability to Procure Food*

Altered ability to procure food is the inability to acquire food because of physical, economic, or sociocultural barriers.

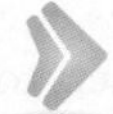

Carp's Cues

These interventions are appropriate for nurses in primary care or in community settings. Consider presenting a short program for older adults living in a community setting on this topic.

Goals

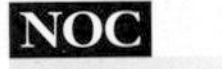

Nutritional Status

The individual will identify a method to acquire food on a regular schedule, as evidenced by the following indicators:

- Describes causative factors when known
- Relates importance of good nutrition

Interventions

NIC

Nutritional Counseling, Nutrition Management, Teaching: Individual, Family, Referral, Environmental Management

Assess Causative Factors

- Inadequate economic resources to obtain adequate nutrition
- Sociocultural barriers
- Physical inability to procure food related to health problem such as COPD, CVA, or quadriplegia

Assess for Food Insecurity

- Refer to Focus Assessment Criteria.
- If indicated, refer to home health nurse to evaluate home environment (e.g., safety issues, cooking facilities, food supply, and cleanliness).
- Access community agencies as indicated (e.g., nutritional programs, community centers, home-delivered grocery services).

For Community/Home Health/Primary Care Nurses

Reduce or Eliminate Contributing Factors, If Possible

Inadequate Economic Resources

- Assess eligibility for food stamps or other government-funded programs for low-income groups; consult with social services.
- Suggest cooperatives or local farmers' markets for shopping.
- Buy foods and meats on sale and freeze; use cheaper cuts and tenderize.
- Suggest foods that are low in cost and high in nutrients; decrease use of prepackaged or prepared items:
  - Beans and legumes as protein sources
  - Powdered milk (alone or mixed half and half with whole milk)
  - Seasonal foods when plentiful
- Encourage growing a small garden or participating in a community plot.

- Freeze or can fruits and vegetables in season (refer to county agricultural agent for information on canning and freezing).

Sociocultural Barriers

- Suggest substitutions of locally available foodstuffs for those to which the individual is accustomed.
- Refer to adult education home economics classes for food preparation.
- Assist to recognize and use additional outlets and sources of food (grocery stores, meat, and fruit markets).
- Encourage peer group meetings among people of similar backgrounds to allow learning and exchange of ideas.
- Acquaint with ethnic food store locations, if available.

Physical/Memory Deficits

- Promote alternative methods of food procurement and preparation.
- Support systems can
  - Purchase or prepare food for individual
  - Take individual to the store to shop
  - Take individual to supermarkets that deliver
  - Arrange Meals on Wheels or similar service
  - Arrange homemaker service
  - Arrange door-to-store bus service
  - List local businesses that offer prepared meals
  - Prepare food for seven meals at once and divide portions onto reusable containers to freeze/microwave. If safety is an issue, remove knobs for controlling stove/oven. Can use microwave, toaster oven with built-in timer.
  - If memory problems are present, call daily to discuss food choices for the day or ask a neighbor to check in to remind him or her of food choices available in their refrigerator/freezer.
- Aid to plan daily activities that allow enough energy for shopping and cooking, such as suggesting rest periods before, during (if needed), and after activity.

R: *People who are impaired either physically or cognitively should receive the necessary support and supervision when selecting foods and self-feeding. Activities needed to procure food depend on skills of cognition, balance, mobility, manual dexterity, and all five senses (Miller, 2015).*

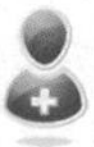

Clinical Alert Sometimes families are too quick to remove an elder relative from their home because of self-care/safety issues. If the individual is high risk for injury or unable to attend to ADLs (activities of daily living) safely, then other living arrangements are probably necessary. However when an individual is not at high risk but is compromised, consider, "Do you want your loved one to be happy or safe?" Encourage the family to creatively adapt to helping their loved one live where they are.

Teach Techniques for Meal Planning and Preparation for One

- Buy small cans of food (they may seem more expensive, but spoiled food is costly).
- When buying fruit, select three stages of ripeness (ripe, medium ripe, green).
- Family-sized packages of meat or fresh vegetables can be broken down and frozen.
- When buying in large quantity, make soups and stews with the extra.
- Use powdered instead of fresh milk in recipes.
- Buy fresh milk in pints or quarts.
- Store large-quantity items (rice, flour, corn meal, dry milk, cereal) in glass jars. Place tightly sealed jars in the freezer for one night to kill any organisms and their eggs.
- Experiment with stir-frying vegetables (e.g., Chinese cabbage, celery) in a little chicken broth.
- If freezer space is available, prepare four to six times as much as you need and freeze in individual portions, dating the packages.
- Use small zip-seal bags to freeze portions. Seal almost completely, and use a straw to suck out air for longer shelf life.
- Store half a loaf of bread well wrapped in the freezer. (It will become stale in the refrigerator.)
- Buy large bags of frozen vegetables, use small amounts, and reclose bags with twist ties.
- Finely chop and freeze fresh herbs (parsley, dill, basil) in small freezer bags. Flatten, so small portions can be broken off after freezing.
- Buy large quantities of meat, and freeze in foil wrap (not freezer paper).

R: *People with difficulty preparing meals can be assisted in reducing daily preparation time through specific planning (*Mahan & Arlin, 1996).*

Initiate Health Teaching and Referrals, as Indicated

- Refer to social worker, occupational therapist, or visiting nurse, as needed.
- Refer to local extension office for information on vegetable gardening, community gardens, and techniques of freezing and canning foods.
- Refer to a dietitian for meal planning.

Impaired Dentition

NANDA-I Definition

Disruption in tooth development/eruption patterns or structural integrity of individual teeth

Defining Characteristics*

Excessive plaque
Asymmetric facial expression
Halitosis
Crown or root caries
Toothache
Tooth enamel discoloration
Excessive calculus
Loose teeth
Malocclusion or tooth misalignment
Incomplete eruption for age (may be primary or permanent teeth)
Premature loss of primary teeth
Tooth fracture(s)
Missing teeth or complete absence
Erosion of enamel

Author's Note

Impaired Dentition describes a multitude of problems with teeth. It is unclear how nurses would use this diagnosis. If the individual had caries, abscesses, misaligned teeth, or malformed teeth, the nurse should refer the person to a dental professional. If problems with teeth are affecting comfort or nutrition, *Impaired Comfort* or *Imbalanced Nutrition* would be the appropriate nursing diagnosis, instead of *Impaired Dentition*.

Impaired Swallowing

NANDA-I Definition

Abnormal functioning of the swallowing mechanism associated with deficits in oral, pharyngeal, or esophageal structure or function

Defining Characteristics (Fass, 2014)

Oral dysfunction
Drooling
Dysarthria
Sialorrhea (hypersalivation)
Food spillage
Piecemeal swallows

Pharyngeal dysfunction
Coughing or choking during food consumption
Dysphonia (defective use of the voice)

Esophageal dysphagia
Difficulty swallowing several seconds after initiating a swallow
Reports a sensation of food getting stuck in the suprasternal notch or behind the sternum

Related Factors

Pathophysiologic

Related to decreased/absent gag reflex, mastication difficulties, or decreased sensations secondary to:

Cerebral palsy*
Muscular dystrophy
Poliomyelitis
Parkinson's disease
Guillain–Barré syndrome
Myasthenia gravis
Amyotrophic lateral sclerosis
CVA
Neoplastic disease affecting brain
Right or left hemispheric brain damage
Vocal cord paralysis
Cranial nerve damage (V, VII, IX, X, XI)

Related to constriction of esophagus secondary to:

Vascular ring anomaly
Large aneurysm of the thoracic aorta

Related to tracheoesophageal tumors, edema

Related to irritated oropharyngeal cavity

Related to decreased saliva

Treatment Related

Related to surgical reconstruction of the mouth, throat, jaw, or nose

Related to decreased consciousness secondary to anesthesia

Related to mechanical obstruction secondary to tracheostomy tube

Related to esophagitis secondary to radiotherapy

Situational (Personal, Environmental)

Related to fatigue

Related to limited awareness, distractibility

Maturational

Infants/Children

Related to decreased sensations or difficulty with mastication

Related to poor suck/swallow/breathe coordination

Older Adult

Related to reduction in saliva, taste

Author's Note

See *Imbalanced Nutrition*.

Errors in Diagnostic Statements

See *Imbalanced Nutrition*.

Key Concepts

- "Dysphagia is an alarm symptom that warrants immediate evaluation to define the exact cause and initiate appropriate therapy. Dysphagia in older adult subjects should not be attributed to normal aging. Aging alone causes mild esophageal motility abnormalities, which are rarely symptomatic" (Fass, 2014).

General Considerations

Physiology

- Swallowing is intellectual, emotional, and physical because it involves the complex process of ingesting liquid or solid food while also protecting the airways for aspiration (Grossman & Porth, 2014; Hickey, 2014).
- The swallowing process occurs in four stages with select cranial nerve involvement (Hickey, 2014):
  - *Stage 1*—**Oral preparatory phase**: Food is placed in the oral cavity and is chewed, forming a bolus.
  - *Stage 2*—**Oral phase**: The bolus of food is centered and moved by the tongue to the posterior pharynx. The tongue maneuvers the food and the soft palate and uvula close off the nasopharynx.
  - *Stage 3*—**Pharyngeal phase**: The food passes the anterior fossa arches and triggers the swallow reflex. The tongue prevents the food from returning the oral cavity by elevation and contraction of the soft palate. Pharyngeal peristalsis begins, causing the food to move downward.
  - *Stage 4*—**Esophageal phase**: Pharyngeal peristalsis pushes the food downward. The larynx elevates and the cricopharyngeal muscles relax, allowing the food to move from the pharynx into the esophagus. The larynx wave pushes the food down the esophagus to the stomach.
- Cranial nerves V, VII, IX, X, and XI are involved in swallowing. Impairment of cranial nerve function (e.g., poststroke, head injury) can cause the following swallowing problems (Hickey, 2014):
  - Trigeminal (V)—loss of sensation and ability to move mandible
  - Facial (VII)—increased salivation; inability to pucker lips, pouching of food
  - Glossopharyngeal (IX)—diminished taste sensation, salivation, and gag reflex
  - Vagus (X)—decreased peristalsis, decreased gag reflex
  - Hypoglossal (XI)—poor tongue control, poor movement of food to the throat
- A cough reflex is essential for rehabilitation, but a gag reflex is not.
- Do not confuse the ability to chew with the ability to swallow. See also *Imbalanced Nutrition*.
- Complications that have been associated with dysphagia poststroke include pneumonia, malnutrition, dehydration, poorer long-term outcome, increased length of hospital stay, increased rehabilitation time and the need for long-term-care assistance, increased mortality, and increased health-care costs (Sura, Madhavan, Carnaby, & Crary, 2012).

Geriatric Considerations

- Approximately, "7% to 10% of adults older than age 50 have been diagnosed with dysphagia; an estimated 14% of adults older than age 60 have dysphagia or another type of swallowing disorder. Dysphagia strikes about 15% of persons in community settings and nearly 40% of long-term-care patients" (Humbert & Robbins, 2008).
- Mortality increased to 63% in 1 year. In addition, adverse events associated with nonoral feeding sources are common and include local wound complications, leakage around the insertion site, tube occlusion, and increased reflux, leading to other complications such as pneumonia.
- Dysphagia can be life-threatening, particularly in elderly patients (Tanner & Culbertson, 2014). Chang et al. (2013) reviewed the death certificates of patients who were described as having died from a stroke; they reported that 5% had died as a result of aspiration pneumonia and 1% had died as a result of choking.

Focus Assessment Criteria

Clinical Alert If impaired swallowing is suspected, hold all PO liquids/foods, and access a swallowing assessment by speech therapist/speech-language pathologists.

Subjective Data

Assess for Defining Characteristics

History of problem with swallowing nasal regurgitation, hoarseness, choking, or coughing? Onset? Problem foods or liquids? Specify?

Assess for Related Factors

- CVA
- Parkinson's disease
- Multiple sclerosis
- Brain lesions
- Head trauma
- Tracheoesophageal tumors
- Oral surgery

Objective Data

Assess for Defining Characteristics

- Decreased or absent swallowing, cough, or gag reflex
- Poor coordination of tongue
- Observed choking or coughing with food or fluid

Assess for Related Factors

- Facial muscle weakness
- Impaired use of tongue
- Chewing difficulties
- Decreased saliva production
- Thick secretions
- Impaired cognition

Goals

NOC
Aspiration Control, Swallowing Status

The individual will report improved ability to swallow, as evidenced by the following indicators:

- Describes causative factors when known
- Describes rationale and procedures for treatment

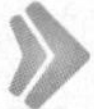

Carp's Cues

Tanner and Culbertson (2014) wrote

The need to preserve life through airway protection is sometimes in tension with the patient's desire to preserve a quality of life that is the same as it was before the onset of current health conditions. Consuming food and liquid includes the pleasures of smelling, tasting, and orally manipulating nutrients.

For this reason nurses and their colleagues in speech-language pathology must consider both the safety of patients and their gustatory wishes. After due consultation, nurses and other providers need to respect the wishes of competent patients, their family members, and/or a patient surrogate if a patient is not competent (American Nurses Association, 2013).

Interventions

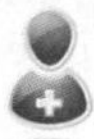

Clinical Alert Despite medical orders for oral fluids or food, the nurse must assess the risks of oral intake for an individual with possible swallowing problems. If the nurse determines that a comprehensive swallowing assessment is needed, all oral fluids and fluids must be prohibited until a specialist evaluation is completed (e.g., speech therapy, nurse specialist).

NIC
Aspiration Precautions, Swallowing Therapy, Surveillance, Referral, Positioning

Assure Individual and/or Family Have Discussed the Advantages and Risks of Dysphagia Management (e.g., Oral Nutrition, Intravenous, Nasogastric, or Percutaneous–Endoscopic–Gastrostomy Tube With a Specialist)

- Document the discussion event and decisions.

R: *Nonoral nutritional treatments reduced the risks of aspiration and choking while providing needed hydration and nutrients (Tanner & Culbertson, 2014). Enteral nutrition has its own risks, including improper tube placement, infection, perforation, hemorrhage, obstruction, necrosis, abscesses, and fistulas. Because NPO status might understandably have a negative impact on a patient's quality of life, the balance between patient safety and quality of life is an important consideration. As noted above, it is necessary to consider the patient's wishes, and if the patient is not competent, consider the wishes of this patient's surrogate, in the decision-making process.*

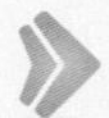

Carp's Cues

If the individual is a candidate for hospice for palliative care, refer to *Risk for Compromised Human Dignity* for interventions directed at assisting the individual/family in decisions regarding sources of nutrition.

Assess for the Presence of Causative or Contributing Factors that Increase the Risk of Impaired Swallowing

- Refer to Focus Assessment Criteria.

Consult with a Speech Therapist for an Evaluation and Recommended Plan of Care

R: *A speech pathologist has the expertise needed to perform the dysphagia evaluation, indicated for the prevention of aspiration pneumonia and improve oral intake (Sura et al., 2012).*

- Alert all staff that individual has impaired swallowing (e.g., alert symbol at bedside, in computer).

R: *Alerting all staff can reduce the risk of aspiration.*

- Consult with swallowing specialist for the best position when taking PO food or fluids (Sura et al., 2012).
- Head posture
  - With food > head extension/chin up > raise chin > better bolus transport

R: *This position propels bolus to back of mouth and widens oropharynx to reduce aspiration.*

  - With liquids > head flexion/chin tuck > tucking chin toward the chest

R: *This position improves airway protection and reduces aspiration with liquids.*

  - Head rotation/head turn > turning head toward the weaker side

R: *Reduces residue after swallow and reduces aspiration with one side facial weakness.*

- Modify the consistency of solid food and/or liquid for individuals with dysphagia. All individuals with dysphagia should be assessed by the dietitian for nutritional support (Sura et al., 2012).

R: *Specialists recommend thickened liquids > for individuals with dysphagia (Sura et al., 2012). However, the overuse of thickened liquids increases the risk of dehydration in elderly individuals with dysphagia (Ibid) (Sura et al., 2012). To standardize modified diets, the National Dysphagia Diet was proposed (Clayton, 2002). The National Dysphagia Diet is comprised of four levels of food modification with specific food items recommended at each level (Ibid).*

Reduce or Eliminate Causative/Contributing Factors in People With

Mechanical Impairment of Mouth

- Assist with moving the bolus of food from the anterior to the posterior part of mouth. Place food in the posterior mouth, where swallowing can be ensured, using soft, moist food of a consistency that can be manipulated by the tongue against the pharynx, such as gelatin, custard, or mashed potatoes.
- Prevent/decrease thick secretions with
  - Frequent mouth care
  - Increased fluid intake—eight glasses of liquid (unless contraindicated)
- Check medications for potential side effects of dry mouth/decreased salivation.

Muscle Paralysis or Paresis

- Plan meals when individual is well rested; ensure that reliable suction equipment is on hand during meals. Discontinue feeding if individual is tired.
- If indicated, use modified supraglottic swallow technique per institution protocol.
- Note the consistency of food that is problematic. Select consistencies that are easier to swallow, such as
  - Viscous foods (e.g., mashed bananas, potatoes, gelatin, gravy)
  - Thick liquids (e.g., milkshakes, slushes, nectars, cream soups)

R: *Some individuals have difficulty with solids, whereas others have difficulty swallowing liquids (Hickey, 2014).*

- If a bolus of food is pocketed in the affected side, teach individual how to use tongue to transfer food or apply external digital pressure to cheek to help remove the trapped bolus (*Emick-Herring & Wood, 1990).

R: *Poor tongue control with impaired oral sensation allows pocketing of food in affected side.*

Impaired Cognition or Awareness

General

- Remove feeding tube during training if increased gag reflex is present.
- Concentrate on solids rather than liquids because liquids usually are less well tolerated.
- Minimize extraneous stimuli while eating (e.g., no television or radio, no verbal stimuli unless directed at task).
- Have individual concentrate on task of swallowing.
- Have individual sit up in chair with neck slightly flexed.
- Instruct to hold breath while swallowing.
- Observe for swallowing and check mouth for emptying.
- Avoid overloading mouth because this decreases swallowing effectiveness.
- Give solids and liquids separately.
- Progress slowly. Limit conversation.
- Provide several small meals to accommodate a short attention span.

Individual With Aphasia or Left Hemispheric Damage

- Demonstrate expected behavior.
- Reinforce behaviors with simple, one-word commands.

Individual With Apraxia or Right Hemispheric Damage

- Divide task into smallest units possible.
- Assist through each task with verbal commands.
- Allow to complete one unit fully before giving next command.
- Continue verbal assistance at each eating session until no longer needed.
- Incorporate written checklist as a reminder to individual.
- *Note:* Individual may have both left- and right-hemispheric damage and require a combination of the above techniques.

R: *A confused individual needs repetitive, simple instructions.*

Reduce the Possibility of Aspiration

- Before beginning any oral intake, assess that the individual is adequately alert and responsive, can control the mouth, has cough/gag reflex, and can swallow saliva.

R: *Impaired reflexes and fatigue increase the risk of aspiration. A bedside swallowing assessment should be done prior to feeding to prevent aspiration.*

- Have suction equipment available and functioning properly.
- Position individual correctly:
  - Sit individual upright (60° to 90°) in chair or dangle his or her feet at side of bed if possible (prop with pillows if necessary).
  - Have individual assume this position 10 to 15 minutes before eating and maintain it for 10 to 15 minutes after finishing eating.
  - Flex his or her head forward on the midline about 45° to keep esophagus patent.

R: *Upright position uses the force of gravity to aid downward motion of food and decreases the risk of aspiration.*

- Keep individual focused on task by giving directions until he or she has finished swallowing each mouthful.
  - "Take a breath."
  - "Move food to middle of tongue."
  - "Raise tongue to roof of mouth."
  - "Think about swallowing."
  - "Swallow."
  - "Cough to clear airway."
- Reinforce voluntary action.

R: *A confused individual needs repetitive, simple instructions.*

- Avoid straws and thin fluids

R: *Straws and thin fluids hasten transit time and increase the risk of aspiration.*

- Start with small amounts and progress slowly as individual learns to handle each step:
  - Ice chips
  - Eyedropper partly filled with water
  - Whole eyedropper filled with water
  - Juice in place of water
  - ¼ teaspoon semisolid food
  - ½ teaspoon semisolid food
  - 1 teaspoon semisolid food
  - vPureed or commercial baby foods
  - One half cracker
  - Soft diet
  - Regular diet; chew food well

R: *Small amounts of fluid with progressive increases can reduce aspiration. Thicker fluids have a slower transit time and allow more time to trigger the swallow reflex.*

- For an individual who has had a CVA, place food at back of tongue and on side of face he or she can control:
  - Feed slowly, making certain individual has swallowed the previous bite.
  - Some individuals do better with foods that hold together (e.g., soft-boiled eggs, ground meat, and gravy).
- If the above strategies are unsuccessful, consultation with nutrition specialist.

R: *Avoid foods that do not form a bolus (e.g., sticky foods, pureed foods, applesauce, dry foods) or do not stimulate the swallowing reflex (e.g., thin liquids).*

Initiate Health Teaching and Referrals, as Indicated

- Advise to continue exercise-based swallow rehabilitation approaches at home.
- Schedule appointments with specialists as indicated.

Ineffective Infant Feeding Pattern

NANDA-I Definition

Impaired ability of an infant to suck or coordinate the suck/swallow response, resulting in inadequate oral nutrition for metabolic needs

Defining Characteristics

Inability to initiate or sustain an effective suck*
Inability to coordinate sucking, swallowing, and breathing*
Regurgitation or vomiting after feeding

Related Factors

Pathophysiologic

Related to increased caloric need secondary to:

Body temperature instability
Tachypnea with increased respiratory effort
Infection
Möbius syndrome
Growth needs
Wound healing
Major organ system disease or failure
Cleft lip/palate

Related to muscle weakness/hypotonia secondary to:

Malnutrition
Congenital defects
Prematurity*
Major organ system disease or failure
Hyperbilirubinemia
Acute/chronic illness
Neurologic impairment/delay*
Lethargy

Treatment Related

Related to hypermetabolic state and increased caloric needs secondary to:

Surgery
Painful procedures
Cold stress
Sepsis
Fever

Related to muscle weakness and lethargy secondary to:

Medications
Muscle relaxants (antiseizure medications, past use of paralyzing agents, sedatives, narcotics)
Sleep deprivation

Related to oral hypersensitivity*

Related to previous prolonged NPO state

Situational (Personal, Environmental)

Related to inconsistent caretakers (feeders)

Related to lack of knowledge or commitment of caretaker (feeder) to special feeding needs or regimen

Related to presence of noxious facial stimuli or absence of oral stimuli

Related to inadequate production of breast milk

Author's Note

Ineffective Infant Feeding Pattern describes an infant with sucking or swallowing difficulties. This infant experiences inadequate oral nutrition for growth and development, which is exacerbated when caloric need increases, as with infection, illness, or stress. Nursing interventions assist infants and their caregivers with techniques to achieve nutritional intake needed for weight gain. In addition, the goal is for the intake eventually to be exclusively oral.

Infants with sucking or swallowing problems who have not lost weight need nursing interventions to prevent weight loss. *Ineffective Infant Feeding Pattern* is clinically useful for this situation.

Errors in Diagnostic Statements

***Risk for Ineffective Infant Feeding Pattern* related to inconsistent oral intake with or without weight loss**

Inconsistent oral intake is a defining characteristic for *Ineffective Infant Feeding Pattern*, not *Risk for Ineffective Infant Feeding Pattern. Ineffective Infant Feeding Pattern* may not be useful as a risk nursing diagnosis, because this actual diagnosis exists whenever an infant has sucking or suck/swallow response difficulties, whether mild or severe. The diagnosis would be appropriate as *Ineffective Infant Feeding Pattern* related to (specify contributing factors, e.g., lethargy) as evidenced by inconsistent oral intake.

Key Concepts

Carp's Cues

For interventions associated with breastfeeding, refer to *Ineffective Breastfeeding* or *Risk for Ineffective Breastfeeding.*

- Usually, infants double their birthweight by 4 to 6 months and triple it by 1 year. On average, infants gain 5 to 7 oz/week in the first 4 to 6 months and 3 to 5 oz/week from 6 to 18 months. Infants usually can increase their length by 50% in the first year, but the rate of increase slows down during the second half of the year. From birth to 6 months, infants gain approximately 1 inch a month, and from 6 to 12 months of age, they gain about ½ inch each month (Hockenberry & Wilson, 2015; Pillitteri, 2014).
- For an infant with an ineffective feeding pattern (with or without a demonstrable oral motor impairment), conversion from a catabolic state to an anabolic state with consistent weight gain from appropriate calories is a prerequisite for goal attainment (Pillitteri, 2014).

- Identification of contributing physiologic factors assists in evaluating and adapting the feeding plan. For example, fever increases caloric needs; mechanical ventilation can decrease caloric needs; infants with impaired renal function or fluid retention can experience weight gain without meeting nutritional metabolic needs; and dysfunction in major organ systems or infection affects feeding patterns adversely and increases caloric needs.
- Some infants with oral motor impairment or weakness feed adequately by mouth when their metabolic need for calories is normal. But in cases of increased caloric need (e.g., congestive heart failure, infection, major organ system dysfunction, wound healing, malnutrition), they cannot take in adequate calories by increasing their volume intake sufficiently because of their ineffective feeding skills. Intervention with these infants is based on providing adequate calories, promoting oral feeding skills, and decreasing (if possible) caloric needs.
- Knowledge of normal infant feeding patterns is necessary to promote effective feeding patterns. For example, a quiet, awake state is ideal for feeding; nonnutritive sucking preceding nutritive sucking can enhance feeding behaviors; and there is a relation between sucking–swallowing–gastric emptying–bowel emptying during feeding. Over time, each infant develops an effective unique feeding pattern.
- High-calorie formulas (up to 32 cal/oz) or calorie-enhanced breast milk can be administered safely to most infants, provided the preparation is consistent with the child's age and needs. For example, concentrating formula to increase calories can increase the protein load disproportionately; therefore, additives (carbohydrate or fat) are often used to increase calories safely. The appropriate use of high-calorie formulas can reduce the target volume per day goal for an infant, making it easier to attain the goal of total oral feedings. Serum protein, albumin, and renal function need to be assessed periodically when high-calorie formulas are used.
- Adapt equipment and feedings for alterations in oral intake, for example, use of a Haberman or comparable nipple for infants with cleft lip/palate or Möbius syndrome; rice cereal for feeding infants with gastroesophageal reflux; and use of cheek/chin support for orally compromised infants.
- Enteral feedings may be required initially to ensure adequate caloric intake, weight gain, and anabolic state. Identifying a total plan for feeding from the beginning that includes both enteral and oral feeding (and oral stimulation if feeding is not possible) is instrumental in promoting the goal of total oral feeding. Infants who are exclusively enterally fed in the first months of life, with no effort to develop oral feeding skills, can become behaviorally disinterested in oral feeding and may remain enterally fed indefinitely.

Focus Assessment Criteria

Subjective and Objective Data

Assess for Defining Characteristics

General

Current weight and height
Weight gain daily/weekly goal
Calories per kilogram daily goal

Feeding History

Previous oral feeding pattern (volume, time interval, duration)
Previous enteral feeding pattern (continuous or bolus, volume, time interval, duration)
GI tolerance of feedings (oral, enteral, emesis, stool pattern)

Assess for Related Factors

Presence/absence of noxious stimuli to face and mouth (including nasogastric/nasojejunal feedings, endotracheal intubation, oral or nasopharyngeal suction, nasal cannula oxygen)

Physiologic Factors

Hyperthermia or hypothermia
Infection
Congestive heart failure
Prematurity
Neurologic dysfunction
Increased respiratory rate and effort
Strength and coordination of nutritive sucking
Irritability
Oral motor developmental delay
Gastroesophageal reflux
Colic
Prolonged NPO state with or without enteral feedings
Elevated body temperature
Strength and coordination of nonnutritive sucking
Impaired sleep patterns
Lethargy

Situational (Personal, Environmental)

Related to inexperienced caregivers

Goals

NOC

Muscle Function, Nutritional Status, Swallowing Status

The infant will receive

- Adequate and appropriate calories (carbohydrate, protein, fat) for age with weight gain at a rate consistent with an individualized plan based on age and needs. Infant caloric intake of 100 to 120 kcal/kg/day for growth
- All feedings orally

The parent will

- Demonstrate increasing skill in infant feeding
- Identify techniques that increase effective feeding

Interventions

NIC

Nonnutritive Swallowing, Swallowing Therapy, Aspiration, Precautions, Bottle Feeding, Parent Education: Infant

Assess the Infant's Feeding Pattern and Nutritional Needs

- Assess volume, duration, and effort during feeding; respiratory rate and effort; and signs of fatigue.
- Assess past caloric intake, weight gain, trends in intake and output, renal function, and fluid retention.
- Identify physiologic ability to feed (Pillitteri, 2014).
  - Can infant stop breathing when sucking and swallowing?
  - Does infant gasp or choke during feedings?
  - What happens to oxygen level, heart rate, and respiratory rate when sucking/swallowing?
  - Does the infant need rest periods? How long? Are there problems in initiating sucking/swallowing again?
- Assess nipple-feeding skills (Pillitteri, 2014).
  - Does the infant actively suck with a bottle?
  - Does the infant initiate a swallow in coordination with suck?
  - Does the infant coordinate sucking, swallowing, and breathing?
  - Is the feeding completed in a reasonable time?

R: *Identification of ineffective feeding patterns should be based on systematic assessment of the infant in collaboration with other professionals. Behaviors that are cues to feeding dysfunction include ineffective coordination of suck/swallow/breathing, low energy or stamina, poor ability or inability to initiate sucking, disorganized rhythm in suck/swallow pattern, inadequate neurobehavioral control, and difficulty shifting back and forth from nonnutritive sucking and nutritive sucking (Pillitteri, 2014).*

- Collaborate with clinical dietitian to set calorie, volume, and weight gain goals.

R: *Close collaboration with a clinical dietitian to assess, plan, set, and evaluate calorie goals, weight gain goals, calorie distribution, and formula preparation is necessary for infants at risk.*

- Collaborate with occupational therapist/speech therapist to identify oral motor skills and planned intervention, if needed.

R: *Close collaboration with a professional skilled in the assessment of infant oral motor skills (e.g., occupational therapist, speech therapist) is necessary to assess, plan, intervene, and evaluate progress toward appropriate oral motor skills in infants with oral motor impairment.*

- Collaborate with parent(s) about effective techniques used with this infant or other children, temperament, and responses to environmental stimuli.

R: *Close collaboration with parents from the beginning about identified needs, negotiation of priorities, and development of interventions is crucial to establishing effective feeding patterns in the infant and strengthening the infant–parent relationship.*

Provide Specific Interventions to Promote Effective Oral Feeding (Hockenberry & Wilson, 2015)

- Ensure a quiet, calm, and dim environment.
- Eliminate painful procedures prior to feeding.

R: *Calm, quiet, dim environments offer less distraction; attempt to decrease the negative effects of painful or very stimulating experiences shortly before or after feedings by timing them.*

- Ensure uninterrupted sleep periods.

R: *Efforts to promote sleep and reduce energy expenditure (primarily by controlling environmental stimuli) can substantially improve the infant's strength and stamina during feeding (Pillitteri, 2014).*

- Encourage nonnutritive sucking not in response to noxious stimuli.
- Ensure nutritive sucking for an identified period.
- Control adverse environmental stimuli and noxious stimuli to face and mouth.

R: *Nonnutritive sucking (pacifier) should not be used exclusively to comfort infants during or after painful procedures or exposure to noxious stimuli. In addition, care and attention to reducing noxious stimuli to the face and mouth (type, frequency, intensity) should be initiated long before attempts to feed orally begin (Pillitteri, 2014).*

- Promote consistency in approach to feeding.
  - Be sensitive to their infants' hunger, satiety, and food preferences, and act promptly and appropriately to meet their feeding needs.
  - It is best to avoid putting the infant on a rigid feeding schedule.
  - An older infant can be offered food at around the time when he or she usually eats, but for infants the caregiver should watch for signs of hunger.

R: *Environmental factors, including light, noise, inconsistent caretakers (feeders), and noxious stimuli, contribute significantly to ineffective feeding patterns. A dysfunctional feeding relationship can result in poor dietary intake and impaired growth.*

- The following actions hinder feeding:
  - Twisting or turning the nipple
  - Moving the nipple up, down, around in the mouth
  - Putting the nipple in and out of the mouth
  - Putting pressure on the jaw or moving the infant's jaw up and down
  - Placing the infant in a head-back position
  - Caregiver anxiousness and impatience

R: *For infants with demonstrable oral motor impairment, early intervention with an identified consistent approach to promoting oral feeding (equipment, body position, jaw and mouth manipulation, volume, time interval, duration) is essential for goal attainment.*

- Refer to *Risk for Aspiration* for interventions for feeding an infant with cleft lip and/or palate.

Establish Partnership With Parent(s) in All Stages of Plan

- Create a supportive environment for the parents to have the primary role in providing feeding-related intervention, when they are present. Whenever possible, nurses use the parents' approach when a parent is not present. In addition, when parents are not present, nurses can support the parents' role by imitating their approach to the infant, and communicate the infant's responses to the parents at a later time.

R: *An infant who receives adequate calories will be more able physically to eat orally; if parents support and value the way calories are delivered and recognize milestones toward the goal, the child will be more likely to receive adequate calories after discharge. In addition, interactions will be more rewarding for both infant and parent during the intervention period (Pilliteri, 2014).*

- Negotiate and identify plans for discharge with parents and incorporate into the overall feeding plan; provide ongoing information about special needs, and assist parents to establish needed resources (equipment, nursing care, and other caretakers) when needed.

R: *Establishing parents as essential participants in the feeding plan gives them a role, place, and reason to be present, so they can develop a closer relationship with the child (Hockenberry & Wilson, 2015).*

OBESITY

Obesity

Overweight
Risk for Overweight

NANDA-I Definition

A condition in which an individual accumulates abnormal or excessive fat for age and gender that exceeds overweight

Defining Characteristics

Adult: BMI of >30
Child <2 years: Term not applicable /not used with infants/children at this age
Child 2 to 18 years: BMI of >30 or >95th percentile for age and gender

Related Factors

Average daily physical activity is less than recommended for gender and age
Consumption of sugar-sweetened beverages
Disordered eating behaviors
Disordered eating perceptions
Economically disadvantaged
Energy expenditure below energy intake based on standard assessment (e.g., WAVE assessment[28])
Excessive alcohol consumption
Fear regarding lack of food supply
Formula- or mixed-fed infants
Frequent snacking
Genetic disorder
Heritability of interrelated factors (e.g., adipose tissue distribution, energy expenditure, lipoprotein lipase activity, lipid synthesis, lipolysis)
High disinhibition and restraint eating behavior score
High frequency of restaurant or fried food
Low dietary calcium intake in children
Maternal diabetes mellitus
Maternal smoking
Overweight in infancy
Parental obesity
Portion sizes larger than recommended
Premature pubarche
Rapid weight gain during childhood
Rapid weight gain during infancy, including the first week, first 4 months, and first year
Sedentary behavior occurring for >2 hr/day
Shortened sleep time
Sleep disorder
Solid foods as major food source at <5 months of age

Author's Note

Given the public health problem of overweight and obesity across the lifespan, the preceding three diagnoses are excellent additions to NANDA-I Classification.

The interventions for these diagnoses will focus on strategies to motivate and engage individuals/families to proceed to a healthy life style.[29]

---

[28]WAVE assessment = weight, activity, variety in diet, excess.
[29]Imbalanced and Risk for Imbalance Nutrition: More than Body Requirement has been deleted from the NANDA-I Classification

Obesity is a complex condition with sociocultural, psychological, and metabolic implications. When the focus is primarily on limiting food intake, as with many weight-loss programs, bariatric surgery, the chance of permanent weight loss is slim. To be successful, in a weight-loss program an individual needs to focus on behavior modification and lifestyle changes, through exercise, decreased intake, and addressing their emotional component of overeating.

If someone is at a healthy weight, but routinely eats foods low in nutrients.

Risk-Prone Health Behavior related to intake of insufficient nutrients and/or inactivity in the presence of a healthy weight that does not meet recommended dietary intake. For some people with dysfunctional eating, *Ineffective Coping* related to increase in eating in response to stressors would be valid and require a referral after discharge.

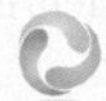

Errors in Diagnostic Statements

Obesity related to depression

This diagnostic statement is incomplete and thus would not direct nursing interventions. With a focused assessment, the nurse can determine activity level, patterns of eating, and types of food/fluids which can be improved. In addition, coping responses and depression need attention.

Key Concepts

- Ogden, Carroll, Kit, and Flegal (2014) reported the following:
  - In 2011 to 2012, 8.1% of infants and toddlers had high weight for recumbent length.
  - More than 23 million 2- to 19-year-olds are overweight or obese.
  - Around 34.9% of adults (age-adjusted) aged 20 or older were obese.
  - No significant change from 2003 to 2004 through 2011 to 2012, obesity in 2- to 19-year-olds, or obesity in adults.
  - A significant decrease in obesity among 2- to 5-year-old children (from 13.9% to 8.4%).
  - A significant increase in obesity among women aged 60 and older (from 31.5% to 38.1%).
- The Incidence of diet-related chronic diseases (U.S. Department of Agriculture & U.S. Department of Health and Human Services, 2010).
  - Cardiovascular disease: 81.1 million Americans—37% of the population—have cardiovascular disease. Major risk factors include high levels of blood cholesterol and other lipids, type 2 diabetes, hypertension (high blood pressure), metabolic syndrome, overweight and obesity, physical inactivity, and tobacco use. About 16% of the US adult population has high total blood cholesterol.
  - Hypertension: 74.5 million Americans—34% of US adults—have hypertension.
  - Hypertension is a major risk factor for heart disease, stroke, congestive heart failure, and kidney disease.
  - Dietary factors that increase blood pressure include excessive sodium and insufficient potassium intake, overweight and obesity, and excess alcohol consumption.
  - 36% of American adults have prehypertension—blood pressure numbers that are higher than normal, but not yet in the hypertension range.
  - Diabetes: Nearly 24 million people—almost 11% of the population—aged 20 years and older have diabetes. The vast majority of cases are type 2 diabetes, which is heavily influenced by diet and physical activity.
  - About 78 million Americans—35% of the US adult population aged 20 years or older—have prediabetes. Prediabetes (also called impaired glucose tolerance or impaired fasting glucose) means that blood glucose levels are higher than normal, but not high enough to be called diabetes.
  - Cancer: Almost one in two men and women—approximately 41% of the population—will be diagnosed with cancer during their lifetime.
  - Dietary factors are associated with risk of some types of cancer, including breast (postmenopausal), endometrial, colon, kidney, mouth, pharynx, larynx, and esophagus.
  - Osteoporosis: One out of every two women and one in four men aged 50 years and older will have an osteoporosis-related fracture in their lifetime.
  - About 85% to 90% of adult bone mass is acquired by the age of 18 in girls and the age of 20 in boys. Adequate nutrition and regular participation in physical activity are important factors in achieving and maintaining optimal bone mass.
- Overeating is a complex problem with physical, social, and psychological components.
- Eighty percent of children of two obese parents will become obese, as opposed to 40% with one obese parent and 7% with no obese parent (*Buiten & Metzger, 2000).

- Body mass index (BMI) is a ratio of weight and height that estimates total body fat. According to 2007 to 2008 National Health and Nutrition Examination Survey (NHANES), 34.2% of Americans 20 years and older are overweight (BMI 25 to 29.9), 55.8% are obese (BMI >30), and 5.7% are extremely obese (BMI >40) (Ogden et al., 2014).
- An excess of 50 to 100 calories each day will cause a 5- to 10-lb gain in 1 year (Dudek, 2014).
- Fluctuations in body weight are common, especially in women. Daily weights can be misleading and disheartening. Body measurements are a better gauge of losses.
- Regular exercise causes lean muscle mass to increase. Because muscle weighs more than fat, the scale may reflect a weight gain.
- Restrictive diets usually do not last and fail to establish healthy eating patterns. A better approach is modifying existing eating habits (*Wiereng & Oldham, 2002).
- WAVE (Weight, Activity, Variety, and Excess) (*Barner, Wylie-Rosett, & Gans, 2001; Gans et al., 2003): Wave is an abbreviated model for addressing nutrition in an individual and achieving healthy weight. With assessment questions and targeted interventions, it was designed to be utilized in health-care settings as a brief intervention to activate an individual to evaluate their nutritional intake and activity level. It also can be useful with the family member responsible for food shopping and preparation, to evaluate food groups served, frequency, and serving sizes eaten. Refer to MyPlate under *Imbalanced Nutrition*. Refer to Tables II.16 and II.17, WAVE Assessment and Recommendations.

Pediatric Considerations

- Results from the 2011 to 2012 National Health and Nutrition Examination Survey (NHANES), using measured heights and weights, indicate that an estimated 16.9% of US children and adolescents aged 2 to 19 are obese and another 14.9% are overweight (Ogden et al., 2014).
- Nonadolescent children should not be put on diets. The goal for growing children is to maintain, not lose, weight. Healthy food choices of fruit, vegetables, and low-fat snacks (e.g., pretzels) can replace foods high in salt, fats, and sugar.
- As BMI increases, so does the prevalence of iron deficiency in overweight children and adolescents (*Nead, Halterman, Kaczorowski, Auinger, & Weitzman, 2004).
- Obesity and overweight rates in children have steadily increased from 1988–2004 to 2007–2008 as follows (National Center for Health Statistics, 2010):
  - From 11.6% to 16.7% among non-Hispanic white boys
  - From 10.7% to 19.8% among non-Hispanic black boys
  - From 14.1% to 26.8% among Mexican-American boys
  - From 8.9% to 14.5% among non-Hispanic white girls
  - From 16.3% to 29.2% among non-Hispanic black girls
  - From 13.4% to 17.4% among Mexican-American girls
- Good weight management for children and adolescents focuses on weight maintenance or a slow weight loss, nutrient and energy needs, hunger prevention, preservation of lean body mass, and increased physical activity and growth.
- In a study of children who were clearly obese (>90th percentile for weight and height), Myers and Vargas (*2000) found that 35% of Hispanic parents did not perceive their child as obese.

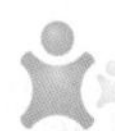

Maternal Considerations

- There has been increasing evidence that maternal obesity is associated with an increased risk of congenital malformations, particularly neural tube defects.
- Recommendations for total weight gain during pregnancy vary (Institute of Medicine, 2009).
  - 25 to 35 lb if you were a healthy weight before pregnancy, with a BMI of 18.5 to 24.9.
  - 28 to 40 lb if you were underweight before pregnancy with a BMI of less than 18.5.
  - 15 to 25 lb if you were overweight before pregnancy with a BMI of 25 to 29.9.
  - 11 to 20 lb if you were obese before pregnancy with a BMI of over 30.
- "American women are now a more diverse group; they are having more twin and triplet pregnancies, and they tend to be older when they become pregnant. Women today are also heavier; a greater percentage of them are entering pregnancy overweight or obese, and many are gaining too much weight during pregnancy. Many of these changes carry the added burden of chronic disease, which can put the mother and her baby's health at risk" (Institute of Medicine, 2009).

Table 11.16 WAVE ASSESSMENT

Weight

Assess patient's BMI.*
Patient is overweight if BMI >25.

Height	Body Weight (lb)	Height	Body Weight (lb)
4′10″	>119	5′8″	>164
4′11″	>124	5′9″	>169
5′0″	>128	5′10″	>174
5′1″	>132	5′11″	>179
5′2″	>136	6′0″	>184
5′3″	>141	6′1″	>189
5′4″	>145	6′2″	>194
5′5″	>150	6′3″	>200
5′6″	>155	6′4″	>205
5′7″	>159		

*Certain patients may require assessment for underweight and/or unintentional weight loss

Activity

Ask patient about any physical activity in the past week: walking briskly, jogging, gardening, swimming, biking, dancing, golf, etc.

1. Does patient do 30 minutes of moderate activity on most days/week?
2. Does patient do "lifestyle" activity like taking the stairs instead of elevators, etc.?
3. Does patient usually watch less than 2 hours of TV or videos/day?

If patient answers *NO* to above questions, assess whether patient is willing to increase physical activity.

Variety

Is patient eating a variety of foods from important sections of the food pyramid?
Grains (6–11 servings)
Fruits (2–4 servings)
Vegetables (3–5 servings)
Protein (2–3 servings)
Dairy (2–3 servings)

Determine Variety and Excess using one of the following methods:

- Do a quick one-day recall.
- Ask patient to complete a self-administered eating pattern questionnaire.

Excess

Is patient eating too much of certain foods and nutrients?

Too much fat, saturated fat, calories

- >6 oz/day of meat
- Ice cream, high-fat milk, cheese, etc.
- Fried foods or foods cooked with fat
- High-fat snacks and desserts
- Eating out >4 meals/week

Too much sugar, calories

- High-sugar beverages
- Sugary snacks/desserts

Too much salt

- Processed meats, canned/frozen meals, salty snacks, added salt

What does patient think are pros/cons of his/her eating pattern?
If patient needs to improve eating habits, assess willingness to make changes.

Source: Brown University School of Medicine Nutrition Academic Award. Used with permission.

Table 11.17 WAVE RECOMMENDATIONS

Weight

If patient is overweight:

1. State concern for the patient (e.g., "I am concerned that your weight is affecting your health.").
2. Give the patient specific advice, that is,
   a) Make one or two changes in eating habits to reduce calorie intake as identified by diet assessment.
   b) Gradually increase activity/decrease inactivity.
   c) Enroll in a weight-management program and/or consult a dietitian.
3. If patient is ready to make behavior changes, jointly set goals for a plan of action and arrange for follow-up.
4. Give patient education materials/resources.

Activity

Examples of moderate amounts of physical activity:

- Walking 2 miles in 30 minutes
- Stair walking for 15 minutes
- Washing and waxing a car for 45–60 minutes
- Washing windows or floors for 45–60 minutes
- Gardening for 30–45 minutes
- Pushing a stroller 1½ miles in 30 minutes
- Raking leaves for 30 minutes
- Shoveling snow for 15 minutes

1. If patient is ready to increase physical activity, jointly set specific activity goals and arrange for a follow-up.
2. Give patient education materials/resources.

Variety

What is a serving?

Grains (6–11 servings)

1 slice bread or tortilla, ½ bagel, ½ roll

1 oz ready-to-eat cereal, ½ cup rice, pasta, or cooked cereal, 3–4 plain crackers

Is patient eating whole grains?

Fruits (2–4 servings)

1 medium fresh fruit, ½ cup chopped or canned fruit, ¾ cup fruit juice

Vegetables (3–5 servings)

1 cup raw leafy vegetables, ½ cup cooked or chopped raw vegetables, ¾ cup vegetable juice

Protein (2–3 servings)

2–3 oz poultry, fish, or lean meat, 1–1 ½ cup cooked dry beans, 1 egg equals 1 oz meat, 4 oz or ½ cup tofu

Dairy (2–3 servings)

1 cup milk or yogurt, 1½ oz cheese

See instructions 1–4 under Excess.

Excess

1. Discuss pros and cons of patient's eating pattern keeping in mind Variety and Excess.
2. If patient is ready, jointly set specific dietary goals and arrange for follow-up.
3. Give patient education materials/resources.
4. Consider referral to a dietitian for more extensive counseling and support.

Suggestions for decreasing excess:

- Eat chicken and fish (not fried) or meatless meals instead of red meat.
- Choose leaner cuts of red meat.
- Choose skim or 1% milk.
- Eat less cheese/choose lower fat cheeses.
- Bake, broil, or grill foods rather than fry.
- Choose low-fat salad dressings, mayo, spreads, etc.
- Eat more whole grains, fruits, and vegetables.
- Drink water instead of sugary drinks.
- Use herbs instead of salt.

Source: Brown University School of Medicine Nutrition Academic Award. Used with permission.

- The emphasis on nutrition and weight gain during pregnancy does not include dieting but instead healthy choices and portions.

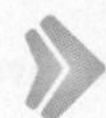

Carp's Cues

Individuals who are very ill are probably not ready for discussions about lifestyle changes.

Provide them with sources of help. Go to ThePoint, and print Getting Started (e.g., smoking, to lose weight), move more and provide it to the individual.

Goals

NOC

Nutritional Status: Nutrient Intake, Weight Control, Exercise Participation, Infant Nutritional Status, Weight Body Mass, Adherence Behavior: Healthy Diet, Weight Loss Behavior

The individual will commit to a weight-loss program, as evidenced by the following indicators:

- Identifies the patterns of eating associated with consumption/energy expenditure imbalance
- Can give examples of nutrient dense foods versus those with "empty calories"
- Can identify three ways to increase his or her activity
- Commits to increasing foods with high nutrient density and less with "empty calories"
- Commits to making 3 to 5 changes in food/fluid choices, which are healthier

The child (over 8) will verbalize what is healthy eating by the following indicators:

- Can describe the "MyPlate"
- Can describe what "empty calories" mean
- Can name "empty calories" beverages and healthier substitutions
- Can name foods high in nutrients
- Can name food high in sugar and "empty calories" and healthier substitutions

The pregnant woman will verbalize healthy eating and recommended weight gain during pregnancy by the following indicators:

- Can describe vitamin, mineral, protein, fat needs during pregnancy
- Can give examples of nutrient dense foods versus those with "empty calories"
- Can identify three ways to increase his or her activity
- Will relate the weight gain appropriate specific to her weight prior to pregnancy
- Can explain why "dieting " is problematic

Interventions

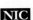

Clinical Alert Individuals can be malnourished even though they are obese or overweight due to intake of foods high in fat and carbohydrates, which are low in nutrients per calorie intake. Individual of a healthy weight may also be undernourished by eating foods high in fat and carbohydrates, which are low in nutrients per calorie intake.

NIC

Self-Efficacy Enhancement, Self-Responsibility Enhancement, Nutritional Counseling, Weight Management, Teaching: Nutrition (age appropriate), Behavioral Modification, Exercise Promotion, Coping Enhancement

- Refer to Appendix D: Strategies to Promote Engagement of Individual/Families for Healthier Outcomes for specific techniques to improve activation and engagement.

Initiate Discussion: "How Can You Be Healthier?"

- Focus on the person's response (e.g., stop smoking, exercise more, eat healthier, and cut down on drinking).
- Refer to index for interventions for the targeted lifestyle change.

R: *The nurse should be cautioned against applying a nursing diagnosis for an overweight or obese person who does not want to participate in a weight-loss program. Motivation for weight loss must come from within.*

Before a Person Can Change, They Must (Martin, Haskard Zolnierek & DiMatteo, 2010)

- Know what change is necessary (information) and why
- Desire the change (motivation)
- Have the tools to achieve and maintain the change (strategy)
- Trust the health-care professional, who has a sympathetic presence (Pelzang, 2010)

R: *Empathic communication involving a thorough understanding of the patient's perspective, improves adherence. Patients who are informed and effectively motivated are also more likely to adhere to their treatment recommendations (*Martin Williams, Haskard, & DiMatteo, 2005).*

If Appropriate, Gently and Expertly Discuss the Hazards of Obesity, but Respect a Person's Right to Choose, the Right of Self-Determination

- "How do you think being overweight affects you?"
- Focus on what the person tells you (e.g., "my sugar is high, my knees hurt"). Do not overload him or her.

If the Person Does Not Identify any Negative Effects of Excess Weight That They Feel, Explain the Effects of Excess Weight are Insidious and Often Not Felt by the Person Until the Effects Threaten Their Health or Cause Pain

To Help to Activate Engagement in an Individual, Ask Them One of the Following Questions. Pick the Best Question That Applies to This Person. Use Language They Understand (e.g., Blood Veins, or Tubes That Carry Blood)

- Do your legs swell during the day and go back to normal during the night?
  - Explain that fat tissue compresses tubes in your legs and prevent fluids from circulating well. Eventually, the swelling will be permanent, 24 hours a day, causing difficulty walking and wearing shoes.
- Do you have high blood pressure or is it getting a little higher each year?
  - Explain that blood vessels are damaged when excess weight puts pressure on them and they stretch, become thinner, and lose their strength. Your heart now has to pump harder, causing high blood pressure. Over time the heart enlarges and cannot pump well. This is heart failure.
- Is your cholesterol levels increasing each year?
  - Explain that the stretching of your blood vessels damages the inside of the blood tubes; cholesterol sticks to the damaged tubes and slows the blood flow to your kidneys, eyes, brain, and legs. This can cause strokes, renal failure, vision problems, and blood clots in your legs.
- You may not feel that anything is wrong, but high blood pressure can permanently damage your heart, brain, eyes, and kidneys before you feel anything. Even losing 10 lb can reduce your blood pressure.
  - Is your blood glucose test getting a little higher each year? Is there diabetes in your family?
  - Explain that the more fatty tissue you have, the more resistant your cells become to insulin.
  - Insulin carries sugar from blood to the cells. When you are overweight, the cells are damaged and will not absorb the insulin. So your blood sugar goes up. High blood sugars damage blood vessels in the eyes, kidneys, and heart.
- Does your back, your knees, or other joints hurt?
  - Explain that extra weight puts pressure on your joints and bones. This pressure wears away the cartilage, the cushion at the ends of your bones. This causes the bone to rub against another bone causing pain.
- Do you think people who are overweight have problem healing from injuries or surgery?
  - Explain that fat tissue has less blood supply, which is needed for healing. The incision has more pressure against, when you are overweight, which can cause the wound to open up. If antibiotics are needed for infection, the medicine does not work well because of poor circulation to the wound.

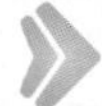

Carp's Cues

It would be wise to mention that individuals, who are thin or of normal weight can have hypertension, arthritis, high cholesterol, and diabetes but not at the high rate as those who are overweight.

Review Usual Daily Intake to Identify Patterns That Contribute to Excess Weight

- Usual breakfast, usual lunch, usual dinner
- Snacks, nighttime eating
- Skipping meals

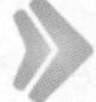

Carp's Cues

"Before you eat or drink something with "empty calories,[30]" ask yourself, "Is this worth it?" If it is, *enjoy* it. There is no such thing as "bad foods" only bad amounts.

Promote Activation to Engage the Individual in Healthier Behavior. Focus on What the Person Wants to Change. Limit to Three Changes

[30]"Empty calories" are foods/drinks that are high in calories but have little or no nutritional value, such as soda, chips, French fries.

R: *"Activation refers to a person's ability and willingness to take on the role of managing their health and health care" (Hibbard & Cunningham, 2008).*

Address What Excesses or Deficiencies Exist, Using the Information He or She Gave, For Example

- I ate fried chicken wings last night for dinner.
- Anything else? No.
- How could you change what you ate to improve nutrients and decrease fat?
- Listen. If no response, suggest
  - One or two piece(s) of fried chicken instead of 12 wings
  - One piece of fried chicken with no batter has 158 calories/thigh or breast of 131 calories
  - One medium fried chicken wing with no batter has 102 calories
  - Ten (10) wings have 1,020 calories
- What could you eat in addition to the fried chicken that is a vegetable (e.g., salad)?

R: *Chicken wings have more fat before frying than a chicken thigh or breast. White meat has less calories than has dark meat.*

Avoid Describing Foods as Bad or Good. Explain Nutrient Density of Foods (*Hunter & Cason, 2006)

R: *The nutrient density of foods can be high, medium, low, or none. Foods with high nutrient density are low in calorie and high in nutrients.*

R: *Nutrient dense foods give the most nutrients for the fewest amounts of calories.*

- Foods that are nutrient dense (low in calories):
  - Fruits and vegetables that are bright or deeply colored
  - Foods that are fortified
  - Lower fat versions of meats, milk, dairy products, and eggs
- Foods that are less nutrient dense (high in calories, low, or no nutrients):
  - Tend to be lighter or whiter in color
  - Contain a lot of refined sugar
  - Tend to be refined products (white bread as compared to whole grains)
  - Contain high amounts of fat for the amount of nutrients compared to similar products (fat-free milk vs. ice cream) For example:
    - An apple is a better choice than a bag of pretzels with the same number of calories, but the apple provides fiber, vitamin C, and potassium.
    - An orange is better than orange juice because it has fiber.
    - Water is better than any sugar drink; even 100% fruit juice.

Overweight

Definition

A condition in which an individual accumulates abnormal or excessive fat for age and gender

Defining Characteristics

Adult: BMI of > 25 kg/m^2
Child < 2 years: Weight-for-length > 95th percentile
Child 2 to 18 years: BMI of > 85th but < 95th percentile, or 25 kg/m^2 (whichever is smaller)

Related Factors

Physiologic

Genetic disorder
Heritability of interrelated factors (e.g., adipose tissue distribution, energy expenditure, lipoprotein lipase activity, lipid synthesis, lipolysis)

Treatment Related

Prolonged steroid therapy
Diminished sense of taste and/or smell (will diminish satiety)

Situational (Personal, Environment)

Economically disadvantaged
Fear regarding lack of food supply
Intake in excess of metabolic requirements
Reported undesirable eating patterns
- Frequent snacking
- High disinhibition and restraint eating behavior score
- High frequency of restaurant or fried food
- Portion sizes larger than recommended
- Consumption of sugar-sweetened beverages
- Disordered eating behaviors (e.g., binge eating, extreme weight control)
- Disordered eating perceptions

Energy expenditure below energy intake based on standard assessment (e.g., WAVE assessment[28])
- Sedentary activity patterns
- Sedentary behavior occurring for > 2 hours/day
- Average daily physical activity is less than recommended for gender and age

Sleep disorder, shortened sleep time
Excessive alcohol consumption
Low dietary calcium intake in children
Obesity in childhood
Parental obesity

Pregnancy
Maternal diabetes mellitus
Maternal smoking

Maturational

Neonates/Infants
Formula- or mixed-fed infants
Premature pubarche
Rapid weight gain during childhood
Rapid weight gain during infancy, including the first week, first 4 months, and first year
Solid foods as major food source at <5 months of age

Goals

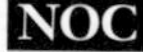

NOC
Nutritional Status: Nutrient Intake, Weight Control, Exercise Participation, Infant Nutritional Status, Weight Body Mass, Adherence Behavior: Healthy Diet, Weight Loss Behavior

The individual will commit to a weight-loss program, as evidenced by the following indicators:

- Identifies the patterns of eating associated with consumption/energy expenditure imbalance
- Can give examples of nutrient dense foods versus those with "empty calories"
- Can identify three ways to increase his or her activity
- Commits to increasing foods with high nutrient density and less with "empty calories"
- Commits to making 3 to 5 changes in food/fluid choices, which are healthier

The child (over 8 years) will verbalize what is healthy eating by the following indicators:

- Can describe the "MyPlate"
- Can describe what "empty calories" mean
- Can name "empty calories" beverages and healthier substitutions
- Can name foods high in nutrients
- Can name food high in sugar and "empty calories" and healthier substitutions

The pregnant woman will verbalize healthy eating and recommended weight gain during pregnancy by the following indicators:

- Can describe vitamin, mineral, protein, fat needs during pregnancy
- Can give examples of nutrient dense foods versus those with "empty calories"

- Can identify three ways to increase his or her activity
- Will relate the weight gain appropriate specific to her weight prior to pregnancy
- Can explain why "dieting" is problematic

Interventions

NIC

Self-Efficacy Enhancement, Self-Responsibility Enhancement, Nutritional Counseling, Weight Management, Teaching: Nutrition (age appropriate), Behavioral Modification, Exercise Promotion, Coping Enhancement

- Refer to *Risk for Overweight* for interventions for overweight individuals.

Risk for Overweight

Definition

Vulnerable to abnormal or excessive fat accumulation for age and gender, which may compromise health

Risk Factors

Adult: BMI approaching > 25 kg/m²
Average daily physical activity is less than recommended for gender and age
Child < 2 years: Weight-for-length approaching 95th percentile
Child 2 to 18 years: BMI approaching 85th percentile, or 25 kg/m² (whichever is smaller)
Children who are crossing BMI percentiles upward
Children with high BMI percentiles
Consumption of sugar-sweetened beverages
Disordered eating behaviors (e.g., binge eating, extreme weight control)
Disordered eating perceptions
Eating in response to external cues (e.g., time of day, social situations)
Eating in response to internal cues other than hunger (e.g., anxiety)
Economically disadvantaged
Energy expenditure below energy intake based on standard assessment (e.g., WAVE assessment[28])
Excessive alcohol consumption
Fear regarding lack of food supply
Formula- or mixed-fed infants
Frequent snacking
Genetic disorder
Heritability of interrelated factors (e.g., adipose tissue distribution, energy expenditure, lipoprotein lipase activity, lipid synthesis, lipolysis)
High disinhibition and restraint eating behavior score
High frequency of restaurant or fried food
Higher baseline weight at beginning of each pregnancy
Low dietary calcium intake in children
Maternal diabetes mellitus
Maternal smoking
Obesity in childhood
Parental obesity
Portion sizes larger than recommended

Premature pubarche
Rapid weight gain during childhood
Rapid weight gain during infancy, including the first week, first 4 months, and first year
Sedentary behavior occurring for >2 hours/day
Shortened sleep time
Sleep disorder
Solid foods as major food source at <5 months of age

Situational (Personal, Environmental)

Related to risk of gaining more than 25 to 30 lb when pregnant

Related to lack of basic nutrition knowledge

Maturational

Adult/Older Adult

Related to decreased activity patterns, decreased metabolic needs

Goals

NOC
Nutritional Status, Weight Control

The person will describe why he or she is at risk for weight gain as evidenced by the following indicators:

- Describes reasons for increased intake with taste or olfactory deficits
- Discusses the nutritional needs during pregnancy
- Discusses the effects of exercise on weight control

Interventions

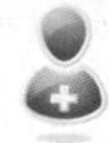

Clinical Alert Individuals can be malnourished even though they are obese or overweight due to intake of foods high in fat and carbohydrates, which are low in nutrients per calorie intake. Individual of a healthy weight may also be nutritionally deficient by eating foods high in fat and carbohydrates. For individual not overweight but have poor nutrition, refer to *Imbalanced Nutrition*.

Getting Started

NIC
Self-Efficacy Enhancement, Self-Responsibility Enhancement, Nutritional Counseling, Weight Management, Teaching: Nutrition (age appropriate), Behavioral Modification, Exercise Promotion, Coping Enhancement

- Refer to Appendix C: Strategies to Promote Engagement of Individual/Families for Healthier Outcomes for specific techniques to improve activation and engagement.

Initiate Discussion: "How Can You Be Healthier?"

- Focus on the person's response (e.g., stop smoking, exercise more, eat healthier, and cut down on drinking).
- Refer to index for interventions for the targeted lifestyle change.

R: *The nurse should be cautioned against applying a nursing diagnosis for an overweight or obese person who does not want to participate in a weight-loss program. Motivation for weight loss must come from within.*

Before a Person Can Change, They Must (Martin et al., 2010)

- Know what change is necessary (information and why)
- Desire the change (motivation)
- Have the tools to achieve and maintain the change (strategy)
- Trust the health-care professional who has a sympathetic presence (Pelzang, 2010)

R: *Empathic communication involving a thorough understanding of the patient's perspective improves adherence. Patients who are informed and effectively motivated are also more likely to adhere to their treatment recommendations (*Martin et al., 2005).*

If Appropriate, Gently and Expertly Teach the Hazards of Obesity But Respect a Person's Right to Choose, the Right of Self-Determination

- "How do you think being overweight affects you?

If the Person Reports No Complaints, Explain That the Effects of Excess Weight Are Insidious and Often Not Felt by the Person Until They Threaten Their Health or Cause Pain

- Focus on what the person tells you (e.g., "My sugar is high, my knees hurt."). Do not overload him or her with

If the Individual Does Not Identify Any Negative Effects of Excess Weight That He or She Feels, Ask Him or Her One of the Following Questions. Pick the Best Question That Applies to The Individual. Use Language He or She Understands

- Do your legs swell during the day and go back to normal during the night?
  - Explain that fat tissue compresses tubes in your legs and prevent fluids from circulating well. Eventually the swelling will be permanent, 24 hours a day, causing difficulty walking and wearing shoes.
- Do you have high blood pressure or is it getting a little higher each year?
  - Explain that blood vessels are damaged when excess weight put pressure on them and they stretch, become thinner, and lose their strength. Your heart now has to pump harder, causing high blood pressure. Over time the heart enlarges and cannot pump well. This is heart failure.
- Is your cholesterol level increasing each year?
  - Explain that the stretching of your blood vessels damages the inside of the blood tubes. Cholesterol sticks to the damaged tubes and slows the blood flow to your kidneys, eyes, brain, and legs. This can cause strokes, renal failure, vision problems, and blood clots in your legs.
- You may not feel that anything is wrong, but high blood pressure can permanently damage your heart, brain, eyes, and kidneys before you feel anything. Even losing 10 lb can reduce your blood pressure.
- Is your blood glucose test getting a little higher each year? Is there diabetes in your family?
  - Explain that the more fatty tissue you have, the more resistant your cells become to insulin.
  - Insulin carries sugar from blood to the cells. When you are overweight, the cells are damaged and will not absorb the insulin. So your blood sugar goes up. High blood sugars damage blood vessels in the eyes, kidneys, and heart.
- Does your back, your knees, or other joints hurt?
  - Explain that extra weight puts pressure on your joints and bones. This pressure wears away the cartilage, the cushion at the ends of your bones. This causes the bone to rub against another bone causing pain.
- Do you think people who are overweight have problems healing from injuries or surgery?
  - Explain that fat tissue has less blood supply, which is needed for healing. The incision has more pressure against, when you are overweight, which can cause the wound to open up. If antibiotics are needed for infection, the medicine does not work well because of poor circulation to the wound.

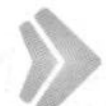

Carp's Cues

It would be wise to mention that individuals, who are thin or of normal weight can have hypertension, arthritis, high cholesterol, and diabetes but not at the high rate as people who are overweight.

- Advise them to focus on a goal of losing 5 lb. Emphasize how heavy 5 lb of sugar is and that every 5 lb lost is less work for their heart and less strain on their joints. A reduction in calories and increase in activity can cause a weight loss of about 2 lb a week.

R: *It can be discouraging to focus on losing 50 lb. Five pounds at a time is more realistic.*

- Refer interested individual to the article, "Do You Know Some of the Health Risks of Being Overweight?" Accessed at the National Institute of Diabetes and Digestive and Kidney Diseases website.

Eating Healthier

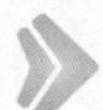

Carp's Cues

"Before you eat or drink something with "empty calories," ask yourself, "Is this worth it?" If it is, *enjoy* it. There is no such thing as "bad foods" only bad amounts.

Promote Activation to Engage the Individual in Healthier Behavior. Focus on What the Person Wants to Change. Limit to Three Changes

R: *"Activation refers to a person's ability and willingness to take on the role of managing their health and health care" (Hibbard & Cunningham, 2008).*

Address What Excesses or Deficiencies Exist, Using the Information He or She Gave, For Example

- I ate fried chicken wings last night for dinner.
- Anything else? No.
- How could you change what you ate to improve nutrients and decrease fat?
- Listen. If no response, suggest
  - One or two piece(s) of fried chicken instead of 12 wings
  - One piece of fried chicken with no batter has 158 calories/thigh or breast of 131calories
  - One medium fried chicken wing with no batter has 102 calories
  - Ten (10) wings have 1,020 calories
- What could you eat in addition to the fried chicken that is a vegetable (e.g., salad)?

R: *Chicken wings have more fat before frying than a chicken thigh or breast. White meat has less calories than dark meat.*

Avoid Describing Foods as Bad or Good. Explain Nutrient Density of Foods (*Hunter & Cason, 2006)

R: *The nutrient density of foods can be high, medium, low, or none. Foods with high nutrient density are low in calorie and high in nutrients.*

R: *Nutrient dense foods give the most nutrients for the fewest amounts of calories.*

- Foods that are nutrient dense (low in calories):
  - Fruits and vegetables that are bright or deeply colored
  - Foods that are fortified
  - Lower fat versions of meats, milk, dairy products, and eggs
- Foods that are less nutrient dense (high in calories, low or no nutrients)
  - Tend to be lighter or whiter in color
  - Contain a lot of refined sugar
  - Tend to be refined products (white bread as compared to whole grains)
  - Contain high amounts of fat for the amount of nutrients compared to similar products (fat-free milk vs. ice cream)
  - For example:
    - Apple is a better choice than a bag of pretzels with the same number of calories, but the apple provides fiber, vitamin C, and potassium.
    - An orange is better than orange juice because it has fiber.
    - Water is better than any sugar drink even 100% fruit juice.

Familiarize With Cues That Often Trigger Eating, Try Not to Eat When You are Not Hungry

- Another activity (e.g., watching TV)
- Everyone else eating
- Boredom or stress

R: *Often, inappropriate response to external cues, including stressors, facilitates or aggravates obesity. This response initiates an ineffective pattern in which the individual eats in response to stress cues rather than physiologic hunger.*

Moving More

Assist to Identify Realistic Exercise Program. Gym Membership is not Required

Discuss the Aspects of Starting the Exercise Program. Advise that a regular exercise program should

- Be enjoyable.
- Be realistic for them.
- Find someone to walk with.
- Start slow and easy. Obtain clearance from primary care provider.
- It is okay to be a little out of breath and you can talk. If you are too short of breath to talk slow down your speed or rest.
- Plan a daily walking program.
- Start at 5 to 10 blocks for 0.5 to 1 mile/day; increase 1 block or 0.1 mile/week.

- Gradually increase the rate and length of walk; remember to progress slowly.
- Avoid straining or pushing too hard and becoming overly fatigued.
- Stop immediately if any of the following occur:
  - Pain in chest (seek emergency treatment)
  - Dizziness
  - Severe breathlessness
  - Loss of muscle control
  - Lightheadedness
  - Nausea
- Refer to the nursing diagnosis *Sedentary Lifestyle* for guidelines to exercising

Initiate Health Teaching as Indicated

- Provide individual with Getting Started to Healthy Eating on thePoint at http://thePoint.lww.com/Carpenito6e.
- Refer to a community weight-loss program (e.g., Weight Watchers, Curves).
- Participate in water aerobics at senior club or gym.
- Advise to consult primary care provider for continued assistance in weight loss.

R: *Strategies are needed after discharge to assist a person initiate/sustain a change in eating patterns and exercise patterns that will focus on why, where, and what is eaten and methods to reduce intake and increase activity.*

Older Adults Interventions

- Refer to the above Intervention under Risk for Overweight—Getting Started & Eating Healthier

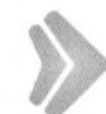

Carp's Cues

Older adults will benefit from specific activities to increase muscle strength, flexibility, and attain a health weight. There are several excellent internet resources written for older adults to start them to move more. Nurses should access them to pass on some simple exercises as standing behind a chair, holding on and lifting heels keeping their toes on the floor. This exercise strengthens the ankle and leg muscles so as to prevent a fall even if the person trips.

Refer to the Following Resource

- Exercise and physical activity—Your everyday guide from the National Institute on Aging accessed at the National Institute on Aging, part of National Institutes of Health website:
  - **Chapter 1: Get Ready** talks about the "why" of exercise and physical activity. It tells you the benefits of being active and describes the different types of exercise.
  - **Chapter 2: Get Set** guides you on getting organized and reviewing your current activity levels, setting short- and long-term goals, and creating a realistic plan for becoming active over time.
  - **Chapter 3: Go!** is all about the "how." The guide offers tips to help you get started. It also has ideas to help you stick with your decision to be active every day and to get you back on track if you have to stop exercising for some reason.
  - **Chapter 4: Sample Exercises** gives you some specific activities and exercises, including exercises to increase your strength, improve balance, become more flexible, and increase endurance. All of the exercises have easy directions to help you do them safely.
  - **Chapter 5: How Am I Doing?** offers you some ways to test your progress and reward your success.
  - **Chapter 6: Healthy Eating** briefly discusses another key to good health—nutritious eating habits.
  - **Chapter 7: Keep Going** includes worksheets to keep track of your progress.
- You'll also find a list of resources for more information. Some of the resources are especially for people with specific health problems or disabilities who want to be active.

Maternal Interventions

Initiate Discussion: "How Can You Be Healthier?"

- Focus on response (e.g., stop smoking, exercise more, eat healthier, and stop drinking alcohol).
- Refer to index for interventions for the targeted lifestyle change.

Discuss Nutritional Intake and Weight Gain During Pregnancy

Discuss the Total Weight Gain Appropriate for the Individual (Institute of Medicine, 2009)

- 25 to 35 lb if you were a healthy weight before pregnancy, with a BMI of 18.5 to 24.9.
- 28 to 40 lb if you were underweight before pregnancy with a BMI of less than 18.5.
- 15 to 25 lb if you were overweight before pregnancy with a BMI of 25 to 29.9.
- 11 to 20 lb if you were obese before pregnancy with a BMI of over 30.

R: *The extra weight gained during pregnancy is needed to nourish the developing fetus. It also stores nutrients for breastfeeding. The amount of weight you should gain depends on your weight and BMI before pregnancy.*

Explain Healthy Weight Gain for Each Trimester (Institute of Medicine, 2009)

- 1 to 4.5 lb during the first trimester
- Approximately 1 to 2 lb/week in the second trimester
- Approximately 1 to 2 lb/week in the third trimester

R: *Obesity related to erratic eating, excess CHO, little fiber and vegetables, >6 hours of TV watching, and eating when sad and/or frustrated as evidenced by BMI of 34.*

R: *Gaining weight at a steady rate within recommended boundaries can also lower your chances of having hemorrhoids, varicose veins, stretch marks, backache, fatigue, indigestion, and shortness of breath during pregnancy.*

Explain the Problems That Can Occur With Too Much Weight Gain During Pregnancy (Institute of Medicine, 2009)

- Gestational diabetes
- Leg pain
- Varicose veins
- High blood pressure
- Backaches
- Increased fatigue
- Increased risk of cesarean delivery

Stress the Importance of Not Dieting, Skipping Meals, but Instead Consume Recommended Portions and Avoid High-Fat/-CHO Foods

R: *Dieting during pregnancy may result in insufficient maternal intake to provide the fetus with the necessary energy for growth. The fetus depends on the mother's dietary intake for growth and development, taking only iron and folate from maternal stores (Pillitteri, 2014).*

- Be aware of rationalization (e.g., a lack of time may be a lack of prioritization).
- Keep a list of positive outcomes and health benefits (e.g., sleep better, lower blood pressure).
- Weight loss in the range of 2 to 4 kg is associated with systolic blood pressure declines in the range of 3 to 8 mm Hg, a clinically significant impact (Harsha & Bray, 2008).

R: *Weight loss is a life-changing event if it is to be sustained. Motivation must be maintained. Weight loss of even 5% to 10% can lower blood pressure and improve glucose lipid profiles (Dennis, 2004).*

Reduce Inappropriate Responses to Stressors

- Distinguish between urge and hunger.
- Use distraction, relaxation, and imagery.
- Use alternative response training:
  - Make a list of external cues/situations that lead to off-target behavior.
  - List constructive behaviors (e.g., take a walk) to replace off-target behaviors.
  - Post the list of alternate constructive behaviors on the refrigerator.
  - Reevaluate every 1 to 2 weeks whether plan is realistic and effective.

R: *Overeating is often associated with boredom and stress.*

Initiate Health Teaching and Referrals, as Indicated

- Refer to support groups (e.g., Weight Watchers, Overeaters Anonymous, TOPS).

R: *Weight-loss strategies are life long and may require assistance from programs and support groups.*

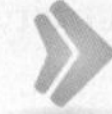

Pediatric Interventions

Carp's Cues

Weight gain in children occurs when intake exceeds energy expenditure (activity). Factors that contribute to the increasing rate of overweight/obesity in children and adolescents are portion sizes, snacking on empty calories, away-from-home eating, sugar-sweetened drinks, and increased sedentary activities (e.g., TV watching, computer games, electronics [e.g., tablets]). Reedy & Kerbes-Smith (2010) reported that 40% of the total calories consumed daily by children and adolescents are empty calories. Frequent sources of empty calories are pizza, soda, fruit drinks, and dairy desserts.

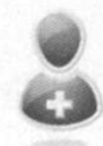

Clinical Alert Children should not be put on diets. The goal for growing children is to maintain, not lose or gain weight. If weight is maintained and the child grows, his or her BMI will decrease. This of course does require different food/beverage choices and increased activity. This is not true for adolescents when they have achieved their lifetime height (e.g., for girls age 13, boys age 18 to 19).

Try to Engage the Child and Family to Realize the Importance of Good Nutrition and Exercise

R: *"Multiple factors influence overweight and obesity rates in children, but, ultimately, an imbalance between energy consumed and energy expended is the determining factor" (Reedy & Kerbes-Smith, 2010, p. 1477).*

- Discuss with family the hazards of being overweight as a child.
- Childhood obesity leads to adult obesity.
- Excess weight elevates blood pressure, heart rate, and cardiac output in children (see Key Concepts, Pediatric Considerations for other health dangers).
- As weight increases, activity decreases.

R: *Refer to Key Concepts.*

Address the Barriers to Parents Taking Action to Help Their Child Eat Better and Exercise More as follows (Dudek, 2014, p. 308)

- A belief that children will outgrow their excess weight.
- Overweight parents feel they do not set a good example.
- A lack of knowledge about how to help their children control their weight.
- A fear that they will cause an eating disorder in their children.

Provide a Color Copy of "MyPlate"

- Refer to *Imbalance Nutrition* for interventions for healthy eating in children and adolescents.

R: *Reedy & Kerbes-Smith (2010, p. 1478) found children and adolescents eat too few vegetables, whole grains, fruits, and milk products. "Therefore, US children and adolescents do not always consume the types and amounts of food they need to support an active, healthy lifestyle."*

Use Creative Methods with Younger Children to Teach Good Nutrition

- Create a felt board with each day of the week on it. Using pictures of food groups, vegetables, grains, milk, meat, cheese, yogurt, and fruits, have the child stick them to the board for that day.
- Read books that emphasize good food that gives more energy, strong muscles and bones, etc.

R: *Children respond favorably to activities that are a bridge between concrete experiences and abstract ideas (Hockenberry & Wilson, 2015).*

The American Academy of Pediatrics Recommends a Few Doable Healthier Behaviors (Barlow, 2007, S. 182)

- Consume five servings of fruits and vegetables every day (ME). Families may subsequently increase to nine servings per day, as recommended by the USDA.
- Reduce sugar-sweetened beverages, such as soda, sports drinks, and punches. Ideally, these beverages will be eliminated from a child's diet, although children who consume large amounts will benefit from reduction to one serving per day; limit "empty high calorie" foods (e.g., chips, cookies, candy, crackers).
- Decrease television viewing (and other forms of screen time) to 2 hr/day. If the child is 2 years of age, then no television viewing should be the goal.

- Be physically active 1 hour each day. Unstructured play is most appropriate for young children. Older children should find physical activities that they enjoy, which may include sports, dance, martial arts, bike riding, and walking. In Structured— play, children can perform several shorter periods of activity over the day.
- Prepare more meals at home rather than purchasing restaurant food.
- Eat at the table as a family at least 5 or 6 times/week (ME).
- Consume a healthy breakfast every day.
- Involve the whole family in lifestyle changes.
- Allow the child to self-regulate his or her meals and avoid overly restrictive feeding behaviors.
- Help families tailor behavior recommendations to their cultural values (suggest).

If Eating "Fast Foods," Point Out Healthier Choices

- Encourage portion control; educate children/adolescents that "large," "extra," "double," or "triple" will be high in calories and fat.
- Recommend smaller portions, since a regular serving is enough for most children, or sharing with a parent or sibling.
- Look for whole grain foods, fruits, vegetables, and calcium-rich foods.
- When planning a fast food meal, select an establishment that promotes healthier options at the point of purchase.
- Address strategies to improve nutrition when eating fast foods:
  - Drink skim milk.
  - Avoid French fries or share one order.
  - Choose grilled foods.
  - Eat salads and vegetables.
  - Explore healthier fast foods at home (e.g., frozen dinners with three food groups).

R: *Fast foods usually contain large amounts of fat and sugar, and often do not offer healthier food choices as whole grains, fruit, baked vs. fried, smaller portions.*

Suggest Healthy Snacks at Home

- Offer fresh fruits, vegetables, cheese and crackers, low-fat milk, calcium-fortified juices, and frozen yogurt as snacks.

R: *Making healthful food available and convenient and increasing healthy snacks reduce the pressure for the child to eat a certain amount at mealtime.*

Initiate Health Teaching and Referrals, as Indicated

- Community programs (YM/WCA, adolescent support groups).
- Access additional information at fast food—www.uptodate.com/contents/fast-food-for-children-and-adolescents.

R: *Community resources may be needed to assist children with lifestyle changes.*

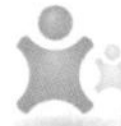

Maternal Interventions

Discuss the Total Weight Gain Appropriate for a pregnant woman (Institute of Medicine, 2009)

- 25 to 35 lb if you were a healthy weight before pregnancy, with a BMI of 18.5 to 24.9.
- 28 to 40 lb if you were underweight before pregnancy with a BMI of less than 18.5.
- 15 to 25 lb if you were overweight before pregnancy with a BMI of 25 to 29.9.
- 11 to 20 lb if you were obese before pregnancy with a BMI of over 30.

R: *The extra weight gained during pregnancy is needed to nourish the developing fetus. It also stores nutrients for breastfeeding. The amount of weight you should gain depends on your weight and BMI before pregnancy.*

Explain Healthy Weight Gain for Each Trimester (Institute of Medicine, 2009)

- 1 to 4.5 lb during the first trimester
- Approximately 1 to 2 lb/week in the second trimester
- Approximately 1 to 2 lb/week in the third trimester

R: *Gaining weight at a steady rate within recommended boundaries can also lower your chances of having hemorrhoids, varicose veins, stretch marks, backache, fatigue, indigestion, and shortness of breath during pregnancy.*

Explain the Problems That Can Occur With Too Much Weight Gain During Pregnancy (Institute of Medicine, 2009)

- Gestational diabetes
- Leg pain
- Varicose veins
- High blood pressure
- Backaches
- Increased fatigue
- Increased risk of cesarean delivery

Stress the Importance of Not Dieting, Skipping Meals, but Instead Consume Recommended Portions and Avoid High-Fat/-CHO Foods

- Refer to *Imbalanced Nutrition* for dietary recommendation for pregnant woman, for example, "MyPlate," vitamins, calcium.

R: *Dieting during pregnancy may result in insufficient maternal intake to provide the fetus with the necessary energy for growth. The fetus depends on the mother's dietary intake for growth and development, taking only iron and folate from maternal stores (Pillitteri, 2014).*

POST-TRAUMA SYNDROME

Post-Trauma Syndrome

Risk for Post-Trauma Syndrome
Rape Trauma Syndrome (Sexual Assault Syndrome)

Definition

Sustained maladaptive response to a traumatic, overwhelming event (NANDA-I)

A response to a horrific, overwhelming event "characterized by intrusive thoughts, nightmares and flashbacks of past traumatic events, avoidance of reminders of trauma, hypervigilance, and sleep disturbance, all of which lead to considerable social, occupational, and interpersonal dysfunction" (Ciechanowski, 2014).

Defining Characteristics

Presence of a Cluster of Actual or Risk Nursing Diagnoses Related to Responses to Traumatic Event(s)

Anxiety (panic, severe, moderate)
Fear
Impaired Social Interactions
Social Isolation
Insomnia
Hopelessness
Self-Care Deficits
Risk for Self-Harm
Chronic Sorrow
Risk for Disabled Family Coping

Diagnostic Criteria for Post-Traumatic Stress Syndrome[31]

Stressor criterion

"Has been exposed to a catastrophic event involving actual or threatened death or injury, or a threat to the physical integrity of him/herself or others (such as sexual violence). Indirect exposure includes learning about the violent or accidental death or perpetration of sexual violence to a loved one" (Friedman, 2016).[31]

Intrusive recollection criterion

Persistent reexperience of the traumatic event through recurrent intrusive recollections of the event, dreams about the event, flashbacks

[31]*DSM-5*, Seven Criteria for PTSD Diagnosis (American Psychiatric Association, 2013; Friedman, 2016)

Avoidance criterion

Avoidance of the stimuli associated with the event, talking about it, avoiding activities, people or places that arouse memories, feeling numb, constricted affect, detachment, alienation[31]

Negative cognitions and mood criterion

Alterations in mood, chronic depression

Alterations in arousal or reactivity criterion

Persistent symptoms of increased arousal, hyperviligence, difficulty sleeping, difficulty concentration

Duration criterion

Symptoms must persist for at least 1 month before Post Traumatic Stress Disorder (PTSD) may be diagnosed.

Functional Significance Criterion

Must experience significant social, occupational, or other distress as a result of these symptoms.

Related Factors

Situational (Personal, Environmental)

Related to exposure to traumatic events of natural origin, including:

Floods
Earthquakes
Volcanic eruptions
Storms
Avalanches
Epidemics*
Disasters*

Related to traumatic events of human origin, such as:

History of criminal victimization*
Concentration camp confinement
Serious accidents (e.g., industrial, motor vehicle)*
Assault
Torture*
Rape
Bombing
Large fires
Witnessing violent death*
Terrorist attacks
Exposure to war*
Witnessing mutilation*
Being held prisoner of war*
Criminal victimization*
Airplane crashes
Abuse (e.g., physical, psychological)*

Related to industrial disasters* (nuclear, chemical, or other life-threatening accidents)

Related to serious threat or injury to loved ones and/or self*

Related to exposure to events involving multiple deaths*

Related to events outside the range of unusual human experience*

Related to sudden destruction of one's home and/or community*

Related to history of abuse (e.g., physical, psychological, sexual)

Author's Note

Post-Trauma Syndrome represents a group of emotional responses to a traumatic event of either natural origin (e.g., floods, volcanic eruptions, earthquakes) or human origin (e.g., war, torture). The emotional responses (e.g., hypervigilance, avoidance, flashbacks, fear, anger) can interfere with interpersonal relationships and daily life responsibilities. This assessment will provide data to formulate nursing diagnoses. It is through these nursing diagnoses that direct nursing interventions, not *Post-Trauma Syndrome*, which is too broad.

From a historical perspective, the significant change ushered in by the PTSD concept was the stipulation that the etiological agent was outside the individual (i.e., a traumatic event) rather than an inherent individual weakness (i.e., a traumatic neurosis). The key to understanding the scientific basis and clinical expression of PTSD is the concept of "trauma" (Friedman, 2016).

Errors in Diagnostic Statements

***Post-Trauma Response* related to expressions of survival guilt and recurring nightmares of auto accident**

Survival guilt and nightmares of a traumatic event represent possible manifestations of post-trauma response, not related factors. The nurse should use Functional Healthy Pattern Assessment to determine how this has negatively *affected the person's and families' lives. The nurse should restate the diagnosis as Post-Trauma Response related to auto accident, as evidenced by recurring nightmares and expressions of survival guilt.*

Key Concepts

General Considerations

- "As a result of research-based changes to the diagnosis PTSD is no longer categorized as an Anxiety Disorder. PTSD is now classified in a new category, Trauma- and Stressor-Related Disorders, in which the onset of every disorder has been preceded by exposure to a traumatic or otherwise adverse environmental event" (Freidman, 2016).
- Freidman (2016) reported the results of multiple studies of the prevalence of PTSD as:
  - Veterans >30.9% for men and 26.9% for woman
  - Gulf War Veterans 13%
  - The lifetime prevalence of PTSD ranges from 6.8% to 12.3% in the general adult population in the United States (US).
  - In postconflict settings such as Algeria (37%), Cambodia (28%), Ethiopia (16%), and Gaza (18%)
  - Using *DSM-IV* criteria for PTSD, the 6-month prevalence was estimated to be 3.7% for boys and 6.3% for girls (Kilpatrick et al., 2003)
- Friedman (2016) writes,

  Like pain, the traumatic experience is filtered through cognitive and emotional processes before it can be appraised as an extreme threat. Because of individual differences in this appraisal process, different people appear to have different trauma thresholds, some more protected from and some more vulnerable to developing clinical symptoms after exposure to extremely stressful situations. Although there is currently a renewed interest in subjective aspects of traumatic exposure, it must be emphasized that events such as rape, torture, genocide, and severe war zone stress are experienced as traumatic events by nearly everyone.

- Trauma is defined in terms of the subjective experience of an event that cannot be dealt with or assimilated in the usual way. Traumatic situations differ from ordinary experiences in that they involve realistic danger of physiologic or psychological destruction, which could mobilize fear of death. A traumatic event may affect only one person or many people at once. It may be of human origin (e.g., rape, wars) or natural origin (e.g., avalanches, volcanoes).
- Generally, traumatic events of natural origin are less severe or long lasting than those of human origin. Those of human origin are often perceived as resulting from indifference, negligence, or malice.
- Horowitz (*1986) conceptualized these phenomena and postulated a phasic tendency in human responses to traumatic events:
  - The initial response to trauma is to survive and to function in the immediate life-threatening situation by using all resources.
  - The powerful coping method of "numbing" reduces psychological and emotional effects.
  - In an attempt to master the traumatic experience, intrusive recollection or reenactment of the trauma erupts into conscious awareness.
  - There is a pattern of oscillation between "numbing" and intrusive reactions peculiar to each person.
  - Gradually, the person works through the trauma by using a broader perception and rationale for the event and the aftermath.
  - Finally, the person assimilates such an experience into a meaningful whole congruent with basic beliefs and values.
- Police officers, firefighters, war veterans, and EMT workers are more vulnerable to PTSD than traditional citizens.
- Individual characteristics, such as early childhood experience, developmental phase, and character strength, may affect the outcome of responses to trauma.
  - The current trauma may reactivate unresolved childhood conflicts.
  - Age can be a crucial factor, because trauma can interrupt a stage of human development.
  - Individual coping resources are important when a person confronts a traumatic situation, and they influence the effectiveness of adaptation.

Substance Abuse and PTSD

- "Among veterans from all eras, symptoms of PTSD have been highly correlated with hazardous drinking, leading to greater decreases in overall health, and greater difficulties readjusting to civilian life. In fact, a diagnosis of co-occurring PTSD and alcohol use disorder has proven more detrimental than a diagnosis of PTSD or alcohol use disorder alone" (Bernardy, Lund, Alexander, & Friedman, 2011).

- Among people with lifetime PTSD, lifetime substance abuse is estimated at 21% to 43%, compared with 8% to 25% in those without PTSD (Jacobsen, Southwick, & Kosten, 2001).

Risk for Suicide

- Health Research Funding.org (2015) reports "Anyone who is suffering from PTSD is at an incredibly high risk for suicide. 22% of people who had suffered PTSD from rape attempted suicide at one point in their lifetime. 23% of individuals with PTSD from a physical assault event also attempted suicide at one point in their lives. 24% of individuals who were confronted with sexual assault as a child attempted suicide throughout their lifetime."

Pediatric Considerations

- Prevalence estimates from studies of this type vary greatly; however, research indicates that children exposed to traumatic events may have a higher prevalence of PTSD than adults in the general population (Gabbay, Oatis, Silva, & Hirsch, 2004).
- Hockenberry and Wilson (2015, p. 643) described three phases of children's responses to a horrific event as:
  - "Following a horrific event, the child's response includes intense fear, helplessness, or horror resulting in behavior that is disorganized, depressed or agitated".
  - In the second phase, the child uses defense mechanisms and appears to have no response. They are numb and can be in denial.
  - In the third phase, the child wants to know what happen? Why? Compared to phase 2 the child appears to be getting worse; they are not. The manifestations of fear, anxiety, phobias, flashbacks, and repetitive playback of the situation are attempts of the child to deal with their fears.
  - Phase 3 can become prolonged and develop into an obsession.
- Individual characteristics, such as early childhood experience, developmental phase, and character strength, may affect the outcome of responses to trauma.
  - The current trauma may reactivate unresolved childhood conflicts.
  - Age can be a crucial factor, because trauma can interrupt a stage of human development.
  - Individual coping resources are important when a person confronts a traumatic situation, and they influence the effectiveness of adaptation.
- A child's response to trauma depends on the nature and the extent of the trauma, developmental age, their social environment, and response of adult caretakers. Coping is a learned response (Hockenberry & Wilson, 2015).
- Children can experience post-traumatic stress symptoms after a friend or acquaintance is killed (*Pfefferbaum et al., 2000).
- Fourth National Incidence Study of Child Abuse and Neglect (NIS-4) (2010) reported the following:
  - The number of children who experienced abuse in the United States is 553,300. The number of sexually abused children is 135,300.
  - The number of children who experienced physical abuse is 323,000.
  - The number of children who experienced emotional abuse is 148,500.
  - Nearly 3 million children (an estimated 2,905,800) experienced endangerment maltreatment.

Focus Assessment Criteria

Subjective and Objective Data

Screen Individuals of All Ages for Abuse, Someone May Be Holding on to This "Secret" for a Lifetime

R: *Individuals, who experience violence and abuse, especially domestic/partner violence often report "Nobody asked me."*

Identify the Traumatic Situation(s)

Explore With Individual and Family Separately

Thoughts, feelings, or behaviors that he or she believes have been different since the traumatic experience.

How these changes have affected his/her life

Discuss Changes in General Lifestyle or Pattern Since the Traumatic Event(s), to Assess Any Readjustment Difficulties for Those Functional Patterns That Are Relevant as

Health Perception–Health Management Pattern

Perceived pattern of health, well-being
Participation in health plan with health-care professional
Knowledge of preventive health practices
Participations in health-promoting activities

Nutritional–Metabolic Pattern
Actual weight, weight loss, or gain
Appetite, preferences

Elimination Pattern
Bowel elimination pattern, changes
Bladder elimination pattern, changes

Activity–Exercise Pattern
Pattern of exercise, activity, leisure, recreation
Ability to perform activities of daily living (self-care, home maintenance, work, eating, shopping, cooking)

Sleep–Rest Pattern
Patterns of sleep, rest
Perception of quality, quantity

Cognitive–Perceptual Pattern
Memory
Decision-making ability, patterns

Self-Perception–Self-Concept Pattern
Attitudes about self, sense of worth
Perception of abilities
Emotional patterns

Role–Relationship Patterns
Patterns of relationships
Role responsibilities
Satisfaction with relationships and responsibilities

Sexuality–Reproductive Pattern
Satisfaction with sexual relationships, sexual identity

Coping–Stress Tolerance Patterns
Ability to manage stress
Knowledge of stress tolerance
Sources of support
Stressful life events in last year
Use of alcohol, misuse of drugs
Thoughts of harming oneself

Value–Belief Pattern
Spiritual beliefs/practices
Perceived conflicts in values

Refer to the Nursing Diagnosis in the Specific Functional Health Pattern for Interventions.

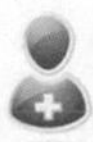

Clinical Alert "For individuals with PTSD, the traumatic event remains, sometimes for decades or a lifetime, a dominating psychological experience that retains its power to evoke panic, terror, dread, grief, or despair" (Friedman, 2016).

Goals

NOC
Abuse Recovery, Coping, Fear Control, Personal Resiliency, Psychosocial Adjustment: Life Change, Social Support, Impulse Self-Control

In the short term, the individual will do the following:

- Acknowledge the traumatic event and begin to work with the trauma.
- Make connections with support persons/resources.
- Engage in activities that reduce stress and improve coping.

As evidenced by the following indicators:

- Talks about the experience and expressing feelings such as fear, anger, and guilt

- Identifies sources of support
- Identifies three coping strategies that may improve their quality of life (e.g., exercise, hobby, nature walks, thought-stopping)

In the long term, the client will assimilate the experience into a meaningful whole and go on to pursue his or her life as evidenced by goal setting and the following indicators:

- Reports a lessening of reexperiencing the trauma or numbing symptoms
- Reports feelings of support and comfort from individuals and/or support groups (Halter, 2014; Varcarolis, 2011)
- Reports engaging in regular activities (daily, weekly) that enhance coping
- Reports cognitive coping strategies that improve their sense of control

Interventions

NIC

Counseling, Anxiety Reduction, Emotional Support, Family Support, Support System Enhancement, Coping Enhancement, Active Listening, Presence, Grief Work, Facilitation, Referral

If This Is Their First Encounter in the Health Setting, Determine the Source(s) of Their Post-Trauma Response

- During the interview, secure a quiet room where there will be no interruptions but easy access to other staff in case of management problems.
- Be aware that talking about a traumatic experience may cause significant discomfort to the person.
- If the person becomes too anxious, discontinue the assessment and help the client regain control of the distress or provide other appropriate interventions.

R: *Short-term crisis intervention should begin as soon as victims are identified.*

Evaluate the Severity of the Responses and Effects on Current Functioning

- Refer to Focus Assessment Criteria.
- If indicated, refer to *Risk for Suicide*. Consult with law enforcement if needed.
- If alcohol/drug abuse is present, refer for counseling.

R: *2,012 over 5,000 suicides in the United States alone occurred as a result of combat-based PTSD. PTSD-related suicide is the 10th leading cause of death in the United States.*

Assist to Decrease Extremes of Reexperiencing or Numbing Symptoms

- Provide a safe, therapeutic environment where the client can regain control.
- Reassure the client that others who have experienced such traumatic events often experienced these feelings/symptoms.
- Stay with the client and offer support during an episode of high anxiety (see *Anxiety* for additional information).
- Assist to control impulsive acting-out behavior by setting limits, promoting ventilation, and redirecting excess energy into physical exercise or activity (e.g., walking, jogging). (See *Risk for Self-Harm* and *Risk for Violence* for additional information.)
- Provide techniques to reduce anxiety (e.g., progressive relaxation, deep breathing).

R: *Attempts to decrease extreme symptoms can help person regain some control. Interventions that focus on helping the person cope can reduce powerlessness (Halter, 2014).*

Assist to Acknowledge and Begin to Work Through the Trauma by Discussing the Experience and Expressing Feelings Such as Fear, Anger, and Guilt

- Provide a safe, structured setting.
- Explain that talking about the traumatic event may intensify the symptoms (e.g., nightmares, flashbacks, painful emotions, numbness).
- Assist the client to proceed at an individual pace.
- Listen attentively with empathy and an unhurried manner.

R: *Providing immediate and ongoing empathy and support prepares victims for referral to more in-depth psychological counseling. The main issues in the acute stage are being in control, fear of being left alone, and having someone listen to them.*

- Assist to talk about trauma, to understand what has occurred, and to validate the reality of personal involvement.

- Help to express feelings associated with the traumatic event and to become aware of the link between the experience and anger, depression, or anxiety.
- Assist to differentiate reality from fantasy and to reflect and talk about the areas of his or her life that have changed.
- Recognize and support cultural and religious values in dealing with the traumatic event.

R: *Assisting to recall and clarify the event puts that event in perspective and helps prevent repression. Clients/victims need to work through trauma at their own pace.*

R: *Anxiety management offers one way to maintain some control over their emotional responses (Boyd, 2012).*

Assist to Identify and Make Connections with Support People and Resources

- Help client to identify his or her strength and resources.
- Explore available support systems.
- Assist client to make connections with support and resources according to his or her needs.

R: *Providing immediate and ongoing empathy and support prepares clients/victims for referral to more in-depth psychological counseling. The main issues in the acute stage are being in control, fear of being left alone, and having someone to listen.*

- Assist to resume old activities and explore some new ones such as exercise, nature walks, and hobbies.

R: *Activities that promote relaxation and confidence can increase self-control of destructive feelings or responses.*

Assist Family/Significant Others

- Assist them to understand what is happening and why.
- Encourage expression of their feelings.
- Provide counseling sessions or link them with appropriate community resources, as necessary.

R: *Strategies focus on assisting significant others to identify how they can be most helpful to prevent client isolation, which can lead to withdrawal and depression.*

Provide Nursing Care Appropriate to Each individual's Traumatic Experience and Needs

Provide or Arrange Follow-up Treatment in Which the Individual Can Continue to Work Through the Trauma and to Integrate the Experience into a New Self-Concept

R: *Follow-up counseling and long-term support therapy in the community should be arranged. Postponing professional help lengthens the time reactions persist and can lengthen recovery (Halter, 2014).*

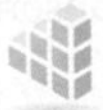

Pediatric Interventions

- Assist children to understand and to integrate the experience in accordance with their developmental stage.
- Respond to the child's present emotions. Avoid forcing the child to share their feelings/fears.

R: *Hockenberry and Wilson (2015) described three phases of children's responses to a horrific event as: Refer to Key Concepts under Pediatric Considerations.*

- Assist them to describe the experience and to express feelings (e.g., fear, guilt, rage) in safe, supportive places, such as play therapy sessions rather than direct inquiries.

R: *Play therapy, such as writing, drawing, telling stories, or playing with dolls, should be offered so children can act out, express feelings, and communicate their experience safely.*

- Provide accurate information and explanations in terms the child can understand.
- Provide family counseling to promote understanding of the child's needs.

R: *Counseling for the parents and child will be needed to assist with evaluating the trauma and assimilating the experience into their lives.*

- Refer to a specialist for ongoing therapy.

R: *Play therapy, such as writing, drawing, telling stories, or playing with dolls, should be offered so children can act out, express feelings, and communicate their experience safely.*

Risk for Post-Trauma Syndrome

Definition

At risk for sustained maladaptive response to a traumatic, overwhelming event (NANDA-I)

At risk for a response to a horrific, overwhelming event "characterized by intrusive thoughts, nightmares and flashbacks of past traumatic events, avoidance of reminders of trauma, hypervigilance, and sleep disturbance, all of which lead to considerable social, occupational, and interpersonal dysfunction" (Ciechanowski, 2015).

Risk Factors

Refer to Related Factors in *Post-Trauma Syndrome.*

Goals

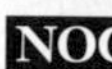

refer to *Post-Trauma Syndrome.*

The individual will continue to cope effectively after the traumatic event and relates she or he will seek professional help as evidenced by the following indicators:

- Identifies signs or symptoms that necessitate professional consultation
- Expresses feelings regarding traumatic event
- Reports any deterioration in his/her ability to cope and function

Interventions

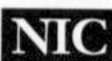

refer to *Post-Trauma Syndrome.*

- Refer to *Post-Trauma Syndrome.*

Rape Trauma Syndrome (Sexual Assault Trauma Syndrome)[32]

Definition

Sustained maladaptive response to a forced, violent sexual penetration against the victim's will and consent (NANDA-I)

State in which an individual experiences a forced, violent sexual assault (vaginal or anal penetration) against his or her will and without his or her consent. The trauma syndrome that develops from this attack or attempted attack includes an acute phase of disorganization of the victim and family's lifestyle and a long-term process of reorganization of lifestyle (*Burgess, 1995).

Defining Characteristics

Reports or evidence of sexual assault.
If the victim is a child, parents may experience similar responses.

Acute Phase

Somatic Responses

Physical trauma (bruises, soreness)
Gastrointestinal irritability (nausea, vomiting, anorexia, diarrhea)
Genitourinary discomfort (pain, pruritus, vaginal discharge)
Skeletal muscle tension (spasms, pain, headaches, sleep disturbances)

Psychological Responses

Overt
Crying, sobbing
Feelings of revenge

[32]Refer to Author' Notes for an explanation of this terminology change.

Change in relationships*
Hyperalertness*
Volatility, anger
Confusion, incoherence, disorientation*

Ambiguous Reaction

Confusion*, incoherence, disorientation*
Masked facies
Calm, numbness
Shock*, numbness, confusion*, or disbelieving
Distractibility and difficulty making decisions

Emotional Reaction

Self-blame
Fear*—of being alone or that the rapist will return (a child victim fears punishment, repercussions, abandonment, rejection)
Denial, shock, humiliation, and embarrassment*
Desire for revenge; anger*
Guilt, shame
Fatigue

Sexual Responses

Mistrust of men (if victim is a woman)
Change in sexual behavior, sexual dysfunction*

Long-Term Phase

Any response of the acute phase may continue if resolution does not occur. In addition, the following reactions can occur 2 or more weeks after the assault.

Psychological Responses

Change in relationship(s) associated with nonsupportive parent, partner, relative, friend (e.g., blames victim for event, "taking too long to get over it")
Intrusive thoughts (anger toward assailant, flashbacks of the traumatic event, dreams, insomnia)
Increased motor activity (moving, taking trips, staying some other place)
Increased emotional lability (intense anxiety, mood swings, crying spells, depression)
Fears and phobias (of indoors, or outdoors, where the rape occurred, of being alone, of crowds, of sexual encounters [with partner or potential partners])

Author's Note

The word *rape* has a history of being viewed as a crime of passion not a crime of violence, Women were (or are) asked what they were wearing or doing prior to the rape. Sexual assault is defined as any sexual activity involving a person who does not or cannot (due to alcohol, drugs, or some sort of incapacitation) consent. The phrase *sexual assault* denotes unprovoked violence, which defines the perpetrator as the criminal and the victim as a "victim of a crime." Rape/sexual assault can be defined differently by states.

Therefore, the nursing diagnosis *Rape Trauma Syndrome* should be revised to *Sexual Assault Trauma Syndrome*. Based on the most recent definition of syndrome nursing diagnoses as a cluster of associated nursing diagnoses, this diagnosis does not represent a syndrome. This diagnosis needs revision. By adding related nursing diagnoses the inclusion of causative or contributing factors with this category is unnecessary, because the etiology is always rape. Thus, the nurse omits the second part of the diagnostic statement; however, he or she can add the individual's report of the rape to the statement. For example, *Sexual Assault Trauma Syndrome as evidenced by the report of a sexual assault and sodomy on June 22 and multiple facial bruises* (refer to ER record for description).

As a family nurse practitioner, this author has interacted with numerous girls and women who have shared their sexual assault, some for the first time in their lives. Two themes are woven into their stories: (1) guilt that they contributed to the assault and (2) profound disappointment with their mother's response. Many mothers blamed their daughter for the event and sometimes refuse to believe their daughter if a relative or paramour is involved; or they suggest their daughter provoked the event. Perhaps that was the only reaction a mother could have at the time, because she could not face the truth. I discussed forgiveness with these women. Forgiveness never means you accept what happened only that you are going to release the pain from yourself. It is a gift you give yourself.

Girls and women shared stories that the rape would not have happened if they had not:

Worn that short skirt
Drank too much
Walked home in the dark
Had engaged in kissing and hugging
Had not gone somewhere alone with him

I share with each girl or woman this scenario: Instead of being sexually assaulted, imagine that you were hit over the head with a shovel. Would it have mattered what you were wearing, doing, or saying at the time? Sexual assault is not sex, it is a violent act like hitting someone with a shovel. I suggest when thoughts of self-blame surface, these women think of the shovel.

Kevin Caruso wrote "And remember that all rapists are cowards, criminals, and losers and belong in prison. There never is an excuse for rape, and it is always a very serious crime" (Accessed at http://www.suicide.org/rape-victims-prone-to-suicide.html).

Errors in Diagnostic Statements

See *Post-Trauma Syndrome*.

Key Concepts

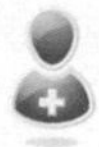

CLINICAL ALERT State laws differ regarding mandatory reporting of abuse or assaults on adults. Some states require reporting of elder abuse to Adult Protective Services (APS) and/or the police. Some states require mandatory reporting of visible evidence of domestic violence. It is important to understand that a health-care professional can report a suspicion of abuse or neglect to the appropriate agency. An investigation will determine if the suspicion is valid. Suspicions should be reported: it is better to be proven wrong rather than for unreported abuse to continue.

General Considerations

- Department of Justice's National Crime Victimization Survey (NCVS)—there is an average of 293,066 victims (aged 12 or older) of rape and sexual assault each year (U.S. Department of Justice, 2014).
- Sexual assault is a crime using sexual means to humiliate or degrade the victim. Someone commits sexual acts against a nonconsenting person. Rape violates the victim's right of privacy, sense of security, safety, and well-being.
- The following statistics are reported about sexual assault: U.S. Department of Justice, *National Crime Victimization Study: 2009 to 2013* (Source: Rape, Abuse and Incest National Network [RAINN], 2009).
  - 44% of victims are under age 18.
  - 80% are under age 30.
  - Approximately four-fifth of assaults are committed by someone known to the victim.
  - 47% of rapists are a friend or acquaintance.
  - 5% are a relative.
  - Approximately 50% of all rape/sexual assault incidents were reported by victims to have occurred within 1 mile of their home or at their home.
- The following were reported: (Department of Health and Human Services, 2012)
  - Persons under 18 years of age account for 67% of all sexual assault victimizations reported to law enforcement agencies. Children under 12 years old account for 34% of those cases, and children under 6 years old account for 14% of those cases.
  - The majority of both female and male victims of rape knew the person who raped them.
  - Rape victims are four times more likely to have contemplated suicide after the rape than noncrime victims, and 13 times more likely than noncrime victims to have attempted suicide.
  - Women who experience rape, stalking, and/or intimate partner violence are significantly more likely to experience asthma, irritable bowel syndrome, diabetes, frequent headaches, chronic pain, difficulty sleeping, activity limitations, poor physical health, and poor mental health than women who have not had such experiences.
  - Men who experience rape, stalking, and/or intimate partner violence are significantly more likely to experience frequent headaches, chronic pain, difficulty sleeping, activity limitations, poor physical health, and poor mental health than men who have not had such experiences.

- Various agencies (Justice Department, National Crime Victimization Survey: 2008 to 2012. FBI, Uniform Crime Reports, Arrest Data: 2006 to 2010, FBI, Uniform Crime Reports, Offenses Cleared Data: 2006 to 2010. Department of Justice, Felony Defendants in Large Urban Counties: 2009. Department of Justice, Felony Defendants in Large Urban Counties: 2009 [accessed at https://rainn.org/get-information/statistics/reporting-rates].) have reported out of every 100 rapes:
  - 32 get reported.
  - 7 lead to arrest.
  - 3 are referred to prosecutors.
  - 2 lead to a felony conviction.
  - 2 rapists will spend a single day in prison.
  - The other 98 will walk free.
- Some myths about rape include the following (*Heinrich, 1987):
  - The rapist is a sexually unsatisfied man who cannot control his urges.
  - Rape is a one-time incident, representing a momentary lapse in judgment.
  - Rapists are strangers.
  - The victim provokes the rape.
  - Only promiscuous women get raped.
  - Rapes happen to women who are out alone at night. If a woman stays home, she will be safe.
  - Women cannot be raped against their will—they can avoid rape by resistance.
  - Most rapes involve black men and white women.
  - Women respect men for overpowering them; they may even enjoy the rape.
  - Rapists are mentally ill or retarded and, therefore, not responsible for their acts.
- Victims, families, society, and caregivers who subscribe to these myths may not view themselves as victims or recognize the criminality of sexual assault, may not seek help, or may be denied supportive interventions (*Heinrich, 1987).
- Rapists can be divided into three broad categories (*Petter & Whitehill, 1998):
  - **Power rapists** (55% of sexual assaults): Attack persons near their age and use intimidation and minimal violence to control. The attack is premeditated.
  - **Anger rapists** (40% of sexual assaults): Target the very young or elderly. They use extreme force and restraints, resulting in physical injury.
  - **Sadistic rapists** (5% of sexual assaults): Attack is premeditated. They derive erotic satisfaction from torturing.

Barriers to Reporting Sexual Assault (U.S. Department of Justice, 2014)

- Individuals who have been sexually assaulted may be reluctant to report the assault to law enforcement and to seek medical attention for a variety of reasons as follows:
  - Blame themselves for the sexual assault and feel embarrassed.
  - Fear of retaliation from assailant(s)
  - Worry about whether they will be believed.
  - May lack the ability or emotional strength to access services
  - May not have their own transportation or access to public transportation
  - May also not speak English well
  - Fear that reporting the assault may jeopardize their immigration status.
  - May lack health insurance and may not be aware that as a crime victim, they are eligible for financial reimbursements for certain services
  - May perceive the medical forensic examination as yet another violation
  - Because of its extensive and intrusive nature in the immediate aftermath of the assault, rather than seek assistance, a sexual assault victim may simply want to go somewhere safe, clean up, and try to forget the assault ever happened.

R: *Sexual assault is a crime of violence against a person's body and will. Sex offenders use physical and/or psychological aggression or coercion to victimize, in the process threatening a victim's sense of privacy, safety, autonomy, and well-being.*

Male-on-Male Sexual Assault

- Male-on-male rape has been heavily *stigmatized*. According to psychologist Dr. Sarah Crome, fewer than 1 in 10 male–male rapes are reported. As a group, male rape victims reported a lack of services and support, and legal systems are often ill equipped to deal with this type of crime (Masho & Anderson, 2009).

- Masho and Anderson (2009) reported that male-to-male sexual assault has a lifetime prevalence of 12.9% among men, with 94% assaulted for the first time before the age of 18. It is also evident that victimized men were more likely to be depressed and ideate suicide and yet did not seek health services. Fewer than 1 in 10 male–male rapes are reported.
- RAINN (2009) reported the following on male-on-male sexual assault:
  - Anxiety, depression, fearfulness, or post-traumatic stress disorder
  - Concerns or questions about sexual orientation
  - Sense of blame or shame over not being able to stop the assault or abuse, especially if you experienced an erection or ejaculation
  - Feeling on edge, being unable to relax, and having difficulty sleeping
  - Feel like "less of a man" or that you no longer have control over your own body
  - Avoiding people or places that are related to the assault or abuse
  - Fear of the worst happening and having a sense of a shortened future
  - Withdrawal from relationships or friendships and an increased sense of isolation
- Male rape victims (including homosexuals) are unlikely to report the rape but are most likely to experience symptoms of rape trauma syndrome (*Carson & Smith-DiJulio, 2006).

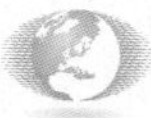

Transcultural Considerations

- The battered woman may come from a culture that accepts domestic violence and may be isolated by cultural dynamics that do not permit her to seek assistance. Additionally, language barriers may interfere with her ability to call 911 or learn about her rights or legal options.
- The professional nurse has an obligation to report injuries and to protect the victim. In situations of spousal rape with no visible injuries, the victim should be informed of options available. State laws differ regarding mandatory reporting.

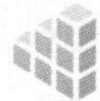

Pediatric Considerations

- Dube et al. (2005) reported "that boys and girls are vulnerable to this form of childhood maltreatment; the similarity in the likelihood for multiple behavioral, mental, and social outcomes among men and women suggests the need to identify and treat all adults affected by childhood sexual abuse."
- In the United States, it is illegal to have sexual intercourse with a child younger than 12. Adolescents are not afforded the same legal protection (Hockenberry & Wilson, 2015).
- Persons under 18 years of age account for 67% of all sexual assault victimizations reported to law enforcement agencies. Children under 12 years old account for 34% of those cases, and children under 6 years old account for 14% of those cases.
- Statuary rape is when the victim is unable to legally give consent because of age (age varies from state to state), mental deficiencies, psychosis, or altered state of consciousness (sleep, drugs, illness, alcohol) (Hockenberry & Wilson, 2015).
- The assailant of a child is most likely someone the child knows, and the assaults usually have occurred for some time within the child's own home or neighborhood. Greater emotional distress and long-term effects have been reported when a child knew and trusted the abuser.
- Adolescents, particularly boys, are more prone to attempt suicide in the aftermath of rape.
- Acquaintance rape is very prevalent among college-aged women and is believed to be underrecognized and underreported.
- Adolescent girls frequently underreport acquaintance rape because they believe they may have contributed to the act in some way (e.g., alcohol use).
- Drug-facilitated sexual assaults are caused by slipping a drug in a drink. "Date rape" drugs are Rohypnol, gamma-hydroxybutyrate (GHB), Burundanga, datura, and ketamine. They cause disinhibition, passivity, relaxation of muscles, and amnesia (Women's Health.org, 2012).

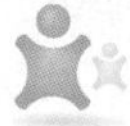

Maternal Considerations

- Refer to *Disabled Family Coping—Domestic Violence*.

Geriatric Considerations

- Elder abuse, including neglect and exploitation, is experienced by 1 out of every 10 people aged 60 and older who lives at home (Acierno et al., 2010). For every one case of elder abuse that is detected or reported, it is estimated that approximately 23 cases remain hidden (Lifespan of Greater Rochester, Inc., 2011).

- Researchers analyzed data from 5,777 adults aged 60 years or older in a randomly selected national sample. One-year prevalence was 4.6% for emotional abuse, 1.6% for physical abuse, 0.6% for sexual abuse, 5.1% for potential neglect, and 5.2% for current financial abuse by a family member. Slightly under 7% reported sexual mistreatment before age 60 (Acierno et al., 2010).
- Only 7% of elder abuse cases are reported, and of these cases less than 1% were sexual (Teaster, Dugar, Mendiondo, Abner, & Cecil, 2006).
- Residents of nursing homes are the most vulnerable to abuse. The failure to address the problem of sexual abuse may be the result of the incomprehensibility of sexual assault of nursing home residents and generalized negative attitudes or hostility toward older and cognitively impaired persons (*Burgess, Dowdell, & Prentley, 2000).
- Burgess et al. (*2000) found that of 20 nursing home victims of sexual assault, 11 died within 1 year of the assault. These victims are not equipped physically, constitutionally, or psychologically to defend themselves or to cope with the aftermath.
- Elder abuse may include physical and sexual abuse, psychological abuse, neglect, exploitation, and medical abuse (*Goldstein, 2005).

Focus Assessment Criteria

Clinical Alert A detailed assessment and examination is necessary for the individual, who has been sexually assaulted. Due to the exceptional, overwhelming emotions that are involved and the possibility of litigation, the nurse should be a Sexual Assault Nurse Examiner (SANE). SANE is a qualification for forensic nurses who have received special training to conduct sexual assault evidentiary examinations for sexual assault victims and may provide expert testimony if a case goes to trial.

Under the SANE model of care, sexual assault victims consistently receive prompt, compassionate, culturally sensitive, and developmentally appropriate services from nurses knowledgeable about victimization issues and expert in assessment and evidence collection that will support future legal proceedings (Stokowski, 2008, p. 1).

The Sexual Assault Response Team (SART) is a community-based team that coordinates the response to victims of sexual assault. The team may be comprised of SANEs, hospital personnel, sexual assault victim advocates, law enforcement, prosecutors, judges, and any other professionals with a specific interest in assisting victims of sexual assault.

Professional nurses, who are not SANE-certified should have available access to a SANE-certified nurse. If it is impossible, then the nurse must proceed following the national guidelines. These guidelines should be available in their health-care settings.

Carp's Cues

Non-SANE nurses can provide sensitive, compassionate, and competent care to the individual, who has been sexually assaulted and their significant others. If the nurse is negative, biased, or judgmental, it is his/her responsibility to step aside and "do no harm," or be asked to do so by a nurse colleague.

Subjective Data (Must Be Recorded)

Refer to Standard of Care for an individual who has been sexually assaulted.

Objective Data

Assess for Injury (Ecchymoses, Lacerations, Abrasions)

Gastrointestinal system (mouth, anus, abdomen)
Skeletal muscle system
Genitourinary system

Assess the Emotional Responses

Crying
Composure
Hysteria
Detachment
Withdrawal

Assess for Change in Behavior in the Cognitively Impaired (*Burgess et al., 2000)

Avoidance behavior with males
Staying near nurses' station
Lying in fetal position
Fear of men
Withdrawal behavior

Goals

NOC

Abused Protection, Abuse Recovery, Coping

The individual, parents, partner/spouse, or significant other will return to precrisis level of functioning, and the child will express feelings concerning the assault and the treatment based on the following indicators:

Short-Term Goals

- Shares feelings
- Describes rationale and treatment procedures
- Identifies members of support system and use them appropriately

Long-Term Goals

- Reports sleeping well
- Reports return to former eating pattern
- Reports occasional somatic reactions or none
- Demonstrates calmness and relaxation

Interventions

NIC

Abuse Protection Support, Coping Enhancement, Rape Trauma Treatment, Support Group, Anxiety Reduction, Presence, Emotional Support, Calming Technique, Active Listening, Family Support, Grief Work Facilitation

Ask the Person: How Can I Help You?

Assist in Identifying Major Concerns (Psychological, Medical, Legal) and Perception of Help Needed

R: *The earlier intervention begins with a rape victim, the less psychological damage she or he will incur. Many victims try to suppress the memory of the assault, so postponing counseling even 1 day may weaken their pursuit of follow-up care. Immediate contact with a counselor may overcome this reluctance.*

Explain the Care and Examination

- Provide interventions in an unhurried manner.
- Do not leave the individual alone.
- Help to meet personal needs (bathing *after* examination and evidence has been acquired).
- Explain every detail before acting and secure permission.

R: *Because the client's right to deny or consent has been violated, it is important to seek permission for care (*Heinrich, 1987). The goal is to establish a safe and empathetic environment.*

- If a family member, partner, or spouse is suspected, request a urine sample and accompany the individual alone to the bathroom. Gently explore who hurt her/him.

Explain the Legal Issues and Police Investigation (*Heinrich, 1987)

Promote a Trusting Relationship

- Stay with the individual during acute stage or arrange for other support.
- Brief on police and hospital procedures during acute stage.
- Explain that the choice to report the rape is the victim's. Explore pros and cons of reporting.

R: *Improved emotional outcomes have been reported by victims who have reported the crime.*

- Refer to Standard of Care or SANE Nurse for guidance in the postassault care.

R: *The evidentiary examination is especially distressing because it can be reminiscent of the assault (*Ledray, 2001). The medical–legal examination serves to assess the condition of the victim and to gather documentary evidence. It consists of a general examination; oral, pelvic, and rectal examinations; a culture for sperm and sexually transmitted diseases; serum pregnancy test; blood typing; and a drug and alcohol screen. Obvious debris is placed in separate envelopes. Dried sperm is collected. The victim's pubic hair and head hair are combed, and samples are placed in separate envelopes. Fingernail scrapings are placed in separate envelopes for each hand (*Heinrich, 1987).*

- If the police interview is permitted:
  - Negotiate with the individual and police for an advantageous time.
  - Explain to the individual what kind of questions will be asked.
  - Remain with the individual during the interview; do not ask questions or offer answers.

Whenever Possible, Provide Crisis Counseling Within 1 Hour of Rape

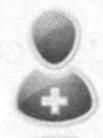

CLINICAL ALERT If the officer is insensitive, intimidating, or offensive, or asks improper questions, discuss this with the officer in private. If the behavior continues, use proper channels and make a complaint.

- Ask permission to contact the rape crisis counselor.
- Be flexible and individualize the approach according to the individual's needs.
- Observe the victim's behavior carefully and record objective data.
- Encourage the victim to verbalize thoughts, feelings, or perceptions of the event.
- Explore available support systems; involve significant others if appropriate.
- Assess stress tolerance.
- Respect the victim's rights; honor wishes to restrict unwanted visitors; offer privacy when appropriate.
- Explain to the victim that this experience will disrupt her or his life, and that feelings that occurred during acute phase may recur; encourage the victim to proceed at her or his own pace.
- Counsel family and friends at their level.
- Share the immediate needs of the victim for love and support.

R: *Rape crisis centers provide rape victims and significant others with information concerning the medical examination, police interrogation, and court procedures; they provide escort service to hospital, police department, and courts; and they provide information about counseling.*

Explain the Risks of Sexually Transmitted Infections (Centers for Disease Control and Prevention, 2013; ***Ledray,** 2001)

- Sexually transmitted diseases (specimens, blood tests): gonorrhea, human immunodeficiency virus (HIV), trichomoniasis, syphilis, hepatitis B, A, C, chlamydia.
- Consult with protocol or physician/nurse practitioner for prophylaxis for chlamydia, HIV, trichomoniasis, gonorrhea.

R: *Certain sexually transmitted infections (STIs) can be treated with medications to eliminate pathogens. The Centers for Disease Control and Prevention (2008) recommend HIV postexposure prophylaxis if began within 48 hours.*

- Vaccinate individuals if needed for tetanus and hepatitis A, B.

R: *An assault outdoors carries the risk for tetanus infection. Hepatitis A and B can be transmitted via body fluids.*

- Determine if the victim is at risk for pregnancy and, if at risk, explain emergency contraceptive pills (ECP).
- No contraceptive use.
- No surgical sterilization.
- Postmenopausal.

Eliminate or Reduce Somatic Symptomatology

Gastrointestinal Irritability

Anorexia

- Offer small, frequent feedings.
- Provide appealing foods.
- Record intake.
- Refer to *Imbalanced Nutrition* if anorexia is prolonged.

Nausea

- Avoid gas-forming foods.
- Restrict carbonated beverages.
- Observe for abdominal distention.
- Offer antiemetic.
- Explain that the side effects of emergency contraceptive pills (ECPs) are nausea and vomiting.

Genitourinary Discomfort

Pain

- Assess for quality and duration.

- Monitor intake and output.
- Inspect urine and external genitalia for bleeding.
- Listen attentively to the victim's description of pain.
- Give pain medication per physician's order (see *Impaired Comfort*).

Discharge

- Assess amount, color, and odor of discharge.
- Allow the victim time to wash and change garments after initial examination has been completed.

Skeletal Muscle Tension

Headaches

- Avoid any sudden change of the victim's position.
- Approach the victim calmly.
- Slightly elevate the bed (unless contraindicated).
- Discuss pain-reducing measures that have been effective in the past.

Generalized Bruising and Edema

- Avoid constrictive garments.
- Handle affected body parts gently.
- Elevate affected body part if edema is present.
- Apply a cool, moist compress to the edematous area for the first 24 hours, then a warm compress after 24 hours.
- Encourage the victim to verbalize discomfort.
- Record any bruises, lacerations, edema, or abrasions.

R: *The interventions for rape trauma syndrome are listed for usefulness under the varied responses for each victim; minimize any further trauma.*

Proceed With Health Teaching to Individual and Family

- Before the individual leaves the hospital, provide a card with information about follow-up appointments and names and telephone numbers of local crisis and counseling centers.
- Plan a home visit or telephone call.
- Arrange for legal or pastoral counseling, if appropriate.
- Recommend and make referrals to a psychotherapist, mental health clinic, citizen action, or community group advocacy-related service.

R: *Some long-term problems can be prevented if the victim's family and friends recognize symptoms as normal. Responses of others can help or hinder recovery greatly. Significant others may also face a crisis and the need for recovery (Adams & Fay, 1989).*

Teach Management of Discomforts

Risks for Individual Sexually Assaulted at College or University

R: *In a survey of college women, 13.3% indicated that they have been forced to have sex in a dating situation (Black, 2011).*

- How to protect yourself from "date rape drugs". (Source: Date rape drugs fact sheet accessed at https://www.womenshealth.gov/publications/our-publications/fact-sheet/date-rape-drugs.html.)

Advise Women and Men to

- Insist on pouring your own drink or watching while your drink is mixed or prepared.
- Do not drink from group drinks such as punch bowls.
- Keep an eye on your drink or open can; Do not trust someone else to watch your drink for you.
- If your opened drink tastes, looks, or smells strange, do not drink it!
- If you think you've been drugged, do not be afraid to seek medical attention immediately.
- Get help for anyone who seems like they may have been drugged—even if you don't know them, stay with them.

Instruct on How One Can Tell He/She Was Drugged

- You feel drunk and haven't drunk any alcohol—or, you feel like the effects of drinking alcohol are stronger than usual.
- You wake up feeling very hung over and disoriented or having no memory of a period of time.
- You remember having a drink, but cannot recall anything after that.

- You find that your clothes are torn or not on right.
- You feel like you had sex, but you cannot remember it.

R: *Most victims don't remember being drugged or assaulted. The victim might not be aware of the attack until 8 or 12 hours after it occurred. These drugs also leave the body very quickly. Once a victim gets help, there might be no proof that drugs were involved in the attack. But there are some signs that you might have been drugged.*

If an Individual Thinks He/She Was Drugged and Sexually Assaulted Advise to

- Get medical care right away. Call 911 or have a trusted friend take you to a hospital emergency room. Don't urinate, douche, bathe, brush your teeth, wash your hands, change clothes, or eat or drink before you go. These things may give evidence of the rape. The hospital will use a "rape kit" to collect evidence.
- Call the police from the hospital. Tell the police exactly what you remember. Be honest about all your activities. Remember, nothing you did—including drinking alcohol or doing drugs—can justify rape.
- Ask the hospital to take a urine (pee) sample that can be used to test for date rape drugs. The drugs leave your system quickly. Rohypnol stays in the body for several hours, and can be detected in the urine up to 72 hours after taking it. GHB leaves the body in 12 hours. Don't urinate before going to the hospital.
- Don't pick up or clean up where you think the assault might have occurred. There could be evidence left behind—such as on a drinking glass or bed sheets.
- Get counseling and treatment. Feelings of shame, guilt, fear, and shock are normal. A counselor can help you work through these emotions and begin the healing process. Calling a crisis center or a hotline is a good place to start. One national hotline is the National Sexual Assault Hotline at 800-656-HOPE.

For Parents of Sexual Assault individuals (Appalachian State University, 2015)

- Refer to the Friends of Sexual Assault Survivors page at http://sexualassault.appstate.edu for a comprehensive, compassionate document on prevention and responses to sexual assault on campus.
- Realize that your initial feelings are valid.
- Spend time with your student, but accept that he or she may need time and space.
- Seek outside resources and support to help yourself get through this difficult time: talk to a counselor, close friend, or other parents of children who have been sexually assaulted.
- Don't make your student feel like they need to take care of you; let another trusted adult be your support person.
- Let your student tell you their needs.
- Tell them you love them and believe them.
- Try to understand as much as you can about sexual assault to best support both your child and yourself.
- Asking questions like "Why did you..." (wear those clothes, get in the car, etc.) may be interpreted as blaming and can be very hurtful.
- Remember the most important message you can give to your student is that you do not blame them.

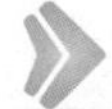

Carp's Cues

Parents may experience a variety of conflicting feelings, guilt, blaming their child, anger in response to sexual abuse. There is no such thing as bad thoughts, only bad words and actions. Their child probably feels she or he may be the cause for the assault; a poor decision does not justify an assault. Their parent's response will be remembered for their lifetime.

Older Adults Interventions

Suspect sexual abuse if the older adult has ecchymoses involving the breasts or genitalia, unexplained vaginal or anal bleeding, stained or torn undergarments, a preoccupation with sex, or a sexually transmitted infection (Lifespan of Greater Rochester, Inc., 2011).

R: *National studies have found that people 50 and older make up 3% of rape/sexual assault victims (Acierno et al., 2010).*

Assess Individuals of All Ages if They Have Ever Been Abused or Assaulted

R: *In a large study of adults over 60, almost 7% reported sexual mistreatment before age 60 (Acierno et al., 2010).*

Carp's Cues

Strong emotions may occur. This may provide the individual with the first opportunity to share their horror. Assumptions that initiating dialogue about past abuse is inappropriate are erroneous. Gentle sympathy with nonjudgmental listening are powerful healers.

Refer the Individual to an Agency to Evaluate Self-Care Ability Living Conditions and the Availability of Social Support

R: *Low social support was associated with more than triple the likelihood that mistreatment of any form would be reported (Acierno. et.al 2010). "Older adults who needed assistance with activities of daily life or who reported poor health were more likely to be targets, a finding that echoes past research on fraud and financial abuse of impaired older adults" (Acierno et al., 2010).*

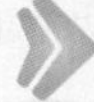

Carp's Cues

In your own community advocate for resources to enhance social support of older adults through a variety of channels, such as reconnection with community resources, improved housing designs for older adults that maximize communal interaction, funding for familial and community programs that bring together the elderly and their neighbors or family members, or—perhaps most important—affordable transportation (Acierno et al., 2010).

POWERLESSNESS

Powerlessness

Risk for Powerlessness

NANDA-I Definition

The lived experience of lack of control over a situation, including a perception that one's actions do not significantly affect an outcome

Defining Characteristics

Overt (anger, apathy) or covert expressions of dissatisfaction over inability to control a situation (e.g., work, illness, prognosis, care, recovery rate) that negatively affects outlook, goals, and lifestyle
Inability to access valued resources (food, shelter, income, education, employment)
Belief that one has little or no control over the cause or the solutions of one's problems

Lack of Information-Seeking Behaviors
Excessive dependence on others
Acting-out behavior
Violent behavior
Inability to effectively problem solve
Passivity
Apathy
Anger
Feelings of alienation
Low self-efficacy
Resignation
Anxiety
Depression
Sense of vulnerability
Feelings of helplessness

Related Factors

Pathophysiologic

Any disease process, acute or chronic, can cause or contribute to powerlessness. Some common sources are as follows:

Related to inability to communicate secondary to:

Stroke
Alzheimer's or Parkinson's disease (dysarthria)
Intubation, mechanical ventilation, or tracheostomy

Related to inability to perform activities of daily living or role responsibilities secondary to surgery, trauma, or arthritis

Related to progressive debilitating disease secondary to such diseases as multiple sclerosis, terminal cancer, or AIDS

Related to substance abuse

Related to cognitive distortions secondary to mental health disorders

Situational (Personal, Environmental)

Related to change from curative status to palliative status

Related to feeling of loss of control and lifestyle restrictions secondary to (specify)

Related to overeating patterns

Related to personal characteristics that highly value control (e.g., internal locus of control)

Related to effects of hospital or institutional limitations

Related to elevated fear of disapproval

Related to consistent negative feedback

Related to long-term abusive relationships

Related to oppressive patriarchal values with women

Related to the presence of an abusive relationships with a history of mental illness (Orzeck, Rokach, & Chin, 2010)

Maturational

Older Adult

Related to multiple losses secondary to aging (e.g., retirement, sensory deficits, motor deficits, money, significant others)

Author's Note

Powerlessness is a feeling that all people experience to varying degrees in various situations. Stephenson (*1979) described two types of powerlessness: (1) *situational powerlessness* occurs in a specific event and is probably short-lived; (2) *trait powerlessness* is more pervasive, affecting general outlook, goals, lifestyle, and relationships.

Hopelessness differs from powerlessness in that a hopeless individual sees no solution to problems or no way to achieve what is desired, even if he or she feels in control. A powerless individual may see an alternative or answer, yet is unable to do anything about it because of perception of lack of control and resources. Prolonged powerlessness may lead to hopelessness.

Errors in Diagnostic Statements

Powerlessness related to hospitalization

Hospitalization evokes varied responses in people and families, including anxiety, fear, and powerlessness. If the hospitalization is expected to be short, the diagnosis of *Anxiety* related to unfamiliar environment, loss of usual routines, and invasion of privacy may be useful to describe situational powerlessness. If the hospitalization is a readmission for a continuing problem, *Powerlessness* may be more appropriate to describe trait powerlessness. The nurse should restate the diagnosis as *Powerlessness* related to readmission for pulmonary infection and effects of illness on career and marriage.

Key Concepts

General Considerations

- An individual's response to loss of control depends on the meaning of the loss, individual coping patterns, personal characteristics (psychological, sociologic, cultural, spiritual), and response of others.
- When an individual does not expect to be able to control outcomes, attention to and retention of information are poor.
- *Powerlessness* is closely related to, but not synonymous with, the concept of external versus internal locus of control. Locus of control is a rather stable personality trait, whereas powerlessness is situationally determined.
- People with an internal locus of control believe they can affect outcomes by actively manipulating themselves or the environment. Examples of internal behavior are participating in regular exercise, acquiring printed literature about a new diagnosis, or learning assertiveness skills.

- People with external locus of control believe that outcomes are outside their control and attribute what happens to them, to others, or to fate. Examples of external behavior are losing weight because of fear of a professional's response and blaming others for present position (e.g., depression, anger).
- Internally controlled people motivate themselves, whereas externally controlled people usually need others to motivate them. Young children are usually internally controlled but can learn to be externally controlled. For example, a child can learn to keep a record of the nutrients needed daily and his intake of them to help him understand the concept of good nutrition and to encourage him to take responsibility for his eating patterns.
- People with an internal locus of control may experience the loss of decision-making ability more profoundly than those with an external locus of control. Individuals with external locus of control seem to be more prone to develop powerlessness.
- *Powerlessness* is part of a continuum with hopelessness and helplessness.

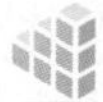

Pediatric Considerations

- Hospitalized children commonly experience powerlessness.
- Differentiating *Powerlessness* from *Anxiety* and *Fear* may be difficult, especially in children. Refer to Key Concepts and Pediatric Considerations under *Anxiety* and *Fear*.
- Children with a more positive self-concept and a higher perceived ability to control their own health were more likely to adhere to treatments (*Burkhart & Rayens, 2005).

Geriatric Considerations

- Older adults are at high risk for powerlessness because multiple losses (previous roles, family, health, and functioning) may accompany the aging process.
- A source of power is gained by being able to control one's own life; however, this can be derailed by powerlessness experienced in negative client–nurse relationships (Haugan, Innstrand, & Moksnes, 2013).
- Personality traits, various effects of diseases, and environmental conditions affect powerlessness. For older adults, disease states might restrict mobility. Changes in environment (e.g., relocating to an extended care facility) can remove opportunities for decision making and autonomy. Institutional policy may require physical or chemical restraints for certain agitated behaviors (Miller, 2015).
- Late-life changes in role, resources, and responsibility can contribute to feelings of loss of control.
- Extensive interactions with caregivers, rather than peers, can lead to a sense of powerlessness. This has implications for the older individual, who, with an increased chance of multiple chronic illnesses, might be in the sick role for an extended period (Miller, 2015).
- In the elderly, perceived control over desirable outcomes is linked to high emotional well-being; conversely, perceived control by others is an emotional risk factor.

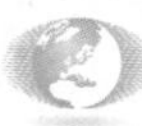

Transcultural Considerations

- The diagnosis of *Powerlessness* can be problematic with individuals from various cultures. In Latin cultures, the concept of fatalism (e.g., what will be, will be) may be a challenge to a nurse who is trying to initiate a lifestyle change for better health (Andrews & Boyle, 2012; Giger, 2013).
- Appropriate language interaction, inclusion of individual and family, and health care provider's ability to show respect and compassion can prevent many health-care-related problems encountered by (*Garrett, Dickson, Young, & Whelan, 2008) individuals with limited English proficiency (Nápoles-Springer, Ortíz, O'Brien, & Díaz-Méndez, 2009).
- Thomas and Gonzalez-Prendes (*2009) found powerlessness experiences by African American women to be associated with oppressive socioeconomic conditions including sexism and racism; in this sense, powerlessness leads to anger and stress and eventually adverse health status.
- Hinton and Earnst (2010) found that the conditions of women's lives in Papua New Guinea exerted a powerful influence on their health. Women interviewed expressed feelings of powerlessness, helplessness, and hopelessness in response to their constant struggle with unequal social relationships, economic constraints, workload demands, and regular abuse and violence.

Focus Assessment Criteria

Because powerlessness is subjective, the nurse must validate with the individual all inferences concerning the individual's feelings of powerlessness. The nurse assesses each individual to determine his or her usual level of control and decision making and the effects that losing elements of control has had. To plan effective interventions, the nurse must determine whether the individual usually seeks to change his or her own behaviors to control problems or whether he or she expects others or external factors to control problems.

Subjective Data

Assess for Defining Characteristics

Decision-Making Patterns

"How would you describe your usual method of making decisions (career, financial, health care)?"

"Do you make your decisions alone?" "Do you consult with others for advice? Whom?"

"Do you allow others to make decisions for you (spouse, children, others)?" "If so, under what circumstances?"

Individual and Role Responsibilities

Ask what responsibilities the individual has

At school

At home

At work

In community and religious organizations

Assess for Related Factors

Perception of Control

"How would you describe your ability—high, moderate, fair, or poor—to control or cure your present health problem (e.g., diabetes mellitus, aphasia, activity intolerance, obesity)?"

"To what do you attribute your (high, moderate, fair, poor) ability to control?"

Objective Data

Assess for Defining Characteristics

Appearance

Participation in Appearance (Grooming and Hygiene) Care (When Indicated)

Actively seeks involvement

Requires reminders or prompts

Reluctant to participate; requires encouragement

Refuses to participate

Information-Seeking Behaviors

Actively seeks information and literature from others concerning condition

Requires encouragement to ask questions

Refuses to receive information

Expresses lack of interest

Response to Limits Placed on Decision-Making and Self-Control Behaviors

Acceptance

Apathy

Depression

Attempts to circumvent limits

Ignores limits

Increases attempts to exercise control

Anger

Withdrawal

Nonverbal Language

Posture

Tone of voice

Eye contact

Gestures

Goals

NOC

Depression Control, Health Beliefs: Perceived Ability to Perform, Health Beliefs: Perceived Control, Participation: Health Care Decisions

The individual will verbalize the ability to control or influence situations and outcomes, as evidenced by the following indicators:

- Identifies the factors that the individual can control
- Makes decisions regarding his or her care, treatment, and future when possible

Interventions

NIC

Mood Management, Teaching: Individual, Decision-Making Support, Self-Responsibility Facilitation, Health System Guidance, Spiritual Support

Assess for Causative and Contributing Factors

- Lack of knowledge
- Previous inadequate coping patterns (e.g., depression; for discussion, see *Ineffective Coping* related to depression)
- Insufficient decision-making opportunities

Eliminate or Reduce Contributing Factors, If Possible

Lack of Knowledge

- Increase effective communication between individual and health care provider.
- Explain all procedures, rules, and options to the individual; avoid medical jargon. Help the individual anticipate situations that will occur during treatments (provides reality-oriented cognitive images that bolster a sense of control and coping strategies).
- Allow time to answer questions; ask the individual to write questions down so he or she does not forget them.
- Provide a specific time (10 to 15 minutes) per shift that the individual knows can be used to ask questions or discuss subjects as desired. Allow individual to verbalize concerns and feelings.
- Anticipate questions and offer information. Help the individual to anticipate events and outcomes.
- While being realistic, point out positive changes in the individual's condition, such as serum enzymes decreasing after myocardial infarction or surgical incision healing well.
- Provide opportunities for the individual and family to identify with a primary nurse to establish continuity in provision of care and implementation of the care plan.

R: *Powerlessness can be ameliorated by implementing coping strategies and by having consistent and reliable nursing care in a patient-centered environment (Haugan, Innstrand, & Moksnes, 2013).*

- If contributing factors are pain or anxiety, provide information about how to use behavioral control techniques (e.g., relaxation, imagery, deep breathing).

R: *Feelings of powerlessness and helplessness are closely associated with incurable diseases (Meeker, Waldrop, Schneider, & Case, 2013).*

Provide Opportunities for the Individual to Control Decisions and to Identify Personal Goals of Care

- Allow the individual to manipulate surroundings, such as deciding what is to be kept where (shoes under bed, picture on window).
- If the individual desires, and as agency policy permits, encourage the individual to bring personal effects from home (e.g., pillows, pictures).
- Do not offer options if there are none (e.g., necessity for turn, cough, and deep breathing after cardiac surgery despite the pain). If there are options, respect and follow the individual's decision.
- Record the individual's specific choices in care plan to ensure that others on staff acknowledge preferences ("dislikes orange juice," "takes showers," "plan dressing change at 7:30 AM before shower").
- Keep promises.
- Shift emphasis from what one cannot do to what one can do.
- Set goals that are short-term, behavioral, practical, and realistic (walk five more feet every day; then in 1 week, individual can walk to the television room).
- Allow the individual to experience outcomes that result from his or her own actions.

R: *People with chronic illness require adjustments in their perceptions of self as their level of autonomy changes. Integrating the limitations that come with chronic illness can assist the individual toward the maximum state of independence possible (Abad-Corpa et al., 2012). People with a sense of hope, self-control, direction, purpose, and identity are better able to meet the challenges of their disease.*

Actively Involve the Individual With External Locus of Control to Monitor Progress

- Have the individual keep a record (e.g., food intake for 1 week; weight loss chart; exercise program; type and frequency of medications taken).
- Provide explicit written directions (e.g., meal plans; exercise regimen—type, frequency, duration; speech practice lessons for aphasia).

R: *Create a learning environment that assists the individual to identify self-management strategies that are meaningful to him or her.*

Assist the Individual in Deriving Power From Other Sources

- Support use of other power sources (e.g., prayer, stress reduction techniques). Provide privacy and support for measures the individual or family may request (e.g., meditation, imagery, special rituals).
- Suggest self-help groups focusing on empowerment.
- Offer referral to faith-based community resources (e.g., religious leaders, faith community nurse, house of worship).

R: *Self-help groups that focused on empowerment issues assisted participants in the direction of valuable progress toward recovery (*Stang & Mittelmark, 2008).*

R: *The individual can be empowered through enhanced educational experiences and opportunities to share their fears and concerns (*Johansson, Salantera, & Katajisto, 2007).*

R: *Setting realistic goals can increase motivation and hope.*

R: *Self-concept can be enhanced when individuals actively engage in decisions regarding health and lifestyle.*

Initiate Health Teaching and Referrals as Indicated (Social Worker, Psychiatric Nurse/Physician, Visiting Nurse, Religious Leader, Self-Help Groups)

Evaluate the Situation with the Individual

- When feelings of powerlessness have subsided, review with the individual what worked best to diminish or alleviate the intensity of the experience.

R: *Self-concept can be enhanced when individuals actively engage in decisions regarding health and lifestyle.*

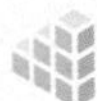

Pediatric Interventions

- Provide opportunities for the child to make decisions (e.g., set time for bath, hold still for injection).
- Engage the child in play therapy before and after a traumatic situation (refer to *Delayed Growth and Development* for specific interventions for age-related development needs).

R: *The goals of nursing interventions to treat powerlessness include modifying the environment to resemble the child's home and providing opportunities for acceptable control. Children can gain mastery over stressful situations by participating in play activities while ill or hospitalized (Hockenberry & Wilson, 2015).*

Risk for Powerlessness

NANDA-I Definition

At risk for the lived experience of lack of control over a situation, including a perception that one's actions do not significantly affect an outcome

Risk Factors

Refer to Related Factors in *Powerlessness*.

Focus Assessment Criteria

Refer to *Powerlessness*.

Goals

Refer to *Powerlessness*.

Interventions

Refer to *Powerlessness*.

INEFFECTIVE PROTECTION

NANDA-I Definition

Decrease in the ability to guard self from internal or external threats, such as illness or injury

Defining Characteristics*

Deficient immunity
Maladaptive stress response
Chilling
Fatigue
Cough
Immobility
Impaired healing
Neurosensory alterations
Insomnia
Dyspnea
Weakness
Restlessness
Altered clotting
Pressure ulcers
Perspiring
Anorexia
Itching
Disorientation

Author's Note

This broad diagnosis describes an individual with compromised ability to defend against microorganisms, bleeding, or both because of immunosuppression, myelosuppression, abnormal clotting factors, or all these. Use of this diagnosis entails several potential problems.

The nurse is cautioned against substituting *Ineffective Protection* for an immune system compromise, AIDS, disseminated intravascular coagulation, diabetes mellitus, or other disorders. Rather, the nurse should focus on diagnoses describing the individual's functional abilities that are or may be compromised by altered protection, such as *Fatigue*, *Risk for Infection*, and *Risk for Social Isolation*. The nurse also should address the physiologic complications of altered protection that require nursing and medical interventions for management, identifying appropriate collaborative problems.

For example, the nurse could use *Ineffective Protection* in each of these three cases: Mr. A, who has leukemia, leukopenia, and no evidence of infection; Mr. B, who is experiencing sickle cell crisis; and Mr. C, who has AIDS. The problem is that this diagnosis does not describe the specific focus of nursing but describes situations in which more specific responses can be diagnosed. For Mr. A, the nursing diagnosis of *Risk for Infection* related to compromised immune system would apply. For Mr. B, the collaborative problem *Risk for Complications of Sickle Cell Crisis* best describes this situation, which the nurse monitors and manages using physician- and nurse-prescribed interventions. The nursing diagnosis *Risk for Infection* and the collaborative problem *Risk for Complications of Opportunistic Infections* would apply for Mr. C. As these examples show, in most cases, the nursing diagnosis *Risk for Infection* and selected collaborative problems prove more clinically useful than *Ineffective Protection*.

Risk Factors

Pathophysiologic

Autoimmune diseases (rheumatoid arthritis, diabetes mellitus, thyroid disease, gout, osteoporosis, etc.)*
Collagen vascular disease
History of allergy*
Structural eyelid problems
Neurologic lesions with sensory or motor reflex loss (lagophthalmos, lack of spontaneous blink reflex due to decreased consciousness, and other medical conditions)*
Ocular surface damage*
Vitamin A deficiency*
Deficient tear-producing glands
Tear gland damage from inflammation
Difficulty blinking due to eyelid problems (e.g., ectropion [turning out]; entropion [turning in])

Treatment Related

Pharmaceutic agents such as angiotensin-converting enzyme inhibitors, antihistamines, diuretics, steroids, antidepressants, tranquilizers, analgesics, sedatives, neuromuscular blockage agents*
Surgical operations*
Anti-inflammatory agents (e.g., ibuprofen, naproxen, birth control pills, decongestants)
After laser eye surgery
Tear gland damage from radiation
After cosmetic eyelid surgery
Oral contraceptives
Mechanical ventilation therapy*

Situational (Personal, Environmental)

Long hours looking at computer screen
Smoking
Heavy drinking
Contact lenses*
Environmental factors (air-conditioning, excessive wind, sunlight exposure, air pollution, low humidity),* hot, dry, windy climate
Place of living*
Female gender*
Lifestyle (e.g., smoking, caffeine use, prolonged reading)*
Air travel

Maturational

Aging
Postmenopause

Risk for Corneal Injury

NANDA-I Definition

Vulnerable to infection or inflammatory lesion of the corneal tissue that can affect superficial or deep layers, which may compromise health

Risk Factors

Pathophysiologic

Glasgow coma scale score <7*
Autoimmune diseases (rheumatoid arthritis, diabetes mellitus, thyroid disease, gout, osteoporosis, etc.)
Collagen vascular disease
History of allergy
Structural eyelid problems
Exposure of the eyeball*
Periorbital edema*
Neurologic lesions with sensory or motor reflex loss (lagophthalmos, lack of spontaneous blink reflex due to decreased consciousness, and other medical conditions)*
Ocular surface damage
Vitamin A deficiency
Deficient tear-producing glands
Tear gland damage from inflammation
Difficulty blinking due to eyelid problems (e.g., ectropion [turning out]; entropion [turning in])
Blinking <5 times a minute*

Treatment Related

Prolonged hospitalization*
Use of supplemental oxygen*
Pharmaceutic agents* such as angiotensin-converting enzyme inhibitors, antihistamines, diuretics, steroids, antidepressants, tranquilizers, analgesics, sedatives, neuromuscular blockage agents*
After laser eye surgery
Tear gland damage from radiation
After cosmetic eyelid surgery
Tracheostomy*
Mechanical ventilation therapy*
Intubation*

Maturational

Aging

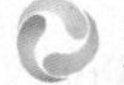

Author's Note

Refer to Author's Notes under *Risk for Dry Eye*.

Key Concepts

- About 20% to 42% of individuals in the intensive care unit develop exposure keratopathy (Rosenberg & Eisen, 2008).
- "Mechanically ventilated patients in the ICU are at risk for exposure keratopathy. This condition predisposes to microbial keratitis, which may lead to corneal perforation and visual loss" (Rosenberg & Eisen, 2008).
- The immune defenses of the eye are a combination of mechanical, anatomical, physiologic, and barrier defense mechanisms. These include an intact corneal epithelium and the constant blinking action of the eyelids. The tear film also has important antimicrobial components such as lactoferrin, beta-lysine, and immunoglobulins (*Ezra Lewis, Healy, & Coombes, 2005; Grossman & Porth, 2014).
- Lagophthalmos is defined as the inability to close the eyelids completely. Blinking covers the eye with a thin layer of tear fluid, thereby promoting a moist environment necessary for the cells of the exterior part of the eye. The tears also flush out foreign bodies and wash them away (Lawrence & Morris, 2008). Mercieca Suresh, Morton, and Tullo (*1999) found that 75% of such patients have lagophthalmos, predisposing them to corneal dryness. In addition, other critically ill patients are unconscious, predisposing to lagophthalmos even without pharmacologic sedation (Rosenberg & Eisen, 2008).

- Individuals "who are mechanically ventilated have high propensity to develop exposure keratitis which may lead to corneal perforation and blindness. In addition to alteration in the protective mechanism of eyes, intensive care environment predisposes exposure of ocular surface to microorganisms and complication of overzealous resuscitation that may end up with chemosis and other eye complications" (Azfar, Khan & Alzeer, 2013).
- The eyes have a naturally occurring blink reflex which facilitates flushing microorganisms out and aids in spreading tears to lubricate the ocular surface. Unfortunately, patients on mechanical ventilation are typically more vulnerable to ocular infection because sedation and the usage of muscle relaxants alter the patient's orbicular muscles of the eye, causing incomplete eyelid closure, decreased blinking, or the loss of the blinking reflex which can result in drying of the ocular surface (Azfar, Khan, & Alzeer, 2013; Rosenberg & Eisen, 2008).

Goals

NOC

Knowledge: Illness Care, Infection Control, Symptom Control, Hydration

The individual will exhibit minimal or no sign/symptoms of eye complications as evidenced by the following indicators:

- Pink conjunctiva
- No increase in drainage or purulent drainage
- Clear cornea
- Eyelid closure (normal or mechanical)

Interventions

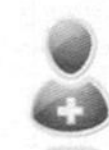

CLINICAL ALERT "It is now a well-known fact that individuals in intensive care areas are at increased risk of developing ophthalmic complications, most commonly as a result of excessive resuscitative effort and exposure of eye surface leading to corneal dryness and ulceration. An intact ocular surface is essential for protection against infection. Dryness and disruption of corneal epithelium can lead to blurring of vision, and it can also place the corneal tissue at risk for infection which can complicate with considerable visual loss. It is obvious that individuals in intensive care units are susceptible to corneal dehydration, abrasion, and corneal perforation; the incidence of which ranges between 3% and 60%" (Azfar, Khan, & Alzeer, 2013).

NIC

Eye Care Infection Protection; Medication Administration: Eye, Comfort Level, Hydration, Anxiety Reduction (Family)

Identify High-Risk Individuals With

- Loss of the blink reflex
- Incomplete eyelid closure
- Decreased tear production, decreased consciousness
- Heavily sedated
- Mechanically intubated

R: *The above conditions prevent eye closure, lack of random eye movements, and diminished or loss of blink reflex. The exposure and drying of the eye can result in superficial keratopathy. This can compromise the integrity of the surface of the cornea, resulting in ulceration, perforation, and scarring. The effects of mechanical ventilation increase intraocular pressure, resulting in edema (Grossman & Porth, 2014; *Joyce, 2002; Leadingham, 2014).*

Follow the Eye Protocol in the Institution or the Dry Eye Prevention Protocol (DEPP) (Leadingham, 2014) as Follows

- Assess high-risk individuals noted above once every 8 hours for loss of blink reflex, and the inability to maintain active eyelid closure. Document findings.

R: *The exposure and drying of the eye can result in superficial keratopathy.*

- Assess for the presence of and for foreign debris and to determine the presences of tent eyelid.

R: *Foreign debris can injure conjunctiva and precipitate infection.*

- If complete eye closure is not present, apply a mechanical eye closure and alignments device to maintain eye integrity and closure.

R: *The application of a mechanical eye closure device prevents eye complications (dry eye, infection, and corneal abrasion).*

- For individuals who demonstrate the inability to reflex blink and maintain independent eyelid closure should receive routine eye care in the form of using a saline solution and gently wiping each eye from inner to outer canthus at least every 2 hours and instilling the prescribed lubricant.

R: *The DEPP describes appropriate nursing assessment, cleaning, and documentation of eye care to prevent the incidence of dry eye from occurring.*

Carp's Cues

The DEPP was developed by Leadingham (2014) as an outcome of quality improvement project. "This quality improvement project was selected because eye care has often been overlooked due to the more acute cardiac, respiratory, and hemodynamic instability of the patients within the intensive care unit" (p. 2). "The utilization of the Iowa Model of Evidence-Based Practice (EBP) was chosen as a framework for this quality improvement project" (p. 3). "This model provided the framework to guide development and implementation of a new eye care protocol based on research in the ICU setting" (p. 3).

- Monitor for keratitis.
  - Red and watery eyes
  - Pain in the eye (if can report)
  - White to gray area on cornea (late sign)

R: *Keratitis is an inflammation of the cornea caused by corneal exposure and a compromise in the normal tear film and/or bacterial or viral infections (*Joyce, 2002).*

- Report any changes in the eye appearance or report of eye pain or blurring (if able) immediately.

R: *Complications of untreated infections can be vision loss.*

- If a prescription for eye care protocol is needed, contact with physician/nurse practitioner (NP) immediately.

R: *Cornea drying can occur quickly in high-risk individuals after 48 hours.*

- Prevent infection.
  - Wear gloves with all eye care.
  - Instruct family not to touch or wipe the eye area of an individual.
  - Avoid any contamination of eye care products. Never touch dropper or tube tip to eyelid. If this occurs, discard the medicine.
  - Shield eyes from respiratory contamination during suctioning etc.
  - Provide a demonstration to a new nurse or student nurse.

R: *Every attempt is made to prevent contamination of the eye. Eye drops can become contaminated when the container is exposed to bacteria.*

Health-Care Providers Who Are Sneezing and Coughing Should Wear Masks

R: *High-risk individuals have an increased chance for contracting a nosocomial ocular infection from health-care providers due to their impaired natural eye protection mechanisms (Leadingham, 2014).*

- Evaluate hydration status frequently.

R: *Mild dehydration can make dry eyes worse (Yanoff & Duker, 2009).*

- Explain to individual and/or significant others the reason for the eye care treatments (e.g., use of shields). Alert family prior to seeing family member.

R: *The individual's appearance with eye patches or polyethylene covers can be very disturbing to significant others.*

Initiate Health Teaching as Indicated

- Advise to see primary care provider or an eye specialist if there are signs and symptoms of dry eyes, infection, and eye pain when at home.

R: *Prolonged dry eyes can cause eye infections, scarring of the cornea surface, and vision problems. Eye complaints must be addressed immediately.*

Risk for Dry Eye

NANDA-I Definition

Vulnerable to eye discomfort or damage to the cornea and conjunctiva due to reduced quantity or quality of tears to moisten the eye, which may compromise health

Risk Factors

Pathophysiologic

Autoimmune diseases (rheumatoid arthritis, diabetes mellitus, thyroid disease, gout, osteoporosis, etc.)*
Collagen vascular disease
History of allergy*
Structural eyelid problems
Neurologic lesions with sensory or motor reflex loss (lagophthalmos, lack of spontaneous blink reflex due to decreased consciousness, and other medical conditions)*
Ocular surface damage*
Vitamin A deficiency*
Deficient tear-producing glands
Tear gland damage from inflammation
Difficulty blinking due to eyelid problems (e.g., ectropion [turning out]; entropion [turning in])

Treatment Related

Pharmaceutic agents such as angiotensin-converting enzyme inhibitors, antihistamines, diuretics, steroids, antidepressants, tranquilizers, analgesics, sedatives, neuromuscular blockage agents*
Anti-inflammatory agents (e.g., ibuprofen, naproxen, birth control pills, decongestants)
After laser eye surgery
Tear gland damage from radiation
After cosmetic eyelid surgery
Oral contraceptives
Mechanical ventilation therapy* (Refer to *Risk for Corneal Injury*)

Situational (Personal, Environmental)

Long hours looking at computer screen
Smoking
Heavy drinking
Contact lenses*
Environmental factors (air-conditioning, excessive wind, sunlight exposure, air pollution, low humidity),* hot, dry, windy climate
Place of living*
Female gender*
Lifestyle (e.g., smoking, caffeine use, prolonged reading)*
Air travel

Maturational

Aging
Perimenopause, menopause

Author's Note

This new NANDA-I nursing diagnosis represents a common problem experienced by most persons acutely or chronically. For some individuals, the problem is annoying, for others it causes a significant chronic discomfort, and for a few individuals dry eye is a serious risk factor that can cause corneal abrasions. Therefore, this diagnosis can be used to prevent or reduce dry eyes.

For those individuals who are at risk for corneal abrasion, such as those with structural eyelid abnormalities or those so debilitated that the natural lubrication system in the eye is compromised (e.g., ventilator support, comatose), *Risk for Corneal Abrasion* would be more clinically useful than *Risk for Dry Eye*. NANDA-I accepted *Risk for Corneal Injury* in 2014.

Errors in Diagnostic Statements

***Risk for Dry Eye* related to inability to close eyes secondary to comatose state**

Individuals who cannot close their eyes completely and are unable to complain of dry eye symptoms need specific interventions to prevent corneal abrasions and conjunctival scarring. The collaborative problem *Risk for Complications of Corneal Injury* would be appropriate.

Key Concepts

General Considerations

- Tears are a complex mixture of water, fatty oils, proteins, and electrolytes. This mixture keeps the surface of the eye smooth and clear and protects them from infection and injury (Grossman & Porth, 2014; Mayo Clinic, 2010).
- Tears are composed of three layers: (1) the outer, oily lipid layer; (2) the middle, watery, lacrimal layer; and (3) the inner, mucous layer (Grossman & Porth, 2014).
- Tears lubricate the eyes and wash away dust and debris by keeping the eye moist. They also contain enzymes that neutralize the microorganisms in the eye (Grossman & Porth, 2014).
- Chronic dry eyes can lead to chronic corneal and conjunctival irritation, which can lead to corneal erosion, scarring, ulceration, thinning, or perforation (Grossman & Porth, 2014).
- Some risk factors result in not enough tear production by the lacrimal gland or associated glands (e.g., rheumatoid arthritis, aging or conditions that cause tears to evaporate too quickly, such as dry environments) (Lin, Tsubota, & Apte, 2016).
- Some dry eye conditions are caused by tears leaving the eye too quickly. Surgery may be indicated to partially or completely close tear ducts to slow tear drainage (Mayo Clinic, 2010).

Geriatric Considerations

- Age-related changes in the eye of decreased elasticity of eyelids and decreased tear production result in dry eyes in older adults (Miller, 2015).

Focus Assessment Criteria

Subjective Data

Assess for Risk Factors *(Mayo Clinic, 2010)*

Refer to Risk Factors.

Assess for Complaints

Dryness
Burning
Irritation
Sensitivity to light
Difficulty wearing contact lens
Scratchiness
Blurred vision, worse at end of day, or after focusing for a prolonged period
Period of excessive tearing

Goals

NOC

Environmental, Health Promotion Behavior, Symptom Control

The individual will report reduction of dry eye symptoms, as evidenced by the following indicators:

- Describe causes of dry eye.
- Identify strategies to prevent dry eyes.

Interventions

NIC

Comfort Level, Hydration, Environmental Management, Nutritional Counseling

Explain Factors That Contribute to Dry Eyes

- Refer to Risk Factors.

Teach to Use Over-the-Counter Artificial Tears or Ocular Lubricants as Needed

- Use drops before reading or other activities that increase eye movements.

- Use preservative-free eye drops if they are used more than four times a day.
- Avoid using drops that "get the red out," which are not effective in lubricating eyes.

R: *Increased eye movements increase the need for lubrication. Preservatives can cause eye irritation (Miller, 2015).*

Increase Environmental Humidity, Especially in the Winter and Dry Climates

- Avoid hot rooms, high winds

R: *Dry climates and windy conditions increase evaporation of tears (Miller, 2015).*

Wear Wraparound Sunglasses or Other Types With Foam or Other Seals; When Swimming, Wear Goggles

R: *These will reduce evaporation of tears (Miller, 2015).*

Avoid Eye Irritants

- Hair sprays
- Tobacco smoke
- Air blowing in eyes (e.g., hair dryer, fans)

R: *Irritants increase the risk of eye damage in the presence of dry eye.*

Use an Air Cleaner/Filter and a Humidifier, If Possible

R: *These additions will reduce dust in the home and increase humidity.*

- Advise the individual of medications that might increase dryness and discomfort. Advise them to discuss the situation with their primary care provider.

R: *Alternative medications may have less or no effect on eye dryness.*

For Contact Lens Wearers

- If eye drops are used, be aware if lens must be removed before instillation of drops and not replaced for 15 minutes.
- Rewetting drops may be effective if eye dryness is mild.
- Wear lens for few hours daily if needed.

R: *Contact lenses interfere with normal lubrication of the eyes.*

Advise of Nutritional and Hydration Effects on Eye Dryness

- Avoid dehydration. Advise to monitor hydration by keeping urine color pale.
- Advise that coffee and tea are diuretics and of the need to increase water intake, unless contraindicated.

R: *Mild dehydration can make dry eyes worse (Yanoff & Duker, 2009).*

- Discuss the relationship of nutritional intake of omega-3 fatty acids such as cold-water fish, sardines, tuna, salmon, cod, herring, flax seed oil, soybean oil, canola oil, fish oil supplements, and vitamin A (e.g., carrots, broccoli supplements).

R: *Diets low in vitamin A and omega-3 fatty acids have been linked to contributing to dry eyes (Mayo Clinic, 2010).*

When Reading or Using a Computer for Long Periods (Mayo Clinic, 2010)

- Take eye breaks, close eyes for a few minutes.
- Blink repeatedly for a few seconds.

R: *These actions help spread tears evenly over the eye. Position computer monitor below eye level.*

R: *This position reduces the width of eye opening and slows the evaporation of tears.*

Advise to See Primary Care Provider or an eye Specialist If There Are Prolonged Signs and Symptoms of Dry Eyes

R: *Prolonged dry eyes can cause eye infections, scarring of the cornea surface, and vision problems (Mayo Clinic, 2010).*

Impaired Tissue Integrity

NANDA-I Definition

Damage to mucous membranes, corneal integumentary, or subcutaneous tissues

Defining Characteristics

Damaged tissue or destroyed tissue (e.g., cornea, mucous membranes, integumentary, subcutaneous)

Related Factors

Pathophysiologic

Related to inflammation of dermal–epidermal junctions secondary to:

Autoimmune alterations
Lupus erythematosus
Scleroderma
Metabolic and endocrine alterations
Diabetes mellitus
Hepatitis
Cirrhosis
Renal failure
Jaundice
Cancer
Thyroid dysfunction
Bacterial
Impetigo
Folliculitis
Cellulitis
Viral
Herpes zoster (shingles)
Gingivitis
Herpes simplex
AIDS
Fungal
Ringworm (dermatophytosis)
Athlete's foot
Vaginitis

Related to decreased blood and nutrients to tissues secondary to:

Diabetes mellitus
Peripheral vascular alterations
Cardiopulmonary disorders
Obesity
Dehydration*
Edema*
Anemia
Venous stasis
Arteriosclerosis
Emaciation
Malnutrition

Treatment Related

Related to decreased blood and nutrients to tissues secondary to:

Therapeutic extremes in body temperature
NPO status
Surgery

Related to imposed immobility secondary to sedation

Related to mechanical trauma

Therapeutic fixation devices
Wired jaw
Casts
Traction
Orthopedic devices/braces

Related to effects of radiation* on epithelial and basal cells

Related to effects of mechanical factors* or pressure secondary to:

Inflatable or foam donuts
Footboards
Dressings, tape, solutions
Nasogastric (NG) tubes
Friction
Oral prostheses/braces
Tourniquets
Restraints
External urinary catheters
Shear
Endotracheal tubes
Contact lenses

Related to the effects of medicines (specify) (e.g., steroids, antibiotics)

Situational (Personal, Environmental)

Related to chemical irritants* secondary to:

Excretions
Secretions
Noxious agents/substances

Related to environmental irritants secondary to:

Radiation/sunburn
Humidity
Bites (insect, animal)
Poisonous plants
Temperature extremes*
Parasites
Inhalants

Related to the effects of pressure of impaired physical mobility* secondary to:

Pain
Fatigue
Motivation
Cognitive, sensory, or motor deficits

Related to inadequate personal habits (hygiene/dental/dietary/sleep)

Related to thin body frame

Maturational

Related to dry, thin skin, and decreased dermal vascularity secondary to aging

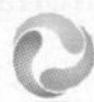

Author's Note

With the newly accepted *Risk for Pressure Ulcer*, *Risk for Cornea Injury*, *Risk for Urinary Tract Injury*, and the addition of *Pressure Ulcer* by this author, *Impaired Tissue Integrity* and *Risk for Impaired Tissue Integrity* are too broad nursing diagnoses for clinical usefulness. When a pressure ulcer is stage IV, necrotic, or infected, it may be more appropriate to label the diagnosis a collaborative problem, such as *Risk for Complications of Stage IV Pressure Ulcer*. This would represent a situation in which a nurse manages with physician, nurse practitioner/physician assistant- and nurse-prescribed interventions. When a stage II or III pressure ulcer needs a dressing that requires a physician's order in an acute care setting, the nurse should continue to label the situation a nursing diagnosis because it would be appropriate and legal for a nurse to treat the ulcer independently in other settings (e.g., in the community).

If an individual is immobile and multiple systems are threatened (respiratory, circulatory, musculoskeletal as well as integumentary), the nurse can use *Disuse Syndrome* to describe the entire situation. If an individual is at risk for damage to corneal tissue, the nurse can use a diagnosis such as *Risk for Corneal Injury* related to corneal drying and lower lacrimal production secondary to unconscious state.

Risk for Impaired Tissue Integrity

Definition

Vulnerable to damage to the mucous membrane, cornea, integumentary system, muscular fascia, muscle, tendon, bone, cartilage, joint capsule, and/or ligament, which may compromise health

Risk Factors

Alteration in metabolism
Alteration in sensation
Chemical injury agent (e.g., burn, capsaicin, methylene chloride, mustard agent)
Excessive fluid volume
Extremes of age
Extremes of environmental temperature
High-voltage power supply
Humidity
Imbalanced nutritional state (e.g., obesity, malnutrition)
Impaired circulation
Impaired mobility
Insufficient fluid volume
Insufficient knowledge about maintaining tissue integrity
Insufficient knowledge about protecting tissue integrity
Mechanical factor
Peripheral neuropathy
Pharmaceutic agent
Radiation therapy
Surgical procedure

Author's Note

Refer to Author's Notes under *Impaired Tissue Integrity*.

Pressure Ulcers • Related to the Effects of Pressure, Friction, Shear, and Maceration

Definition

A pressure ulcer is a localized injury to the skin and/or underlying tissue, usually over a bony prominence, as a result of pressure, or pressure in combination with shear (e.g., sacrum, calcaneus, ischium) (National Pressure Ulcer Advisory Panel, 2014).

Defining Characteristics (National Pressure Ulcer Advisory Panel, 2014)

Category/Stage I: Nonblanchable Erythema

Intact skin with nonblanchable redness of a localized area usually over a bony prominence. The area may be painful, firm, soft, warmer, or cooler as compared to adjacent tissue.

Category/Stage II: Partial Thickness

Partial thickness loss of dermis presenting as a shallow open ulcer with a red pink wound bed, without slough. May also present as an intact or open/ruptured serum-filled or serosanguineous filled blister. Presents as a shiny or dry shallow ulcer without slough or bruising. Bruising indicates deep tissue injury.*

Author's Note

Category/Stage III and IV, Unstageable/Unclassified, Suspected Deep Tissue Injury require complex medical and nursing treatments. These pressure ulcer would be more appropriate as collaborative problems as Risk for Sepsis. Appropriate nursing diagnoses are *Risk for Infection*, *Impaired Physical Mobility*, *Imbalanced Nutrition*, and *Risk for Health Management*.

Category/Stage III: Full Thickness Skin Loss

Full thickness tissue loss. Subcutaneous fat may be visible but bone, tendon, or muscle is *not* exposed. Slough may be present but does not obscure the depth of tissue loss. *May* include undermining and tunneling. Bone/tendon is not visible or directly palpable.

The depth of a Category/Stage III pressure ulcer varies by anatomical location.

Category/Stage IV: Full Thickness Tissue Loss

Full thickness tissue loss with exposed bone, tendon, or muscle. Slough or eschar may be present. Often includes undermining and tunneling. The depth of a Category/Stage IV pressure ulcer varies by anatomical location. Category/Stage IV ulcers can extend into muscle and/or supporting structures (e.g., fascia, tendon, or joint capsule) making osteomyelitis or osteitis likely to occur. Exposed bone/muscle is visible or directly palpable.

Additional Categories/Stages for the USA

Unstageable/Unclassified: Full thickness skin or tissue loss—depth unknown

Full thickness tissue loss in which actual depth of the ulcer is completely obscured by slough (yellow, tan, gray, green, or brown) and/or eschar (tan, brown, or black) in the wound bed. Until enough slough and/or eschar are removed to expose the base of the wound, the true depth cannot be determined; but it will be either a Category/Stage III or IV.

Suspected Deep Tissue Injury—depth unknown

Purple or maroon localized area of discolored intact skin or blood-filled blister due to damage of underlying soft tissue from pressure and/or *shear*. The area may be preceded by tissue that is painful, firm, mushy, boggy, warmer, or cooler as compared to adjacent tissue. Deep tissue injury may be difficult to detect in individuals with dark skin tones. Evolution may include a thin blister over a dark wound bed. The wound may further evolve and become covered by thin eschar. Evolution may be rapid exposing additional layers of tissue even with optimal treatment.

Related Factors

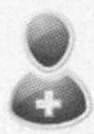

Clinical Alert Coleman et al. (2013) reported "overall there is no single factor which can explain pressure ulcer risk, rather a complex interplay of factors which increase the probability of pressure ulcer development."

Pathophysiologic

Related to decreased blood and nutrients to tissues secondary to:

Peripheral vascular alterations
Obesity
Anemia
Venous stasis
Cardiopulmonary disorders
Arteriosclerosis
Dehydration
Malnutrition
Edema*
Emaciation

Treatment Related

Related to decreased blood and nutrients to tissues secondary to:

Therapeutic extremes in body temperature
Surgery
Obesity
NPO status

Related to imposed immobility secondary to sedation

Related to mechanical trauma

Therapeutic fixation devices
Wired jaw
Casts
Traction
Orthopedic devices/braces

Related to effects of radiation* on epithelial and basal cells

Related to effects of mechanical irritants* or pressure secondary to:

Inflatable or foam donuts
Tourniquets
Footboards
Restraints
Dressings, tape, solutions
External urinary catheters
NG tubes
Shear
Friction
Endotracheal tubes
Oral prostheses/braces
Contact lenses

Situational (Personal, Environmental)

Related to chemical irritants* secondary to:

Excretions
Secretions
Noxious agents/substances

Related to environmental irritants secondary to:

Radiation/sunburn
Humidity
Bites (insect, animal)
Poisonous plants
Temperature extremes*
Parasites
Inhalants

Related to the effects of pressure of impaired physical mobility* secondary to:

Pain
Fatigue
Motivation
Cognitive, sensory, or motor deficits

Related to dry, thin skin and decreased dermal vascularity secondary to aging

Errors in Diagnostic Statements

Pressure Ulcer stage II related to immobility

The development of pressure ulcers is usually the result of several contributing factors. For healing to occur interventions must focus on optimal nutrition, hydration, and relief from pressure and shear forces. In addition individual risk factors as smoking, hyperglycemia, and incontinence must be addressed. A more clinically useful diagnosis would be *Pressure Ulcer stage II related to compromised nutrition, decreased mobility secondary to obesity, and stress incontinence.*

Key Concepts

General Considerations

- Pressure ulcers are among the most common conditions encountered in acutely hospitalized individuals (0% to 46%), in critical care (13.1% to 45.5%) or those requiring long-term institutional care (4.1% to 32.2%). An estimated 2.5 million pressure ulcers are treated each year in acute care facilities in the United States alone (National Pressure Ulcer Advisory Panel, 2014).
- According to the Agency for Healthcare Research & Quality (AHRQ) (2011), pressure ulcers cost the US health-care system an estimated $9.1 to $11.6 billion annually.
- The average hospital treatment cost associated with stage IV pressure ulcers and related complications was $129,248 for hospital-acquired ulcers during one admission, and $124,327 for community-acquired ulcers over an average of four admissions (Brem et al., 2010).
- Studies have shown that the development of a pressure ulcer independently increases the length of a patient's hospital stay by 4 to 10 days. These prolonged hospital stays are also associated with an increased incidence of nosocomial infections and other complications.
- In the fourth quarter of 2011, on average, nursing homes had 6.9% of their long-stay high-risk residents with pressure ulcers and (Berlowitz, 2015; Ling & Mandl, 2013):
  - The 10% of nursing homes who performed the best had 2% or less prevalence of pressure ulcers among their high-risk residents.
  - The 10% of nursing homes who performed the poorest had 12% or more prevalence of pressure ulcers among their high-risk residents.
  - 6.9% of facilities reported no pressure ulcers.
- Among short-stay nursing home residents, the following risk factors for pressures ulcers were identified at admission (Link & Mandl, 2013):
  - 89.2% had an impairment in bed mobility.
  - 34.5% had bowel incontinence (occasional or more).
  - 42.4% had diabetes or peripheral vascular disease.
  - 9.8% had a low body mass index.
- Tissues are groupings of specialized cells that unite to perform specific functions. The human body is composed of four basic types of tissues: epithelial, connective (including skeletal tissue and blood), muscle, and nervous.
- The external covering of the body is composed of epithelial tissue, called the integument. Wherever the body exposes large openings to the outside (e.g., the mouth), its outer covering changes from integument to an inner lining called the mucous membrane. Each layer of the integument has its counterpart in a complete mucous membrane. The integument includes both the skin and the subcutaneous tissue.
- The skin is a complex organ consisting of two layers: the outer epidermis and the deeper dermis. The epidermis is approximately 0.04 mm thick, and the dermis is about 0.5 cm thick (Grossman & Porth, 2014).
- The epidermis functions as a barrier to protect inner tissues (from injury, chemicals, organisms); as a receptor for a range of sensations (touch, pain, heat, cold); as a regulator of body temperature through radiation (giving off heat), conduction (transfer of heat), and convection (movement of warm air molecules away from the body); as a regulator of water balance by preventing water and electrolyte loss; and as a receptor for vitamin D from the sun (*Maklebust & Sieggreen, 2006).
- A water-soluble mitotic inhibitor called *chalone* depresses epidermal regeneration. Chalone levels are high during daytime stress and activity and lower during sleep. Therefore, healing is promoted during rest and sleep (Maklebust & Sieggreen, 2006).
- Beneath the avascular epidermis lies the highly vascularized dermis. The dermis contains epithelial tissue, connective tissue, muscle, and nervous tissue. The dermis is rich in collagen, which imparts toughness to the skin. Hair follicles extend into the dermis and serve as islands of cells for rapid reepithelialization of minor wounds. Sweat glands in the dermis contribute to control of body water and temperature. Small muscles within the dermis serve to produce goose pimples. Specialized dermal nerve endings for pain, touch, heat, and cold cannot be replaced once destroyed (Maklebust & Sieggreen, 2006).
- The subcutaneous tissue, which lies beneath the dermis, stores fat for temperature regulation and contains the remainder of the sweat glands and hair follicles (Grossman & Porth, 2014).
- Causes of tissue destruction can be mechanical, immunologic, bacterial, chemical, or thermal. Mechanical destruction includes physical trauma and surgical incision. Immunologic destruction occurs as an allergic response. Bacterial destruction results from an overgrowth of organisms. Chemical destruction results when a caustic substance contacts unprotected tissue. Thermal destruction occurs when tissue is exposed to temperature extremes that are incompatible with cell life (Grossman & Porth, 2014).

- Wound healing is a complex sequence of events initiated by injury to the tissues. The components are coagulation of bleeding, inflammation, epithelialization, fibroplasia and collagen metabolism, collagen maturation, scar remodeling, and wound contraction (Grossman & Porth, 2014; Guo & DiPietro, 2010).
- A wound must be considered in relation to the entire person. Major factors that affect wound healing are nutrition(vitamins, minerals,) anemia, blood volume and tissue oxygenation, steroids and anti-inflammatory drugs, diabetes mellitus, chemotherapy, radiation, infection, age and sex hormones, stress, obesity, alcoholism, and smoking, and nutrition (Guo & DiPietro, 2010).
- The presence of necrotic tissue, foreign material, and bacteria results in the abnormal production of metalloproteases, which alter the balance of inflammation and impair the function of the cytokines. Cytokines are produced by a broad range of cells, including immune cells like macrophages, B lymphocytes, T lymphocytes and mast cells, as well as endothelial cells, fibroblasts, and various stromal cells, which serve to reduce inflammation and promote healing (are anti-inflammatory) (Armstrong & Meyr, 2014).
- The depth of a Category/Stage III pressure ulcer varies by anatomical location. The bridge of the nose, ear, occiput, and malleolus do not have (adipose) subcutaneous tissue and Category/Stage III ulcers can be shallow. In contrast, areas of significant adiposity can develop extremely deep Category/Stage III pressure ulcers. Bone/tendon is not visible or directly palpable (National Pressure Ulcer Advisory Panel, 2014).

Nutritional Requirements and Pressure Ulcers

- Individuals with pressure ulcers are in a chronic catabolic state. Optimizing both protein and total caloric intake is critical for healing (Berlowitz, 2015).
- Adequate calories, protein, fluids, vitamins, and minerals are required by the body for maintaining tissue integrity and preventing tissue breakdown (Dorner, Posthauer, & Thomas, 2009).
- Nutritional risk factors for pressure ulcers are unintentional weight loss, undernutrition, protein energy malnutrition (PEM), dehydration, low body mass index (BMI), reduced food intake, and impaired ability to eat independently (Dorner et al., 2009).

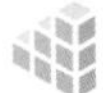

Pediatric Considerations

- A newborn commonly exhibits normal skin variations, such as Mongolian spots, milia, and stork bites, which can be upsetting to parents but are clinically insignificant.
- Several common skin conditions affect children in specific age groups. These include atopic, seborrheic, and diaper dermatitis in infancy and acne in adolescence.
- Infants and young children have a thin epidermis and require special protection from the sun.

Geriatric Considerations

- The skin changes as the result of aging and repeated exposure to ultraviolet light that increase the risk of pressure ulcers and delayed healing (*Fore, 2006; Grossman & Porth 2014).
- "Skin aging involves chronological or intrinsically aged skin and photoaged skin changes. A majority of the skin changes associated with aging are due to intrinsic aging rather than photodamage or lifestyle. Ultraviolet exposure will speed up chronological skin changes, suggesting similar molecular mediators and some similar outcomes of damage. With increasing age, the impact of photoaging increases and the effect of the underlying genetic tendencies decreases" (*Fore, 2006).
- The epidermis becomes 20% thinner with aging and turnover rate generally slows (Grossman & Porth, 2014).
- "The overall thickness of the skin decreases with a decline in the thickness of the stratum spinosum and a significant decrease in the maximum thickness of skin. The usual 28-day turnover time for skin increases approximately 30% to 50% by age 80" (*Fore, 2006).
- Elastin, which gives the skin flexibility, elasticity, and tensile strength, decreases with age. It is found in tissues associated with body movement, such as the walls of major blood vessels, heart, lungs, and skin. The decreased turgor results in dry, wrinkled skin, increasing the incidence of bruising and skin hemorrhages (Grossman & Porth, 2014).
- Collagen, found in all connective tissues such as blood, lymph, and bone, binds together and supports other tissues. The extracellular matrix of connecting tissue is composed primarily of collagen and elastin, and approximately 80% of the dermis consists of collagen. With aging, skin strength decreases because of age-related loss of collagen from the dermis and the degeneration of the elastic properties of the remaining collagen.
- Some older adults exhibit shiny, loose, thin, transparent skin, primarily on the backs of the hands and the forearms. Subcutaneous fat decreases with aging, reducing the cushioning of bony prominences and putting older adults at increased risk for pressure ulcers (Miller, 2015).

- Vascularity also decreases within the subcutaneous tissue, delaying the absorption of medication administered via this route, and is then complicated by increased healing time (Grossman & Porth, 2014).
- Aging causes diminished immunocompetence and decreased angiogenesis, which delays wound healing (Grossman & Porth, 2014).
- Age-related decreases in perspiration, sebum secretion, and the number of sebaceous glands cause drier, coarser skin that is more prone to fissures and cracks (Miller, 2015).
- In older adults, cells are larger and proliferate more slowly, fibroblasts decrease in number, and dermal vascularity decreases. All these factors contribute to slower wound healing (Grossman & Porth, 2014).

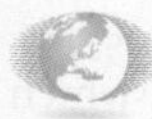

Transcultural Considerations

- All skin colors have an underlying red tone. Pallor in black-skinned people is seen as an ashen or gray tone. Pallor in brown-skinned people appears as a yellowish-brown color. Pallor can be assessed in mucous membranes, lips, nail beds, and conjunctiva of the lower eyelids (Weber & Kelly, 2014).
- Mongolian spots are dark blue or black areas of pigmentation seen on the skin of Black, Asian, Native American, or Mexican American newborns. They are often mistaken for bruises. By adulthood, they are lighter but still visible (Giger, 2013).
- Some folk remedies may be misdiagnosed as injuries. Three folk practices of Southeast Asians leave marks on the body that can be assumed as signs of violence or abuse. Cao gio is rubbing of the skin with a coin to produce dark blood or ecchymotic strips; it is done to treat colds and flu-like symptoms. Bat gio is pinching skin on the temples to treat headaches or on the neck for a sore throat; if petechiae or ecchymoses appear, the treatment is a success. Poua is the burning of the skin with the tip of a dried weed-like grass; it is believed the burning will cause the noxious element that causes the pain to exude (Giger, 2013).

Focus Assessment Criteria Subjective/Objective Data

Medical, surgical, and dental history
Use of tobacco, alcohol
Current drug therapy
What drugs? How often? When was last dose taken?

Assess For Factors Contributing to the Development or Extension of Pressure Ulcers

Advanced age

Skin deficits

Dryness	Obesity	Excessive perspiration
Edema	Thinness	

Sensory Perception

Diabetic neuropathy	Diminished response	Acuity of illness
Spinal cord injury	Mental capacity	

Activity Level-Related Variables

Immobile	Chairfast	Walking with no limitations
Bedfast	Walking with limitations	Ability to eat independently

Perfusion-Related Variables

Diabetes	Circulation	Smoking, edema
Vascular disease	Blood pressure	

Laboratory Tests to Assess Risk Factors for Pressure Ulcers

Urea	Albumin	Hemoglobin (Hgb)
Electrolytes protein	Lymphopenia	

Compromised Oxygen Transport

Peripheral vascular disorders	Anemia	Cardiopulmonary disorders
Venous stasis	Arteriosclerosis	

Chemical/Mechanical Irritants

Radiation	Casts, splints, braces	Incontinence (feces, urine)

Nutritional deficiencies

Protein	Trace elements	Hydration
Minerals	Vitamins	

Systemic disorders
Refer to Related Factors—Pathophysiologic

Skin
Color Turgor Moisture
Texture Vascularity Temperature

Lesions
Location Size Color
Distribution Shape Drainage
Type

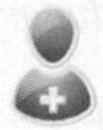

CLINICAL ALERT A picture of any skin abnormalities should be taken according to institution's policies.

Circulation
Do capillaries refill within 3 seconds after blanching?
Does erythema subside within 30 minutes after pressure is removed?
Edema
Note degree and location
Palpate over bony prominences for sponginess (indicates edema)

Goals

NOC
Tissue Integrity

The individual's pressure ulcer will demonstrate as evidenced by the following indicators:

- Progressive healing of pressure ulcer
- Participates in risk reduction (specify)

The individual/family will accurately

- Demonstrates pressure ulcer care
- Identifies signs of improvement and/or deterioration
- Explains rationale for interventions

Interventions

Ensure Assessment and Documentation of Skin and Tissue Condition at Intervals Depending on Individual's Risk (National Pressure Ulcer Advisory Panel, 2014)

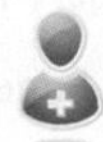

CLINICAL ALERT The superficial skin is less susceptible to pressure-induced damage than deeper tissues, and thus, the external appearance may underestimate the extent of pressure-related injury. Pressure ulcers are typically related to immobility (i.e., bed-bound or chair-bound individual), but can also result from poorly fitting casts or other medical equipment (Berlowitz, 2015).

NIC
Teaching Interventions, Surveillance, Nutritional Management, Pressure Prevention, Positioning, Incontinence, Pressure Ulcer Care

- Blanching response
- Localized heat
- Edema
- Induration (hardness)
- Localized pain

R: *Studies reported that pain over the site was a precursor to tissue breakdown (National Pressure Ulcer Advisory Panel, 2014).*

- Ask the individual if they have any areas of discomfort or pain that could be attributed to pressure damage.
- Observe the skin for pressure damage caused by medical devices (for example, catheters and cervical collars).

R: *This provides a baseline for diagnosis or evidence of healing or deterioration.*

For Individuals with Darkly Pigmented Skin, Consider (*Bennett, 1995; Clark, 2010, p. 17)

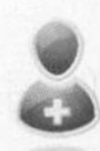

CLINICAL ALERT Researchers have reported that the failure to identify early stages of pressure damage results in greater numbers of people with darkly pigmented skin developing more severe forms of pressure damage (Baumgarten et al., 2009; National Pressure Ulcer Advisory Panel, 2014; *Rosen et al., 2006).

- The color of intact dark pigmented skin may remain unchanged (does not blanch) when pressure is applied over a bony prominence.
- Local areas of intact skin that are subject to pressure may feel either warm or cool when touched. This assessment should be performed without gloves to make it easier to distinguish differences in temperature after any body fluids are cleansed before making this direct contact.
- Areas of skin subjected to pressure may be purplish/bluish/violet in color. This can be compared with the erythema seen in people with lighter skin tones.
- Complains of, or indicate, current or recent pain or discomfort at body sites where pressure has been applied.

R: *Stage I pressure ulcers are underdetected in individuals with darkly pigmented skin. Visual cues for changes in skin appearance may be relatively easy to observe in Caucasian skin, but with darker pigmentation it may be harder to spot visual signs of early changes due to pressure damage (Clark, 2010; National Pressure Ulcer Advisory Panel, 2014).*

- Ensure a nutritional assessment is completed by a registered dietician/nutritionist using the MNA if possible.

R: *MNA is the only nutritional screening tool that has been specifically validated in individuals with pressure ulcers (National Pressure Ulcer Advisory Panel, 2014).*

- Report to prescribing provider when food and/or fluid intake is decreased.

R: *Fortified foods and/or high-calorie, high-protein oral nutrition supplements between meals may be needed (National Pressure Ulcer Advisory Panel, 2014).*

Advise Family/Friends the Importance of Nutritionally Dense Foods/Beverages Versus Calories-Dense Foods/Beverages

- Calorie-dense foods, also called energy-dense foods, contain high levels of calories per serving in fat and carbohydrates. Many processed foods are considered calorie-dense, such as cakes, cookies, snacks, doughnuts, and candies.
- Nutrient-dense foods contain high levels of nutrients, such as protein, carbohydrates, fats, vitamins, and minerals, but with fewer calories. Some nutrient-dense foods are fresh fruits, vegetables, berries, melons, dark-green vegetables, sweet potatoes, tomatoes, and whole grains, including quinoa, barley, bulgur, and oats. Lean beef and pork are high in protein and contain high levels of zinc, iron, and B-vitamins.

R: *Individuals with pressure ulcers need 30 to 35 kcal/kg body weight, 1.25 to 1.5 g protein/kg of body weight daily, and vitamins and minerals (National Pressure Ulcer Advisory Panel, 2014). Calorie-dense foods do not provide the needed nutrients and can replace the needed nutrient-dense foods when the individual's appetite is poor.*

- Refer to *Imbalance Nutrition* for interventions related to promoting optimal intake of required nutrients.

R: *Malnutrition is associated with impaired wound healing (National Pressure Ulcer Advisory Panel, 2014).*

Monitor Hematology Laboratories' Results as (National Pressure Ulcer Advisory Panel, 2014)

- Electrolyte imbalances
- Elevated urea
- Elevated creatinine
- Elevated C-reactive protein
- Lymphopenia
- Low hemoglobin

R: *A systematic review of primary research laboratory abnormalities as risk factors for pressure ulcer development (Coleman et al., 2013; de Souza & de Gouveia Santos, 2010)*

Follow the Wound Care Procedure as Prescribed by a Wound Specialist or Prescribing Professional (Physician, Nurse Practitioner, Physician Assistant)

- Wound bed preparation (tissue management, infection/inflammation control, moisture barrier, epithelial edge advancement) (National Pressure Ulcer Advisory Panel, 2014)

R: *Wound bed preparation promotes a wound environment as well vascularized area, free from nonviable tissue and excess exudate, that will enhance normal progression toward wound healing. A warm, moist wound bed stimulates growth factor activity and promotes accelerated reepithelialization. This does not promote infection (National Pressure Ulcer Advisory Panel, 2014).*

- Wound cleansing: use of fluids to remove surface contaminants, remnants of previous dressings, and bacteria.

R: *The choice of fluids, for example, sterile, antimicrobial is dependent on the condition of the individual, for example, immunocompromised and/or presence of infection.*

- Wound debridement of devitalized tissue within the wound bed and the edges

R: *Devitalized tissue is nonviable or necrotic. It is normally moist, yellow, green, tan, or gray with or without black/brown eschar.*

- Prevention, assessment, treatment of infection:
  - Suspect an infection when:
    - Lack of signs of healing for 2 weeks
    - Friable (easily bleeds) granulation tissue
    - Malodor
    - Increased pain in ulcer
    - Increased heat in area around ulcer
    - Increased drainage
    - Unsatisfactory change in character of drainage (e.g., bloody, purulent)
    - Increase in necrotic tissue in the wound bed and/or
    - Pocketing or bridging in the wound bed.

R: *Wound healing is delayed and/or may be abnormal when there are significant bacteria.*

- Suspect biofilm in pressure ulcer when:
  - Ulcer is present more than 4 weeks
  - Lacks signs of any healing in the previous 2 weeks
  - Has clinical signs and symptoms of inflammation
  - Does not respond to antimicrobial therapy

R: *Bacterial biofilms cause 60% of chronic skin wounds with enhanced resistance to endogenous antibiotics and phagocytic cells as well as antibiotics and antiseptics.*

- Wound dressings: should keep wound moist, contain exudate, protect periulcer skin, comply with the size and location, presence of tunneling
  - When the dressing does not address the characteristics of the ulcer or the ulcer has deteriorated, consult with specialist.

R: *As the ulcer heals or deteriorates the type of dressing needed may change.*

Consider Pressure-Dispersing Devices, Microclimate Manipulations and Fabrics, for Example, Silk-Like Texture Designed to Reduce Shear/Friction As Appropriate (National Pressure Ulcer Advisory Panel, 2014)

R: *Microclimate control devices provide constant air flow to cool the skin and promote evaporation of moisture from skin surface. Increased levels of moisture reduce skin tensile strength and intracellular structure of stratum corneum and increase friction (National Pressure Ulcer Advisory Panel, 2014).*

Consider Applying Polyurethane Foam Dressing to Bony Prominences (e.g., Heel, Elbows, Sacrum). Avoid Dressing That Cannot Be Easily Removed (National Pressure Ulcer Advisory Panel, 2014)

R: *Multiple layers in dressings reduce shear force. Easily removed dressing will reduce injury to fragile skin (National Pressure Ulcer Advisory Panel, 2014).*

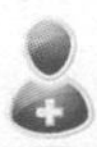

CLINICAL ALERT Repositioning regularly is done to prevent pressure ulcers and reduce interface pressures is the standard of care, yet prior work has found that standard repositioning does not relieve all areas of at-risk tissue in nondisabled subjects.

Encourage Highest Degree of Mobility to Avoid Prolonged Periods of Pressure: Exercise and Mobility Increase Blood Flow to all Areas

- Principles of pressure ulcer prevention include reducing or rotating pressure on soft tissue. If pressure on soft tissue exceeds intracapillary pressure (approximately 32 mm Hg), capillary occlusion and resulting hypoxia can cause tissue damage. The greater the duration of immobility, the greater the likelihood of the development of small vessel thrombosis and subsequent tissue necrosis (National Pressure Ulcer Advisory Panel, 2014).
- Do not position person on reddened and/or tender areas.

R: *Pressure on compromised tissue will decrease circulation and increase tissue injury.*

- Avoid all inflatable donuts or rings.

R: *These devices reduce circulation to the compromised tissue.*

Immobility

- Encourage range-of-motion exercises and weight-bearing mobility, when possible, to increase blood flow to all areas.
- Promote optimal circulation when in bed.
- Use repositioning schedule that relieves vulnerable area most often (e.g., if the vulnerable area is the back, the turning schedule would be left side to back, back to right side, right side to left side, and left side to back); post "turn clock" at bedside.
- Turn or instruct them turn or shift weight every 30 minutes to 2 hours, depending on other causative factors and the ability of the skin to recover from pressure. Install an overhead trapeze to allow for increased mobility.

Assess Dependent Skin Areas With Every Position Turn

- Use finger or transparent disk to assess whether skin is blanchable or nonblanchable.

R: *"Blanchable erythema is visible skin redness that become white when pressure is applied and reddens when pressure relieved" (National Pressure Ulcer Advisory Panel, 2014, p. 63). It may result from normal reactive hyperemia that should disappear within several hours or it may result from inflammatory erythema with intact capillary bed. Nonblanchable erythema is visible redness that persists with the application of pressure, which indicates structural damage to microcirculation. This represents Category/Stage I pressure ulcer (National Pressure Ulcer Advisory Panel, 2014, p. 63).*

- Assess skin temperature, edema, and change in tissue consistency as compared to surrounding tissue.

R: *Localized heat, edema, and change in tissue consistency as induration/hardness as compared to surrounding tissue are warning signs for pressure ulcer development (National Pressure Ulcer Advisory Panel, 2014).*

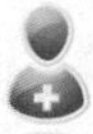

Clinical Alert Do not wear gloves when assessing skin temperature and changes in tissue consistency. As indicated cleanse skin prior to assessing and follow usual hand-washing procedures.

Increase frequency of the turning schedule if any nonblanchable erythema is noted. Consult with prescribing professional for the utilization of pressure-dispersing devices and microclimate manipulation devices in addition to repositioning.

R: *Peterson, Gravenstein, Schwab, van Oostrom, and Caruso (2013) reported using pressure mapping devices to measure pressure on skin/tissue, when high-risk individuals were positioned on their back, left side, and right side. Bedridden individuals at risk for pressure ulcer formation exhibit high skin–bed interface pressures on specific skin areas that are likely always at risk (i.e., triple-jeopardy and always-at-risk areas) for the vast majority of the time they are in bed despite routine repositioning care. Triple jeopardy were skin areas that were consistently compressed in all three positions. "Healthcare providers are unaware of the actual tissue-relieving effectiveness (or lack thereof) of their repositioning interventions, which may partially explain why pressure ulcer mitigation strategies are not always successful. Relieving at-risk tissue is a necessary part of pressure ulcer prevention, but the repositioning practice itself needs improvement."*

- Place the individual in normal or neutral position with body weight evenly distributed. Use 30° laterally inclined position when possible.

R: *Pressure is a compressing downward force on a given area. If pressure against soft tissue is greater than intracapillary blood pressure (approximately 32 mm Hg), the capillaries can be occluded, and the tissue can be damaged as a result of hypoxia.*

- Keep the bed as flat as possible to reduce shearing forces; limit semi-Fowler's position to only 30 minutes at a time.

R: *Keeping the bed as flat as possible (lower than 30°) and supporting the feet with a footboard help prevent shear; the pressure created when two adjacent tissue layers move in opposition. If a bony prominence slides across the subcutaneous tissue, the subepidermal capillaries may become bent and pinched, resulting in decreased tissue perfusion.*

- Alternate or reduce the pressure on the skin with an appropriate support surface.
- Suspend heels off bed surface.
- Use enough personnel to lift the individual up in bed or a chair rather than pull or slide skin surfaces.

R: *A lift sheet will minimize the friction caused by dragging and pulling.*

- To reduce shearing forces, support the feet with a footboard to prevent sliding.

R: *Shear is a parallel force in which one layer of tissue moves in one direction and another layer moves in the opposite direction. If the skin sticks to the bed linen and the weight of the body makes the skeleton slide down inside the skin (as with semi-Fowler's positioning), the subepidermal capillaries may become angulated and pinched, resulting in decreased perfusion of the tissue (Grossman & Porth, 2014).*

Promote Optimal Circulation When the Person Is Sitting

- Limit sitting time for those at high risk for ulcer development.
- Instruct to lift self using chair arms every 10 minutes, if possible, or assist in rising up off the chair at least every hour, depending on risk factors present.
- Do not elevate the legs unless calves are supported to reduce the pressure over the ischial tuberosities.
- Pad the chair with pressure-relieving cushion.
- Inspect areas at risk of developing ulcers with each position change.
    - Ears
    - Elbows
    - Occiput
    - Trochan
    - Scrotum
    - Heels
    - Ischia
    - Sacrum
    - Scapula
- Do not rub reddened areas.

R: *Massaging can damage the capillaries and impair circulation.*

Protect Skin Near Feeding Tubes or Endotracheal Tubes With a Protective Barrier

- Change skin barrier when loose or leaking.
- Instruct to report discomforts.

R: *An NG tube can irritate skin and mucosa. Gastric juices can cause severe skin breakdown.*

R: *The detrimental effect of smoking on wound healing is multifactorial with mechanisms that include vasoconstriction causing a relative ischemia of operated tissues, a reduced inflammatory response, impaired bacteriocidal mechanisms, and alterations of collagen metabolism (Armstrong, & Meyr, 2014).*

Initiate Health Teaching and Referrals as Needed

- Teach the individual/family appropriate measures to prevent pressure, shear, friction, and maceration and to not use inflatable donuts or rings (*Bergstrom et al., 1994; National Pressure Ulcer Advisory Panel, 2014; *Wound Ostomy Continence Nursing [WOCN], 2003).
- If indicated, observe family member perform wound care.
- Ensure a home health evaluation is scheduled for the day the individual return to home.

R: *The complexity of care involved in pressure ulcers requires nursing expertise as soon as possible in their home.*

- If this is problematic use the Mini Nutritional Assessment access at http://www.mna-elderly.com/forms/mini/mna_mini_english.pdf.

Risk for Pressure Ulcer

NANDA-I Definition

Vulnerable to localized injury to the skin and/or underlying tissue usually over a bony prominence as a result of pressure, or pressure in combination with shear (National Pressure Ulcer Advisory Panel, 2014).

Risk Factors

Pathophysiologic

Adult: Braden scale score of <18
Alteration in cognitive functioning

Alteration in sensation
American society of anesthesiologists (ASA) physical status classification score ≥2
Anemia
Cardiovascular disease
Child: Braden Q scale of ≤16
Decrease in serum albumin level
Electrolyte imbalances, elevated urea, elevated creatinine above 1 mg/dL, lymphopenia, elevated C-reactive protein*
Decrease in tissue oxygenation
Decrease in tissue perfusion* (e.g., hypertension, hypotension, CVA, diabetes mellitus, renal disease, peripheral vascular disease)
Dehydration
Diabetes mellitus*
Edema
Elevated skin temperature by 1° C to 2° C
History of cerebral vascular accident
History of pressure ulcer
History of trauma
Hyperthermia
Impaired circulation
Low score on Risk Assessment Pressure Sore (RAPS) scale
Lymphopenia
New York Heart Association (NYHA) Functional Classification ≥2
Hip fracture
Nonblanchable erythema (Author's Note: This is not a risk factor but instead represents Stage I pressure ulcer)

Treatment Related

Pharmaceutic agents (e.g., general anesthesia, vasopressors, antidepressant, norepinephrine)
Extended period of immobility on hard surface (e.g., surgical procedure ≥2 hours)
Shearing forces
Surface friction
Use of linen with insufficient moisture wicking property

Situational (Personal, Environmental)

Extremes of weight
Inadequate nutrition
Incontinence
Insufficient caregiver
Knowledge of pressure ulcer prevention
Physical immobilization
Pressure over bony prominence
Reduced triceps skinfold thickness
Scaly skin
Dry skin
Self-care deficit
Skin moisture
Smoking
Female gender
Decreased cognition[33]
Dibilitated[33]

Maturational

Extremes of age

Author's Note

Refer to *Pressure Ulcer*.

Key Concepts

Refer to *Pressure Ulcer*.

[33]Added by author source: National Pressure Ulcer Advisory Panel (2014).

Focus Assessment Criteria

Braden Scale for Predicting Pressure Sore Risk (© Copyright Barbara Braden and Nancy Bergstrom, 1988 All rights reserved)

SENSORY PERCEPTION ability to respond meaningfully to pressure-related discomfort			
1. Completely Limited Unresponsive (does not moan, flinch, or grasp) to painful stimuli, due to diminished level of consciousness or sedation OR limited ability to feel pain over most of body.	**2. Very Limited** Responds only to painful stimuli. Cannot communicate discomfort except by moaning or restlessness OR has a sensory impairment which limits the ability to feel pain or discomfort over half of body.	**3. Slightly Limited** Responds to verbal commands, but cannot always communicate discomfort or the need to be turned OR has some sensory impairment which limits ability to feel pain or discomfort in 1 or 2 extremities.	**4. No Impairment** Responds to verbal commands. Has no sensory deficit which would limit ability to feel or voice pain or discomfort.

MOISTURE degree to which skin is exposed to moisture			
1. Constantly Moist Skin is kept moist almost constantly by perspiration, urine, etc. Dampness is detected every time patient is moved or turned.	**2. Very Moist** Skin is often, but not always, moist. Linen must be changed at least once a shift.	**3. Occasionally Moist** Skin is occasionally moist, requiring an extra linen change approximately once a day.	**4. Rarely Moist** Skin is usually dry, linen only requires changing at routine intervals.

ACTIVITY degree of physical activity			
1. Bedfast Confined to bed.	**2. Chairfast** Ability to walk severely limited or nonexistent. Cannot bear own weight and/or must be assisted into chair or wheelchair.	**3. Walks Occasionally** Walks occasionally during day, but for very short distances, with or without assistance. Spends majority of each shift in bed or chair.	**4. Walks Frequently** Walks outside room at least twice a day and inside room at least once every 2 hours during waking hours.

MOBILITY ability to change and control body position			
1. Completely Immobile Does not make even slight changes in body or extremity position without assistance.	**2. Very Limited** Makes occasional slight changes in body or extremity position but unable to make frequent or significant changes independently.	**3. Slightly Limited** Makes frequent though slight changes in body or extremity position independently.	**4. No Limitation** Makes major and frequent changes in position without assistance.

NUTRITION usual food intake pattern			
1. Very Poor Never eats a complete meal. Rarely eats more than one-third of any food offered. Eats two servings or less of protein (meat or dairy products) per day. Takes fluids poorly. Does not take a liquid dietary supplement OR is NPO and/or maintained on clear liquids or IVs for more than 5 days.	**2. Probably Inadequate** Rarely eats a complete meal and generally eats only about half of any food offered. Protein intake includes only three servings of meat or dairy products per day. Occasionally will take a dietary supplement OR receives less than optimum amount of liquid diet or tube feeding.	**3. Adequate** Eats over half of most meals. Eats a total of four servings of protein (meat, dairy products) per day. Occasionally will refuse a meal, but will usually take a supplement when offered OR is on a tube feeding or TPN regimen which probably meets most of nutritional needs.	**4. Excellent** Eats most of every meal. Never refuses a meal. Usually eats a total of four or more servings of meat and dairy products. Occasionally eats between meals. Does not require supplementation.

Friction & Shear		
1. Problem Requires moderate to maximum assistance in moving. Complete lifting without sliding against sheets is impossible. Frequently slides down in bed or chair, requiring frequent repositioning with maximum assistance. Spasticity, contractures, or agitation leads to almost constant friction.	**2. Potential Problem** Moves feebly or requires minimum assistance. During a move skin probably slides to some extent against sheets, chair, restraints, or other devices. Maintains relatively good position in chair or bed most of the time but occasionally slides down.	**3. No Apparent Problem** Moves in bed and in chair independently and has sufficient muscle strength to lift up completely during move. Maintains good position in bed or chair.

Scoring: The Braden scale is a summated rating scale made up of six subscales scored from 1 to 3 or 4, for total scores that range from 6 to 23. A lower Braden scale score indicates a lower level of functioning and, therefore, a higher level of risk for pressure ulcer development. A score of 19 or higher, for instance, would indicate that the patient is at low risk, with no need for treatment at this time. The assessment can also be used to evaluate the course of a particular treatment.

Total Score ____________

Goals

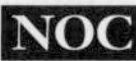

Tissue Integrity: Skin and Mucous Membrane

The individual demonstrate skin integrity free of pressure ulcers (if able), as evidenced by the following indicators:

- Describes etiology and prevention measures
- Participates in risk reduction
- Consumes recommended daily dietary intake

Interventions

NIC

Pressure Management, Skin Surveillance, Positioning, Teaching Interventions, Surveillance, Nutritional Management, Pressure Prevention, Positioning, Incontinence

Use a Formal Risk Assessment Scale to Identify Individual Risk Factors in Addition to Activity and Mobility Deficits

- Refer to Focus Assessment Criteria.

Perform Regular Skin Assessments as Frequently as Indicated

- Skin inspection should include assessment for localized heat, edema, or induration (hardness), especially in individuals with darkly pigmented skin.
- Inspect areas at risk of developing ulcers with each position change.
  - Ears
  - Elbows
  - Occiput
  - Trochanter[34]
  - Heels
  - Ischia
  - Sacrum
  - Scapula
  - Scrotum

Assess Dependent Skin Areas With Every Position Turn

- Use finger or transparent disk to assess whether skin is blanchable or nonblanchable.

R: *"Blanchable erythema is visible skin redness that become white when pressure is applied and reddens when pressure relieved" (National Pressure Ulcer Advisory Panel, 2014, p. 63). It may result from normal reactive hyperemia that should disappear within several hours or it may result from inflammatory erythema with intact capillary bed. Nonblanchable erythema is visible redness that persists with the application of pressure, which indicates structural damage to microcirculation. This represents Category/Stage I pressure ulcer (National Pressure Ulcer Advisory Panel, 2014, p. 63).*

- Assess skin temperature, edema, and change in tissue consistency as compared to surrounding tissue.

R: *Localized heat, edema, and change in tissue consistency as induration/hardness as compared to surrounding tissue are warning signs for pressure ulcer development (National Pressure Ulcer Advisory Panel, 2014).*

- Observe the skin for pressure damage caused by medical devices (e.g., catheters and cervical collars).

Clinical Alert Do not wear gloves when assessing skin temperature and changes in tissue consistency. As indicated cleanse skin prior to assessing and follow usual hand-washing procedures.

- Ask individuals to identify any areas of discomfort or pain that could be attributed to pressure damage.
- Document all skin assessments, noting details of any pain possibly related to pressure damage.

R: *The frequency of inspection may need to be increased in response to any deterioration in overall condition.*

- Ask the individual if they have any areas of discomfort or pain that could be attributed to pressure damage.

R: *Studies reported that pain over the site was a precursor to tissue breakdown (National Pressure Ulcer Advisory Panel, 2014).*

---

[34]Areas with little soft tissue over a bony prominence are at greatest risk.

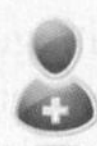

Clinical Alert Researchers have reported that the failure to identify early stages of pressure damage results in greater numbers of people with darkly pigmented skin developing more severe forms of pressure damage (Baumgarten et al., 2009; National Pressure Ulcer Advisory Panel, 2014; *Rosen et al 2006).

For Individuals with Darkly Pigmented Skin, Consider (*Bennett, 1995; Clark, 2010, p. 17)

- The color of intact dark pigmented skin may remain unchanged (does not blanch) when pressure is applied over a bony prominence.
- Local areas of intact skin that are subject to pressure may feel either warm or cool when touched. This assessment should be performed without gloves to make it easier to distinguish differences in temperature after any body fluids are cleansed before making this direct contact.
- Areas of skin subjected to pressure may be purplish/bluish/violet in color. This can be compared with the erythema seen in people with lighter skin tones.
- Complains of, or indicate, current or recent pain or discomfort at body sites where pressure has been applied.

R: *Stage I pressure ulcers are underdetected in individuals with darkly pigmented skin. Visual cues for changes in skin appearance may be relatively easy to observe in Caucasian skin, but with darker pigmentation it may be harder to spot visual signs of early changes due to pressure damage (Clark, 2010; National Pressure Ulcer Advisory Panel, 2014).*

- Increase frequency of the turning schedule if any nonblanchable erythema is noted. Consult with prescribing professional for the utilization of pressure-dispersing devices and microclimate manipulation devices in addition to repositioning.

R: *Principles of pressure ulcer prevention include reducing or rotating pressure on soft tissue. If pressure on soft tissue exceeds intracapillary pressure (approximately 32 mm Hg), capillary occlusion and resulting hypoxia can cause tissue damage. The greater the duration of immobility, the greater the likelihood of the development of small vessel thrombosis and subsequent tissue necrosis (National Pressure Ulcer Advisory Panel, 2014).*

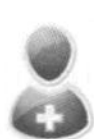

Clinical Alert Peterson et al. (2013) reported using pressure mapping devices to measure pressure on skin/tissue when high-risk individuals were positioned on their back, left side, and right side. Bedridden individuals at risk for pressure ulcer formation exhibit high skin–bed interface pressures on specific skin areas that are likely always at risk (i.e., triple-jeopardy and always-at-risk areas) for the vast majority of the time they are in bed despite routine repositioning care. Triple jeopardy were skin areas that were consistently compressed in all three positions. "Healthcare providers are unaware of the actual tissue-relieving effectiveness (or lack thereof) of their repositioning interventions, which may partially explain why pressure ulcer mitigation strategies are not always successful. Relieving at-risk tissue is a necessary part of pressure ulcer prevention, but the repositioning practice itself needs improvement."

- Repositioning should be undertaken using the 30° tilted side-lying position (alternately, right side, back, left side) or the prone position if the individual can tolerate this, and if her or his medical condition allows. Avoid postures that increase pressure, such as the 90° side-lying position, or the semi-recumbent position.
- Ensure that the heels are free of the surface of the bed. Position knee in slight flexion. Uses a pillow under the calves so that heels are elevated (i.e., "floating").

R: *Heel protection devices should elevate the heel completely (offload them) in such a way as to distribute the weight of the leg along the calf without putting pressure on the Achilles tendon.*

- Use transfer aids to reduce friction and shear. Lift—don't drag—the individual while repositioning.

R: *Shear is a parallel force in which one layer of tissue moves in one direction and another layer moves in the opposite direction. If the skin sticks to the bed linen and the weight of the body makes the skeleton slide down inside the skin (as with semi-Fowler's positioning), the subepidermal capillaries may become angulated and pinched, resulting in decreased perfusion of the tissue (Grossman & Porth, 2014).*

R: *Friction is the physiologic wearing away of tissue. If the skin is rubbed against the bed linens, the epidermis can be denuded by abrasion.*

- Avoid positioning the individual directly onto medical devices, such as tubes or drainage systems.
- Avoid positioning the individual on bony prominences with existing nonblanchable erythema.
- If sitting in bed is necessary, avoid head-of-bed elevation or a slouched position that places pressure and shear on the sacrum and coccyx.

R: *Reposition the individual in such a way that pressure is relieved or redistributed.*

Repositioning the Seated Individual

- Position the individual so as to maintain his or her full range of activities.
- Select a posture that is acceptable for the individual, and minimizes the pressures and shear exerted on the skin and soft tissues. Place the feet of the individual on a footstool or footrest when the feet do not reach the floor.
- Limit the time an individual spends seated in a chair without pressure relief.

R: *Prevention in individuals at risk should be provided on a continuous basis during the time that they are at risk.*

Use of Support Surfaces to Prevent Pressure Ulcers

- Use a pressure-redistributing seat cushion for individuals sitting in a chair whose mobility is reduced.
- Limit the time an individual spends seated in a chair without pressure relief.
- Use alternating pressure active support overlays or mattress as indicated.

R: *A pressure-reducing surface must not be able to be fully compressed by the body. To be effective, a support surface must be capable of first being deformed and then redistributing the weight of the body across the surface. Comfort is not a valid criterion for determining adequate pressure reduction. A hand check should be performed to determine if the product is effectively reducing pressure. The palm is placed under the pressure-reducing mattress; if the individual can feel the hand or the caregiver can feel the individual, the pressure is not adequate.*

Attempt to Modify Contributing Factors to Lessen the Possibility of a Pressure Ulcer Developing

Incontinence of Urine or Feces

- Determine the etiology of the incontinence.
- Maintain sufficient fluid intake for adequate hydration (approximately 2,500 mL daily, unless contraindicated); check oral mucous membranes for moisture and check urine specific gravity.
- Establish a schedule for emptying the bladder (begin with every 2 hours).
- If the individual is confused, determine what his or her incontinence pattern is and intervene before incontinence occurs.
- Explain problem to the individual; secure his or her cooperation for the plan.
- When incontinent, wash the perineum with a liquid soap.
- Apply a protective barrier to the perineal region (incontinence film barrier spray or wipes).
- Check the individual frequently for incontinence when indicated.
- For additional interventions, refer to *Impaired Urinary Elimination.*

R: *Maceration is a mechanism by which the tissue is softened by prolonged wetting or soaking. If the skin becomes waterlogged, the cells are weakened and the epidermis is easily eroded. Bowel incontinence is more damaging than urinary incontinence, due to the additional digestive enzymes found in stool. Care must be taken to prevent excoriation (National Pressure Ulcer Advisory Panel, 2014).*

Skin Care

- Do not turn the individual onto a body surface that is still reddened from a previous episode of pressure loading.
- Do not use massage for pressure ulcer prevention or do not vigorously rub skin that is at risk for pressure ulceration.

R: *Massage is contraindicated in the presence of acute inflammation and where there is the possibility of damaged blood vessels or fragile skin.*

- Use skin emollients to hydrate dry skin in order to reduce risk of skin damage. Protect the skin from exposure to excessive moisture with a barrier product.

R: *Excessive moisture will contribute to maceration when tissues are softened by prolonged wetting, which breaks down the protective layer of epidermis/dermis.*

- Avoid use of synthetic sheepskin pads; cutout, ring, or donut-type devices; and water-filled gloves.

R: *These products are irritating and create pressure, which compromises circulation.*

- Monitor serum prealbumin levels.
  - Less than 5 mg/dL predicts a poor prognosis.
  - Less than 11 mg/dL predicts high risk and requires aggressive nutritional supplementation.
  - Less than 15 mg/dL predicts an increased risk of malnutrition (Dudek, 2014).

R: *Laboratory values, such as albumin, prealbumin, and transferrin, may not reflect the current nutritional state, especially in the critically ill individual. Other assessment factors such as weight loss, illness severity, comorbid conditions, and gastrointestinal function should be considered for a nutrition plan of care (Doley, 2010).*

Nutrition

- Ensure a nutritional assessment is completed by a registered dietician/nutritionist using the MNA if possible.

R: *MNA is the only nutritional screening tool that has been specifically validated in individuals with pressure ulcers (National Pressure Ulcer Advisory Panel, 2014).*

- Report to prescribing provider when food and/or fluid intake is decreased.

R: *Fortified foods and/or high-calorie, high-protein oral nutrition supplements between meals may be needed (National Pressure Ulcer Advisory Panel, 2014).*

- Advise family/friends the importance of nutritionally dense foods/beverages versus calories-dense foods/beverages.
  - Calorie-dense foods, also called energy-dense foods, contain high levels of calories per serving in fat and carbohydrates. Many processed foods are considered calorie-dense, such as cakes, cookies, snacks, doughnuts, and candies.
  - Nutrient-dense foods contain high levels of nutrients, such as protein, carbohydrates, fats, vitamins and minerals, but with fewer calories. Some nutrient-dense foods are fresh fruits, vegetables, berries, melons, dark-green vegetables, sweet potatoes, tomatoes, and whole grains, including quinoa, barley, bulgur, and oats. Lean beef and pork are high in protein and contain high levels of zinc, iron, and B-vitamins.

R: *Individuals with pressure ulcers need 30 to 35 kcal/kg body weight, 1.25 to 1.5 g protein/kg of body weight daily, and vitamins and minerals (National Pressure Ulcer Advisory Panel, 2014). Calorie-dense foods do not provide the needed nutrients and can replace the needed nutrient-dense foods when the individual's appetite is poor.*

- Refer to *Imbalance Nutrition* for interventions related to promoting optimal intake of required nutrients.

R: *Malnutrition is associated with impaired wound healing (National Pressure Ulcer Advisory Panel, 2014).*

Initiate Health Teaching as Indicated

- Instruct the individual/family in specific techniques to use at home to prevent pressure ulcers.
- Teach how to use their finger to assess whether skin is blanchable or nonblanchable and when to notify primary care provider.
- Stress prevention and early identification of nonblanchable redness.
- Consider the use of long-term pressure-relieving devices for permanent disabilities.
- Initiate a referral to a home health nurse for an in home assessment.

R: *Pressure reduction is the one consistent intervention that must be continued at home.*

Impaired Skin Integrity

NANDA-I Definition

Altered epidermis and/or dermis

Defining Characteristics*

Destruction of skin layers
Disruption of skin surface

Invasion of body structures

Author's Note

Impaired Skin Integrity has limited clinical use, since *Risk for Pressure Ulcer* (approved By NANDA-I) and *Pressure Ulcer* were added in this edition by the author.

Related Factors

Refer to *Pressure Ulcer*.

Key Concepts

Refer to *Pressure Ulcer*.

Focus Assessment Criteria

Refer to *Pressure Ulcer*.

Goals

NOC
Refer to Pressure Ulcer

Refer to *Pressure Ulcer*.

Interventions

Refer to *Pressure Ulcer*.

Risk for Impaired Skin Integrity

NANDA-I Definition

At risk for alteration in epidermis and/or dermis

Risk Factors

Refer to Related Factors under *Impaired Skin Integrity*.

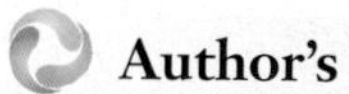

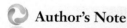

Author's Note

Risk for Impaired Skin Integrity has little clinical usefulness since NANDA-I accepted *Risk for Pressure Ulcer*. Refer to *Risk for Pressure Ulcer* for interventions.

Impaired Oral Mucous Membrane

Definition

Disruption of the lips, soft tissues, buccal cavity, and/or oropharynx

Defining Characteristics

Disrupted tissue on lips, buccal cavity, and/or oropharynx
Color changes—erythema, pallor, white patches, lesions, and ulcers

Moisture changes—increased or decreased saliva
Cleanliness changes—debris, malodor, and discoloration of the teeth
Mucosal integrity changes—difficulty swallowing, decreased taste, and difficulty weaning
Perception changes—difficulty swallowing, decreased taste, difficulty wearing dentures, burning, pain, and change in voice quality

Related Factors

Pathophysiologic

Related to inflammation secondary to:

Diabetes mellitus
Periodontal disease
Oral cancer
Infection

Treatment Related

Related to drying effects of:

NPO more than 24 hours
Radiation to head or neck
Prolonged use of steroids or other immunosuppressive agents and other medications including opioids, antidepressants, phenothiazines, antihypertensives, antihistamines, diuretics, and sedatives.
Use of antineoplastic drugs
Oxygen therapy
Mouth breathing
Fever
Blood and marrow stem cell transplant

Related to mechanical irritation secondary to:

Endotracheal tube
NG tube

Situational (Personal, Environmental)

Related to chemical irritants* secondary to:

Acidic foods
Drugs
Noxious agents
Alcohol
Tobacco
High sugar intake

Related to mechanical trauma secondary to:

Broken or jagged teeth
Ill-fitting dentures
Braces

Related to malnutrition*

Related to inadequate oral hygiene

Related to lack of knowledge of oral hygiene

Author's Note

See *Impaired Tissue Integrity*.

Errors in Diagnostic Statements

See *Impaired Tissue Integrity*.

Key Concepts

General Considerations

- Oral health directly influences many activities of daily living (eating, fluid intake, breathing) and interpersonal relations (appearance, self-concept, communication).
- Many oral diseases begin quietly and are painless until significant involvement has taken place.
- Common causes of decreased salivation are dehydration, anemia, radiation treatment to head and neck, vitamin deficiencies, removal of salivary glands, allergies, and side effects of drugs (e.g., antihistamines, anticholinergics, phenothiazine, narcotics, chemotherapy, and other antineoplastic medications).
- Mucosal damage usually occurs 7 to 14 days after the start of radiation and 3 to 9 days after the start of chemotherapy.
- Gibson et al. (2013) estimates that 40% of chemotherapy patients, 80% of stem cell transplant patients, and 100% of patients receiving radiation to the head and neck will develop oral mucositis.
- Consequences of mucositis include increased risk for mortality, delaying treatment, increased need for nutritional support, increased fatigue and bleeding, increased risk for infection, pain, and decreased quality of life.
- Initiating oral care protocols have decreased both ventilator-associated pneumonia (Feider, Mitchell, & Bridges, 2010) and nonventilator acquired pneumonia (Quinn et al., 2014).
- When the mucosa is damaged, the treatment includes the principles of wound management: moisture, cleansing, and promoting healing.
- Alcohol and tobacco are chronic irritants to oral mucosa and may lead to oral carcinoma.
- Oral mucositis and stomatitis do not have identical processes. Oral mucositis is the inflammation of the oral mucosa resulting from chemotherapy, other antineoplastic agents, and ionizing radiation that is manifested by erythema or ulcerations, whereas stomatitis refers to any inflammation of the oral tissues (dentition/periapices, periodontium), including infections of the oral cavity and oral mucositis (National Cancer Institute [NCI], 2014).
- Mucous membranes are highly susceptible to toxicity because of their rapidly proliferating cells. Individuals exposed to multiple therapies or who have predisposing risk factors such as poor oral hygiene, dental caries, and tobacco or alcohol use are more likely to develop mucositis.
- Chemotherapy or direct radiation also can cause xerostomia, which is a decrease in the quality and quantity of saliva (NCI, 2014).
- Cryotherapy, lower-level laser therapy, oral care protocols, and palifermin are interventions recommended for practice that have strong evidence regarding treatment of oral mucositis, while prophylactic chlorhexidine mouth rinses for prevention, lactobacillus lozenges for patients with head and neck cancer receiving chemotherapy and radiation, and benzydamine rinses for patients with head and neck cancer are mucositis interventions that are likely to be effective (Eilers, Harris, Henry, & Johnson, 2014).
- Palifermin, a keratinocyte growth factor, may prevent chemotherapy-induced oral mucositis in individuals with a hematologic malignancy and who is receiving a stem cell transplant. Another advantage is that palifermin reduces the incidence and duration of mucositis (NCI, 2014).
- The cost of mucositis is usually doubled when classified as severe because of the increased length of stay (Carlotto, Hogsett, Maiorini, Razulis, & Sonis, 2013).

Pediatric Considerations

- Oral candidiasis (thrush) is common in newborns. It can be acquired via person-to-person transmission, from a maternal vaginal infection during delivery, or from use of contaminated nipples or other articles (Pillitteri, 2014).
- Teething may cause discomfort and make gums appear red and swollen.

Geriatric Considerations

- Age-related changes in oral mucosa include loss of elasticity, atrophy of epithelial cells, and diminished blood supply to connective tissue (Chan, Lee, Poh, & Prabhakaran, 2011).
- Dry mouth and vitamin deficiencies in older adults increase vulnerability to oral ulcerations and infection (Chan et al., 2011).
- Older adults commonly exhibit increased saliva viscosity and diminished saliva quantity (Chan et al., 2011).

Focus Assessment Criteria

Subjective Data

Assess for Defining Characteristics

Refer to Defining Characteristics.

Assess for Related Factors

Refer to Related Factors.

Objective Data and Physical Assessment

Use a standardized oral assessment/measurement tool.

Gather equipment to use to assess oral cavity. Equipment includes a good light source, tongue blade, nonsterile gloves, and gauze to retract the tongue as well as suction equipment if needed. Systemically examine oral cavity for change in oral mucosa, moisture level, cleanliness, presence of ulcers or lesions, integrity of lips, and quality of speech and voice.

Assess for Defining Characteristics

Lips
- Color
- Blisters
- Ulcers/lesions
- Edema
- Cracks
- Fissures
- Bleeding

Tongue
- Color
- Cracks, dryness
- Edema
- Lesions
- Hairy extensions
- Masses
- Ulcers
- Bleeding
- Exudates
- Blisters

Oral Mucosa (Gums, Floor of Mouth, Inner Cheeks, Palate)
- Color
- Bleeding
- Swelling (along gumline)
- Moisture
- Plaques
- Ulcers

Saliva
- Watery
- Absent
- Thick
- Color

Teeth
- Sharp edges
- Chips
- Cracks
- Looseness
- Missing teeth
- Plaque or debris

Dentures/Prosthetics
- Condition
- Sharp edges
- Loose parts
- Fit
- Cracks
- Chips

Gingiva
- Color
- Edema
- Bleeding

Swallowing
- Ability to swallow
- Pain

Voice
- Difficulty talking
- Deeper raspy voice

Goals

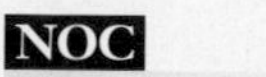

Oral Tissue Integrity

The individual will be free of oral mucosa irritation or exhibit signs of healing with decreased inflammation, as evidenced by the following indicators:

- Describes factors that cause oral injury
- Demonstrates knowledge of optimal oral hygiene
- Be free of oral discomfort during food and fluid intake

Interventions

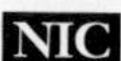

Oral Health Restoration, Chemotherapeutic Management, Oral Health Maintenance, Oral Health Promotion

Assess for Causative or Contributing Factors

- Assess with a valid and reliable tool as a first step to preventing and treating oral mucositis (Eilers et al., 2014).

R: *Researchers have reported that for individuals with mechanical ventilation, only 32% had suctioning to manage oral secretions, 33% had their teeth brushed, 65% had swab cleansing, and 63% had a moisturizer applied to the oral mucosal tissues. In addition, nurses reported performing oral care than actually completing (*Cutler & Davis, 2005; Fields, 2008; Goss, Coty, & Myers, 2011).*

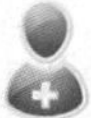

Clinical Alert Too often, oral care and assessment are omitted in individual care.

- Refer to Related Factors.
- Evaluate person's ability to perform oral hygiene. Allow person to perform as much oral care as possible. For high-risk individuals, inspect the oral cavity for lesions (e.g., white patches, broken teeth, and signs of infection).

R: *A focused assessment will be indicated.*

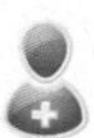

Clinical Alert Advise staff/student to report any complaints of mouth sores, white patches, broken and/or sharp teeth, and problems with swallowing.

Teach Preventive Oral Hygiene to Individuals at Risk for Development of Mucositis

- Refer to impaired oral mucous membrane related to inadequate oral hygiene for specific instructions on brushing and flossing.

Instruct Individual to

- Perform the regimen including brushing, flossing, rinsing, and moisturizing after meals and before sleep.
- Avoid mouthwashes with alcohol content, lemon/glycerin swabs, or prolonged use of hydrogen peroxide.

R: *These solutions can cause mucosal abnormalities, dryness, and discomfort (*Meurman et al., 1996; NCI, 2014).*

- Rinse mouth with saline or saline and bicarbonate solution.
- Apply lubricant to lips every 2 hours and PRN (e.g., lanolin, A&D ointment).
- Inspect mouth daily for lesions and inflammation and report alterations.
- Avoid foods that are spicy, salty, hot, rough, or acidic.
- Report following symptoms: temperature greater than 101° F, new lesions or sores in mouth, bleeding from gums, difficulty swallowing or inability to take in fluids, and pain in the mouth.
- Keep mouth clean and moist.

R: *Factors that contribute to oral disease include inadequate hygiene and dry mucous membranes.*

Consult With Physician for Possible Need for Prophylactic Antifungal or Antibacterial Agent for Immunocompromised Individuals at Risk for Mucositis (Freifeld et al., 2011)

- Instruct individual to see a dentist 2 to 3 weeks before therapy begins for diagnosis and treatment of infections and to ensure adequate time for healing.
- Consult with dentist for a regimen of daily fluoride treatments and oral hygiene.
- Instruct individual to see a dentist during treatment as needed and 2 months after treatment.

- Refer any suspicious oral lesions to health-care provider for culture to identify organism.
- Administer antibiotics, antifungals, or antivirals as prescribed.
- Monitor temperature every 4 hours and report abnormal readings to health-care provider.
- Replace toothbrush after treatment of suspected or documented oral infection.

R: *Dental disease is a reservoir of infections and requires careful management by knowledgeable professionals.*

Promote Healing and Reduce Progression of Mucositis

- Inspect oral cavity two times a day with tongue blade and light; if mucositis is severe, inspect mouth every 4 hours.
- Ensure that oral hygiene regimen is done every 1 to 2 hours while awake and every 4 hours during the night for patients with severe mucositis.
- Use normal saline solution as a mouthwash.
- Floss teeth only once in 24 hours.
- Omit flossing if bleeding is excessive.

R: *Systematically applied protocols may significantly decrease the incidence, severity, and duration of oral problems (Eilers et al., 2014).*

R: *Salt and soda rinses are effective and the least costly selection for the prevention of treatment of mucositis. Foam brushes are not equal to toothbrushes for removing plaque and bacteria for cavity prevention. The effectiveness of mouthwash preparations over normal saline has not been supported in the literature (Eilers et al., 2014; ONS, 2007).*

R: *Proper hydration must be maintained to liquefy secretions and prevent drying of oral mucosa.*

Reduce Oral Pain and Maintain Adequate Food and Fluid Intake

- Assess individual's ability to chew and swallow.
- Administer mild analgesic every 3 to 4 hours as ordered by physician.
- Instruct individual to:
  - Avoid commercial mouthwashes, citrus fruit juices, spicy foods, extremes in food temperature (hot, cold), crusty or rough foods, alcohol, and mouthwashes with alcohol.
  - Eat bland, cool foods (e.g., sherbets).
  - Drink cool liquids every 2 hours and PRN.
- Consult with dietitian for specific interventions.
- Refer to *Impaired Nutrition: Less Than Body Requirements* related to anorexia for additional interventions.
- Consult with physician for an oral pain relief solution.
  - Xylocaine viscous 2% oral: swish and expectorate every 2 hours and before meals. (If throat is sore, the solution can be swallowed; if swallowed, Xylocaine produces local anesthesia and may affect the gag reflex.) The dose of the viscous Xylocaine is not to exceed 25 mm per day (National Comprehensive Cancer Network [NCCN], 2008).
  - A protective barrier may be applied and requires frequent applications because of limited duration (e.g., Episil, Gelclair, Mugard). Prophylaxis is not recommended (Eilers, 2014).
  - Topical morphine provides a reduction in pain severity and duration of pain. If the morphine is in an alcohol-based formula, it may cause burning.

R: *Proper hydration must be maintained to liquefy secretions and prevent drying of oral mucosa.*

R: *Dry oral mucosa causes discomfort and increases the risk of breakdown and infection.*

Initiate Health Teaching and Referrals, as Indicated

- Teach individual and family the factors that contribute to stomatitis and its progression.
- Teach diet modifications to reduce oral pain and to maintain optimal nutrition.
- Have individual describe or demonstrate home care regimen.

R: *The frequency of oral health maintenance varies according to an individual's health status and self-care ability. All individuals should have their teeth and mouth cleaned at least once after meals and at bedtime. High-risk individuals (e.g., NG tubes, cancer, poorly nourished) should have oral care done at least every 4 hours.*

Risk for Impaired Oral Mucous Membrane • Related to Inadequate Oral Hygiene or Inability to Perform Oral Hygiene

NANDA-I Definition

Vulnerable to injury to the lips, soft tissues, buccal cavity, and/or oropharynx

Risk Factors

Refer to Related Factors under Impaired Oral Mucous Membrane.

Goals

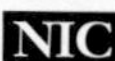
Oral Tissue Integrity

The individual will demonstrate integrity of the oral cavity, as evidenced by the following indicators:

- Be free of harmful plaque to prevent secondary infection
- Be free of oral discomfort during food and fluid intake
- Demonstrates optimal oral hygiene

Interventions

NIC
Oral Health Restoration, Chemotherapeutic Management, Oral Health Maintenance, Oral Health Promotion

Assess for Causative or Contributing Factors

- Refer to Related Factors.

Discuss the Importance of Daily Oral Hygiene and Periodic Dental Examinations

- Explain the relationship of plaque to dental and gum disease.
- Evaluate individual's ability to perform oral hygiene.
- Allow individual to perform as much oral care as possible.

R: *Plaque, microbial flora found in the mouth, is the primary cause of dental cavities and periodontal disease. Daily removal of plaque through brushing and flossing can help prevent dental decay and disease.*

Teach Correct Oral Care

- Have individual sit or stand upright over sink (if he or she cannot get to a sink, place an emesis pan under the chin or have suction set up at bedside).
- Remove and clean dentures and bridges daily.
  - Brush dentures inside and outside daily with a denture brush or stiff, hard toothbrush; rinse in cool water before replacing.
  - Individuals who are intubated, unconscious, or have severe mucositis should not have dentures replaced into mouth. Store dentures in a cleaning solution and change solution daily to prevent bacterial growth.
  - Have family discard any ill-fitting dentures.

R: *Unclean or ill-fitting dentures can contribute to infection.*

- Floss teeth (every 24 hours).
  - With a piece of dental floss approximately 25 inches long, floss each tooth by wrapping the floss around the second and third fingers of each hand.
  - Begin with the back teeth; insert the floss between each tooth gently to avoid injuring the gum.
  - Wrap floss around tooth, making a C, and gently pull floss up and down over the back of each tooth.
  - Repeat this in reverse to floss the front of the tooth.
  - Remove the floss either by pulling straight up or by releasing one end and pulling the floss through (minor bleeding may occur).
  - Rinse.
  - Floss holders can make flossing easier (back teeth cannot be reached with a floss holder).

R: *Flossing removes plaque from gumline and is recommended by the American Dental Association as part of a daily oral hygiene plan (American Dental Association, 2014).*

- Brush teeth (after meals and before sleep).

- Use a soft-bristled toothbrush (avoid hard brushes) with a nonabrasive toothpaste with fluoride or sodium bicarbonate (1 teaspoon in 8 ounces of water; may be contraindicated in people with sodium restrictions). Air dry toothbrush between uses.
- Brush back and forth or in a small circle, starting at the back of the mouth and brushing one or two teeth at a time.
- Gently brush tongue and inner sides of cheeks.
- Rinse with water, normal saline, or sterile water for 30 seconds.
- Apply moisturizer to lips and inside of mouth.

R: *Daily removal of plaque can prevent dental disease.*

- Inspect mouth for lesions, sores, or excessive bleeding

Perform Oral Hygiene on the Individual Who Is Unconscious or at Risk for Aspiration as Often as Needed

Preparation

- Gather equipment: soft-bristled toothbrush, toothpaste, cup of water, suction setup, light source, emesis basin, towel, wash cloth, and gloves (may use a kit that contains all supplies).
- Tell individual what you are going to do.
- Turn individual to the side, supporting his or her back with a pillow (protect bed with an absorbent pad).
- Place a tongue blade or bite block if necessary to keep mouth open.
- Wear gloves to protect self.

Brushing Procedure

- For people with their own teeth, brush following the procedure outlined above. Use sodium bicarbonate (1 teaspoon:8 ounces water), water, or normal saline solution (may be contraindicated in people with sodium restrictions).
- Place emesis basin against individual's mouth and use the suction to remove secretions from the mouth.
- For people with dentures, remove dentures and clean as above. Leave dentures out for people who are semicomatose and store in water (in denture cup).
- Use toothettes if patient does not tolerate brushing.

R: *The bristles of a toothbrush are much more effective at removing plaque than foam toothettes (Quinn et al., 2014).*

- Use a bulb syringe to rinse mouth; aspirate rinse with suction or use an aspirating toothbrush.
- Move tongue blade or bite block, if necessary, for access to other areas; do not put fingers on tops or edges of teeth.
- Brush tongue and inner cheek tissue gently.
- Apply lip lubricant and mouth moisturizer.

Perform Oral Hygiene on Individuals Who Are Intubated and/or Mechanically Ventilated

- Gather equipment (same as for unconscious individual).
- Position individual head of bed higher than 30° unless medically contraindicated.

R: *Providing comprehensive oral care to decrease the bacterial load in the mouth and keeping the head of the bed elevated greater than 30° help decrease aspiration and may prevent pneumonia (Quinn et al., 2014).*

- Brush teeth, tongue, and gums as described above twice a day.
- Swab oral cavity every 2 to 4 hours and as needed with normal saline or mouth rinse solution.

R: *Recommendations for oral care include routine brushing of teeth, oral cleansing every 2 to 4 hours and as needed, use of antiseptic oral rinse (no alcohol), routine suctioning, and application of oral mouth moisturizer (Goss, Coty, & Myers, 2011).*

- Use oral chlorhexidine gluconate rinses or gels as per protocols or orders.
- Apply mouth moisturize to mouth and lips.
- Remove excess oral secretions by using the suction.

R: *Use of chlorhexidine gluconate is associated with a reduction in the development of ventilatory-associated pneumonia (Shi et al., 2013). Further studies are needed to determine what mouth care solutions are the most effective.*

R: *Factors that contribute to oral disease are excessive use of alcohol and tobacco, microorganisms, inadequate nutrition (quantity, quality), inadequate hygiene, and trauma (NG tubes, ill-fitting dentures, sharp-edged teeth, sharp-edged prostheses, improper use of cleaning devices).*

R: *Oral health is influenced by microorganisms that grow in the plaque. With ventilators the microorganisms can transfer to the lungs and cause ventilator-associated pneumonia (Needleman et al., 2012).*

R: *The NCCN (2008) recommend that bone marrow and stem cell transplant individuals should receive dental evaluation and treatment before transplant. Oral care should include daily flossing, brushing teeth with a soft-bristled toothbrush at least twice a day, and using toothettes if individual cannot tolerate the toothbrush, and oral rinses four to six times a day with normal saline, sterile water, or sodium bicarbonate.*

Initiate Health Teaching and Referrals, as Indicated

- Teach person and family the factors that contribute to stomatitis and its progression.
- Teach diet modifications to reduce oral pain and to maintain optimal nutrition.
- Have individual describe or demonstrate home care regimen.

R: *The frequency of oral health maintenance varies according to a person's health status and self-care ability, but minimum is in AM and at bedtime. High-risk individuals (e.g., NG tubes, cancer, poorly nourished) should have an oral assessment daily.*

- Explain factors that contribute to oral disease are excessive use of alcohol, tobacco, microorganisms, inadequate nutrition (quantity, quality), inadequate hygiene, and trauma (ill-fitting dentures, sharp-edged teeth, sharp-edged prostheses, improper use of cleaning devices).
- Refer individuals with tooth and gum disorders to dentist.

Identify Individuals Who Need Toothbrush Adaptations to Perform Own Mouth Care

- For individuals with difficulty closing hands tightly, refer to occupational therapy.
- For individuals with limited hand mobility, enlarge toothbrush handle with a spongy hair roller, wrinkled aluminum foil, or a bicycle handlebar grip attached with a small amount of plaster of Paris.
- For individuals with limited arm movement, extend handle of standard toothbrush by attaching handle of an old toothbrush (after cutting off bristle end) to a new toothbrush with strong cord or plastic cement, or by attaching toothbrush to a plastic rod. (The toothbrush can be curved by gently heating and then bending it.)
- Refer the individual to occupational therapy.

Refer Individuals With Tooth and Gum Disorders to a Dentist

Pediatric Interventions

Teach Parents to

- Provide their child with fluoride supplements if not present in concentrations higher than 0.7 parts per million in drinking water.
- Avoid taking tetracycline drugs during pregnancy or giving them to children younger than 8 years.
- Refrain from putting an infant to bed with a bottle of juice or milk.
- Provide child with safe objects for chewing during teething.
- Replace toothbrushes frequently (every 3 months).
- Schedule dental checkups every 6 months after 2 years of age.
- Supervise and assist preschool child with brushing and flossing in front of mirror.
  - Talk to child when brushing.
  - "Ask child to 'tweet like a bird' to brush front teeth and 'roar like a lion' to brush back teeth" (Perry et al., 2014).
  - Incorporate brushing and flossing teeth into bedtime rituals.

Teach Child

- Why tooth care is important
- To avoid highly sugared liquids, foods, and chewing gum
- To drink water and extra fluid
- To brush teeth using fluoride toothpaste

R: *The objective of oral hygiene is to remove plaque, which causes decay and periodontal disease (Needleman et al., 2012).*

R: *Flossing removes plaque from gumline.*

Maternal Interventions

- Stress the importance of good oral hygiene and continued dental examinations. Advise women to increase intake of vitamin C.
- Remind individual to advise dentist of her pregnancy.
- Explain that gum hypertrophy and tenderness are normal during pregnancy.

R: *Gum hypertrophy, tenderness, and bleeding during normal pregnancy may be the result of vascular swelling called epulis of pregnancy (Clocheret, Dekeyser, Carels, & Willems, 2014).*

Geriatric Interventions

Explain High-Risk, Age-Related Factors (Chan et al., 2011)

- Degenerative bone disease
- Diminished oral blood supply
- Dry mouth
- Vitamin deficiencies

R: *Age-related changes and nutritional deficiencies increase vulnerability to oral ulcerations and infection (Chan et al., 2011).*

Explain That Some Medications Cause Dry Mouth

- Laxatives
- Antibiotics
- Antidepressants
- Anticholinergics
- Analgesics
- Iron sulfate
- Cardiovascular medications

R: *Dry mouth contributes to tissue injury.*

Determine Any Barriers to Dental Care

- Financial
- Mobility
- Dexterity

INEFFECTIVE RELATIONSHIP*

Ineffective Relationship

Risk for Ineffective Relationship

NANDA-I Definition

A pattern of mutual partnership that is insufficient to provide for each other's needs

Defining Characteristics*

No demonstration of mutual respect between partners
No demonstration of mutual support in daily activities between partners
No demonstration of understanding of partner's insufficient (physical, social, psychological) functioning
No demonstration of well-balanced autonomy between partners
No demonstration of well-balanced collaboration between partners
No identification of partner as a key person
Inability to communicate in a satisfying manner between partners
Report of dissatisfaction with complementary relation between partners

Report of dissatisfaction with fulfilling emotional needs by one's partner
Report of dissatisfaction with fulfilling physical needs by one's partner
Report of dissatisfaction with the sharing of ideas between partners
Report of dissatisfaction with the sharing of information between partners
Does not meet development goals appropriate for family life-cycle stage

Related Factors*

Cognitive changes in one partner
Developmental crises
History of domestic violence
Poor communication skills
Stressful life events
Substance abuse
Unrealistic expectations

Author's Note

This NANDA-I diagnosis represents problems or situations that can disrupt partner relationships. The list of related factors presents substantial different foci for interventions. For example, the interventions for relationship problems associated with substance abuse versus domestic violence and incarceration versus stressful life events are very different.

This book contains assessment and interventions with rationale for all of the related factors listed above, for example:

- Related to domestic violence, refer to *Dysfunctional Family Processes*.
- Related to substance abuse, refer to *Disturbed Self-Concept*, *Ineffective Denial*, and/or *Dysfunctional Family Processes*.
- Related to unrealistic expectations, refer to *Compromised Family Processes*.
- Related to poor communication skills and stressful life events, refer to *Compromised Family Processes* and *Readiness for Enhanced Relationships*.
- Related to cognitive changes, refer to *Chronic Confusion* and *Altered Thought Processes*.

Thus, when *Ineffective or Risk for (Partner) Relationship* is validated, the nurse can find goals and interventions/rationale in sections listed above or can use one of the above diagnoses instead if found to be more descriptive.

Risk for Ineffective Relationship

NANDA-I Definition

Vulnerable to developing a pattern that is insufficient for providing a mutual partnership to provide for each other's needs

Risk Factors

Cognitive changes in one's partner
Developmental crises
Domestic violence
Incarceration of one's partner
Poor communication skills
Stressful life events
Substance abuse
Unrealistic expectations

RELOCATION STRESS [SYNDROME]

Relocation Stress [Syndrome]

Risk for Relocation Stress [Syndrome]

Relocation Stress [Syndrome] • Related to Changes Associated With Health-Care Facility Transfers or Admission to Long-Term–Care Facility

NANDA-I Definition

Physiologic and/or psychological disturbance following transfer from one environment to another

Note: Other terms found in the literature that describe relocation stress include admission stress, post-relocation crisis, relocation crisis, relocation shock, relocation trauma, transfer stress, transfer trauma, translocation syndrome, and transplantation shock.

Defining Characteristics (*Barnhouse, Harkulich, & Brugler, 1992)

Responds to transfer or relocation with
- Loneliness
- Depression
- Anger

Change in former eating habits
Decrease in self-care activities
Decrease in leisure activities
Change in former sleep patterns
Gastrointestinal disturbances
Increased verbalization of needs
Demonstration of dependency
Need for excessive reassurance
Demonstration of insecurity
Restlessness
Apprehension
Anxiety
Increased confusion (older adult population)
Demonstration of lack of trust
Withdrawal
Hypervigilance
Allergic symptoms
Weight change
Sad affect
Unfavorable comparison of posttransfer to pretransfer staff
Verbalization of being concerned/upset about transfer
Verbalization of insecurity in new living situation

Related Factors

Pathophysiologic

Related to compromised ability to adapt to a unit transfer, for example, ICU, relocation, living condition changes secondary to:

Decreased physical health status*
Physical difficulties
Decreased psychosocial health status
Increased/perceived stress before relocation

Situational (Personal, Environmental)

Related to little or no preparation for the impending move

Related to insufficient finances, foreclosures

Related to high degree of changes associated with admission to a care facility

Related to relocation of a family unit secondary to:

Loss of social and familial ties
Change in relationship with family members
Abandonment

Maturational

School-Aged Children and Adolescents

Related to foster home placement or transfer into another foster home

Related to losses associated with moving secondary to:

Fear of rejection, loss of peer group, or school-related problems
Decreased security in new adolescent peer group and school

Older Adult

Related to the need to be closer to family members for assistance

Related to inability to continue to live in present housing

Author's Note

NANDA has accepted *Relocation Stress* as a syndrome diagnosis. It does not fit the criterion for a syndrome diagnosis, which is a cluster of actual or risk nursing diagnoses as defining characteristics. The defining characteristics associated with *Relocation Stress* are observable or reportable cues consistent with *Relocation Stress*, not *Relocation Stress Syndrome*. The author recommends deleting "Syndrome" from the label.

Relocation represents a disruption for all parties involved. It can accompany a transfer from one unit to another or from one facility to another. It can involve a voluntary or forced permanent move to a long-term–care facility or new home. Since 2009, 4.4 million housing units have been foreclosed on in the United States. In 2013, the rate trended down 18%. In December 2015, 9.3 million properties, or 19% of all homes, were reported to be "deeply underwater," meaning borrowers owed at least 25% more on their mortgage than the homes were worth (Chrisitie, 2014). This explosion of foreclosures in the United States and abroad has severely compromised individuals and families. The relocation disturbs all age groups involved. When physiologic and psychological disturbances compromise functioning, the nursing diagnosis *Relocation Stress Syndrome* is appropriate.

The optimal nursing approach to relocation stress is to initiate preventive measures, using *Risk for Relocation Stress* as the diagnosis. Therefore, the interventions to prevent *Relocation Stress Syndrome* are emphasized, even if *Relocation Stress* occurs.

Errors in Diagnostic Statements

Relocation Stress related to apprehension and sadness associated with impending family move

Apprehension and sadness are appropriate responses for children involved in a family move. Adolescents are especially disrupted because of peer relationships. Apprehension and sadness are not related factors but rather manifestations. The nurse should write the diagnosis as *Relocation Stress related to perceived negative effects of family move as evidenced by statements of apprehension and sadness.*

Key Concepts

General Considerations

- According to a 2013 Gallup survey, nearly a quarter of the adult US population moved during the previous 5 years.
- Relocation stress can accompany any type of move, including previous home to new home (house, apartment), home to college, home to institution (hospital, long-term–care nursing facility), institution to home (especially after an extended illness), moves within an institution (from one bed to another in the same room, from one room to another on the same unit/floor, from one room to another on different units/floors), and moves between institutions (hospital to long-term–care facility or one long-term nursing care facility to another) (*Davies & Nolan, 2004).
- Relocation stress typically occurs shortly before and after the move. Not all relocated people experience relocation stress, because the related factors are not present to the same degree in all those experiencing relocation.
- When a move results from a husband's change of employment, a relocated husband often finds satisfaction with his new job. The relocated wife seeks new neighbors, friends, home, and community activities as a primary source of satisfaction. If previously employed, she often feels isolated because of the possible unavailability of jobs in the new environment (*Puskar, 1990). Relocated wives who coped well

demonstrated active behaviors (problem solving, support seeking from family and friends, volunteer activities); wives who coped poorly showed passive behaviors (eating, sleeping, crying, watching television, becoming angry at self and others; *Puskar, 1990).

- Transfers from intensive care units:
  - One study reported that 28% of medical ICU transfer reports contained at least one critical or serious error, with eight or more discharge medications being predictive of such errors (*Perren, Arber, & Davidson, 2008).
  - The risk of errors has also been found to be associated with discharge time, particularly night (Beck & Luine, 2002; Goldfrad & Rowan, 2000; Priestap & Martin, 2006) and weekend discharges.
  - Researchers reported that 30.7% of individuals had adverse events after transfer from an ICU (*Chaboyer, Thalib, Foster, Ball, & Richards, 2008). The three most common adverse events are hospital-incurred infection or sepsis ($n = 32$, 21.8%), hospital-incurred accident or injury ($n = 17$, 11.6%), and other complication such as deep vein thrombosis, pulmonary edema, or myocardial infarction ($n = 17$).
  - It was found that the positive effect of the liaison nurse role in reducing the discharge delay remained after adjusting for potential confounders. We conclude that the liaison nurse role is effective in reducing the discharge delay in ICU transfer.
- Relocation stress has been compared with separation anxiety as a result of separation from monitors and nurse and physician surveillance, which results in an inability to cope.
- Houser (*1974) reported the following in a study of 12 individuals transferred from a coronary care unit: 6 of 12 individuals required readmission for cardiovascular complications, and 5 of the 6 had a high anxiety rating when transferred. Those who did not discuss their feelings were most likely to experience complications after transfer. After instituting a program aimed at reducing transfer stress, there were fewer complications, and observed complications were less dangerous than those that the control group experienced.

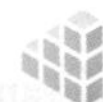

Pediatric Considerations

- When families need to relocate, their social attachment systems may be disrupted, thus producing slight changes in health status, daily functioning, and loneliness (*Puskar, 1986).
- Because of age and maturation, children of different ages experience relocation in different ways.
- A relocated child's stress and frustration may lead to aggression, withdrawal, and deterioration in schoolwork, which may lead to future adjustment problems if the child is not well socialized in the new environment.
- When relocated, toddlers and preschoolers often demonstrate changes in eating and sleeping patterns along with minor disabilities (*Puskar & Dvorsak, 1991).
- During interviews of 15 parents of premature infants transferred between level 1, 2, and 3 nurseries and home, Gibbins and Chapman (1996) documented the following parental responses:
  - Sources of parental stress included lack of information about their infants' condition and events of the transfer between units and discharge home, insecurity about their own comfort in a new unit, inconsistencies in care within the different nurseries, and dependency on particular caregivers within the neonatal ICU (NICU).
  - Parents had ambivalent feelings about transfer from a NICU (level 3 nursery) to an intermediate care unit (level 2 nursery). Parents also became more judgmental about the NICU care near the time of transfer to the level 2 nursery and rationalized the transfer from the NICU.
  - Forty-one mothers of infants transferred from a tertiary-care NICU to a community hospital nursery reported mild to moderate stress with the transfer and perceived the transfer as fairly positive. The higher the mothers viewed the quality of the transfer, the less stress they reported with this transfer (*Flanagan, Slattery, Chase, Meade, & Cronenwett, 1996).
- "School mobility is associated with increased risk of psychotic-like symptoms, both directly and indirectly. The findings highlight the potential benefit of strategies to help mobile students to establish themselves within new school environments to reduce peer difficulties and to diminish the risk of psychotic-like symptoms. Awareness of mobile students as a possible high-risk population, and routine inquiry regarding school changes and bullying experiences, may be advisable in mental health care settings" (Singh, Winsper, Wolke, & Bryson, 2014). Singh et al. (2014) reported the results of several studies that support the theory that psychosis exists on a continuum and that subclinical psychotic-like symptoms in childhood significantly increase the risk of psychotic disorder and suicide in adulthood.
- Singh et al. reported that school mobility, involvement in bullying, urbanity, and family adversity were all independently associated with definite psychotic-like symptoms.

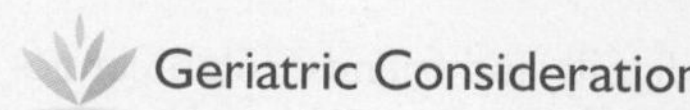

Geriatric Considerations

- In 2012, about 58,500 paid, regulated long-term–care services providers served about 8 million people in the United States. Long-term–care services were provided by 4,800 adult day services centers, 12,200 home health agencies, 3,700 hospices, 15,700 nursing homes, and 22,200 assisted living and similar residential care communities (Harris-Kojetin, Sengupta, Park-Lee & Valverde, 2013).
- Older adults have three types of moves (*Longino & Bradley, 2006):
  - Voluntary move to a desirable geographic area (amenity-driven moves)
  - Move closer to family because of widowhood and moderate disability (assistive moves)
  - Move to an institution because of health problems
- Older adults moved from their family home experience (*Johnson & Tripp-Reimer, 2001; Miller, 2015):
  - Loss of spouse
  - Chronic conditions and declining functional abilities
  - Lack of available assistive services
  - Lack of caregiver
  - Cognitive impairments
  - Psychiatric illness
  - Change in neighborhood (e.g., unsafe, socially isolated)
- Relocating rural older adults frequently identified perceived choice, environmental predictability, and social support from family, residential neighbors, and friends as factors associated with positive adjustment (*Armer, 1996).

Suicide in Nursing Homes

- Rates of death by suicide among LTC facility residents have been reported ranging from 16.5 to 34.8 per 100,000 residents per year (O'Riley, Nadorff, Conwell, & Edelstein 2013). In comparison, the rate of death by suicide in community-dwelling adults in the United States aged 65 years and older was 14.9 per 100,000 in 2010 (O'Riley et al., 2013).
- Most common means of suicide in nursing homes include jumping from buildings, cutting, taking an overdose of medication, and hanging (Substance Abuse and Mental Health Services Administration, 2011).
- The greatest incidence of relocation stress typically occurs shortly before and up to 3 months after the move (*Beirne, Patterson, Galie, & Goodman, 1995;*Reinardy, 1995).
- In a study conducted by Rodgers (*1986), the process of nursing home placement began with families recognizing and ultimately accepting the need to admit their loved ones to a nursing home. Concerns over safety provided a means to justify, rather than an initial incentive to seek the placement.

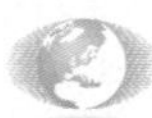

Transcultural Considerations

- Immigration to another country can be planned, forced or unexpected. The responses to immigration are complex. Frequently, families are separated. *Relocation Stress Syndrome* does not adequately address the experiences and stressors experienced by immigrants. Nursing diagnoses related to the immigration experience are presently in development.

Focus Assessment Criteria

Subjective Data

Assess for Defining Characteristics

The Relocated Individual/Family Members Complains of

Dissatisfaction with new environment	Loneliness
Increased family conflicts	Problems adjusting
Loss of control	Feelings of insecurity
Anger at loss of control over own life	Anger toward people responsible for placement

Changes in

Sleep patterns	Nutritional intake
Socialization	Cognition
Orientation	

Assess for Related Factors

History of
One or more changes in environment in the last 3 months
Multiple moves in the last 5 years
Traumatic experiences after previous moves
Being in the same environment for more than 40 years

Risk Factors
Moderate-to-severe confusion/disorientation
Perceived poor health
Lack of support/family/friends/staff
Low self-esteem
Functional deterioration
Involuntary move
Communication difficulties
Lack of continuity of care
Expression of dissatisfaction with life
Lack of preparation for move(s)
Lack of choices or input on the part of the relocating individual
Multiple chronic illnesses
Lack of familiarity with nursing home before relocation
Nursing home location far from previous residence

Objective Data

Assess for Defining Characteristics

Change in weight
Increased medical visits
Sleep problems
Change in cognition
Change in eating patterns
Decline in self-care activities

Goals

Refer to *Risk Relocation Stress Syndrome.*

Interventions/Rationale

Refer to *Risk for Relocation Stress Syndrome.*

Risk for Relocation Stress [Syndrome]

NANDA-I Definition

At risk for physiologic and/or psychological disturbance following transfer from one environment to another

Risk Factors

Refer to *Relocation Stress Syndrome.*

Key Concepts

Refer to *Relocation Stress Syndrome.*

Focus Assessment Criteria

Refer to *Relocation Stress Syndrome.*

Goals

NOC

Anxiety Self-Control, Coping, Loneliness, Psychosocial Adjustment: Life Change, Quality of Life, Fear Control

The individual/family members will report adjustment to the new environment with minimal disturbances, as evidenced by the following indicators:

- Shares in decision-making activities regarding the new environment
- Expresses concerns regarding the move to a new environment
- Verbalizes one positive aspect of the relocation
- Establishes new bonds in the new environment
- Becomes involved in activities in the new environment

Interventions

NIC

Anxiety Reduction, Coping Enhancement, Counseling, Family Involvement Promotion, Support System Enhancement, Anticipatory Guidance, Family Integrity Promotion, Transfer, Relocation Stress Reduction

Determine the Reason for the Move

- Voluntary Move: usually related to a move by parents/caregivers. Usually positive, however the new job may a less desirable. These moves are typically the least stressful of the three for adolescents.
- Forced Move: can be the result of eviction, fleeing, and migratory work or going back to live with extended family. These situations are almost always negative with numerous stressors on the family unit.
- Legal Move: is enforced and bound by law. Examples are relocation under witness protection, a foster child or steward of the state and most frequently child custody with divorce.
- Refer to Moving With Teens access at http://www.parenthood.com/article/moving_with_teens.html#.VwF6aqQrJKM

Advise Parents/Caregiver to Access Scroll Personnel Before School Starts

- If desired, share with teacher if this is a planned move, forced, or legal.

R: *Most persons assume all moves are welcomed by the family.*

- Is there a program for welcoming new students?
- Ask if an appropriate student be assigned to buddy with the new student.
- Ask about clubs, organizations, etc., that may be of interest to the new student.
- Suggest each student introduce themselves in addition to the new student.

R: *Strategies can give the new student a good, welcoming, first impression. Early peer rejection was associated with declining classroom participation and increasing school avoidance (Buhs, Ladd & Herald, 2009).*

Encourage Each Family Member to Share Feelings About the Move

- Provide privacy for each person.
- Encourage family members to share feelings with one another.
- Discuss the possible and different effects of the move on each family member.
- Inform parents regarding potential changes in children's conduct with relocation, such as regression, withdrawal, acting out, and changes with eating (breast/bottle-feeding).
- Instruct parents to obtain all pertinent documents regarding children's medical/dental history (e.g., immunizations, communicable diseases, dental work).
- Allow for some ritual(s) when leaving the old environment. Encourage reminiscing, which will bring closure for many family members.

R: *A lack of choice, or even the sense that their choice is limited, may increase stubbornness, fear of loss, and apprehension about the many components of an imminent change (Buhs, Ladd & Herald, 2008).*

Teach Parents Techniques to Assist Their Children With the Move

- Remain positive about the move before, during, and after accepting that the child may not be optimistic.
- Explore various options with children on how to communicate with friends/families in previous environment. Children's relationships with friends in the previous community are important, especially for "peer reassurance" after relocation.
- Keep regular routines in the new environment; establish them as soon as possible.
- Acknowledge the difficulty of peer losses with the adolescent.

R: *"Mobility, especially when linked to school change, may hinder key developmental outcomes. The inevitable breaking of social ties may create psychosocial stress and increase the risk of antisocial behavior, friendship problems, and bully victimization" (Singh et al., 2014).*

- Join the organizations to which the child previously belonged (e.g., Scouts, sports).
- Assist children to focus on similarities between old and new environments (e.g., clubs, Scouts, church groups).
- Plan a trip to school during a class and lunch period to reduce fear of unknown.
- Allow children some choices regarding room arrangements, decorating, and the like.
- Ask teacher or counselor at the new school to introduce the adolescent to a student who recently relocated to that school.
- Allow children to mourn their losses as a result of the move.

R: *Children need early notification, predictability, and decision-making opportunities when an upcoming relocation is planned.*

Advise Parents/Caregivers to Routinely Discuss Their School Experience

- Avoid asking "How is school?
- Ask instead, "Who did you eat lunch with? What did you do at recess?"
- What do you like about this new school?
- What do you not like?

R: *Singh et al. (2014) found a significant association between bullying involvement and psychotic-like symptoms; involvement in bullying was the strongest predictor of psychotic-like symptoms, leading to an approximately 2.5 times increased risk.*

Assess the Following Areas When Counseling a Relocated Adolescent

- Perceptions about the move
- Concurrent stressors
- Usual and present coping skills
- Support (family, peers, and community)

R: *The adolescent has a developmental task of becoming independent, which is challenged with relocation (*Puskar & Rohay, 1999). Peer networks are important during adolescence because the relocated adolescent needs additional parental and peer reassurance.*

Initiate Health Teaching and Referrals, as Indicated

- Alert the family to the possible need for counseling before, during, or after the move.
- Furnish a written directory of relevant community organizations such as area churches, children's groups, parents without partners, senior citizens' groups, and Welcome Wagon or other local new-neighbor groups.
- Instruct the family about appropriate community services.
- Consult the school nurse regarding school programs for new students.

R: *Early relocation planning is paramount to ensuring a smooth transfer for all involved individuals.*

Relocation Stress [Syndrome] • Related to Changes Associated with Health-Care Facility Transfers or Admission to Long-Term–Care Facility

Goals

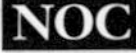
NOC

See also *Relocation Stress*, Adaptation to New Environment

The individual will describe realistic expectations of the new environment, as evidenced by the following indicators:

- Participate in decision-making activities regarding the new environment.
- Voice concerns regarding the move to a new environment.
- Describe realistic expectations of the new environment.

Interventions

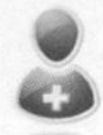

CLINICAL ALERT "During the past few decades the numbers of ICUs and beds has increased significantly, but so too has the demand for intensive care . Currently large, and increasing, numbers of critically ill patients require transfer between critical care units. Inter-unit transfer poses significant risks to critically ill patients, particularly those requiring multiple organ support" (Droogh, Smit, Absalom, Ligtenberg, & Zijlstra, 2015).

NIC

See also *Relocation Stress.*

Provide Family and Individual With the Relocation or Transfer Plans as Soon as Possible. Use Simple Explanations if Indicated

- Elicit discussions with concerns and questions.

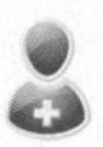

CLINICAL ALERT Unfortunately, ill individuals may not able to express and communicate their own will, due to sedation, altered mental status, or other barriers. Discharge planning in general is described as a process which should provide continuity of care.

R: *The most important strategy for families and individuals when transferring from an ICU was information prior to the actual transfer (*Mitchell, Courtney, & Coyer, 2003).*

Expect Challenges to the Transfer. Use Clinical Data to Support Rationale for the Transfer

R: *"Individuals sometimes struggle with feelings of abandonment, vulnerability, helplessness, and unimportance. Ambivalent feelings about the upcoming transfers are also shown to be common; both positive and negative emotions have been reported" (Häggström & Bäckström, 2014).*

Assess for Factors That May Contribute to Relocation Stress

- See Related Factors and Focus Assessment Criteria.

In Intensive Care Units, Implement an Orderly, Planned Transition to Reduce Stress and Adverse Events

R: *Transition planning often lacks guidelines and tends to be ad hoc and influenced by the individual's acuity (Häggström & Bäckström, 2014).*

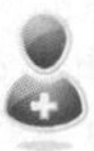

CLINICAL ALERT Priorities in ICU may be necessary to enable admission for the most ill individuals, causing unplanned discharges even during night which are related to higher risks (Häggström & Bäckström, 2014). A study by Goldfrad and Rowan (2000) found that the overall ICU mortality is 2 to 5 times higher if the individual is discharged at night. In their study, the staff estimated that only 44% of these patients were fully ready for the transfer, compared with over 80% of patients who were transferred during the day.

- Gradually decrease the frequency of nursing assessments, for example, frequency of vital signs before ICU transfer, when possible.
- Present transfer from a critical care unit as an indicator of improvement.
- Inform of signs of daily progress.
- Transfer in an unhurried manner.

R: *The most important strategy for families and individuals when transferring from an ICU was information prior to the actual transfer (*Mitchell et al. 2003). There should be a visible, gradual transition from critical care monitoring to usual nursing unit monitoring to reduce fears.*

- Evaluate the individual's pulse and respiratory rate prior to transfer.

R: *Possible significant predictors of adverse events prior to transfer are a respiratory rate less than 10 per minute or greater than or equal to 25 per minute and pulse rate exceeding 110 per minute (*Chaboyer et al., 2008).*

- In residential settings, design a program to prepare relocated residents and staff for the move, orienting them to the physical layout many times until they feel familiar with the new environment.
- Initially maintain t at the same activity level and diet through pretransfer and posttransfer units.
- Transfer to similar, proximal area when possible.
- Wean any monitoring equipment gradually before transfer.
- Transfer during daytime hours.
- Maintain people in familiar groups at mealtimes and in living arrangements.

- Allow time for discussions regarding living spaces in old and new environments.
- Gradually decrease nursing attention before ICU transfer, when possible.

R: *Open communication with older adults both before and after a move is necessary, assessing their experiences with change and adjustment, coping history and style, and decisional control.*

Involuntary Relocation/Lack of Control in Decision Making

- Offer decision-making opportunities throughout the relocation experience.
- Elicit the person's input regarding the new environment when possible, such as use of decorations and arrangement of furniture.
- Present transfer from a critical care unit as an indicator of improvement.
- Inform the hospitalized individual of signs of daily progress.
- Transfer the individual in an unhurried manner.
- Establish mutual goals before relocation to a nursing home.
- Provide opportunities for questions/answers with relocation preparation.
- Hold regular staff/resident meetings after relocation, encouraging new members to be involved with the facility's rules and regulations (*Wilson, 1997).

R: *Wilson (*1997) and Meacham and Brandriet (1997) found older adults made an effort to protect their significant others by hiding their feelings about relocation and attempting to maintain a sense of normalcy. Therefore, it is critical for new residents to develop trusting relationships with others to discuss the stressors of relocation.*

Reduce the Physiologic Effects of Relocation

Assess

- Blood pressure, temperature
- Respiratory function
- Orientation
- Signs of infection
- Level of discomfort
- Provide adequate rest and aggressively reduce exposure to infection during first few weeks. Prepare visitors for visits (e.g., hand washing, masks if indicated).

R: *Adaptation to relocation can negatively affect physical status, leading to increased risk of infection. Natural killer cell activity is reduced for at least 2 weeks after relocation (*Lutgendoef et al., 2001).*

Prevent or Reduce Confusion

- Refer to *Confusion* for additional interventions.

Promote Integration after Admission/Transfer Into a Long-Term–Care Nursing Facility

R: *The less control older people perceive they have over the move and the less predictable the new environment seems, the greater the stress of relocation (Kaplan, Barbara, & Berkman, 2013).*

R: *Residents who were allowed choice regarding room location and favorite objects had an increased sense of control and less stress (*Mitchell, 1999).*

- Allow as many choices as possible regarding physical surroundings and daily routines.
- Encourage the individual or family to bring familiar objects from the individual's home.
- Orient to the physical layout of the environment.
- Introduce relocated individuals to new staff and fellow residents.
- Encourage interaction with other people in the new facility.
- Assist the individual in maintaining previous interpersonal relationships.
- Clearly state smoking rules and orient the individual to areas where smoking is permitted.
- Promote the development or maintenance of a relationship with a confidante.
- Reestablish normal routines, while initially increasing staffing and lighting, when a large number of long-term–care residents are involved in a secondary relocation.
- Assist nursing home residents to meet people from their previous geographic area.
- Arrange frequent contacts by a volunteer or staff member with each newly admitted resident. Also, match a successfully relocated resident with the new resident to begin the networking process.

R: *Older adults may use a variety of coping strategies, ranging from aggressive anger to passive resignation, when relocated to a nursing home. Any nursing interventions related to relocation stress should reflect the resident's effective coping strategies.*

Ensure That Each Resident Is Screened for Depression and Suicide

R: *Nursing home residents may be at a higher risk of suicide than community-dwelling older adults because they possess many of the characteristics that are known to influence risk in the general population, including psychiatric illness, social isolation, and functional impairment.*

- If a resident says "I wish I were dead," do not assume the person is suicidal. Assume they are distressed. Access an assessment for depression and risk for suicide.

R: *Long-term–care facilities are required to screen their residents for suicide risk and to implement protocols to effectively manage residents' responses (O'Riley et al., 2013).*

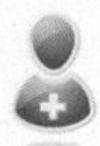

CLINICAL ALERT Studies on the rates of suicidal ideation in the LTC population have demonstrated frequency rates ranging from 11% to 43%. The rate of suicide in nursing homes is more than double for the same age group living in the community (O'Riley et al., 2013). Individuals who commit suicide in LTC give fewer warnings of intent, do more planning, are more determined and use more violent means.

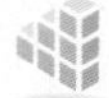

Pediatric Interventions

- Include parents in the care of their hospitalized premature infant as much as possible.
- Promote the use of support systems both inside and outside the hospital for parents of hospitalized infants.

R: *Parents of children facing transfer from the ICU to a general unit who were given a verbal explanation 1 to 2 hours before the transfer had significantly less anxiety than parents who were informed immediately before the transfer (Hockenberry & Wilson, 2015).*

For Infants Who Require Transfer to Another Unit or Health-Care Facility (Häggström & Bäckström, 2014)

- Assess the perceptions of parents of hospitalized infants regarding an upcoming transfer and their interest in related information.
- Maintain at least daily communication with parents about their hospitalized infant (e.g., condition, timing of transfer, mechanisms for continuity of care between the pre- and posttransfer nurseries) and their concerns.
- Suggest that parents of hospitalized infants visit the nursery to which their child will be transferred before the event.
- Develop and use a mechanism for a thorough exchange of information between pre- and posttransfer nurseries.

R: *Parents of preterm infants want to protect their child during hospitalization in addition to wanting to receive information about each new environment where their child will be transferred (Gibbins & Chapman, 1996).*

Initiate Health Teaching and Referrals, as Indicated

- If relocation is being considered to a family member's home, skilled care, or nursing home, advise the family to slowly prepare the person for the move:
  - Elicit a conversation to explore his or her feelings about the possible relocation.
  - Point out the advantages and disadvantages. Avoid arguing.
  - Plan a visit to the facility.
- Notify the individual about relocation as early as possible to increase the predictability of his or her reaction.
- Make appropriate professional referrals as needed, as well as suggesting a telephone monitoring system such as "Lifeline."

R: *Open communication with older adults both before and after a move is necessary, assessing their experiences with change and adjustment, coping history and style, and decisional control.*

- Refer relocated families to community agencies related to newcomers and to mental health agencies when at risk for relocation stress syndrome.

R: *With the influx of people who have chronic mental illness into the community, it is important that their needs and problems be assessed accurately so interventions and services that ensure successful relocation and adjustment can be planned and implemented.*

RISK FOR COMPROMISED RESILIENCE

NANDA-I Definition

At risk for decreased ability to sustain a pattern of positive responses to an adverse situation or crisis

Risk Factors*

Chronicity of existing crises
Multiple coexisting adverse situations
Presence of additional new crisis (e.g., unplanned pregnancy, death of spouse, loss of job, illness, loss of housing, death of family member)

Author's Note

This NANDA-I diagnosis is not a response but an etiology of a coping problem. Resilience is a strength that can be taught to and nurtured in children. Resilient individuals and families can cope in adverse situations and crises. They problem-solve and adapt their functioning to the situation. For example, when a mother of a family of five had to undergo chemotherapy, the family formulated a plan together to divide the responsibilities previously managed by the mother.

When an individual or family is experiencing chronic, multiple adverse situations or a new crisis, refer to *Risk for Ineffective Coping*. In situations involving the loss of family member, significant other, or friend, refer to *Grieving* for Key Concepts, Goals, and Interventions/Rationale.

IMPAIRED INDIVIDUAL RESILIENCE

NANDA-I Definition

Decreased ability to sustain a pattern of positive responses to an adverse situation or crisis

Defining Characteristics*

Decreased interest in academic activities
Decreased interest in vocational activities
Depression, guilt, shame
Isolation
Low self-esteem
Lower perceived health status
Renewed elevation of distress
Social isolation
Using maladaptive coping skills (e.g., drug use, violence)

Related Factors*

Demographics that increase chance of maladjustment
Drug use
Inconsistent parenting
Low intelligence
Low maternal education
Large family size
Minority status
Parental mental illness
Poor impulse control
Poverty, violence
Psychological disorders
Vulnerability factors that encompass indices that exacerbate the negative effects of the risk condition

Author's Note

This NANDA-I diagnosis does not represent a nursing diagnosis. The defining characteristics are not defining resilience but in fact a variety of coping problems or mental disorders. Most of the related factors are prejudicial, pejorative, and cannot be changed by interventions. One related factor listed—poor impulse control—is a sign and symptom of hyperactivity disorders and some mental disorders. Resilience is a strength that can be taught to and nurtured in children. Resilient individuals and families can cope in adverse situations and crises. They problem-solve and adapt their functioning to the situation. For example, when a mother of a family of five had to undergo chemotherapy, the family formulated a plan together to divide the responsibilities previously managed by the mother. When an individual or family has inadequate resilience, they are at risk for ineffective coping. Refer to *Ineffective Coping* and *Compromised or Disabled Family Coping* for Key Concepts, Goals, and Interventions/Rationale.

RISK FOR INEFFECTIVE RESPIRATORY FUNCTION[35]

Risk for Ineffective Respiratory Function

Dysfunctional Ventilatory Weaning Response
Risk for Dysfunctional Ventilatory Weaning Response
Ineffective Airway Clearance
Ineffective Breathing Pattern
Impaired Gas Exchange
Impaired Spontaneous Ventilation

Definition

At risk for experiencing a threat to the passage of air through the respiratory tract and/or to the exchange of gases (O_2–CO_2) between the lungs and the vascular system

Risk Factors

Presence of risk factors that can change respiratory function (see Related Factors)

Related Factors

Pathophysiologic

Related to excessive or thick secretions secondary to:

Infection
Inflammation
Allergy
Cardiac or pulmonary disease

Related to immobility, stasis of secretions, and ineffective cough secondary to:

Diseases of the nervous system (e.g., Guillain–Barré syndrome, multiple sclerosis, myasthenia gravis)
Central nervous system (CNS) depression/head trauma
Cerebrovascular accident (stroke)
Quadriplegia

Situational (Personal Environmental)

Related to immobility secondary to:

Surgery or trauma
Fatigue
Pain
Perception/cognitive impairment
Fear
Anxiety

[35]This diagnosis is not currently on the NANDA-I list but has been included for clarity or usefulness.

Related to effects of smoking

Related to exposure to noxious chemical

Related to extremely high or low humidity:

For infants, related to placement on stomach to sleep
Exposure to cold, laughing, crying, allergens, smoke

Treatment Related

Related to immobility secondary to:

Sedating or paralytic effects of medications, drugs, or chemicals (specify)
Anesthesia, general or spinal

Related to suppressed cough reflex secondary to (specify)

Related to effects of tracheostomy (altered secretions)

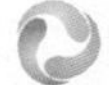

Author's Note

Nurses' responsibilities associated with problems of respiratory function include identifying and reducing or eliminating risk (contributing) factors, anticipating potential complications, monitoring respiratory status, and managing acute respiratory dysfunction.

The author has added *Risk for Ineffective Respiratory Function* to describe a state that may affect the entire respiratory system, not just isolated areas, such as airway clearance or gas exchange. Allergy and immobility are examples of factors that affect the entire system; thus, it is incorrect to say *Impaired Gas Exchange* is related to immobility, because immobility also affects airway clearance and breathing patterns. The nurse can use the diagnoses *Ineffective Airway Clearance* and *Ineffective Breathing Patterns*, when nurses can definitely alleviate the contributing factors influencing respiratory function (e.g., ineffective cough, stress).

The nurse is cautioned not to use this diagnosis to describe acute respiratory disorders, which are the primary responsibility of medical providers and nursing together (i.e., collaborative problems). Such problems can be labeled *Risk for Complications of Acute Hypoxia* or *Risk for Complications of Pulmonary Edema*. When an individual's immobility is prolonged and threatens multiple systems—for example, integumentary, musculoskeletal, vascular, as well as respiratory—the nurse should use *Disuse Syndrome* to describe the entire situation.

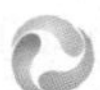

Errors in Diagnostic Statements

***Ineffective Breathing Patterns* related to respiratory compensation for metabolic acidosis**

This diagnosis represents the respiratory pattern associated with diabetic ketoacidosis. Related nursing responsibilities would include monitoring, early detection of changes, and rapid initiation of nursing and medical interventions. This does not represent a situation for which nurses diagnose and are accountable to prescribe treatment. Rather, the collaborative problem *Risk for Complications of Ketoacidosis* represents the nursing accountability for the situation.

***Ineffective Airway Clearance* related to mucosal edema and loss of ciliary action secondary to thermal injury**

After sustaining burns of the upper airway, an individual is at risk for pulmonary edema and respiratory distress. This potentially life-threatening situation requires both nurse- and physician-prescribed interventions. The collaborative problem *Risk for Complications of Respiratory secondary to thermal injury* would alert nurses that close monitoring for respiratory complications and management, if they occur, are indicated.

***Ineffective Airway Clearance* related to decreased cough and gag reflexes secondary to anesthesia**

The nursing focus for the above problem is on preventing aspiration through proper positioning and good oral hygiene, not on teaching effective coughing. Thus, the nurse should restate the diagnosis as *Risk for Aspiration* related to decreased cough and gag reflexes secondary to anesthesia.

Key Concepts

General Considerations

- Ventilation requires synchronous movement of the walls of the chest and abdomen. With inspiration, the diaphragm moves downward, the intercostal muscles contract, the chest wall lifts up and out, the pressure inside the thorax lowers, and air is drawn in. Expiration occurs as air is forced out of the lungs by the elastic recoil of the lungs and the relaxation of the chest and diaphragm. Expiration is diminished in older adults and those with chronic pulmonary disease, increasing the likelihood of CO_2 retention (Grossman & Porth, 2014).

- Pulmonary function depends on the following:
  - Adequate perfusion (passage of blood through pulmonary vessels)
  - Satisfactory diffusion (movement of oxygen and carbon dioxide across alveolar capillary membrane)
- Successful ventilation (exchange of air between alveolar spaces and the atmosphere)
- Oxygenation depends on the ability of the lungs to deliver oxygen to the blood and on the ability of the heart to pump enough blood to deliver the oxygen to the microcirculation of the cells.
- Although arterial blood gases and oxygen saturation studies are helpful in diagnosing problems with oxygenation, vital signs and mental function are key guides to determining the seriousness of the problem; some individuals can tolerate oxygen problems better than others.
- A cough ("the guardian of the lungs") is accomplished by closure of the glottis and the explosive expulsion of air from the lungs by the work of the abdominal and chest muscles. Although most coughing serves a beneficial purpose, the following may be signs of a medical problem requiring medical intervention (Grossman & Porth, 2014):
  - Coughs lasting longer than 2 weeks or associated with high fever
  - Coughs consistently triggered by something (may actually be allergic bronchial asthma)
  - Barking cough, especially in a child
  - Breath holding can result in a Valsalva maneuver: a marked increase in intrathoracic and intra-abdominal pressure, with profound circulatory changes (decreased heart rate, cardiac output, and blood pressure).
- The terms tachypnea, hyperpnea, hyperventilation, bradypnea, hypoventilation, and hypopnea are frequently confused (Grossman & Porth, 2014).
  - Tachypnea: rapid, shallow respiratory rate
  - Hyperpnea: rapid respiratory rate with increased depth
  - Hyperventilation: increased rate or depth of respiration causing alveolar ventilation that is above the body's normal metabolic requirements
  - Bradypnea: slow respiratory rate
  - Hypoventilation: decreased rate or depth of respiration, causing a minute alveolar ventilation that is less than the body's requirements
  - Hypopnea: underbreathing; slower and/or shallower than normal
- Hypoxia and hypoxemia contribute to increased intracranial pressure, brain swelling, brain damage, and shock. Oxygen demand is greater during febrile illness, exercise, pain, and physical and emotional stress.
- Nicotine is one of the most toxic and addicting of all poisonous substances. Education, preventive health practices, interventions to enhance tobacco cessation, treatment for nicotine dependence, and relapse prevention should be standard nursing practice.
- Nurses must be persistent in helping their individuals to stop smoking by encouraging efforts to quit as often as needed (in many cases, at each individual encounter). Refer to *Ineffective Health Maintenance related to insufficient knowledge of effects of tobacco use.*

Pediatric Considerations

- The characteristics of normal respiration in the newborn differ from those of older infants and children (Hockenberry & Wilson, 2015).
- Respirations are irregular and abdominal; to be accurate, count respirations for 1 full minute.
- The rate is between 30 and 50 breaths/min.
- Periods of apnea, lasting less than 15 seconds, may occur.
- Obligate nasal breathing occurs through the first 3 weeks of life.
- Characteristics of the respiratory system of the infant and young child include the following:
  - Abdominal breathing continues until the child is about 5 years of age.
  - Smaller airway diameter increases the risk of obstruction.
  - Infants and small children swallow sputum when it is produced.
- Huckabay and Daderian (*1989) noted that pediatric individuals who were given a choice in the selection of the color of water in blow bottles performed significantly more breathing exercises than those who were not given a choice.
- Studies show that the past common practice of placing infants on their stomach for sleep increases the incidence of sudden infant death syndrome, making placement on back or side a safer option.

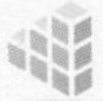

Maternal Considerations

- Increased levels of estrogen and progesterone increase tidal volume by decreasing pulmonary resistance (Pillitteri, 2014).
- During pregnancy, oxygen consumption increases by 14%: half is for fetus development and the rest is for other increased needs (e.g., uterus, breasts; Pillitteri, 2014).

Geriatric Considerations

- Age-related changes in the respiratory system have little effect on function in healthy adults unless they interact with risk factors such as smoking, immobility, or compromised immune system (Miller, 2015).
- The following age-related changes in the respiratory system are typical (Miller, 2015):
  - No change in total volume
  - 50% increase in residual volume
  - Compromised gas exchange in lower lung regions
  - Reduced compliance of the bony thorax
  - Decreased strength of the respiratory muscles and diaphragm
  - Age-related kyphosis and diminished immune response compromise respiratory function and increase the risk of pneumonia and other respiratory infections.
  - Swallowing disorders are common. Elderly are at higher risk for aspiration (which could lead to pneumonia) (Miller, 2015).
- Adults aged 65 and older have a yearly death rate from pneumonia or influenza of 9 per 100,000. When smoking, exposure to air pollutants, or occupational exposure to toxic substances is present; the rate increases to 217 per 100,000. If two or more risk factors are present, the rate rises to 979 per 100,000 (Miller, 2015).

Focus Assessment Criteria

Subjective Data

Assess History of Symptoms (e.g., Pain, Dyspnea, Cough)

Onset: Precipitated by what? Relieved by what?
Description: Relieved by what?

Assess for Risk Factors

Smoking ("pack-years": number of packs per day multiplied by the number of smoking years)
Smoking within the 8 weeks before anesthesia or surgery
Allergy (medication, food, environmental factors—dust, pollen, other)
Trauma, blunt or overt (chest, abdomen, upper airway, head)
Surgery/pain
  Incision of chest/neck/head/abdomen
  Recent intubation
Environmental factors
  Toxic fumes (cleaning agents, smoke)
  Extreme heat or cold
  Daily inspired air at work and in the home (humid, dry, level of pollution, level of pollens)

For Infant, History of
Placement on stomach to sleep
Prematurity
Low birth weight
Cesarean birth
Complicated delivery
Breastfeeding formula

Objective Data

Assess for Defining Characteristics

Mental Status

Respiratory Status
Rate (per minute)

Rhythm
Depth
Symmetric

Cough
Effective/productive (brings forth sputum and clears lungs)
Ineffective/nonproductive (does not bring forth mucus or clear lungs)
Triggered by what? Relieved by what?
Needs assistance with coughing

Sputum
Color
Character
Amount
Odor

Breath Sounds
Detected by auscultation: compare right upper and lower regions to left upper and lower regions
Listen to all four quadrants of the chest

Circulatory Status
Pulse
Blood pressure
Skin color

Goals

NOC
Aspiration Control, Respiratory Status

The individual will have a respiratory rate within normal limits compared with baseline, as evidenced by the following indicators:

- Expresses willingness to be actively involved in managing respiratory symptoms and maximizing respiratory function
- Relates appropriate interventions to maximize respiratory status (varies depending on health status)
- Has satisfactory pulmonary function, as measured by pulmonary function tests

Interventions

NIC
Airway Management, Cough Enhancement, Respiratory Monitoring, Positioning

Determine Causative Factors

- Refer to Related Factors.

Eliminate or Reduce Causative Factors, If Possible

- Encourage ambulation as soon as consistent with the medical plan of care.
- If the individual cannot walk, establish a regimen for being out of bed in a chair several times a day (e.g., 1 hour after meals and 1 hour before bedtime).
- Increase activity gradually. Explain that respiratory function will improve and dyspnea will decrease with practice.

R: *Lying flat causes the abdominal organs to shift toward the chest, thereby crowding the lungs and making it more difficult to breathe.*

- For neuromuscular impairment:
  - Vary the position of the bed, thereby gradually changing the horizontal and vertical position of the thorax, unless contraindicated.
  - Assist to reposition, turning frequently from side to side (hourly if possible).
  - Encourage deep breathing and controlled coughing exercises five times every hour.
  - Teach to use a blow bottle or incentive spirometer every hour while awake. (With severe neuromuscular impairment, the individual may have to be wakened during the night as well.)
  - For a child, use colored water in a blow bottle; have him or her blow up balloons.

R: *Exercises and movement promote lung expansion and mobilization of secretions. Incentive spirometry promotes deep breathing by providing a visual indicator of the effectiveness of the breathing effort.*

- Ensure optimal hydration status and nutritional intake.

R: *Adequate hydration and humidity liquefy secretions, enabling easier expectoration and preventing stasis of secretions, which provide a medium for microorganism growth (Halm & Krisko-Hagel, 2008). Hydration also helps decrease blood viscosity, which reduces the risk of clot formation.*

For the Individual With a Decreased Level of Consciousness

- Position the individual from side to side with a set schedule (e.g., left side on even hours, right side on odd hours); do not leave the individual lying flat on his or her back.
- Position the individual on the right side after feedings (nasogastric tube feeding, gastrostomy) to prevent regurgitation and aspiration.

R: *Lying flat causes the abdominal organs to shift toward the chest, thereby crowding the lungs and making it more difficult to breathe.*

- Keep the head of the bed elevated 30° unless contraindicated (Institute for Healthcare Improvement, 2008).

Identify Individuals Who Are Unsuccessful in Attempts to Clear Secretions and Who May Require Suctioning (Nance-Floyd, 2011)

- Assess for:
  - Increased work of breathing
  - Changes in respiratory rate
  - Decreased oxygen saturation
  - Copious secretions, wheezing
- Proceed to suction (Sharma, Sarin, & Bala, 2014):
  - Place the person in supine position with head slightly extended.
  - Place the person on pulse oximeter to assess oxygenation.
  - Hyperoxygenate for 30 to 60 seconds before suctioning.
  - Make sure not to apply suction while inserting the suction catheter.
  - Apply continuous suction by covering the suction control hole.
  - Remove catheter in rotating movement.
  - The single episode of suctioning from removing of ventilator to reattachment of ventilator should not exceed 10 to 15 seconds.
  - Monitor O_2 saturation level of patient between each episode of suctioning.
  - Follow age-related protocols for suction pressure for newborns, infants, children, and adolescents.
- Do not use normal saline solution or normal saline bullets routinely to loosen tracheal secretions because this practice (Nance-Floyd, 2011)
  - May reach only limited areas
  - May flush particles into the lower respiratory tract
  - May lead to decreased postsuctioning oxygen saturation
  - Increases bacterial colonization
  - Damages bronchial surfactant

R: *The optimal methods to liquefy secretions are to use a humidifier and maintain hydration of the person.*

- See also *Risk for Aspiration*.
- Consult with physical therapy and respiratory therapy as indicated.

R: *Interventions that can enhance pulmonary function include exercise conditioning to improve lung compliance, relaxation and breathing training, chest percussion, postural drainage, and psychosocial rehabilitation.*

Prevent the Complications of Immobility

- See *Disuse Syndrome*.

Dysfunctional Ventilatory Weaning Response

Risk for Dysfunctional Ventilatory Weaning Response

NANDA-I Definition

Inability to adjust to lowered levels of mechanical ventilator support that interrupts and prolongs the weaning process

Defining Characteristics*

Dysfunctional ventilatory weaning response is a progressive state, and experienced nurses have identified three levels (*Logan & Jenny, 1990): mild, moderate, and severe. The defining characteristics occur in response to weaning.

Mild

Restlessness
Slight increase of respiratory rate from baseline
Expressed feelings of increased oxygen need, breathing discomfort, fatigue, and warmth
Queries about possible machine dysfunction
Increased concentration on breathing

Moderate

Slight increase from baseline blood pressure (<20 mm Hg)*
Slight increase from baseline in heart rate (<20 beats/min)*
Increase from baseline in respiratory rate (<5 breaths/min)
Hypervigilance to activities
Inability to respond to coaching
Decreased air entry heard on auscultation
Inability to cooperate
Apprehension
Diaphoresis
Wide-eyed look
Color changes: pale, slight cyanosis
Slight respiratory accessory muscle use

Severe

Agitation*
Deterioration in arterial blood gases from current baseline
Increase from baseline blood pressure (<20 mm Hg)
Increase from baseline heart rate (<20 beats/min)
Shallow breaths
Cyanosis
Gasping breaths
Paradoxical abdominal breathing
Decreased level of consciousness
Adventitious breath sounds
Full respiratory accessory muscle use
Profuse diaphoresis
Asynchronized breathing with the ventilator
Paradoxical abdominal breathing

Related Factors

Pathophysiologic

Related to muscle weakness and fatigue secondary to:

Unstable hemodynamic status
Decreased level of consciousness
Chronic neuromuscular disability
Metabolic/acid–base abnormality
Severe disease process
Chronic respiratory disease
Multisystem disease
Fluid/electrolyte imbalance
Anemia
Infection
Chronic nutritional deficit
Debilitated condition
Pain

Related to ineffective airway clearance*

Treatment Related

Related to obstructed airway

Related to muscle weakness and fatigue secondary to:

Excess sedation, analgesia
Uncontrolled pain

Related to inadequate nutrition (deficit in calories, excess carbohydrates, inadequate fats, and protein intake)*

Related to prolonged ventilator dependence (more than 1 week)

Related to previously unsuccessful ventilator weaning attempt(s)

Related to too-rapid pacing of the weaning process

Situational (Personal, Environmental)

Related to insufficient knowledge of the weaning process*

Related to excessive energy demands (self-care activities, diagnostic, and treatment procedures, visitors)

Related to inadequate social support*

Related to insecure environment (noisy, upsetting events, busy room)

Related to fatigue secondary to interrupted sleep patterns

Related to inadequate self-efficacy

Related to moderate to high anxiety related to breathing efforts

Related to fear of separation from ventilator

Related to feelings of powerlessness*

Related to feelings of hopelessness*

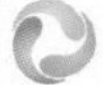

Author's Note

Dysfunctional Ventilatory Weaning Response is defined as the inability to adjust to lowered levels of mechanical ventilator support that interrupts and prolongs the weaning process. When this occurs, the ventilator support continues. When readiness to wean is confirmed, the diagnosis of *Risk for Dysfunctional Ventilatory Weaning Response* would be correct with unsatisfactory attempts as related factors and other factors that contributed to the unsuccessful weaning. Thus this diagnosis should be *Risk for Dysfunctional Ventilatory Weaning Response*, defined as vulnerable to experiencing an inability to adjust to lowered levels of mechanical ventilator support that interrupts and prolongs the weaning process, which may compromise health. The related factors listed above would become risk factors for this risk diagnosis. The process of weaning is an art and a science. Because weaning is a collaborative process, the nurse's ability to gain the individual's trust and willingness to work is an important determinant of the weaning outcomes, especially with long-term individuals. This trust is fostered by the knowledge and self-confidence nurses display and by their ability to deal with individuals' specific concerns (*Jenny & Logan, 1991).

Errors in Diagnostic Statements

***Dysfunctional Ventilatory Weaning Response* related to increased blood pressure, heart rate, respiratory rate, and agitation during weaning**

This diagnosis does not indicate the reasons for weaning problems. The related factors are evidence of *Dysfunctional Ventilatory Weaning Response*, not causative and contributing factors. The nurse should write the diagnosis with the related factors if they are known, or "unknown etiology," if not known.

Key Concepts

General Considerations

- Weaning is the process of assisting individuals to breathe spontaneously without mechanical ventilation. Weaning success has been defined as spontaneous breathing for 24 hours without ventilatory support, with or without an artificial airway.
- Ventilator weaning is a multidisciplinary effort in which the presence of knowledgeable nurses affects the outcomes positively. Experienced nurses agree that weaning is a collaborative process shared with the individual who has both a physical and a psychological aspect. For ventilator-dependent individuals, it can be a very stressful experience (*Logan & Jenny, 1990; *Rose, Dainty, Jordan, & Blackwood, 2014).
- In a review of 42 qualitative studies of health-care providers, individuals, and individuals' families involved in weaning, "important issues identified were perceived importance of interprofessional collaboration and communication, need to combine subjective knowledge of the individuals with objective clinical

data, balancing of weaning systematization with individual needs, and appreciation of the physical and psychological work of weaning" (*Rose et al., 2014, p. e54).

- Although weaning as soon as possible is important to avoid muscle deconditioning and complications related to prolonged endotracheal intubation and tracheostomy, premature attempts may be counterproductive because of adverse physiologic and psychological effects.
- Because weaning is a collaborative process, the nurse's ability to gain the individual's trust and willingness to work is an important determinant of outcomes, especially with long-term individuals. This trust is fostered by the knowledge and self-confidence nurses display and by their ability to deal with the individual's specific concerns (*Jenny & Logan, 1991).
- Dysfunctional ventilatory weaning is usually multifactorial. Marini (*1991) notes that, at the bedside, the subjective assessment of the weaning trial by an experienced clinician remains the most reliable predictor of weaning success or failure. Close monitoring of the individual's weaning work is needed to prevent serious respiratory fatigue, which can require up to 24 to 48 hours of recovery before the individual can proceed (*Rose, Nelson, Johnston, & Presneill, 2007).
- Readiness testing has two major purposes. The first is to identify individuals who are ready to wean from mechanical ventilation. This is important because clinicians tend to underestimate the capacity of individuals to breathe independently. Unnecessary mechanical ventilation needlessly increases the risk of complications related to mechanical ventilation (Epstien, 2015).
- Required criteria—The following are required criteria (*Macintyre et al., 2001; *Krieger, Ershowsky, Becker, & Gazeroglu, 1989; *Meade et al., 2001; cited in Epstein, 2015):
  - The cause of the respiratory failure has improved.
  - Adequate oxygenation—This may be indicated by either a ratio of arterial oxygen tension to fraction of inspired oxygen (PaO_2/FiO_2) ≥ 150 mm Hg or an oxyhemoglobin saturation (SpO_2) ≥ 90% while receiving an FiO_2 ≤ 40% and a positive end-expiratory pressure (PEEP) ≤ 5 cmH_2O. For patients who have chronic hypoxemia, a PaO_2/FiO_2 ≥ 120 mm Hg may be used instead. These thresholds are empiric, since no study has established a minimal acceptable PaO_2, PaO_2/FiO_2, SpO_2, or alveolar-arterial oxygen gradient for weaning.
  - Arterial pH > 7.25
  - Hemodynamic stability, without myocardial ischemia—The blood pressure thresholds below or above which it is unsafe for a patient to wean have not been established. However, it seems reasonable to require that the systolic blood pressure be >90 mm Hg or <180 mm Hg to begin weaning. The use of vasopressors to maintain the systolic blood pressure >90 mm Hg is acceptable, but only low doses should be necessary (e.g., dopamine <5 μg/kg/min).
  - The individual is able to initiate an inspiratory effort.
- Optional criteria—In contrast, the following criteria are optional:
  - Hemoglobin level ≥ 7 to 10 mg/dL—Previously, any degree of anemia was considered a contraindication to weaning because it reduces oxygen-carrying capacity. However, only severe anemia is currently considered a contraindication to weaning. The change is largely due to a secondary analysis of a randomized trial that compared a restrictive blood transfusion strategy (i.e., maintain hemoglobin level of 7 to 10 g/dL) to a liberal strategy (i.e., maintain a hemoglobin level of 10 to 12 g/dL).The analysis found that the strategies had no effect on the rate of successful weaning (78% vs. 82%).
  - Core temperature ≤ 38° C to 38.5° C—The rationale for this criterion is that the presence of fever makes successful weaning less likely because it increases the minute ventilation and, thus, the load on the respiratory system. It is also associated with rapid breathing. Individual whose fever is caused by sepsis may also have diminished respiratory muscle function. A temperature threshold above which weaning is unsafe has not been identified.
  - A mental status that is either awake and alert or easily arousable—This criterion is considered optional because although an awake or easily arousable patient is ideal for weaning, an abnormal mental status (i.e., Glasgow coma scale score < 8 or the inability to follow simple commands) does not appear to be associated with a higher rate of extubation failure. Thus, as long as an individual can protect the airway, an abnormal mental status does not preclude extubation. Evaluation of the ability to protect the airway is described separately.
- The physiologic inspiratory work of breathing includes three components (Grossman & Porth, 2014):
  - Compliance work to expand the elastic forces of the lung
  - Tissue resistance work to overcome the viscosity of the lung and thoracic cage
  - Airway resistance work to overcome the resistance to the flow of air into and out of the lungs
- Mechanical ventilation increases the work of breathing by decreasing airway diameter and increasing its length, thus increasing resistance. During weaning, the clinician manipulates pressure–volume

changes to promote reconditioning of the respiratory muscles without causing excessive fatigue (Grossoman & Porth, 2014).

- Dysfunctional ventilatory weaning response can involve respiratory inspiratory muscle fatigue, which can take up to 24 to 48 hours for recovery. The fatigue increases dyspnea, which in turn creates anxiety, triggering more fatigue and increased breathlessness.

Focus Assessment Criteria

Subjective Data

Assess for Defining Characteristics

Concerns about starting or continuing weaning process
Readiness
Previous experience
Expectations
Possibility of failure
Feelings about comfort, rest, and energy status
Knowledge of weaning process

Assess for Related Factors

Medication history
Tobacco and alcohol use

Objective Data

Assess for Defining Characteristics

Respiratory status: Complete respiratory assessment (see Focus Assessment Criteria in *Risk for Ineffective Respiratory Function*)
Level of consciousness
Baseline skin color
Airway clearance
Secretions (type and amount)
Adventitious breath sounds
Arterial blood gases
Use of accessory muscles
Vital signs

Assess for Related Factors

Respiratory disease, acute and chronic diseases
Mechanical ventilator information
  Ventilator settings and size of endotracheal or tracheostomy tube
  Ventilation history, including reason for ventilation
  Length of time on the ventilator
  Whether weaning has been attempted before, and if so, with what results
Current hemodynamic, nutritional, infection, and pain status

Goals

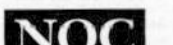

NOC

Anxiety Control, Respiratory Status, Vital Signs Status, Knowledge: Weaning, Energy Conservation

The individual will achieve progressive weaning goals, as evidenced by the following indicators:

- Spontaneous breathing for 24 hours without ventilatory support
- Demonstrates a positive attitude toward the next weaning trial
- Collaborates willingly with the weaning plan
- Communicates comfort status during the weaning process
- Attempts to control the breathing pattern
- Tries to control emotional responses
- Becomes tired from the work of weaning, but not exhausted

Interventions

NIC
Anxiety Reduction, Preparatory Sensory Information, Respiratory Monitoring, Ventilation Assistance, Presence, Endurance

If Applicable, Assess Causative Factors for Previous Unsuccessful Weaning Attempts

- Refer to Related Factors.

Determine Readiness for Weaning (Morton et al., 2005)

R: *Discontinuing mechanical ventilation is a two-step process that consists of readiness testing and weaning (Epstein, 2015).*

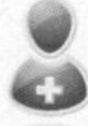

Clinical Alert Mechanically ventilated individuals should have their readiness to wean assessed daily. It is recommended that weaning be initiated on the basis of objective clinical criteria alone, rather than using a weaning predictor or the clinician's subjective impression (Epstein, 2015). In review of studies of numerous weaning predictors, none appear to be superior to objective clinical criteria in predicting a patient's readiness to wean (Epstein, 2015). A dysfunctional weaning response to a weaning trial also can influence the individual's motivation and self-efficacy, creating doubt about the ability to wean and weakening the resolve to work (*Jenny & Logan, 1991).

Required Criteria

- The cause of the respiratory failure has improved.
- $PaO_2/FiO_2 \geq 150$ or $SpO_2 \geq 90\%$ on $FiO_2 \leq 40\%$ and positive end-expiratory pressure (PEEP) ≤ 5 cmH_2O. A threshold of $PaO_2/FiO_2 \geq 120$ can be used for patients with chronic hypoxemia. pH > 7.25 (Some individuals require higher levels of PEEP to avoid atelectasis during mechanical ventilation.)
- Hemodynamic stability (no or low-dose vasopressor medications)
- Able to initiate an inspiratory effort

Additional Criteria (Optional Criteria)

- Hemoglobin $\geq$ 8 to 10 mg/dL
- Core temperature $\leq$ 38° C to 38.5° C
- Mental status awake and alert or easily arousable

R: *"The purpose of readiness testing is to identify individuals who are ready to wean, since clinicians tend to underestimate the capacity of individuals to breathe independently. "It is also intended to identify individuals who are not ready for weaning, thereby protecting them against the potential risks of premature weaning" (Epstien, 2015).*

Clinical Alert The nurse responsible for educating and supporting the individual/family through the weaning process must be experienced, as not to project their inexperience to the individual/family. Episodes of unsuccessful weaning will heighten the individual's anxiety and negatively affect subsequent attempts.

If Readiness for Weaning Is Present, Engage the Individual in Establishing the Plan

- Explain the weaning process.

R: *Weaning may involve either a period of breathing without ventilator support (i.e., a spontaneous breathing trial [SBT]) or a gradual reduction in the amount of ventilator support (Epstien, 2015).*

- Negotiate progressive weaning goals.
- Create a visual display of goals that uses symbols to indicate progression (e.g., bar or line graph to indicate increasing time-off ventilator).
- Explain that these goals will be reexamined daily.
- Refer to unit protocols for specific weaning procedures.

R: *An initial step in the weaning plan is the careful preparation of individuals. This includes teaching them about their collaborative weaning role, maximizing their energy resources and physical rest, enhancing their psychological willingness to proceed, and reinforcing their belief that they can perform the work of weaning (*Jenny & Logan, 1998). Individuals may have difficulty expressing their thoughts, so nurses must use multiple communication methods and persist until an effective method is found.*

Explain the Individual's Role in the Weaning Process

R: *Weaning collaboration involves specific roles for both the nurse and the individual. The nurse must know the individual, conserve his or her energy, and assist with the work of weaning. The individual's collaborative work requires a trust relationship and the belief that he or she will be protected during weaning (*Jenny & Logan, 1991).*

- From initial intubation, promote the understanding that mechanical ventilation is temporary if appropriate.
- Share nurses' expectations of their collaborative work role when the individual is judged ready to wean.
- Help the individual to understand the importance of communicating comfort status and trying to reach the current weaning goals, and that rest will be allowed throughout the process.

R: *The strategies can increase psychological readiness.*

Strengthen Feelings of Self-Esteem, Self-Efficacy, and Control

- Reinforce self-esteem, confidence, and control through normalizing strategies such as grooming, dressing, mobilizing, and conversing socially about things of interest to the individual.
- Permit as much control as possible by informing the individual of the situation and his or her progress, permitting shared decision making about details of care, following the individual's preferences as far as possible, and improving comfort status.
- Increase confidence by praising successful activities, encouraging a positive outlook, and reviewing positive progress to date. Explain that people usually succeed in weaning; reassure the individual you will be with him or her every step of the way.
- Demonstrate confidence in the individual's ability to wean.
- Maintain the individual's confidence by adopting a weaning pace that ensures success and minimizes setbacks.
- Explain what you are doing and why to reduce the individual's need for heightened vigilance and feelings of uncertainty.
- Note concerns that hinder comfort and confidence (family members, topics of conversation, room events, previous weaning failures); discuss them openly, if possible.

R: *Successful weaning is both an art and a science. The art depends on using subjective clinical judgment about the individual situation. The science involves the theories of oxygen exchange, carbon dioxide exchange, and mechanical efficiency (*Henneman, 2001). Nurses are a critical factor in imparting a positive outlook, creating a secure environment, enhancing feelings of self-esteem and self-confidence, and helping individuals deal with setbacks through their ability to combine the art and science of weaning (*Jenny & Logan, 1994; *Rose et al., 2007).*

Reduce Negative Effects of Anxiety and Fatigue

R: *A qualitative study reported individuals during the weaning process disclosed "being dependent for survival on other people and technical medical equipment created a sense of being vulnerable in an anxious situation and a feeling of uncertainty about one's own capacity to breathe. Having lines and tubes in one's body was stressful" (Engström, Nyström, Sundelin, & Rattray, 2013).*

- Monitor status frequently to avoid undue fatigue and anxiety. Use a systematic, comprehensive tool. A pulse oximeter is a noninvasive and unobtrusive way to monitor oxygen saturation levels.
- Provide regular periods of rest before fatigue advances.
- Reduce activities.
- Maintain or increase ventilator support and/or oxygen in consultation with a physician.
- During a rest period, dim lights, post "do not disturb" signs, and play instrumental music with 60 to 80 beats/min. Allow the individual to select type of music (*Chan, 1998).
- Encourage calmness and breath control by reassuring the individual that he or she can and will succeed.
- Consider use of alternative therapies such as music, hypnosis, and biofeedback.
- If the individual is becoming agitated, calm him or her down while remaining at the bedside, and coach him or her to regain breathing control. Monitor oxygen saturation and vital signs closely during this intervention.
- If the weaning trial is discontinued, explore the individual's perceptions of weaning failure. Reassure the individual that the trial was good exercise and a useful form of training. Remind the individual that the work is good for the respiratory muscles and will improve future performance.

R: *Successful weaning depends on adequate energy resources, careful use of available energy, and skilled withdrawal of the ventilator support within the limits of the individual's ability to tolerate additional breathing work. Altered or depleted energy reserve enhances fatigue. Thus, energy-conservation techniques are crucial to all weaning approaches (*Jenny & Logan, 1998; *Logan & Jenny, 1990).*

Create a Positive Weaning Environment That Increases Feelings of Security

R: *Chen, Lin, Tzeng, and Hsu (2009) reported that participants disclosed that the professionalism of nurses and concern from family members were essential sources of support for successful weaning.*

- Provide a room with a quiet atmosphere, low activity, soft music, and no chatter within the individual's hearing.

R: *Music with 60 to 80 beats/min decreases arousability of the CNS and exerts a hypnotic, relaxed state (*Chan, 1998).*

- Delegate the most skilled staff to wean individual who have experienced moderate to severe responses or who are at high risk for doing so. Delay weaning if nurses experienced in weaning are not available.
- Remain visible in the room to reinforce feelings of safety.
- Reassure the individual that help is immediately available, if needed.
- Monitor visitors' effects on the individuals; help visitors understand how they can best assist. Explore their feelings of the situation.
- Encourage supportive visitors when possible during the weaning process. Visits from people who upset the individuals should be postponed.
- Ensure that individuals are included in discussions that they are likely to overhear.

R: *Weaning setbacks are common and require individual support. During prolonged weaning, the individual must be psychologically motivated to wean. Music therapy seems to have a beneficial effect in promoting relaxation in mechanically ventilated individuals (*Chan, 1998). Feelings of powerlessness, hopelessness, and depression are combated with active decision making with the individual, explanation of sensations experienced, positive feedback, and conveyance of hopefulness, encouragement, and support (*Logan & Jenny, 1991).*

Promote Optimal Energy Resources

- Assist the individual to cough and deep-breathe regularly, and use prescribed bronchodilators, humidification, and suctioning to improve air entry.
- Ensure that nutritional support falls within current guidelines for ventilated and weaning individuals.
- Provide sufficient rest periods to prevent undue fatigue.
- Use ventilator support at night if necessary to increase sleep time, and try to avoid unnecessary awakening.

R: *To maintain adequate energy levels, nutritional support is necessary. It should avoid creating the complications of lipogenesis, overfeeding, and excessive carbohydrate loading to prevent excessive levels of carbon dioxide and respiratory acidosis (Dudek, 2014).*

Control Activity Demands

- Coordinate necessary activities to promote adequate time for rest or relaxation.
- Ensure that all staff follow the individualized care plan.
- Coach the individual in breath control by regular demonstrations of slow, deep, rhythmic patterns of breathing. Help the individual to synchronize breathing with the ventilator.
- If the individual's concentration creates tension and increases anxiety, provide distraction in the form of supportive visitors, radio, television, or conversation.

R: *As ventilator support is withdrawn, individuals have to work harder. Their work of weaning involves controlling their breathing, communicating their comfort status, cooperating with the therapeutic regimen, and trying to control their emotional responses to feelings of fatigue and anxiety (*Jenny & Logan, 1991).*

Follow the Institution's Multidiscipline Weaning Protocol

- Document the specifics of the plan with a timetable.
- Establish predetermined criteria for terminating the weaning process.
- Outline each discipline's responsibilities.
- Review goals and progress at each shift. Document response.
- Collaborate if revisions are needed.

R: *Collaborative weaning plans with clear goals and responsibilities and timetable have decreased ventilator and ICU days.*

Risk for Dysfunctional Ventilatory Weaning Response

NANDA-I Definition

Inability to adjust to lowered levels of mechanical ventilator support during the weaning process, related to physical and/or psychological unreadiness to wean

Risk Factors

Pathophysiologic

Related to airway obstruction

Related to muscle weakness and fatigue secondary to:

Impaired respiratory functioning
Metabolic abnormalities
Dysrhythmia
Fluid and/or electrolyte
Decreased level of consciousness
Fever
Anemia
Severe disease
Unstable hemodynamic status
Acid–base abnormalities
Mental confusion
Infection
Multisystem disease

Treatment Related

Related to ineffective airway clearance

Related to excess sedation, analgesia

Related to uncontrolled pain

Related to fatigue

Related to inadequate nutrition (deficit in calories, excess carbohydrates, inadequate fat and protein intake)

Related to prolonged ventilator dependence (more than 1 week)

Related to previous unsuccessful ventilator weaning attempt(s)

Related to too-rapid pacing of the weaning process

Situational (Personal, Environmental)

Related to muscle weakness and fatigue secondary to:

Chronic nutritional deficit
Obesity
Ineffective sleep patterns

Related to knowledge deficit related to the weaning process

Related to inadequate self-efficacy related to weaning

Related to moderate to high anxiety related to breathing efforts

Related to fear of separation from ventilator

Related to feelings of powerlessness

Related to depressed mood

Related to feelings of hopelessness

Related to uncontrolled energy demands (self-care activities, diagnostic and treatment procedures, visitors)

Related to inadequate social support

Related to insecure environment (noisy, upsetting events, busy room)

Author's Note

See *Dysfunctional Ventilatory Weaning Response*.

Errors in Diagnostic Statements

See *Dysfunctional Ventilatory Weaning Response*.

Key Concepts

- Clients at high risk for unsuccessful ventilator weaning are those who, for one reason or another, do not meet the traditional criteria for readiness to wean, such as (Morton et al., 2005):
  - Respiratory rate less than 25 to 35 breaths per minute
  - Oxygen concentration of 40% or less on the ventilator
  - Negative inspiratory pressure less than –29 to –30 cm H_2O
  - Positive expiratory pressure greater than +20 to +30 cm H_2O
  - Spontaneous tidal volume 2-6 mL/kg
  - Vital capacity greater than 10 to 15 mL/kg
  - Adequate arterial blood gases for client
  - Rested, controlled discomfort
- Although weaning as soon as possible is important to avoid muscle deconditioning and complications related to prolonged endotracheal intubation and tracheostomy, premature attempts may be counterproductive because of adverse physiologic and psychological effects.
- Because weaning is a collaborative process, the nurse's ability to gain the client's trust and willingness to work is an important determinant of outcomes, especially with long-term clients. This trust is fostered by the knowledge and self-confidence nurses display and by their ability to deal with the client's specific concerns (Jenny & Logan, 1991).
- Weaning collaboration involves specific roles for both the nurse and the client. The nurse must know the client, manage his or her energy, and assist with the work of weaning. The client's collaborative work requires a trust relationship and the belief that he or she will be protected during weaning.
- Respiratory muscles must be stressed to a certain point of fatigue and then allowed to rest. The critical point of fatigue and duration of rest have not been documented in the literature, and this judgment depends on clinical expertise (Slutsky, 1993).
- Dysfunctional ventilatory weaning is usually multifactorial. Marini (1991) notes that, at the bedside, the subjective assessment of the weaning trial by an experienced clinician remains the most reliable predictor of weaning success or failure. Close monitoring of the client's weaning work is needed to prevent serious respiratory fatigue, which can require up to 24 to 48 hours of recovery before the client can proceed (Rose et al., 2007).
- A dysfunctional weaning response to a weaning trial also can influence the client's motivation and self-efficacy, creating doubt about the ability to wean and weakening the resolve to work (Jenny & Logan, 1991).

Focus Assessment Criteria

See *Dysfunctional Ventilatory Weaning Response*.

Goals

NOC

Anxiety Reduction, Preparatory Sensory Information, Respiratory Monitoring, Ventilation Assistance, Presence, Endurance

The client will:

- Demonstrate a willingness to start weaning.
- Demonstrate a positive attitude about the ability to succeed.
  - Maintain emotional control.
  - Collaborate with planning of the weaning.

Interventions

NIC

Refer to *Dysfunctional Ventilatory Weaning Response*

Refer to *Dysfunctional Ventilatory Weaning Response*.

Ineffective Airway Clearance

NANDA-I Definition

State in which a client experiences inability to clear secretions or obstructions from the respiratory tract to maintain a clear airway

Defining Characteristics

Ineffective or absent cough
Inability to remove airway secretions
Abnormal breath sounds
Abnormal respiratory rate, rhythm, and depth

Related Factors

See *Risk for Ineffective Respiratory Function.*

Key Concepts

See *Risk for Ineffective Respiratory Function.*

Focus Assessment Criteria

See *Risk for Ineffective Respiratory Function.*

Goals

NOC
Aspiration Control, Respiratory Status

The individual will not experience aspiration, as evidenced by the following indicators:

- Demonstrates effective coughing
- Demonstrates increased air exchange

Interventions

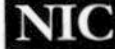
Cough Enhancement, Airway Suctioning, Positioning, Energy Management

The nursing interventions for the diagnosis *Ineffective Airway Clearance* represent interventions for any individual with this nursing diagnosis, regardless of the related factors.

Assess for Causative or Contributing Factors

- Refer to Related Factors.

Assess and Evaluate

- Sputum (color, volume, odor)
- Respiratory status before and after coughing exercises (breath sounds, rate, rhythm)

R: *These assessments can detect abnormal sputum (green, yellow, bloody, and retained secretions).*

Supervise or Provide Oral Care as Indicated

- If on ventilator, every 2 hours or 12 times in 24 hours.
- Brush teeth at 8 AM and 8 PM with chlorhexidine.
- Cleanse the mouth with tooth sponges 10 times/day.

R: *Oral care with a toothbrush reduces plaque and bacteria. Optimal oral care can improve appetite and promote positive interactions by reducing odor. Chlorhexidine reduces bacterial colonization and prevents ventilator-associated pneumonia (VAP) (*Munro & Grap, 2004; Sedwick, Lance-Smith, Reeder, & Nardi, 2012).*

- Refer to *Risk for Oral Mucous Membrane* for additional interventions.

Reduce or Eliminate Barriers to Airway Clearance

Inability to Maintain Proper Position

- Assist with positioning frequently; monitor for risk for aspiration (see *Risk for Aspiration*).

Ineffective Cough

- Instruct on the proper method of controlled coughing.
  - Breathe deeply and slowly while sitting up as high as possible.

R: *Sitting upright shifts the abdominal organs away from the lungs, enabling greater expansion.*

  - Use diaphragmatic breathing.

R: *Diaphragmatic breathing reduces the respiratory rate and increases alveolar ventilation.*

  - Hold the breath for 3 to 5 seconds, then slowly exhale as much of this breath as possible through the mouth (lower rib cage and abdomen should sink down).
  - Take a second breath; hold, slowly exhale, and cough forcefully from the chest (not from the back of the mouth or throat), using two short, forceful coughs.
  - Increase fluid intake if not contraindicated.

R: *Deep breathing dilates the airways, stimulates surfactant production, and expands the lung tissue surface, thus improving respiratory gas exchange. Coughing loosens secretions and forces them into the bronchus to be expectorated or suctioned. In some individuals, "huffing" breathing may be effective and is less painful.*

Pain or Fear of Pain Related to Surgery or Trauma

- Assess present analgesic regimen.
  - Administer pain medications as needed.
  - Coordinate analgesic doses with coughing sessions (e.g., give doses 30 to 60 minutes before coughing sessions).
  - Assess medication's effectiveness: Is the individual too lethargic? Is he or she still in pain?
  - Note the time when the individual seems to have the best pain relief with optimal level of alertness and physical performance. This is the time for active breathing and coughing exercises.
- Provide emotional support.
  - Explain the importance of coughing after pain relief.
  - Reassure that suture lines are secure and that splinting by hand or pillow will minimize pain of movement.
- Use appropriate comfort measures for the site of pain.
  - Splint abdominal or chest incisions with hand, pillow, or both.
- For Sore Throat
  - Provide humidity unless contraindicated.
  - Consider a warm saline gargle every 2 to 4 hours.
  - Consider use of an anesthetic lozenge or gargle, especially before coughing sessions.
  - Examine the throat for exudate, redness, and swelling; note if it is associated with fever.
  - Explain that a sore throat is common after anesthesia and should be a short-term problem.
- Maintain good body alignment to prevent muscular pain and strain.
  - Acquire and use extra pillows on both sides, especially the affected side, for support.
  - Position the individual to prevent slouching and cramping positions of the thorax and abdomen; reassess positioning frequently.
- Assess understanding of the use of analgesia to enhance breathing and coughing effort.
  - Teach during periods of optimal level of consciousness.
  - Continually reinforce the rationale for the plan of nursing care. ("I will be back to help you cough when the pain medicine is working and you can be most effective.")

R: *Pain or fear of pain can inhibit participation in coughing and breathing exercises. Adequate pain relief is essential.*

R: *Coughing exercises are fatiguing and painful. Emotional support provides encouragement.*

Viscous (Thick) Secretions

- Maintain adequate hydration (increase fluid intake to 2 to 3 quarts a day if not contraindicated by decreased cardiac output or renal insufficiency).

R: *Secretions must be sufficiently liquid to enable expulsion.*

- Maintain adequate humidity of inspired air.

R: *Thick secretions are difficult to expectorate and can cause mucous plugs, leading to atelectasis.*

Fatigue, Weakness, and Drowsiness

- Plan and bargain for rest periods. ("Work to cough well now; then I can let you rest.")
- Vigorously coach and encourage coughing, using positive reinforcement. ("You worked hard; I know it's not easy, but it is important.")
- Be sure the coughing session occurs at the peak comfort period after analgesics, but not peak level of sleepiness.
- Allow for rest after coughing and before meals.
- For lethargy or decreased level of consciousness, stimulate the individual to breathe deeply hourly. ("Take a deep breath.")

R: *Coughing exercises are fatiguing and painful. Emotional support provides encouragement.*

For Chronic, Unrelieved Coughing

- Minimize irritants in the inspired air (e.g., dust, allergens).
- Provide periods of uninterrupted rest.
- Administer prescribed medications—cough suppressant, expectorant—as ordered by the physician/nurse practitioner (withhold food and drink immediately after administration of medications for best results).

R: *Uncontrolled coughing is tiring and ineffective and may contribute to bronchitis.*

Provide Health Teaching and Referrals, as Indicated

- Teach the individual and family:
  - Hydration requirements
  - Mouth care
  - Effective coughing techniques
  - Signs of infection (change in sputum color, fever)
  - Refer to home health nursing if needed.

R: *Instructions to continue effective coughing at home are needed to prevent retention of secretions and infection.*

 Pediatric Interventions

- Instruct parents on the need for the child to cough, even if it is painful.
- Allow an adult and older child to listen to the lungs and describe if clear or if rales are present.
- Consult with a respiratory therapist for assistance, if needed.

R: *Explaining and demonstrating the benefits of coughing can increase parent and child cooperation.*

Ineffective Breathing Pattern

NANDA-I Definition

Inspiration and/or expiration that does not provide adequate ventilation

Defining Characteristics*

Tachypnea, hyperpnea
Panic and anxiety
Complaints of headache, dyspnea, numbness and tingling, lightheadedness, chest pain, palpitations, and, occasionally, syncope, bradycardia
Decreased expiratory pressure
Decreased inspiratory pressure
Alterations in depth of breathing
Orthopnea
Dysrhythmic respirations
Assumption of three-point position
Decreased minute ventilation
Dyspnea
Increased anterior–posterior diameter
Prolonged expiration phase
Altered chest excursion
Use of accessory muscles to breathe
Splinted/guarded respirations
Nasal flaring
Pursed-lip breathing

Related Factors

See *Risk for Ineffective Respiratory Function.*

Author's Note

Hypoventilation represents a collaborative problem as *Risk for Complications of Hypoxia*. Refer to the collaborative section for interventions. This diagnosis will focus on hyperventilation, which are more amenable to nursing interventions.

Errors in Diagnostic Statements

See *Risk for Ineffective Respiratory Function.*

Key Concepts

- Hyperventilation is breathing that is deeper and more rapid than normal. It causes a decrease in carbon dioxide (CO_2), and respiratory alkalosis (Grossman & Porth, 2014).
- Causes of hyperventilation syndrome are organic (drug effects, CNS lesions); physiologic (response to high altitude, heat, exercise); emotional (anxiety, hysteria, anger, depression); and habitual faulty breathing habits (rapid, shallow breathing; (Grossman & Porth, 2014).
- The prevalence of hyperventilation syndrome has been reported to range from 25% to 83% in individuals with an anxiety disorder and up to 11% in individuals with nonpsychiatric medical comorbidities (Schwartzstein & Richards, 2014).
- Symptoms of hyperventilation are headache, dyspnea, numbness and tingling, lightheadedness, chest pain, palpitations, and, occasionally, syncope (Grossman & Porth, 2014).
- Panic and anxiety can manifest with hyperventilation.
- Nurses involved in caring for individuals with chronic obstructive pulmonary disease must be skilled at teaching pursed-lip breathing, a critical survival skill that these individuals must learn to maintain function. Studies show that pursed-lip breathing decreases respiratory rate, increases tidal volume, decreases arterial CO_2, increases arterial oxygen, and improves exercise performance.

Goals

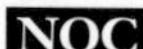

NOC

Respiratory Status, Vital Signs Status, Anxiety Control

The individual achieves improved respiratory function as evidenced by the following indicators:

- Demonstrates respiratory rate within normal limits, compared with baseline (8 to 24 breaths/min)
- Expresses relief of or improvement in feelings of shortness of breath
- Relates causative factors
- Demonstrates rebreathing techniques

Interventions

NIC

Respiratory Monitoring, Progressive Muscle Relaxation, Teaching, Anxiety Reduction

Assess History of Hyperventilating, Symptoms, and Causative Factors

- Previous episodes—when, where, circumstances
- Organic and physiologic
- Emotional (e.g., panic/anxiety disorder)
- Faulty breathing habits

Consider Other Medical Conditions That Can Present with Hyperventilation (Schwartzstein & Richards, 2014)

- Metabolic disorders (ketoacidosis, less frequently hypoglycemia or hypocalcemia)
- Acute coronary syndrome
- Arrhythmia
- Heart failure
- Pulmonary embolism
- Pneumothorax
- Asthma exacerbation
- Chronic obstructive pulmonary disease exacerbation

- Seizure disorder
- Hyperthyroidism

R: *"Multiple serious and potentially-emergent medical conditions may present with symptoms also common in experiencing with hyperventilation" (Schwartzstein & Richards, 2014).*

Explain the Signs and Symptoms the Person May be Experiencing (Schwartzstein & Richards, 2014)

- Feeling anxious, nervous, or tense
- Sense of impending doom
- Frequent sighing or yawning
- Feeling that you can't get enough air (air hunger) or need to sit up to breathe
- A pounding and racing heartbeat
- Problems with balance, lightheadedness, or vertigo
- Numbness or tingling in the hands, feet, or around the mouth
- Chest tightness, fullness, pressure, tenderness, or pain
- Carpopedal spasm (tetany)

R: *It has also been proposed that paresthesias or tetany in individuals with an acute episode of hyperventilation may be due to local vasoconstriction, leading to tissue hypoxemia and/or cerebral vasoconstriction (Schwartzstein & Richards, 2014).*

- Headache
- Gas, bloating, or burping
- Twitching
- Sweating
- Vision changes, such as blurred vision or tunnel vision
- Problems with concentration or memory
- Loss of consciousness (fainting)

R: *The signs and symptoms are the result of increasing carbon dioxide levels (Schwartzstein & Richards, 2014).*

During an Acute Episode, Instruct the Person to Breathe With You (WebMD, 2012)

- Breathe through pursed lips, as if you are whistling, or pinch one nostril and breathe through your nose. It is harder to hyperventilate when you breathe through your nose or pursed lips, because you can't move as much air.
- Slow your breathing to 1 breath every 5 seconds, or slow enough that symptoms gradually go away.
- Try belly-breathing, which fills your lungs fully, slows your breathing rate, and helps you relax.
- Place one hand on your belly just below the ribs. Place the other hand on your chest. You can do this while standing, but it may be more comfortable while you are lying on the floor with your knees bent.
- Take a deep breath through your nose. As you inhale, let your belly push your hand out. Keep your chest still.
- As you exhale through pursed lips, feel your hand go down. Use the hand on your belly to help you push all the air out. Take your time exhaling.
- Repeat these steps 3 to 10 times. Take your time with each breath.
- Instruct to always try measures to control their breathing or belly-breathe first. If these techniques don't work and there are no other health problems as heart or lung problems, such as coronary artery disease, asthma, chronic obstructive pulmonary disease (COPD, emphysema), or a history of deep vein thrombosis, stroke, or pulmonary embolism., try breathing in and out of a paper bag (WebMD, 2014).

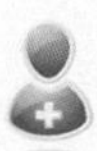

Clinical Alert "Having individual rebreathe into a paper bag may be tried so long as it is clear that the patient is not experiencing an acute hypoxic or cardiac event; when possible, however, there are **very rare** case reports of post-hyperventilation apnea that have been associated with severe hypoxemia and even death" (Schwartzstein & Richards, 2014)

- Take 6 to 12 easy, natural breaths, with a small paper bag held over your mouth and nose. Then remove the bag from your nose and mouth and take easy, natural breaths (WebMD, 2012).
- Next, try belly-breathing (diaphragmatic breathing).
- Alternate these techniques until your hyperventilation stops.
- If hyperventilation continues for longer than 30 minutes, instruct to seek emergency care (e.g., call 911); do not drive yourself to the hospital.

Remove or Control Causative Factors

- Explain the cause, if known.
- Stay with the person.
- If fear or panic has precipitated the episode
  - Remove the cause of the fear, if possible.
  - Reassure that measures are being taken to ensure safety.
  - Distract the individual from thinking about the anxious state by having him or her maintain eye contact with you (or perhaps with someone else he or she trusts); say, "Now look at me and breathe slowly with me, like this."
  - Reassure the individual that he or she can control breathing; tell him or her that you will help.

R: *Interventions focus on slowing the breathing pattern and educating the individual to control response.*

R: *Calming an individual with shortness of breath by telling him or her that actions are being taken to improve the situation (e.g., "I'm here, and I will get you through this") is an essential intervention to reduce panic and decrease symptoms (WebMD, 2012).*

Initiate Health Teaching and Referrals as Needed

- Explain a high altitude (above 6,000 feet [1,829 m]) rapid breathing faster than normal.

R: *Increased respiration is a natural response to an increased altitude where there is less oxygen in the air (Schwartzstein & Richards, 2014).*

- Refer to pulmonary rehabilitation for breathing retraining.

R: *Breathing retraining, which focuses on enhancing a person's awareness of breathing pattern and strategies to normalize the pattern when symptoms occur, is most commonly performed in the setting of pulmonary rehabilitation (Schwartzstein & Richards, 2014).*

- Refer to mental health if panic or anxiety disorder is suspected.

R: *Breathing retraining, which focuses on enhancing a patient's awareness of breathing pattern and strategies to normalize the pattern when symptoms occur, is also a component of psychiatric and cognitive-behavioral therapy (Schwartzstein & Richards, 2014).*

Impaired Gas Exchange

See also *Risk for Complications of Hypoxemia*.

NANDA-I Definition

State in which a person experiences an actual or potential decreased passage of gases (oxygen and carbon dioxide) between the alveoli of the lungs and the vascular system

Defining Characteristics

Major (Must Be Present)

Dyspnea on exertion

Minor (May Be Present)

Tendency to assume three-point position (sitting with one hand on knee and bending forward)
Pursed-lip breathing
Lethargy and fatigue
Decreased oxygen content, decreased oxygen saturation
Cyanosis

Related Factors

See Related Factors for *Ineffective Respiratory Function*.

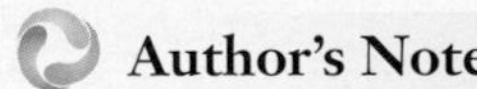

Respiratory problems that nurses can treat as nursing diagnoses are *Ineffective Airway Clearance*, *Ineffective Breathing Patterns*, and *Risk for Ineffective Respiratory Function*. If gas exchange does not improve when these nursing diagnoses are treated, then the problem is a collaborative problem. This should be labeled *Risk for Complications of Hypoxia*. In addition, the nurse should assess the individual's function health patterns to determine the effects of decreased oxygenation on sleep, emotional status, fatigue, and nutrition, and formulate the appropriate nursing diagnoses.

Impaired Spontaneous Ventilation

NANDA-I Definition

Decreased energy reserves resulting in an inability to maintain independent breathing that is adequate to support life

Defining Characteristics*

Major (Must Be Present)

Dyspnea
Increased metabolic rate

Minor (May Be Present)

Increased restlessness
Increased heart rate
Reports apprehension
Decreased PO_2
Increased use of accessory muscles
Increased PCO_2
Decreased tidal volume
Decreased cooperation
Decreased SaO_2

Author's Note

This diagnosis represents respiratory insufficiency with corresponding metabolic changes that are incompatible with life. This situation requires rapid nursing and medical management, specifically resuscitation and mechanical ventilation. *Inability to Sustain Spontaneous Ventilation* is not appropriate as a nursing diagnosis; it is hypoxemia, a collaborative problem. Hypoxemia is insufficient plasma oxygen saturation from alveolar hypoventilation, pulmonary shunting, or ventilation–perfusion inequality. As a collaborative problem, physicians prescribe the definitive treatments; however, both nursing- and medical-prescribed interventions are required for management. The nursing accountability is to monitor status continuously and to manage changes in status with the appropriate interventions using protocols. For interventions, refer to *Risk for Complications of Hypoxemia* in Section 3 in Carpenito, L. J. (2013). *Nursing diagnosis: Application to clinical practice* (14th ed.). Philadelphia, PA: Lippincott Williams & Wilkins.

INEFFECTIVE ROLE PERFORMANCE

NANDA-I Definition

Patterns of behavior and self-expression that do not match environmental context, norms, and expectations

Defining Characteristics*

Altered role perceptions
Anxiety

Inadequate adaptation to change
Role ambivalence
Role conflict, confusion, denial, dissatisfaction
Uncertainty
Role strain

Related Factors

Knowledge
Unrealistic role expectations
Inadequate role preparation (e.g., role transition, skill, rehearsal, validation)
Lack of education
Lack of role model

Physiologic
Body image alteration
Low self-esteem
Neurologic defects

Social
Conflict
Inadequate support system
Inappropriate linkage with the health care system
Job schedule demands
Young age
Cognitive deficits
Depression, mental illness
Pain
Developmental level
Domestic violence
Inadequate role socialization
Lack of resources
Lack of rewards
Low socioeconomic status
Stress

Author's Note

The nursing diagnosis *Ineffective Role Performance* has a defining characteristic of "conflict related to role perception or performance." All people have multiple roles. Some are prescribed, such as gender and age; some are acquired, such as parent and occupation; and some are transitional, such as elected office or team member.

Various factors affect an individual's role, including developmental stage, societal norms, cultural beliefs, values, life events, illness, and disabilities. When an individual has difficulty with role performance, it may be more useful to describe the effect of the difficulty on functioning, rather than to describe the problem as *Ineffective Role Performance*. For example, an individual who has experienced a cerebrovascular accident (CVA) may undergo a change from being the primary breadwinner to becoming unemployed. In this situation, the nursing diagnosis *Interrupted Family Processes* and/or *Fear* related to loss of role as financial provider secondary to effects of CVA would be appropriate. In another example, if a woman could not continue her household responsibilities because of illness and other family members assumed these responsibilities, the situations that may arise would better be described as *Risk for Disturbed Self-Concept* related to recent loss of role responsibility secondary to illness and *Risk for Impaired Home Maintenance Management* related to lack of knowledge of family members.

A conflict in a family regarding others meeting role obligations or expectations can represent related factors for the diagnosis *Ineffective Family Processes* related to conflict regarding expectations of members meeting role obligations.

Until clinical research defines this diagnosis and the associated nursing interventions, use *Ineffective Role Performance* as a related factor for another nursing diagnosis (e.g., *Anxiety*, *Grieving*, *Stress Overload*, or *Disturbed Self-Concept*).

SELF-CARE DEFICIT SYNDROME

Self-Care Deficit Syndrome[36]

Feeding Self-Care Deficit
Bathing Self-Care Deficit
Dressing Self-Care Deficit
Instrumental Self-Care Deficit[36]
Toileting Self-Care Deficit

[36]These diagnoses are not currently on the NANDA-I list but have been included by the author for clarity or usefulness.

Definition[36]

State in which an individual experiences an impaired motor function or cognitive function, causing a decreased ability in performing each of the five self-care activities

Defining Characteristics

Major (One Deficit Must Be Present in Each Activity)

Feeding Self-Care Deficit
Inability (or unwilling) to[37]
- Bring food from a receptacle to the mouth
- Complete a meal
- Place food onto utensils
- Handle utensils
- Ingest food in a socially acceptable manner
- Open containers
- Pick up cup or glass
- Prepare food for ingestion
- Use assistive device

Self-Bathing Deficits (Include Washing Entire Body, Combing Hair, Brushing Teeth, Attending to Skin and Nail Care, and Applying Makeup)[37]
Inability (or unwilling) to[37]
- Access bathroom
- Get bath supplies
- Wash body
- Dry body
- Obtain a water source
- Regulate bath water

Self-Dressing Deficits (Including Donning Regular or Special Clothing, Not Nightclothes)[37]
Inability or unwillingness to[37]
- Choose clothing or put clothing on lower body
- Put clothing on upper body
- Put on necessary items of clothing
- Maintain appearance at a satisfactory level
- Pick up clothing
- Put on shoes/remove shoes
- Put on/remove socks
- Use assistive devices
- Use zippers
- Fasten, unfasten clothing
- Obtain clothing

Self-Toileting Deficits
Unable or unwillingness to[37]
- Get to toilet or commode
- Carry out proper hygiene
- Manipulate clothing for toileting
- Rise from toilet or commode
- Sit on toilet or commode
- Flush toilet or empty commode

Instrumental Self-Care Deficits[37]
- Difficulty using telephone
- Difficulty accessing transportation
- Difficulty laundering, ironing
- Difficulty managing money
- Difficulty preparing meals
- Difficulty with medication administration
- Difficulty shopping

---

[37]This characteristic has been included by the author for clarity or usefulness.

Related Factors

Pathophysiologic

Related to lack of coordination secondary to (specify)

Related to spasticity or flaccidity secondary to (specify)

Related to muscular weakness secondary to (specify)

Related to partial or total paralysis secondary to (specify)

Related to atrophy secondary to (specify)

Related to muscle contractures secondary to (specify)

Related to visual disorders secondary to (specify)

Related to nonfunctioning or missing limb(s)

Related to regression to an earlier level of development

Related to excessive ritualistic behaviors

Related to somatoform deficits (specify)

Treatment Related

Related to external devices (specify: casts, splints, braces, intravenous [IV] equipment)

Related to postoperative fatigue and pain

Situational (Personal, Environmental)

Related to cognitive deficits

Related to fatigue

Related to pain

Related to decreased motivation

Related to confusion

Related to disabling anxiety

Maturational

Older Adult

Related to decreased visual and motor ability, muscle weakness

Author's Note

Self-care encompasses the activities needed to meet daily needs, commonly known as activities of daily living (ADLs), which are learned over time and become lifelong habits. Self-care activities involve not only what is to be done (hygiene, bathing, dressing, toileting, feeding), but also how much, when, where, with whom, and how (Miller, 2015).

In every individual, the threat or reality of a self-care deficit evokes panic. Many people report that they fear loss of independence more than death. A self-care deficit affects the core of self-concept and self-determination. For this reason, the nursing focus for self-care deficit should be not on providing the care measure, but on identifying adaptive techniques to allow the individual the maximum degree of participation and independence possible.

The diagnosis *Total Self-Care Deficit* once was used to describe an individual's inability to complete feeding, bathing, toileting, dressing, and grooming (*Gordon, 1982). The intent of specifying "Total" was to describe an individual with deficits in several ADLs. Unfortunately, sometimes its use invites, according to M. A. Magnan (Personal Communication, 1989), "preconceived judgments about the state of an individual and the nursing interventions required." The individual may be viewed as in a vegetative state, requiring only minimal custodial care. *Total Self-Care Deficit* has been eliminated because its language does not denote potential for growth or rehabilitation.

Currently not on the NANDA list, the diagnosis *Self-Care Deficit Syndrome* has been added here to describe an individual with compromised ability in all five self-care activities. For this individual, the nurse assesses functioning in each area and identifies the level of participation of which the individual is capable. The goal is to maintain current functioning, to increase participation and independence, or both. The syndrome distinction clusters all five self-care deficits together to enable grouping of interventions when indicated, while also permitting specialized interventions for a specific deficit.

The danger of applying a *Self-Care Deficit* diagnosis lies in the possibility of prematurely labeling an individual as unable to participate at any level, eliminating a rehabilitation focus. It is important that the nurse classify the individual's functional level to promote independence. (Refer to the functional level classification scale in Focus Assessment Criteria.) Use this scale with the nursing diagnosis (e.g., *Toileting Self-Care Deficit* 2 = minimal help). Continuous reevaluation is also necessary to identify changes in the individual's ability to participate in self-care.

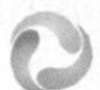

Errors in Diagnostic Statements

Toileting Self-Care Deficit related to insufficient knowledge of ostomy care

The diagnosis *Toileting Self-Care Deficit* describes an individual who cannot get to, sit on, or rise from the toilet or perform clothing and hygiene activities related to toileting. Insufficient knowledge of ostomy care does not apply. Depending on the risk factors or signs and symptoms, the diagnosis of *Ineffective Management of Therapeutic Regimen* related to insufficient knowledge of ostomy care would apply.

Dressing Self-Care Deficit related to inability to fasten clothing

Inability to fasten clothing represents a sign or symptom of *Dressing Self-Care Deficit*, not a related factor. Using a focus assessment, the nurse needs to determine the contributing factors (e.g., insufficient knowledge of adaptive techniques needed).

Self-Care Deficit Syndrome related to cognitive deficits

As a syndrome diagnosis, no related factors are indicated and, in fact, they are not very useful for treatment. Instead, the nurse should write the diagnosis as *Self-Care Deficit Syndrome: Feeding (1), Bathing (4), Dressing (4), Toileting (5), Instrumental (2)*. The number code indicates the present level of functioning needed. The goals or outcome criteria should represent improved or increased functioning.

Key Concepts

General Considerations

- The concept of self-care emphasizes each individual's right to maintain individual control over his or her own pattern of living. (This applies to both the ill and the well individuals.)
- Neglect of an extremity refers to the memory loss of the presence of an extremity (e.g., an individual who has had a stroke or brain injury resulting in partial paralysis may ignore the arm or leg on the affected side of the body). Refer to *Unilateral Neglect.*
- The following key elements promote relearning of self-care tasks:
  - Providing a structured, consistent environment and routine
  - Repeating instructions and tasks
  - Teaching and practicing tasks during periods of least fatigue
  - Maintaining a familiar environment and teacher
  - Using patience, determination, and a positive attitude (by both learner and teacher)
  - Practice, practice, practice

Endurance

- The endurance or ability of the individual to maintain a given level of performance is influenced by the ability to use oxygen to produce energy (related to the optimal functioning of the heart and respiratory and circulatory systems) and the functioning of the neurologic and musculoskeletal systems. Thus, individuals with alterations in these systems have increased energy demands or decreased ability to produce energy.
- Stress consumes energy; the more stressors an individual has, the more fatigue he or she experiences. Stressors can be personal, environmental, disease related, and treatment related. Examples of possible stressors follow:

Personal	*Environmental*	*Disease Related*	*Treatment Related*
Age	Isolation	Pain	Walker
Support system	Noise	Anemia	Medications
Lifestyle	Unfamiliar setting	Diagnostic studies	

- Signs and symptoms of decreased oxygen in response to activity (e.g., self-care, mobility) are as follows:
  - Sustained increased heart rate 3 to 5 minutes after ceasing the activity or a change in the pulse rhythm
  - Failure of systolic blood pressure reading to increase with activity or a decrease in value
  - Decrease or excessive increase in respiratory rate and dyspnea
  - Weakness, pallor, or cerebral hypoxia (confusion, incoordination)
  - Refer to Key Concepts under *Activity Intolerance* for additional information.

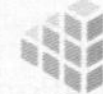

Pediatric Considerations

- Parents/caregivers can facilitate a child's mastery of self-care skills. The desired outcome is that the child participates in his or her care to the maximum of ability (Hockenberry & Wilson, 2015).
- The nurse should assess each child's unique ability to engage in self-care activities to promote control over self and environment.
  - Children with cancer with higher self-concept scores performed more self-care practices and received less dependent care from their mothers (*Mosher & Moore, 1998).

Geriatric Considerations

- Age-related changes do not in themselves cause self-care deficits. Older adults do, however, have an increased incidence of chronic diseases that can compromise functional ability (e.g., arthritis, cardiac disorders, visual impairments).
- Older adults with dementia have varying degrees of difficulty with self-care activities depending on memory deficits, ability to follow directions, and judgment (Miller, 2015).

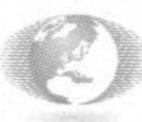

Transcultural Considerations

- In some cultures, family members may show their concern for the sick relative by doing as much as possible for him or her (e.g., feeding, bathing). This practice may prevent the individual from actively participating in a rehabilitation program (Giger, 2013).
- All cultures have rules, often unspoken, about who touches whom, when, and where. For example, in Afghan culture touching the opposite sex is discouraged even by nurses and doctors. In the Japanese culture, individuals are uncomfortable with overuse of personal contact. With Mexican women, a female nurse should always assist a male physician, when examining a woman (Giger, 2013).

Focus Assessment Criteria

Subjective and Objective Data

Evaluate Each ADL Using the Following Scale

0 = Is completely independent
1 = Requires use of assistive device
2 = Needs minimal help
3 = Needs assistance and/or some supervision
4 = Needs total supervision
5 = Needs total assistance or unable to assist

Assess for Defining Characteristics

Self-Feeding Abilities
Refer to Defining Characteristics.

Self-Bathing Abilities
Refer to Defining Characteristics.

Self-Dressing/Grooming Abilities
Refer to Defining Characteristics.

Self-Toileting Abilities
Refer to Defining Characteristics.

Instrumental ADLs

Telephone
Ability to dial

Ability to talk, hear
Ability to answer

Transportation
Ability to drive
Access to transportation

Laundry
Availability of washer
Ability to wash, iron
Ability to put away

Food Procurement and Preparation
Ability to cook
Ability to select foods
Ability to shop

Medications
Ability to remember
Ability to administer

Finances
Ability to write checks and pay bills
Ability to handle cash transactions (simple, complex)

Assess for Related Factors

Ability to remember
Judgment
Ability to follow directions
Ability to identify/express needs
Ability to anticipate needs (food, laundry)
Social supports:
- Support people.
- Availability of help with transportation, shopping, money management, laundry, housekeeping, and food preparation
- Community resources

Motivation
Endurance

Goals

NOC
See Bathing, Feeding, Dressing, Toileting, and/or Instrumental Self-Care Deficit

The individual will participate in feeding, dressing, toileting, and bathing activities, as evidenced by the following indicators (specify what the individual can perform with and without assistance):

- Identifies preferences in self-care activities (e.g., time, products, location)
- Demonstrates optimal hygiene after assistance with care

Interventions

NIC
See Feeding, Bathing, Dressing, Toileting, and/or Instrumental Self-Care Deficit

Assess for Causative or Contributing Factors

- Refer to Related Factors.

Use the Following Scale to Rate the Individual's Ability to Perform

- 0 = Is completely independent
- 1 = Requires use of assistive device
- 2 = Needs minimal help
- 3 = Needs assistance and/or some supervision
- 4 = Needs total supervision
- 5 = Needs total assistance or unable to assist

R: *This coding allows for establishing a baseline from which to evaluate progress.*

Promote Optimal Participation

- Consult with a physical therapist to assess present level of participation and for a plan.
  - Determine areas for potentially increased participation in each self-care activity.
  - Explore the individual's goals and determine what the individual perceives as his or her own needs.
  - Compare what the nurse believes are the individual needs and goals, and then work to establish mutually acceptable goals.
  - Allow ample time to complete activities without help. Promote independence, but assist when the individual cannot perform an activity.

R: *Offering choices and including the individual in planning care reduces feelings of powerlessness; promotes feelings of freedom, control, and self-worth; and increases his or her willingness to comply with therapeutic regimens. Optimal education promotes self-care.*

Promote Self-Esteem and Self-Determination

- Determine preferences for:
  - Schedule
  - Products
  - Methods
  - Clothing selection
  - Hair styling
- During self-care activities, provide choices and request preferences.
- Do not focus on disability.
- Offer praise for independent accomplishments.

R: *Inability to care for oneself produces feelings of dependency and poor self-concept. With increased ability for self-care, self-esteem increases.*

Evaluate one's Ability to Participate in Each Self-Care Activity (Feeding, Dressing, Bathing, Toileting)

- Reassess ability frequently and revise code as appropriate.

R: *Coding each self-care ability provides a baseline to evaluate progress.*

Refer to Interventions Under Each Diagnosis—Feeding, Bathing, Dressing, Toileting, and Instrumental Self-Care Deficit—as Indicated

R: *Enhancing an individual's self-care abilities can increase his or her sense of control and independence, promoting overall well-being.*

Feeding Self-Care Deficit

NANDA-I Definition

Impaired ability to perform or complete self-feeding activities

Defining Characteristics*

Inability (or unwilling) to[38]

- Bring food from a receptacle to the mouth
- Complete a meal
- Get food onto utensils
- Handle utensils
- Ingest food in a socially acceptable manner
- Open containers
- Pick up cup or glass
- Prepare food for ingestion
- Use assistive device

[38]These characteristics have been added by the author for clarity and usefulness.

Related Factors

Refer to *Self-Care Deficit Syndrome.*

Author's Note

This diagnosis is appropriate for an individual who has difficulty with the activities of self-feeding. Individuals who have difficulty chewing and ingesting sufficient calories need an additional diagnosis of Imbalanced Nutrition.

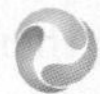

Errors in Diagnostic Statements

Refer to *Self-Care Deficit Syndrome.*

Key Concepts

Refer to *Self-Care Deficit Syndrome.*

Focus Assessment Criteria

Refer to Self-Care Deficit Syndrome.

Goals

NOC

Nutritional Status, Self-Care: Eating, Swallowing Status

The individual will demonstrate increased ability to feed self or report that he or she needs assistance, as evidenced by the following indicators:

- Demonstrates ability to make use of adaptive devices, if indicated
- Demonstrates increased interest and desire to eat
- Describes rationale and procedure for treatment
- Describes causative factors for feeding deficit

Interventions

NIC

Feeding, Self-Care Assistance: Feeding, Swallowing Therapy, Teaching, Aspiration Precautions

Assess Causative Factors

- Refer to Related Factors.

Use the Following Scale to Rate the Individual's Ability to Perform

- 0 = Is completely independent
- 1 = Requires use of assistive device
- 2 = Needs minimal help
- 3 = Needs assistance and/or some supervision
- 4 = Needs total supervision
- 5 = Needs total assistance or unable to assist

R: *This coding allows for establishing a baseline from which to evaluate progress.*

Provide Opportunities to Relearn or Adapt to Activity

Common Nursing Interventions for Feeding

- Ascertain from the individual or family members what foods the person likes or dislikes.
- Provide meals in the same setting with pleasant surroundings that are not too distracting.
- Maintain correct food temperatures (hot foods hot, cold foods cold).
- Provide pain relief because pain can affect appetite and ability to feed self.
- Provide good oral hygiene before and after meals.
- Encourage to wear dentures and eyeglasses.
- Assist to the most normal eating position suited to his or her physical disability (best is sitting in a chair at a table).
- Provide social contact during eating.

R: *These strategies attempt to normalize mealtime to increase participation and intake.*

Specific Interventions for People With Sensory/Perceptual Deficits

- Encourage to wear prescribed corrective lenses.
- Describe the location of utensils and food on the tray or table.
- Describe food items to stimulate appetite.
- For perceptual deficits, choose different colored dishes to help distinguish items (e.g., red tray, white plates).
- Ascertain usual eating patterns and provide food items according to preference (or arrange food items in clock-like pattern); record on the care plan the arrangement used (e.g., meat, 6 o'clock; potatoes, 9 o'clock; vegetables, 12 o'clock).
- Encourage eating of "finger foods" (e.g., bread, bacon, fruit, hot dogs) to promote independence.
- Avoid placing food to the blind side of the field cut until visually accommodated to surroundings; then encourage him or her to scan the entire visual field.

R: *Enhancing an individual's self-care abilities can increase his or her sense of control and independence, promoting overall well-being.*

Specific Interventions for People With Missing Limbs

- Provide an eating environment that is not embarrassing to the individual; allow sufficient time for eating.
- Provide only the supervision and assistance necessary for relearning or adaptation.
- To enhance independence, provide necessary adaptive devices:
  - Plate guard to avoid pushing food off the plate
  - Suction device under the plate or bowl for stabilization
  - Padded handles on utensils for a more secure grip
  - Wrist or hand splints with clamp to hold eating utensils
  - Special drinking cup
  - Rocker knife for cutting
- Assist with setup if needed, opening containers, napkins, condiment packages; cutting meat; and buttering bread.
- Arrange food that there is enough space to perform the task of eating.

R: *Assistive devices can improve self-care abilities.*

Specific Interventions for People With Cognitive Deficits

- Provide an isolated, quiet atmosphere until the individual can attend to eating and is not easily distracted from the task.
- Supervise the feeding program until there is no danger of choking or aspiration.
- Orient to location and purpose of feeding equipment.
- Avoid external distractions and unnecessary conversation.
- Place the individual in the most normal eating position he or she can physically assume.
- Encourage to attend to the task, but be alert for fatigue, frustration, or agitation.
- Provide one food at a time in usual sequence of eating until the individual can eat the entire meal in normal sequence.
- Encourage to be tidy, to eat in small amounts, and to put food in the unaffected side of the mouth if paresis or paralysis is present.
- Check for food in cheeks.
- Refer to *Impaired Swallowing* for additional interventions.

R: *Strategies are needed to reduce environmental distractions and to increase attention to the task.*

Initiate Health Teaching and Referrals, as Indicated

- Ensure that both individual and family understand the reason and purpose of all interventions.
- Proceed with teaching as needed.
  - Maintain safe eating methods.
  - Prevent aspiration.
  - Use appropriate eating utensils (avoid sharp instruments).
  - Test the temperature of hot liquids and wear protective clothing (e.g., paper bib).
  - Teach the use of adaptive devices.

R: *Eating has physiologic, psychological, social, and cultural implications. Increasing one's control over meals promotes overall well-being.*

Bathing Self-Care Deficit

NANDA-I Definition

Impaired ability to perform or complete bathing activities for self

Defining Characteristics*

Self-bathing deficits (including washing the entire body, combing hair, brushing teeth, attending to skin and nail care, and applying makeup)[39]

Inability (or unwilling) to[39]

- Access bathroom
- Get bath supplies
- Wash and/or dry body
- Obtain a water source
- Regulate bath water

Related Factors

Refer to *Self-Care Deficit Syndrome*.

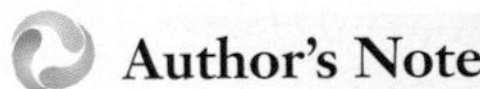

Author's Note

Refer to *Self-Care Deficit Syndrome*.

Errors in Diagnostic Statements

Refer to *Self-Care Deficit Syndrome*.

Key Concepts

Refer to *Self-Care Deficit Syndrome*.

Focus Assessment Criteria

Refer to *Self-Care Deficit Syndrome*.

Goals

NOC

Self-Care: Activities of Daily Living, Self-Care: Bathing

The individual will perform bathing activities at expected optimal level or report satisfaction with accomplishments despite limitations, as evidenced by the following indicators:

- Relates a feeling of comfort and satisfaction with body cleanliness
- Demonstrates the ability to use adaptive devices
- Describes causative factors of the bathing deficit

Interventions

NIC

Self-Care Assistance: Bathing, Teaching: Individual

Assess Causative Factors

- Refer to Related Factors.

Use the Following Scale to Rate the individual's Ability to Perform

- 0 = Is completely independent
- 1 = Requires use of assistive device
- 2 = Needs minimal help

[39]These characteristics have been added by the author for clarity and usefulness.

- 3 = Needs assistance and/or some supervision
- 4 = Needs total supervision
- 5 = Needs total assistance or unable to assist

R: *This coding allows for establishing a baseline from which to evaluate progress.*

Provide Opportunities to Relearn or Adapt to Activity

General Nursing Interventions for Inability to Bathe

- Bathing time and routine should be consistent to encourage optimal independence.
- Encourage to wear prescribed corrective lenses or hearing aid.
- Keep the bathroom temperature warm; ascertain referred water temperature.
- Provide for privacy during bathing routine.
- Elicit his or her usual bathing routine.
- Keep the environment simple and uncluttered.
- Observe skin condition during bathing.
- Provide all bathing equipment within easy reach.
- Provide for safety in the bathroom (nonslip mats, grab bars).
- When the individual is physically able, encourage the use of either a tub or shower stall, depending on which he or she uses at home. (The individual should practice in the hospital in preparation for going home.)
- Provide for adaptive equipment as needed:
  - Chair or stool in bathtub or shower
  - Long-handled sponge to reach back or lower extremities
  - Grab bars on bathroom walls where needed to assist in mobility
  - Bath board for transferring to tub chair or stool
  - Safety treads or nonskid mat on floor of bathroom, tub, and shower
  - Washing mitts with pocket for soap
  - Adapted toothbrushes
  - Shaver holders
  - Handheld shower spray
- Provide for relief of pain that may affect one's ability to bathe self.[40]

R: *Offering choices and including the individual in planning care reduces feelings of powerlessness; promotes feelings of freedom, control, and self-worth; and increases the individual's willingness to comply with therapeutic regimens. Assistive devices can improve self-care abilities.*

Specific Bathing Interventions for People With Visual Deficits

- Place bathing equipment in a location most suitable to the individual. Ensure his or her ability to locate all bathing utensils.
- Avoid placing bathing equipment to the blind side the of individual with the field cut.
- Keep the call bell within reach.
- Give the individual with visual impairment the same degree of privacy and dignity as any other person.
- Announce yourself before entering or leaving the bathing area.
- Observe his or her ability to perform mouth care, hair combing, and shaving.
- Provide place for clean clothing within easy reach.

R: *Inability to perform self-care produces feelings of dependency and poor self-concept. With increased ability for self-care, self-esteem increases.*

Specific Bathing Interventions for People With Cognitive Deficits

- Provide a consistent time for bathing as part of a structured program to help decrease confusion.
- Keep instructions simple and avoid distractions; orient to the purpose of bathing equipment and put toothpaste on the toothbrush.
- If the individual cannot bathe the entire body, have him or her bathe one part until he or she does it correctly; give positive reinforcement for success.
- Supervise activity until the individual can safely perform the task unassisted.
- Encourage attention to the task, but be alert for fatigue that may increase confusion.

[40]May require a primary care professional's order.

- Preserve dignity and decrease agitation.
- Provide verbal warning prior to doing anything (e.g., touching, spraying with water).
- Apply firm pressure to the skin when bathing; it is less likely to be misinterpreted than a gentle touch.
- Use a warm shower or bath to help a confused or agitated individual to relax.
- Add lavender oil to bath water if desired.
- Determine the best method to bathe the individual (e.g., towel bath, shower, tub bath).

R: *Aggression may be precipitated by baths or showers. Soap and towels in a warm environment have been found to reduce aggression.*

Initiate Health Teaching and Referrals, as Indicated

- Communicate to staff and family members the individual's ability and willingness to learn.
- Teach the use of adaptive devices.
- Ascertain bathing facilities at home and assist in determining if there is any need for adaptations; refer to occupational therapy or social service for help in obtaining needed home equipment.
- Teach to use the tub or shower stall, depending on what is used at home.
- If the individual is paralyzed, instruct family to demonstrate complete skin check of key areas for redness (buttocks, bony prominences).
- Teach the family to maintain a safe bathing environment.

R: *Cleanliness is important for comfort, positive self-esteem, and social interactions.*

R: *Inability to care for oneself produces feelings of dependency and poor self-concept. With increased ability for self-care, self-esteem increases.*

Dressing Self-Care Deficit

NANDA-I Definition

Impaired ability to perform or complete dressing activities for self

Defining Characteristics

Self-dressing deficits (including donning regular or special clothing, not nightclothes)[41]
Inability (or unwillingness) to[41]
Choose clothing
Put clothing on lower or upper body
Maintain appearance at a satisfactory level
Pick up clothing
Put on/remove shoes
Put on/remove socks
Use assistive devices
Use zippers
Fasten, unfasten clothing
Obtain clothing

Related Factors

Refer to *Self-Care Deficit Syndrome*.

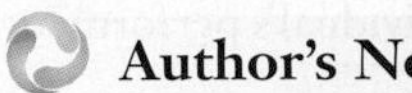

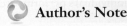

Author's Note

Refer to *Self-Care Deficit Syndrome*.

[41]These characteristics have been added by the author, for clarity and usefulness.

Errors in Diagnostic Statements

Refer to *Self-Care Deficit Syndrome*.

Key Concepts

Refer to *Self-Care Deficit Syndrome*.

Focus Assessment Criteria

Refer to *Self-Care Deficit Syndrome*.

Goals

NOC

Self-Care: Activities of Daily Living, Self-Care: Dressing

The individual will demonstrate increased ability to dress self or report the need to have someone else assist him or her to perform the task, as evidenced by the following indicators:

- Demonstrates ability to use adaptive devices to facilitate independence in dressing
- Demonstrates increased interest in wearing street clothes
- Describes causative factors for dressing deficits
- Relates rationale and procedures for treatments

Interventions

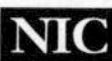

NIC

Self-Care Assistance: Dressing/Grooming, Teaching: Individual, Dressing

Assess Causative Factors

- Refer to Related Factors.

Use the Following Scale to Rate the Individual's Ability to Perform

- 0 = Is completely independent
- 1 = Requires use of assistive device
- 2 = Needs minimal help
- 3 = Needs assistance and/or some supervision
- 4 = Needs total supervision
- 5 = Needs total assistance or unable to assist

R: *This coding allows for establishing a baseline from which to evaluate progress.*

General Nursing Interventions for Self-Dressing

- Obtain clothing that is larger-sized and easier to put on, including clothing with elastic waistbands, wide sleeves, and pant legs, dresses that open down the back for women in wheelchairs, and dresses with Velcro fasteners or larger buttons.
- Encourage to wear prescribed corrective lenses or hearing aid.
- Promote independence in dressing through continual and unaided practice.
- Allow sufficient time for dressing and undressing because the task may be tiring, painful, or difficult.
- Plan for the individual to learn and demonstrate one part of an activity before progressing further.
- Lay clothes out in the order in which the individual will need them to dress.
- Provide dressing aids as necessary (some commonly used aids include dressing stick, Swedish reacher, zipper pull, buttonhook, long-handled shoehorn, and shoe fasteners adapted with elastic laces).
- If needed, increase participation in dressing by medicating for pain 30 minutes before it is time to dress or undress, if indicated.[42]
- Provide for privacy during dressing routine.
- Provide for safety by ensuring easy access to all clothing and by ascertaining the individual's performance level.

R: *Inability to care for oneself produces feelings of dependency and poor self-concept. With increased ability for self-care, self-esteem increases. Optimal personal grooming promotes psychological well-being.*

---

[42]May require a primary care professional's order.

Specific Dressing Interventions for People With Visual Deficits

- Allow to select the most convenient location for clothing and adapt the environment to accomplish the task best (e.g., remove unnecessary barriers).
- Announce yourself before entering or leaving the dressing area.
- If he or she has a field cut, avoid placing clothing to the blind side until he or she is visually accommodated to the surroundings; then encourage him or her to turn the head to scan the entire visual field.

R: *Strategies used include consistent placement of items needed for dressing.*

Specific Dressing Interventions for People With Cognitive Deficits (Miller, 2015)

- Keep verbal communication simple.
  - Ask yes/no questions.
  - Use one-step requests (e.g., "put your sock on").
  - Praise after each step.
  - Be specific and concise.
  - Call the person by name.
  - Use the same word for the same thing (e.g., "shirt").
  - Dress the bottom half, and then the top half.
- Prepare an uncluttered environment.
  - Ensure good lighting.
  - Make bed; minimize visual clutter.
  - Lay clothes face down.
  - Place clothes in the order that they will be used.
  - Allow a choice from only two pieces.
  - Place matching clothes together on hangers.
  - Remove dirty clothes from the dressing area.
- Provide nonverbal cues.
  - Hand one clothing item at a time in correct order.
  - Place shoes beside the correct foot.
  - Use gestures to explain.
  - Point or touch the body part to be used.
  - If he or she cannot complete all the steps, always allow him or her to finish the dressing step, if possible—zipper pants, buckle belt.
  - Decrease assistance gradually.

R: *Strategies are needed to reduce environmental distractions and to increase attention to the task.*

Initiate Health Teaching and Referrals, as Indicated

- Access a home health nurse for an in-home evaluation.

R: *An in-home health nurse assessment is critical for self-care activities to be maintained and/or progressed to a higher level.*

Instrumental Self-Care Deficit[43]

Definition

Impaired ability to perform certain activities or access certain services essential for managing a household

Defining Characteristics

Observed or reported difficulty with one or more of the following:

Using a telephone
Accessing transportation

[43]This diagnosis is not currently on the NANDA-I list but has been included by the author for clarity or usefulness.

Laundering and ironing
Preparing meals
Shopping (food, clothes)
Managing money
Administering medication

Related Factors

Refer to *Self-Care Deficit Syndrome.*

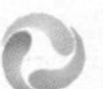

Author's Note

Instrumental Self-Care Deficit is not currently on the NANDA-I list but has been added here for clarity and usefulness. This diagnosis describes problems with performing certain activities or accessing certain services needed to live in the community (e.g., phone use, shopping, money management). This diagnosis is important to consider when planning individual discharge and during home visits by community nurses.

Errors in Diagnostic Statements

***Instrumental Self-Care Deficit* related to possible inability to plan meals and manage laundry**

When a nurse suspects that an individual or family may have compromised ability to engage in certain activities needed to live in and run a household, the nurse should label the diagnosis Possible *Instrumental Self-Care Deficit* and add related factors representing why he or she suspects the diagnosis (e.g., related to difficulty remembering routine tasks or related to poor planning skills). The nurse detecting evidence of memory or judgment difficulties could interpret this as a risk factor for *Risk for Instrumental Self-Care Deficit*.

Key Concepts

- Instrumental ADLs include housekeeping, preparing and procuring food, shopping, laundering, ability to self-medicate safely, ability to manage money, and access to transportation (Miller, 2015). Instrumental ADLs require more complex tasks than ADLs.
- Maintaining people in the community, rather than in nursing homes, also maintains autonomy, strengthens family life, and affirms the value of older adults in our society.

Focus Assessment Criteria

Refer to *Self-Care Deficit Syndrome*.

Goals

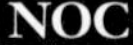

NOC
Self-Care: Instrumental Activities of Daily Living (IADL)

The individual or family will report satisfaction with household management, as evidenced by the following indicators:

- Demonstrates use of adaptive devices (e.g., telephone, cooking aids)
- Describes a method to ensure adherence to medication schedule
- Reports ability to make calls and answer the telephone
- Reports regular laundering by self or others
- Reports daily intake of at least two nutritious meals
- Identifies transportation options to stores, primary care provider, house of worship, and social activities
- Demonstrates management of simple money transactions
- Identifies people who will assist with money matters

Interventions

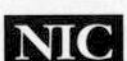

Teaching: Individual, Referral, Family Involvement Promotion

Assess for Causative and Contributing Factors

- Refer to Related Factors.

Use the Following Scale to Rate the Person's Ability to Perform

- 0 = Is completely independent
- 1 = Requires use of assistive device
- 2 = Needs minimal help
- 3 = Needs assistance and/or some supervision
- 4 = Needs total supervision
- 5 = Needs total assistance or unable to assist

R: *This coding allows for establishing a baseline from which to evaluate progress.*

Assist the Individual in Identifying Self-Help Devices

Grooming/Dressing Aids

- Refer to *Impaired Physical Mobility*.

Kitchen/Eating Aids

- Dishes with one side built up
- Built-up handles on cutlery (use plastic foam curlers)
- Bulldog clip to secure a straw in a glass
- Built-up corner of a cutlery board to hold and anchor food or pot (e.g., to butter toast, mash potatoes)
- Mounted jar opener
- Nonskid material applied under dishes (same strips used to prevent slipping in bathtub)
- Two-sided suction holder to hold dishes in place

R: *A variety of assistive devices are available for use in the kitchen.*

Communication/Security

- Motion-activated lights near walkway/entrance
- Nightlight for path to the bathroom
- Light next to the bed
- Specially adapted telephones (amplified, big buttons)
- Specially adapted safety devices (bracelet alarm)

R: *A variety of assistive devices is available to prevent injury and to call for assistance.*

Promote Self-Care and Safety for the Person With Cognitive Deficit

Evaluate Activities That Are Achievable

- Turn on lights before dark.
- Use nightlights.
- Keep the environment simple and uncluttered.
- Use clocks and calendars as cues.
- Mark on calendar (using picture symbols) reminders for shopping, laundry, cleaning, doctor's appointments, and the like.

R: *Interventions focus on assisting the individual and family to maintain safely as much functional independence as possible (Miller, 2015).*

For Laundry, Teach to

- Separate dark and light clothes
- Use pictures to illustrate steps for washing clothes
- Mark cup with line to indicate amount of soap needed
- Minimize ironing
- Use an iron with automatic shutoff mechanism

R: *Interventions focus on assisting the individual and family to maintain safely as much functional independence as possible (Miller, 2015).*

Evaluate the Person's Ability to Select, Procure, and Prepare Nutritious Food Daily

- Prepare a permanent shopping list with cues for essential foods and products.
- Teach to review the list before shopping, check items needed, and, in the store, check off items selected. (Use a pencil that can be erased to reuse list.)
- Teach how to shop for single-person meals (refer to *Imbalanced Nutrition* for specific techniques).
- If possible, teach to use a microwave to reduce the risk of heat-related injuries or accidents.

R: *Interventions focus on assisting the individual and family to maintain as much functional independence as possible (Miller, 2015).*

Offer Hints to Improve Adherence to Medication Schedule

- Have someone place medications in a commercial pill holder divided into 7 days.
- Take out the exact amount of pills for the day. Divide them in small cups, each labeled with time of day.
- If needed, draw a picture of the pills and the quantity on each cup.
- Teach the individual to transfer the pills from cup to small plastic bag when planning to be away from home.
- Tell the individual whom to call for instructions if he or she misses a dose.

R: *Simple strategies can be used to remember the medication schedule and prevent errors.*

R: *Interventions focus on assisting the individual and family to maintain as much functional independence as possible (Miller, 2015).*

Initiate Health Teaching and Referrals, as Indicated

- Discuss the importance of identifying the need for assistance.
- Discuss the possibility of bartering for services (e.g., wash the neighbor's clothes in exchange for shopping help).
- Identify a person who can provide immediate help (e.g., neighbor, friend, hotline).
- Identify sources for help with laundry, shopping, and money matters.

Determine Available Sources of Transportation (Neighbors, Relatives, Community Centers)

- Church groups or social service agency
- Refer the individual to community agencies for assistance (e.g., Department of Social Services, area agency on aging, senior neighbors, public health nursing, Meals on Wheels).

R: *Community resources, neighbors, religious groups, or all three can assist the individual when caregivers are unavailable or nonexistent (Miller, 2015).*

Toileting Self-Care Deficit

NANDA-I Definition

Impaired ability to perform or complete toileting activities for self

Defining Characteristics*

Unable (or unwilling) to[44]

Get to toilet or commode
Carry out proper hygiene
Manipulate clothing for toileting
Rise from toilet or commode
Sit on toilet or commode
Flush toilet or empty commode

[44]These characteristics have been added by the author for clarity and usefulness.

Related Factors

Refer to *Self-Care Deficit Syndrome.*

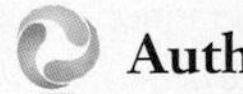

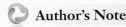

Author's Note

Refer to *Self-Care Deficit Syndrome.*

Errors in Diagnostic Statements

Refer to *Self-Care Deficit Syndrome.*

Key Concepts

Refer to *Self-Care Deficit Syndrome.*

Focus Assessment Criteria

Refer to *Self-Care Deficit Syndrome.*

Goals

NOC

Self-Care: Activities of Daily Living, Self-Care: Hygiene, Self-Care: Toileting

The individual will demonstrate increased ability to toilet self or report the need to have someone assist him or her to perform the task, as evidenced by the following indicators (specify when assistance is needed):

- Demonstrates the ability to use adaptive devices to facilitate toileting
- Describes causative factors for toileting deficit
- Relates the rationale and procedures for treatment

Interventions

NIC

Self-Care Assistance: Toileting, Self-Care Assistance: Hygiene, Teaching Individual, Mutual Goal Setting

Assess Causative Factors

- Refer to Related Factors.

Use the Following Scale to Rate His or Her Ability to Perform

- 0 = Is completely independent
- 1 = Requires use of assistive device
- 2 = Needs minimal help
- 3 = Needs assistance and/or some supervision
- 4 = Needs total supervision
- 5 = Needs total assistance or unable to assist

R: *This coding allows for establishing a baseline from which to evaluate progress.*

Common Nursing Interventions for Toileting Difficulties

- Encourage to wear prescribed corrective lenses or hearing aid.
- Obtain bladder and bowel history from the individual or family (see *Impaired Bowel Elimination* or *Impaired Urinary Elimination*).
- Ascertain the communication system the individual uses to express the need to toilet.
- Maintain a bladder and bowel record to determine toileting patterns.
- Provide adequate fluid intake and a balanced diet to promote adequate urinary output and normal bowel evacuation.
- Promote normal elimination by encouraging activity and exercise within the individual's capabilities.
- Avoid development of "bowel fixation" by less frequent discussion and inquiries about bowel movements.

- Be alert to the possibility of falls when toileting (be prepared to ease him or her to the floor without injuring either of you).
- Achieve independence in toileting by continual and unaided practice.
- Allow sufficient time for the task of toileting to avoid fatigue. (Lack of sufficient time to toilet may cause incontinence or constipation.)
- Avoid the use of indwelling and condom catheters to expedite bladder continence (if possible).

R: *The person's maximum involvement in toileting activities can reduce the embarrassment associated with needing assistance with toileting.*

R: *These strategies provide a structured, consistent environment and routine for achieving individual goals.*

Specific Toileting Interventions for People With Visual Deficits

- Keep the call bell easily accessible so the individual can quickly obtain help to toilet; answer the call bell promptly to decrease anxiety.
- If the bedpan or urinal is necessary for toileting, be sure it is within the person's reach.
- Avoid placing toileting equipment to the side of the field cut. (When he or she is visually accommodated to surroundings, you may suggest he or she search the entire visual field for equipment.)
- Announce yourself before entering or leaving the toileting area.
- Observe his or her ability to obtain equipment or get to the toilet unassisted.
- Provide for a safe and clear pathway to toilet area.

R: *These strategies provide a structured, consistent environment and routine for achieving individual goals.*

Specific Toileting Interventions for People With Affected or Missing Limbs

- Provide only the supervision and assistance necessary for relearning or adapting to the prosthesis.
- Encourage to look at the affected area or limb and use it during toileting tasks.
- Encourage useful transfer techniques taught by occupational or physical therapy. (The nurse becomes familiar with the planned mode of transfer.)
- Provide the necessary adaptive devices to enhance independence and safety (commode chairs, spill-proof urinals, fracture bedpans, raised toilet seats, side support rails for toilets).
- Provide for a safe and clear pathway to toilet area.

R: *A variety of assistive devices and techniques are available to prevent injury and promote self-care.*

Specific Toileting Interventions for People With Cognitive Deficits

- Offer toileting reminders every 2 hours, after meals, and before bedtime.
- When the individual can indicate the need to toilet, begin toileting at 2-hour intervals, after meals, and before bedtime.
- Answer the call bell immediately to avoid frustration and incontinence.
- Encourage wearing ordinary clothes. (Many confused people are continent while wearing regular clothing.)
- Avoid the use of bedpans and urinals; if physically possible, provide a normal atmosphere of elimination in bathroom. (The toilet used should remain constant to promote familiarity.)
- Give verbal cues as to what is expected of him or her and positive reinforcement for success.
- Work to achieve daytime continence before expecting nighttime continence. (Nighttime incontinence may continue after daytime continence has returned.)
- Refer to *Impaired Urinary Elimination* for additional information on incontinence.

R: *Interventions focus on assisting the individual and family to maintain safely as much functional independence as possible (Miller, 2015).*

Initiate Health Teaching and Referrals, as Indicated

- Assess the understanding and knowledge of the individual and family of foregoing interventions and rationales.
- Ensure an in-home evaluation by a home health nurse.

R: *Community resources, neighbors, religious groups, or all three can assist the person in maintaining self-care even when caregivers are unavailable or nonexistent (Miller, 2015).*

DISTURBED SELF-CONCEPT

Disturbed Self-Concept

Disturbed Body Image
Disturbed Personal Identity
Risk for Disturbed Personal Identity
Disturbed Self-Esteem
Chronic Low Self-Esteem
Risk for Chronic Low Self-Esteem
Situational Low Self-Esteem
Risk for Situational Low Self-Esteem

Definition[45]

A negative state of change about the way a person feels, thinks, or views himself or herself or their total beliefs about three interrelated dimensions of self: body image, self-esteem, or personal identity (Boyd, 2012)

Defining Characteristics

This diagnosis reflects a broad diagnostic category that can be used initially until more specific assessment data can support a more specific nursing diagnosis, such as *Disturbed Body Image* or *Disturbed Self-Esteem*.

Some examples of signs and symptoms (observed or reported) are as follows:

- Verbal or nonverbal negative response to actual or perceived change in structure, function, or both (e.g., shame, embarrassment, guilt, revulsion)
- Expression of shame or guilt
- Rationalization or rejection of positive feedback and exaggeration of negative feedback about self
- Hypersensitivity to slight criticism
- Episodic occurrence of negative self-appraisal in response to life events in an individual with a previously positive self-evaluation
- Verbalization of negative feelings about self (helplessness, uselessness)

Related Factors

A disturbed self-concept can occur as a response to a variety of health problems, situations, and conflicts. Some common sources follow.

Pathophysiologic

Related to change in appearance, lifestyle, role, response of others secondary to:

Chronic disease
Loss of body parts
Loss of body functions
Severe trauma
Pain

Situational (Personal, Environmental)

Related to feelings of abandonment or failure secondary to:

Divorce, separation from, or death of a significant other
Loss of job or ability to work

Related to immobility or loss of function

Related to unsatisfactory relationships (parental, spousal)

Related to sexual preferences (homosexual, lesbian, bisexual, abstinent)

[45]This definition has been added by the author for clarity and usefulness.

Related to teenage pregnancy

Related to gender differences in parental child-rearing

Related to experiences of parental violence

Related to change in usual patterns of responsibilities

Maturational

Middle-Aged
Loss of role and responsibilities

Older Adult
Loss of role and responsibilities

Author's Note

Self-concept reflects self-view, encompassing body image, esteem, role performance, and personal identity. Self-concept develops over a lifetime and is difficult to change. It is influenced by interactions with the environment and others and by the individual's perceptions of how others view him or her.

Disturbed Self-Concept represents a broad diagnostic category under which fall more specific nursing diagnoses. Initially, the nurse may not have sufficient clinical data to validate a more specific diagnosis, such as *Chronic Low Self-Esteem* or *Disturbed Body Image*; thus, he or she can use *Disturbed Self-Concept* until data can support a more specific diagnosis.

Self-esteem is one of the four components of self-concept. *Disturbed Self-Esteem* is the general diagnostic category. *Chronic Low Self-Esteem* and *Situational Low Self-Esteem* represent specific types of *Disturbed Self-Esteem* and thus involve more specific interventions. Initially, the nurse may not have sufficient clinical data to validate a more specific diagnosis, such as *Chronic Low Self-Esteem* or *Situational Low Self-Esteem*; thus, *Disturbed Self-Esteem* may be appropriate to use. Refer to the Defining Characteristics under these categories for validation.

Situational Low Self-Esteem is an episodic event that challenges one's usual affirmative self-esteem; repeated occurrence, continuous negative self-appraisals over time, or both may lead to *Chronic Low Self-Esteem*, abusive relationship, repeated unsuccessful employment.

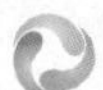

Errors in Diagnostic Statements

Disturbed Self-Concept related to substance abuse

Although a relationship exists between negative self-concept and alcohol and/or drug abuse, listing substance abuse as a related factor does not describe the nursing focus. If the individual acknowledged a substance abuse problem and expressed a desire for assistance, the diagnosis *Ineffective Coping* related to inability to constructively manage stressors without alcohol or drugs could be appropriate. If the individual denies a problem, the diagnosis *Ineffective Denial* related to lack of acknowledgment of substance abuse/dependency would apply—if the nurse will address the denial. A nurse with data that suggest or confirm *Disturbed Self-Concept* should explore contributing factors (e.g., guilt influenced by social stigma). The nurse can use "unknown etiology" until focus assessment identifies contributing factors.

Disturbed Body Image related to mastectomy

Mastectomy can produce various responses, including grief, anger, and negative feelings about self. A woman undergoing breast surgery for cancer is at high risk for both *Disturbed Body Image* and *Disturbed Self-Esteem*. Thus, the diagnosis *Risk for Disturbed Self-Concept* related to possible negative effects of changed appearance and diagnosis of cancer would be most appropriate. A nurse with data to support *Disturbed Self-Concept* should record it as a problem diagnosis with these same related factors and include "as evidenced by" to specify signs and symptoms of or manifestations (e.g., *Disturbed Self*-Concept related to perceived negative effects of changed appearance and diagnosis of cancer, as evidenced by reports of negative feelings about "new self" and determination not to let husband see her).

Key Concepts

General Considerations

- Both the individual and the nurse have their own personal self-concept. To deal effectively with others, the nurse must be aware of his or her own behavior, feelings, attitudes, and responses.
- Self-concept involves a person's feelings, attitudes, and values and affects his or her reactions to all experiences.
- A person's self-concept evolves from infancy through old age. With aging, new skills and challenges emerge. Successful completion of developmental tasks contributes to a positive self-concept (Boyd, 2012).
- Interactions with others, the sociocultural milieu, and developmental task completion influence self-concept (Boyd, 2012).
- The concept of self includes components of body image, self-esteem, and personal identity (Boyd, 2012).
  - *Body Image:* The sum of the conscious and unconscious attitudes the individual has toward his or her body. It includes present and past perceptions.
  - *Self-Esteem:* The individual's personal judgment of his or her own worth obtained by analyzing how well his or her behavior conforms to self-ideals. High self-esteem is rooted in unconditional acceptance of self, despite mistakes, defeats, and failures, as an innately worthy and important being.
  - *Personal Identity:* The organizing principle of the personality that accounts for the unity, continuity, consistency, and uniqueness of the individual. It connotes autonomy and includes self-perceptions of sexuality. Identity formation begins in infancy and proceeds throughout life, but it is the major task of adolescence.
- Disturbances in the components of self-concept are described as follows:
  - *Body Image:* Viewing oneself differently as a result of actual or perceived changes in body appearance or function
  - *Self-Ideal:* A change in self-expectations/striving
  - *Self-Esteem:* Lack of confidence in ability to accomplish that which is desired
  - *Role Performance:* Inability to perform those functions and activities expected of a particular role in a given society
  - *Personal Identity:* Disturbance in perception of self ("Who am I?")

Loss of Body Part/Function

- People have a concept of self that includes feelings about self-worth, attractiveness, worth of love, and capabilities. A physical injury assaults one's mental image of one's own body and person. This injury or loss involves the grieving process.
- Facial disfigurement causes the most changes in body image and self-concept.
- Factors that influence successful reimaging are the individual's perspective on value of lost function, nature of change, prior life experiences, self-esteem, social support, others' attitudes, and access to medical technology.

Cancer Treatments and Body Image

- The treatments for cancer can influence one's view of one's body. Some treatments are visible, as a tracheostomy, hair loss; some are covered, as a mastectomy or colostomy, and some affect sexual functions, as erectile problems after prostate cancer treatment or infertility. Visible or not, negative changes related to cancer treatments can negatively impact one's image of themselves and how they interact with others.
- Fatigue, pain, and other discomforts, for example, nausea and pruritus can interfere with activities that have been very important to the person and can negatively affect their self-esteem and/or body image.

Self-Esteem

- Self-esteem evolves from a comparison between self-concept and self-ideal. The greater the congruency, the higher the self-esteem.
- Self-esteem derives from the individual's own perceptions of competency and efficacy and from appraisals of others. In general, people hold positive self-enhancing beliefs about themselves, the world, and the future. These biased perceptions are considerably more positive than objective evidence indicates.
- As self-esteem declines, so does an individual's belief that he or she can exert control over the environment. Likewise, as personal control is perceived to decrease, so does self-esteem. Attributing failure to a lack of ability (internal cause) leads to decreased expectations and motivation.

- In response to a threat to individual's self-concept, three cognitive processes protect self-esteem:
  - Searching for meaning in the experience
  - Regaining mastery over the event; exerting personal control
  - Self-enhancement ("How am I managing compared with others?")
- The following behaviors are associated with low self-esteem: rigidity; procrastination; repetitive, unnecessary apologies; minimizing one's abilities; emphasizing deficits; expecting failure; self-destructive behaviors; approval-seeking behavior; inability to accept compliments; disregard for one's own opinions; difficulty in forming close relationships; and inability to say "no" when appropriate (Miller, 2015).
- Low self-esteem has been regarded as an important cause of violence; however, the opposite view is theoretically viable. Violence appears often as a result of threatened egotism (i.e., highly favorable views of self that some person or circumstance disputes). This is the dark side of high self-esteem.

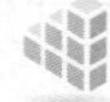

Pediatric Considerations

- Self-concept is learned. A child's concept of self, for example, emerges as a result of changes during earlier developmental stages.
- To develop and maintain self-esteem, a child needs to feel worthwhile, different in some way, and superior to and more lovable than any other child (Hockenberry & Wilson, 2015).
- Self-esteem increases as a child develops meaningful relationships and masters developmental tasks. Early adolescence is a time of risk to self-esteem as the adolescent strives to define an identity and sense of self within a peer group (Boyd, 2012).
- Present and past perceptions of his or her body, physiologic functioning, developmental maturation, and responses from others influence a child's development of body image. Adolescence is probably the critical period of development for body image formation, as pubertal changes force alteration of the adolescent's body image. The development of a positive body image by age is charted below (Boyd, 2012):

Age	*Developmental Task*
Birth to 1 year	Learns to tolerate small frustrations
	Learns to trust
1 to 3 years	Learns to like body
	Learns mastery of
	Motor skills
	Language skills
	Bowel training
3 to 6 years	Learns initiative
	Learns sex typing
	Identifies with parent models
	Increases skills (motor, language)
6 to 12 years	Develops a sense of industry
	Has a clear sex role identification
	Learns peer interaction
	Develops academic skills
Adolescence	Establishes self-identity and sexual role
	Uses abstract thought
	Develops personal value system

- Children learn to see themselves in the way that parents and significant others see them.
- To develop a healthy personality, a child needs a positive and accurate body image, realistic self-ideal, positive self-concept, and high self-esteem.
- Although obese children and adolescents may be at particular risk for developing body image or self-esteem disturbance, lower self-esteem is more likely in children who believe they are responsible for their excess weight compared with those who attribute their excess weight to an external cause. Lower self-esteem is also found in those children who believe that their excess weight hinders their social interaction (*Pierce & Wardle, 1997).
- Negative self-concepts have been associated with self-destructive health behaviors in children and adolescents, such as overeating, alcoholism, smoking, and drug abuse (*Winkelstein, 1989).
- Mastery describes positive coping with stress. Successful coping enhances self-esteem.

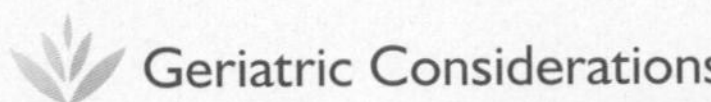

Geriatric Considerations

- Enrique Peon Lobato (2013) wrote, "Strengthen your autonomy, not admitting more help than needed; accept your limitations with realistic goals that can be achieved, reward yourself with your success, feeling realized, continue assuming decisions that affect your life; go out, do not confine yourself, there is a whole world out there, keep on being useful with small and simple domestic tasks and think about life in your realm, have intimacy, since it is important to have your own space. Self-esteem is part of our life. If we feed it daily through diverse activities and attitudes we will achieve a satisfactory ageing. Acting positively will become a habit and will improve your image."
- According to Miller (2015), self-esteem is "one of the characteristics most highly associated with both depression and happiness" in older adults.
- Self-esteem depends on interactions with others and on others' opinions. In Western societies, a generally negative view of aging can contribute to an older adult's decreased self-esteem.
- Many variables interact to produce a decline in self-esteem in older adults, including negative societal attitudes, decreased social interactions, and decreased power and control over the environment.
- Environmental factors in long-term care facilities that can influence self-esteem of older residents include decor, social roles, choices available, architectural design, space, and privacy (Miller, 2015).

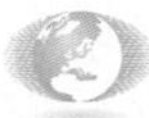

Transcultural Considerations

- In the Latin culture, the man is the head of the household and has authority over his family. He must provide for and protect his family. This concept is described as *machismo*. Loss of self-esteem or authority is incompatible with machismo. Anything that challenges his ability to provide for his family challenges his very core or self-concept (Giger, 2013).

Focus Assessment Criteria

Disturbed Self-Concept is manifested in a variety of ways. An individual may respond with an unacceptable change in another life process (see *Spiritual Distress, Fear, Ineffective Coping*). The nurse should be aware of this and use the assessment data to ascertain the dimensions affected. The assessment should focus on deficits, dysfunction, and strengths (Froggart & Liersch-Sumkis, 2014).

It may be difficult for the nurse to identify the cues and make the inferences necessary to diagnose a self-concept disturbance. Each individual reacts differently to loss, pain, disability, and disfigurement. Therefore, the nurse should determine an individual's usual reactions to problems and feelings about himself or herself before attempting to diagnose a change.

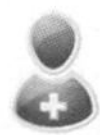

Clinical Alert "The key to effective mental health assessment is the nurse's ability to develop a therapeutic relationship with the person and others within her or his supportive network, as early as possible" (Froggart & Liersch-Sumkis, 2014, p. 92). Be careful not to fall victim to the pressure to complete a preestablished assessment form at the expense of projecting insensitivity and intimidating an distressed individual to disclose personal information that glossed over because of time.

Froggart and Liersch-Sumkis (2014, p. 94) address the situation of asking personal questions because of intense pressure and agency compelling demands by posing these questions for the nurse to ask themselves as follows:

- What do you think you might be feeling or experiencing at this time?
- What do you think the consumer might be feeling or experiencing at this time?
- What steps can you take to respond to this situation? What options do you have?
- What might be the longer-term implications of these actions you take at this time?

Attitude to interview (engaged, reluctant, avoidance, hostile, suspicious) (Froggart & Liersch-Sumkis, 2014)

Subjective Data

Assess for Defining Characteristics

Self-View/ Insight

"Describe yourself."

Awareness of being unwell? Denial? Blames others?

"What do you like most/about yourself?"

"What do you/others want to change about you?"

"What do you enjoy?"
"Has being ill affected how you see yourself?"

Identity
"What personal achievements have given you satisfaction?"
"What are your future plans?"

Role Responsibilities
"What do you do for a living? Job responsibilities? Home responsibilities?"
"Are these satisfying?"
If the person has had a role change, how has it affected lifestyle and relationships?

Affect and Mood
"How do you feel now?"
"How would you describe your usual mood?"
"What things make you happy/upset?"

Body Image
"What do you like least about your body?"
"What do you like most about your body?"
"Has there been change in the way you feel about yourself or the way others respond to you?"
Children may be able to draw self-portraits.

Assess for Related Factors

Stress Management
"How do you manage stress?"
"To whom do you go for help with a problem?"

Support System
"Any problems in current relationships?"
"Does your family regularly discuss problems?"
"What other supports do you have? Spiritual? Social?"

Objective Data

Assess for Defining Characteristics

General Appearance
Eye contact
Facial expression
Body posture/language (eye contact, head and shoulder flexion, gait/stride)
Dress (tidy, appropriate, disheveled, unkempt) (Froggart & Liersch-Sumkis, 2014)

Thought Processes/Content
Orientation
Difficulty concentrating
Slowed thought processes
Poor memory or may even be missing large portions of personal history\
Impaired judgment

Risks for Self-Harm or Harm to Others
Suspicious
Homicidal/suicidal ideation
Impaired judgment
Rambling
Sexual preoccupation
Delusions (grandeur, persecution, reference, influence, or bodily sensations)
Difficulty concentrating
Slowed thought processes
Poor memory or may even be missing large portions of personal history

Behavior
School problems (truancy, low/drop in grades)
Problems on job (lateness, decreased productivity, accident-prone, burnout symptoms)

Social withdrawal
Sexual behavior (increase, decrease, promiscuity)

Communication Patterns
With significant others:
- Relates well
- Dependent
- Hostile
- Demanding

Nutritional Status
Appetite
Eating patterns
Episodes of dysphagia, choking
Weight (gain/loss)

Rest–Sleep Pattern
Recent change

Goals

NOC

Quality of Life, Depression Level, Depression, Self-Control, Self-Esteem, Coping

The individual will demonstrate healthy adaptation and coping skills, as evidenced by the following indicators:

- Appraises self and situations realistically without distortions
- Verbalizes and demonstrate increased positive feelings

Interventions

NIC

Hope Instillation, Mood Management, Values Clarification, Counseling, Referral, Support Group, Coping Enhancement

Nursing interventions for the various problems that might be associated with a diagnosis of *Disturbed Self-Concept* are similar.

Contact the Individual Frequently and Treat Him or Her With Warm, Positive Regard

R: *Frequent contact by the caregiver indicates acceptance and may facilitate trust. They may be hesitant to approach the staff because of negative self-concept.*

Encourage the Individual to Express Feelings and Thoughts About the Following:

- Condition
- Progress
- Prognosis
- Effects on lifestyle
- Support system
- Treatment

R: *Encouraging the individual to share feelings can provide a safe outlet for fears and frustrations and can increase self-awareness. "Understanding is gained through engaging in a series of continuing and evolving conversations" (McCormack, 2007 in Froggart & Liersch-Sumkis, 2014, p. 104).*

Document the Person's Own Words Not an Interpretation of the Words

R: *This will preserve the person's meaning, not reinterpretation in medical or technical language (Froggart & Liersch-Sumkis, 2014).*

Provide Reliable Information and Clarify Any Misconceptions

R: *Misconceptions can increase anxiety and damage self-concept needlessly.*

Help to Identify Positive Attributes and Possible New Opportunities

Assist With Hygiene and Grooming, as Needed

R: *Participation in self-care and planning can aid positive coping.*

Encourage Visitors

R: *Frequent visits by support people can help the individual feel that he or she is still a worthwhile, acceptable person, which should promote a positive self-concept.*

Help to Identify Strategies to Increase Independence and to Maintain Role Responsibilities

R: *A strong component of self-concept is the ability to perform functions expected of one's role, thus decreasing dependency and reducing the need for others' involvement.*

Promote the Most Involvement in Self-Care as Possible

- Prioritizing activities
- Using mobility aids and assistive devices, as needed

R: *Participation in self-care and planning can aid positive coping.*

- Research has reported, "Elderly people with sound balance skills and upper limb strength have a high level of autonomy in the performance of BADL and IADL" (Candela, Zucchetti, Magistro, Ortega, & Rabaglietti, 2014, p. 356)
- "The perception of physical functioning also has a strong relationship with autonomy in ADL. That is, elderly people who perceive their body as highly functioning are more autonomous" (Candela et al., 2014, p. 356)

Discuss With His or Her Family the Importance of Communicating the Person's Value and Importance to Them

- Use their name, no mom or pop.
- Use the same tone of voice as one would use with colleague.
- Do not raise your voice unless the person is hard of hearing and not wearing a hearing aid.

R: *Communication as to an adult rather as to a child enhances self-esteem and promotes adjustment.*

- Provide person with choices when the choice is feasible.
- Do not promote unnecessary dependence even if convenient for caregivers.

R: *Strategies that increase one's sense of control reduce the treat to self-esteem (Miller, 2015).*

Initiate Health Teaching, as Indicated

- Teach what community resources are available, if needed (e.g., mental health centers, self-help groups such as Reach for Recovery, Make Today Count).
- Refer to specific health teaching issues under *Disturbed Body Image* and *Disturbed Self-Esteem* (*Chronic* and *Situational*).

R: *Addressing spiritual issues within the counseling process involves an accurate assessment of spiritual functioning and relevant interventions used with discretion and respect for individual beliefs.*

R: *Nurses must receive adequate education and keep their knowledge updated. Nurses should receive regular clinical supervision and support to ensure that they can provide therapeutic care for individuals with self-concept disturbances.*

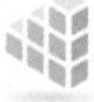

Pediatric Interventions

- Allow the child to bring his or her own experiences into the situation (e.g., "Some children say that an injection feels like an insect sting; some say they don't feel anything. After we do this, you can tell me how it feels"; *Johnson, 1995).

R: *Allowing the child to describe the experience supports that he or she is unique.*

- Avoid using "good" or "bad" to describe behavior. Be specific and descriptive (e.g., "You really helped me by holding still. Thank you for helping"; *Johnson, 1995).

R: *It is more helpful to be specific and descriptive when praising a child rather than describing behavior as "good" or "bad."*

- Connect previous experiences with the present one (e.g., "The X-ray camera will look different from the last time. You will have to hold real still again. The table will move, too"; *Johnson, 1995).

R: *The nurse can provide information that helps the child make sense of the situation by linking the present or future experience to past experience.*

- Convey optimism with positive self-talk (e.g., "I am so busy today. I wonder if I will get all my work done? I bet I can." or "When you come back from surgery you will need to stay in bed. What would you like to do when you come back?").

R: *Positive self-talk denotes optimism to the child.*

- Help the child plan playtime with choices. Encourage crafts that produce an end product.

R: *Allowing the child choices and productive play can enhance self-concept.*

- Encourage interactions with peers and supportive adults.
- Encourage child to decorate room with crafts and personal items.

R: *Skill building and positive social relationships increase a child's sense of value and worth.*

Disturbed Body Image

NANDA-I Definition

Confusion in mental picture of one's physical self

Defining Characteristics

Verbal or nonverbal negative response to actual or perceived change in structure and/or function (e.g., shame, embarrassment, guilt, revulsion)
Not looking at body part*
Not touching body part*
Intentional hiding or overexposing body part*
Change in social involvement*
Negative feelings about body; feelings of helplessness, hopelessness, powerlessness, vulnerability
Preoccupation with change or loss
Refusal to verify actual change
Depersonalization of part or loss
Self-destructive behaviors (e.g., mutilation, suicide attempts, overeating/undereating)

Related Factors

Pathophysiologic

Related to changes in appearance secondary to:

Chronic disease
Illness*
Aging
Severe trauma
Loss of body part or body function

Related to unrealistic perceptions of appearance secondary to:

Psychosis
Anorexia nervosa
Bulimia

Treatment Related

Related to changes in appearance secondary to:

Hospitalization
Surgery*
Chemotherapy
Radiation
Treatment regimen*

Situational (Personal, Environmental)

Related to physical trauma* secondary to:

Sexual abuse
Rape (perpetrator known or unknown)
Accidents
Assault

Related to effects of (specify) on appearance:
Obesity

Related to cognitive/perceptual factors*

Related to morbid fear of obesity (Varcarolis, 2011)

Maturational

Related to developmental changes*

Immobility
Pregnancy

Author's Note

See *Disturbed Self-Concept*.

Errors in Diagnostic Statements

See *Disturbed Self-Concept*.

Key Concepts

- An amputation results in several limitations in performing professional, leisure, and social activities. It reduces mobility, pain, and physical integrity, which disturbs the integrity of the human body and lowers the quality of life (QoL). Psychological issues range from depression, anxiety, and to suicide in severe cases (*Atherton & Robertson, 2006; Holzer et al., 2014). The loss of a body part also affects the perception of someone's own body and its appearance (Holzer et al., 2014).
- Holzer et al. (2014) reported that individuals "with lower-limb amputations have lower levels of body image perception and QoL. Self-esteem seems to be an independent aspect, which is not affected by lower-limb amputation. However, self-esteem is influenced significantly by phantom pain sensation."
- Refer also to *Disturbed Self-Concept*.

Goals

NOC

Body Image, Child Development: (Specify Age), Grief Resolution, Psychosocial Adjustment: Life Change, Self-Esteem

The person will implement new coping patterns and verbalize and demonstrate acceptance of appearance (grooming, dress, posture, eating patterns, presentation of self) as evidenced by the following indicators:

- Acknowledges his or her feelings regarding his or her loss
- Demonstrates a willingness and ability to resume self-care/role responsibilities
- Initiates new or reestablish contacts with existing support systems

Interventions

NIC

Self-Esteem Enhancement, Counseling, Presence, Active Listening, Body Image Enhancement, Grief Work Facilitation, Support Group, Referral

Establish a Trusting Nurse–Individual Relationship

- Encourage person to express feelings, especially about the way he or she feels, thinks, or views self.
- Acknowledge feelings of hostility, grief, fear, and dependency; teach strategies for coping with emotions.
- Explore belief system (e.g., does pain, suffering, loss mean punishment?).
- Encourage individual to ask questions about health problem, treatment, progress, and prognosis.
- Provide reliable information and reinforce information already given.
- Clarify any misconceptions about self, care, or caregivers.
- Avoid criticism.
- Provide privacy and a safe environment.
- Use therapeutic touch, with person's consent.
- Encourage individual to connect with spiritual beliefs and values regarding a higher power.

R: *Frequent contact by the caregiver indicates acceptance and may facilitate trust. The individual may be hesitant to approach the staff because of negative self-concept; the nurse must reach out.*

Promote Social Interaction

- Assist to accept help from others, when necessary.
- Avoid overprotection, but limit the demands made.
- Encourage movement.
- Prepare significant others for physical and emotional changes.
- Support family as they adapt.
- Encourage visits from peers and significant others.
- Encourage contact (letters, telephone) with peers and family.
- Encourage involvement in unit activities.
- Provide opportunity to share with people going through similar experiences.
- Discuss the importance of communicating the individual's value and importance to them with his or her support system.

R: *Social interactions can reaffirm that the person is acceptable and that previous support system is still intact. Isolation can increase feelings of guilt, fear, and embarrassment.*

Provide Specific Interventions in Selected Situations

Loss of Body Part or Function

- Assess the meaning of the loss for the individual and significant others, as related to visibility of loss, function of loss, and emotional investment.
- Explore and clarify misconceptions and myths regarding loss or ability to function with loss.
- Expect the person to respond to the loss with denial, shock, anger, and depression.
- Be aware of the effect of the responses of others to the loss; encourage sharing of feelings between significant others.
- Validate feelings by allowing the individual to express his or her feelings and to grieve.
- Explore realistic alternatives and provide encouragement.
- Explore strengths and resources with person.
- Assist with the resolution of a surgically created alteration of body image:
  - Replace the lost body part with prosthesis as soon as possible.
  - Encourage viewing of site.
  - Encourage touching of site.
  - Encourage activities that encompass new body image (e.g., shopping for new clothes).
- Teach about the health problem and how to manage.
- Begin to incorporate person in care of operative site.
- Gradually allow individual to assume full self-care responsibility, if feasible.

R: *Participation in self-care and planning promotes positive coping with the change.*

R: *Identifying personal attributes and strengths can help the person focus on the positive characteristics that contribute to the whole concept of self rather than only on the change in body image. The nurse should reinforce these positive aspects and encourage the individual to reincorporate them into the new self-concept.*

Changes Associated With Chemotherapy (*Camp-Sorrell, 2007)

- Discuss the possibility of hair loss, absence of menses, temporary or permanent sterility, decreased estrogen levels, vaginal dryness, and mucositis.
- Encourage to share concerns, fears, and perception of the effects of these changes on life.
- Explain where hair loss may occur (head, eyelashes, eyebrows; axillary, pubic, and leg hair).
- Explain that hair will grow back after treatment but may change in color and texture.
- Encourage to select and wear a wig before hair loss. Suggest consulting a beautician for tips on how to vary the look (e.g., combs, clips).
- Encourage the wearing of scarves or turbans when wig is not on.
- Teach to minimize the amount of hair loss by:
  - Cutting hair short
  - Avoiding excessive shampooing, using a conditioner twice weekly
  - Patting hair dry gently
  - Avoiding electric curlers, dryers, and curling irons
  - Avoiding pulling hair with bands, clips, or bobby pins
  - Avoiding hair spray and hair dye
  - Using wide-tooth comb, avoiding vigorous brushing
- Refer to American Cancer Society for information about new or used wigs.

R: *Open, honest discussions—expressing that changes will occur but that they are manageable—promote feelings of control. Participation in self-care and planning promotes positive coping with the change.*

- Discuss the difficulty that others (spouse, friends, coworkers) may have with visible changes.
- Encourage to initiate calls and contacts with others who may be having difficulty.
- Encourage to ask for assistance of friends, relatives. Ask person if the situation were reversed, what he or she would want to do to help a friend.
- Allow significant others opportunities to share their feelings and fears.
- Assist significant others to identify positive aspects of the individual and ways this can be shared.
- Provide information about support groups for couples.

R: *Increased social interaction through involvement in groups enables a person to receive social and intellectual stimulation, which enhances self-esteem.*

Anorexia Nervosa, Bulimia Nervosa

- Differentiate between body image distortion and body image dissatisfaction.
- Provide factual feedback on low weight and determents to health. Do not argue or challenge their distorted perceptions (Varcarolis, 2011).
- Know that the person's distorted image is their reality (Varcarolis, 2011).
- Assist to identify their positive traits (Varcarolis, 2011).
- Refer individuals for psychiatric counseling.

R: *Acknowledgment of their perceptions projects understanding and avoids power struggles (Varcarolis, 2011).*

Psychoses

- Refer to *Confusion* for specific information and interventions.

Sexual Abuse

- Refer to *Disabled Family Coping* for specific information and interventions.

Sexual Assault

- Refer to *Rape-Trauma Syndrome* for specific information and interventions.

Assault

- Refer to *Post-Trauma Response* for specific information and interventions.

Initiate Health Teaching, as Indicated

- Teach what community resources are available, if needed (e.g., mental health centers, self-help groups such as Reach for Recovery, Make Today Count).

R: *Professional counseling is indicated for an individual with poor ego strengths and inadequate coping resources.*

R: *Increased social interaction through involvement in groups enables a person to receive social and intellectual stimulation, which enhances self-esteem.*

- Teach wellness strategies.

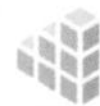

Pediatric Interventions

For Hospitalized Child

- Prepare child for hospitalization, if possible, with an explanation and a visit to the hospital to meet personnel and examine the environment.
- Provide familiarities/routines of home as much as possible (e.g., favorite toy or blanket, story at bedtime).
- Provide nurturance (e.g., hug).

R: *Attempts to retain the normality of the child's world can help to increase security (Hockenberry & Wilson, 2015).*

- Provide child with opportunities to share fears, concerns, and anger:
  - Provide play therapy.
  - Correct misconceptions (e.g., that the child is being punished; that parents are angry).
  - Encourage family to stay with or visit child, despite the child's crying when they leave; teach them to provide accurate information about when they will return to reduce fears of abandonment.
  - Allow parents to help with care.
  - Ask child to draw a picture of self, and then ask for a verbal description.

R: *Play therapy puts the child in control by providing opportunities to make choices (Hockenberry & Wilson, 2015).*

- Assist child to understand experiences:

- Provide an explanation ahead of time, if possible.
- Explain sensations and discomforts of condition, treatments, and medications.
- Encourage crying.

R: *Interventions that provide expressive outlets for tension and fear can help maintain the child's integrity (Hockenberry & Wilson, 2015).*

Discuss With Parents How Body Image Develops and What Interactions Contribute to Their Child's Self-Perception

- Teach the names and functions of body parts.
- Acknowledge changes (e.g., height).
- Allow some choices for what to wear.

R: *Opportunities for choices and success enhance self-esteem and coping.*

For Adolescents

- Discuss with parents the adolescent's need to "fit in":
  - Do not dismiss concerns too quickly.
  - Be flexible and compromise when possible (e.g., clothes are temporary, tattoos are not).
  - Negotiate a time period to think about options and alternatives (e.g., 4 to 5 weeks).
  - Provide with reasons for denying a request. Elicit adolescent's reasons. Compromise if possible (e.g., parents want curfew at 11:00 PM; adolescent wants 12:00 PM; compromise at 11:30 PM).
  - Provide opportunities to discuss concerns when parents are not present.
  - Prepare for impending developmental changes.

R: *Opportunities for open dialogue, choices, and success enhance self-esteem and coping.*

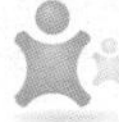

Maternal Interventions

- Encourage the woman to share her concerns.
- Attend to each concern, if possible, or refer her to others for assistance.
- Discuss the challenges and changes that pregnancy and motherhood bring.
- Encourage her to share expectations: her own and those of her significant others.
- Assist her to identify sources for love and affection.

R: *Open, honest discussions—expressing that changes will occur but that they are manageable—promote feelings of control.*

- Provide anticipatory guidance to both parents-to-be concerning. (Pillitteri, 2014)
  - Fatigue and irritability
  - Appetite swings
  - Gastric disturbances (nausea, constipation)
  - Back and leg aches
  - Changes in sexual desire and activity (e.g., sexual positions as pregnancy advances)
  - Mood swings
  - Fear (for self, for unborn baby, of loss of attractiveness, of inadequacy as a parent)
  - Encourage sharing of concerns between spouses

R: *Support can be given more freely and more realistically if others are prepared.*

Disturbed Personal Identity

NANDA-I Definition

Inability to maintain an integrated and complete perception of self

Defining Characteristics (Varcarolis, 2011)

Appears unaware of or uninterested in others or their activities
Unable to identify parts of the body or body sensations (e.g., enuresis)

Excessively imitates other's activities or words
Fails to distinguish parent/caregiver as a whole person
Becomes distressed with bodily contact with others
Spends long periods of time in self-stimulating behaviors (self-touching, sucking, rocking)
Needs ritualistic behaviors and sameness to control anxiety
Cannot tolerate being separated from parent/caregiver

Related Factors (Varcarolis, 2011)

Pathophysiologic

Related to biochemical imbalance

Related to impaired neurologic development or dysfunction

Maturational

Related to failure to develop attachment behaviors resulting in fixation at autistic phase of development

Related to interrupted or uncompleted separation/individualization process resulting in extreme separation anxiety

Author's Note

Disturbed Personal Identity in the nursing literature is utilized to label autism or schizophrenia. It does not direct nursing interventions. It is more clinically useful to identify how a disorder affects Functional Health Patterns. From this data nursing diagnoses that can direct nursing intervention can be confirmed as *Impaired Social Interactions, Risk for Violence to others, Self-Care Deficits,* or *Risk for Disabled Family Coping.*

Risk for Disturbed Personal Identity

NANDA-I Definition

Risk for the inability to maintain an integrated and complete perception of self

Risk Factors*

Chronic low self-esteem
Psychiatric disorders (e.g., psychoses, depression, dissociative disorder)
Cult indoctrination
Situational crises
Situational low self-esteem
Cultural discontinuity
Social role change
Discrimination
Stages of development
Dysfunctional family processes
Stages of growth
Ingestion/inhalation of toxic chemicals
Use of psychoactive pharmaceutical agents
Manic states
Multiple personality disorder
Organic brain syndromes
Perceived prejudice

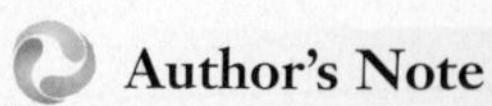

Author's Note

Refer to *Disturbed Personal Identity*.

Disturbed Self-Esteem[46]

Definition

State in which a person experiences or is at risk of experiencing negative self-evaluation about self or capabilities

Defining Characteristics (*Leuner, Coler, & Noris, 1994; *Norris & Kunes-Connell, 1987)

Major (Must Be Present, One or More)

Observed or Reported
Self-negating verbalization
Expressions of shame or guilt
Evaluates self as unable to deal with events
Rationalizes away or rejects positive feedback and exaggerates negative feedback about self
Lack of or poor problem-solving ability
Hesitant to try new things or situations
Rationalizes personal failures
Hypersensitivity to slight criticism

Minor (May Be Present)

Lack of assertion
Overly conforming
Indecisiveness
Passive
Seeks approval or reassurance excessively
Lack of culturally appropriate body presentation (posture, eye contact, movements)
Denial of problems obvious to others
Projection of blame or responsibility for problems

Related Factors

Disturbed Self-Esteem can be either episodic or chronic. Failure to resolve a problem or multiple sequential stresses can result in chronic low self-esteem (CLSE). Those factors that occur over time and are associated with CLSE are indicated by "CLSE" in parentheses.

Pathophysiologic

Related to change in appearance secondary to:

Loss of body parts
Loss of body functions
Disfigurement (trauma, surgery, birth defects)

Related to biochemical/neurophysiologic imbalance

Situational (Personal, Environmental)

Related to unmet dependency needs

Related to feelings of abandonment secondary to:

Death of significant other
Separation from significant other
Child abduction/murder

Related to feelings of failure secondary to:

Loss of job or ability to work
Financial problems
Increase/decrease in weight
Premenstrual syndrome
Unemployment
Relationship problems

[46]This diagnosis is not presently on the NANDA-I list, but has been added for clarity and usefulness.

Marital discord
In-laws
Separation
Stepparents

Related to assault (personal, or relating to the event of another's assault—e.g., same age, same community)

Related to failure in school

Related to history of ineffective relationship with parents (CLSE)

Related to history of abusive relationships (CLSE)

Related to unrealistic expectations of child by parent (CLSE)

Related to unrealistic expectations of self (CLSE)

Related to unrealistic expectations of parent by child (CLSE)

Related to parental rejection (CLSE)

Related to inconsistent punishment (CLSE)

Related to feelings of helplessness and/or failure secondary to institutionalization:

Mental health facility
Orphanage
Jail
Halfway house

Related to history of numerous failures (CLSE)

Maturational

Infant/Toddler/Preschool

Related to lack of stimulation or closeness (CLSE)

Related to separation from parents/significant others (CLSE)

Related to continual negative evaluation by parents

Related to inability to trust significant others (CLSE)

School-Aged

Related to failure to achieve grade-level objectives

Related to loss of peer group

Related to repeated negative feedback

Related to loss of independence and autonomy secondary to (specify)

Related to disruption of peer relationships

Related to scholastic problems

Related to loss of significant others

Middle-Aged

Related to changes associated with aging

Older Adult

Related to losses (people, function, financial, retirement)

Author's Note

See *Disturbed Self-Concept*.

Errors in Diagnostic Statements

See *Disturbed Self-Concept*.

Key Concepts

See *Disturbed Self-Concept*.

Focus Assessment Criteria

See *Disturbed Self-Concept*.

Interventions

Refer to *Disturbed Self-Concept*.

Chronic Low Self-Esteem

NANDA-I Definition

Long-standing negative self-evaluating/feelings about self or self-capabilities

Defining Characteristics (*Leuner et al., 1994; Norris & *Kunes-Connell, 1987)

Major (80% to 100%)

Long-Standing or Chronic
Self-negating verbalization
Reports feelings of shame/guilt*
Evaluates self as unable to deal with events*
Rationalizes away/rejects positive feedback and exaggerates negative feedback about self*
Hesitant to try new things/situations*
Exaggerating negative feedback about self*

Minor (50% to 79%)

Frequent lack of success in work or other life events*
Overly conforming, dependent on others' opinions*
Lack of culturally appropriate body presentation (eye contact, posture, movements)
Nonassertive/passive*
Indecisive
Excessively seeks reassurance*

Related Factors

See *Disturbed Self-Esteem*.

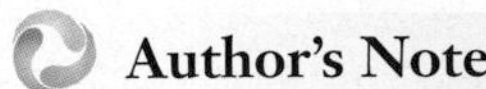

Author's Note

See *Disturbed Self-Concept*.

Errors in Diagnostic Statements

See *Disturbed Self-Concept*.

Goals

NOC
Depression Level, Depression Self-Control, Anxiety Level, Quality of Life, Self-Esteem

The individual will identify positive aspects of self and a realistic appraisal of limitations as evidenced by the following indicators (Halter, 2014; Varcarolis, 2011):

- Identifies two strengths
- Identifies two unrealistic expectations and modify more realistic life goals
- Verbalizes acceptance of limitations
- Ceases self-abusive descriptions of self (e.g., I am stupid)

Interventions

NIC
Hope Instillation, Anxiety Reduction, Self-Esteem Enhancement, Coping Enhancement, Socialization Enhancement, Referral

Assist the Person to Reduce Present Anxiety Level

- Be supportive, nonjudgmental.
- Accept silence, but let him or her know you are there.
- Orient as necessary.
- Clarify distortions; do not use confrontation.
- Be aware of your own anxiety and avoid communicating it to the person.
- Refer to *Anxiety* for further interventions.

R: *People with low self-esteem are usually anxious, fearful people. Anxiety levels must be mild or moderate before other interventions can be effective (Halter, 2014).*

Enhance the Person's Sense of Self

- Be attentive.
- Respect personal space.
- Validate your interpretation of what he or she is saying or experiencing ("Is this what you mean?").
- Help him or her to verbalize what he or she is expressing nonverbally.
- Assist individual to reframe and redefine negative expressions (e.g., not "failure," but "setback").
- Use communication that helps to maintain his or her individuality ("I" instead of "we").
- Pay attention to person, especially new behavior.
- Encourage good physical habits (healthy food and eating patterns, exercise, proper sleep).
- Provide encouragement as he or she attempts a task or skill.
- Provide realistic positive feedback on accomplishments.
- Teach person to validate consensually with others.
- Teach and encourage esteem-building exercises (self-affirmations, imagery, mirror work, use of humor, meditation/prayer, relaxation).

R: *Strategies focus on helping the person reexamine negative feelings about self and identifying positive attributes.*

R: *Persons with low self-esteem have difficulty asking appropriately for what they need or want (Varcarolis, 2011).*

Promote Use of Coping Resources

- Identify the individual's areas of personal strength:
  - Sports, hobbies, crafts
  - Health, self-care
  - Work, training, education
  - Imagination, creativity
  - Writing skills, math
  - Interpersonal relationships
- Share your observations with the individual.
- Provide opportunities for individual to engage in the activities.

R: *Individual collaboration is necessary for him or her to assume ultimate responsibility for behavior.*

Assist to Identify Cognitive Distortions That Increase Negative Self-Appraisal (Halter, 2014)

- *Overgeneralization*: Teach to focus on each event as separate.
- *Self-Blame*: Teach to evaluate if she or he is really responsible and why.
- *Mind-Reading*: Advise to clarify verbally what he or she thinks is happening.
- *Discounting positive responses of others*: Teach to respond with only "thank you."

R: *These cognitive distortions reinforce negative inaccurate perception of self and the world (Halter, 2014).*

Provide Opportunities for Positive Socialization

- Encourage visits/contact with peers and significant others (letters, telephone).
- Be a role model in one-to-one interactions.

R: *Role modeling positive socialization can decrease feelings of isolation and can encourage a more realistic appraisal of self (Varcarolis, 2011).*

- Involve in activities, especially when strengths can be used.
- Do not allow person to isolate self (refer to *Social Isolation* for further interventions).

- Involve the individual in supportive group therapy.
- Teach social skills as required (refer to *Impaired Social Interaction* for further interventions).
- Encourage participation with others sharing similar experiences.

R: *Opportunities for the person to be successful increases self-esteem (Varacolis, 2011).*

Set Limits on Problematic Behavior Such as Aggression, Poor Hygiene, Ruminations, and Suicidal Preoccupation

- Refer to *Risk for Suicide* and/or *Risk for Violence* if these are assessed as problems.

Provide for Development of Social and Vocational Skills

- Refer for vocational counseling.
- Involve the individual in volunteer organizations.
- Encourage participation in activities with others of same age.
- Arrange for continuation of education (e.g., literacy class, vocational training, art/music classes).

R: *Opportunities for success can increase self-esteem.*

Risk for Chronic Low Self-Esteem

NANDA-I Definition

At risk for long-standing negative self-evaluating/feelings about self or self-capabilities

Risk Factors*

Ineffective adaptation to loss
Lack of affection
Lack of membership in group
Perceived discrepancy between self and cultural norms
Perceived discrepancy between self and spiritual norms
Perceived lack of belonging
Perceived lack of respect from others
Psychiatric disorder
Repeated failures
Repeated negative reinforcement
Traumatic event
Traumatic situation

Goals

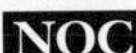
NOC
Depression Level, Depression Self-Control, Anxiety Level, Quality of Life, Self-Esteem

The person will identify positive aspects of self and a realistic appraisal of limitations as evidenced by the following indicators (Varcarolis, 2011):

- Identifies two strengths
- Identifies two unrealistic expectations and modify more realistic life goals
- Verbalizes acceptance of limitations
- Ceases self-abusive descriptions of self (e.g., I am stupid, etc.)

Interventions

NIC
Hope Instillation, Anxiety Reduction, Self-Esteem Enhancement, Coping Enhancement, Socialization Enhancement, Referral

Refer to *Disturbed Self-Concept* for intervention to promote positive self-worth.

Situational Low Self-Esteem

NANDA-I Definition

Development of a negative perception of self-worth in response to a current situation

Defining Characteristics (*Leuner et al., 1994; *Norris & Kunes-Connell, 1987)

Major (80% to 100%)

Episodic occurrence of negative self-appraisal in response to life events in a person with a previously positive self-evaluation
Verbally reports current situational challenge to self-worth*
Verbalization of negative feelings about self (helplessness, uselessness)*

Minor (50% to 79%)

Self-negating verbalizations*
Expressions of shame/guilt
Evaluates self as unable to handle situations/events*
Difficulty making decisions

Related Factors

See *Disturbed Self-Esteem*.

Author's Note

See *Disturbed Self-Esteem*.

Errors in Diagnostic Statements

See *Disturbed Self-Esteem*.

Key Concepts

- Mulla describes the characteristics of a healthy personality including (Mulla, 2010) the following:
  - Realistic self-appraisals (The gap between the real and the ideal self-concept is very much smaller among the well-adjusted.)
  - Realistic appraisal of situations (approaches situations with a realistic attitude accepting the bad with the good)
  - Realistic evaluation of achievements (A well-adjusted person is able to evaluate his achievements realistically and to react to them in a rational way without feeling superiority over others)
  - Acceptance of reality (learns to accept his limitations, either physical or psychological, if he cannot change them)
  - Acceptance of responsibility (When wrong, accepts the blame and is willing to admit that he made a mistake)
  - Autonomy (In decision-making, he is able to make important decisions with a minimum of worry, conflict, advice seeking and other types of running away behavior)
  - Acceptable emotional control (has developed, over a period, a degree of stress tolerance, anxiety tolerance, depression tolerance, and pain tolerance)
  - Goal orientation (The well-adjusted person set realistic goals and well-adjusted make it their business to acquire the knowledge and skills needed to reach their goals.)
  - Outer orientation (He is willing to respond in any way he can to the needs of others and does not regard it as an imposition)
  - Social acceptance (He can be natural, at ease and friendly in his relationships with others and all this increases his social acceptance)

- Philosophy-of-life-directed (As well-adjusted people are goal-oriented, so do they direct their lives by a philosophy which helps them to formulate plans to meet their goals in a socially approved way)
- Happiness (In a well-adjusted person happiness outway unhappiness and the person is an essentially happy person.)
- People with healthy personalities can experience a change in their positive self-perception in response to a profound event or a series of negative experiences.
- Responses to a situation that challenges a person's previously positive view of self are feelings of being weak, helpless, or hopeless; fear; vulnerability; and feelings of being fragile, incomplete, worthless, and inadequate (*Stuart & Sundeen, 2008).

Goals

NOC

Decision-Making, Grief Resolution, Psychosocial Adjustment: Life Change, Self-Esteem

The individual will express a positive outlook for the future and resume previous level of functioning as evidenced by the following indicators:

- Identifies source of threat to self-esteem and work through that issue
- Identifies positive aspects of self
- Analyzes his or her own behavior and its consequences
- Identifies one positive aspect of change

Interventions

NIC

Active Listening, Presence, Counseling, Cognitive Restructuring, Family Support, Support Group, Coping Enhancement

Carp's Cues

Under Key Concepts are Dr. Mulla's characteristics of healthy personalities. Nurses can use foster and reinforce these positive attributes. For example, when person is unsuccessful, explore with the person if they should have accept the responsibility. Were they prepared? Were they overcommitted? This focus may reduce the person questioning their fundamental competencies.

Assist the Individual to Identify and to Express Feelings

- Be empathic, nonjudgmental.
- Listen. Do not discourage expressions of anger, crying, and so forth.
- Ask what was happening when he or she began feeling this way.
- Clarify relationships between life events.

R: *Self-acceptance can be increased with clarification of feelings and thoughts.*

Assist the Individual to Identify Positive Self-Evaluations

- Are there individuals who trigger negative feelings? Do they think they can change the behaviors of others?
- Limit exposure to "Toxic" people.

R: *Attempt to clarify that one does not change the behavior of others, but one can change their own response.*

- How does he or she manage anxiety—through exercise, withdrawal, drinking/drugs, talking?
- Reinforce adaptive coping mechanisms.
- Examine and reinforce positive abilities and traits (e.g., hobbies, skills, school, relationships, appearance, loyalty, industriousness).
- Listen carefully to their reasons for the negative feeling about themselves. Are they realistic? How could he or she respond differently to reduce negative feelings?
- Do not confront defenses.
- Communicate confidence in the individual's ability.
- Involve in mutual goal setting.
- Have the person write positive true statements about self (for his or her eyes only); have him or her read the list daily as a part of normal routine.
- Reinforce use of esteem-building exercises (self-affirmations, imagery, meditation/prayer, relaxation, use of humor).

Assist to Identify Cognitive Distortions That Increase Negative Self-Appraisal (Varcarolis, 2011)

- Overgeneralization.
- Teach to focus on each event as separate.

- Self-blame.
- Teach to evaluate if he or she is really responsible and why.
- Mind-reading.
- Advise to clarify verbally what he or she thinks is happening.
- Discounting positive responses of others.
- Teach to respond with only "Thank you."

R: *These cognitive distortions reinforce negative, inaccurate perception of self and the world (Varcarlois, 2011).*

Assess and Mobilize Current Support System

- Does he or she live alone? Is he or she employed?
- Does he or she have available friends and relatives?
- Is religion a support?
- Has he or she previously used community resources?
- Refer individual to vocational rehabilitation for retraining.
- Support returning to school for further training.
- Assist individual to involve local volunteer organizations (senior citizens employment, foster grandparents, local support groups).
- Arrange continuation of school studies for students.

R: *Social support increases resourcefulness, self-esteem, and well-being (Halter, 2014)*

Assist to Learn New Coping Skills

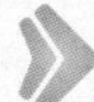

Carp's Cues

For a practical, short guideline to positive self-talk refer to Martin, B. (2013). Challenging negative self-talk. *Psych Central*. Retrieved on August 26, 2015, from http://psychcentral.com/lib/challenging-negative-self-talk

- Practice positive self-talk (Martin, 2013; *Murray, 2000):
  - Avoid jumping to negative conclusions? (Martin, 2013).
  - Write a brief description of the change and its consequence (e.g., My work evaluation was poor evaluation was terrible.).
  - Review each negative comment. Is it true? If yes how can you improve this.
  - If not true, tell yourself why it is not true. Is it partially true?
  - Are there any other ways that I could look at this situation? (Martin, 2013)
- Challenge to imagine positive futures and outcomes.
- Encourage a trial of new behavior.
- Reinforce the belief that the individual does have control over the situation.
- Obtain a commitment to action.

R: *Self-talk does not imply that one likes the situation, however, it helps one find potential benefits of the situation (*Murray, 2000).*

- Stop destructive self-talk as soon as it starts.

R: *Destructive self-talk is full of self-criticism. The thinking patterns of individuals with clinical depression find that their self-talk tends toward frequently and relentless form of destructive self-talk.*

Assist to Manage Specific Problems

- Rape—Refer to *Rape-Trauma Syndrome.*
- Loss—Refer to *Grieving.*
- Hospitalization—Refer to *Powerlessness and Parental Role Conflict.*
- Ill family member—Refer to *Interrupted Family Processes.*
- Change or loss of body part—Refer to *Disturbed Body Image.*
- Depression—Refer to *Ineffective Coping and Hopelessness.*
- Domestic violence—Refer to *Disabled Family Coping.*

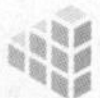

Pediatric Interventions

- Provide opportunities for child to be successful and needed.
- Personalize the child's environment with pictures, possessions, and crafts he or she made.
- Provide structured and unstructured playtime.

- Ensure continuation of academic experiences in the hospital and home. Provide uninterrupted time for schoolwork.

R: *See Disturbed Self-Concept.*

Risk for Situational Low Self-Esteem

NANDA-I Definition

At risk for developing a negative perception of self-worth in response to a current situation

Risk Factors

See *Situational Low Self-Esteem.*

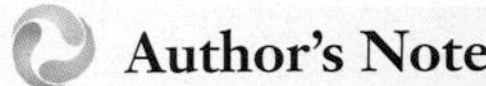

Author's Note

See *Situational Low Self-Esteem.*

Errors in Diagnostic Statements

See *Situational Low Self-Esteem.*

Key Concepts

See *Situational Low Self-Esteem.*

Goals

NOC

Refer to Situational Low Self-Esteem

The individual will continue to express a positive outlook for the future to identify positive aspects of self as evidenced by the following indicators:

- Identifies threats to self-esteem
- Identifies one positive aspect of change

Interventions

See *Situational Low Self-Esteem.*

RISK FOR SELF-HARM[47]

Risk for Self-Harm

Self-Mutilation
Risk for Self-Mutilation
Risk for Suicide

Definition

State in which a individual is at risk for inflicting direct harm on himself or herself. This may include one or more of the following: self-abuse, self-mutilation, suicide.

[47]This diagnosis is not presently on the NANDA-I list but has been added for clarity and usefulness.

Defining Characteristics

Expresses desire or intent to harm self
Expresses desire to die or commit suicide
Past history of attempts to harm self

Reported or Observed

Depression	Hopelessness	Poor self-concept
Helplessness	Hallucinations/delusions	Lack of support system
Substance abuse	Emotional pain	Poor impulse control
Hostility	Agitation	

Related Factors

Risk for Self-Harm can occur as a response to a variety of health problems, situations, and conflicts. Some sources are listed next.

Pathophysiologic

Related to feelings of helplessness, loneliness, or hopelessness secondary to:

Disabilities
Terminal illness
Chronic illness
Chronic pain
Chemical dependency
Substance abuse
New diagnosis of positive HIV status
Mental impairment (organic or traumatic)
Psychiatric disorder
- Schizophrenia
- Personality disorder
- Bipolar disorder
- Adolescent adjustment disorder
- Posttrauma syndrome
- Somatoform disorders

Treatment Related

Related to unsatisfactory outcome of treatment (medical, surgical, psychological)

Related to prolonged dependence on:

Dialysis	Insulin injections
Chemotherapy/radiation	Ventilator

Situational (Personal, Environmental)

Related to:

Incarceration	Ineffective coping skills	Substance abuse in family
Depression	Parental/marital conflict	Child abuse

Real or perceived loss secondary to:

Finances/job	Separation/divorce	Status/prestige	Natural disaster
Death of significant others	Threat of abandonment	Someone leaving home	

Related to wish for revenge on real or perceived injury (body or self-esteem)

Maturational

Related to indifference to pain secondary to autism

Adolescent

Related to feelings of abandonment

Related to peer pressure

Related to unrealistic expectations of child by parents

Related to depression

Related to relocation

Related to significant loss

Older Adult

Related to multiple losses secondary to:

Retirement
Social isolation
Significant loss
Illness

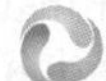

Author's Note

Risk for Self-Harm (added by this author) represents a broad diagnosis that can encompass self-abuse, self-mutilation, and/or risk for suicide. Although initially they may appear the same, the distinction lies in the intent. Self-mutilation and self-abuse are pathologic attempts to relieve stress temporarily, whereas suicide is an attempt to die to relieve stress permanently (J. S. Carscadden, Personal Communication, 1998).

Risk for Self-Harm also can be a useful early diagnosis when insufficient data are present to differentiate one from the other. In some clinical situations, the person may have delirium or dementia. This person is at risk of harming themselves (e.g., pulling out a Foley catheter or IV). *Risk for Injury* would be clinically useful.

Risk for Suicide has been in this author's work for more than 20 years. *Risk for Suicide* was added to the NANDA-I list in 2006. Previously, *Risk for Violence to Self* was included under *Risk for Violence.* The term violence is defined as a swift and intense force or a rough or injurious physical force. As the reader knows, suicide can be either violent or nonviolent (e.g., overdose of barbiturates). Using the term violence in this diagnostic context, unfortunately, can lead to nondetection of an individual at risk for suicide because of the perception that the person is not capable of violence.

Risk for Suicide clearly denotes an individual at high risk for suicide and in need of protection. Treatment of this diagnosis involves validating the risk, contracting with the person, and providing protection. Treatment of the underlying depression and hopelessness should be addressed with other applicable nursing diagnoses (e.g., *Ineffective Coping, Hopelessness*).

Errors in Diagnostic Statements

Risk for Suicide related to recent diagnosis of cancer

In this situation, the recent diagnosis of cancer in itself is not a risk factor for suicide. The individual may be depressed, severely stressed, and/or exhibiting suicidal intentions. All *Risk for Self-Harm* diagnostic statements should contain both verbal and nonverbal cues to suicidal intent (e.g., *Risk for Suicide* related to remarks about life being unbearable and reports of giving belongings away).

Key Concepts

General Considerations

- In 2013, the most recent year for which data is available, 494,169 people visited a hospital for injuries due to self-harm behavior, suggesting that approximately 12 people harm themselves (not necessarily intending to take their lives) for every reported death by suicide.
- Violence, whether directed toward oneself or others, can elicit strong reactions from people. Nurses, whose profession encompasses caregiving, health promotion, and nurturance, must examine their own attitudes, responses, and behavior toward violence.
- Because much of the practice of self-mutilation is a "shame-based" problem, the condition is more likely to be underreported rather than overreported. Identification is difficult, because so many who engage in self-harm become extremely adept at hiding the causes of their injuries.

- Self-harm is found in people from all economic and educational backgrounds, and in both men and women. It usually appears in the early teenage years, although it may commence before adolescence. It frequently is associated with long-term effects of physical, psychological, and sexual abuse during childhood.
- Many people who harm themselves are given a psychiatric diagnosis of personality disorder or, more specifically, borderline personality disorder, although other psychiatric diagnoses may be associated with self-harm (see the Pathophysiologic section). An important consideration is that not all people with these diagnoses harm themselves, and not all self-injurers qualify for these diagnoses. Treatment will differ depending on the diagnosis (*Carscadden, 1997).
- Self-mutilation may also be prevalent with mentally challenged people, and management in this particular population will differ again, owing to the cognition level of the self-injurer.
- Often repetitive and chronic in nature, self-harm frequently distorts or disrupts the individual–therapist relationship and increases the need for a length of hospitalizations. These hospitalizations often exacerbate the problem further. Hospitalization usually increases the individual's dependency and decreases his or her accountability.

Self-Mutilation

- There are various levels or stages in impending self-harm. The transition from one level to another may be rapid or slowly progressive. The individual may or may not be aware of the stages and the transition. Awareness of each stage and its characteristics facilitates intervention. The earlier the stage, the clearer the thinking, the less intense the feelings, and the more control the individual has. An individual can easily identify stages once he or she learns the defining characteristics (*Carscadden, 1993a).
- Although self-harm may create a sense of urgency, imminent disaster, and a strong and immediate sense of responsibility in the listener or observer, one must be careful not to be caught up in this and feel compelled to do something. (This excludes the psychotic and mentally challenged population.) The very act of trying to intervene or prevent the behaviors may increase the likelihood of more serious harm, including completed suicide. The risk increases because of the following:
  - The more often intervention takes place, the more likely death by mistake will occur (wrong pills, too many, the expected rescue being thwarted)
  - There may be a need to use increasingly dangerous methods to get the same result
  - Before long, countertransference hate sets in. In an empathic, yet matter-of-fact manner, the nurse must convey that the individual's actions are in his or her hands alone and that no one can be his or her guardian or savior.

    This is the hardest thing for anyone to say; however, for the self-injurer to survive and mature, he or she must become responsible for his or her own actions. If someone else takes control, the self-injurer will not progress (Carscadden, 1998).
- Families are often the forgotten sufferers in the self-harm syndrome. They are caught in the same shame-based system as the self-injurer, and this often precludes their reaching out for help with the bewilderment, frustration, and helplessness experienced in day-to-day living with the self-injurer. They need assistance in demystifying self-harm, identifying how it has affected them, and examining some coping methods for supporting themselves and the self-injurer on the road to recovery. Educational and support groups as well as family counseling are good ways to begin this process (*Carscadden, 1997).

Focus Assessment Criteria

The nurse must be able to differentiate between the diagnoses of *Risk for Suicide* and *Risk for Self-Mutilation* or *Self-Abuse*. Although initially they may appear (in action) or sound (in statements) the same, the distinction lies in the intent. Self-mutilation and self-abuse are pathologic attempts to relieve stress (temporary reprieve), whereas suicide is an attempt to die (to relieve stress permanently). The nurse will be able in the assessment to gather data that enable him or her to distinguish which diagnosis is appropriate for the individual. It is prudent to remember that some individuals may become so self-harmful that they eventually die, even though they are not intentionally suicidal.

Subjective Data

Assess for Risk Factors

Psychological Status
Present concerns:

Have you experienced a severe stressor recently?
How are you feeling?
Do you want to hurt yourself?
Can you tell me the reason?

Assess for risks of suicide:

Age: Is the individual 19 years or younger or 45 years old or older (especially older than age 65)?
Gender: Is the individual a man?
Emotional state: Is the individual depressed? Does the individual abuse alcohol? Chemical dependency/substance abuse?
Social supports: Does the individual have significant relatives, friends, meaningful employment, and spiritual or religious supports?
Previous attempt: Has the individual attempted suicide before?
Method: Is there a specific plan (e.g., pills, wrist slashing, shooting)? Plans for rescue?
Availability: Is the method accessible? Is access easy or difficult?
Specificity: How specific is the plan?
Lethality: How lethal is the method?

History of psychiatric problems

Acute or chronic illness—how is it affecting life?

Prescribed drugs:

Assessment of the awareness of self-harm activities
Acknowledgment or denial

Self-Harm/Mutilation

Can the person identify specifics in the process?

Personal triggers
Situations
Particular types of people or places
Flashbacks or nightmares

Does the individual disassociate or "numb out?"

Support System

Who is relied on during periods of stress?
Are they available?

Objective Data

Behavior During Interview

Agitated
Restless
Withdrawn
Hostile
Cooperative
Disassociated

Communication Pattern

Hopeless/helpless (subjective)
Denial
Allusive
Suicidal expressions

Evidence of Self-Harm

Be highly suspicious if

There have been repeated accidents
Wears long sleeves in hot weather
Is reluctant to uncover parts of body

Look for

Scars
Lumps/bumps
Open cuts
Reddened, irritated areas
Sores
Burn marks
Areas that do not heal as expected
Clumps/patches of missing hair
Noncompliance with treatment for serious physical or medical conditions (e.g., diabetes)

Goals

NOC
Aggression Self-Control, Impulse Self-Control

The individual will choose alternatives that are not harmful as evidenced by the following indicators:

- Acknowledges self-harm thoughts
- Admits to use of self-harm behavior if it occurs
- Be able to identify personal triggers
- Learns to identify and tolerate uncomfortable feelings

Interventions

NIC
Presence, Anger Control, Environmental Management: Violence Prevention, Behavior Modification, Security Enhancement, Therapy Group, Coping Enhancement, Impulse Control Training, Crisis Intervention

Establish a Trusting Nurse–Individual Relationship

- Demonstrate acceptance of the person as a worthwhile person through nonjudgmental statements and behavior.
- Ask questions in a caring, concerned manner.
- Encourage expression of thoughts and feelings.
- Actively listen or provide support by just being there if the individual is silent.
- Be aware of the supersensitivity.
- Label the behavior, not the individual.
- Be honest in your interactions.
- Assist the individual in recognizing hope and alternatives.
- Provide reasons for necessary procedures or interventions.
- Maintain the individual's dignity throughout your therapeutic relationship.

R: *Frequent contact by the caregiver indicates acceptance and may facilitate trust. The individual may be hesitant to approach the staff because of negative self-concept; the nurse must reach out.*

Help Reframe Old Thinking/Feeling Patterns (*Carscadden, 1993a)

- Encourage the belief that change is possible.
- Help to assess payoffs and drawbacks to self-harm.
- Rename words that have a negative connotation (e.g., "setback," not "failure").
- Encourage identification of personal triggers.
- Assist in exploring viable alternatives.
- Encourage the individual to become comfortable with and to use sad or negative feelings.

R: *Expressing feelings and perception increases self-awareness and helps the nurse plan effective interventions to address his or her needs. Validating perceptions provides reassurance and can decrease anxiety.*

Facilitate the Development of New Behavior

- Validate good coping skills already in existence.
- Encourage journaling: keeping a diary of triggers, thoughts, feelings, and alternatives that work or do not work.
- Assist to develop body awareness as a method of ascertaining triggers and determining levels of impending self-harm.

R: *Expressing feelings and perception increases the individual's self-awareness and helps the nurse plan effective interventions to address his or her needs. Validating the individual's perceptions provides reassurance and can decrease anxiety.*

- Follow policies/procedures to prevent and/or intervene in self-harm attempts.

R: *It is important not to reward the act of self-harm with reinforcements (negative or positive). Treatment of the injury should be done matter-of-factly, much like removing a splinter, but also respond to the person with dignity. Returning to activities/schedules as quickly as possible restores responsibility to the person.*

Reduce Excessive Stimuli

- Provide a quiet, serene atmosphere.
- Establish firm, consistent limits while giving the individual as much control/choice as possible within those boundaries.
- Intervene at the earliest stages to assist the individual in regaining control, prevent escalation, and allow treatment in the least restrictive manner.
- Keep communication simple. Agitated people cannot process complicated communication.

- Provide an area where the individual can retreat to decrease stimuli (e.g., time-out room, quiet room; individuals on hallucinogens need a darkened, quiet room with a nonintrusive observer).
- Remove potentially dangerous objects from the environment (if the individual is in crisis stage).

R: *A quiet environment reduces reactivity, enhances calm feelings, and decreases the likelihood of confusion and fear.*

Promote the Use of Alternatives

- Stress that there are always alternatives.
- Stress that self-harm is a choice, not something uncontrollable. Tell me about a time you resisted the urge to hurt yourself?
- Relieve pent-up tension and purposeless hyperactivity with physical activity (e.g., brisk walk, dance therapy, aerobics).
- Provide acceptable physical outlets (e.g., yelling, pounding pillow, tearing up newspapers, using clay or Play-Doh, taking a brisk walk).
- Provide for less physical alternatives (e.g., relaxation tapes, soft music, warm bath, diversional activities).

R: *Self-destructive behavior can be the result of anger or sadness turned inward.*

Determine Present Level of Impending Self-Harm, If Indicated

Beginning Stage (Thought Stage)

- Remind that this is an "old tape" and to replace it with new thinking and belief patterns.
- Provide nonintrusive, calming alternatives.

Climbing Stage (Feeling Stage)

- Remind to consider alternatives.
- Give as much control to the person as possible to support his or her accountability.
- Are you in control? How can I help? Would you like me to assist?
- Provide more intense interventions at this stage.

Crisis Stage (Behavior Stage)

- Give positive feedback if the individual chooses an alternative and does not harm himself or herself.
- Ask to put down any object of harm if he or she possesses one.
- Continue to emphasize there are always alternatives.
- As soon as possible to give responsibility back to him or her. "Are you in control now?" "Are you feeling safe?"
- Attend to practical issues in a nonpunitive, nonjudgmental manner.

R: *Control of environment is a basic, but not to be discounted, intervention. A structured schedule provides boundaries and security, enhancing the sense of safety. A quiet environment reduces reactivity, enhances calm feelings, and decreases the likelihood of confusion and fear. Gross motor activity in a protected environment can lessen aggressive drives, whereas rest periods promote opportunities for relaxation, calm the emergency response, and reconnect body/mind/heart.*

Post-crisis Stage

- Give positive reinforcements if the person did not harm himself or herself.
- Assist in problem solving on how to divert himself before the crisis stage.
- Assess the degree of injury/harm if the person did not choose the alternative.
- Pay as little attention as possible to the act of self-harm and focus on prior stages (e.g., "Can you remember what triggered you?" "What kinds of things were going through your mind?" "What do you think you might have done instead?").
- Return the person to normal activities/routine as soon as possible.

R: *Maladaptive behaviors can be replaced with healthy ones to manage stress and anxiety* (Halter, 2014)

Initiate Support Systems to Community, When/Where Indicated

Teach Family

- Constructive expression of feelings.
- How to recognize levels of impending self-harm.
- How to assist with appropriate interventions.
- How to deal with self-harm behavior/results.

Supply Phone Number of 24-hour Emergency Hotlines

Provide Referral to

- Individual therapist

- Family counseling
- Peer support group
- Leisure/vocational counseling
- Halfway houses
- Other community resources

R: *Many mental health conditions are chronic and require ongoing access to resources for family and individual.*

Self-Mutilation

NANDA-I Definition

Deliberate self-injurious behavior causing tissue damage with the intent of causing nonfatal injury to attain relief of tension

Defining Characteristics*

Expresses desire or intent to harm self[48]
Past history of attempts to harm self, including:
- Cuts on body
- Scratches on body
- Picking at wounds
- Abrading
- Constricting a body part
- Biting
- Self-inflicted burns
- Severing
- Inhalation of harmful substances
- Insertion of object into body orifice
- Hitting
- Ingestion of harmful substances

Related Factors

See *Risk for Self-Harm*.

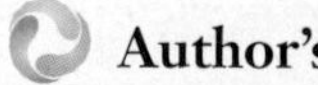

Author's Note

See *Risk for Self-Harm*.

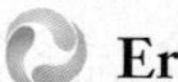

Errors in Diagnostic Statements

See *Risk for Self-Harm*.

Key Concepts

See *Risk for Self-Harm*.

Focus Assessment Criteria

See *Risk for Self-Harm*.

Interventions

See *Risk for Self-Harm*.

[48]This has been added by the author for clarity and usefulness.

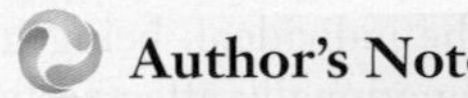

Self-Mutilation is an event; when the event is over the individual continues to be at risk for self-mutilation. Therefore Risk for Self-Mutilation is the correct nursing diagnosis

Risk for Self-Mutilation

NANDA-I Definition

At risk for deliberate self-injurious behavior causing tissue damage with the intent of causing nonfatal injury to attain relief of tension

Related Factors (Varcarolis, 2011)

Pathophysiologic

Related to biochemical/neurophysiologic imbalance secondary to:

Bipolar disorder
Psychotic states
Autism
Mentally impaired

Situational (Personal, Environmental)

Related to:

History of self-injury
Desperate need for attention
History of physical, emotional, or sexual abuse
Ineffective coping skills
Eating disorders
Inability to verbally express tensions
Impulsive behavior
Feelings of depression, rejection, self-hatred, separation anxiety, guilt, and/or depersonalization

Maturational

Children/Adolescents

Related to emotional disturbed or battered children

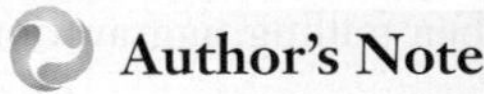

See Risk for Self-Harm.

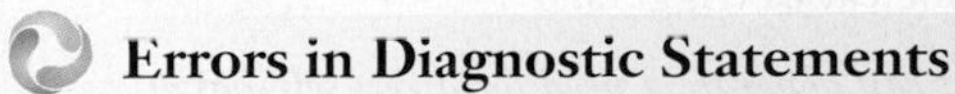

See Risk for Self-Harm.

Key Concepts

- Researchers have found that unqualified nursing staff report more negativity and worry in working with individuals who display self-harm than qualified staff (Wheatley & Austin-Payne, 2009). Nursing attitudes toward self-harm can be improved through nursing education and supervision (Tofthagen, Talsethand, & Fagerström, 2014).

- The first main category contained four subcategories: caring attitude toward the individual, being in a reflective dialogue to promote the individual's verbal expressions, and being emotionally affected by individuals that self-harm (Tofthagen et al., 2014).
- Individuals who self-injure have been mentally harmed previously in life and who because of this are vulnerable in relationships with other people (Tofthagen et al., 2014). This inhibits healthy relationships from forming. See also *Risk for Self-Harm*.

Goals

NOC
Impulse-Self Control, Self-Mutilation Restraint

The individual will identify persons to contact if thoughts of self-harm occur as evidenced by the following indicators.

Long-Term (Varcarolis, 2011)

- Demonstrate a decrease in frequency and intensity of self-inflicted injury by (date)
- Participate in therapeutic regimen
- Demonstrate two new coping skills that work when tension mounts and impulse is present instead of acting-out behaviors by (date)

Short-Term

- Respond to external limits
- Express feelings related to stress and tension instead of acting-out behaviors by (date)
- Discuss alternative ways the person can meet demands of current situation by (date)

Interventions (Varcarolis 2011)

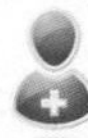

Clinical Alert Nurses reported "being emotionally affected by individuals who, self-harm. They described that relapses could be experienced as a 'defeat'". Nurses can become discouraged or experience a sense of powerlessness. They fear projecting their frustrations to the individual (Tofthagen et al., 2014).

NIC
Active Listening, Coping Enhancement, Impulse Control Training, Behavior Management: Self-Harm, Hope Instillation, Contracting, Surveillance: Safety

Convey Confidence That the Person Can Change Their Behavior With a Caring Attitude

R: *"The implication for clinical practice is that mental health nurses are in a position where they can promote patients' recovery processes, by offering individuals alternative activities and by working in partnership with patients to promote their individual strengths and life knowledge" (Tofthagen et al., 2014).*

- Initiate agency procedure to identify and remove all sources of potential harm (e.g., person search, belongings search). Limit personal belongings.
- Try to learn about the person (e.g., interests, goals).

R: *Nurses reported they wanted to understand and see the person behind "the suffering human being"*

- Assess history of self-mutilation (Varcarolis, 2011).

R: *The more individuals injure themselves, the more likely they will become addicted to self-harm (Tofthagen et al., 2014; Ystgaard, 2003)*

- Types of mutilating behaviors (e.g., cutting, burning, self-hitting, strangulation, hair pulling, aggravation of chronic wounds, and/or insertion of objects into the body)
- Frequency of behaviors
- Triggers preceding events (e.g., being alone, rejection, conversations with a physician or nurse, evenings, and/or private circumstances). Some individuals may be unclear of triggers.

R: *Triggers can include situations, thoughts, and/or feelings that can generate a need for direct self-harm.*

Explore for Feeling Before the Act of Mutilation and What They Mean (e.g., Gain Control Over Others, Attention, Method to Feel Alive, Expression of Guilt, or Self-Hate)

R: *Exploring feeling can help gain insight into self-mutilation, guiding the person's recovery as a process or a learning situation for her/him (Tofthagen et al., 2014).*

If a Self-Injury Occurs

- Respond to self-mutilation episodes matter-of-fact; maintain the belief that the person can improve.

R: *A neutral approach decreases blaming and discourages special attention for the episode.*

- Collaborate on alternative behaviors to self-mutilation.
- Avoidance of certain activities that trigger behavior.
- Discussion of their feelings before self-mutilation.
- Clearly establish limits on behavior.

R: *"Consistency can establish a sense of security" (Varcarolis, 2011).*

Be Vigilant for Signs of Worsening and Increased Risk for Suicide

- Refer to *Risk for Suicide.*

R: *"Individuals can be ambivalent to whether they live or die, so the harm they cause themselves can fluctuate between self-harm and attempted suicide" (Tofthagen et al., 2014).*

Initiate Referrals as Needed

- Connect with community resources (therapist, support groups).

R: *"Self-harm can thus be described as a long-term illness and, consequently, many people suffering from self-harm must learn how to cope with their illness" (Tofthagen et al., 2014).*

Risk for Suicide

NANDA-I Definition

At risk for self-inflicted, life-threatening injury

Risk Factors

Suicidal behavior (ideation, talk, plan, available means) (Varcarolis, 2011)
Persons high risk for suicide (refer to Key Concepts under Suicide)
Poor support system*
Family history of suicide*
Hopelessness/helplessness*
Poor support system
History of prior suicidal attempts*
Alcohol and substance abuse*
Legal or disciplinary problems*
Grief/bereavement (loss of person, job, home)
Suicidal cues (Varcarolis, 2011)
Overt ("No one will miss me," "I am better off dead," "I have nothing to live for")
Covert (making out a will, giving valuables away, writing forlorn love notes, acquiring life insurance)

Key Concepts

- American Foundation for Suicide Prevention (2015) using Centers for Disease Control and Prevention (CDC) statistics reported:
  - In 2013, the highest suicide rate (19.1) was among people 45 to 64 years old. The second highest rate (18.6) occurred in those 85 years and older. The third highest rate (15%) is among persons 65 to 83 years old. Younger groups have had consistently lower suicide rates than middle-aged and older adults. In 2013, adolescents and young adults aged 15 to 24 had a suicide rate of 10.9 (American Foundation for Suicide Prevention, 2015).
  - Of those who died by suicide in 2013, 77.9% were male and 22.1% were female (American Foundation for Suicide Prevention, 2015).
  - In 2013, the highest U.S. suicide rate (14.2) was among Whites and the second highest rate (11.7) was among American Indians and Alaska Natives. Much lower and roughly similar rates were found among Asians and Pacific Islanders (5.8), Blacks (5.4), and Hispanics (5.7).
  - In 2013, firearms were the most common method of death by suicide, accounting for a little more than half (51.4%) of all suicide deaths. The next most common methods were suffocation (including hangings) at 24.5% and poisoning at 16.1%.

Suicide

- Suicidal behavior is an attempt to escape from intolerable life stressors that have accumulated over time. It is accompanied by intense feelings of hopelessness, little social support, and insufficient coping skills to manage extreme stressors that are present (Boyd, 2012).
- Depression, low self-esteem, helplessness, and hopelessness are related to suicide. The greater the degree of hopelessness, the greater is the risk for suicide. Loss clearly increases the risk of suicide. Cumulative losses increase the risk dramatically (Halter, 2014).
- People exhibiting poor reality testing, delusions, and poor impulse control are at high risk. Alcohol and drugs tend to lower impulse control.
- Changes in behavior (e.g., giving away possessions) may signal an increase in risk. An individual may appear to be better just before an attempt. This may result from feelings of relief after making a decision.
- The more resources that are available, the more likely it is that the crisis can be managed effectively. Resources include personal support systems, employment, physical and mental abilities, finances, and housing.
- Some people use suicide attempts as a way to cope with stress. The more frequent the attempts and the more lethal, the higher the current risk. Suicidal ideation moves from the general to the specific, with more detailed plans representing a higher risk. An event may precipitate an attempt. The difference between a negative life event and one that may lead to a suicide attempt is that with the latter, the individual already has engaged in 26%.
- Lethality describes "the probability that a client will successfully complete suicide." It is determined by the "seriousness of the intent and the likelihood that the planned method of death will succeed" (Boyd, 2012).
- Ninety (90%) of adults who commit suicide have an associated psychiatric disorder as Major Depression, Bipolar Disorder, Substance Abuse, Conduct Disorder, Anxiety Disorders Borderline Personality Disorders, Schizophrenia, Eating Disorders (Fowler, 2012).
- Twenty-six (26%) of individual with HIV reported attempting suicide since their HIV diagnosis with 27% attempting within the first week of diagnosis—47%within the first month after diagnosis (Fowler, 2012).
- Prediction of suicide risk is not an exact science. Some errors that can be made result from the following:
    - Overreliance on mood as an indicator; not all people who commit suicide are clinically depressed.
    - Reliance on intuition; many people can totally conceal their intention.
    - Failure to assess support system.
    - Countertransference, particularly the failure of the therapist to acknowledge negative feelings that are aroused.
- The AIDS-related multiple losses that HIV-negative gay men may experience can result in repetitive overwhelming emotions, physical exhaustion, and spiritual demoralization. If coupled with shunning and isolation, despair is increased and chronic (*Mallinson, 1999).

Pediatric Considerations

- The preteen and early adolescent years are often when self-harm begins to manifest itself. Adults must be in tune with changes in behavior and changes in apparel and be highly suspicious of multiple "accidents."
- Of adolescent suicides, almost 50% had made previous attempt (Hockenberry & Wilson, 2015).
- Important indicators of suicide risks are psychiatric conditions and alcohol use. These teens seek release from their psychiatric and social problems (Hockenberry & Wilson, 2015).
- Suicide in children (5 to 14 years of age) tends to be more impulsive than in other age groups. Hyperactivity also seems to contribute to the impulsive nature.
- Recognition of depression in adolescents is often difficult because they mask their feelings with bored and angry behavior. Some symptoms include being sad or blue, withdrawal from social activities, trouble concentrating, somatic complaints, changes in sleep or eating patterns, and feelings of guilt or inadequacy.
- Suicide is the leading cause of death among Gay and Lesbian youth nationally. Thirty (30%) of Gay youth attempt suicide near the age of 15 (CDC, 2012). Supportive friends, family, and relatives can be protective factors to prevent suicide (Saewyc et al., 2007).
- Suicide is the third leading cause of death among adolescents. A frequent factor is lack of or loss of a meaningful relationship (Hockenberry & Wilson, 2015).

Geriatric Considerations

- The "baby Boomers" have had a consistently higher rate of suicide during each stage of life (Morbidity and Mortality Weekly Report, 2013).

- White men older than 65 years have twice the rate of suicide of all other age groups. They constitute 18.5% of the population but commit 23% of all suicides (Miller, 2015).
- Retirement, loss of vigor, and loss of a meaningful role negatively affect the self-esteem of older men.
- Older adults tend to complete suicide when they attempt it. The ratio of attempts to completion is 4:1, whereas for younger people it is approximately 25:1 (Miller, 2015).
- Alcohol contributes to depression. Depression increases alcohol use. Both are significant risk factors for suicide in older adults.
- Depressed older adults usually talk less about suicide than younger adults but use more violent means and are more often successful (Miller, 2015).
- Suicide potential often is overlooked because of the prevalent view that older adults are generally passive and nonviolent. In addition, complaints about depression and hopelessness may be subtle and thus easily ignored in older adults (Miller, 2015).

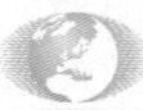

Transcultural Considerations

- Acceptance of sudden, violent death is difficult for family members in most societies (Andrews & Boyle, 2012).
- Islamic law strictly forbids suicide. Some religions (e.g., Catholicism) do not permit church funerals for suicide victims.
- The Northern Cheyenne Indians believe suicide or any violent death prevents the spirit from entering the spirit world (Andrews & Boyle, 2012).
- Suicide of elderly Eskimos, who could no longer contribute to the sustenance of the tribe, was expected (Giger, 2013).

Focus Assessment Criteria

Refer to *Risk for Self-Harm.*

Goals

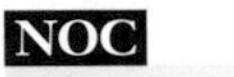

NOC

Impulse-Self Control, Suicide Self-Restraint

The individual will identify persons to contact if suicidal thoughts occur, and he or she will not commit suicide as evidenced by the following indicators.

Long-Term (Varcarolis, 2011)

- State the desire to live
- Name two people he or she can call if thoughts of suicide recur before discharge
- Name at least one acceptable alternative to his or her situation
- Identify at least one realistic goal for the future

Short-Term

- Remain safe while in the hospital
- Stay with a friend or family if person has a potential for suicide (if in the community)
- Keep an appointment for the next day with a crisis counselor (if in the community)
- Join family in crisis family counseling
- Have links to self-help groups in the community

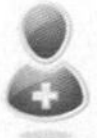

Clinical Alert After cancer and heart disease, suicide accounts for more years of life lost than any other cause of death (American Foundation for Suicide Prevention, 2015).

Protective factors buffer individuals from suicidal thoughts and behavior (CDC, 2014; U.S. Public Health Service 1999).

- Effective clinical care for mental, physical, and substance abuse disorders
- Easy access to a variety of clinical interventions and support for help-seeking
- Family and community support (connectedness)
- Support from ongoing medical and mental health care relationships
- Skills in problem solving, conflict resolution, and nonviolent ways of handling disputes
- Cultural and religious beliefs that discourage suicide and support instincts for self-preservation

Interventions

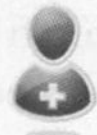

CLINICAL ALERT Talking to someone about suicide does not give them the idea. It validates that the nurse suspects the person is suffering alone.

Assist the Individual in Reducing His or Her Present Risk for Self-Destruction

Assess Level of Present Risk (Refer to Table II.18)

Table II.18 ASSESSING THE DEGREE OF SUICIDAL RISK (Varcarolis, 2011; Halter, 2014; Hockenberry & Wilson, 2015)

Behavior or Symptom	Intensity of Risk		
	Low	*Moderate*	*High*
Anxiety	Mild, moderate	High, or panic state	
Depression	Mild	Moderate	Severe or a sudden change to a happy or peaceful state
Isolation/withdrawal	Some feelings of isolation, no withdrawal	Some feelings of hopelessness, and withdrawal	Hopeless, withdrawn, and self-deprecating, isolation
Daily functioning	Effective	Moody	Depressed
	Good grades in school[a]	Some friends	Poor grades[a]
	Close friends	Prior suicidal thoughts	Few or no close friends
	No prior suicide attempt		Prior suicide attempts
	Stable job		Erratic or poor work history
Lifestyle	Stable	Moderately stable	Unstable
Alcohol/drug use	Infrequently to excess	Frequently to excess	Continual abuse
Previous suicide attempts	None or of low lethality (few pills)	One or more (pills, superficial wrist slash)	One or more (entire bottle of pills, gun, hanging)
Associated events	None or an argument	Disciplinary action[a]	Relationship breakup
		Failing grades[a]	Death of a loved one
		Work problems	Loss of job
		Family illness	Pregnancy[a]
Purpose of act	None or not clear	Relief of shame or guilt	Wants to die
		To punish others	Escape to join deceased
		To get attention	Debilitating disease
Family's reaction and structure	Supportive	Mixed reaction	Angry and unsupportive
	Intact family	Divorced/separated	Disorganized
	Good coping and mental health	Usually copes and understands	Rigid/abusive
	No history of suicide		Prior history of suicide in family
Suicide plan (method, location, time)	No plan	Frequent thoughts, occasional ideas about a plan	Specific plan
Lethality of suicide attempts		Wrist slashing	Firearms
		Overdose of nonprescription drugs except aspirin and acetaminophen	Hanging
			Jumping
			Carbon monoxide
			Overdose of antidepressants, barbiturates, aspirin, acetaminophen

[a]Applies only to children and adolescents.

NIC

Active Listening, Coping Enhancement, Suicide Prevention, Impulse Control Training, Behavior Management: Self-Harm, Hope Instillation, Contracting, Surveillance: Safety

- High
- Moderate
- Low

Assess Level of Long-Term Risk

- History of an attempted suicide (highest risk predictor)
- Lifestyle
- Lethality of plan
- Usual coping mechanisms
- Support available

Provide a Safe Environment Based on Level of Risk; Notify All Staff That the individual Is at Risk for Self-Harm; Use Both Written and Oral Communication (Varcarolis, 2011)

- When the person is being constantly observed, he or she is not to be allowed out of sight, even though privacy is lost.
- Arm's length is the most appropriate space for high-risk individuals.
- Initiate suicide observation for risk persons.
- Provide 15-minute visual check of mood, behaviors, and verbatim statements.

R: *The level of protection of the individual will be determined by his or her risk for suicide. High-risk suicidal persons should be admitted to a closely supervised environment and should not be allowed access to certain items.*

- Restrict glass, nail files, scissors, nail polish remover, mirrors, needles, razors, soda cans, plastic bags, lighters, electric equipment, belts, hangers, knives, tweezers, alcohol, and guns.
- Provide meals in a closely supervised area, usually on the unit or in individual's room:
- Ensure adequate food and fluid intake.
- Use paper/plastic plates and utensils.
- Check to be sure all items are returned on the tray.
- When administering oral medications, check to ensure that all medications are swallowed.
- Designate a staff member to provide checks on the individual as designated by the institution's policy. Provide relief for the staff member.
- Restrict to the unit unless specifically ordered by physician/nurse practitioner. When the individual is off unit, provide a staff member to accompany him or her.
- Instruct visitors on restricted items (e.g., ensure they do not give food in a plastic bag).
- The use of restricted items in the presence of staff, depending on the level of risk.
- For acutely suicidal individual, provide a hospital gown to deter the person from leaving the facility. As risk decreases, the individual may be allowed own clothing.
- Conduct room searches periodically according to institution policy.
- Use seclusion and restraint if necessary (refer to Risk for Violence for discussion).
- Notify the police if the individual leaves the facility and is at risk for suicide.
- Keep accurate and thorough records of the individual's behaviors and all nursing assessments and interventions.

R: *High-risk suicidal persons should be admitted to a closely supervised environment and should not be allowed access to certain items.*

Emphasize the Following (Varcarolis, 2011)

- The crisis is temporary.
- Unbearable pain can be survived.
- Help is available.
- You are not alone.

R: *"These statements give perspective to the person and help offer hope for the future" (Varcarolis, 2011).*

Observe for a Sudden Change in Emotions from Sad, Depressed to Elated, Happy, or Peaceful

R: *A sudden change in emotions can indicate the risk of suicide is very high as the individuals seek a way to lose the emotional pain.*

Carp's Cues

Read "If You Are Thinking About Suicide. Read This First" found at www.metanoia.org/suicide. Refer individuals who are at risk to this site.

Help Build Self-Esteem and Discourage Isolating Behaviors

- Be nonjudgmental and empathic.
- Be aware of own reactions to the situation.
- Encourage interactions with others.
- Divert attention to the external world (e.g., odd jobs).
- Convey a sense that the person is not alone (use group or peer therapy).
- Seek out the individual for interactions.
- Provide planned daily schedules for people with low impulse control.

R: *Suicidal individuals are usually ambivalent about the decision. Staff can work with the positive goals to effect a change in attitude and to promote socialization.*

Assist to Identify and Contact Support System

- Inform family and significant others.
- Enlist support.
- Do not provide false reassurance that behavior will not recur.
- Encourage an increase in social activity.

R: *Caregivers can become immobilized or drained by the acutely suicidal individual. Feelings of hopelessness are often communicated to the individual.*

Assist in Developing Positive Coping Mechanisms

- Encourage appropriate expression of anger and hostility.
- Set limits on ruminations about suicide or previous attempts.
- Assist the individual in recognizing predisposing factors: "What was happening before you started having these thoughts?"
- Facilitate examination of life stresses and past coping mechanisms.
- Explore alternative behaviors.
- Anticipate future stresses and assist in planning alternatives.
- Help to identify negative thinking patterns and direct the individual to practice altering them.
- Refer to Anxiety, Ineffective Coping, and Hopelessness for further interventions.

R: *The person's participation in their plan of care can increase their sense of responsibility and control (Halter, 2014).*

Initiate Health Teaching and Referrals, When Indicated

- Refer for ongoing psychiatric follow-up.
- Refer for peer or group therapy.
- Refer for family therapy, especially when a child or adolescent is involved.
- Instruct significant others in how to recognize an increase in risk: change in behavior, verbal or nonverbal communication, withdrawal, or signs of depression.
- Supply the phone number of 24-hour emergency hotline.

R: *Interventions are based on the type of risk the individual presents. Long-term treatment is often more difficult to institute than emergency care in some communities.*

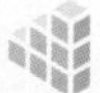

Pediatric Interventions

Take all Suicide Threats Seriously. Listen Carefully

R: *All threats or gestures to hurt oneself must be taken seriously regardless of the child's developmental age. Suicide attempts or threats may not represent a true desire to die, but they definitely represent a cry for help.*

Determine Whether the Child Understands the Finality of Death (e.g., "What Does it Mean to Die?")

- "Have you ever seen a dead animal on the road? Can it get up and run?"
- Explore feelings and reason for suicidal feelings.

R: *Suicidal threats and ideation signal a crisis that requires specific care.*

Consult with a Psychiatric Expert Regarding the Most Appropriate Environment for Treatment

R: *Treatment strategies depend on the child's living situation, psychiatric history, and support system available.*

Participate in Programs in School to Teach About the Symptoms of Depression and Signs of Suicidal Behavior

R: *Children who attempt suicide may have marked depression (Varcarolis, 2011).*

With Adolescents, Explore (Hockenberry & Wilson, 2015) **the Following**

- Chronic mental disorders (e.g. conduct disorders, autistic spectrum disorders, depression)
- Physical, emotional, and/or sexual abuse
- Family problems
- Strength of support systems
- Disruption of friendship or romantic relationship
- Presence of performance failure (e.g., examination, course)
- Recent or upcoming change (change of school, relocation)
- Sexual orientation (LGBT)

Convey Empathy Regarding Problems and/or Losses

- Do not minimize the loss; instead focus on their disappointment.

R: *Certain stressors are especially significant for adolescents, who are developmentally preoccupied with status, peers, and appearances (Varcarolis, 2011).*

INEFFECTIVE SEXUALITY PATTERNS

Ineffective Sexuality Patterns

Related to Prenatal and Postpartum Changes
Sexual Dysfunction

NANDA-I Definition

Expressions of concern regarding own sexuality

Defining Characteristics

Actual concerns regarding sexual behaviors, sexual health, sexual functioning, or sexual identity.
Expression of concern about the impact a medical diagnosis or treatment for a medical condition may have on sexual functioning or sexual desirability.

Related Factors

Ineffective sexual patterns can occur as a response to various health problems, situations, and conflicts. Some common sources are as follows:

Pathophysiologic

Related to biochemical effects on energy and libido secondary to:

Endocrine

Diabetes mellitus
Hyperthyroidism
Addison's disease
Decreased hormone production
Myxedema
Acromegaly

Genitourinary

Chronic renal failure

Neuromuscular and Skeletal

Arthritis
Amyotrophic lateral sclerosis
Multiple sclerosis
Disturbances of nerve supply to brain, spinal cord, sensory nerves, or autonomic nerves

Cardiorespiratory

Peripheral vascular disorders
Cancer
Myocardial infarction
Congestive heart failure
Chronic respiratory disorders

Related to fears associated with (sexually transmitted diseases [STDs])* (specify):

Human immunodeficiency virus (HIV)/Acquired immunodeficiency syndrome (AIDS)
Human papilloma virus
Herpes
Gonorrhea
Chlamydia
Syphilis

Related to effects of alcohol on performance

Related to decreased vaginal lubrication secondary to (specify)

Related to fear of premature ejaculation

Related to pain during intercourse

Treatment Related

Related to effects of:

Medications (Table II.19)
Radiation therapy

Related to altered self-concept from change in appearance (trauma, radical surgery)

Related to knowledge/skill deficit about alternative responses to health-related transitions, altered body function or structure, illness or medical treatment*

Situational (Personal, Environmental)

Related to fear of pregnancy*

Related to lack of significant other*

Related to conflicts with sexual orientation preferences*

Related to conflicts with variant preferences

Related to partner problem (specify):

Unwilling
Not available
Uninformed
Conflicts
Abusive
Separated, divorced

Related to lack of privacy*

Related to ineffective role model*

Related to stressors secondary to:

Job problems
Value conflicts
Financial worries
Relationship conflicts

Related to misinformation or lack of knowledge

Related to fatigue

Related to fear of rejection secondary to obesity

Related to fear of sexual failure

Related to fear of pregnancy

Related to depression

Related to anxiety

Related to guilt

Related to history of unsatisfactory sexual experiences

Related to multiple issues associated with transgender, lesbian, or gay identification

Related to inadequate social programs targeted on and/or appropriate for LGBT youth, adults, and elders

Table II.19 DRUGS THAT AFFECT SEXUALITY

Drug	Effect on Sexuality
Alcohol	In small amounts, may increase libido and decrease sexual inhibitions In large amounts, impairs neural reflexes involved in erection and ejaculation Chronic use causes impotence and sterility in men; decreased desire and orgasmic dysfunction in women
Amyl nitrate	Peripheral vasodilator reputed to cause intensified orgasms when inhaled at time of orgasm May cause loss of erection, hypotension, and syncope
Antidepressants	Peripheral blockage of nervous innervation to sex organs Significant percentage of impotence and ejaculatory dysfunction in men Decreased libido in both genders
Antihistamines	Block parasympathetic innervation of sex organs Sedative effect may decrease desire Decrease in vaginal lubrication
Antihypertensives	Libido may be decreased in both genders Some cause impotence and ejaculatory problems in up to 50% of men See specific class of medications
Antispasmodics	Inhibit parasympathetic innervation of sex organs May cause impotence
Chemotherapeutics	Combination therapy may cause azoospermia or oligospermia in men and temporary or permanent menopause in women; fertility may be temporarily or permanently altered; libido may be decreased and body image altered
Cocaine	Short-term use is reported to enhance sexual experience Chronic use causes loss of desire and sexual dysfunction in both sexes
Hormones	Estrogen suppresses sexual function in men Testosterone may increase libido in both sexes but causes virilization in women Chronic use of anabolic steroids causes testicular atrophy, decreased testosterone, and decreased sperm production; may cause permanent sterility
Marijuana	May decrease sexual inhibitions Chronic use may cause decreased libido and impotence
Narcotics	Chronic use causes decreased libido in both sexes Testosterone levels and amount of semen decreased Erectile and ejaculatory dysfunction common
Oral contraceptives	Removes fear of pregnancy May cause decreased libido
Sedatives/tranquilizers	Initially and in low doses may enhance sexual pleasure due to relaxation and decrease of inhibitions Long-term use decreases libido and may cause orgasmic dysfunction and impotence
Diuretics	May cause erectile, ejaculatory, and libido problems, especially at higher doses
Anxiolytics	Altered libido in both genders; erectile problems and delayed ejaculation in men
Sildenafil citrate (Viagra)	Enhances erectile ability in men with impaired potency

Maturational

Adolescent

Related to ineffective/absent role models*

Related to negative sexual teaching

Related to absence of sexual teaching

Adult

Related to adjustment to parenthood

Related to effects of menopause on libido and vaginal tissue atrophy

Related to values conflict

Related to effects of pregnancy on energy levels and body image

Related to effects of aging on energy levels and body image

Related to the challenges and barriers for sexual expression of residents in care environments

Author's Note

The diagnoses *Ineffective Sexuality Patterns* and *Sexual Dysfunction* are difficult to differentiate. *Ineffective Sexuality Patterns* represents a broad diagnosis, of which sexual dysfunction can be one part. *Sexual Dysfunction* may be used most appropriately by a nurse with advanced preparation in sex therapy. Until *Sexual Dysfunction* is well differentiated from *Ineffective Sexuality Patterns*, most nurses should not use it.

Errors in Diagnostic Statements

***Ineffective Sexuality Patterns* related to reports of absent libido**

Report of absent libido represents a symptom of *Ineffective Sexuality Patterns*, not a "related to" statement. If further assessment revealed the individual's dissatisfaction with present sexual patterns, the nurse could record the diagnosis *Ineffective Sexuality Patterns* related to unknown etiology as evidenced by reports of absent libido. The use of "unknown etiology" in this diagnostic statement prompts focus assessments to determine contributing factors (e.g., stress, medication side effects).

***Sexual Dysfunction* related to impotence secondary to spinal cord injury**

How would the nurse treat this diagnosis? The impotence will not change. A nurse can focus on exploring feelings, providing information regarding alternative methods for achieving sexual satisfaction and referrals to experts. Thus, the focus is on improving both partners' satisfaction with the nursing diagnosis *Ineffective Sexual Patterns* related to insufficient knowledge of alternative methods for sexual expression.

Key Concepts

General Considerations

- Sexual health is the integration of somatic, emotional, intellectual, physical, and social aspects of a sexual being in ways that are enriching and that enhance personality, communication, and love.
- Sexual behaviors are the behaviors an individual uses to communicate feelings and attitudes about their sexuality. They include behaviors used in release of sexual tension, either alone or with a partner to attain intimate sexual satisfaction and/or procreation.
- All people are sexual beings. Sexuality is an integral part of identity regardless of age.
- Sexuality encompasses how a person feels about himself or herself and how an individual interacts with others.
- Sexual function refers to psychological and physiologic ability to perform in a sexually satisfying manner, with or without a partner, old or young.
- The characteristics of a sexually healthy individual are as follows:
  - Positive body image
  - Acceptance of sexual and body functions as normal and natural
  - Accurate knowledge about human sexuality and sexual functioning
  - Recognition and acceptance of own sexual feelings
  - Capacity for intimacy in relationships
  - Acceptance of mistakes/imperfections in self and others
  - Prevention of pregnancy when it is not desired
  - Protection of self from STDs

Medications and Sexuality

- Drugs can influence sexual functioning positively and negatively (see Table II.19).
- The individual has the right to be educated about all medication side effects, including those affecting sexuality.

The Nurse's Role in Discussing Sexuality

- The nurse must become educated regarding sexuality and sexual health throughout the life span. It is important for the nurse to examine his or her own beliefs and feelings concerning sexuality, sexual function, and what is considered sexually normal and abnormal.
- Many nurses have difficulty providing care in the area of sexuality and do not address sexual concerns unless the individual asks specific questions. Research indicates, however, that many individuals wish nurses and other health-care professionals would initiate discussion of sexuality and satisfaction with sexual function.

- The PLISSIT model (*Annon, 1976) is helpful for the nurse generalist providing care in the area of sexuality:
- *Permission:* Convey to the individual and significant other a willingness to discuss sexual thoughts and feelings (e.g., "Some people with your diagnosis have concerns about how it will affect sexual functioning. Is this a concern for you or your partner?").
- *Limited Information:* Provide the individual and significant other with information on the effects certain situations (e.g., pregnancy), conditions (e.g., cancer), and treatments (e.g., medications) can have on sexuality and sexual function.
- *Specific Suggestions:* Provide specific instructions that can facilitate positive sexual functioning (e.g., changes in coital positions).
- *Intensive Therapy:* Refer people who need more help to an appropriate health-care professional (e.g., sex therapist, surgeon).

- Giving a person "permission" to discuss sexual concerns is by far the most important aspect of nursing care in the area of sexuality. The nurse should give permission by:
  - Including sexuality in the initial health history and addressing questions on sexuality in a manner similar to questions on bowel and bladder function. This helps the individual see that nurses view sexuality as a routine part of human health.
  - Offering to discuss sexual concerns at appropriate times during the individual's hospitalization/visit (Wilmoth, 1994)
  - The nurse should assure the individual of the confidentiality of all data on sexuality and obtain permission from the individual before making a referral for a sexual problem.

Contraception and STDs

- Research has shown that the use of mechanical barrier methods (condom, diaphragm, vaginal sponge, cervical cap) and/or chemical barriers containing nonoxynol-9 (foam, jelly, cream) are effective in reducing the transmission of HIV and other STDs.
- Use of the intrauterine device, oral contraceptives, Norplant, Depo-Provera, or sterilization provides no protection from STDs. Individuals using these methods must be counseled to use a chemical or mechanical barrier method to protect them from disease.

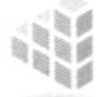

Pediatric Considerations

- The Youth Risk Behavior Surveillance System (YRBSS) monitors six categories of priority health-risk behaviors among youth and young adults: (1) behaviors that contribute to unintentional injuries and violence; (2) tobacco use; (3) alcohol and other drug use; (4) sexual behaviors that contribute to unintended pregnancy and sexually transmitted infections (STIs), including HIV infection; (5) unhealthy dietary behaviors; and (6) physical inactivity. In addition, YRBSS monitors the prevalence of obesity and asthma. YRBSS includes a national school-based Youth Risk Behavior Survey (YRBS) conducted by Centers for Disease Control and Prevention (CDC) and state and large urban school district school-based YRBSs conducted by state and local education and health agencies. This report summarizes results for 104 health-risk behaviors plus obesity, overweight, and asthma from the 2013 national survey, 42 state surveys, and 21 large urban school district surveys conducted among students in grades 9 to 12 (CDC, 2015).
- The Youth Risk Behavior Surveillance System (YRBSS) findings related to Sexual Behavior/Birth Control are (CDC, 2015):
  - 46.8% of students had had sexual intercourse.
  - 5.6% of students had had sexual intercourse for the first time before age 13 years.
  - 15.0% of students had had sexual intercourse with four or more persons during their life.
  - 34.0% of students had had sexual intercourse with at least one person during the 3 months before the survey.
    - Of the 34.0% of currently sexually active student nationwide, 59.1% reported that either they or their partner had used a condom during last sexual intercourse.
    - Of the 34.0% of currently sexually active students nationwide, 19.0% reported that either they or their partner had used birth control pills to prevent pregnancy before last sexual intercourse.
    - Of the 34.0% of currently sexually active students nationwide, 25.3% reported that either they or their partner had used birth control pills; an IUD (such as Mirena or ParaGard) or implant (such as Implanon or Nexplanon); or a shot (such as Depo-Provera), patch (such as OrthoEvra), or birth control ring (such as NuvaRing) to prevent pregnancy before last sexual intercourse.
    - Of the 34.0% of currently sexually active students nationwide, 13.7% reported that neither they nor their partner had used any method to prevent pregnancy during last sexual intercourse.
    - Of the 34.0% of currently sexually active students nationwide, 22.4% had drunk alcohol or used drugs before last sexual intercourse.

- Sex role identification begins in infancy and is determined by adolescence.
  - Infants can identify body parts by the end of the first year.
  - Toddlers learn gender differentiation.
  - Preschoolers frequently engage in masturbation and sex play with peers (e.g., comparing genitals).
  - School-aged children continue to gain awareness about their sex role identity. Although masturbation and sex play are common in the young school-aged child, the older school-aged child becomes involved in purposeful sexual behavior (e.g., hugging, kissing members of the opposite sex) (Hockenberry & Wilson, 2015).
  - Adolescents experience altered body image in response to the physical changes of puberty. The key developmental task of adolescence is identity formation, which is influenced by sexual maturation and assuming a sex role (Hockenberry & Wilson, 2015).
- Parents are the primary force in sex education in a child's life. This includes what is not said as well as what is said.
- Formal sex education, presented from a life span approach, is best offered during middle childhood. Topics should include sexual maturation and the process of reproduction.
- STDs continue to be a major cause of morbidity among adolescents and young adults. The highest rates of chlamydial infections in females occur in adolescents (CDC, 2015).
- Risky behavior by adolescents and young adults increases their vulnerability to STDs, pelvic inflammatory disease, infertility, AIDS, and chronic incurable conditions such as hepatitis B or C virus infection, human papilloma virus (HPV) infection, and genital herpes.
- Half of ninth through 12th graders report having had sexual intercourse (CDC, 2015).
- About 16% of high school students report having four or more sexual partners (CDC, 2015).
- Only 58% of high school students reported using a condom. Only 16% reported using birth control (CDC, 2015).
- Katsufrakis & Nusbaum (2011) reported:
  - Fifty percent of boys and 24% of girls report having sex because of curiosity.
  - Forty-eight percent of girls and 25% of boys report having sex for affection.
  - Another reason for having sex, yet reluctantly is peer pressure (30%).

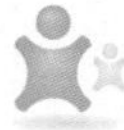

Maternal Considerations

- Pregnant women have varying degrees of sexual desire during pregnancy. Some women are very sexually excitable and some women are not.
- Libido changes by large degrees during different stages of pregnancy.
- Vasocongestion of the lower pelvis during pregnancy may cause increase orgasm for some women during their first trimester (Pillitteri, 2014).
- A woman's body image affects her sexuality. (If thinness is an attribute, then many pregnant women are confused about changing size.)
- A woman's attitude toward her body can influence her partner's sexual attraction toward her.
- The postpartum period is a time of self-doubt. For the first 6 weeks, a new mother feels lost, overwhelmed, tired, depressed, ignorant, and isolated. Her self-esteem as well as her sexuality may suffer.
- Polomeno (1999) found the postnatal sexual concerns of men and women (M, men; W, women) to be:
  - Having time for each other (M, W)
  - Sexual intercourse the first time (M, W)
  - Separating oneself from the baby (W)
  - Contraception (M, W)
  - Reactivating the passion, fun, and romance (M, W)
  - To be desired (W)
  - Fatigue and its impact on sexual desire (W)
  - Postpartum depression (M)
  - Balancing intimacy and the baby (W)
  - Time required for healing (W)
  - Fear of pain (M, W)
  - His perception of her and her body (W)

Geriatric Considerations

- "Sexuality is a broad multi-dimensional construct which encompasses relationships, romance, intimacy (ranging from simple touching and hugging, to sexually explicit contact), gender, grooming, dress and styling. Being able to express our sexuality is known to be important to health, well-being, quality of life, and furthermore, human rights. The desire or need to express one's sexuality does not expire with age and for many older people including those living in aged care facilities, sexuality continues to be important" (Bauer, Fetherstonhaugh, Tarzia, Nay, & Beattie, 2014).

- Older adults are psychologically and physically capable of engaging in sexual activity regardless of age-related changes in sexual anatomy and physiology.
- Sexual activity is often beneficial for older adults, reducing anxiety while providing intimacy and improving quality of life.
- With aging, woman experience decreased breast tone, thinning and loss of elasticity of the vaginal wall, decreased vaginal lubrication, and shortening of vaginal length from loss of circulating estrogen (Miller, 2015).
- With aging, men experience decreased production of spermatozoa, decreased ejaculatory force, and smaller, less-firm testicles. Direct stimulation may be required to achieve an erection; however, the erection may be maintained for a longer time (Miller, 2015).
- The need for intimacy and touch is especially important for older adults, who may be experiencing diminishing meaningful relationships.
- Past sexual function (enjoyment, interest, frequency) serves as a predictor of sexual activity in older adults. To be capable of sexual activity in old age, the individual must participate in sexual activity throughout life.
- Adult children and caregivers commonly view sexual activities of older adults as immoral, inappropriate, and negative (Miller, 2015).
- The sexual functioning of older adults is most influenced by myths and misunderstanding. According to Miller (2015), because sex is so closely identified with youthfulness, the stereotype of "sexless seniors" is widely believed.

Transcultural Considerations

- People of some cultures (e.g., Hispanic, Native American) are very hesitant to discuss sexuality.
- Some cultures view the postpartum period as a state of impurity. Certain foods and practices are taboo (e.g., intercourse). The woman may be secluded during postpartum bleeding. Some cultures end seclusion with a ritual bath (e.g., Navajo, Hispanic, Orthodox Jewish; Andrews & Boyle, 2012).
- Native American women believe in the importance of monthly menstruation to maintain physical well-being and harmony (Andrews & Boyle, 2012).

Focus Assessment Criteria

Guidelines for Taking a Sexual History

Discuss sexuality in a private, relaxed setting to ensure confidentiality.
Do not judge the individual by your own beliefs/practices.
Permit the individual to refuse to answer.
Clarify your vocabulary; use slang terms if needed to convey meaning.
Assess only those areas pertinent for this individual at this time.
Strive to be open, warm, objective, unembarrassed, and reassuring.
Keep in mind that it is more appropriate to assume that the individual has had some sexual experience than to assume none.
Several sessions may be necessary to complete the interview.

Subjective Data

Determine History

Age, sex, marital/relationship status
Sexual orientation/preference
Number of children and siblings
Sexual abuse
Depression
Medications
Communication patterns with significant others
Quality of relationship with significant other
Religious and cultural background
Job and financial status
Medical and surgical history
Drug and alcohol use (present and past)

Assess Concerns and Sexuality Patterns

How has your health problem affected your ability to function as a wife/mother/partner/father/husband? (Wilmoth, 1994)
How has your health problem affected the way you feel about yourself as a man/woman? (Wilmoth, 1994)
How has your health problem affected your ability to function sexually? (Wilmoth, 1994)

Sexual Function
Usual pattern
Present pattern
Satisfaction (individual, partner)
Desire (individual, partner)
Erection problems for man (attaining, sustaining)
Ejaculation problems for man (premature, retarded, retrograde)
Decreased lubrication for woman
Decreased orgasm for woman

Sexual Problem
Description
Onset (when, gradual/sudden)
Pattern over time (increased, decreased, unchanged)
Individual's concept of cause
Knowledge of problem by others (partner, physician, others)
Expectations

School-Aged Child
Knowledge:
"What is the difference between boys and girls?"
"What do you know about having babies?"
"Who taught you? At what age?"
Body changes:
"Is your body changing in any way? How? Why?"
"How do you feel about these changes?"
Masturbation:
"Almost everyone touches their body; how do you feel about this?"

Adolescent
Knowledge and attitudes:
"What are your parents' attitudes toward sex, nudity, and touching?"
"How are subjects discussed in your home?"
"How does pregnancy occur?"
"What are some methods of birth control?"
"What do you know about sexually transmitted diseases?"
Body changes:
"Is your body changing in any way? How? Why?"
"How do you feel about these changes?"
Sexual activity:
"Some young people are sexually active and others choose not to be sexually active; what are your beliefs about this?"
"Are you sexually active? If so, describe the type of birth control and safe sex practices you use."
"Have you ever been touched inappropriately or forced to have sex?"
"Some teens are attracted to people of their gender; have you experienced these feelings?" (Smith, 1993)

Senior Citizens
Knowledge:
"How do you feel when you hear that older adults have little interest in sexuality?"
"What do you know about sexually transmitted diseases?"
Body changes:
"How do you feel about the way your body has aged?"
"What do you do to make yourself feel good about yourself sexually?"
Sexual activity:
"Do you feel loved, valued by others?"
"How are your needs for touching and intimacy met?"
"Have you been able to maintain your sexual activity?"

Assess for Related Factors

Refer to Related Factors.

Goals

NOC

Body Image, Self-Esteem, Role Performance, Sexual Identity

The individual will resume previous sexual activity or engage in alternative satisfying sexual activity as evidenced by the following indicators:

- Identifies effects of stressors, loss, or change on sexual functioning
- Modifies behavior to reduce stressors
- Identifies limitations on sexual activity caused by a health problem
- Identifies appropriate modifications in sexual practices in response to these limitations
- Reports satisfying sexual activity

Interventions

NIC

Behavioral Management, Sexual Counseling, Emotional Support, Active Listening, Teaching: Sexuality

Assess for Causative or Contributing Factors

- Refer to Related Factors.

Explore the Individual's Patterns of Sexual Functioning Using the PLISSITT Model (*Annon, 1976)

- Encourage him or her to share concerns; assume that individuals of all ages have had some sexual experience, and convey a willingness to discuss feelings and concerns.

R: *A time-tested model for the nurse generalist providing care in the area of sexuality in any setting*

- *Permission:* Convey to the individual and significant other a willingness to discuss sexual thoughts and feelings (e.g., "Some people with your diagnosis have concerns about how it will affect sexual functioning. Is this a concern for you or your partner?").
- *Limited Information:* Provide the individual and significant other with information on the effects certain situations (e.g., pregnancy), conditions (e.g., cancer), and treatments (e.g., medications) can have on sexuality and sexual function.
- *Specific Suggestions:* Provide specific instructions that can facilitate positive sexual functioning (e.g., changes in coital positions).
- *Intensive Therapy:* Refer people who need more help to an appropriate health-care professional (e.g., sex therapist, surgeon).

R: *Many individuals are reluctant to discuss sexuality issues. A relaxed approach can encourage the individual to share feelings and concerns.*

Discuss the Relationship Between Sexual Functioning and Life Stressors

- Clarify the relation between stressors and problem in sexual functioning.
- Explore options available for reducing the effects of the stressor on sexual functioning (e.g., increase sleep, increase exercise, modify diet, explore stress reduction methods).

R: *Explaining that impaired sexual functioning has a physiologic basis can reduce feelings of inadequacy and decreased self-esteem; this actually may help improve sexual function.*

Reaffirm the Need for Frank Discussion Between Sexual Partners

- Explain how the individual and the partner can use role playing to discuss concerns about sex.

R: *Role playing helps an individual gain insight by placing himself or herself in another's position, and allows more spontaneous sharing of fears and concerns.*

- Reaffirm the need for closeness and expressions of caring through touching, massage, and other means.
- Suggest that sexual activity need not always culminate in vaginal intercourse, but that the partner can reach orgasm through noncoital manual or oral stimulation.

R: *Sexual pleasure and gratification are not limited to intercourse. Other expressions of caring may prove more meaningful.*

Address Factors for Individuals With Acute or Chronic Illness

- Eliminate or reduce causative or contributing factors, if possible, and teach the importance of adhering to medical regimen designed to reduce or control disease symptoms.
- Provide limited information and specific suggestions.
  - Provide appropriate information to individual and partner concerning actual limitations on sexual functioning caused by the illness (limited information).

- Teach possible modifications in sexual practices to assist in dealing with limitations caused by illness. See Table II.20 for more details.

TABLE II.20 DISORDERS THAT ALTER SEXUALITY

Health Problem	Sexual Complication	Nursing Intervention
Diabetes mellitus	*Men:* Erectile difficulties due to diabetic neuropathies or microangiopathy	LI: Encourage proper metabolic control.
	Women: Decreased desire; decreased vaginal lubrication	LI: Encourage proper metabolic control; teach signs and symptoms of vaginitis.
	SS: Eventually may require penile implant; refer to urologist.	SS: Suggest use of water-soluble lubricating jelly.
Chronic obstructive pulmonary disease	Activity intolerance due to exertional dyspnea; coughing and expectoration	LI: Teach controlled breathing; plan intercourse for time of peak effect from medications; avoid sex after large meal or physical exertion, or immediately after awakening; plan for nonhurried, relaxed, low-stress encounters, for losses.
	Anxiety	SS: Suggest positions that minimize chest pressure (sitting or side-lying); explain that waterbeds also help decrease exertion during sex.
Arthritis	Pain, joint stiffness, fatigue	LI: Explain that arthritis has no effect on physiologic aspects of sexual functioning. SS: Suggest that the couple plan intercourse for time of peak medication effects; promote joint relaxation by taking warm bath/shower alone/with partner; perform mild range-of-motion exercises.
	Decreased libido from steroid medications	LI: Teach that decreased desire is a common side effect of medication.
Transurethral resection of the prostate (TURP) to treat benign prostatic hypertrophy	Retrograde ejaculation due to damage to internal bladder sphincter	LI: Explain that erection and orgasm will still occur, but ejaculate will be decreased or absent; urine will be cloudy.
Cardiovascular disease	Anxiety, fear of performance, fear of chest pain, death, decreased desire, decreased arousal, decision of partner to stop sexual activity	LI: Explain that infarction has no direct effect on physiologic sexual functioning; activity usually is safe 5–8 weeks postinfarction, based on Index of Sexual Readiness (ability to take brisk walk, climb two flights of stairs without chest pain). Teach to avoid sexual activity after large meal, drinking alcohol, or in room with extremes in temperature. Point out that some medications may cause sexual dysfunction (see Table II.19). SS: Encourage nonsexual touching; suggest positions that conserve energy (side-to-side lying, supine lying position, or sitting in chair with partner on top); explore option of masturbation; assure that oral–genital sex does not place additional strain on heart. Warn to avoid anal sex because anal penetration stimulates vagus nerve and decreases cardiac function.
Chronic renal failure (CRF)	Chronic/recurrent uremia can produce state of depression, decreased sexual desire and arousal	LI: Acknowledge that stress of disease and dialysis may cause decreased desire; encourage nonsexual touching without pressure to perform.
	Untreated CRF causes cessation of ovulation and menses in women and causes atrophy of testicles, decreased spermatogenesis, decreased plasma testosterone, and erectile dysfunction in men. Dialysis may restore ovulation and menses in women and return testosterone levels to normal in men; sexual desire may return to predisease levels with treatment.	Reassure that these problems are usually reversible with dialysis. Warn that birth control should be continued because fertility may return. Explain that sexual dysfunction may be a product of emotional stress and the physiologic components of the disease. SS: Explain that measurement of nocturnal penile tumescence can distinguish between organic and psychological causes of sexual dysfunction in men.
Total abdominal hysterectomy with bilateral salpingo-oophorectomy	Loss of circulating estrogen	LI: Teach signs and symptoms of menopause, use of water-soluble vaginal lubricants.
	Postoperative psychological adjustment or change in sexual identity, grieving, loss of reproductive capacity Explore the meaning of uterine and ovarian loss to the woman. Assure her that the surgery will not change her ability to respond and function sexually.	Encourage discussion with physician about estrogen replacement creams. Explain that in most cases intercourse may be resumed after 6-week postoperative visit.

TABLE II.20 DISORDERS THAT ALTER SEXUALITY (*continued*)

Health Problem	Sexual Complication	Nursing Intervention
Enterostomal surgery		
Anterior–posterior resection	*Women:* Loss of uterus and ovaries; shortening of vagina *Men:* Erectile dysfunction, decrease in amount/force of ejaculate or retrograde ejaculation due to interruption of sympathetic and parasympathetic nerve supply *Note:* Amount of rectal tissue removed appears to determine degree of dysfunction.	LI: See above. SS: Suggest coital positions that decrease depth of penetration (e.g., side-to-side lying, man on top with legs outside the woman's, woman on top). LI: Explain that erectile dysfunction may be temporary or permanent. Encourage use of touch and other noncoital means of sexual communication.
Colostomy/ileostomy	Alteration in sexual self-concept, body image	LI: Allow the individual to express feelings about change in body appearance; encourage communication with partner.
	Decrease in desire, arousal, and orgasm	LI: Teach that fatigue and decreased desire are common after surgery. Discuss ways to increase sexual attractiveness; suggest wearing sexy lingerie or other clothing to hide appliance.
	Anxiety over spillage, odor	Teach to empty bag before sexual activity; encourage to maintain a sense of humor, because accidents will sometimes occur.
Spinal cord injury	Erectile dysfunction in men (varies with age and type of surgery)	Encourage alternative ways to express sexuality if intercourse is not possible.
	Sexual disability depends on level and type of cord injury: after injury, separation of genital sexual functioning and cerebral eroticism	LI: Discuss sexual options available depending on extent of injury (e.g., a waterbed to amplify pelvic movements). Encourage continued use of contraceptives, as appropriate.
	Men with complete upper motor neuron injury may not be able to ejaculate.	SS: Discuss alternate positions (e.g., partner on top). Encourage experimentation with vibrators, massage, and other means of sexual expression. May be a candidate for a penile implant. May have urinary tract infection. Refer to a urologist.
Note: Much information is available on the sexual implications of spinal cord injury. The reader is referred to available literature on this subject.		
Cancer	Sexual implications depend on site of disease and treatment.	LI: Encourage expression of anxiety and fear; encourage grieving for losses.
	May feel guilty about desiring touch, need for sexual activity	Assure that sexual expression, even when one has cancer, is natural, and that the need for intimacy often increases during this time.
	Changes in role function and sexually defined gender roles	Encourage discussion between partners about this; encourage negotiation about role changes, which may be temporary.
	Fear of being contagious	Assure the individual and partner that the disease cannot be transmitted through sexual activity.
	Change in body image	Discuss purchase of wig, false eyelashes before hair loss; suggest sexy lingerie, other ways to pamper oneself to increase feelings of sexual desirability and attractiveness.
	Fatigue	Explain that severe fatigue may hinder sexual desire and that fatigue does not indicate rejection of partner. Encourage verbal and nonverbal communication between the individual and partner.
Chemotherapy	*Alkylating agents, antimetabolites, and antitumor antibiotics:* Amenorrhea, oligospermia, azoospermia, decreased desire, ovarian dysfunction, erectile dysfunction *Vinca alkaloids:* Retrograde ejaculation, erectile dysfunction, decreased desire, ovarian dysfunction, temporary decrease in sexual desire/arousal	LI: Encourage discussion about changes in body appearance/function. Explore option of sperm banking. Urge to continue use of contraceptives. False-positive Pap smear possible. Encourage nonsexual touching; rest; avoidance of alcoholic beverages, narcotics, and sedatives before sexual activity; use of water-soluble lubricants to decrease vaginal irritation; avoidance of oral and anal sex during periods of neutropenia.
	Genetic teratogenicity and mutagenicity	Encourage the couple to seek genetic counseling before conception.

(*continued*)

TABLE II.20 DISORDERS THAT ALTER SEXUALITY *(continued)*

Health Problem	Sexual Complication	Nursing Intervention
Radiation therapy	Most side effects are site dependent; however, side effects such as fatigue, neutropenia, anorexia generally are present in all people.	LI: Teach to plan sexual activity after rest periods and to use positions that require less exertion for the individual. Encourage nonsexual touching and communication. Teach that individual is not radioactive during external treatment. Teach site-specific side effects and impact on sexual functioning.

LI, limited informatio n; SS, specific suggestion.

R: *Both partners probably have concerns about sexual activity. Repressing these feelings hurts the relationship.*

Facilitate Adaptation to Change in or Loss of Body Part

- Assess the stage of adaptation of the individual and partner to the loss (denial, depression, anger, resolution; see *Grieving*).
- Encourage adherence to the medical regimen to promote maximum recovery.
- Encourage the couple to discuss the strengths of their relationship and to assess the influence of the loss on these strengths.
- Clarify the relationship between loss or change and the problem in sexual functioning.

R: *Providing accurate information on the effect of cord injury on sexual functioning can prevent false hope or give real hope, as appropriate.*

- Refer also to *Risk for Disturbed Body Image*.

Provide Referrals as Indicated

- Enterostomal therapist
- Physician
- Nurse specialist
- Sex therapist

R: *Specialist interventions may be needed.*

Older Adults Interventions

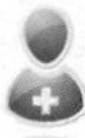

CLINICAL ALERT Lindau et al. (2007) revealed that in a study of the prevalence of sexual activity, behaviors, and problems in a national probability sample of 3,005 US adults (1,550 women and 1,455 men) 57 to 85 years of age, current sexual activity was reported in 73% of adults aged 57 to 64, 53% of adults aged 65 to 74, and 26% of adults aged 75 to 84.

- Multiple publications have reported the challenges and difficulties for older people with respect to the expression of their sexuality in the care environment (Bauer et al., 2014). Complicating the problem are the negative and judgmental staff attitudes; inadequate knowledge; and training (Bauer et al., 2014), including around the needs of people who identify as gay, lesbian, bisexual, transgender, or intersex (GLBTI) (a problem-based view of sexuality for people with dementia); the prioritization of other aspects of a resident's well-being over sexuality and a lack of privacy.
- Use the PLISSIT model to assess sexual concerns and issues with older adults. See above for specifics (Kazer, 2012a).
- The PLISSIT model and the questions suggested may be used with older adults in a variety of clinical settings. Despite the findings that sexuality continues throughout all phases of life, little material, scientific or otherwise, exists in the literature to guide nurses toward assessing the sexuality of older adults (Kazer, 2012b).

Carp's Cues

It is common for health-care professionals to feel uncomfortable with assessing the sexual desires and functions of all individuals. Comfortable confidence will only come first with the nursing professional's appreciation of the importance of sexual expression for many individuals and partners and second by initiating discussions/assessments. Consider why are nurses comfortable asking detailed questions about bowel movements, for example, frequency, color, consistency, quantity, and not sexual concerns.

Prove Factual Information of Treatment-Related Negative Effects on Sexual Desire/Function

- Discuss normal age-related physiological changes.
  - Women experience decreased breast tone, thinning and loss of elasticity of the vaginal wall, decreased vaginal lubrication, and shortening of vaginal length from loss of circulating estrogen (Miller, 2015).
  - Men experience decreased production of spermatozoa, decreased ejaculatory force, and smaller, less-firm testicles. Direct stimulation may be required to achieve an erection; however, the erection may be maintained for a longer time (Miller, 2015).
- Address how the effects of medications and medical conditions may affect one's sexual function. Refer to Table II.19.

Facilitate Communication with Older Adults and Their Families Regarding Sexual Health as Desired, Including the Following (Kazer, 2012a)

- Encourage family meetings with open discussion of issues if desired.
- Teach about safe sex practices.
- Discuss use of condoms to prevent transmission of sexually transmitted infections (STIs) and HIV.
- Ensure privacy and safety among long-term care and community-dwelling residents.

R: *High quality of life as measured by a standardized quality of life assessment*

- Privacy, dignity, and respect surrounding their sexuality
- Communication and education regarding sexual health as desired
- Ability to pursue sexual health free of pathologic and problematic sexual behaviors

R: *When sexual concerns are discussed and opportunities for sexual expression provided, problematic sexual behaviors can be reduced.*

Ensure the Residential Community Facility Has a Program for

- Provision of education on the ongoing sexual needs of older adults and appropriate interventions to manage these needs with dignity and respect
- Inclusion of sexual health questions in routine history and physical
- Frequent reassessment of individuals for changes in sexual health
- Provision of needed privacy for individuals to maintain intimacy and sexual health (e.g., in long-term care)

R: *This is critical to ensure empathetic and correct approaches to sexuality and expression.*

Pediatric Interventions

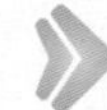

Carp's Cues

This section represents samples of practical advice on discussing sex and sexual activity with older children/adolescents. Refer to Ginsburg, K. R. (2015). *Talking to your child about sex*. Retrieved from Healthy Children website of the American Academy of Pediatrics.

Age-related teaching about menstruation, sexual functioning, pregnancy, birth control etc. is appropriate under the nursing diagnosis *Risk for Ineffective Health Maintenance* or *Risk Prone Behavior.*

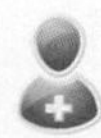

Clinical Alert Be clear that safety is nonnegotiable. Think about your bottomline priorities for your children. Chances are nothing matters more to you than their safety. Be very clear, and repeat often, that nothing matters more than knowing they are going to be okay. Establish a code word they can use to get your attention and help when they need to get out of a potentially dangerous or uncomfortable situation. Set a standard for protecting themselves from disease and unwanted pregnancy regardless of whether you agree with their decision-making about sex. Make sure that they know they can come to you for help if something goes wrong (Ginsburg, 2015).

- To reduce the tension, have the conversation in the car or while cooking to reduce the need for eye contact and reduce the early termination of the dialogue.

- Don't abstain from educating your own children (Ginsburg, 2015).
- Right time, right place (Ginsburg, 2015)
- Avoid sexuality conversations that are all *"don'ts"* (Ginsburg, 2015).
- Find out what your child is thinking when talking about their relationships or sexual experiences (Ginsburg, 2015).
- Talking about sex is difficult. When necessary, identify and encourage them to ask for help from other trusted adults; it doesn't always have to be you.
- Emphasize no means no to female and male adolescents.

Risk for Ineffective Sexuality Patterns • Related to Prenatal and Postpartum Changes

Goals

NOC
Self-Esteem, Body Image, Role Performance

The will express increased satisfaction with sexual patterns as evidenced by the following indicators:

- Identifies factors that can hinder sexuality
- Shares concerns

Interventions

NIC
Sexual Counseling, Anticipatory Guidance, Teaching: Sexuality, Body Image Enhancement, Support System Enhancement

Assess Sexual Patterns Before, During, and After Pregnancy

Prenatal

- Has the pregnancy made any changes in your life and sexual relationship? Increased/ decreased?
- Are there any concerns or worries engaging in sexual activity during pregnancy or afterward?
- What has your physician/nurse midwife said about sex during pregnancy?
- How does the pregnancy make you feel? (Ask both partners.)
- How do you feel about one another's experience of the pregnancy?
- What are your feelings about sex during pregnancy? Cultural influences?
- What have you heard about what you should or should not do sexually during pregnancy?
- Have you experienced any physical difficulties with intercourse during pregnancy?
- How do you think having a baby will change your life? How do you plan to manage these changes?
- What medications do you take?
- Have you had any recent changes in your health?

R: *Preparation of the woman and her partner for the changes associated with pregnancy, labor, delivery, and postpartum can reduce anxiety.*

Postpartum

- Are you still bleeding?
- Have you resumed sexual activity?
- Are you concerned about conceiving again?
- Has breastfeeding altered your sexual relationship?
- How has having a baby affected your sexuality?
- Is your episiotomy healed and comfortable during intercourse?
- Have you experienced a lack of lubrication since delivery?
- Do you ever have time alone with your partner?

R: *Exploring sexual patterns, concerns, and fears can provide opportunities to correct misinformation and to open dialogue between partners.*

Provide Facts Regarding the Effects of Sexual Activity on Pregnancy and Fetus (Pillitteri, 2014)

- Orgasm will not cause spontaneous miscarriage or premature labor.
- Foreplay involving the breasts (e.g., massaging) may release oxytocin. It may be contraindicated in a woman with a history of premature labor.
- Vasoconstriction and new growth of blood vessels during pregnancy may increase sexual pleasure during and after pregnancy.

- In woman with previous miscarriage or if vaginal bleeding is present, sexual intercourse may be contraindicated.

Reduce or Eliminate Contributing Factors

Body Changes

- Provide literature or suggested reading list to establish knowledge about pregnancy and changes.
- Refer to community resources.
- Refer to early pregnancy classes.
- Refer to childbirth preparation classes.
- View video about sex during pregnancy.
- Suggest alternative sexual positions for later pregnancy to prevent abdominal pressure:
  - Side-lying
  - Woman on hands and knees
  - Woman kneeling
  - Woman on top
  - Woman standing
  - Woman astride man
- Discuss postpartum changes.
- Provide literature.
- Give reassurance about these changes:
  - Episiotomy
  - Lochia—how long it will last, how it will change
  - Lubrication
  - Uterine resolution
  - Flabby abdominal musculature
  - Breast engorgement
  - Breast leakage during lovemaking
- Reassure the woman that this state is temporary and will resolve in 2 to 3 months.
- Refer her to a postpartum exercise class.

R: *Pregnancy is a time of stress for both man and woman; to deny physical closeness at a time when both partners are struggling can add to tension and alienation.*

R: *Preparation of the woman and her partner for the changes associated with pregnancy, labor, delivery, and postpartum can reduce anxiety.*

Change in Sex Drive

- Reassure the woman that sexual attitudes change throughout pregnancy from feeling very desirous of sex to wanting only to be cuddled.
- Support acceptance of whatever pleasuring may be desired. Encourage flexibility and alternative sexual patterns (e.g., oral sex, mutual masturbation, fondling, stroking, massage, vibrators).
- Encourage honest communication with her partner concerning desires or changes in interest.

R: *The woman may worry about her partner's acceptance; the man may be afraid of hurting the woman and needs to know that sexual activity does not harm the fetus.*

Fatigue

- Acknowledge this as a factor, especially during first trimester and again during the last month.
- Fatigue can be a major contributor to postpartum sexual problems.
- Encourage the individual to make time for her relationship, in sexual as well as other contexts.
- Encourage the individual to ask for help, hire a sitter, and so forth.

R: *Helping the couple understand what factors affect libido (e.g., fatigue) can reduce feelings of rejection.*

Emotional Liability

- Encourage the woman and/or partner to discuss emotions:
  - Postpartum emotional changes can be intense. They can be hormonally influenced but are aggravated by fatigue and loss of identity.
  - Conflicting feelings are common. Woman and partner need an opportunity to discuss.
  - Resentment of partner is common; this will certainly affect sexual rapport.
  - Resentment of the infant can create intense guilt and may cause the woman to cling more to the child and reject others. Or she may become depressed and less responsive to infant and partner.
  - Expression and acceptance of feelings are imperative.

- Listen—allow time for the individual to elaborate on feelings.
- Reassure that these feelings are normal.
- Recommend reading material.
- Refer to other pregnant couples for verification.
- Relate your own experiences, if appropriate.
- Refer to therapy, if indicated.

R: *Communication problems are the most common type of marital problems. Couples are encouraged to share their sexual needs and preferences.*

Fear of Damaging Fetus

- Reassure that, unless problems exist (preterm labor, previous early loss, bleeding or rupture of membranes), intercourse is allowed until labor begins.
- Refer to a physician for reassurance.
- Explore misinformation. Use anatomic charts to show protection of the baby in the uterus.
- Inform the couple that orgasm causes contractions that are not harmful and will subside.

R: *Barring complications, a pregnant woman is free to engage in sexual activity with her partner to the extent that it is comfortable and desired.*

Dyspareunia in Pregnancy

- Explore what pain is experienced and when.
- Suggest alternative positions:
  - Woman on top
  - Posterior–vaginal entry
  - Side-lying
- Suggest use of water-soluble lubricant.
- Refer to a physician/nurse midwife or nurse practitioner if pain continues.

R: *Alternative sexual positions can prevent abdominal pressure or deep penetration.*

Dyspareunia Postpartum

- Explore what pain is experienced and under what circumstances.
- Assess healing of the episiotomy:
  - The incision heals on the surface after 1 week.
  - Dissolvable stitches can take up to 1 month to resolve; there may be tenderness and swelling until then.
  - Nerves can remain sensitive and tender for as long as 6 months.
- Suggest varied positions.
- Suggest use of water-soluble lubricant (nursing women report reduced vaginal lubrication during the entire nursing experience).
- Teach the woman to identify her pelvic floor muscles and strengthen them with exercise:
  - "For posterior pelvic floor muscles, imagine you are trying to stop the passage of stool, and tighten your anus muscles without tightening your legs or your abdominal muscles."
  - "For anterior pelvic floor muscles, imagine you are trying to stop the passage of urine; tighten the muscles (back and front) for 4 seconds, and then release them; repeat ten times, four times a day" (can be increased to four times an hour if indicated).
- Instruct the woman to stop and start the urinary stream several times during voiding.
- Refer the woman to a physician, nurse midwife, or nurse practitioner if pain continues.

R: *Discomfort with sexual activity will decrease libido in women.*

Guilt Over Baby

- Encourage discussion; reassure that these feelings are normal; allow time to elaborate.
- Expression of these feelings often creates a release and relaxation.
- Include partner in discussion. (Both may have similar feelings they have not felt free to express to each other.)
- Refer to postpartum support groups.
- Refer to psychological or social assistance if pathology is observed.
- Encourage the couple to allow themselves to get help in caring for the infant. They need time alone. Suggest they arrange a "date" where they can be alone, with no threat of intrusion of a crying baby. They may then be able to rediscover or renew their intimacy.

Initiate Discussion With Her Partner Private

- Engage the partner alone to explore concerns, questions, life after a child.
- Advise to access online information on pregnancy, birth, and beyond for dads and partners is an excellent resource for partners during pregnancy, accessed at the National Health Service UK website.

R: *Fathers/partners need to make their own adjustment, both pre- and postnatally. They may feel lost, displaced, or left out. They may have confusing feelings of resentment, especially as the infant suckles the breast (Pillitteri, 2014).*

Fear of Pregnancy

- Encourage discussion.
- Explore contraceptive choices.
- Refer the woman to a nurse midwife, nurse practitioner, or physician for contraception.
- Inform the woman that breastfeeding does not provide effective contraception and that prepregnancy contraceptive devices may no longer fit.
- Warn that, although some oral contraceptives can be used while nursing, they usually significantly reduce milk supply.

R: *Fear of pregnancy can diminish libido in men and women.*

Teach Techniques to Increase the Couple's Connectedness (*Polomeno, 1999)

- Explore fears and anxieties (separately).
- Discuss barriers to disclosing fears and anxieties.
- Role-play disclosure of fears and anxieties.
- Encourage the couple to share the "little things" that represent caring.

R: *For women, "little things" that represent caring have the same value, whether it is helping with household chores or planning a dinner out. For men, small acts earn small points whereas big gifts earn big points (*Gray, 1995).*

- Instruct on "heart talks." One partner talks for 5 minutes with no interruption or arguing. The other partner then has a chance to talk. At the end, the couple hugs and says, "I love you" (*Polomeno, 1999).
- Instruct on "sexual conversation" (*Gray, 1995). Useful questions are:
  - What do you like about having sex with me?
  - Would you like more sex?
  - Would you like more or less foreplay?
  - Is there a way that you would like me to touch you?
- Talk regarding keeping romance alive.
- Set aside regular time with each other.
- Hold hands.
- Send messages that the other partner is appreciated.

R: *"Romance is important in keeping love, passion, and sex alive in a couple's relationship" (*Polomeno, 1999). Romance conveys to a woman that she is important and respected. When a woman appreciates her male partner's efforts, he feels more loved and encouraged to be more romantic (*Gray, 1995).*

Initiate Health Teaching and Referrals

- Teach couples to abstain from intercourse and seek the advice of their health-care provider if any of the following are present (Gilbert & Harmon, 1998):
  - Vaginal bleeding
  - Premature dilation
  - Multiple pregnancy
  - Engaged fetal head or lightening
  - Placenta previa
  - Rupture of membranes
  - History of premature delivery
  - History of miscarriage
- If any of the above is present, the couple should not engage in any sex play. Couples should be instructed to ask very specific questions about what is allowed and what is not allowed.

R: *Intercourse and orgasm are safe for most women, except those with high-risk pregnancies. Semen contains prostaglandin, which may hasten cervical thinning (Gilbert & Harmon, 1998). Orgasm even without intercourse is contraindicated in high-risk pregnancies in most circumstances.*

Sexual Dysfunction

NANDA-I Definition

The state in which an individual experiences a change in sexual function during the sexual response phases of desire, excitation, and/or orgasm, which is viewed as unsatisfying, unrewarding, or inadequate

Defining Characteristics*

Alterations in achieving sexual satisfaction and/or perceived sex role
Actual or perceived limitations imposed by disease and/or therapy
Change in interest in others and/or in self
Inability to achieve desired satisfaction
Perceived alteration in sexual excitement
Perceived deficiency of sexual desire
Seeking confirmation of desirability
Verbalization of problem

Related Factors

See *Ineffective Sexuality Patterns*.

Author's Note

See *Ineffective Sexuality Patterns*.

RISK FOR SHOCK

See also *Risk for Complications of Hypovolemia*.

NANDA-I Definition

At risk for inadequate blood flow to the body's tissues, which may lead to life-threatening cellular dysfunction

Risk Factors*

Hypertension
Hypovolemia
Hypoxemia
Hypoxia
Infection
Sepsis
Systemic inflammatory response syndrome

Author's Note

This NANDA-I diagnosis represents several collaborative problems. In order to decide which of the following collaborative problems is appropriate for an individual individual, determine what you are monitoring for. Which of the following describes the focus of nursing for this individual?

- *Risk for Complications of Hypertension*
- *Risk for Complications of Hypovolemia*
- *Risk for Complications of Sepsis*
- *Risk for Complications of Decreased Cardiac Output*
- *Risk for Complications of Hypoxemia*
- *Risk for Complications of Allergic Reaction*
- Refer to Section 3 for Goals and Interventions for the diagnoses listed above.

DISTURBED SLEEP PATTERN

Disturbed Sleep Pattern

Insomnia
Sleep Deprivation

NANDA-I Definition

Time-limited interruptions of sleep amount and quality due to external factors

Defining Characteristics

Adults
Difficulty falling or remaining asleep
Fatigue on awakening or during the day
Dozing during the day
Agitation
Mood alterations

Children
Reluctance to retire
Persists in sleeping with parents
Frequent awakening during the night

Related Factors

Many factors can contribute to disturbed sleep patterns. Some common factors follow.

Pathophysiologic

Related to frequent awakenings secondary to:

Impaired oxygen transport
  Angina
  Respiratory disorders
  Peripheral arteriosclerosis
  Circulatory disorders
Impaired elimination; bowel or bladder
  Diarrhea
  Retention
  Constipation
  Dysuria
  Incontinence
  Frequency
Impaired metabolism
  Hyperthyroidism
  Hepatic disorders
  Gastric ulcers

Treatment Related

Related to interruptions (e.g., for therapeutic monitoring, laboratory tests)*

Related to physical restraints*

Related to difficulty assuming usual position secondary to (specify)

Related to excessive daytime sleeping or hyperactivity secondary to (specify medication):

Tranquilizers
Sedatives
Amphetamines
Monoamine oxidase inhibitors
Hypnotics
Barbiturates
Antidepressants
Corticosteroids
Antihypertensives

Situational (Personal, Environmental)

Related to lack of sleep privacy/control*

Related to lighting, noise, noxious odors*

Related to sleep partner (e.g., snoring)*

Related to unfamiliar sleep furnishings*

Related to ambient temperature, humidity*

Related to caregiving responsibilities*

Related to change in daylight–darkness exposure*

Related to excessive hyperactivity secondary to:

Bipolar disorder
Attention-deficit disorder
Panic anxiety
Illicit drug use

Related to excessive daytime sleeping

Related to depression

Related to inadequate daytime activity

Related to pain

Related to anxiety response

Related to discomfort secondary to pregnancy

Related to lifestyle disruptions

Occupational
Sexual
Social
Emotional
Financial

Related to environmental changes (specify)

Hospitalization (noise, disturbing roommate, fear)
Travel

Related to fears

Related to circadian rhythm changes

Maturational

Children

Related to fear of dark

Related to fear

Related to enuresis

Related to inconsistent parenteral responses

Related to inconsistent sleep rituals

Adult Women

Related to hormonal changes (e.g., perimenopausal)

Author's Note

Sleep disturbances can have many causes or contributing factors. Some examples are asthma, tobacco use, stress, marital problems, and traveling. *Disturbed Sleep Pattern* describes a situation that is probably transient due to a change in the individual or environment (e.g., acute pain, travel, hospitalization). *Risk for Disturbed Sleep Pattern* can be used when an individual is at risk due to travel or shift work. *Insomnia* describes an individual with a persistent problem falling asleep or staying asleep because of chronic pain and multiple chronic stressors. It may be clinically useful to view sleep problems as a sign or symptom of another nursing diagnosis such as *Stress Overload*, *Pain*, *Ineffective Coping*, *Dysfunctional Family Coping*, or *Risk-Prone Health Behavior*.

Errors in Diagnostic Statements

Insomnia related to apnea

This diagnosis requires monitoring and comanagement by nurses and physicians; thus, the nurse should write it as the collaborative problem *RC of Sleep Apnea*.

Disturbed Sleep Pattern related to hospitalization

This diagnosis does not reflect the treatment needed. The effects of hospitalization on sleep should be specified, such as in *Disturbed Sleep Pattern* related to changes in usual sleep environment, unfamiliar noises, and interruptions for assessments.

Key Concepts

General Considerations

- Chronic sleep insufficiency is common in modern society and may result from a variety of factors, including work demands, social and family responsibilities, medical conditions, and sleep disorders. As sleep debt accumulates, individuals may experience reduced performance, increased risk for accidents and death, and detrimental effects on both psychological and physical health (Cirelli & Tononi, 2015).
- Sleep has two dimensions: duration (quantity) and depth (quality). When individuals fail to obtain adequate duration or quality of sleep, daytime alertness and function suffer. In response to sleep deprivation, sleep is often both longer and deeper. In many cases, however, sleep intensity can change without major changes in sleep duration. Sleep duration alone is therefore not a good indicator of how much sleep is needed to feel refreshed in the morning and function properly.
- Sleep involves two distinct stages: rapid eye movement (REM) and nonrapid eye movement (NREM). NREM sleep constitutes about 75% of total sleep time; REM sleep accounts for the remaining 25% (Grossman & Porth, 2014).
- The entire sleep cycle is completed in 70 to 100 minutes; this cycle repeats itself four or five times during the course of the sleep period.
- Sleep is a restorative and recuperative process that facilitates cellular growth and repair of damaged and aging body tissues. During NREM sleep, metabolic, cardiac, and respiratory rates decrease to basal levels and blood pressure decreases. There is profound muscle relaxation, bone marrow mitotic activity, and accelerated tissue repair and protein synthesis. During REM sleep, the sympathetic nervous system accelerates, with erratic increases in cardiac output and heart and respiratory rate. Perfusion to gray matter doubles, and cognitive and emotional information is stored, filtered, and organized (Boyd, 2004).
- The active phase of the sleep cycle, REM sleep, is characterized by increased irregular vital signs, penile erections, flaccid musculature, and release of adrenal hormones. REM sleep occurs approximately four or five times a night and is essential to an individual's sense of well-being. REM sleep is instrumental in facilitating emotional adaptation; an individual needs substantially more REM sleep after periods of increased stress or learning (Blissitt, 2001).
- Percentage of time in bed at night actually spent asleep, or *sleep efficiency*, influences perception of the quality of sleep. Studies report that younger people typically report sleep efficiency of 80% to 95%, whereas older people report 67% to 70% (Hayashi & Endo, 1982).
- Sleep deprivation results in impaired cognitive functioning (memory, concentration, judgment) and perception, mental fatigue, reduced emotional control, behavioral manifestations similar to those experienced in psychosis, increased suspicion, irritability, depression, and disorientation. It also lowers the pain threshold and decreases production of catecholamines, corticosteroids, and hormones (Boyd, 2004; Hickey, 2014).
- National Sleep Foundation (2015) recommends the sleep needed according to age as follows:
  - Newborns (0 to 3 months): Sleep range narrowed to 14 to 17 hours each day (previously it was 12 to 18)
  - Infants (4 to 11 months): Sleep range widened 2 hours to 12 to 15 hours (previously it was 14 to 15)
  - Toddlers (1 to 2 years): Sleep range widened by 1 hour to 11 to 14 hours (previously it was 12 to 14)
  - Preschoolers (3 to 5): Sleep range widened by 1 hour to 10 to 13 hours (previously it was 11 to 13)
  - School-age children (6 to 13): Sleep range widened by 1 hour to 9 to 11 hours (previously it was 10 to 11)
  - Teenagers (14 to 17): Sleep range widened by 1 hour to 8 to 10 hours (previously it was 8.5 to 9.5)
  - Younger adults (18 to 25): Sleep range is 7 to 9 hours (new age category)
  - Adults (26 to 64): Sleep range did not change and remains 7 to 9 hours
  - Older adults (65+): Sleep range is 7 to 8 hours (new age category)
- Hammer (1991) identified three subcategories of *Disturbed Sleep Pattern*: latency, or difficulty falling asleep; interrupted; and early-morning awakening.
- People with depression report early-morning awakenings and inability to return to sleep. People with anxiety complain of insomnia and multiple awakenings (Boyd, 2005).

- Hypnotics contribute to sleep disturbances through the following mechanisms:
  - Requiring increasing dosage as a result of tolerance
  - Depressing central nervous system (CNS) function
  - Producing paradoxic effects (nightmares, agitation)
  - Interfering with REM and deep sleep stages
  - Causing daytime somnolence because of a long half-life
- Sleep disturbances are reported by 50% to 100% of peri- and postmenopausal women. These sleep disturbances are caused by hot flashes and sweating caused by hormonal changes (Landis & Moe, 2004).
- Sleep disturbances in peri- and postmenopausal women are caused by the reregulation of neuroendocrine hypothalamic function and changes in the amount and type of sex steroid hormones. These changes affect mood, cognition, stress reactivity, body temperature, and sleep–wake cycles (Landis & Moe, 2004).

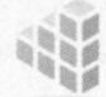 Pediatric Considerations

- Children exhibit wide variations in amount and distribution of sleep (National Sleep Foundation, 2015). Refer to age-related sleep requirements described earlier.
- Sleep affects a child's growth and development as well as the family unit as a whole.
- As children mature, the number of hours spent in sleep decreases. Moreover, the quality of sleep changes with maturity. Sleep is characterized as being deep and restful 50% of the time in an infant versus 80% of the time in the older child (Hockenberry & Wilson, 2015).

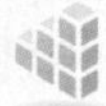 Maternal Considerations

- The activity of the fetus can interfere with sleep late in pregnancy. Dyspnea can occur if the mother is lying flat (Pillitteri, 2014).
- The effects of maternal rest/sleep deprivation may negatively affect the woman's ability to acquire and sustain her new role (Larkin & Butler, 2000).

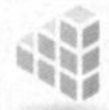 Geriatric Considerations

- Research has found that sleep efficiency declines with advancing age, so more time is needed in bed to achieve restorative sleep. Sleep time decreases with age (e.g., 6 hours by 70 years). Stages 3 and 4 and REM sleep decrease with aging (Hammer, 1991).
- Sleep pattern disturbances are the most frequent complaint among older adults (Hammer, 1991).
- Older adults have more difficulty falling asleep, are more easily awakened, and spend more time in the drowsiness stage and less time in the dream stage than do younger people (Miller, 2015).
- Miller (2015) reports that approximately 70% of older adults complain of sleep disturbances, usually involving daytime sleepiness, difficulty falling asleep, and frequent arousals.

Focus Assessment Criteria

Subjective Data

Assess for Defining Characteristics

Sleep Patterns (Present, Past)

Rate sleep on a scale of 1 to 10 (10 = rested, refreshed)

Usual bedtime and arising time

Difficulty getting to sleep, staying asleep, or awakening (number)

Naps

Observe vigilance by nursing staff in observing patients for snoring, apneas during sleep, excessive leg movements during sleep, and difficulty staying awake during normal daytime activities.

Sleep Requirements

To establish the amount of sleep an individual needs, have him or her go to bed and sleep until waking in the morning (without an alarm clock). The individual should do this for a few days. Calculate the average of the total sleeping hours, subtracting 20 to 30 minutes, which is the time most people need to fall asleep.

History of Symptoms

Complaints of

Sleeplessness

Fear (nightmares, dark, maturational situations)
Depression
Anxiety
Irritability

Assess for Related Factors

Refer to Related Factors.

Objective Data

Assess for Defining Characteristics

Physical characteristics
Drawn appearance (pale, dark circles under eyes, puffy eyes)
Yawning
Dozing during the day
Decreased attention span
Irritability

Goals

NOC
Rest, Sleep, Well-Being, Parenting Performance

The individual will report an optimal balance of rest and activity, as evidenced by the following indicators:

- Describes factors that prevent or inhibit sleep
- Identifies techniques to induce sleep

Interventions

NOC
Energy Management, Sleep Enhancement, Relaxation Therapy, Exercise Promotion, Environmental Management, Parent Education: Childrearing Family

Because various factors can disrupt sleep patterns, the nurse should consult the index for specific interventions to reduce certain factors (e.g., pain, anxiety, fear). The following suggests general interventions for promoting sleep and specific interventions for selected clinical situations.

Discuss the Reasons for Differing Individual Sleep Requirements, Including Age, Lifestyle, Activity Level, and Other Possible Factors

R: *Although many believe that a person needs 8 hours of sleep each night, no scientific evidence supports this. Individual sleep requirements vary greatly. Generally, a person who can relax and rest easily requires less sleep to feel refreshed. With aging, less time is spent in the sleep cycle stages 3 and 4, which are the most restorative stages of sleep. The results are difficulty falling asleep and staying asleep (Cole & Richards, 2007).*

Explain Sleep Insufficiency May be a Consequence of a Reduced Amount of Duration and/or Sleep Quality

R: *Sleep quality is determined by the number of arousals (or awakenings) from sleep during the night, as well as the percentage, duration, and type of sleep stages. It is possible for an individual to sleep eight or more hours and still be sleep deprived. In such cases, the sleep deprivation is usually due to disturbances in the quality of sleep.*

Explain the Effects of Sleep Deprivation (e.g., Cognition, Stress Management)

R: *Sleep deprivation results in impaired cognitive functioning (e.g., memory, concentration, and judgment) and perception, reduced emotional control, increased suspicion, irritability, and disorientation. It also lowers the pain threshold and decreases production of catecholamines, corticosteroids, and hormones. Sleep disturbance is the leading cause of hospital complications, such as falls, delirium (Colten & Altevogt, 2006).*

Explain the Need for Sleep Cycle

R: *Sleep cycle—An individual typically goes through four or five complete sleep cycles each night. Awakening during a cycle may cause him or her to feel poorly rested in the morning.*

Ask About Their Usual Bedtime Routine—Time, Hygiene Practices, Rituals Such as Reading—and Adhere to It as Closely as Possible

R: *Sleep is difficult without relaxation, which the unfamiliar hospital environment can hinder.*

Encourage or Provide Evening Care

- Bathroom or bedpan
- Personal hygiene (mouth care, bath, shower, partial bath)
- Clean linen and bedclothes (freshly made bed, sufficient blankets)

R: *A familiar bedtime ritual may promote relaxation and sleep.*

R: *Sleep is difficult without relaxation, which the unfamiliar hospital environment can hinder.*

Increase Daytime Activities in Assisted Living, Nursing Home, or at Home, as Indicated

- Establish with the individual a schedule for a daytime program of activity (walking, physical therapy).
- Discourage naps longer than 90 minutes.
- Encourage naps in the morning.
- Limit the amount and length of daytime sleeping if excessive (i.e., more than 1 hour).
- Encourage others to communicate with the individual and stimulate wakefulness.

R: *Early-morning naps produce more REM sleep than do afternoon naps. Naps that are longer than 90 minutes decrease the stimulus for longer sleep cycles in which REM sleep is obtained.*

Sleep Apnea

- All patients benefit from positive reinforcement while trying to acclimate to nightly use of a positive airway pressure device.

Promote a Sleep Ritual or Routine. Reduce Barriers to Sleep.

R: *Sleep rituals prepare the mind, body, and spirit for rest and decrease cortical responses.*

- Consume a desired bedtime snack (avoid highly seasoned and high-roughage foods) and warm milk.

R: *Warm milk contains L-tryptophan, which is a sleep inducer.*

- Avoid alcohol, caffeine, and tobacco at least 4 hours before retiring.

R: *Caffeine and nicotine are CNS stimulants that lengthen sleep latency and increase nighttime wakening. Alcohol induces drowsiness but suppresses REM sleep and increases the number of awakenings (Miller, 2015).*

Use Pillows for Support

R: *Pillows can support a painful limb, pregnant or obese abdomen, or the back.*

Explain the Need to Avoid Sedative and Hypnotic Drugs

R: *Sleep medications can increase awakenings and fewer total sleep hours (LaReau, Benson, Watcharotone, & Manguba, 2008). These medications begin to lose their effectiveness after a week of use, requiring increased dosages and leading to the risk of dependence.*

- Cluster procedures to minimize the times you need to wake the individual at night. If possible, plan for at least 4 periods of 90-minute uninterrupted sleep.

R: *To feel rested, a person usually must complete an entire sleep cycle (70 to 90 minutes) four or five times a night.*

- If the individual is being awoken for monitoring, use SBAR with prescribing professional.

SBAR

Situation: Mr. Nelo has slept only _ hours in the last 24 hours.

Background: He is not sleeping because ….

Assessment: He is complaining of more pain, wants a sleeping pill.

Recommendation: It would be useful to… (e.g., stop vital signs 10 PM–6 AM) unless needed, change the times for medication administration.

Provide Treatments Before 10 PM and After 6 AM When Possible

- Discuss with physician/NP/PA the use of a "Sleep Protocol." This will allow the nursing staff the authority not to wake a person for blood draws or vital signs if appropriate (Bartick, Thai, Schmidt, Altaye, & Solet, 2010):
  - Close the door to the room or pull the curtains.
  - Designate "quiet time" between 10 PM and 6 AM.
  - Lullabies were played over public address system.
  - Overhead hallway lights went off on a timer at 10 PM.

- Mute phones close to individual rooms, avoid intercom use except in emergencies.
- Vital signs were taken at 10 PM, and started again at 6 AM unless otherwise indicated.
- Medications are ordered bid, tid, qid, not "q" certain hours when possible.
- No administering a diuretic after 4 PM.
- Avoiding blood transfusions during "quiet time" due to frequent monitoring.

R: *A small study reported that "Sleep Protocol" can reduce the number of individuals reporting disturbed sleep to 38% and a 49% reduction in individuals needing sedatives (Bartick et al., 2010). Implementation of the sleep hygiene protocol permitted acutely injured or ill patients in our intensive*

care unit to fall asleep more quickly and to experience fewer sleep disruptions (Faraklas et al., 2013).

Advice Ancillary Staff/Student to Report the Amount of Time Spent Sleeping, Including Naps, Nighttime

R: *The quality and amount of sleep time with at least 4 periods of 90 minutes of uninterrupted sleep is the goal.*

Initiate Health Teaching as Indicated

- If poor sleep is contributing to daytime fatigue and pain, try the following tips to improve sleep at home (Arthritis Foundation, 2012):
  - Maintain a regular daily schedule of activities, including a regular sleep schedule.
  - Exercise, but not late in the evening.
  - Set aside an hour before bedtime for relaxation.
  - Eat a light snack before bedtime. You should not go to bed hungry, nor should you feel too full.
  - Make your bedroom as quiet and as comfortable as possible. Maintain a comfortable room temperature. Invest in a comfortable mattress and/or try a body-length pillow to provide more support.
  - Use your bedroom only for sleeping and for being physically close to your partner.
  - Arise at the same time every day, even on weekends and holidays.
  - Avoid long naps. If a nap is needed to get you through the day, keep it short, and schedule it well in advance of your bedtime. Try exercising in the afternoon rather than napping.
  - Avoid sleeping pills.
  - Avoid drinking alcohol near bedtime and caffeine-containing foods/drinks, coffee, tea, chocolate.
  - Don't smoke. If you must smoke, don't smoke before bedtime.
  - Use a clock radio with an automatic shutoff to play soft music at bedtime. If you are not a heavy sleeper, wake up to music rather than a clanging alarm.
  - Take a warm bath before going to bed.
  - Listen to soothing music or a relaxation tape.
  - Read before bedtime if you like, but avoid suspenseful, action-filled novels or work-related material that can preoccupy your thoughts and cause a poor night's sleep.
  - Use earplugs or white noise to block distracting noises.
  - Before going to bed, write down your worries and make a "things to do" list. Then put it away for tomorrow so you can stop thinking about them.
  - If you don't go to sleep within 30 minutes after going to bed, or if you wake up in the middle of the night and can't get back to sleep, get up and go to a different room. Try a relaxation technique, read, or listen to soothing music.
- Refer to thePoint: Getting Started to Sleep Better.

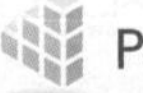

Pediatric Interventions

Explain the Sleep Differences of Infants and Toddlers (*Murray, Zentner, & Yakimo, 2009)

15 months	Shorter morning nap, needs afternoon nap
17–24 months	Has trouble falling asleep
18 months	Has a favorite sleep toy, pillow, or blanket
19 months	Tries to climb out of bed
20 months	May awake with nightmares
21 months	Sleeps better, shorter afternoon naps
24 months	Wants to delay bedtime, needs afternoon nap, sleeps less time
2–3 years	Can change to bed from crib, needs closely spaced side rails

R: *There are age-related sleep requirements and behavior.*

- Explain night to the child (stars and moon).
- Discuss how some people (nurses, factory workers) work at night.
- Explain that when night comes for them, day is coming for other people elsewhere in the world.

- If a nightmare occurs, encourage the child to talk about it, if possible. Reassure the child that it is a dream, even though it seems very real. Share with the child that you have dreams too.

R: *Children need to understand nighttime and be assisted to prepare for it. Preparation for bedtime involves switching the child from activity to bedtime gradually. It is a time for calmness, reassurance, and closeness.*

Stress the Importance of Establishing a Sleep Routine (*Murray et al., 2009)

- Set a definite time and bedtime routine. Begin 30 minutes before bedtime. Try to prevent the child from becoming overtired and agitated.
- Establish a bedtime ritual with bath, reading a story, and soft music.
- Ensure that the child has his or her favorite bedtime object/toy, pillow, blanket, and so forth.
- Quietly talk and hold the child.
- Avoid TV and videos.
- If the child cries, go back in for a few minutes and reassure for less than a minute. Do not pick up the child. If crying continues, return in 5 minutes and repeat the procedure.
- "If extended crying continues, lengthen the time to return to the child to 10 minutes" (*Murray et al., 2009). Eventually the child will fatigue and fall asleep.
- "The child should remain in his or her bed rather than co-sleep for part or all of the night with parents" (*Murray et al., 2009). Occasional exceptions can be made for family crises, trauma, and illness.

R: *"Bedtime rituals become a precedent for other separations and help the child strengthen a sense of trust and build autonomy" (*Murray et al., 2009). Co-sleeping with parents interferes with parental restorative sleep and promotes the child as in charge.*

- Provide a night light or a flashlight to give the child control over the dark.
- Reassure the child that you will be nearby all night.

R: *Children can be helped to learn that their beds are safe places. Bedtime is often difficult with sleep problems commonly related to resistance to separation and normal fears.*

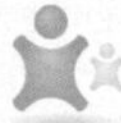

Maternal Interventions

- Discuss reasons for sleeping difficulties during pregnancy (e.g., leg cramps, backache, fetal movements).
- Teach to position pillows in side-lying position (one between legs, one under abdomen, one under top arm, one under head).

R: *Interventions that reduce discomfort of enlarging the uterus can promote sleep (Pillitteri, 2014).*

- Refer to Interventions for *Sleep Promotion Strategies*.

Geriatric Interventions

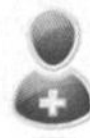

CLINICAL ALERT Excessive sleepiness may be caused by difficulty initiating sleep, impaired sleep maintenance, waking prematurely, sleep disorders, or sleep fragmentation (Chasens & Umlauf, 2012).

Older adults report obstructive sleep apnea (OSA), insomnia, and restless legs syndrome (Chasens & Umlauf, 2012).

Older adults report excessive sleepiness as a common symptom; unfortunately is often ignored. A focused assessment on this reported symptom is indicated to determine contributing factors and treatment (Chasens & Umlauf, 2012).

Refer Also to the Generic Intervention Discussed Earlier

Explain the Effects of Aging on Sleep Efficiency. Younger People Have 80% to 90% Sleep Efficiency and Older Adults Have 50% to 70% (Miller, 2015)

R: *Sleep efficiency is the percentage of time asleep during the time in bed (Miller, 2015).*

Explain the Age-Related Effects on Sleep

R: *Older adults have more difficulty falling asleep, are more easily awakened, and spend more time in the drowsiness stage and less time in the dream stage than do younger people (Miller, 2015).*

Consult with Primary Care Provider for Treatment on Medical Complaints That Interfere With Sleep

R: *Management of medical conditions, psychological disorders, and symptoms that interfere with sleep, such as depression, pain, hot flashes, anemia, or uremia (Chasens & Umlauf, 2012).*

Explain That Medications (Prescribed, Over the Counter) Should Be Avoided Because of Their Risk for Dependence and the Risks of Drowsiness

- If the individual needs sleeping pills occasionally, advise him or her to consult primary care provider for a type with a short half-life.

R: *Over-the-counter sleep aids contain antihistamines, which can cause dizziness and risk for falls.*

Insomnia

NANDA-I Definition

A disruption in amount and quality of sleep that impairs functioning

Defining Characteristics*

Observed changes in affect
Increased absenteeism (e.g., school, work)
Reports:
- Changes in mood
- Dissatisfaction with sleep (current)
- Lack of energy
- Observed lack of energy
- Decreased health status
- Increased accidents
- Waking up too early

Decreased quality of life
Difficulty concentrating
Difficulty falling or staying asleep
Nonrestorative sleep
Sleep disturbances that produce next-day consequences

Related Factors

Refer to *Disturbed Sleep Pattern*.

Interventions

NOC
Refer to Ineffective sleep Patterns

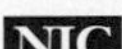

NIC
Refer to Ineffective sleep Patterns

- Have the individual keep a sleep–awake diary for 1 month to include bedtime, arising time, difficulty getting sleep, number of awakenings (reason), and naps.

R: *Sleep diaries provide data to improve the validity of assessment. Review the diary with the individual.*

R: *Examining the diary can identify if a sleep problem exists.*

- Evaluate if there is a physiologic condition or medication that is interfering with sleep. Refer to Related Factors under Pathophysiologic and Treatment Related under *Disturbed Sleep Pattern*. Refer to the primary care provider for management.
- Evaluate if a psychological state is interfering with sleep. Refer to Situational under Related Factors. Refer to mental health professions.
- Determine if the lifestyle or life events are interfering with sleep. Refer to other nursing diagnoses if appropriate: *Grieving*, *Stress Overload*, *Ineffective Coping*, or *Risk-Prone Health Behavior*.

R: *Sleep disturbances can have many causes with varied interventions.*

Refer to *Disturbed Sleep Pattern* for Interventions to Establish a Sleep Ritual or Routine

Sleep Deprivation

NANDA-I Definition

Prolonged periods of time without sleep (sustained natural, periodic suspension of relative unconsciousness)

Author's Note

This diagnostic label represents a situation in which the individual's sleep is insufficient. It is difficult to differentiate this diagnosis from the others. Refer to *Disturbed Sleep Pattern* for interventions.

Defining Characteristics

Refer to *Disturbed Sleep Pattern.*

Related Factors

Refer to *Disturbed Sleep Pattern.*

Goals/Interventions

Refer to *Disturbed Sleep Pattern.*

IMPAIRED SOCIAL INTERACTION

NANDA-I Definition

Insufficient or excessive quantity or ineffective quality of social exchange

Defining Characteristics

Social isolation is a subjective state. Thus, the nurse must validate all inferences about an individual's feelings of aloneness because the causes vary and people show their aloneness in different ways.

Discomfort in social situations*
Dysfunctional interaction with others*
Family report of changes in interaction (e.g., style, pattern)*
Impaired social functioning*
Dissatisfaction with social engagement (e.g., belonging, caring, interest, shared history)*
Use of unsuccessful social interaction behaviors

Related Factors*

Impaired social interactions can result from a variety of situations and health problems related to the inability to establish and maintain rewarding relationships. Some common sources include the following.

Pathophysiologic

Related to embarrassment, limited physical mobility,* or energy secondary to:

Disfigurement
Loss of body part
Post cerebral vascular accident (stroke)
Loss of body function
Terminal illness

Related to communication barriers* secondary to:

Hearing deficits
Mental retardation
Visual deficits
Speech impediments
Chronic mental illness

Treatment Related

Related to surgical disfigurement

Related to therapeutic isolation*

Situational (Personal, Environmental)

Related to alienation from others secondary to:

- Constant complaining
- High anxiety
- Rumination
- Impulsive behavior
- Overt hostility
- Delusions
- Manipulative behaviors
- Hallucinations
- Mistrust or suspicion
- Disorganized thinking
- Illogical ideas
- Dependent behavior
- Egocentric behavior
- Strong unpopular beliefs
- Emotional immaturity
- Depressive behavior
- Aggressive responses

Related to language/cultural barriers

Related to lack of social skills

Related to change in usual social patterns secondary to:

- Divorce
- Relocation
- Death

Maturational

Child/Adolescent

Related to inadequate sensory stimulation

Related to altered appearance

Related to speech impediments

Related to Autism spectrum disorders

Adult

Related to loss of ability to practice vocation

Older Adult

Related to change in usual social patterns secondary to:

- Loss of friends, relatives (relocation, death disability)
- Death of spouse
- Functional deficits
- Retirement

Author's Note

Social competence refers to an individual's ability to interact effectively with others. Interpersonal relationships assist one through life experiences, both positive and negative. Positive relationships with others require positive self-concept, social skills, social sensitivity, and acceptance of the need for independence. To interact satisfactorily with others, an individual must acknowledge and accept his or her limitations and strengths (*Maroni, 1989).

An individual without positive mental health usually does not have social sensitivity and thus is uncomfortable with the interdependence necessary for effective social interactions. An individual with poor self-concept may constantly sacrifice his or her needs for those of others or may always put personal needs before the needs of others (*Maroni, 1989).

The diagnosis *Impaired Social Interaction* describes an individual who exhibits ineffective interactions with others. If extreme, prolonged, or both, this problem can lead to a diagnosis of *Social Isolation*. The nursing focus for *Impaired Social Interaction* is increasing the individual's sensitivity to the needs of others and teaching reciprocity.

Errors in Diagnostic Statements

***Impaired Social Interaction* related to verbalized discomfort in social situations**

In this diagnosis, the individual's report of discomfort represents a diagnostic cue, not a related factor. The nurse performs a focus assessment to determine reasons for the individual's discomfort; until he or she knows these reasons, the nurse can record the diagnosis *Impaired Social Interaction* related to unknown etiology as evidenced by expressed discomfort in social situations.

Key Concepts

General Considerations

- Blumer (*1969) described three premises of human conduct and interactions:
  - Life experiences have different meanings for each person. People respond to situations and others on the basis of these meanings or significance.
  - People learn meanings from social interactions with others.
  - During encounters, people interpret and apply or modify their previous meanings.
- Social competence is one's ability to interact effectively with his or her environment.
- Effective reality testing, ability to solve problems, and various coping mechanisms are necessary for an individual to be socially competent.
- Both the individual and the environment contribute to impaired functioning. An individual may be able to function in one environment or situation but not in others.
- Adequate social functioning is associated most often with conjugal living and a stable occupation.

Chronic Mental Illness

- Chronic mental illness is characterized by recurring episodes over a long period. The extent to which role performance is impaired varies. The extent of impairment is related to social inadequacy.
- Disturbed thought processes may interfere with the individual's ability to engage in appropriate social or occupational role behavior.
- Dependency is one of the most consistent features presented. It may be seen through multiple readmissions requiring a large amount of clinician's time, resistance to discharge, resistance to any change including medication, and refusal to leave home.
- The origins of impaired social interactions in people with chronic mental illness vary. For some, it is the result of poor reality testing. If an individual cannot perceive reality accurately, it is difficult to manage everyday problems. For others, it may be the result of social isolation or the loss of interpersonal skills because of long-term institutionalization.
- The individual with chronic mental illness usually has no friends, is socially isolated, and engages in little community activity (Varcarolis, 2011).
- Deinstitutionalization has decreased the number of institutionalized people and the median length of hospital stay, thus changing the character of today's chronically ill population. An emerging group of people 18 to 35 years of age is distinctly different from older institutionalized adults in that their lives reflect a transient existence and multiple hospital admissions versus perhaps a safer, stable, long-term residence in a state hospital.
- People with chronic mental illness often lose their jobs, not because of an inability to do tasks but because of deficits in emotional and interpersonal functions. Social skills training has shown that skill-building programs improve posthospital adjustment (Halter, 2014).

Pediatric Considerations

- A child is significantly affected when a parent is emotionally disturbed. Emotionally disturbed parents may not be able to meet the physical or safety needs of their children.
- Young children depend on their parents to interpret the world for them. Parents with *Impaired Social Interaction*, *Confusion*, or both may not interpret experiences for the child accurately (Varcarolis, 2011).
- Impaired social interaction may result in social isolation. Also, see the nursing diagnosis *Impaired Parenting*.
- Adolescents with substance abuse problems use the substance to achieve popularity, to reduce stress, or both. Poor personal and social competence are also present (Johnson, 1995).
- Young people with chronic mental illness exhibit problems with impulse control (e.g., suicidal gestures, legal problems, alcohol/drug intoxication); disturbances in affect (e.g., anger, argumentativeness, belligerence); and poor reality testing, especially when under stress. The population varies from system-dependent, poorly motivated people to system-resistant people with low frustration tolerance and refusal to acknowledge problems (Varcarolis, 2011).
- Despite variations, children and adolescents with chronic mental illness share several factors (Varcarolis, 2011).
  - Difficulty maintaining stable, supportive relationships—most have transient, unstable relationships with marginally functional people.
  - Repeated errors in judgment—they seem unable to learn from their experiences or to transfer knowledge from one situation to another.
  - Vulnerability to stress—those experiencing stress are at greater risk for relapse.

- Patterns of social interaction are demanding, hostile, and manipulative, producing negative reactions among caregivers.
- Effective social interactions depend on positive self-esteem. No data suggest that older adults have diminished self-esteem compared with younger adults (Miller, 2015).
- In older adults, common threats to self-esteem include devaluation, dependency, functional impairments, and decreased sense of control (Miller, 2015).
- Depression-related affective disturbances of daily life occur in 27% of older adults. Major depression occurs in 2% of community-living older adults and in 12% of older people living in nursing homes (Varcarolis, 2011).
- Depressed older adults lose interest in social activities and do not display positive interactions when they do interact.

Focus Assessment Criteria

Subjective Data

Assess for Defining Characteristics

Relationships

Does he or she have friends or family?
Does he or she initiate friendships?
Does he or she initiate contact or wait for friends to make contact?
Is he or she satisfied with social interactions?
What is the reason for dissatisfaction with his or her social network?

Coping Skills

How does the individual respond to stress, conflict?
Substance abuse (drugs, alcohol, food)
Aggression (verbal or physical)
Withdrawal
Suicidal ideation or gestures

Legal History (Arrests, Convictions)

Assess for Related Factors

Interaction Patterns and Skills

Job Related

Job-seeking and interviewing skills
- Can identify own job-related assets
- Dresses appropriately
- Asks appropriate questions
- Identifies employment sources
- Can complete an application
- Has realistic employment expectations

Employment history
- Length of employment
- Reasons for leaving (problems with coworkers or supervisors)
- Frequency of job changes

Interactions with coworkers
- Contacts outside work

Living Arrangements

Residential patterns
- Where? Family, group home, boardinghouse, institution?
- How long?
- Frequency of relocation
- Reasons for relocation

Obstacles to community functioning
- Poor personal hygiene
- Legal problems
- Expects self-reliance

Unemployed
Lacks leisure activities
Unstable, transient residences
Inappropriate behavior in public
Social isolation

Leisure/Recreation
"What do you do with your free time?"
What interferes with participating in recreational activities?
Preference for individual or group activity

Objective Data

Assess for Related Factors

General Appearance
Facial expression (e.g., sad, hostile, expressionless)
Dress (e.g., meticulous, disheveled, seductive, eccentric)
Personal hygiene
- Cleanliness
- Clothes (appropriateness, condition)
- Grooming

Communication Pattern

Content
Appropriate
Worthlessness
Denial of problem
Homicidal or suicidal plans
Religiosity
Suspicious
Obsessions
Sexually preoccupied
Rambling
Delusions
Exaggerated

Pattern of Speech
Appropriate
Circumstantial (cannot get to point)
Jumps from one topic to another
Indecisive
Blocking (cannot finish idea)
Neologisms
Word salad

Rate of Speech
Appropriate
Reduced
Excessive
Pressured

Relationship Skills
Can listen and respond appropriately
Has conversational skills
Is withdrawn/preoccupied with self
Shows dependency or passivity
Is demanding/pleading
Is hostile
Has barriers to satisfactory relationships
- Social isolation
- Thought disturbances
- Severe depression
- Chronic mental illness
- Panic attacks
- Preoccupation with illness

Goals

NOC
Family Functioning, Social Interaction Skills, Social Involvement

The individual/family will report increased satisfaction in socialization, as evidenced by the following indicators:

- Identifies problematic behavior that deters socialization
- Substitutes constructive behavior for disruptive social behavior (specify)
- Describes strategies to promote effective socialization

Interventions

NIC

Anticipatory Guidance, Behavior Modification, Family Integrity Promotion, Counseling, Behavior Management, Family Support, Self-Responsibility Facilitation

> **Clinical Alert** Halter (2014) writes, "Individuals with serious mental illness are at risk for multiple physical, emotional and social problems: they are more likely to be victims of crime, be medically ill, have undertreated untreated physical illnesses, die prematurely, be homeless, be incarcerated, be unemployed, or underemployed, engage in binge substance abuse, live poverty, and report lower quality of life than persons without such illnesses (p. 585). They 'live in a "parallel universe" separate from "the normals."'"

Provide Support to Maintain Basic Social Skills and Reduce Social Isolation

- See *Risk for Loneliness* or Further Interventions.

Provide an Individual, Supportive Relationship

- Assist the individual to manage present stresses.
- Focus on present and reality.
- Help to identify how stress precipitates problems.
- Support healthy defenses.
- Help the individual to identify alternative courses of action.
- Assist the individual to analyze approaches that work best.

R: *The individual needs continual encouragement to test new social skills and to explore new social situations. In situations when assertive behavior is indicated, for example, state your requests or dissatisfaction, prepare them that aggression may be the response (Halter, 2014).*

Promote Participation in Supportive Group Therapy

- Focus on the here and now.
- Establish group norms that discourage inappropriate behavior.
- Encourage testing of new social behavior.
- Use snacks or coffee to decrease anxiety during sessions.
- Model certain accepted social behaviors (e.g., respond to a friendly greeting instead of ignoring it).
- Foster development of relationships among members through self-disclosure and genuineness.
- Use questions and observations to encourage people with limited interaction skills.
- Encourage members to validate their perception with others.
- Identify strengths among members and ignore selected weaknesses.
- Activity groups and drop-in socialization centers can be used for some individuals.

R: *The nurse models appropriate social skills and uses group therapy as other examples of social skills.*

Hold People Accountable for Their Own Actions

- Contact the individual when he or she fails to attend a scheduled appointment, job interview, and so forth.
- Do not wait for an individual to initiate participation.
- Treat individuals as responsible citizens.
- Allow decision-making, but outline limits as necessary.
- Discourage using their illness as an excuse for their unacceptable behavior.
- Set consequences and enforce when necessary, including encounters with the law.
- Help to see how his or her behaviors or attitudes contribute to their frequent interpersonal conflicts.

R: *Passivity or lack of motivation is a part of the illness; thus, caregivers should not simply accept it. Caregivers must use an assertive approach in which the treatment is "taken to the client" rather than waiting for him or her to participate (Varcarolis, 2011).*

Provide for Development of Social Skills

- Identify the environment in which social interactions are impaired: living, learning, and working.
- Provide instruction in the environment where the person is expected to function, when possible (e.g., accompany to a job site, work with the person in his or her own residence).
- Develop an individualized social skill program. Examples of some social skills are grooming and personal hygiene, posture, gait, eye contact, beginning a conversation, listening, and ending a conversation. Include modeling, behavior rehearsal, and homework.
- Combine verbal instructions with demonstration and practice.
- Be firm in setting parameters of appropriate social behaviors, such as punctuality, attendance, managing illnesses with employers, and dress.

- Use the group as a method of discussing work-related problems.
- Use sheltered workshops and part-time employment depending on level at which success can best be achieved.
- Give positive feedback; make sure it is specific and detailed. Focus on no more than three behavioral connections at a time; too lengthy feedback adds confusion and increases anxiety.

R: *Effective social skills can be learned with guidance, demonstration, practice, and feedback (Halter, 2014).*

- Convey a "can-do" attitude.
- Role play aspects of social interactions (*McFarland, Wasli, & Gerety, 1996):
  - How to initiate a conversation
  - How to continue a conversation
  - How to terminate a conversation
  - How to refuse a request
  - How to ask for something
  - How to interview for a job
  - How to ask someone to participate in an activity (e.g., going to the movies)

R: *Role playing provides an opportunity to rehearse problematic issues and to receive feedback. The nurse models appropriate social skills and uses group therapy as other examples of social skills.*

Assist Family and Community Members in Understanding and Providing Support

- Provide facts concerning mental illness, treatment, and progress to family members. Gently help family accept the illness.
- Validate family members' feelings of frustration in dealing with daily problems.
- Provide guidance on overstimulating or understimulating environments.
- Allow families to discuss their feelings and how their behavior affects the individual. Refer to a family support group, if available.
- Develop an alliance with family.
- Arrange for periodic respite care.

R: *Both individuals and families are under stress, and both may suffer from insufficiencies in empathy and understanding (Hasson-Ohayon et al., 2012). The individual's behaviors that strain the family include excessively demanding behavior, social withdrawal, lack of conversation, and minimal leisure interests. The family also affects the individual's ability to survive in the community by either supportive or unsupportive behaviors.*

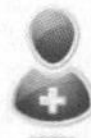

Clinical Alert "The rapidly growing body of research on internalized stigma has shown that self-stigma is associated with low self-esteem, low sense of empowerment, low social support, low hope, poor adherence to treatment and low subjective quality of life (QoL)" (Mashiach-Eizenberg Hasson-Ohayon, Yanos, Lysaker, & Roe, 2013).

Avoid Stigmatization and Stereotyping Individuals With Mental Illness and Participating in Discussions That Promote it (Corrigan et al., 2009)

R: " *Internalized stigma (or self-stigma) within the context of mental health refers to the process by which a person with a serious mental illness (SMI) loses previously held or hoped for identities (e.g., self as student or worker) and adopts stigmatizing views held by many members of the community (e.g., self as dangerous, self as incompetent)". Approximately, a third of people with serious mental illness experience high levels of internalized stigma that constitute a significant barrier to recovery (Mashiach-Eizenberg et al., 2013). Persons with SMI experience internalized stigma, reduced self-esteem, and self-efficacy, which might lead them to the "why try" model, thus avoid pursuing life goals (Corrigan Larson & Rüsch 2009; Mashiach-Eizenberg et al., 2013).*

Explore Strategies for Handling Difficult Situations (e.g., Disrupted Communications, Altered Thoughts, Alcohol and Drug Use Without Shaming, Excessive Criticism and Any Reinforcement That the Unsatisfactory Behavior Was Expected)

R: *Mashiach-Eizenberg et al. (2013) reported results that are consistent with previous research indicating that internalized stigma may lead to negative outcomes such as feelings of shame, diminished sense of meaning in life, and lessened sense of empowerment, social support, and quality of life (QoL). "Positive self-esteem affects the level of hope one has toward the future."*

Role Play With Family Members in Different Problem Situations

R: *This nonthreatening strategy can boost confidence for success in the family and project this expectation to the individual, which can increase his or her sense of "I can." Mashiach-Eizenberg et al. (2013) reported results that are consistent with previous research indicating that internalized stigma may lead to negative outcomes such as feelings of shame, diminished sense of meaning in life, and lessened sense of empowerment, social support and quality of life (QoL). "Positive self-esteem affects the level of hope one has toward the future."*

Refer to *Disabled Family Coping* or *Confusion* for Additional Interventions

R: *Helping the family learn strategies to handle problem behavior provides a sense of control over their lives (Stuart & Sundeen, 2002).*

Initiate Health Teaching and Referrals, as Indicated

- Teach the individual (*McFarland et al., 1996) with an emphasis on how they can be successful:
  - Responsibilities of role as individual (making requests clearly known, participating in therapies)
  - To outline activities of the day and to focus on accomplishing them
  - How to approach others to communicate
  - To identify which interactions encourage others to give him or her consideration and respect
  - To identify how he or she can participate in formulating family roles and responsibility to comply
  - To recognize signs of anxiety and methods to relieve them
  - To identify positive behavior and to experience self-satisfaction in selecting constructive choices
- Refer to a variety of social agencies; however, one agency should maintain coordination and continuity (e.g., job training, anger management).
- Refer for supportive family therapy as indicated.
- Refer families to local self-help groups.
- Provide numbers for crisis intervention services.

R: *Passivity or lack of motivation is a part of the illness; thus, caregivers should not simply accept it. Caregivers must use an assertive approach in which the treatment is "taken to the person" rather than waiting for him or her to participate (Varcarolis, 2011).*

R: *Community resources are vital to successful management and support.*

Pediatric Interventions

If Impulse Control Is a Problem

- Set firm, responsible limits.
- Do not lecture.
- State limits simply and back them up.
- Maintain routines.
- Limit play to one playmate to learn appropriate play skills (e.g., relative, adult, quiet child).
- Gradually increase the number of playmates.
- Provide immediate and constant feedback.
- Change your interactions with the child. Instead of long-winded explanations and cajoling, use clear, brief directions to remind your child of responsibilities.

R: *Failure to control impulses disrupts socialization (e.g., family, peers, school; Johnson, 1995).*

Discuss Selective Parenting Skills

- Reward small increments of desired behavior.
- Discipline effectively. Instead of yelling or spanking, contract appropriate age-related consequences (e.g., time out, loss of activity [use of car, bicycle, removal of privileges]).
- Avoid harsh criticism.
- *Do not* disagree in front of child.
- Establish eye contact before giving instructions and ask child to repeat back what was said.
- Teach older child to self-monitor target behaviors and to develop self-reliance.
- Help the child discover a talent. Finding out what your child does well—whether it's sports, art, or music.

R: *All kids need to experience success to feel good about themselves and can boost social skills and self-esteem. Families can be helped to learn effective parenting skills to enhance the child's success (Hockenberry & Wilson, 2015).*

If Antisocial Behavior Is Present, Help to

- Discuss realistic behavioral goals (Halter, 2014).
- Describe behaviors that interfere with socialization.
- Role play alternative responses.
- Limit social circle to a manageable size.
- Elicit peer feedback for positive and negative behavior.
- Consistently follow through with consequences of rule-breaking (Halter, 2014).
- Evaluate safety for the individual and for others.

R: *Skills that reduce social deficits can increase responsibility for personal actions and decrease blaming of others (Halter, 2014).*

R: *Failure to control impulses disrupts socialization (e.g., family, peers, school) (Johnson, 1995).*

Assist the Adolescent to Decrease Social Deficits With More Effective Social Skills as

- Assertiveness
- Anger management
- Problem solving
- Refusal skills
- Stress management
- Clarification of values

R: *Skills that reduce social deficits can increase social acceptance, control, and self-esteem.*

Role Play With Parents Different Problem Situations

R: *This nonthreatening strategy can boost confidence for success in the parents and project this expectation to the child/adolescent, which can increase his or her sense of "I can." Mashiach-Eizenberg et al. (2013) reported results that are consistent with previous research indicating that internalized stigma may lead to negative outcomes such as feelings of shame, diminished sense of meaning in life, and lessened sense of empowerment, social support, and quality of life (QoL). "Positive self-esteem affects the level of hope one has toward the future" (Eizenberg et al., 2013).*

SOCIAL ISOLATION

NANDA-I Definition

Aloneness experienced by the individual and perceived as imposed by others and as a negative or threatening state

Defining Characteristics

Absence of support system
Desires to be alone
Cultural incongruence
Developmental delay
Developmentally inappropriate interests
Disabling condition
Aloneness imposed by others and/or rejection*
Inability to meet expectations of others*
Insecurity in public*
Withdrawn
History of rejection
Feeling different than others
Illness
Meaningless actions
Member of a subculture
Purposelessness
Repetitive actions
Hostility*
Withdrawn*
Sad, affect*
Flat affect
Poor eye contact
Preoccupied with own thoughts
Values incongruent with cultural norms

Related Factors

Alteration in mental status
Alteration in physical appearance

Alteration in wellness
Developmentally inappropriate interests
Factors impacting satisfying personal relationships (e.g., developmental delay)
Inability to engage in satisfying personal relationships
Insufficient personal resources (e.g., poor achievement, poor insight); affect unavailable and poorly controlled
Social behavior incongruent with norms
Values incongruent with cultural norms

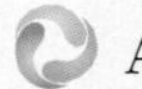

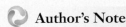

Author's Note

In 1994, NANDA added a new diagnosis: *Risk for Loneliness*. It more accurately adheres to the NANDA definition of "response to." In addition, an individual can experience loneliness even with many people around. In reviewing the defining characteristics and related factors listed above, some are repeated in both categories. This author recommends deleting *Social Isolation* from clinical use and using *Loneliness* or *Risk for Loneliness* instead. An individual with difficulty with communicating one to one or in group may avoid social interactions or experience negative responses from others. *Impaired Social Interactions* can be used to describe this person.

CHRONIC SORROW

Definition

Cyclical, recurring, and potentially progressive pattern of pervasive sadness experienced (by parent, caregiver, individual with chronic illness or disability) in response to continual loss throughout the trajectory of an illness or disability (NANDA-I)

State in which an individual experiences, or is at risk to experience, permanent pervasive psychic pain and sadness, variable in intensity, in response to a loved one forever changed by an event or condition and the ongoing loss of normalcy (*Teel, 1991)

Defining Characteristics

Lifelong episodic sadness to loss of a loved one or loss of normalcy in a loved one who has been changed by an event, a disorder, or disability
Variable intensity
Expresses feelings that interfere with ability to reach highest level of personal and/or social well-being*
Negative feelings of variable intensity, periodic, recurrent*
Anger
Loneliness
Sadness
Frustration
Guilt
Self-blame
Fear
Overwhelmed
Emptiness
Helplessness
Confusion
Disappointment

Related Factors

Situational (Personal, Environmental)

Related to the chronic loss of normalcy secondary to a child's or adult child's condition, for example:

Asperger's syndrome
Autism
Mental retardation
Spina bifida

Severe scoliosis
Chronic psychiatric condition
Down syndrome
Sickle cell disease
Type I diabetes mellitus
Human immunodeficiency virus

Related to lifetime losses associated with infertility

Related to ongoing losses associated with a degenerative condition (e.g., multiple sclerosis, Alzheimer's disease)

Related to loss of loved one

Related to losses associated with caring for a child with fatal illness

Author's Note

They coexist; they do not blend into one color or feeling. Because ours is such a "can do" society, there is pressure on families to quickly put their feelings of sadness away or deny them. Families are told to "think positively" and to "get on with your lives." They are told that God has "selected" them to receive this special child because they are such strong people. These kinds of comments, while well meant, deny the validity of parental long-term grieving. The discomfort of observing pain in those we care about can be part of the reason that others make such comments. Grieving is a process that takes time, often years.

Olshansky identified *Chronic Sorrow* in 1962. Chronic sorrow differs from grieving, which is time-limited and results in adaptation to the loss. *Chronic sorrow* varies in intensity but persists as long as the individual with the disability or chronic condition lives (*Burke, Hainsworth, Eakes, & Lindgren, 1992). *Chronic sorrow* can also accompany the loss of a child with heightened sorrow as time passes and events of birthdays, graduations, marriage are notably missing. *Chronic Sorrow* can also occur in an individual who suffers from a chronic disease that regularly impairs his or her ability to live a "normal life" (e.g., paraplegic, AIDS, sickle cell disease).

"Chronic sorrow does not mean that the families don't love or feel pride in their children. These feelings, and many other feelings, exist alongside the sadness. It is as if many threads are woven side-by-side, bright and dark, in the fabric of the parents/caregivers' lives" (Rhode Island Department of Health, 2011, p. 22).

Errors in Diagnostic Statements

***Chronic Sorrow* related to recent death of sister**

Chronic Sorrow is related to ongoing losses secondary to loss of normalcy and participation in events that hallmark our lives as holidays, scholastic achievements, being grandparent. This loss of normalcy can be related to a loved one with a condition that makes a certain relationship impossible. Death of a parent, sibling, or child can affect an individual, through his or her lifetime. The response to this loss initially can be grieving; however, over time the individual may continue to experience pervasive psychic pain. This response can be either *Chronic Sorrow* or *Complicated Grieving*. Careful assessment and discussion can help the nurse differentiate the two.

Key Concepts

- Chronic sorrow is cyclic or recurrent. It is triggered by situations that bring to mind the individual's losses, disappointments, or fears (*Lindgren, Burke, Hainsworth, & Eakes, 1992).
- Chronic mental illness produces a situation with no predictable end and thus can be a lifelong disruption for the family members (*Eakes, 1995; Halter, 2014).
- The usual grieving process is linear in nature with a final goal of acceptance and adaptation. "Prolonged chronic grief or mourning results when adaptation is not made; it is considered an abnormal response. These models of grief contrasted with Olshansky's (*1962) theory, which described chronic sorrow as ongoing yet periodic, as well as normal" (Gordon, 2009).
- Chronic sorrow is a functional coping response. It is normal, unlike pathologic grief or depression (*Burke et al., 1992; Gordon, 2009).
- Response to the death of a loved one could be chronic sorrow. For example, the death of a woman in her 30s could evoke a chronic sorrow response in a surviving sister.
- When a child is disabled, the initial response from the parent will be anxiety, family disorganization, denial, and grief. Then the parent will seek outside help. Unlike grief responses to death, which have some

form of closure, parents with *Chronic Sorrow* reexperience the grief response periodically (*Kearney & Griffin, 2001).

- When a loved one becomes inaccessible emotionally or cognitively, there are daily reminders of the lost relationship (*Teel, 1991). Many situations can trigger recognition of the loss of a hoped-for relationship, such as a school play, school dances, family vacations, dating, marriages, and grandchildren.
- Mallow and Bechtel (*1999) found mothers of disabled children responded with chronic sorrow, whereas fathers responded with resignation.
- Mallow and Bechtel (*1999) reported most fathers in this study depicted their adjustment as steady and gradual, while a majority of the mothers depicted their adjustment as having peaks and valleys.
- Parents of children with a developmental disability experience joy and sorrow, hope and no hope, and defiance and despair (*Kearney & Griffin, 2001).
- "Quality of life of children with cancer cannot be promoted without adequate support for families and caregivers. As mothers are the main caregivers in Iranian families (Rassouli & Sajjadi, 2014), it is essential to identify the psychological components that affect mothers' capability to deal with and adjust to their child's disease" (Nikfarid, Rassouli, Borimnejad, & Alavimajd, 2015, p. 4).
- Researchers found chronic sorrow frequency in mothers of children with cancer as "No chronic sorrow present," "likely chronic sorrow present," and "chronic sorrow present" were found in 2.3% (n = 6), 63.6% (n = 168), and 34.1% (n = 90) of mothers, respectively (Nikfarid et al., 2015).

Focus Assessment Criteria

Subjective Data

The Situation or Source of Sorrow
Perception/coping
Perception of child's abilities, language skills, motor skills, social skills, friendships, self-care abilities, past/recent illnesses (*Melnyk, Feinstein, Moldenhouer, & Small, 2001)
Milestones that increase chronic sorrow
Barriers to coping (*Melnyk et al., 2001)
Interfamily relationships
Social support
Financial issues and employment
Changes/stressors in family

Goals

NOC

Depression Level, Coping, Mood Equilibrium Acceptance: Health Status

The individual will be assisted in anticipating events that can trigger heightened sadness, as evidenced by the following indicators:

- Expresses sadness
- Discusses the loss(es) periodically

Interventions

NIC

Anticipatory Guidance, Coping Enhancement, Referral, Active Listening, Presence, Resiliency Promotion

Explain Chronic Sorrow

- Normal response
- Focus on loss of normalcy
- Not time-limited
- Episodic
- Persists throughout life

R: *Olshansky (1962) observed that parents of children with mental disabilities may suffer from chronic sorrow throughout their lives as a reaction to both the loss of the expectations they had for the perfect child and the day-by-day reminders of dependency (Gordon, 2009). He also encouraged professionals to recognize chronic sorrow as a natural response to a tragic situation in order to assist parents in achieving greater comfort living with and managing a child with a mental disability (Gordon, 2009). Emotions of chronic sorrow occur periodically and are ongoing (*Gamino, Hogan, & Sewell, 2002).*

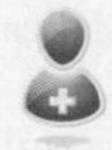

CLINICAL ALERT Gordon (2009) so perfectly writes:

On a busy workday, it may be difficult to take the time to listen to parents, so instead of ignoring the parents' feelings, the nurse can say, "I have five minutes to talk if you are free," or "Your feelings are very important to me, please give me ten minutes so I can have another nurse cover my patients, and we can talk." After five minutes, the nurse may conclude the conversation by saying, "I appreciate you sharing your feelings with me, and I think it is important that you continue to talk to someone about this. Would you like to talk to a counselor or pray with someone from pastoral care?"

Carp's Cues

Nurses who carve out 5 minutes of specific empathetic, dialoguing *thrive*. Nurses who do not simply survive. In the end both the nurse and the individual either triumph or not. Beware of believing you never have the time. Perhaps you feel that you need solutions if you initiate a conversation. Giving advice or solutions is not the purpose or productive, it is listening, clarifying, and validating. Never underestimate the power of 1, 2, 3, 4, or 5 minutes of caring!

Encourage to Share Feelings Since the Change (e.g., Birth of Child, Accident)

R: *Professionals recognize chronic sorrow as a natural response to a tragic situation in order to assist parents in achieving greater comfort living with and managing a child with a mental disability. Families report that open, honest communication is beneficial (Gordon, 2009). They need to know what to expect to help reduce life-span crises (*Eakes, 1995).*

Helpful Responses (Gordon, 2009)

- "You look like you have been crying; would you like to talk about it?"
- "It's okay to feel sad."
- "It sounds like attending the wedding triggered feelings of sadness related to your child not being able to marry/have children due to his/her disability."

Nonhelpful Responses

- "Getting married is not that important."
- "Your other children will get married."
- "At least your child is alive."

R: *By validating the parents' feelings, they are reassured that what they are experiencing is a normal response to a living grief (Gordon, 2009). Nonhelpful responses dismiss the person's feelings.*

Promote Hopefulness (Hockenberry & Wilson, 2015)

R: *Health-care professional may project the situation as hopeless and may interpret parent expressions of optimism as maladaptive (Gordon, 2009; *Kearney & Griffin, 2001). Hopefulness is an internal quality that mobilizes humans into goal-directed action (Hockenberry & Wilson, 2015).*

- Advise of age-related health promotion needs.
- Provide anticipatory guidance for maturational stages (e.g., puberty).
- Discuss possible age-related self-care responsibilities.
- Advise how to negotiate self-care activities between parent and child.

Explore Activities That the Child and/or the Parent Enjoy Doing

R: *Living with someone with a disability can include pain, suffering, and sorrow, but also joy, hope, and optimism (Gordon, 2009; *Kearney & Griffin, 2001).*

Acquire a Consult with Play Therapist

R: *Parents can receive "training in play therapy methods, and direct supervision from a play therapist" (Gordon, 2009). Through play therapy, children learn to communicate with others, modify behaviors, and express feelings (Gordon, 2009).*

Convey an Interest of Each Individual and Family

R: *Getting to know the family can help dispel stereotyping and gain an appreciation of "this family unit."*

Prepare for Subsequent Crises Over the Life Span

- Gently encourage the involved individuals to share lost dreams or hopes.

- Assist to identify developmental milestones that will exacerbate the loss of normalcy (e.g., school play, sports, prom, dating).
- Clarify that feelings will fluctuate (intense, diminished) over the years, but the sorrow will not disappear.
- Advise that these crises may feel like the first response to the "news."
- Provide siblings opportunities to share their feelings.

R: *An empathetic presence that focuses on feelings can reduce feelings of isolation (*Eakes, Burke, & Hainsworth, 1998).*

Explore Activities That Can Improve Coping on a Day-to-Day Basis as (Gordon, 2009)

- Accessing resources to learn more about condition, for example, library, Internet
- Regular stress-reducing activities, for example, exercising (yoga at home, walking, reading, crafts)
- Keeping a journal

R: *"Journaling may be beneficial in allowing parents to recognize, vent, express, and/or process their feelings" (Gordon, 2009).*

- Help plan how to have "a night out."

Encourage Participation in Support Groups With Others Experiencing Chronic Sorrow and Expression of Grief

- Stress the importance of maintaining support systems and friendships.
- Share the difficulties of the following (*Monsen, 1999):
  - Living worried
  - Treating the child like other children
  - Staying in the struggle

R: *Parents can learn successful coping mechanisms and prevent social isolation from other parents undergoing a similar experience. Researchers have reported mothers had a higher frequency of chronic sorrow than fathers (*Damrosch & Perry, 1989; Hobdell et al., 2007).*

- Professional approaches that involved encouraging/allowing expressions of sadness, and positive feedback on how they handled certain situations was appreciated (*Damrosch & Perry, 1989).

R: *Monsen (*1999) reported that parents of children with spina bifida had a pattern of coping that encompassed living worried, trying to treat the child like other children, and staying strong over the long haul.*

Acknowledge That Parent(s) Is the Child's Expert Caregiver (*Melnyk et al., 2001)

- Elicit routines from the parents.
- Prepare the family for transition to another health-care provider (e.g., child to adult providers).
- Differentiate between chronic sorrow and depression. If depression is suspected, parents should be referred to a psychiatrist/psychiatric nurse practitioner for proper assessment and diagnosis (Gordan, 2009).

R: *Major depressive disorder is considered a depressed mood or diminished interest in almost all usual activity for at least 2 weeks. "Roos (*2002) believes depression is a complication related to stressors that influence people who experience chronic sorrow, while Hobdell et al. (2007) suggests depression is a component of chronic sorrow" (Gordon, 2009).*

Link the Family With Appropriate Services (e.g., Home Health, Respite Counselor) (Gordon, 2009)

- Spiritual support to assist with grieving
- Social services, government services, for example, financial support, medical equipment needs, respite care, volunteers
- Refer individuals with children diagnosed with autism spectrum disorders to the "Resource Guide for Families of Children with Autism Spectrum Disorders," accessed at the Rhode Island Department of Health website; search for *resource guide autism*.

Carp's Cues

The above resource is full of first-person stories of caregivers that reflect reality, hope, and inspiration. Even if the affected individual does not have autism spectrum disorders, caregivers of individuals with unending needs will find these stories have remarkable insight.

R: *As needs change, new resources may be needed.*

Refer to *Caregiver Role Strain* for Additional Interventions

SPIRITUAL DISTRESS

Spiritual Distress

Related to Conflict Between Religious or Spiritual Beliefs and Prescribed Health Regimen
Risk for Spiritual Distress
Impaired Religiosity
Risk for Impaired Religiosity

NANDA-I Definition

A state of suffering related to impaired ability to experience meaning in life through connections with self, others, the world, or a superior being.

Defining Characteristics

Questions meaning of life, death, and suffering
Reports no sense of meaning and purpose in life
Lacks enthusiasm for life, feelings of joy, inner peace, or love
Demonstrates discouragement or despair
Feels a sense of emptiness
Experiences alienation from spiritual or religious community
Expresses need to reconcile with self, others, God, or Creator
Presents with sudden interest in spiritual matters (reading spiritual or religious books, watching spiritual or religious programs on television)
Displays sudden changes in spiritual practices (rejection, neglect, doubt, fanatical devotion)
Verbalizes that family, loved ones, peers, or health-care providers opposed spiritual beliefs or practices
Questions credibility of religion or spiritual belief system
Requests assistance for a disturbance in spiritual beliefs or religious practice

Related Factors

Pathophysiologic

Related to challenge in spiritual health or separation from spiritual ties secondary to:

Hospitalization
Pain
Terminal illness
Loss of body part or function
Trauma
Debilitating disease
Miscarriage, stillbirth

Treatment Related

Related to conflict between (specify prescribed regimen) and beliefs:

Abortion
Isolation
Surgery
Blood transfusion
Medications
Dietary restrictions
Medical procedures
Dialysis

Situational (Personal, Environmental)

Related to death* or illness of significant other

Related to embarrassment of expressions of spirituality or religion, such as prayers, meditation, or other rituals

Related to barriers to practicing spiritual rituals:

Restrictions of intensive care
Lack of privacy
Unavailability of special foods/diet or ritual objects
Confinement to bed or room

Related to spiritual or religious beliefs opposed by family, peers, or health-care providers

Related to divorce, separation from loved one, or other perceived loss

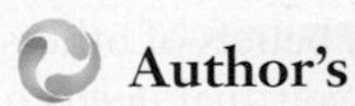

Author's Note

Wellness represents a response to an individual's potential for personal growth, involving use of all of an individual's resources (social, psychological, cultural, environmental, spiritual, and physiologic).

To promote positive spirituality the nurse can assist people with spiritual concerns or distress by providing resources for spiritual help, by listening nonjudgmentally, and by providing opportunities to meet spiritual needs (O'Brien, 2010; *Wright, 2004).

Spirituality and religiousness are two different concepts. Burkhart and Solari-Twadell (*2001) define spirituality as the "ability to experience and integrate meaning and self; others, art, music, literature, nature, or a power greater than oneself." Religiousness is "the ability to exercise participation in the beliefs of a particular denomination of faith community and related rituals" (*Burkhart & Solari-Twadell, 2001). Although the spiritual dimension of human wholeness is always present, it may or may not exist within the context of religious traditions or practices.

Impaired Religiousness was approved by NANDA in 2004. This diagnosis can be used for *Spiritual Distress* when a person has a barrier to practicing his or her religious rituals that the nurse can assist by decreasing or removing. *Impaired Religiosity* would be appropriate.

Errors in Diagnostic Statements

***Spiritual Distress* related to critical illness and doubts about religious beliefs statements of "My God has abandoned me"**

Statements of "My God has abandoned me" do not represent related factors but is evidence of *Spiritual Distress* (Defining Characteristics). Until related factors are known, the nurse can record the diagnosis as *Spiritual Distress* related to unknown etiology as expressed by statements of "My God has abandoned me."

For example, critical illness can challenge a person's spiritual beliefs and evoke feelings of guilt, anger, disappointment, and helplessness. If, after further assessments, critical illness is contributing to spiritual distress, then the diagnosis *Spiritual Distress* related to critical illness and doubts about religious beliefs statements of "My God has abandoned me" would be appropriate.

Key Concepts

General Considerations

- All people have a spiritual dimension, regardless of whether they participate in formal religious practices (O'Brien, 2010; Puchalski & Ferrell, 2010; *Wright, 2004). An individual is a spiritual person even when disoriented, confused, emotionally ill, irrational, or cognitively impaired.
- The nurse must consider the person's spiritual nature as part of total care, along with the physical and psychosocial dimensions. Research indicates that most persons feel religion is important in times of crisis (*Kendrick & Robinson, 2000; Puchalski & Ferrell, 2010).
- The spiritual may include, but is not limited to, religion; spiritual needs include finding meaning, hope, relatedness, forgiveness or acceptance, or transcendence (*Kemp, 2006, *Mauk & Schmidt, 2004). Other descriptions of spirituality include inner strengths, meaning and purpose, and knowing and becoming (*Burkhart, 1994; O'Brien, 2010), and by connection to self/others/God or a higher power (Puchalski & Ferrell, 2010).
- Health-care systems often give spiritual concerns low priority in care planning and delivery. This is less true in hospice organizations, where the spiritual component of care is more likely to be recognized and included (*Kemp, 2006; O'Brien, 2010).
- Religion influences attitudes and behavior related to right and wrong, family, child-rearing, work, money, politics, and many other functional areas.
- To deal effectively with a person's spiritual needs, the nurse must recognize his or her own beliefs and values, acknowledge that these values may not be applicable to others, and respect the person's beliefs when helping him or her to meet perceived spiritual needs.
- The value of prayers or spiritual rituals to the believer is not affected by whether they can be scientifically "proved" to be beneficial.

- Research indicates that many nurses feel inadequately prepared to provide spiritual care, and that fewer than 15% include spirituality in nursing care (*Piles, 1990). "Among the reasons that nurses fail to provide spiritual care are the following: (1) They view religious and spiritual needs as a private matter concerning only an individual and his or her Creator; (2) they are uncomfortable about their own religious beliefs or deny having spiritual needs; (3) they lack knowledge about spirituality and the religious beliefs of others; (4) they mistake spiritual needs for psychosocial needs; and (5) they view meeting the spiritual needs of persons as a family or pastoral responsibility, not a nursing responsibility" (Andrews & Boyle, 2012).

Pediatric Considerations

- James Fowler's *Stages of Faith Development* (*1995) includes "Undifferentiated Faith" (infancy) in which the nurse must be concerned with issues of parent–infant bonding as the infant struggles to establish trust, courage, hope, and love.
- In the "Intuitive-Projective Faith" stage (3 to 6 years; *Fowler, 1995), pediatric nurses are encouraged to acknowledge that the child's faith development is influenced by examples, moods, actions, and stories of their faith tradition.
- The "Mythic-Literal Faith" stage (7 to 12 years) of development includes the child's internalization of their faith's stories, beliefs, and observances (*Fowler, 1995).
- "Synthetic–Conventional Faith" (13 to 20 years) stage describes the adolescent's faith development outside of the family context in which faith is included as part of one's identity and outlook (*Fowler, 1995). This provides an understanding for the nurse of how the person interacts with family members and external peers.

Geriatric Considerations

- National Council on Aging defines spiritual well-being as "the affirmation of life in relationship with God, self, community, and environment that nurtures and celebrates wholeness" (*Thorson & Cook, 1980).
- There is disagreement among scholars whether older adults (older than 65 years) become more or less involved in religious or spiritual issues as they age (*O'Brien, 2010).
- Older adults tend to view the practice of religion as more important than younger adults (Nelson-Becker, Nakashima, & Canda, 2008).
- Although some of the physical and psychosocial deficits of older age may hinder one's religious practices, personal spirituality may deepen (*Kelcourse, 2004).
- Studies of religiosity among older adults demonstrate common religious practices among denominations: prayer, meditation, church membership, participation in religious worship services, study of religious teachings, and spiritual reading (*Halstead, 2004).
- For cognitively impaired older adults, traditional prayers learned in one's youth are sometimes remembered and can provide comfort (O'Brien, 2010).
- Factors that contribute to spiritual distress and put older adults at risk include questions concerning life after death as the person ages, separation from formal religious community, and a value–belief system that is continuously challenged by losses and suffering (*Nelson-Becker, 2004).
- Approximately 75% of all older adults are members of religious organizations. This does not necessarily mean that they attend formal services and meetings regularly (*Nelson-Becker, 2004).
- James Fowler's *Stages of Faith Development* (*1995) for adults include the Conjunctive Faith stage (midlife and beyond) in which the older adult may start to reincorporate earlier religious beliefs and traditions that were previously discarded. In this instance the nurse acknowledges the individual's more mature spirituality, which aids the person in finding meaning in his or her illness (O'Brien, 2010).
- As a common coping method for older adults, prayer increases feelings of self-worth and hope by reducing sense of aloneness and abandonment. In addition to private prayer and meditation, television and radio often provide adjunct stimuli for spiritual life (*Kelcourse, 2004).
- Older adults may rely on spiritual life more than most young people because of other limitations in their lives. The spiritual realm allows for satisfying connectedness with others. An older person can counterbalance some of the negative, isolating aspects of aging by identifying with tradition and institutional values. Private religion can help to motivate and provide purpose to life.

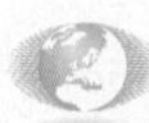

Transcultural Considerations

- Religious beliefs, an integral component of culture, may influence a person's explanation of the causes of illness, perception of its severity, and choice of healer. In times of crisis, such as serious illness and impending death, religion may be a source of consolation for the person and family and may influence the course of action believed to be appropriate (Andrews & Boyle, 2012; *Tinoco, 2006).

- Belonging to a specific cultural group does not imply that the person subscribes to that culture's dominant religion. In addition, even when a person identifies with a particular religion, he or she may not accept all its beliefs or practices (Andrews & Boyle, 2012; *Lipson & Dibble 2006; *Tinoco, 2006).
- The nurse's role is not "to judge the religious virtues of individuals but rather to understand" those aspects related to religion that are important to the person and family members (Andrews & Boyle, 2012). Box II.6 was compiled with the intent to assist nurses with this understanding.

Focus Assessment Criteria

Most spiritual assessment tools reflect a Christian theology rather than nonreligious spiritual practices. Assessment tools vary by discipline (chaplain, nurse, social worker, physician) and each may identify a particular aspect of spirituality upon which to focus. A comprehensive spiritual assessment should be completed by a professional spiritual care provider, but reassessment of spiritual needs should be performed routinely as the illness experience changes or progresses. A more comprehensive spiritual assessment may only be possible once a trusted nurse–individual relationship has been established. When assessing:

- Use open-ended questions.
- Assess for congruency between affect, behavior, and communication.
- Take note of any objects in the environment that bring the individual meaning, such as paintings, religious symbols, photos of nature, or music.
- Initiate assessment by acknowledging that questions may be of a personal or sensitive nature and assess the person's comfort level in answering.
- Note the language of the person's response and adapt questions accordingly.

Subjective Data

Assess for Defining Characteristics

What is your source of spiritual strength or meaning?
What is your source of peace, comfort, faith, well-being, hope, or worth?
How do you practice your spiritual beliefs?
What practices are important for your spiritual well-being?
Do you have a spiritual leader? If yes, would you like to contact him or her?
How has being ill or hurt affected your spiritual beliefs?
What influence does your faith or beliefs have on how you take care of yourself?
How have your beliefs influenced your behavior during this illness?
What role do your beliefs play in regaining your health?

Assess for Related Factors

How can I help you maintain your spiritual strength (e.g., contact spiritual leader, provide privacy at special times, request reading materials)?

Objective Data

Assess for Defining Characteristics

Current Practices
Any religious or spiritual articles (clothing, medals, texts)
Visits from spiritual leader
Visits to place of worship or meditation
Requests for spiritual counseling or assistance

Response to Interview on Spiritual Needs
Fear
Doubt
Anxiety
Anger

Participation in Spiritual Practices
Rejection or neglect of previous practices
Increased interest in spiritual matters

Box II.6 OVERVIEW OF RELIGIOUS BELIEFS

Agnostic

Beliefs

It is impossible to know if God exists (specific moral values may guide behavior)

Amish

Illness

Usually taken care of within family

Texts

Bible; Ausbund (16th-century German hymnal)

Beliefs

Rejection of all government aid; rejection of modernization

Legally exempt from immunizations

Armenian

See Eastern Orthodox

Atheist

Beliefs

God does not exist (specific moral values may guide behavior)

Baha'i

Illness

Religion and science are both important

Usual hospital routines and treatments are usually acceptable

Death

Burial mandatory; interment near place of death

Beliefs

Purpose of religion is to promote harmony and peace

Education very important

Baptist, Churches of God, Churches of Christ, and Pentecostal (Assemblies of God, Foursquare Church)

Illness

Some practice laying on of hands, divine healing through prayer

May request Communion

Some prohibit medical therapy

May consider illness divine punishment or intrusion of Satan

Diet

No alcohol (mandatory for most); no coffee, tea, tobacco, pork, or strangled animals (mandatory for some)

Some fasting

Birth

Oppose infant baptism

Text

Bible

Beliefs

Some practice glossolalia (speaking in tongues)

Buddhism

Illness

Considered trial that develops the soul

May wish counseling by priest

May refuse treatment on holy days (1/1, 1/16, 2/15, 3/21, 4/8, 5/21, 6/15, 8/1, 8/23, 12/8, 12/31)

Diet

Strict vegetarianism (mandatory for some)

Use of alcohol, tobacco, and drugs discouraged

Death

Last-rite chanting by priest

Death leads to rebirth; may wish to remain alert and lucid

Texts

Buddha's sermon on the "eightfold path"; the Tripitaka, or "three baskets" of wisdom

Beliefs

Cleanliness is of great importance

Suffering is universal

Christian Science

Illness

Caused by errors in thought and mind

May oppose drugs; intravenous fluid; blood transfusions; psychotherapy; hypnotism; physical examinations; biopsies; eye, ear, and blood pressure screening; and other medical and nursing interventions

Accept only legally required immunizations

May desire support from a Christian Science reader or treatment by a Christian Science nurse or practitioner (a list of these nonmedical practitioners and nurses may be found in the *Christian Science Journal*)

Healing is spiritual renewal

Death

Autopsy permitted only in cases of sudden death

Text

Bible; *Science and Health With Key to the Scriptures*, by Mary Baker Eddy

Church of Christ

See Baptist

Church of God

See Baptist

Confucian

Illness

The body was given by one's parents and should therefore be well cared for

May be strongly motivated to maintain or regain wellness

Beliefs

Respect for family and older people important

Cults (Variety of Groups, Usually With Living Leader)

Illness

Most practice faith healing

May reject modern medicine and condemn health personnel as enemies

Therapeutic compliance and follow-up are usually poor

Illness may represent wrong thinking or inhabitation by Satan

Beliefs

Expansion of cult through conversions important

May depend on cult environment for definition of reality

(continued)

Box II.6 OVERVIEW OF RELIGIOUS BELIEFS (*continued*)

Eastern Orthodox (Greek Orthodox, Russian Orthodox, Armenian)

Illness

May desire Holy Communion, laying on of hands, anointing, or sacrament of Holy Unction
Most oppose euthanasia and favor every effort to preserve life
Russian Orthodox men should be shaved only if necessary for surgery

Diet

May fast Wednesdays, Fridays, during Lent, before Christmas, or for 6 hours before Communion (seriously ill are exempted)
May avoid meat, dairy products, and olive oil during fast (seriously ill are exempted)

Birth

Baptism 8–40 days after birth, usually by immersion (mandatory for some)
May be followed immediately by confirmation; Greek Orthodox only: If death of infant is imminent, nurse should baptize infant by touching the forehead with a small amount of water three times.

Death

Last rites and administration of Holy Communion (mandatory for some)
May oppose autopsy, embalming, and cremation

Texts

Bible; prayer book

Religious Articles

Icons (pictures of Jesus, Mary, saints) are important
Holy water and lit candles
Russian Orthodox wears cross necklace that should be removed only if necessary

Other

Greek Orthodox opposes abortion
Confession at least yearly (mandatory for some)
Holy Communion four times yearly: Christmas, Easter, 6/30, and 8/15 (mandatory for some)
Dates of holy days may differ from Western Christian calendar

Episcopal

Illness

May believe in spiritual healing
May desire confession and Communion

Diet

May abstain from meat on Fridays
May fast during Lent or before Communion

Birth

Infant baptism is mandatory (Nurse may baptize infant when death is imminent by pouring water on forehead and saying, "I baptize you in the name of the Father, the Son, and the Holy Spirit.")

Death

Last rites optional

Texts

Bible; prayer book

Friends (Quaker)

No minister or priests; direct, individual, inner experience of God is vital

Diet

Most avoid alcohol and drugs and favor practice of moderation

Death

Many do not believe in afterlife

Beliefs

Pacifism important; many are conscientious objectors to war

Greek Orthodox

See Eastern Orthodox

Hinduism

Illness

May minimize illness and emphasize its temporary nature
Viewed as result of karma (actions/fate) from previous life
Caused by body and spirit not being in harmony or by tension in interpersonal relationships
Believe in healing responses triggered by treatment
Strong belief in alternative healing practices (e.g., herbal treatments, faith healing)

Diet

Various doctrines, many vegetarian; many abstain from alcohol (mandatory for some); beef and pork are forbidden; prefer fresh, cooked foods

Death

Believe in immortality of the soul
Seen as rebirth; may wish to be alert; chant prayer
Priests may tie sacred thread around neck or wrist, or body—do not remove
Water is poured into mouth, and family washes body
Cremation preferred—must be soon after death

Beliefs

Physical, mental, and spiritual discipline and purification of body and soul emphasized
Believe in the world as a manifestation of Brahman, one divine being pervading all things

Texts

Vedas	Ramayana
Upanishads	Mahabharata
Bhagavad-Gita	Puranas

Worship

Daily prayers, usually in home; quiet meditation
Rituals may include use of water, fire, lights, sounds, natural objects, special postures, and gestures

Jehovah's Witness

Illness

Oppose blood transfusions and organ transplantation (mandatory)
May oppose other medical treatments and all modern science
Oppose faith healing; oppose abortion

(*continued*)

Box II.6 OVERVIEW OF RELIGIOUS BELIEFS (*continued*)

Diet

Refuses foods to which blood has been added; may eat meats that have been drained

Text

Bible

Judaism

Illness

Medical care emphasized
Rabbinical consultation necessary for donation and transplantation of organs
May oppose surgical procedures on the Sabbath (sundown Friday to sundown Saturday; seriously ill are exempted)
May prefer burial of removed organs or body tissues
May oppose shaving
May wear skull cap and socks continuously, believing head and feet should be covered

Diet

Fasting for 24 hours on holy days of Yom Kippur (in September or October) and Tishah-b'Ab (in August)
Matzo replaces leavened bread during Passover week (in March or April)
May observe strict Kosher dietary laws (mandatory for some) that prohibit pork, shellfish, and the eating of meat and dairy products at same meal or with same dishes (milk products, served first, can be followed by meat in a few minutes; reverse is not Kosher; seriously ill are exempted)

Birth

Ritual circumcision 8 days after birth (mandatory for some); fetuses are buried

Death

Ritual burial; society members wash body
Burial as soon as possible
May oppose cremation
Many oppose autopsy and donation of body to science
Most do not believe in afterlife
Generally oppose prolongation of life after irreversible brain damage

Texts

Torah (first five books of Old Testament)
Talmud
Prayer book

Religious Articles

Menorah (seven-branched candlestick)
Yarmulke (skull cap, may be worn continuously)
Tallith (prayer shawl worn for morning prayers)
Tefillin, or phylacteries (leather boxes on straps containing scripture passages)
Star of David (may be worn around neck)

Beliefs

Observation of the Sabbath (Friday evening to Saturday evening) may require not writing, traveling, using electrical appliances, or receiving treatment

Krishna

Diet

Vegetarian diet; no garlic or onions
No drugs, alcohol; herbal tea only

Death

Cremation mandatory

Texts

Vedas
Srimad-Bhagavatam

Beliefs

Continual practice of mantra (chant)
Belief in reincarnation

Lutheran, Methodist, Presbyterian

Illness

May request Communion, anointing and blessing, or visitation by minister or elder
Generally encourages use of medical science

Birth

Baptism by sprinkling or immersion of infants, children, or adults

Death

Optional last rites or scripture reading

Texts

Bible; prayer book

Mennonite

Illness

Opposes laying on of hands; may oppose shock treatment and drugs

Texts

Bible; 18 articles of the Dordrecht Confession of Faith

Beliefs

Shun modernization; no participation in government, pensions, or health plans

Methodist

See Lutheran

Mormon (Church of Jesus Christ of Latter-Day Saints)

Illness

May come through partaking of harmful substances such as alcohol, tobacco, drugs, and so forth
May be seen as a necessary part of the plan of salvation
May desire Sacrament of the Lord's Supper to be administered by a Church Priesthood holder
Divine healing through laying on of hands
Church may provide financial support during illness

Diet

Prohibits alcohol, tobacco, and hot drinks (tea and coffee); sparing use of meats

Birth

No infant baptism; infants are born innocent

(continued)

Box II.6 OVERVIEW OF RELIGIOUS BELIEFS *(continued)*

Death

Cremation is opposed

Texts

Bible

Book of Mormon

Beliefs

Special undergarment may be worn by both men and women and should not be removed except during serious illness, childbirth, emergencies, and so forth

Beliefs

Abortion is opposed

Vicarious baptism for deceased who were not baptized in life

Muslim (Islamic, Moslem) and Black Muslim

Illness

Opposes faith healing; favors every effort to prolong life

May be noncompliant because of fatalistic view (illness is God's will)

Group prayer may be helpful—no priests

Diet

Pork is prohibited

May oppose alcohol and traditional black American foods (corn bread, collard greens)

Fasts sunrise to sunset during Ramadan (ninth month of Muslim year—falls different time each year on Western calendar; seriously ill are exempted)

Birth

Circumcision practiced with accompanying ceremony

Aborted fetus after 30 days is treated as human being

Death

Confession of sins before death, with family present if possible; may wish to face toward Mecca

Family follows specific procedure for washing and preparing body, which is then turned to face Mecca

May oppose autopsy and organ transplantation

Funeral usually within 24 hours after death

Texts

Koran (scriptures); Hadith (traditions)

Prayer

Five times daily—on rising, midday, afternoon, early evening, and before bed—facing Mecca and kneeling on prayer rug

Ritual washing after prayer

Beliefs

All activities (including sleep) restricted to what is necessary for health

Personal cleanliness very important

All Muslims: Gambling and idol worship prohibited

Pentecostal

See Baptist

Presbyterian

See Lutheran

Quakers

See Friends

Roman Catholic

Illness

Allowed by God because of man's sins, but not considered personal punishment

May desire confession (penance) and Communion

Anointing of sick for all seriously ill individuals (some individuals may equate this with "Last Rites" and assume they are dying)

Donation and transplantation of organs permitted

Burial of amputated limbs (mandatory for some)

Diet

Fasting or abstaining from meat mandatory on Ash Wednesday and Good Friday (seriously ill are exempted); optional during Lent and on Fridays

Fasts from solid food for 1 hour and abstains from alcohol for 3 hours before receiving Communion (mandatory; seriously ill are exempted)

Birth

Baptism of infants and aborted fetuses mandatory (nurse may baptize in case of imminent death by sprinkling water on the forehead and saying, "I baptize you in the name of the Father, of the Son, and of the Holy Ghost")

Death

Anointing of sick (mandatory)

Extraordinary artificial means of sustaining life are unnecessary.

Texts

Bible; prayer book

Religious Articles

Rosary, crucifix, saints' medals, statues, holy water, lit candles

Other

Attendance at mass required (seriously ill are exempted) on Sundays or late Saturday and on holy days (1/1, 8/15, 11/1, 12/8, 12/25, and 40 days after Easter)

Sacrament of Penance at least yearly (mandatory)

Opposes abortion

Russian Orthodox

See Eastern Orthodox

Seventh-Day Adventist (Advent Christian Church)

Illness

May desire baptism or Communion

Some believe in divine healing

May oppose hypnosis

May refuse treatment on the Sabbath (sundown Friday to sundown Saturday)

Healthful diet and lifestyle are stressed

Diet

No alcohol, coffee, tea, narcotics, or stimulants (mandatory)

Some abstain from pork, other meat, and shellfish

Birth

Opposes infant baptism

Text

Bible, especially Ten Commandments and Old Testament

(continued)

Box II.6 OVERVIEW OF RELIGIOUS BELIEFS *(continued)*

Shinto

Illness

May believe in prayer healing
Great concern for personal cleanliness
Physical health may be valued because of emphasis on joy and beauty of life
Family extremely important in giving care and providing emotional support

Beliefs

Worships ancestors, ancient heroes, and nature
Traditions emphasized; aesthetically pleasing area for worship important

Sikhism

Diet

Frequently vegetarian; may exclude eggs and fish

Religious Articles

Men may wear uncut hair, a wooden comb, an iron wrist band, a short sword, and short trousers. These symbols should not be disturbed.

Death

Cremation mandatory, usually within 24 hours after death

Text

Guru Granth Sahib

Taoist

Illness

Illness is seen as part of the health/illness dualism
May be resigned to and accepting of illness
May consider medical treatment as interference

Death

Seen as natural part of life; body is kept in house for 49 days
Mourning follows specific ritual patterns

Text

Tao-te-ching by Lao-tzu

Beliefs

Aesthetically pleasing area for meditation important

Unitarian Universalist

Illness

Reason, knowledge, and individual responsibility are emphasized, so may prefer not to see clergy

Birth

Most do not practice infant baptism

Death

Prefer cremation

Zen

Meditation using lotus position (many hours and years are spent in meditation and contemplation): Goal is to discover simplicity.

Illness

May wish consultation with Zen master

Goals

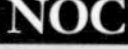

Hope, Spiritual Well-Being

The person will find meaning and purpose in life, even during illness, as evidenced by the following indicators:

- The person expresses his or her feelings related to beliefs and spirituality.
- The person describes his or her spiritual belief system as it relates to illness.
- The person finds meaning and comfort in religious or spiritual practice.

Interventions

NIC

Spiritual Growth Facilitation, Hope Instillation, Active Listening, Presence, Emotional Support, Spiritual Support

Create an Environment of Trust (Puchalski & Ferrell, 2010)

- Be open to listening to the patient's story, not just the medical facts.
- Listen for the content, emotion and manner, and spiritual meanings.
- Give "permission" to discuss spiritual matters with the nurse by bringing up the subject of spiritual welfare, if necessary.
- Be fully present.

R: *The nurse should practice with a confidence to initiate spiritual dialogues and as an advocate in recognizing and respecting the person's spiritual needs (*Mauk & Schmidt, 2004).*

Eliminate or Reduce Causative and Contributing Factors, If Possible

Feeling Threatened and Vulnerable Because of Symptoms or Possible Death

- Inform individuals and families about the importance of finding meaning in illness.
- Suggest using prayer, imagery, and meditation to reduce anxiety and provide hope and a sense of control.

Failure of Spiritual Beliefs to Provide Explanation or Comfort During Crisis of Illness/Suffering/Impending Death

- Use questions about past beliefs and spiritual experiences to assist the person in putting this life event into wider perspective.
- Offer to contact the usual or a new spiritual leader.
- Offer to pray/meditate/read with the person if you are comfortable with this, or arrange for another member of the health-care team if more appropriate.
- Provide uninterrupted quiet time for prayer/reading/meditation on spiritual concerns.

R: *The nurse should practice with a confidence to initiate spiritual dialogues and as an advocate in recognizing and respecting the person's spiritual needs (*Mauk & Schmidt, 2004).*

Conflict Between Religious or Spiritual Beliefs and Prescribed Health Regimen

Reduce or Eliminate for Causative and Contributing Factors

- Lack of information about or understanding of spiritual restrictions
- Lack of information about or understanding of health regimen
- Informed, true conflict
- Parental conflict concerning treatment of their child
- Lack of time for deliberation before emergency treatment or surgery
- Practice as an advocate for the person and family.

Doubting Quality of Own Faith to Deal with Current Illness/Suffering/Death

- Be available and willing to listen when person expresses self-doubt, guilt, or other negative feelings.
- Silence, touch, or both may be useful in communicating the nurse's presence and support during times of doubt or despair.
- Offer to contact usual or new spiritual leader.

R: *Research shows that people with higher levels of spiritual well-being tend to experience lower levels of anxiety. For many people, spiritual activities provide a direct coping action and may improve adaptation to illness (Puchalski & Ferrell, 2010).*

Anger Toward God/Supreme Deity or Spiritual Beliefs for Allowing or Causing Illness/Suffering/Death

- Express that anger toward God/Supreme Deity is a common reaction to illness/suffering/death.
- Help to recognize and discuss feelings of anger.

R: *The individual may view anger at God and a religious leader as "forbidden" and may be reluctant to initiate discussions of spiritual conflicts (*Kemp, 2006).*

- Allow to problem-solve to find ways to express and relieve anger.
- Offer to contact the usual spiritual leader or offer to contact another spiritual support person (e.g., pastoral care, hospital chaplain) if the person cannot share feelings with the usual spiritual lead.

R: *The nurse should be the link between the family and other members of the health-care team.*

Lack of Information About Spiritual Restrictions

- Have the spiritual leader discuss restrictions and exemptions as they apply to those who are seriously ill or hospitalized.
- Provide reading materials on religious and spiritual restrictions and exemptions.
- Encourage the person to seek information from and discuss restrictions with spiritual leader and/or others in the spiritual group.
- Chart the results of these discussions.

R: *Interventions focus on providing information about all alternatives and the consequences of each option.*

Informed, True Conflict

- Encourage the person and physician/nurse practitioner to consider alternative methods of therapy.
- Support the person making an informed decision—even if the decision conflicts with nurse's own values.

R: *Interventions focus on providing information about all alternatives and the consequences of each option.*

Parental Conflict Over Treatment of the Child

- If parents refuse treatment of the child, follow the interventions under informed conflict discussed earlier.
- If parents still refuse treatment, the physician or hospital administrator may obtain a court order appointing a temporary guardian to consent to treatment.

R: *Court orders to save a child's life remove the parent's right to refuse (Hockenberry & Wilson, 2015).*

- Call the spiritual leader to support the parents (and possibly the child).
- Encourage expression of negative feelings.

R: *The nurse should be the link between the family and other members of the health-care team.*

Spiritual Distress • Related to Conflict Between Religious or Spiritual Beliefs and Prescribed Health Regimen

Goals

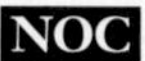

NOC Refer to *Spiritual Distress*.

The person will find meaning and purpose in life, including the illness experience, as evidenced by the following indicators:

- Expresses decreased feelings of guilt and fear
- Relates that the person is supported in decisions about his or her health regimen
- States that conflict has been eliminated or reduced

Interventions

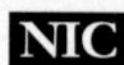

NIC Refer to *Spiritual Distress*.

Assess for Causative and Contributing Factors (See Box II.6)

- Lack of information about or understanding of spiritual restrictions
- Lack of information about or understanding of health regimen
- Informed, true conflict
- Parental conflict concerning treatment of their child
- Lack of time for deliberation before emergency treatment or surgery

R: *The nurse's role is as an advocate for the family.*

R: *Interventions focus on providing information about all alternatives and the consequences of each option.*

R: *The nurse should be the link between the family and other members of the health-care team.*

R: *Court orders to save a child's life remove the parents' right to refuse (Hockenberry & Wilson, 2015).*

Eliminate or Reduce Causative and Contributing Factors, If Possible

Lack of Information About Spiritual Restrictions

- Have the spiritual leader discuss restrictions and exemptions as they apply to those who are seriously ill or hospitalized.
- Provide reading materials about religious and spiritual restrictions and exemptions.
- Encourage the person to seek information from and discuss restrictions with others in the spiritual group.
- Chart the results of these discussions.

R: *The nurse's role is as an advocate for the family.*

R: *Interventions focus on providing information about all alternatives and the consequences of each option.*

R: *The nurse should be the link between the family and other members of the health-care team.*

Lack of Information About Health Regimen

- Provide accurate information about health regimen, treatments, and medications.
- Explain the nature and purpose of therapy.
- Discuss possible outcomes without therapy; be factual and honest, but do not attempt to frighten or force the person to accept treatment.

R: *The nurse's role is as an advocate for the family.*

R: *Interventions focus on providing information about all alternatives and the consequences of each option.*

Informed, True Conflict

- Encourage the person and physician to consider alternative methods of therapy.*
- Support the person making an informed decision—even if the decision conflicts with nurse's own values.
- Nurse can consult own spiritual leader.
- Change assignment so a nurse with compatible beliefs can care for the person.
- Arrange for discussions among health-care team to share feelings.

R: *The nurse's role is as an advocate for the family.*

R: *Interventions focus on providing information about all alternatives and the consequences of each option.*

Parental Conflict Over Treatment of the Child

- If parents refuse treatment for the child, follow the interventions under Informed, True Conflict.
- If parents still refuse treatment, the physician or hospital administrator may obtain a court order appointing a temporary guardian to consent to treatment.
- Call the spiritual leader to support the parents (and possibly the child).
- Encourage expression of negative feelings.

R: *The nurse's role is as an advocate for the family.*

R: *Interventions focus on providing information about all alternatives and the consequences of each option.*

R: *The nurse should be the link between the family and other members of the health-care team.*

R: *Court orders to save a child's life remove the parents' right to refuse (Hockenberry & Wilson, 2015).*

Emergency Treatment

- Consult the family if possible.
- Delay treatment, if possible, until spiritual needs have been met (e.g., receiving last rites before surgery)[49]; send the spiritual leader to the treatment room or operating room, if necessary.
- Anticipate reaction and provide support when the person chooses or is forced to accept spiritually unacceptable therapy.
  - Depression, withdrawal, anger, and fear
  - Loss of will to live
  - Reduced speed and quality of recovery

R: *The nurse's role is as an advocate for the family.*

R: *Interventions focus on providing information about all alternatives and the consequences of each option.*

Risk for Spiritual Distress

NANDA-I Definition

At risk for an impaired ability to experience and integrate meaning and purpose in life through connectedness with self, others, art, music, literature, nature, and/or a power greater than oneself

Risk Factors

Refer to *Spiritual Distress.*

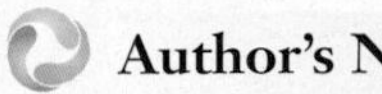

Author's Note

Refer to *Spiritual Distress.*

Errors in Diagnostic Statements

Refer to *Spiritual Distress.*

[49]May require a primary care professional's order.

Key Concepts

Refer to *Spiritual Distress.*

Goals

NOC

Refer to *Spiritual Distress.*

The person will find meaning and purpose in life, including during illness, as evidenced by the following indicators:

- Practices spiritual rituals
- Expresses comfort with beliefs

Interventions

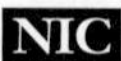

Refer to *Spiritual Distress.*

Refer to *Spiritual Distress.*

Impaired Religiosity

NANDA-I Definition

Impaired ability to exercise reliance on beliefs and/or participate in rituals of a particular faith tradition

Defining Characteristics

Individuals experience distress because of difficulty with adhering to prescribed religious rituals such as the following:

Religious ceremonies
Dietary regulations
Certain clothing
Prayer
Request to worship
Holiday observances
Separation from faith community*
Emotional distress regarding religious beliefs, religious social network, or both
Need to reconnect with previous belief patterns and customs
Questioning of religious belief patterns and customs*

Related Factors

Pathophysiologic

Related to sickness/illness*

Related to suffering

Related to pain*

Situational (Personal, Environmental)

Related to personal crisis* secondary to activity

Related to fear of death*

Related to embarrassment at practicing spiritual rituals

Related to barriers to practicing spiritual rituals

Intensive care restrictions

Confinement to bed or the room
Lack of privacy
Lack of availability of special foods/diets
Hospitalization

Related to crisis within the faith community, which causes distress in the believer

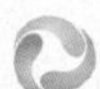

Author's Note

Refer to *Spiritual Distress*.

Key Concepts

- Refer to *Spiritual Distress*.
- To assist people in spiritual distress, the nurse must know certain beliefs and practices of various spiritual groups. Box II.6 provides information about the beliefs and practices that relate most directly to health and illness. It is intended as a reference only. Major religions, denominations, and spiritual groups are arranged alphabetically. Denominations with similar practices and restrictions are grouped together. Not every member of each religion adheres to all practices and beliefs set forth. It is important to verify with the person his or her unique practices and traditions when asking questions about religious preference. No attempt is made to discuss the broad beliefs and philosophies of the selected groups; see Bibliography for texts supplying such in-depth information.

Focus Assessment Criteria

Refer to *Spiritual Distress*.

Goals

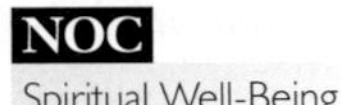

Spiritual Well-Being

The person will express satisfaction with ability to practice or exercise beliefs and practices, as evidenced by the following indicators:

- Continues spiritual practices not detrimental to health
- Expresses decreasing feelings of guilt and anxiety

Interventions

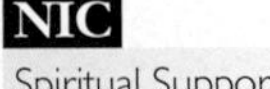

Spiritual Support

Explore Whether the Person Desires to Engage in an Allowable Religious or Spiritual Practice or Ritual; If So, Provide Opportunities to Do So

R: *For an individual who places a high value on prayer or other spiritual practices, these practices can provide meaning and purpose and can be a source of comfort and strength (*Carson, 1999).*

R: *Privacy and quiet provide an environment that enables reflection and contemplation.*

R: *These measures can help the person maintain spiritual ties and practice important rituals.*

Express Your Understanding and Acceptance of the Importance of the Individual's Religious or Spiritual Beliefs and Practices

R: *Conveying a nonjudgmental attitude may help reduce the person's uneasiness about expressing his beliefs and practices.*

R: *The nurse—even one who does not subscribe to the same religious beliefs or values of the person—can still help the person meet his or her spiritual needs.*

Assess for Causative and Contributing Factors

- Hospital or nursing home environment
- Limitations related to disease process or treatment regimen (e.g., cannot kneel to pray because of traction; prescribed diet differs from usual religious diet)
- Fear of imposing on or antagonizing medical and nursing staff with requests for spiritual rituals
- Embarrassment over spiritual beliefs or customs (especially common in adolescents)

- Separation from articles, texts, or environment of spiritual significance
- Lack of transportation to spiritual place or service
- Spiritual leader unavailable because of emergency or lack of time

R: *Privacy and quiet provide an environment that enables reflection and contemplation.*

R: *The nurse—even one who does not subscribe to the same religious beliefs or values of the person—can still help the person meet his or her spiritual needs.*

R: *These measures can help the person maintain spiritual ties and practice important rituals.*

Eliminate or Reduce Causative and Contributing Factors, If Possible

Limitations Imposed by the Hospital or Nursing Home Environment

- Provide privacy and quiet as needed for daily prayer, visit by spiritual leader, and spiritual reading and contemplation.
  - Pull the curtains or close the door.
  - Turn off the television and radio.
  - Ask the desk to hold calls, if possible.
  - Note the spiritual interventions on Kardex and include in the care plan.
- Contact the spiritual leader to clarify practices and perform religious rites or services, if desired.
  - Communicate with the spiritual leader concerning the person's condition.
  - Address Roman Catholic, Orthodox, and Episcopal priests as "Father," other Christian ministers as "Pastor," and Jewish rabbis as "Rabbi."
- Prevent interruption during the visit, if possible.
- Offer to provide a table or stand covered with a clean white cloth.
- Inform the person about religious services and materials available within the institution.

R: *Conveying a nonjudgmental attitude may help reduce the person's uneasiness about expressing his or her beliefs and practices.*

R: *Privacy and quiet provide an environment that enables reflection and contemplation.*

R: *The nurse—even one who does not subscribe to the same religious beliefs or values of the person—can still help the person meet his or her spiritual needs.*

Limitations Related to Disease Process or Treatment Regimen

- Encourage spiritual rituals not detrimental to health (see Box II.6):
  - Assist individuals with physical limitations in prayer and spiritual observances (e.g., help to hold rosary; help to kneeling position, if appropriate).
  - Assist in habits of personal cleanliness.
  - Avoid shaving if beard is of spiritual significance.
  - Allow the person to wear religious clothing or jewelry whenever possible.
  - Make special arrangements for burial of respected limbs or body organs.
  - Allow the family or spiritual leader to perform ritual care of the body.
  - Make arrangements as needed for other important spiritual rituals (e.g., circumcisions).
- Maintain diet with spiritual restrictions when not detrimental to health (see Box II.6):
  - Consult with a dietitian.
  - Allow fasting for short periods, if possible.
  - Change the therapeutic diet as necessary.
  - Have family or friends bring in special food, if possible.
  - Have members of the spiritual group supply meals to the person at home.
  - Be as flexible as possible in serving methods, times of meals, and so forth.

R: *For an individual who places a high value on prayer or other spiritual practices, these practices can provide meaning and purpose and can be a source of comfort and strength (*Carson, 1999).*

R: *These measures can help the person maintain spiritual ties and practice important rituals.*

R: *Many religions prohibit certain behaviors; complying with restrictions may be an important part of the person's worship.*

Fear of Imposing or Embarrassment

- Communicate acceptance of various spiritual beliefs and practices.
- Convey a nonjudgmental, respectful attitude.
- Acknowledge the importance of spiritual needs.

- Express the willingness of the health-care team to help the person meet spiritual needs.
- Provide privacy and ensure confidentiality.

R: *Conveying a nonjudgmental attitude may help reduce the person's uneasiness about expressing his or her beliefs and practices.*

R: *The nurse—even one who does not subscribe to the same religious beliefs or values of the person—can still help the person meet his or her spiritual needs.*

Separation From Articles, Texts, or Environment of Spiritual Significance

- Question the person about missing religious or spiritual articles or reading material (see Box II.6).
- Obtain missing items from the clergy in the hospital, spiritual leader, family, or members of the spiritual group.
- Treat these articles and books with respect.
- Allow the person to keep spiritual articles and books within reach as much as possible or where they can be easily seen.
- Protect articles from loss or damage (e.g., a medal pinned to a gown can be lost in the laundry).
- Recognize that articles without overt religious meaning may have spiritual significance for the person (e.g., wedding band).
- Use spiritual texts in large print, in Braille, or on tape when appropriate and available.
- Provide an opportunity for the person to pray with others or be read to by members of his or her own religious group or a member of the health-care team who feels comfortable with these activities.

Suggested Readings

- Jews and Seventh-Day Adventists would find Psalms 23, 34, 42, 63, 71, 103, 121, and 127 appropriate.
- Christians would also appreciate I Corinthians 13, Matthew 5:3–11, Romans 12, and the Lord's Prayer.

R: *For a person who places a high value on prayer or other spiritual customs, these practices can provide meaning and purpose and can be a source of comfort and strength (*Carson, 1999).*

R: *Privacy and quiet provide an environment that enables reflection and contemplation.*

R: *These measures can help the person maintain spiritual ties and practice important rituals.*

Lack of Transportation

- Take the person to the chapel or quiet environment on hospital grounds.
- Arrange transportation to the church or synagogue for the person at home.
- Provide access to spiritual programming on radio and television when appropriate.

R: *Privacy and quiet provide an environment that enables reflection and contemplation.*

Spiritual Leader Unavailable Because of Emergency or Lack of Time

- Baptize the critically ill newborn of Greek Orthodox, Episcopal, or Roman Catholic parents (see Box II.6).
- Perform other mandatory spiritual rituals, if possible.
- Offer a visit from the hospital spiritual care professional.

R: *For an individual who places a high value on prayer or other spiritual customs, these practices can provide meaning and purpose and can be a source of comfort and strength (*Carson, 1999).*

R: *The nurse—even one who does not subscribe to the same religious beliefs or values of the person—can still help the person meet his or her spiritual needs.*

R: *These measures can help the person maintain spiritual ties and practice important rituals.*

Risk for Impaired Religiosity

NANDA-I Definition

At risk for an impaired ability to exercise reliance on religious beliefs and/or participate in rituals of a particular faith tradition

Related Factors

Refer to *Impaired Religiosity*.

Goals

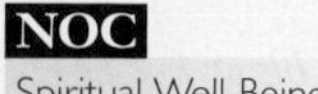
Spiritual Well-Being

The person will express continued satisfaction with religious activities, as evidenced by the following indicators:

- Continues to practice religious rituals
- Describes increased comfort after assessment

Interventions

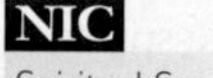
Spiritual Support

Refer to *Impaired Religiosity* for interventions.

STRESS OVERLOAD

NANDA-I Definition

Excessive amounts and types of demands that require action

Defining Characteristics

Reports excessive situational stress (e.g., rates stress level as 7 or above on a 10-point scale)*
Reports negative impact from stress (e.g., physical symptoms, psychological distress, feeling of being sick or of going to get sick)*

Physiologic

Headaches	Fatigue	Restlessness
Sleep difficulties	Indigestion	

Emotional

Crying	Feeling of pressure*	Easily upset
Edginess	Increased anger*	Feeling sick
Nervousness	Increased impatience*	Feeling of tension*
Overwhelmed		

Cognitive

Memory loss	Problems with decision-making*	Loss of humor
Forgetfulness	Constant worry	Trouble thinking clearly

Behavioral

Isolation	Difficulty functioning*	Compulsive eating
Lack of intimacy	Intolerance	Resentment
Excessive smoking		

Related Factors

The Related Factors of *Stress Overload* represent the multiple coexisting stressors that can be pathophysiologic, maturational, treatment related, situational, environmental, personal, or all of these. An individual may be able to reduce or eliminate some stressors, while others that are chronic require new strategies to manage these stressors.

Pathophysiologic

Related to coping with:

Acute illness (myocardial infarction, fractured hip)
Chronic illness* (arthritis, depression, chronic obstructive pulmonary disorder)
Terminal illness*
New diagnosis (cancer, genital herpes, HIV, multiple sclerosis, diabetes mellitus)
Disfiguring condition

Situational (Personal, Environmental)

Related to actual or anticipated loss of a significant other secondary to:

Death, dying
Moving
Divorce
Military duty

Related to coping with:

Dying
War
Assault

Related to actual or perceived change in socioeconomic status secondary to:

Unemployment
New job
Promotion
Illness
Foreclosure
Destruction of personal property

Related to coping with:

Family violence*
New family member
Substance abuse
Relationship problems
Declining functional status of older relative

Maturational

Related to coping with:

Retirement
Financial changes
Loss of residence
Functional losses

Author's Note

This diagnosis represents an individual in an overwhelming situation influenced by multiple varied stressors. If stress overload is not reduced, the individual will deteriorate and may be in danger of injury and illness.

Key Concepts

- *Health People 2020* has the following goals, which can influence stress and stress management (U.S. Department of Health and Human Service, 2015):
  - Improve health-related quality of life and well-being for all individuals.
  - Improve mental health through prevention and by ensuring access to appropriate, quality mental health services.
  - Reduce illness, disability, and death related to tobacco use and secondhand smoke exposure.
  - Reduce substance abuse to protect the health, safety, and quality of life for all, especially children.
  - Improve health, fitness, and quality of life through daily physical activity.
  - Improve the health and well-being of women, infants, children, and families.
- Stress is present in all persons. Stress is the physical, psychological, social, or spiritual effect of life's pressures and events (Edelman, Kudzma, & Mandle, 2014).
- Stress is a psychological, emotional state experienced by an individual in response to a specific stressor or stressors or demand that results in harm, either temporary or permanent, to the individual (*Ridner, 2004).
- Excessive stress requires recognition, perception, and adaptation (*Cahill, Gorski, & Le, 2003).
- A chronic state of stress or repeated episodes of psychological stress (depression, anger, hostility, anxiety) can lead to cardiovascular disease, arteriosclerosis, headaches, and gastrointestinal disorders (Edelman et al., 2014).

Focus Assessment Criteria

Subjective/Objective

Ask Individual to Rate His or Her Usual Level of Stress (0 to 10)

0 = little
>10 = overwhelming

Ask to Describe How His or Her Stress Is Affecting Their Ability to Function

Work
Sleep
Relationships

Assess for (Edelman et al., 2014)

Emotional State

Feeling out of control	Unhappy	Depressed
Impatient	Overwhelmed	Irritable
Unable to relax or agitated	Lonely	Moody
Easily upset	Isolated	

Physical

Indigestion	A clenched jaw	Diarrhea or constipation
Fatigue	Nausea	Headaches
Restlessness	Dizziness	Back problems/pain
Aches and pains	Rapid heartbeat	Frequent colds
Tight muscles	Chest pain	

Behavioral

Sleeping too much or too little	Domineering, interrupting others
Eating too much or too little	Procrastinating or neglecting responsibilities
Speaking and eating quickly	Use or overuse of alcohol, cigarettes, or drugs to relax

Cognitive

Poor judgment, constant worrying	Forgetfulness
Anxious or racing thoughts	Constant worry
Inability to concentrate	Memory problems or seeing only the negative

Relationships

Isolation	Nagging	Loneliness
Lashing out	Loss of sex drive	Loss of sense of humor

Assess for Overuse of

Sleep	Food
Tobacco	Drugs (prescription, street)
Alcohol	

Goals

NOC

Well-Being: Health Beliefs, Anxiety Reduction, Coping, Knowledge: Health Promotion, Knowledge: Health Resources

The individual will verbalize intent to change two behaviors to decrease or manage stressors, as evidenced by the following indicators:

- Identifies stressors that can be controlled and those that cannot
- Identifies one successful behavior change to increase stress management
- Identifies one behavior to reduce or eliminate that will increase successful stress management

Interventions

NIC

Anxiety Reduction, Behavioral Modification, Exercise Promotion

Clinical Alert At the website, Peaceful Parenting Institute (2015), the effects of chronic stress overload is described:

The person who grew up in a relatively relaxed and emotionally safe environment will generally be better able to identify that their stress levels are too high and will be less tolerant of living with such discomfort on an ongoing basis, hence likely to be more proactive about meeting their self-care needs.

However, when someone grows up in an emotionally stifling, demanding, or chaotic environment, their body becomes accustomed to the regular high peaks of stress and anxiety and rushes of adrenalin. Eventually the child's physiologic resting state, even when there isn't an apparent threat, remains in a state of heightened stress and low (or high)-level anxiety.

The result is always living on the edge to one extent or another, but because this was normal as a child, it's difficult for the person, as an adult, to recognize that they need and deserve to generally live in a more relaxed state.

Assist to Recognize His or Her Thoughts, Feelings, Actions, and Physiologic Responses

- Refer to Focus Assessment Criteria.

R: *Self-awareness can help the individual reframe and reinterpret their experiences (Edelman et al., 2014).*

Teach How to Break the Stress Cycle and How to Decrease Heart Rate, Respirations, and Strong Feelings of Anger (Edelman et al., 2014)

- Purposefully distract yourself by thinking of something pleasant.
- Engage in a diversional activity.
- Teach to use mini-relaxation techniques (Edelman et al., 2014).
  - Inhale through nose for 4 seconds, exhale through mouth for 4 seconds.
  - Repeat this controlled breathing and think about something that makes you smile, for example, a child, your pet.
- Refer to resources to learn relaxation techniques such as audiotapes, printed material, and yoga.

R: *Faced with overwhelming multiple stressors, the person can be assisted to differentiate which stressors can be modified or eliminated (Edelman & Mandel, 2010).*

Ask to List One or Two Changes They Would Like to Make in the Next Week

- Diet (eat one vegetable a day)
- Exercise (walk one to two blocks each day)

R: *In a person who is already overwhelmed, small changes in lifestyle may have a higher chance for success and will increase confidence (*Bodenheimer, MacGregor, & Shariffi, 2005).*

If Sleep Disturbances Are Present, Refer to *Insomnia*

If Spiritual Needs Are Identified as Deficient, Refer to *Spiritual Distress*

- Ask what activity brings the individual feelings of peace, joy, and happiness. Ask them to incorporate one of these activities each week.

R: *Overwhelmed individuals usually deny themselves such activities. Leisure can break the stress cycle (Edelman et al., 2014).*

- Ask the individual what is important, and if change is needed in their life.

R: *Values clarification assists the overwhelmed individual to identify what is meaningful and valued and if it is present in their actual living habits (Edelman et al., 2014).*

Assist to Set Realistic Goals to Achieve a More Balanced Health-Promoting Lifestyle

- What is most important?
- What aspects of your life would you like to change most?
- What is the first step?
- When?

R: *Setting realistic goals will increase confidence and success (*Bodenheimer et al., 2005).*

Initiate Health Teaching and Referrals, as Necessary

- If the individual is engaged in substance or alcohol abuse, refer for drug and alcohol abuse.
- If the individual has severe depression or anxiety, refer for professional counseling.
- If family functioning is compromised, refer for family counseling.

RISK FOR SUDDEN INFANT DEATH SYNDROME

NANDA-I Definition

Vulnerable to unpredicted death of infant

Risk Factors

There is no single risk factor. Several risk factors combined may be contributory (refer to Related Factors).

Related Factors (American Association of Pediatrics, 2011; Corwin, 2015)

Pathophysiologic

Related to increased vulnerability secondary to:

Cyanosis
Hypothermia
Fever
Poor feeding
Irritability
Respiratory distress
Tachycardia
Tachypnea
Low birth weight*
Small for gestational age*
Prematurity*
Low Apgar score (less than 7)
History of diarrhea, vomiting, or listlessness 2 weeks before death

Related to increased vulnerability secondary to prenatal maternal:

Anemia*
Urinary tract infection
Poor weight gain
Sexually transmitted infections

Situational (Personal, Environmental)

Related to increased vulnerability secondary to maternal:

Cigarette smoking*
Drug use during pregnancy
Lack of breastfeeding*
Inadequate prenatal care*
Low educational levels*
Single mother*
Multiparity with first
Young age (younger than 20)*
Young age during pregnancy*

Related to increased vulnerability secondary to:

Crowded living conditions*
Sleeping on stomach*
Poor family financial status
Cold environment
Low socioeconomic status

Related to increased vulnerability secondary to:

Male gender*
Native Americans*
Previous sudden infant death syndrome (SIDS) death in family
African descent*
Multiple births

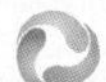

Errors in Diagnostic Statements

Risk for Sudden Infant Death Syndrome related to low-income parents

Although poor living conditions have been linked to SIDS, the wording of this diagnosis is problematic. The following diagnosis would be more clinically useful: *Risk for Sudden Infant Death Syndrome* related to insufficient knowledge of caregivers about causes and prevention of SIDS.

Key Concepts

- Each year in the United States, there are about 3,500 sudden unexpected infant deaths (SUIDs). These deaths occur among infants less than 1 year old and have no immediately obvious cause (Centers for Disease Control and Prevention [CDC], 2015).
- The three commonly reported types of SUID:
  - SIDS—About 1,500 infants died of SIDS in 2013.
  - Unknown cause
  - Accidental suffocation and strangulation in bed
- SIDS is the third cause of death of infants between 7 and 365 days of age (CDC, 2015).
- SIDS rates declined considerably from 130.3 deaths per 100,000 live births in 1990 to 39.7 deaths per 100,000 live births in 2013, since the American Academy of Pediatrics (AAP) advised sleeping position on the back for infants in 1996.
- SIDS has similar risk factors to other sleep-related infant deaths, including those attributed to suffocation, asphyxia, and entrapment (Corwin, 2015).
- Although etiology is unknown, autopsies show consistent pathologic findings as pulmonary edema and intrathoracic hemorrhages.
- "SIDS usually occurs between the second and fourth months of life, a period of remarkable developmental changes in cardiac, ventilatory, and sleep/wake patterns in otherwise normal infants. This coincidence of timing suggests that SIDS infants are vulnerable to sudden death during a critical period of autonomic maturation" (Corwin, 2015).
- The risk of SIDS is even stronger when a baby shares a bed with a smoker. To reduce risk, advice women not smoke during pregnancy, and do not smoke or allow smoking around your baby (CDC, 2015).
- No evidence is available that confirms apnea monitors prevent SIDS (Corwin, 2015; *Sherratt, 1999).

Focus Assessment Criteria

Refer to Related Factors.

Goals

NOC

Knowledge: Maternal–Child Health, Risk Control: Tobacco Use, Risk Control, Knowledge: Infant Safety

The caregiver will reduce or eliminate risk factors that are modifiable, as evidenced by the following indicators:

- Positions the infant on the back or lying on the side
- Eliminates smoking in the home, near the infant, and during pregnancy
- Participates in prenatal and newborn medical care
- Improves maternal health (e.g., treats anemia, promotes optimal nutrition)
- Enrolls in drug and alcohol programs, if indicated

Interventions

NIC

Teaching: Infant Safety, Risk Identification

Explain SIDS to Caregivers and Identify Risk Factors Present

R: *The primary focus of nursing with parents caring for an infant at risk for SIDS is emotional support.*

Reduce or Eliminate Risk Factors That Can Be Modified (Corwin, 2015)

- Maternal factors:
  - Young maternal age <20
  - Maternal smoking during pregnancy
  - Late or no prenatal care
- Infant and environmental factors:
  - Preterm birth and/or low birth weight
  - Prone sleeping position
  - Sleeping on a soft surface and/or with bedding accessories such as loose blankets and pillows
  - Bed-sharing (e.g., sleeping in parents' bed)
  - Overheating

R: *More than 95% of SIDS cases are associated with one or more risk factors, and in many cases, the risk factors are modifiable (Corwin, 2015).*

Teach Environmental Practices to Reduce SIDS

- Position infant on his or her back.
- Use a pacifier.

R: *American Association of Pediatrics (2011) suggests offering a pacifier during sleep because it is associated with less SIDS as long as it does not interfere establishment of breastfeeding.*

- Avoid overheating the infant during sleep, (e.g., excessive clothing, bedding, hot room).
- Avoid loose or soft bedding (e.g., mattresses).
- Avoid pillows, sleep positioners.
- Avoid sleeping with the infant (Anderson, 2000).
- Avoid tobacco smoke.

R: *Sleeping on the abdomen has been linked to SIDS (Hockenberry & Wilson, 2015).*

R: *Maternal smoking during pregnancy and exposure to smoke after birth has been associated with SIDS (American Academy of Pediatrics [AAP], 2000).*

- Avoid using car seats to sleep outside the car. Car seats, strollers, or swings should not be routinely used for sleep.

R: *Young infants do not breathe as well in the sitting position. Use of a car seat for car travel has safety benefits that clearly outweigh the small risk of SIDS associated with sleep in these devices.*

Initiate Health Teaching and Referrals, as Indicated

- Refer the parent(s) to drug and alcohol treatment programs, as indicated.
- Discuss strategies to stop smoking (refer to index—*smoking*).
- Provide emergency numbers, as indicated.
- Refer to social agencies, as indicated.

DELAYED SURGICAL RECOVERY

Delayed Surgical Recovery

Risk for Delayed Surgical Recovery

NANDA-I Definition

Extension of the number of postoperative days required to initiate and perform activities that maintain life, health, and well-being

Defining Characteristics

Postpones resumption of work/employment recover*
Requires help to complete self-care*
Loss of appetite with or without nausea*
Fatigue*
Perceives that more time is needed to activities*
Evidence of interrupted healing of surgical area (e.g., red, indurated, draining, immobilized)*
Difficulty moving about*
Venous obstruction/pooling

Author's Note

This diagnosis represents an individual who has not achieved recovery from a surgical procedure within the expected time. Based on the defining characteristics from NANDA-I, some confusion exists regarding the difference between defining characteristics (signs and symptoms) and related factors. A possible use of this diagnosis is as a risk diagnosis. Persons who are at high risk for *Delayed Surgical Recovery*, for example, the obese, those with diabetes mellitus, or cancer, could be identified. Interventions to prevent this state could be implemented. The diagnosis has not been developed sufficiently for clinical use. This author recommends using other nursing diagnoses, such as *Self-Care Deficit*, *Acute Pain*, or *Imbalanced Nutrition*.

Risk for Delayed Surgical Recovery

Definition

Vulnerable to an extension of the number of postoperative days required to initiate and perform activities that maintain life, health, and well-being, which may compromise health

Risk Factors

American Society of Anesthesiologist (ASA) Physical Status classification score ≥3
Diabetes mellitus
Edema at surgical site
Extensive surgical procedure
Extremes of age
History of delayed wound healing
Impaired mobility
Malnutrition
Obesity
Pain
Perioperative surgical site infection
Persistent nausea
Persistent vomiting
Pharmaceutical agent
Postoperative emotional response
Prolonged surgical procedure
Psychological disorder in postoperative period
Surgical site contamination
Trauma at surgical site

Author's Note

Risk for Delayed Surgical Recovery is a clinically useful nursing diagnosis to designate individuals who are at risk for delayed transition to home. Factors that increase an individual's risk for infection are usually associated with delayed transition. Nursing care needs to be more aggressive in reducing factors that contribute to infection, such as uncontrolled diabetes mellitus, tobacco use. In addition, strict environmental control to prevent transfer of infection to the compromised individual is imperative.

Errors in Diagnostic Statements

Risk for Delayed Surgical Recovery related to homeless status

A homeless person often stays in an institution for extended time, even though they are clinically stable. The social and housing barriers should be addressed using *Ineffective Health Maintenance* related to lack of housing, family conflicts, and insufficient social support. This situation would be better described with *Risk for Delayed Transition*. This diagnosis is very relevant in the current health-care environment, which focuses on reducing time spent in hospitals. This diagnosis is presently not on the NANDA-I list.

Key Concepts

- "A wound is a disruption of the normal structure and function of the skin and underlying soft tissue. Acute wounds in normal, healthy individuals heal through an orderly sequence of physiological events that include hemostasis, inflammation, epithelialization, fibroplasia, and maturation. When this process is altered or stalled, a chronic wound may develop and this is more likely to occur in patients with underlying disorders such as peripheral artery disease, diabetes, venous insufficiency, nutritional deficiencies, and other disease states" (Armstrong & Meyt, 2014).

- "SSIs remain a substantial cause of morbidity, prolonged hospitalization, and death. SSI is associated with a mortality rate of 3%, and 75% of SSI-associated deaths are directly attributable to the SSI" (Centers for Disease Control and Prevention [CDC], 2015).
- Surgical wounds are classified according to the degree of bacterial load or contamination of the surgical wound, as clean, clean-contaminated, contaminated, and dirty. The majority of clean and clean-contaminate wounds are closed primarily at the completion of the surgery. Contaminated and dirty wounds (e.g., fecal contamination, debridement for wound infection) are typically packed open (Armstrong & Meyt, 2014).
- Reestablishment of skin integrity following a surgical wound in individuals, without risk factors, is usually complete within 2 to 4 weeks (Armstrong & Meyt, 2014). The quality of the healed tissue after dehiscence depends upon the severity of tissue trauma, the suture material used in repair, and the presence of factors that may delay healing or reduce the tensile strength of the final scar.
- Optimal nutrition is imperative for the prevention of infection which has deleterious effects on wound healing.
- The detrimental effect of smoking on wound healing is multifactorial with mechanisms that include vasoconstriction, causing a relative ischemia of operated tissues, a reduced inflammatory response, impaired bactericidal mechanisms, and alterations of collagen metabolism. These are postulated to impair wound healing and cause wound dehiscence and incisional hernia.
- A mild degree of perioperative hypothermia (less than 36° C [96.8° F]) can be associated with significant morbidity and mortality. Research reports a threefold increase in the frequency of surgical site infections is reported in colorectal surgery patients who experience perioperative hypothermia (Hart Bordes, Hart, Corsino, & Harmon 2011).
- Certain medications can impair the healing process (anticoagulants, aspirin, colchicines, systemic corticosteroids, penicillamine, cyclosporine, metronidazole, cytotoxic chemotherapeutics).

Focus Assessment Criteria

Assess for Risk Factors for Surgical Site Infection

Refer to Interventions.

Goals

The individual will:

- Have surgical site that shows evidence of healing.
- Increase mobility and participation in self-care activities
- Report pain is relieved to their satisfaction
- Resume pre-surgery intake

Interventions

Assess for the following risk factors. Total the number of risk factors from (1 to 10) in the (). The higher the score, the greater their risk. For example, an individual, who smokes, has diabetes mellitus and is obese has a total score of 15. The diagnosis can be written as *High Risk for Delayed Surgical Healing* (15) or add the risk factors, for example, as *High Risk for Delayed Surgical Healing related to obesity, diabetes mellitus, and tobacco use.*

- Infection colonization of microorganisms (1)

R: *Preoperative nares colonization with Staphylococcus aureus noted in 30% of most healthy populations, and especially methicillin-resistant S. aureus (MRSA), predisposes individuals to have higher risk of SSI (Price et al., 2008).*

- Preexisting remote body site infection (1)
- Preoperative contaminated or dirty wound (e.g., post-trauma) (1)

R: *The Risk of Surgical Site Infection is influenced by the amount and virulence of the microorganism and the ability of the individual to resist it (Pear, 2007).*

- Glucocorticoid steroids (2)

R: *Systemic glucocorticoids (GC), which are frequently used as anti-inflammatory agents, are well-known to inhibit wound repair via global anti-inflammatory effects and suppression of cellular wound responses, including* *fibroblast proliferation and collagen synthesis. Systemic steroids cause wounds to heal with incomplete granulation tissue and reduced wound contraction (Armstrong & Meyt, 2014; Franz et al., 2008).*

- Tobacco use (3)

R: *Smoking has a transient effect on the tissue microenvironment and a prolonged effect on inflammatory and reparative cell functions, leading to delayed healing and complications. Quitting smoking 4 weeks before surgery restores tissue oxygenation and metabolism rapidly (Sørensen, 2012).*

- Malnutrition (4)

R: *Malnourished individuals have been found to have less-competent immune response to infection and decreased nutritional stores that will impair wound healing (Armstrong & Meyt, 2014; Speaar, 2008).*

- Obesity (5)

R: *An obese individual may experience a compromise in wound healing due to poor blood supply to adipose tissue. In addition, antibiotics are not absorbed well by adipose tissue. Despite excessive food intake, many obese individuals have protein malnutrition, which further impedes the healing (Armstrong & Meyt, 2014; Cheadle, 2006).*

- Perioperative hyperglycemia (6)

R: *There are two primary mechanisms that place individuals experiencing acute perioperative hyperglycemia at increased risk for SSI. The first mechanism is the decreased vascular circulation that occurs, reducing tissue perfusion and impairing cellular-level functions. A clinical study by Akbari et al. (1998) noted that when healthy, nondiabetic subjects ingested a glucose load, the endothelial-dependent vasodilatation in both the micro- and macrocirculations were impaired similar to that seen in diabetic patients. The second affected mechanism is the reduced activity of the cellular immunity functions of chemotaxis, phagocytosis, and killing of polymorphonuclear cells as well as monocytes/macrophages that have been shown to occur in the acute hyperglycemic state.*

- Diabetes mellitus (7)

R: *Postsurgical adverse outcomes related to DM are believed to be related to the preexisting complications of chronic hyperglycemia, which include vascular atherosclerotic disease and peripheral as well as autonomic neuropathies (Armstrong & Meyt, 2014; *Geerlings et al., 1999).*

- Altered immune response (8)

R: Suppression of the immune system by disease, medication, or age can delay wound healing (Cheadle, 2006).

- Chronic alcohol use/acute alcohol intoxication (9)

R: *Chronic alcohol exposure causes impaired wound healing and enhanced host susceptibility to infections. Wounds from trauma in the presence of acute alcohol exposure have a higher rate of postinjury infection due to decreased neutrophil recruitment and phagocytic function (Guo & DiPietro, 2010).*

Monitor the Surgical Site for Bleeding, Dehiscence, Hematoma, and Inadequate Incisional Closure

R: *Wound dehiscence is the partial or complete separation of the outer layers of the joined incision and evisceration. Evisceration is the protrusion of the intestines through the open incision. The seepage of serosanguineous fluid through a closed abdominal wound is an early sign of abdominal wound dehiscence with possible evisceration. When this occurs, the surgeon should remove one or two sutures in the skin and explore the wound manually, using a sterile glove. If there is separation of the rectus fascia, the individual may be taken to the operating room for primary closure. Wound dehiscence may or may not be associated with intestinal evisceration. When the latter complication is present, the mortality rate is dramatically increased and may reach 30% (Pear, 2007).*

Monitor for Signs of Paralytic Ileus

- Absent bowel sounds
- Nausea, vomiting
- Abdominal distention

R: *Intraoperative manipulation of abdominal organs and the depressive effects of narcotics and anesthetics on peristalsis can cause paralytic ileus, usually between the third and fifth postoperative day. Pain typically is localized, sharp, and intermittent.*

Explain the Effects of Nicotine (Cigarettes, Cigars, Smokeless) on Circulation

- If the individual quit before the surgery, stress the importance of continued smoking cessation to reduce the risk of infection. Refer to Getting Started to Quit Smoking on thePoint at and print guideline for individual.

R: *Nicotine can cause vasoconstriction and hypercoagulable state which contributes to poor circulation and clot formation (Giardina, 2015). Smoking cessation for at least 4 weeks before surgery reduces surgical site infections, but not other healing complications.*

Refer to Specific Nursing Diagnoses to Reduce the Risk Factors If Amenable to Nursing Care as

- *Imbalanced Nutrition*
- *Obesity*
- *Risk Prone Behaviors*, for example, alcohol, tobacco use
- *Ineffective Health Management* related to .... as evidenced by uncontrolled glucose levels
- *Nonengagement* related to .... as evidenced by inadequate management of disease (specify)

Initiate Health Teaching and Referrals as Needed

- Demonstrate wound care, observe a relative or the individual doing wound care.
- Refer to drug/alcohol program if indicated.
- Arrange for home nursing consultation.
- Refer to diabetic education program.

INEFFECTIVE TISSUE PERFUSION[50]

Ineffective Tissue Perfusion

Risk for Decreased Cardiac Tissue Perfusion
Risk for Ineffective Cerebral Tissue Perfusion
Risk for Ineffective Gastrointestinal Tissue Perfusion
Ineffective Peripheral Tissue Perfusion
Risk for Ineffective Peripheral Tissue Perfusion
Risk for Peripheral Neurovascular Dysfunction
Risk for Ineffective Renal Perfusion

Definition

Decrease in oxygen resulting in failure to nourish tissues at capillary level

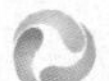

Author's Note

The use of any *Ineffective Tissue Perfusion* diagnosis other than *Peripheral* merely provides new labels for medical diagnoses, labels that do not describe the nursing focus or accountability.

When using these diagnoses, nurses cannot be accountable for prescribing the interventions for outcome achievement. Instead of using *Ineffective Tissue Perfusion*, the nurse should focus on the nursing diagnoses and collaborative problems that are present or at risk for because of altered renal, cardiac, cerebral, pulmonary, or gastrointestinal (GI) tissue perfusion. Refer to Section 3 for specific collaborative problems, for example, *Risk for Complications of Increased Intracranial Pressure, Risk for Complications of GI Bleeding, Risk for Decreased Cardiac Output, Risk for Renal Insufficiency, Risk for Hypoxemia*.

Ineffective Peripheral Tissue Perfusion can be a clinically useful nursing diagnosis if used to describe chronic arterial or venous insufficiency or potential thrombophlebitis. In contrast, acute embolism and thrombophlebitis represent collaborative problems as *Risk for Complications of Pulmonary Embolism* or *RC of Deep Vein Thrombosis*. A nurse focusing on preventing deep vein thrombosis in a postoperative individual would write the diagnosis *Risk for Ineffective Peripheral Tissue Perfusion related to postoperative immobility and dehydration*.

[50]This diagnosis is presently not on the NANDA-I list but has been added by this author for clarity and usefulness.

Errors in Diagnostic Statements

***Ineffective GI Tissue Perfusion* related to esophageal varices**

Because this diagnosis actually represents a situation that nurses monitor and manage with nursing and medical interventions, the diagnosis should be rewritten as the collaborative problem *Risk for Complications of Esophageal varices*.

***Ineffective Cerebral Tissue Perfusion* related to cerebral edema secondary to intracranial infections**

This diagnosis represents a new label for encephalitis, meningitis, or abscess. Instead, the nurse should specify collaborative problems to clearly describe and designate the nursing accountability: *Risk for Complications of Increased Intracranial Pressure* and *Risk for Complications of Sepsis*. In addition, certain nursing diagnoses may be indicated (e.g., *Risk for Infection Transmission, Acute Pain*).

***Ineffective Peripheral Tissue Perfusion* related to deep vein thrombosis**

Deep vein thrombosis is a medical diagnosis that evokes responses for which nurses are accountable: Monitoring for and managing, with physician- and nurse-prescribed interventions, physiologic complications (e.g., embolism, venous ulcers). This situation would be represented by collaborative problems such as *Risk for Complications of Embolism*. In addition, the nurse would intervene independently to prevent complications of immobility and teach how to prevent recurrence, applying nursing diagnoses such as *Disuse Syndrome* and *Risk for Ineffective Health Maintenance related to insufficient knowledge of risk factors*.

Risk for Decreased Cardiac Tissue Perfusion

NANDA-I Definition

Vulnerable to a decrease in cardiac (coronary) circulation, which may compromise health

Risk Factors*[51]

Pharmaceutical agent* (medication side effect of combination pills)
Cardiovascular surgery* (treatment)
Cardiac tamponade* (clinical emergency)
Coronary artery spasm* (clinical emergency)
Diabetes mellitus* (medical diagnosis with multiple complications with associated modifiable risk lifestyles)
Drug abuse* (clinical situations with multiple complications)
Elevated C-reactive protein* (positive laboratory test)
Family history of coronary artery disease* (factor with associated modifiable risk lifestyles)
Hyperlipidemia* (medical diagnosis with associated modifiable risk lifestyles)
Hypertension* (medical diagnosis with multiple complications with associated modifiable risk lifestyles)
Hypoxemia* (complication)
Hypovolemia* (complication)
Hypoxia* (complication)
Substance abuse (medical diagnosis)
Insufficient knowledge of modifiable risk factors (e.g., smoking, sedentary lifestyle, obesity)
(These related factors are more appropriate to the nursing diagnoses of *Risk Prone Health Behavior* and/or *Ineffective Health Management*)

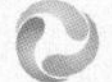

Author's Note

This NANDA-I nursing diagnosis represents a collection of risk factors or that have different clinical implications. Some include a collection of physiologic complications that relate to the situation and can be labeled as *Risk for Complications of Cardiac Surgery*, *Risk for Complications of Acute Coronary Syndrome*, and *Risk for Complications of Diabetes Mellitus*. Some are single complications such as *Risk for Complications of Hypovolemia* and *Risk for Complications of Hypoxia*.

---

[51] Text in parentheses has been added by author to indicate that nursing diagnosis is not the clinical terminology to communicate clinical emergencies or to direct medical treatment for complications.

For example, *Risk for Complications of Cocaine Abuse* would describe monitoring and management of complications such as cardiac/vascular shock, seizures, coma, respiratory insufficiency, stroke, and hyperpyrexia. These complications are different from *Risk for Complications of Alcohol Abuse,* which describes the monitoring and management of complications of delirium tremors, seizures, autonomic hyperactivity, hypovolemia, hypoglycemia, alcohol hallucinosis, and cardiovascular shock.

Some complications are medical emergencies such as cardiac tamponade, coronary artery spasm or occlusion, all of which have protocols for medical interventions.

If a diagnosis is needed for this clinical situation, use *Risk for Complications of Medication Therapy Adverse Effects*, specifically *Risk for Complications of Oral Combination Contraception Therapy*.

Risk for Ineffective Cerebral Tissue Perfusion

NANDA-I Definition

Vulnerable to a decrease in cerebral tissue circulation that may compromise health

Risk Factors*

Abnormal partial thromboplastin time
Akinetic left ventricular segment
Arterial dissection
Atrial myxoma
Carotid stenosis
Coagulopathies (e.g., sickle cell anemia)
Disseminated intravascular coagulation
Head trauma
Hypertension
Left atrial appendage thrombosis
Mitral stenosis
Recent myocardial infarction
Substance abuse
Treatment-related side effects
(cardiopulmonary bypass, pharmaceutical agents)
Abnormal prothrombin time
Aortic atherosclerosis
Atrial fibrillation
Brain Tumor
Cerebral aneurysm
Dilated cardiomyopathy
Embolism
Hypercholesterolemia
Endocarditis
Mechanical prosthetic valve
Neoplasm of the brain
Sick sinus syndrome
Thrombolytic therapy

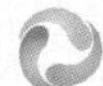

Author's Note

This NANDA-I nursing diagnosis represents a collection of risk factors that have very different clinical implications. Some are physiologic complications that are related to a medical diagnosis or treatment and can be labeled as *Risk for Complications of Head Trauma, Risk for Complications of Brain Tumor,* or *Risk for Complications of Thrombolytic Therapy*. These clinical situations have both nursing diagnoses and collaborative problems that require interventions.

For example, *Risk for Complications of Cranial Surgery* would have the following collaborative problems:

- *Risk for Complications of Increase Intracranial Pressure*
- *Risk for Complications of Hemorrhage, Hypovolemia/Shock*
- *Risk for Complications of Thromboembolism*
- *Risk for Complications of Cranial Nerve Dysfunction*
- *Risk for Complications of Cardiac Dysrhythmias*
- *Risk for Complications of Seizures*
- *Risk for Complications of Sensory/Motor Alterations*

Nursing diagnoses associated with this clinical situation*:

- *Anxiety* to impending surgery and fear of outcomes
- *Acute Pain* related to compression/displacement of brain tissue and increased intracranial pressure
- *Risk for Ineffective Self Heath Management* related to insufficient knowledge of wound care signs and symptoms of complications, restrictions, and follow-up care

Goals/Interventions

Refer to Section 3 for specific collaborative problems under *Risk for Complications of Neurologic Dysfunction.*

Risk for Ineffective Gastrointestinal Tissue Perfusion

NANDA-I Definition

Vulnerable to a decrease in gastrointestinal circulation, which may compromise health

Risk Factors*

Abdominal aortic aneurysm
Abnormal partial thromboplastin time

Acute gastrointestinal hemorrhage
Age >60 years
Coagulopathy (e.g., sickle cell anemia)
Diabetes mellitus
Disseminated intravascular coagulation in female gender
Ulcer, ischemic colitis, ischemic pancreatitis
Cerebral vascular accident; decrease in left ventricular performance
Impaired liver function (e.g., cirrhosis, hepatitis)
Poor left ventricular performance

Hemodynamic instability
Myocardial infarction renal disease (e.g., polycystic kidney, renal artery stenosis, failure)
Trauma
Treatment regimen
Vascular disease

Abdominal compartment syndrome

Anemia
Gastrointestinal condition

Smoking

Author's Note

This diagnosis is too general for clinical use because it represents a variety of physiologic complications related to GI perfusion. These complications are collaborative problems and should be separated to more specific complications, for example, as

- *Risk for Complications of GI Bleeding*
- *Risk for Complications of Paralytic Ileus*
- *Risk for Complications of Hypovolemia/Shock*

Goals/Interventions

Refer to Section 3 for goals and interventions/rationale for *Risk for Complications of GI Bleeding or Paralytic Ileus or Hypovolemia/Shock*.

Ineffective Peripheral Tissue Perfusion

NANDA-I Definition

Decrease in blood circulation to the periphery that may compromise health

Defining Characteristics

Presence of one of the following types (see Key Concepts for definitions):

Claudication (arterial)*
Rest pain (arterial)
Skin color changes*
Reactive hyperemia (arterial)
Skin temperature changes
Warmer (venous)
Capillary refill longer than 3 seconds (arterial)*
Edema* (venous)
Change in motor function (arterial)
Hard, thick nails

Loss of hair
Aching pain (arterial or venous)
Diminished or absent arterial pulses* (arterial)
Pallor (arterial)
Cyanosis (venous)
Cooler (arterial)
Decreased blood pressure (arterial)
Change in sensory function (arterial)
Trophic tissue changes (arterial)
Nonhealing wound

Related Factors

Pathophysiologic

Related to compromised blood flow secondary to:

Vascular disorders
- Arteriosclerosis
- Raynaud's disease/syndrome
- Arterial thrombosis
- Sickle cell crisis
- Rheumatoid arthritis
- Leriche's syndrome
- Aneurysm
- Buerger's disease
- Collagen vascular disease
- Alcoholism
- Venous hypertension
- Varicosities
- Deep vein thrombosis
- Cirrhosis

Diabetes mellitus
Hypotension
Blood dyscrasias
Renal failure
Cancer/tumor

Treatment Related

Related to immobilization

Related to presence of invasive lines

Related to pressure sites/constriction (elastic compression bandages, stockings, restraints)

Related to blood vessel trauma or compression

Situational (Personal, Environmental)

Related to pressure of enlarging uterus on pelvic vessels

Related to pressure of enlarged abdomen on pelvic vessels

Related to vasoconstricting effects of tobacco

Related to decreased circulating volume secondary to dehydration

Related to dependent venous pooling

Related to hypothermia

Related to pressure of muscle mass secondary to weight lifting

Author's Note

See *Ineffective Peripheral Tissue Perfusion*.

Key Concepts

General Considerations

- Adequate cellular oxygenation depends on the following processes (Grossman & Porth, 2014):
  - The ability of the lungs to exchange air adequately (O_2–CO_2)
  - The ability of the pulmonary alveoli to diffuse oxygen and carbon dioxide across the cell membrane to the blood
  - The ability of the red blood cells (hemoglobin) to carry oxygen
  - The ability of the heart to pump with enough force to deliver the blood to the microcirculation
  - The ability of intact blood vessels to deliver blood to the microcirculation
- Hypoxemia (decreased oxygen content of the blood) results in cellular hypoxia, which causes cellular swelling and contributes to tissue injury.
- Arterial blood flow is enhanced by a dependent position and inhibited by an elevated position. (Gravity pulls blood downward, away from the heart.)

- When an alteration in peripheral tissue perfusion exists, the nurse must consider its nature. The two major components of the peripheral vascular system are the arterial and the venous systems. Signs, symptoms, etiology, and nursing interventions are different for problems in each of these two systems and therefore are addressed separately.
- Changes in arterial walls increase the incidence of stroke and coronary artery disease (stroke) (Grossman & Porth, 2014).
- High levels of circulating lipids increase the risk of coronary heart disease, peripheral vascular disease, and stroke (Grossman & Porth, 2014).

 Geriatric Considerations

- Age-related vascular changes include stiffened blood vessels, which cause increased peripheral resistance, impaired baroreceptor functioning, and diminished ability to increase organ blood flow (Miller, 2015). These age-related changes cause the veins to become more dilated and less elastic. Valves of the large leg veins become less efficient. Age-related reductions in muscle mass and inactivity further reduce peripheral circulation (Miller, 2015).
- Physical deconditioning or lack of exercise accentuates the functional consequences of age-related cardiovascular changes. Contributing factors to deconditioning include acute illness, mobility limitations, cardiac disease, depression, and lack of motivation (Miller, 2015).

Focus Assessment Criteria

See Tables II.21 and II.22.

Table II.21 ARTERIAL INSUFFICIENCY VS VENOUS INSUFFICIENCY: A COMPARISON OF SUBJECTIVE DATA

Symptom	Arterial Insufficiency	Venous Insufficiency
Pain		
Location	Feet, muscles of legs, toes	Ankles, lower legs
Quality	Burning, shocking, prickling, throbbing, cramping, sharp	Aching, tightness
Quantity	Increase in severity with increased muscle activity or elevation	Varies with fluid intake, use of support hose, and decreased muscle activity
Chronology	Brought on predictably by exercise	Greater in evening than in morning
Setting	Use of affected muscle groups	Increases during course of day with prolonged standing or sitting
Aggravating factors	Exercise Extremity elevation	Immobility Extremity dependence
Alleviating factors	Cessation of exercise Extremity dependence	Extremity elevation Compression stockings or Ace wraps
Paresthesia	Numbness, tingling, burning, decreased touch sensation	No change unless arterial system or nerves are affected

Table II.22 ARTERIAL INSUFFICIENCY VS VENOUS INSUFFICIENCY: A COMPARISON OF OBJECTIVE DATA

Sign	Arterial Insufficiency	Venous Insufficiency
Temperature	Cool skin	Warm skin
Color	Pale on elevation, dependent rubor (reactive hyperemia)	Flushed, cyanotic
		Typical brown discoloration around ankles
Capillary filling	<3 seconds	Nonapplicable
Pulses	Absent or weak	Present unless there is concomitant arterial disease, or edema may obscure them
Movement	Decreased motor ability with nerve and muscle ischemia	Motor ability unchanged unless edema is severe enough to restrict joint mobility
Ulceration	Occurs on foot at site of trauma or at tips of toes (most distal to be perfused)	Occurs around ankle (area of greatest pressure from chronic venous stasis due to valvular incompetence)
	Ulcers are deep with well-defined margins	Ulcers shallow with irregular edges
	Surrounding tissue is shiny and taut with thin skin	Surrounding tissue edematous with engorged veins

Subjective Data

Assess for Defining Characteristics

Pain (associated with, time of day)
Temperature change
Pallor, cyanosis, paresthesias
Change in motor function

Assess for Related Factors

Medical History
Refer to Related Factors.

Risk Factors
Smoking (never, quit, years)
Immobility
Stress
History of phlebitis
Sedentary lifestyle
Family history of heart disease, vascular disease, stroke, kidney disease, or diabetes mellitus

Medications
Type Side effects Dosage

Objective Data

Assess for Defining Characteristics

Skin
Temperature (cool, warm)
Color (pale, dependent rubor, flushed, cyanotic, brown discolorations)
Ulcerations (size, location, description of surrounding tissue)
Bilateral pulses (radial, femoral popliteal, posterior tibial, dorsalis pedis)
Rate, rhythm
Volume
Absent, nonpalpable
Weak
Normal, easily palpable
Aneurysmal
Paresthesia (numbness, tingling, burning)
Edema (location, pitting)
Capillary refill (normal less than 3 seconds)
Motor ability (normal, compromised)

Goals

NOC
Sensory Functions; Cutaneous, Tissue Integrity, Tissue perfusion: Peripheral

The individual will report a decrease in pain as evidenced by the following indicators:

- Defines peripheral vascular problem in own words
- Identifies factors that improve peripheral circulation
- Identifies necessary lifestyle changes
- Identifies medical regimen, diet, medications, activities that promote vasodilation
- Identifies factors that inhibit peripheral circulation
- States when to contact physician or health-care professional

Interventions

NIC
Peripheral Sensation Management, Circulatory Care: Venous Insufficiency, Circulatory Care: Arterial Insufficiency, Positioning, Exercise Promotion

Assess Causative and Contributing Factors

- Underlying disease
- Inhibited arterial blood flow
- Inhibited venous blood flow
- Fluid volume excess or deficit
- Hypothermia or vasoconstriction
- Activities related to symptom/sign onset

Promote Factors That Improve Arterial Blood Flow

- Keep extremity in a dependent position.

R: *Arterial blood flow is enhanced by a dependent position and inhibited by an elevated position (gravity pulls blood downward, away from the heart).*

- Keep extremity warm (do not use heating pad or hot water bottle).

R: *Peripheral vascular disease will reduce sensitivity. The individual will not be able to determine if the temperature is hot enough to damage tissue; the use of external heat may also increase the metabolic demands of the tissue beyond its capacity.*

Reduce Risk for Trauma

- Change positions at least every hour.
- Avoid leg crossing.
- Reduce external pressure points (inspect shoes daily for rough lining).
- Avoid sheepskin heel protectors (they increase heel pressure and pressure across dorsum of foot).
- Encourage range-of-motion exercises.
- Discuss smoking cessation (see Ineffective Health Maintenance related to tobacco use).

R: *Cellular nutrition and function depend on adequate blood flow through the microcirculation.*

R: *Tight garments and certain leg positions constrict leg vessels, further reducing circulation.*

Promote Factors That Improve Venous Blood Flow

- Elevate extremity above the level of the heart (may be contraindicated if severe cardiac or respiratory disease is present).

R: *Venous blood flow is enhanced by an elevated position and inhibited by a dependent position. (Gravity pulls blood downward, away from the heart.)*

- Avoid standing or sitting with legs dependent for long periods.
- Consider the use of elastic compression stockings.

R: *Compression stockings increase venous return and the rate of venous flow and decrease venous pooling.*

Teach to

- Avoid pillows behind the knees or Gatch bed, which is elevated at the knees.
- Avoid leg crossing.
- Change positions, move extremities, or wiggle fingers and toes every hour.
- Avoid garters and tight elastic stockings above the knees.
- Measure baseline circumference of calves and thighs if the individual is at risk for deep venous thrombosis, or if it is suspected.

R: *Reduce or remove external venous compression that impedes venous flow.*

Plan a Daily Walking Program

- Refer to Sedentary Lifestyle for specific interventions.

Initiate Health Teaching, as Indicated

- Teach individual to:
  - Avoid long car or plane rides (get up and walk around at least every hour).
  - Keep dry skin lubricated (cracked skin eliminates the physical barrier to infection).
  - Wear warm clothing during cold weather.
  - Wear cotton or wool socks.
  - Use gloves or mittens if hands are exposed to cold (including home freezers).
  - Avoid dehydration in warm weather.

R: *These measures can increase circulation and prevent injuries.*

- Give special attention to feet and toes:
  - Wash feet and dry well daily.
  - Do not soak feet.
  - Avoid harsh soaps or chemicals (including iodine) on feet.
  - Keep nails trimmed and filed smooth.
  - Inspect feet and legs daily for injuries and pressure points.

- Wear clean socks.
- Wear shoes that offer support and fit comfortably.
- Inspect the inside of shoes daily for rough lining.

R: *Daily foot care can reduce tissue damage and help prevent or detect early further reducing circulation.*

Explain the Relation of Certain Risk Factors to the Development of Atherosclerosis

- Smoking
- Vasoconstriction
- Elevated blood pressure
- Decreased oxygenation of the blood
- Increased lipidemia
- Increased platelet aggregation

R: *The effects of nicotine on the cardiovascular system contribute to coronary artery disease, stroke, hypertension, and peripheral vascular disease (Grossman & Porth, 2014).*

- Hypertension/hyperlipidemia

R: *Constant increased pressure causes damage to the vessel lining, which promotes plaque formation and narrowing. Hyperlipidemia promotes atherosclerosis.*

- Sedentary lifestyle

R: *Inactivity decreases muscle tone and strength and decreases circulation.*

- Excess weight (greater than 10% of ideal)

R: *Obesity increases peripheral resistance and venous pooling; excess weight increases cardiac workload, causing hypertension (Grossman & Porth, 2014).*

- Refer to community resources for lifestyle changes.

R: *Community resources can assist the individual with weight loss, smoking cessation, diet, and exercise programs.*

Risk for Ineffective Peripheral Tissue Perfusion

NANDA-I Definition

Vulnerable to a decrease in blood circulation to the periphery, which may compromise health

Risk Factors*

Age >60 years
Deficient knowledge of aggravating factors (e.g., smoking, sedentary lifestyle, trauma, obesity, salt intake, immobility)
Deficient knowledge of disease process (e.g., diabetes mellitus, hyperlipidemia)
Diabetes mellitus
Endovascular procedures
Hypertension
Sedentary lifestyle
Smoking

Goals

Refer to *Ineffective Peripheral Tissue Perfusion.*

Interventions

Refer to *Ineffective Peripheral Tissue Perfusion.*

Risk for Peripheral Neurovascular Dysfunction

See also *Risk for Complications of Compartment Syndrome* in Section 3.

Definition

At risk for disruption in the circulation, sensation, or motion of an extremity

Risk Factors

Pathophysiologic

Related to increased volume of (specify extremity) secondary to:

Bleeding (e.g., trauma*, fractures*)
Venous obstruction*/pooling
Arterial obstruction
Coagulation disorder

Related to increased capillary filtration secondary to:

Allergic response (e.g., insect bites)
Trauma
Severe burns (thermal, electrical)
Frostbite
Nephrotic syndrome
Venomous bites (e.g., snake)
Hypothermia

Related to restrictive envelope secondary to circumferential burns

Treatment Related

Related to increased capillary filtration secondary to:

Total knee replacement
Total hip replacement

Related to restrictive envelope secondary to:

Tourniquet
Ace wraps
Brace
Restraints
Antishock trousers
Excessive traction
Air splints
Circumferential dressings
Cast
Premature or tight closure of fascial defects

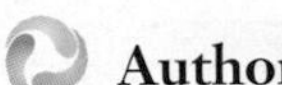

Author's Note

This diagnosis represents a situation that nurses can prevent complications by identifying who is at risk and implementing measures to reduce or eliminate causative or contributing factors. *Risk for Peripheral Neurovascular Dysfunction* can change to compartment syndrome. *Risk for Complications of Compartment Syndrome* is inadequate tissue perfusion in a muscle, usually an arm or leg, caused by edema, which obstructs venous and arterial flow and compresses nerves. The nursing focus for compartment syndrome is diagnosing early signs and symptoms and notifying the physician. The medical interventions required to abate the problem are surgical, such as evacuation of hematoma, repair of damaged vessels, or fasciotomy. Refer to *Risk for Complications of Compartment Syndrome* in Section 3 for specific interventions for either diagnosis. Students should consult with their faculty for direction to use either *Risk for Peripheral Vascular Dysfunction* or *Risk for Complications of Compartment Syndrome*.

Risk for Ineffective Renal Perfusion

NANDA-I Definition

At risk for a decrease in blood circulation to the kidney that may compromise health

Risk Factors*

Abdominal compartment syndrome
Burns
Diabetes mellitus
Hyperlipidemia
Hypoxemia
Malignancy
Multitrauma
Renal disease (polycystic kidney)
Systemic inflammatory response syndrome
Treatment-related side effects (e.g., pharmaceutical agents, surgery)
Vascular embolism vasculitis
Advance age
Cardiac surgery
Exposure to toxins
Hypertension
Hypoxia
Malignant hypertension
Polynephritis
Smoking
Bilateral cortical necrosis
Cardiopulmonary bypass
Female glomerulonephritis
Hypovolemia
Infection (e.g., sepsis, localized infection)
Metabolic acidosis
Renal artery stenosis

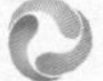

Author's Note

This NANDA-I diagnosis represents a potential complication which is a collaborative problem, *Risk for Complications of Renal Insufficiency*.

If the situation is a medical diagnosis of Acute Kidney Failure or Chronic Renal Disease, using *Risk for Complications of Acute Kidney Failure* would include the following collaborative problems*:

- *Risk for Complications of Fluid Overload*
- *Risk for Complications of Metabolic Acidosis*
- *Risk for Complications of Acute Albuminemia*
- *Risk for Complications of Hypertension*
- *Risk for Complications of Pulmonary Edema*
- *Risk for Complications of Dysrhythmias*
- *Risk for Complications of Gastrointestinal Bleeding*

Nursing diagnoses associated with this clinical situation:

- *Risk for Infection* related to invasive procedures
- *Imbalanced Nutrition:* Related to anorexia, nausea, vomiting, loss of taste, loss of smell, stomatitis, and dietary restrictions
- *Risk for Impaired Tissue Integrity* related to retention of metabolic wastes, increased capillary fragility, and platelet dysfunction

Goals/Interventions

- Refer to Section 3 for Goals and Interventions for *Risk for Complications of Renal Insufficiency.*
- Refer to Section 2 for Goals and Interventions for specific related nursing diagnoses.

IMPAIRED URINARY ELIMINATION

Impaired Urinary Elimination

Maturational Enuresis
Functional Urinary Incontinence
Reflex Urinary Incontinence
Stress Urinary Incontinence
Continuous Urinary Incontinence
Urge Urinary Incontinence
Overflow Urinary Incontinence

NANDA-I Definition

Dysfunction in urinary elimination

Defining Characteristics

Major (Must Be Present, One or More)

Reports or experiences a urinary elimination problem, such as:

- Urgency*
- Dribbling
- Frequency*
- Bladder distention
- Hesitancy*
- Large residual urine volumes
- Retention*
- Enuresis
- Dysuria*
- Incontinence*
- Nocturia*

Related Factors

Pathophysiologic

Related to incompetent bladder outlet secondary to:

Refer to *Overflow Urinary Incontinence.*

Related to decreased bladder capacity or irritation to bladder secondary to (refer to Urge Incontinence):

- Infection*
- Glucosuria
- Trauma
- Carcinoma
- Urethritis

Related to diminished bladder cues or impaired ability to recognize bladder cues secondary to (refer to Impaired Urinary Elimination):

- Cord injury/tumor/infection
- Diabetic neuropathy
- Brain injury/tumor/infection
- Alcoholic neuropathy
- Cerebrovascular accident
- Autonomic Neuropathies
- Tabes dorsalis
- Demyelinating diseases
- Parkinsonism
- Multiple sclerosis
- Alpha adrenergic agents

Related to sensory motor impairment* (refer to Reflex Incontinence)

Related to multiple causality*

Related to anatomic obstruction* (refer to Urinary Retention)

Related to urethral stricture

Treatment Related

Related to effects of surgery on bladder sphincter secondary to:

- Postprostatectomy
- Extensive pelvic dissection

Related to diagnostic instrumentation

Related to decreased muscle tone secondary to:

- General or spinal anesthesia
- Drug therapy (iatrogenic)
  - Antihistamines
  - Immunosuppressant therapy
  - Epinephrine
  - Diuretics
  - Anticholinergics
  - Tranquilizers
  - Sedatives
  - Muscle relaxants
  - After use of indwelling catheters

Situational (Personal, Environmental)

Related to weak pelvic floor muscles secondary to:

Obesity
Childbirth
Aging
Recent substantial weight loss

Related to inability to communicate needs

Related to diet (refer to Urge Incontinence)

Related to bladder outlet obstruction secondary to:

Fecal impaction
Chronic constipation
Benign prostatic hyperplasia

Related to decreased bladder muscle tone secondary to:

Dehydration

Related to decreased attention to bladder cues secondary to:

Depression
Delirium/altered mental status
Intentional suppression (self-induced deconditioning)
Confusion

Related to environmental barriers to bathroom secondary to:

Distant toilets
Poor lighting
Unfamiliar surroundings
Medical equipment that is attached
Urinal not within reach

Related to inability to access bathroom on time secondary to:

Refer to *Functional Incontinence*.

Maturational

Child

Related to small bladder capacity
Related to lack of motivation

Author's Note

Impaired Urinary Elimination is too broad a diagnosis for effective clinical use; however, it is clinically useful until additional data can be collected. With more data the nurse can use a more specific diagnosis, such as *Stress Urinary Incontinence*, whenever possible. When the etiologic or contributing factors for incontinence have not been identified, the nurse could write a temporary diagnosis of *Impaired Urinary Elimination* related to unknown etiology, as evidenced by incontinence.

Under the Related Factors, the reader is directed to a more specific urinary nursing diagnosis, if indicated.

The nurse performs a focused assessment to determine whether the incontinence is transient, in response to an acute condition (e.g., infection, medication side effects), or established in response to various chronic neural or genitourinary conditions (Miller, 2015). In addition, the nurse should differentiate the type of incontinence: functional, reflex, stress, or urge.

Errors in Diagnostic Statements

Impaired Urinary Elimination related to surgical diversion

This diagnosis represents a new label for urostomy and does not focus on the nursing accountability. The nurse should assess an individual with a urostomy for its effect on functional patterns and physiologic functioning. For this individual, the collaborative problems *Risk for Complications of Stoma Obstruction* and *Risk for Complications of Internal*

Urine Leakage, as well as nursing diagnoses such as *Risk for Impaired Tissue Integrity* and *Risk for Ineffective Health Maintenance*, could apply.

***Impaired Urinary Elimination* related to renal failure**

This nursing diagnosis renames renal failure and is incorrect. This diagnostic statement does not direct nursing interventions. Interventions required are collaborative (medical and nursing). For this reason, the diagnosis *Excess Fluid Volume* related to acute renal failure also would be incorrect. Renal failure causes or contributes to various problem or potential nursing diagnoses, such as *Risk for Infection* and *Risk for Imbalanced Nutrition*, and collaborative problems, such as *Risk for Complications of Fluid/Electrolyte Imbalances* and *Risk for Complications of Metabolic Acidosis*.

***Impaired Urinary Elimination* related to effects of aging**

The physiologic effects of aging on the urinary tract system can influence functioning negatively when other risk factors (e.g., mobility problems, dehydration, side effects of medications, decreased awareness of bladder cues) are also present. This nursing diagnosis projects a biased view of anticipated incontinence in an older adult, with associated use of indwelling catheters, incontinence briefs, bed pads, or all of these. When this equipment is used, the nurse is not treating incontinence, but rather managing urine. The use of such equipment is a short-term solution. For these situations, *Risk for Infection* and *Risk for Pressure Ulcer* would apply. When an older adult has an incontinent episode, the nurse should proceed cautiously before applying the nursing diagnosis label of "incontinence." If factors exist that increase the likelihood of recurrence and the individual is motivated, the diagnosis *Risk for Functional/Urge Incontinence* related to (specify—e.g., dehydration, mobility difficulties, decreased bladder capacity) could apply. This diagnosis would focus nursing interventions on preventing incontinence, rather than expecting it as inevitable. For an older individual with the combination of functional and urge incontinence, the nurse would focus on assisting him or her to increase bladder capacity and to reduce barriers to bathrooms, using the diagnosis *Functional/Urge Incontinence* related to age-related effects on bladder capacity, self-induced fluid limitations, and unstable gait.

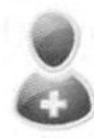

CLINICAL ALERT As with other embarrassing or uncomfortable symptoms, those affected with incontinence will be hesitant to speak up or ask questions about their condition, even at their primary care provider office. Buckley and Lapitan (2010) reported that some degree of urinary incontinence was reported by 25% to 45% of women. Urinary incontinence becomes more common as woman age (20 to 39) with 7% to 37% of women reporting experiencing some degree of incontinence. Woman over 50 reported having incontinence on a daily basis of 9% to 39%. The prevalence of incontinence in older men was reported to be approximately half that in women, with 11% to 34% reporting symptoms of incontinence.

Key Concepts

General Considerations

- The three components of the lower urinary tract that assist to maintain continence are as follows (Grossman & Porth, 2014):
  - Detrusor muscle in the bladder wall, which allows bladder expansion to increase with volume of urine
  - Internal sphincter or proximal urethra, which, when contracted, prevents urine leakage
  - External sphincter, which by voluntary control provides added support during stressed situations (e.g., overdistended bladder)
- Innervation of the bladder arises from the spinal cord at the levels of S2 to S4. The bladder is under parasympathetic control. The cortex, midbrain, and medulla influence voluntary control over urination (Hickey, 2014).
- The female urethra is 3 to 5 cm long. The male urethra is approximately 20 cm long. The urethra primarily maintains continence, but the cerebral cortex is the principal area for suppression of the desire to micturate (Grossman & Porth, 2014).
- Capacity of the normal bladder (without experiencing discomfort) is 250 to 400 mL. The desire to void occurs when 150 to 250 mL of urine is in the bladder.
- Bladder tissue tone can be lost if the bladder is repeatedly distended to 1,000 mL (atonic bladder) or continuously drained (Foley catheter).
- Mechanisms to stimulate the voiding reflex or Credé's method may be ineffective if the bladder capacity is less than 200 mL.
- Caffeinated beverages/foods (e.g., coffee, tea, chocolate), carbonated beverages, alcohol, red wine, highly acidic foods, and foods high in potassium can irritate the bladder, causing urgency and frequency (Griebling, 2009).
- Injury to the spinal cord above S2 to S4 produces a spastic or reflex bladder tone. Injury to the spinal cord below S2 to S4 produces a flaccid or atonic bladder.

Infection

- Stasis or pooling of urine and alkaline urine contributes to bacterial growth. Bacteria can travel up the ureters to the kidney (ascending infection).
- Recurrent bladder infections cause fibrotic changes in the bladder wall, with a resultant decrease in bladder capacity.
- Urinary stasis, infections, alkaline urine, and decreased urine volume contribute to the formation of urinary tract calculi.

Incontinence

- Of noninstitutionalized persons aged 65 and over, 50.9% reported a urinary leakage and/or accidental bowel leakage of mucus, liquid stool, or solid stool; of them, 43.8% reported a urinary leakage and 17.3% reported an accidental bowel leakage (Gorina, Schappert, Bercovitz, Elgaddal, & Kramarow, 2014).
- Among residential care facilities residents, 39.0% had had an episode of urinary and/or bowel incontinence during the 7 days prior to the survey, with 36.6% reported to have had an episode of urinary incontinence and 20.4% reported to have had an episode of bowel incontinence (Gorina et al., 2014).
- Urinary incontinence affects people of all ages, but most commonly the elderly. Urinary incontinence remains underdiagnosed and underreported primarily due to embarrassment (DeMaagd & Davenport, 2012).
- In the United States, 17 million people have urinary incontinence, creating a financial burden of over $76 million dollars to both individuals as well as the health-care system (Testa, 2015).
- The prevalence of urinary incontinence is higher in women than it is in men up until the age of 80 in which both women and men are affected to equal degrees. Incidence in women is highest in Caucasians followed by Asians and the African Americans (Khandelwal & Kistler, 2013; Townsend, Curhan, Resnick, & Grodstein, 2010).
- An estimated 423 million people worldwide will suffer from urinary incontinence by 2018 (Irwin, Kopp, Agatep, Milsom, & Abrams 2011).
- Causes of transient incontinence include acute confusion, urinary tract infection, atrophic vaginitis, side effects of medications, metabolic imbalance, impaction, mobility problems, urosepsis, depression, and pressure sores.
- Controllable incontinence cannot be cured, but urine removal can be planned.
- Certain medications are associated with incontinence. Narcotics and sedatives diminish awareness of bladder cues. Adrenergic agents cause retention by increasing bladder outlet resistance. Anticholinergics (antidepressants, some antiparkinsonian medications, antispasmodics, antihistamines, antiarrhythmics, opiates) cause chronic retention with overflow. Diuretics rapidly increase urine volume and can cause incontinence if voiding cannot be delayed (Miller, 2015).
- Social isolation of people with incontinence can be self-imposed because of fear and embarrassment or imposed by others because of odor and aesthetics.
- Depression can prevent the individual from recognizing or responding to bladder cues and, thus, contributes to incontinence.
- Management of urinary incontinence should first include nonpharmacologic interventions such as weight loss, proper nutrition, avoiding constipation, and regular, moderate intensity physical activity (*Peterson, 2008; Townsend, Danforth, Curhan, Resnick, & Grodstein 2007).
- Advancing age, greater parity, higher body mass index, low physical activity, and medical conditions including stoke, type 2 diabetes, and history of a hysterectomy are all associated with greater odds of having urinary incontinence (Devore, Minassian, & Grodstein, 2013).

Intermittent Catheterization

- This method maintains the tonicity of the bladder muscle, prevents overdistention, and provides for complete emptying of the bladder. As a rule of thumb, bladder volume should not exceed 500 mL, although some clinicians prefer to not exceed 400 mL. Intermittent catheterization is then continued as needed typically 4 to 6 times a day (Newman & Willson, 2011).
- The initial removal of more than 500 mL of urine from a chronically distended bladder can cause severe hemorrhage, which results when bladder veins, previously compressed by the distended bladder, rapidly dilate and rupture when bladder pressure is abruptly released. (After the initial release of 500 mL of urine, alternate the release of 100 mL of urine with 15-minute catheter clamps.)
- In individuals with spinal injuries at the T4 level or above, it is necessary to empty the bladder completely regardless of high volumes (>500 mL) because of the risk of autonomic dysreflexia. Interruption of the sympathetic nervous system causes the veins not to dilate rapidly.
- Refer to *Risk for Infection* for an extensive nursing intervention related to incontinence and evaluating the use of indwelling catheters.

Continuous Incontinence

- A cognitively impaired individual with continuous incontinence requires caregiver-directed treatment. In institutional settings, indwelling and external catheters or disposable or washable incontinence briefs or pads are beneficial to the caregivers but detrimental to the incontinent individual. Aids and equipment should be considered only after other means have been attempted. In the home setting, the caregiver's needs may take precedence over those of the cognitively impaired individual. Urinary incontinence is cited as the major reason for seeking institutional care for people living at home (Miller, 2015).

Geriatric Considerations

- Reports regarding how many elderly patients suffer from incontinence vary, most probably because it may be overlooked and not adequately evaluated by professionals; as a result, appropriate treatment is denied. Older individuals may not admit to the problem because of attitudes about the inevitability of such complications.
- Age-related physiologic changes result in decreased bladder capacity, incomplete emptying, contractions during filling, and increased residual urine (Miller, 2015).
- Urinary incontinence is associated with increased occurrence of falls, dermatitis, pressure sores, and urinary tract infections (*Wenger et al., 2009; Long, Reed, Dunning & Ying, 2012; Jackson et al., 2004).
- Another aspect to consider is loss of dignity and psychosocial distress. Patients who are incontinent are more likely to have depression and limited sexual and social interactions, and rely on the care provided by caregivers (Coyne et al., 2008).
- Older adults not only have a decreased ability to inhibit bladder contractions, but they can comfortably store only a limited 250 to 300 mL of urine compared with a storage capacity of 350 to 400 mL in younger adults.
- The sensation to void is delayed in older adults, which shortens the interval between the initial perception of the urge and the actual need to void, resulting in urgency (Miller, 2015). Any factor that interferes with the older adult's perception to void (e.g., medications, depression, limited fluid intake, neurologic impairments) or delays his or her ability to reach the toilet can cause incontinence.
- Other physiologic components of aging that contribute to incontinence are the diminished ability of kidneys to concentrate urine, decreasing muscle tone of the pelvic floor muscles, and the inability to postpone urination.
- Frequent voiding out of habit or limiting fluids may contribute to urgency by impairing the neurologic mechanisms that signal the need to void because the bladder is rarely fully expanded.
- The diminished vision, impaired mobility, and decreased energy level that may accompany aging mean that increased time is needed to locate the toilet, which also requires the individual to be able to delay urination.
- Pelvic floor muscle training and bladder training are most beneficial in resolving urinary incontinence in younger women mostly suffering from stress incontinence (Choi, Palmer, & Park, 2007).

Focus Assessment Criteria

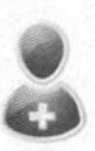

Clinical Alert It is important to determine the natural history of the incontinent pattern. A new onset of incontinence is likely to be the result of a precipitating factor outside the urinary tract (e.g., medications, acute illness, inaccessible toilets, impaired mobility that prevents getting to the toilet on time), which usually can be easily corrected. Incontinence can be either transient (reversible) or established (controllable).

Subjective Data

Assess for Defining Characteristics

"Do you have a problem with controlling your urine (or going to the bathroom)?"
"When did this start?

History of Symptoms

Lack of control	Burning	Urgency
Pain or discomfort	Hesitancy	Retention
Dribbling	Change in voiding pattern	Frequency

Restrictions on Lifestyle

Social	Occupational
Sexual	Role responsibilities

Adult Incontinence

Onset and Duration (Day, Night, Just Certain Times)

Factors That Increase Incidence

Delay in getting to bathroom
Coughing
Laughing
When excited
Standing
Leaving bathroom
Turning in bed
Running

Perception of Need to Void

Present
Absent
Diminished

Ability to Delay Urination After Urge

Present (How long?)
Absent

Sensations Before or During Micturition

Difficulty starting stream
Need to force urine out
Difficulty stopping stream
Lack of sensation to void

Relief After Voiding

Complete
Continued desire to void after emptying bladder

Use of Catheters, Incontinence

Childhood Enuresis
Onset and pattern (day, night)
Toilet-training history
Family history of bed-wetting
Response of others to child (parents, siblings, peers)

Briefs, Bed Pads

Environmental Barriers
Location of bathroom within 40 feet
Stairs, narrow doorways
Dim lighting
Ability to locate bathroom in social settings

Assess for Related Factors

Voiding and Fluid Intake Patterns
Record for 2 to 4 days to establish a baseline.
What is daily fluid intake?
When does incontinence occur?

Muscle Tone
Abdomen firm, or soft and pendulous?
History of recent significant weight loss or gain?

Reflexes
Presence or absence of cauda equina reflexes
Anal
Bulbocavernosus

Bladder
Distention (palpable)
Can it be emptied by external stimuli? (Credé's method, gentle suprapubic tapping, or warm water over the perineum, Valsalva maneuver, peppermint oil, running tap water)
Capacity (at least 400 to 500 mL)
Residual urine
None
Present (in what amount?)

Functional Ability

Get in/out of chair	Maintain balance
Walk alone to bathroom	Manipulate clothing

Cognitive Ability

Asks to go to bathroom	Aware of incontinence
Initiates toileting with reminders	Expects to be incontinent

Assess for Any:

Constipation	Mobility disorders
Depression	Dehydration
Fecal impaction	Sensory disorders

Maturational Enuresis[52]

Definition

State in which a child/adolescent experiences involuntary voiding during sleep that is not pathophysiologic in origin

Defining Characteristics

Reports or demonstrates episodes of involuntary voiding during sleep

Related Factors

Situational (Personal, Environmental)

Related to stressors (school, siblings)

Related to inattention to bladder cues

Related to unfamiliar surroundings

Maturational

Child

Related to small bladder capacity

Related to lack of motivation

Related to attention-seeking behavior

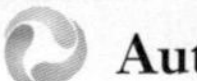

Author's Note

Enuresis can result from physiologic or maturational factors. Certain etiologies, such as strictures, urinary tract infection, constipation, nocturnal epilepsy, and diabetes, should be ruled out when enuresis is present. These situations do not represent nursing diagnoses.

When enuresis results from small bladder capacity, failure to perceive cues because of deep sleep, inattention to bladder cues, or is associated with a maturational issue (e.g., new sibling, school pressures), the nursing diagnosis *Maturational Enuresis* is appropriate. Psychological problems usually are not the cause of enuresis but may result from lack of understanding or insensitivity to the problem. Interventions that punish or shame the child must be avoided.

Errors in Diagnostic Statements

Maturational Enuresis related to stressors and conflicts

[52]This diagnosis is not presently on the NANDA-I list but has been included for clarity and usefulness.

Rather than focus on etiology for maturational enuresis, the nurse should focus on teaching the child and parents management strategies. The nurse also should encourage parents to share their concerns and direct them away from punishing behaviors. Given this nursing focus, the nurse could restate the diagnosis as *Maturational Enuresis* related to unknown etiology, as evidenced by reported episodes of bed-wetting.

Ask about the pattern of bed-wetting, including questions such as:

- How many nights a week does bed-wetting occur?
- How many times a night does bed-wetting occur?
- Does there seem to be a large amount of urine?
- At what times of night does the bed-wetting occur?
- Does the child or young person wake up after bed-wetting?

Ask about the presence of daytime symptoms in a child or young person with bed-wetting, including the following:

- Daytime frequency (that is, passing urine more than seven times a day)
- Daytime urgency
- Daytime wetting
- Passing urine infrequently (fewer than four times a day)
- Abdominal straining or poor urinary stream
- Pain passing urine

Ask about daytime toileting patterns in a child or young person with bed-wetting, including the following:

- Whether daytime symptoms occur only in some situations
- Avoidance of toilets at school or other settings
- Whether the child or young person goes to the toilet more or less frequently than his or her peers

Assess whether the child or young person has any comorbidities or there are other factors to consider, in particular

- Constipation and/or soiling
- Developmental, attention, or learning difficulties
- Diabetes mellitus
- Behavioral or emotional problems
- Family problems or a vulnerable child or young person or family

Recent change or stressor; school, peers, new family member, relocation, family problems (financial, illness, separation, divorce)

- Consider maltreatment (for the purposes of the child mistreatment guideline, to consider maltreatment means that maltreatment is one possible explanation for the alerting feature or is included in the differential diagnosis) if
  - A child or young person is reported to be deliberately bed-wetting
  - Parents or caregivers are seen or reported to punish a child or young person for bed-wetting despite professional advice that the symptom is involuntary

Key Concepts

- The newborn may void up to 20 times per day because of small bladder capacity. As the child grows, bladder capacity increases and frequency of urination decreases (Hockenberry & Wilson, 2015).
- Most children have complete neuromuscular control of urination by 4 or 5 years of age. Enuresis is defined as urinary incontinence at any age when urinary control would be expected (Hockenberry & Wilson, 2015).
- "At five years of age, 15 percent of children are incompletely continent of urine. Most of these children have isolated nocturnal enuresis" (Tu, Baskin, & Amhym, 2014). "Enuresis (synonymous with intermittent nocturnal incontinence) refers to discrete episodes of urinary incontinence during sleep in children ≥5 years of age" (Tu, Baskin, & Amhym, 2014).
- The etiology of enuresis is complex and not well understood. The following factors have been implicated (National Clinical Guideline Centre, 2010; Tu et al., 2014):
  - Developmental/maturational delay (e.g., small functional bladder capacity, deep sleep, mental retardation)
  - Organic factors (e.g., infection, sickle cell anemia, diabetes, neuromuscular disorders)
  - Psychological/emotional factors (e.g., stressors such as birth of sibling, hospitalization, divorce of parents; Kelleher, 1997).
- Children at risk for overflow retention include those who (Hockenberry & Wilson, 2015)
  - Have congenital anomalies of the urinary tract
  - Are neurologically impaired

- Have undergone surgery
- Enuresis is primarily a maturational problem and usually ceases between 6 and 8 years of age. It is more common in boys. By adolescence, 99% become continent (National Clinical Guideline Centre, 2010; Tu et al., 2014).
- There is a high frequency of bed-wetting in children whose parents or other near relatives were bed-wetters (National Clinical Guideline Centre, 2010; Tu et al., 2014).
- Most children with nocturnal enuresis have neither a psychiatric nor an organic illness (National Clinical Guideline Centre, 2010; Tu et al., 2014).

Focus Assessment Criteria (National Clinical Guideline Centre, 2010)

Ask about the pattern of bed-wetting, including questions such as:
- How many nights a week does bed-wetting occur?
- How many times a night does bed-wetting occur?
- Does there seem to be a large amount of urine?
- At what times of night does the bed-wetting occur?
- Does the child or young person wake up after bed-wetting?

Ask about the presence of daytime symptoms in a child or young person with bed-wetting, including
- Daytime frequency (that is, passing urine more than seven times a day)
- Daytime urgency
- Daytime wetting
- Passing urine infrequently (fewer than four times a day)
- Abdominal straining or poor urinary stream
- Pain passing urine

Ask about daytime toileting patterns in a child or young person with bed-wetting, including
- Whether daytime symptoms occur only in some situations
- Avoidance of toilets at school or other settings
- Whether the child or young person goes to the toilet more or less frequently than his or her peers

Assess whether the child or young person has any comorbidities or there are other factors to consider, in particular
- Constipation and/or soiling
- Developmental, attention, or learning difficulties
- Diabetes mellitus
- Behavioral or emotional problems
- Family problems or a vulnerable child or young person or family

Recent change or stressor
- School
- Relocation
- Peers
- Family problems
- New sibling

Inattention to bladder cues

Sexual abuse

Goals

NOC

Urinary Continence, Knowledge: Enuresis, Family Functioning

The child will have reduction in number of wet nights, as evidenced by the following indicators:

- Will list the factors that decrease enuresis
- Will relate that bed-wetting is not their fault
- Will relate optimism about the prospects of stopping bed-wetting

Interventions

NIC

Urinary Incontinence Care: Enuresis, Urinary Habit Training, Anticipatory Guidance, Family Support

Ascertain That Physiologic Causes of Enuresis Have Been Ruled Out

- Examples include infections, meatal stenosis, fistulas, pinworms, epispadias, ectopic ureter, and minor neurologic dysfunction (hyperactivity, cognitive delay).

Determine Contributing Factors

- Refer to Related Factors.

Promote a Positive Parent–Child Relations

- Inform children and young people with bed-wetting that it is not their fault. Do not exclude younger children (for example, those under 7 years) from the management of bed-wetting on the basis of age alone (National Clinical Guideline Centre, 2010).

R: *The most important reason for treating enuresis is to minimize the embarrassment and anxiety of the child and the frustration experienced by the parents. Most children with enuresis feel very much alone with their problem (National Clinical Guideline Centre, 2010; Tu et al., 2014).*

- Inform the parents or caregivers that bed-wetting is not the child or young person's fault and that punitive measures should not be used in the management of bed-wetting (National Clinical Guideline Centre, 2010; Tu et al., 2014).

R: *"Surveys indicate that between one-fourth and one-third of parents punish their child for wetting the bed, and sometimes the punishment is physically abusive" (Tu & Baskin, 2014).*

- Explore with family members if there is a history of bed-wetting in the family (e.g., parents, aunts, uncles).

R: *Family members with a history of enuresis should be encouraged to share their experiences and offer moral support to the child. The knowledge that another family member had and outgrew the problem can be therapeutic (Rittig et al., 2013).*

- Offer support, assessment, and treatment tailored to the circumstances and needs of the child or young person and parents or caregivers.
- Explain to the parents and the child the physiologic development of bladder control.

R: *This can help to relieve feelings of guilt or blame (National Clinical Guideline Centre, 2010; Tu & Baskin, 2014).*

- Explain to parents that disapproval (shaming, punishing) is useless in stopping enuresis but can make child shy, ashamed, and afraid.

R: *Anger, punishment, and rejection by parents and peers contribute to feelings of shame, embarrassment, and low self-esteem (Carpenter, 1999; Tu & Baskin, 2014).*

- Address excessive or insufficient fluid intake or abnormal toileting patterns before starting other treatment for bed-wetting in children and young people.
- Advice parents or caregivers to try a reward system alone (as described above) for the initial treatment of bed-wetting in young children who have some dry nights. For example, rewards may be given for (National Clinical Guideline Centre, 2010).
  - Drinking recommended levels of fluid during the day
  - Using the toilet to pass urine before sleep
  - Engaging in management (for example, taking medication or helping to change sheets)

Reduce Contributing Factors, If Possible

Small Bladder Capacity

- After child drinks fluids, encourage him or her to postpone voiding to help stretch the bladder.

Sound Sleeper

- Have child void before retiring.
- Restrict fluids at bedtime.
- If child is awakened later (about 11 PM) to void, attempt to awaken child fully for positive reinforcement.

Too Busy to Sense a Full Bladder (If Daytime *Wetting Occurs*)

- Teach child awareness of sensations that occur when it is time to void.
- Teach child the ability to control urination (have him or her start and stop the stream; have him or her "hold" the urine during the day, even if for only a short time).
- Bladder retraining can help control dysfunctional voiding.

R: *Choosing scheduled intervals to empty bladder helps to lessen the sense of urgency.*

- Have child keep a record of how he or she is doing; emphasize dry days or nights (e.g., stars on a calendar).
- If child wets, have him or her explain or write down (if feasible) why he or she thinks it happened.

R: *These strategies engage the child in the treatment plan and increase awareness that the problem can be controlled.*

- With school age children, assess if the child is using the bathroom at school. Do they get sufficient bathroom breaks? Can a reminder device be used (vibrating watch, cell phone)?

R: *Arrangements may need to be made with the teacher for extra bathroom time). The use of devices, such as a vibrating watch, cell phone, may help remind the child when it is time to use the bathroom (*Ball & Bindler, 2008).*

If Indicated, Discuss a Bed Alarm System and Refer Them to Their Primary Care Provider
(National Clinical Guideline Centre, 2010)

R: *Inform the child or young person and their parents or caregivers that the aims of alarm treatment for bed-wetting are to train the child or young person to recognize the need to pass urine, wake to go to the toilet or hold on, and learn over time to hold on or to wake spontaneously and stop wetting the bed (National Clinical Guideline Centre, 2010).*

- Encourage children and young people with bed-wetting and their parents or caregivers to discuss and agree on their roles and responsibilities for using the alarm and the use of rewards.
- Offer an alarm as the first-line treatment to children and young people whose bed-wetting has not responded to advice on fluids, toileting, or an appropriate reward system.
- An alarm is considered inappropriate, particularly if (National Clinical Guideline Centre, 2010).
  - Bed-wetting is very infrequent (that is, less than 1 to 2 wet beds per week).
  - The parents or caregivers are having emotional difficulty coping with the burden of bed-wetting.
  - The parents or caregivers are expressing anger, negativity, or blame toward the child or young person.
  - Continue alarm treatment in children and young people with bed-wetting who are showing signs of response until a minimum of 2 weeks' uninterrupted dry nights has been achieved. Stop treatment only if there are no early signs of response.

Initiate Health Teaching and Referrals, as Indicated

- Teach child and parents the facts about enuresis.
- Teach family techniques to control the adverse effects of enuresis (e.g., plastic mattress covers, use of sleeping bag [machine-washable] when staying overnight away from home).
- Advice to avoid all caffeine-containing drinks all together. Avoid fluids 2 hours before going to bed.

R: *Foods that can irritate the bladder include coffee, tea, chocolate, and sodas or other carbonated beverages containing caffeine.*

R: *Although nighttime incontinence can be cured, it may take as long as 6 months to a year. Reassure the parents and the child. Without implying punishment, involve the child in bed changing for nocturnal enuresis (*Ball & Bindler, 2008).*

R: *Interventions for nocturnal enuresis must focus on reducing social and emotional stigma. Seek opportunities to teach the public about enuresis and incontinence (e.g., school and parent organizations, self-help groups).*

Functional Urinary Incontinence

NANDA-I Definition

Inability of a usually continent person to reach the toilet in time to avoid unintentional loss of urine

Defining Characteristics

Incontinence before or during an attempt to reach the toilet

Related Factors

Pathophysiologic

Related to diminished bladder cues and impaired ability to recognize bladder cues secondary to:

Brain injury/tumor/infection
Alcoholic neuropathy
Cerebrovascular accident
Parkinsonism
Demyelinating diseases
Progressive dementia
Multiple sclerosis
encephalopathy

Treatment Related

Related to decreased bladder tone secondary to:

Antihistamines
Immunosuppressant therapy
Epinephrine
Diuretics
Anticholinergics
Tranquilizers
Sedatives
Muscle relaxants

Situational (Personal, Environmental)

Related to impaired mobility

Chronic or acute pain
Medical equipment

Related to decreased attention to bladder cues

Depression
Intentional suppression (self-induced deconditioning)
Confusion

Related to environmental barriers to using bathroom

Distant toilets/seat height
Bed too high
Poor lighting
Side rails
Unfamiliar surroundings
Clothing
Medical equipment including sequential compression devices (SCDs), IV poles, and other medical devices
Lack of timely help from staff
No call light within reach
No urinal at the bedside

Maturational

Older Adult

Related to motor and sensory losses

Key Concepts

- Functional incontinence is the inability or unwillingness of the individual with a normal bladder and sphincter to reach the toilet in time.
- Functional incontinence may be caused by conditions affecting physical and emotional abilities to manage the act of urination.
- Underlying psychological problems can be a functional etiology of incontinence.
- Among residential care facilities residents, 39.0% had had an episode of urinary and/or bowel incontinence during the 7 days prior to the survey, with 36.6% reported to have had an episode of urinary incontinence and 20.4% reported to have had an episode of bowel incontinence (Gorina et al., 2014).
- For individuals with dementia-induced functional incontinence, timed and prompted voiding is the most successful approach to incontinence management (*Yap & Tan, 2006).

Focus Assessment Criteria

See *Impaired Urinary Elimination.*

Goals

NOC

Tissue Integrity, Urinary Continence, Urinary Elimination

The individual will report no or decreased episodes of incontinence, as evidenced by the following indicators:

- Removes or minimizes environmental barriers at home
- Uses proper adaptive equipment to assist with voiding, transfers, and dressing
- Describes causative factors for incontinence

Interventions

NIC

Perineal Care, Urinary Incontinence Care, Prompted Voiding, Urinary Habit Training, Urinary Elimination Management, Teaching: Procedure/Treatment

Assess Causative or Contributing Factors

Obstacles to Toilet

- Lack of timely response for help from caregivers
- Poor lighting, slippery floor, misplaced furniture and rugs, inadequate footwear, toilet too far, bed too high, side rails up
- Inadequate toilet (too small for walkers, wheelchair, seat too low/high, no grab bars)
- Inadequate signal system for requesting help
- Lack of privacy

Sensory/Cognitive Deficits

- Visual deficits (blindness, field cuts, poor depth perception)
- Cognitive deficits as a result of aging, trauma, stroke, tumor, infection

Motor/Mobility Deficits

- Limited upper and/or lower extremity movement/strength (inability to remove clothing)
- Barriers to ambulation (e.g., vertigo, fatigue, altered gait, hypertension, pain)

R: *Barriers can delay access to the toilet and cause incontinence if the individual cannot delay urination. A few seconds' delay in reaching the bathroom can make the difference between continence and incontinence.*

Factors that increase urgency

- Caffeine, carbonated beverages, overhydration, dehydration, artificial sweeteners, tobacco use

R: *Causal associations with tobacco use and carbonated drinks are confirmed for bladder disorders associated with incontinence (Dallosso, McGrother, Matthews, & Donaldson, 2003).*

Reduce or Eliminate Contributing Factors, If Possible

Environmental Barriers

- Assess path to bathroom for obstacles, lighting, and distance.
- Assess adequacy of toilet height and need for grab bars.
- Assess adequacy of room size.
- Assess if individual can remove clothing easily.
- Provide a commode between bathroom and bed, if necessary.
- Provide a urinal at the bedside.

Sensory/Cognitive Deficits

- For all patients with any sensory or cognitive deficit:
  - Keep call bell easily accessible.
  - Assess for patient safety in the bathroom and remain as close as possible while maintaining privacy.
  - Allow sufficient time for the task.
- For an individual with diminished vision:
  - Ensure adequate lighting.
  - Encourage individual to wear prescribed corrective lens.
  - Provide clear, safe pathway to bathroom.
  - If bedpan or urinal is used, make sure it is within easy reach in the same preferred location at all times.
- For an individual with cognitive deficits:
  - Offer toileting reminders every 2 hours or more often if indicated, after meals, and before bedtime.
  - Establish appropriate means to communicate need to void.
  - Answer call bell immediately.
  - Encourage wearing of ordinary clothes and assess need for adaptive devices on clothing to make dressing and undressing easier.
  - Provide a normal environment for elimination (use bathroom, if possible), and assume the natural position for urination as possible.

R: *The sitting position for the female and the standing position for the male allow optimal relaxation of the external urinary sphincter and perineal muscles.*

- Reorient to where he or she is and what task he or she is doing.
- Be consistent in your approach.

- Give simple step-by-step instructions; use verbal and nonverbal cues.
- Give positive reinforcement for success.
- Assess his or her ability to provide self-hygiene.

R: *An individual with a cognitive deficit needs constant verbal cues and reminders to establish a routine and to reduce incontinence.*

Provide for Factors That Promote Continence

Maintain Optimal Hydration

- Drink most fluids during the daytime. Drink no more than 2 L (about 2 quarts) of fluid a day but at least 1 L. Avoid or limit bladder irritants: Individuals who increased their fluid intake to 3,700 mL or more per day demonstrated an increased incidence of urinary incontinence than with an intake of 2,400 mL/day (Miller, Guo, & Rodseth, 2011).
- Decrease fluid intake after 7 PM; provide only minimal fluids during the night.

R: *Dehydration can prevent the sensation of a full bladder and can contribute to loss of bladder tone. Spacing fluids helps promote regular bladder filling and emptying. Dehydration irritates the bladder lining, making the urgency worse (Griebling, 2009).*

Explain Foods/Fluids That Increase Bladder Irritation and/or Volume Increasing Urgency (Davis et al., 2013; Derrer, 2014; Gleason et al., 2013; Lukacz, 2015)

- Caffeinated beverages/foods (e.g., coffee, tea, chocolate), alcohol, red wine, highly acidic foods, and foods high in potassium can irritate the bladder, causing urgency and frequency (Griebling, 2009).
- Carbonated beverages should be eliminated or decreased because they may increase bladder activity and urgency (Wilson et al., 2005).
  - Excessive fluid intake overfills bladder.
  - Insufficient fluid Intake irritates the bladder.
  - Spicy foods irritate the bladder.
  - Artificial sweeteners irritate the bladder.
- Encourage intake of 16 oz of unsweetened/or reduced sugar blueberry or cranberry juice.

R: *Acidic urine deters the growth of most bacteria implicated in cystitis.*

Maintain Adequate Nutrition to Ensure Bowel Elimination at Least Once Every 3 Days

- Minimize constipation.

R: *Constipation may increase the risk of urinary retention as well as exacerbate any incontinence (Wood & Anger, 2014).*

Promote Personal Integrity and Provide Motivation to Increase Bladder Control

- Encourage to share feelings about incontinence and determine its effect on his or her social patterns.
- Convey that incontinence can, at the very least, be controlled to maintain dignity.
- Use protective pads or garments only after conscientious reconditioning efforts have been completely unsuccessful after 6 weeks.
- Work to achieve daytime continence before expecting nighttime continence.
- Encourage socialization. If fear or embarrassment is preventing socialization, instruct individual to use sanitary pads or briefs temporarily until control is established.
- Discourage the use of bedpans.
- If hospitalized, provide opportunities to eat meals outside bedroom (day room, lounge).
- Change clothes as soon as possible when wet to avoid indirectly sanctioning wetness.
- Refer to *Social Isolation* and *Ineffective Coping* for additional interventions, if indicated.

R: *Wearing normal clothing or nightwear helps simulate the home environment, where incontinence may not occur. A hospital gown may reinforce incontinence. Use of bathroom rather than bedpans simulates the home environment.*

Promote Skin Integrity

- Identify individuals at risk for development of pressure ulcers.
- Avoid harsh soaps and alcohol products. Gently cleanse the skin, moisturize, and apply a skin protectant or moisture barrier (Beekman et al., 2012).
- Avoid the use of briefs or adult diapers as they trap heat and moisture and can lead to redness and inflammation and subsequently skin erosion (Chatham & Carls, 2012).

- Keep moisture away from the skin.
- Refer to *Risk for Pressure Ulcers* for additional information.

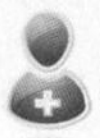

CLINICAL ALERT "Normal skin pH is acidic at 4 to 6.5, which helps protect the skin against microorganism invasion. Frequent use of soap can alter skin pH to an alkaline state, leaving it more vulnerable to microorganism invasion. Exposure to urine or diarrhea damages the skin and increases the risk of Pressure Ulcers. Urine is absorbed by keratinocytes (outermost layer of skin), and when these cells are softened, they cannot provide protection from pressure injury. Urine contains urea, and ammonia can damage the skin. In an incontinent individual with a urinary tract infection, urine will also be alkaline and injurious to the skin" (Langemo & Black, 2010, p. 61).

Teach Prevention of Urinary Tract Infections

- Encourage regular, complete emptying of the bladder.
- Ensure adequate fluid intake at least 2,000 mL daily.
- Keep urine acidic; avoid citrus juices, dark colas, coffee, tea, and alcohol, which act as irritants. It has been demonstrated that an increase in bladder irritants can lead to increased urinary leakage (Miller et al., 2011).
- Teach to recognize abnormal changes in urine properties.
  - Increased mucus and sediment
  - Blood in urine (hematuria)
  - Change in color (from normal straw-colored) or odor
- Teach individual to monitor for signs and symptoms of infection.
  - Elevated temperature, chills, and shaking
  - Painful urination
    - Urgency
    - Frequent small voids or frequent small incontinences
    - Nausea/vomiting
    - Lower back, flank pain, or both
    - Suprapubic pain

R: *Bacteria multiply rapidly in stagnant urine retained in the bladder. Moreover, overdistention hinders blood flow to the bladder wall, increasing the susceptibility to infection from bacterial growth. Regular, complete bladder emptying greatly reduces the risk of infection.*

- Changes in urine properties: The urine dipstick test is the most reliable tool for detecting a urinary tract infection by measuring presence of nitrites and leukocytes (Medina-Bombardo & Jover-Palmer, 2011).

Explain Age-Related Effects on Bladder Function and That Urgency and Nocturia Do Not Necessarily Lead to Incontinence

Initiate Health Teaching Referral, When Indicated

- Refer to home health nurse (occupational therapy department) for assessment of bathroom facilities at home.

Geriatric Interventions

- Emphasize that incontinence is not an inevitable age-related event.

R: *Explaining the cause can motivate the individual to participate.*

- Explain not to restrict fluid intake because of fear of incontinence.

R: *Dehydration can cause incontinence by eliminating the sensation of a full bladder (the signal to urinate) and by reducing the individual's alertness to the sensation.*

R: *Studies have shown that mild dehydration impairs cognitive abilities and contributes to increased anxiety and fatigue in adults (Ganio et al., 2011). This may be even more problematic for someone of advanced age.*

- Teach older adults not to depend on thirst sensations but to drink liquids even when not thirsty every 2 hour, especially in hot weather or when exercising.

R: *The hypothalamus regulates body temperature, sleep, and appetite, monitors the blood's concentration of sodium and other substances, and receives inputs from sensors in the blood vessels that monitor blood volume and pressure (hydration). As one ages, the function of the hypothalamus diminishes (Grossman & Porth, 2014).*

- To reduce nocturia, limit fluids after dinner. Emphasize the need to have easy access to bathroom at night. Use a night light. If needed, consider commode chair or urinal.

R: *This is to prevent falls.*

Reflex Urinary Incontinence

NANDA-I Definition

Involuntary loss of urine at somewhat predictable intervals when a specific bladder volume is reached

Defining Characteristics

Major (Must Be Present)*

Inability to voluntarily inhibit voiding or imitate voiding
Incomplete emptying with lesion above pontine micturition center
Incomplete emptying with lesion above sacral micturition
Predictable pattern of voiding
Sensation of urgency without voluntary inhibition of bladder contraction
Sensations associated with full bladder (e.g., sweating, restlessness, abdominal discomfort)
No sensation of bladder fullness, urge to void or voiding

Related Factors

Pathophysiologic

Related to impaired conduction of impulses above the reflex arc level secondary to:

Cord injury/tumor/infection

Related to postoperative dribbling and incontinence secondary to:

Transurethral resection of the prostate
Prostate surgery

Key Concepts

- The three main centers responsible for the inhibition and facilitation of micturition include the sacral micturition center at S2 to S4, the cerebral cortex, and the pontine micturition center.
- A lesion above the sacral cord segments (above T12) involving both motor and sensory tracts of the spinal cord results in a reflex bladder. Other common names for this type of bladder dysfunction are spastic, supraspinal, hypertonic, automatic, and upper motor neuron bladder.
- A lesion that does not completely transect the spinal cord can produce variable findings.
- Control from higher cerebral centers is removed in the reflex neurogenic bladder. Therefore, the individual cannot start or stop micturition in a voluntary manner.
- The simple spinal reflex arc takes over the control of micturition.
- A positive bulbocavernosus reflex suggests that the voiding reflex (spinal reflex arc) is intact.
- If the opening of the urinary sphincter and the relaxation of the striated muscle surrounding the urinary sphincter are uncoordinated, there is a potential for large residual urine volumes after triggered voiding.
- Autonomic dysreflexia is an abnormal hyperactive reflex activity that occurs only in people with spinal cord injury with a lesion above T8. Most often, these individuals have an upper motor neuron bladder (reflex incontinence). This is a life-threatening situation in which the blood pressure rises to lethal levels. Autonomic hyperreflexia is most often caused by bladder or bowel distension.
- Urinary incontinence is one of the most common side effects after having a prostatectomy. A study of 405 men showed that 59% were incontinent post prostatectomy even 6 weeks after surgery, but only

22% reported incontinence at 58 weeks. The best outcomes were in nonobese and physically active men (Wolin, Luly, Sutcliffe, Andriole, & Kibel, 2010).

- There is no evidence that pelvic floor muscle training exercises before prostate surgery improve outcomes, decreasing the chance of incontinence, except to give men a sense of control (Wilson et al., 2005).

Focus Assessment Criteria

See *Impaired Urinary Elimination*.

Goals

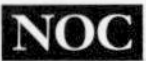

See *Functional Urinary Incontinence*.

The individual will report a state of dryness that meets personal satisfaction, as evidenced by the following indicators:

- Has a residual urine volume of less than 50 mL
- Uses triggering mechanisms to initiate reflex voiding

Interventions

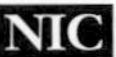

See also *Functional Urinary Incontinence*, Pelvic Muscle Exercises, Weight Management

Assess for Causative and Contributing Conditions

- Refer to Related Factors.
- Explain rationale for treatment(s).

Develop a Bladder-Retraining or Reconditioning Program

- See Interventions under *Continuous Incontinence*.

Teach Techniques to Stimulate Reflex Voiding

- Cutaneous triggering mechanisms
- Repeated deep, sharp suprapubic tapping (most effective)
- Instruct individual to
    - Place self in a half-sitting position
    - Tap directly at bladder wall at a rate of seven or eight times for 5 seconds (35 to 40 single blows)
    - Use only one hand
    - Shift site of stimulation over bladder to find most successful site
    - Continue stimulation until a good stream starts
    - Wait approximately 1 minute; repeat stimulation until bladder is empty
- One or two series of stimulations without response signify that nothing more will be expelled.
- If the preceding measures are ineffective, instruct individual to perform each of the following for 2 to 3 minutes, waiting 1 minute between attempts:
    - Stroking glans penis
    - Lightly punching abdomen above inguinal ligaments
    - Stroking inner thigh
- Encourage individual to void or trigger at least every 3 hours.
- Indicate on intake and output sheet which mechanism was used to induce voiding.
- People with abdominal muscle control should use the Valsalva maneuver during triggered voiding.
- Teach that if he or she increases fluid intake, he or she also needs to increase the frequency of triggering to prevent overdistention.
- Schedule intermittent catheterization program (see *Continuous Incontinence*).

R: *Stimulating the reflex arc replaces the internal sphincter of the bladder, allowing urination. Stimulating the bladder wall or cutaneous sites (e.g., suprapubic, pubic) can trigger the reflex arc.*

R: *Preferred cutaneous triggering methods are light, rapid suprapubic tapping, light pulling of pubic hair, massage of the abdomen, and digital rectal stimulation.*

R: *Use of Credé's maneuver should be avoided with a reflex bladder because the urethra may be damaged or vesicoureteral reflux may occur if the external sphincter is contracted.*

R: *Contraction of abdominal muscles compresses the bladder to empty it.*

Initiate Health Teaching, as Indicated

Arrange an At-Home Assessment by a Home Health Nurse

- Teach bladder reconditioning program (see *Continuous Incontinence*).
- Teach intermittent catheterization (see *Continuous Incontinence*).
- Teach prevention of urinary tract infections (see *Continuous Incontinence*).

R: *Strategies to control urination must be continued at home.*

- If individual is at high risk for dysreflexia, refer to *Dysreflexia*.

Stress Urinary Incontinence

NANDA-I Definition

Sudden leakage of urine with activities that increase in intra-abdominal pressure

Defining Characteristics*

Observed or reported involuntary leakage of small amounts of urine:

In the absence of detrusor contraction
In the absence of an overactive bladder
On physical exertion
With coughing, laughing, sneezing, or all of these

Related Factors

Pathophysiologic

Related to incompetent bladder outlet secondary to:

Congenital urinary tract anomalies

Related to degenerative changes in pelvic muscles* and structural supports secondary to:

Estrogen deficiency

Related to intrinsic urethral sphincter*

Situational (Personal, Environmental)

Related to high intra-abdominal pressure* and weak pelvic muscles* secondary to:

Obesity
Pregnancy
Smoking
Sex
Poor personal hygiene

Related to weak pelvic muscles and structural supports secondary to:

Recent substantial weight loss
Childbirth

Maturational

Older Adult

Related to loss of muscle tone

Key Concepts

General Considerations

- "'Pelvic floor health' is the physical and functional integrity of the pelvic floor unit through the life stages of an individual (male or female), permitting an optimal quality of life through its multifunctional role, where the individual possesses or has access to knowledge, which empowers the ability to prevent or manage dysfunction" (Pierce, Perry, Gallagher, & Chiarelli, 2015).

- Lukacz (2015) defines stress incontinence occurs when the muscles and tissues around the urethra (where urine exits) do not stay closed properly when there is increased pressure (stress) in the abdomen, leading to urine leakage. Increased pressure occurs with coughing, sneezing, laughing, or running. Stress incontinence is a common reason for incontinence in women, especially those who are obese or have had vaginal deliveries.
- The incidence of stress urinary incontinence was reported in 15% of women and urgency incontinence/overactive bladder in 13% (Lawrence, Lukacz, Nager, Hsu, & Luber, 2008; Lukacz, 2015).
- Menopausal decrease in elasticity of the perineal tissue usually worsening stress incontinence.
- Urinary incontinence is twice as common in women as in men (Zaccardi, Wilson, & Mokrzycki, 2010).
- A trial of vaginal estrogen cream in the postmenopausal woman who exhibits a pale, atrophic vaginal vault may help to reduce the incidence of incontinence.

Maternal Considerations

- Pressure of the uterus can cause stress incontinence, which can be misinterpreted as amniotic fluid and vice versa.

Focus Assessment Criteria

Refer to *Impaired Urinary Elimination.*

Goals

NOC

Refer to *Functional Urinary Incontinence.*

The individual will report a reduction or elimination of stress incontinence, as evidenced by the following indicator:

- Be able to explain the cause of incontinence and rationale for treatments

Interventions

NIC

See also *Functional Incontinence*, Pelvic Muscle Exercise, Weight Management

Routinely Assess Women of All Ages for Their Knowledge of Pelvic Floor Health and Stress Incontinence. Specifically Ask If They Experience Leaking of Urine

R: *Nygaard et al. (*1994) reported in a "study of elite nulliparous college athletes that 32% of the athletes leaked urine during their sports, 13% beginning in junior high". "Gymnastic athletes had the highest incidence of urinary leakage at 67%, with basketball close behind at 66%, and tennis at 50%" (*Nygaard et al., 1994; *Smith, 2004).*

Determine Contributing Factors That Can Be Reduced (*Smith, 2004)

- Obesity refers also to *Obesity/Overweight* nursing diagnoses.
- Lack of knowledge of pelvic muscle structures and effects of weakness caused by, for example, obesity, vaginal childbirth, sports, loss of estrogen (perimenopause, menopause)
- With aging, a stretching or sagging of the pelvic floor may result in hernia-like positions of the bladder, the uterus, or the rectum.
- Chronic constipation-frequent straining and bearing down to have a bowel movement stretches the pelvic muscles.
- Hysterectomy—the removal of the uterus removes one of the support structures for the other pelvic organ.
- Situational—prolonged standing, lifting, or carrying weight for a job or exercise
- Smoking and chronic coughing add extra stress to the pelvic floor muscles and ligaments.

R: *The above situations are important times to keep the pelvic muscles exercised, increasing the blood supply to the muscles and providing strength and tone of the fibers for support. Pelvic floor weakness with incontinence or pelvic organ prolapse can interfere with social, recreational, and career activities (*Smith, 2004).*

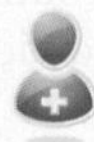

Clinical Alert The following myths held by health-care professional and women are barriers to discussions and successful management of stress incontinence (*Smith, 2004):

- Underappreciation and the lack of knowledge of the complex nature of the pelvic floor and its function
- That it is difficult to isolate pelvic muscles
- That pelvic floor weakness is a natural result of aging.
- That women are not comfortable discussing pelvic floor dysfunction symptoms.

Explain the Effect of Incompetent Floor Muscles on Continence (See Key Concepts)

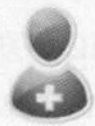

CLINICAL ALERT "Effective and consistent pelvic muscle exercises can provide many benefits across the lifespan of women. Beginning in young healthy women, strengthening the pelvic floor muscles provides support for the bladder and urethra against the forces of increased intra-abdominal pressures from activity or exertion; provides increased sensation and control during sexual activity; and prepares the pelvic floor for pregnancy and childbirth" (*Smith, 2004).

Teach Pelvic Muscle Exercises

- Explain that it will take 4 to 6 months before results can be noted (Mayo Clinic, 2012; *Smith, 2004).

R: *Like other muscles in the body, the muscles in the pelvic floor are subject to fatigue and injury. They can also be actively exercised to increase their tone and size to prevent fatigue and injury (*Smith, 2004).*

Teach How to Self-Assess Whether Exercises Are Being Done Correctly

- Stand with one foot elevated on a stool, insert finger in vagina, and feel the strength of the contraction. Evaluate the strength of the contraction on a scale of 0 to 5 (Sampselle & DeLancey, 1998):
  - 0 = No palpable contraction
  - 1 = Very weak, barely felt
  - 2 = Weak but clearly felt
  - 3 = Good but not maintained when moderate finger pressure is applied
  - 4 = Good but not maintained when intense finger pressure is applied
  - 5 = Maximum strength with strong resistance
- Consult an incontinence specialist for use of vaginal weights for pelvic floor strengthening if indicated.

Provide Instructions for Pelvic Muscle Exercises (Kegel Exercises)

Explain

- Pelvic floor muscle rehabilitation is an important treatment for strengthening perineal muscles and is an effective exercise to prevent stress and urgency incontinence (Domoulin, Hay-Smith, & Mac Habee-Segui, 2014).

R: *Pelvic floor muscle training should be encouraged and taught to all young women and older and for all incontinence episodes mixed, urge, or stress (Wilson et al., 2005).*

- To learn which muscles to tighten to stop urination as you are urinating; this includes tightening the rectal muscles.

R: *This will indicate if you are tightening the correct muscles.*

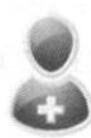

CLINICAL ALERT Don't make a habit of using Kegel exercises to start and stop your urine stream. Doing Kegel exercises while emptying your bladder can actually weaken the muscles, as well as lead to incomplete emptying of the bladder—which increases the risk of a urinary tract infection.

- Empty your bladder before doing Kegel exercises.
- Hold the contractions for 5 to 10 seconds and release. Relax between contractions taking care to keep contraction and relaxation times equal. Gradually increase the time of contracting from 2 seconds to 10 seconds. If you contract for 10 seconds, relax for 10 seconds before next contraction.
- Perform 40 to 60 contractions divided in 2 to 4 sessions each time. These should be spread out through the day and incorporate different positions (sitting, standing, and lying).
- For best results, focus on tightening only your pelvic floor muscles. Be careful not to flex the muscles in your abdomen, thighs, or buttocks. Avoid holding your breath. Instead, breathe freely during the exercises (Mayo Clinic, 2012).
- A good way to help to remember to do exercises is to incorporate them into daily routine, such as stopping at a traffic light or washing dishes (Wilkinson & Van Leuven, 2007). Refer individuals to "How to do Kegel exercises," accessed under women's health at the Mayo Clinic website.

R: *In stress incontinence, childbirth, trauma, menopausal atrophy, or obesity has weakened or stretched the pelvic floor muscles (pubococcygeus) and levator ani muscles.*

Initiate Referrals for Individuals Who Continue to Remain Incontinent After Attempts at Bladder Reconditioning or Muscle Retraining

- Refer to a urogynecology specialist for a comprehensive workup.
- Schedule intermittent catheterization program, if appropriate (see *Continuous Incontinence*).

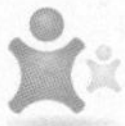

Maternal Interventions

- For increased abdominal pressure during pregnancy:
  - Teach individual to avoid prolonged standing.
  - Teach individual the benefit of frequent voiding (at least every 2 hours).
  - Teach pelvic muscle exercises after delivery.

R: *Pressure of the uterus on the bladder can cause involuntary loss of urine.*

Continuous Urinary Incontinence[53]

Definition

State in which an individual experiences continuous, unpredictable loss of urine* without distention or awareness of bladder fullness

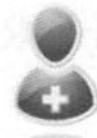

Clinical Alert Incontinence-associated dermatitis is associated with both fecal and urinary incontinence and has been identified as a risk factor leading to hospital-acquired pressure ulcers (HAPU). As such, the Centers for Medicare and Medicaid Services have limited reimbursement for institutions that report HAPUs.

Defining Characteristics

Constant flow of urine at unpredictable times without uninhibited bladder contractions/spasm or distention
Lack of bladder filling or perineal filling
Nocturia
Unawareness of incontinence
Incontinence refractory to other treatments

Related Factors

Refer to *Impaired Urinary Elimination*.

Key Concepts

Refer to *Impaired Urinary Elimination*.

Focus Assessment Criteria

Refer to *Impaired Urinary Elimination*.

Goals

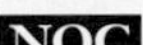

NOC
Refer to Functional Urinary Incontinence.

The individual will be continent (specify during day, night, 24 hours), as evidenced by the following indicators:

- Identifies the cause of incontinence and rationale for treatments
- Identifies daily goal for fluid intake

[53]This diagnosis is not presently on the NANDA-I list but has been included for clarity and usefulness.

Interventions

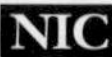

See also *Functional Incontinence*, Pelvic Muscle Exercise, Weight Management

Develop a Bladder-Retraining or Reconditioning Program, Which Should Include Communication, Assessment of Voiding Pattern, Scheduled Fluid Intake, and Scheduled Voiding Times

Promote Communication Among All Staff Members and Among Individual, Family, and Staff

- Provide all staff with sufficient knowledge concerning the program planned.
- Assess staff's response to program.

Assess the Individual's Potential for Participation in a Bladder-Retraining Program

- Cognition
- Desire to change behavior
- Ability to cooperate
- Willingness to participate

R: *Continence training programs are either self-directed or caregiver-directed. Self-directed programs of bladder training, retraining, and exercises are for motivated, cognitively intact individuals (Miller, 2015). Caregiver-directed programs of scheduled toileting or habit training are appropriate for motivated caregivers of individuals with cognitive impairment.*

R: *Education of caregivers increases preparedness, decreases burden, and reduces role strain, thereby reducing overall stress when caring for an incontinent individual or family member.*

Provide Rationale for Plan and Acquire Informed Consent With Individual If Possible

Encourage to Continue Program by Providing Accurate Information Concerning Reasons for Success or Failure

Assess Voiding Pattern

- Monitor and record:
  - Intake and output
  - Time and amount of fluid intake
  - Type of fluid
  - Amount of incontinence; measure if possible or estimate amount as small, moderate, or large
  - Amount of void, whether it was voluntary or involuntary
  - Presence of sensation of need to void
  - Amount of retention (amount of urine left in the bladder after an unsuccessful attempt at manual triggering or voiding)
  - Amount of residual (amount of urine left in the bladder after either a voluntary or manual triggered voiding; also called a *postvoid residual*)
  - Amount of triggered urine (urine expelled after manual triggering [e.g., tapping, Credé's method])
- Identify certain activities that precede voiding (e.g., restlessness, yelling, exercise).
- Record in appropriate column.

Schedule Fluid Intake and Voiding Times

- Provide fluid intake of 2,000 mL each day unless contraindicated.
- Discourage fluids after 7 PM.
- Provide caregiver education.
- Initially, bladder emptying is done at least every 2 hours and at least twice during the night; goal is 2- to 4-hour intervals.
- If the individual is incontinent before scheduled voids, shorten the time between voids.

Reduce Incontinence-Associated Dermatitis

- Decrease the alkalizing effect of urine on the skin.
- Use a no-rinse perineal cleanser instead of soap and water (Beekman et al., 2011).
- Avoid fragrances, alcohol, and alkaline agents (found in many commercial soaps).
- Apply moisturizer immediately after bathing, to dry skin, when pores are open.
- Select a moisturizer that is occlusive (white petroleum, lanolin, emollients).
- Decrease injury with washing, for example, use soft premoistened wipes instead of abrasive towels.
- Do not try to remove all of the ointment with cleansing.

- Dry skin gently by patting, not rubbing.
- Use a moisture barrier product (e.g., Curity Moisture Barrier Cream; No Sting Barrier Film).

R: *Incontinence-associated dermatitis has been defined as "skin inflammation and erythema, with or without erosion or denudation, due to irritants of urine and/or fecal incontinence" (Gray et al., 2007).*

R: *In a study of 608 acute care patients from medical-surgical and intensive care units, 42.5% of incontinent patients had varying degrees of skin injury (Junkin & Selekof, 2007).*

R: *The essential components of any continence training program (self-directed or caregiver-directed) include motivation, assessment of voiding and incontinence patterns, a regular fluid intake of 2,000 to 3,000 mL/day, timed voiding of 2- to 4-hour intervals in an appropriate place, and ongoing assessment (Miller, 2015).*

R: *Dehydration can cause incontinence by eliminating the sensation of a full bladder (the signal to urinate) and by reducing the individual's alertness to the sensation.*

Teach About the Bladder Reconditioning Program

- Explain rationale and treatments (see Key Concepts).
- Explain the schedule of fluid intake, voiding attempts, manual triggering, and catheterization to control incontinence.
- Teach the importance of positive reinforcement and adherence to program for best results.
- Refer to community nurses for assistance in bladder reconditioning if indicated.

Initiate Health Teaching

- If appropriate, teach intermittent catheterization.
- Instruct in prevention of urinary tract infection.
- For people living in the community, initiate a referral to the visiting nurse for follow-up and/or regular changes of an indwelling catheter.

R: *Chronic catheterization requires use of community nurses.*

Urge Urinary Incontinence

NANDA-I Definition

Involuntary passage of urine occurring soon after a strong sense of urgency to void

Defining Characteristics*

Observed or reported inability to reach toilet in time to avoid urine loss
Reports urinary urgency
Reports involuntary loss of urine with bladder contractions or bladder spasms

Related Factors

Pathophysiologic

Related to decreased bladder capacity secondary to:

Infection	Demyelinating diseases	Neurogenic disorders or injury/tumor/infection injury
Cerebrovascular accident	Urethritis	Alcoholic neuropathy
Trauma	Diabetic neuropathy	Parkinsonism

Treatment Related

Related to decreased bladder capacity secondary to:

Abdominal surgery
After use of indwelling catheters

Situational (Personal, Environmental)

Related to irritation of bladder stretch receptors secondary to:

Alcohol
Caffeine
Excess fluid intake

Related to decreased bladder capacity* secondary to:

Frequent voiding

Maturational

Child

Related to small bladder capacity

Older Adult

Related to decreased bladder capacity

Key Concepts

- University of Texas at Austin, School of Nursing, Family Nurse Practitioner Program, Recommendations for the management of urge urinary incontinence in women (Austin, TX, University of Texas at Austin, School of Nursing, 2010, May 9, p. 24):
  - Urge incontinence is an involuntary loss of urine associated with a strong desire to void. It is characterized by loss of large volumes of urine and may be triggered by emotional factors, body position changes, or the sight and sound of running water. This type of incontinence is commonly called *bladder detrusor instability* or *vesical instability* (Halter, 2014).
  - Detrusor instability is characterized by uninhibited detrusor contractions sufficient to cause urinary incontinence. Common causes include central nervous system disease, hyperexcitability of the afferent pathways, and deconditioned voiding reflexes.
  - An individual with an uninhibited neurogenic bladder has damage to the cerebral cortex (e.g., cerebrovascular accident, Parkinson's disease, brain injury/tumor), affecting the ability to inhibit urination. Sensation of bladder fullness is also limited; this is manifested by urgency. There is little time between the sensation to void and the uninhibited contraction.
  - Warning time is the time an individual can delay urination after feeling the urge to void. Diminished warning time can cause incontinence if the individual cannot reach a toilet in time.

Focus Assessment Criteria

Refer to *Impaired Urinary Elimination*.

Goals

NOC

Refer to *Functional Urinary Incontinence*.

The individual will report no or decreased episodes of incontinence (specify), as evidenced by the following indicators:

- Able to explain their unique cause of incontinence
- Describes bladder irritants

Interventions

NIC

See also *Functional Incontinence*, Environmental Management, Urinary Catheterization, Teaching: Procedure/Treatment, Tube Care: Urinary, Urinary Bladder Training

Assess for Causative or Contributing Factors

- Refer to Related Factors.
- Weight loss: recommended as noninvasive therapy. Outcomes were better when looking at stress versus urge incontinence and obese versus overweight, but still effective. Formerly obese patients were shown to have improved outcomes after weight loss (Grade A, Evidence Fair) (DuBeau, 2015; Holroyd-Leduc, Tannenbaum, Thorpe, & Straus, 2004; *Morant, 2005).
- Dietary changes: recommended as noninvasive therapy. The elimination of bladder irritants from the diet has not been rigorously evaluated (Grade A, Evidence Fair) (DuBeau, 2014, 2015; *Morant, 2005).

Assess Pattern of Voiding/Incontinence and Fluid Intake

- Maintain optimal hydration (see *Continuous Incontinence*).
- Assess voiding pattern (see *Continuous Incontinence*).

Reduce or Eliminate Causative and Contributing Factors, When Possible

Bladder Irritants

- Initiate bladder reconditioning program (see *Continuous Incontinence*).
- Caffeinated beverages/foods (e.g., coffee, tea, chocolate), alcohol, red wine, highly acidic foods, and foods high in potassium can irritate the bladder, causing urgency and frequency (Griebling, 2009).
- Carbonated beverages should be eliminated or decreased because they may increase bladder activity and urgency (Wilson et al., 2005).
- Understand and explain the risk of insufficient fluid intake and its relation to infection and concentrated urine.

R: *Optimal hydration is needed to prevent urinary tract infection and renal calculi.*

Diminished Bladder Capacity

- Determine time between urge to void and need to void (record how long individual can delay urination).
- Teach an individual with difficulty prolonging waiting time to communicate to personnel the need to respond rapidly to his or her request for assistance for toileting (note on care plan).
- Teach the individual to increase waiting time by increasing bladder capacity.
- Determine volume of each void.
- Ask the individual to "hold off" urinating as long as possible.
- Give positive reinforcement.
- Discourage frequent voiding that is the result of habit, not need.
- Develop bladder reconditioning program (see *Continuous Incontinence*).

R: *Deconditioning of the voiding reflex can result in incontinence through self-induced or iatrogenic causes. Frequent toileting (more than every 2 hours) causes chronic low-volume voiding, which reduces bladder capacity and increases detrusor tone and bladder wall thickness, which in turn potentiate incontinent episodes.*

Overdistended Bladder

- Explain that diuretics are given to help reduce the water in the body; they work by acting on the kidneys to increase the flow of urine.
- Explain that in diabetes mellitus, insulin deficiency causes high levels of blood sugar. The high level of blood glucose pulls fluid from body tissues, causing osmotic diuresis and increased urination (polyuria).
- Explain that because of the increased urine flow, regular voiding is needed to prevent overdistention of the bladder.
- Smoking cessation is recommended.

R: *Risk for urge incontinence is greatest for current smokers and less but still present for former smokers (University of Texas at Austin, School of Nursing, 2010).*

- Assess voiding pattern (see *Continuous Incontinence*).
- Check postvoid residual; if greater than your institutions' policy, include intermittent catheterization in bladder reconditioning program.
- Initiate bladder reconditioning program (see *Continuous Incontinence*).

R: *Overdistention results in loss of bladder sensation, which causes incontinence episodes.*

- Pelvic floor muscle rehabilitation (PFMR): recommended as a noninvasive therapy. It appears to be an effective treatment for women with urge incontinence.

Uninhibited Bladder Contractions

- Assess voiding pattern (see *Continuous Incontinence*).
- Establish method to communicate urge to void (document on care plan).
- Teach individual to communicate to personnel the need to respond rapidly to a request to void.
- Establish a planned-voiding pattern.
- Provide an opportunity to void on awakening; after meals, physical exercise, bathing, and drinking coffee or tea; and before going to sleep.
- Begin by offering use of bedpan, commode, or toilet every half hour initially, and gradually lengthen the time to at least every 2 hours.
- If the individual has incontinent episode, reduce the time between scheduled voidings.

- Document behavior/activity that occurs with void or incontinence (see *Continuous Incontinence*).
- Encourage the individual to try to "hold" urine until time to void, if possible.
- Consult primary care professional for pharmacologic and alternative interventions.
- Refer to *Continuous Incontinence* for additional information on developing a bladder reconditioning program.

R: *The essential components of any continence training program (self-directed or caregiver-directed) include motivation, assessment of voiding and incontinent patterns, a regular fluid intake of 2,000 to 3,000 mL/day, timed voiding of 2- to 4-hour intervals in an appropriate place, and ongoing assessment (Miller, 2015).*

Initiate Health Teaching

- Instruct about prevention of urinary tract infections (refer to *Functional Incontinence*).

Overflow Urinary Incontinence[54]

NANDA-I Definition

Involuntary loss of urine associated with overdistention of the bladder

Defining Characteristics*

Bladder distention
High residual volume observed after void
Observed or reported involuntary leakage of small volumes of urine
Nocturia

Related Factors

Pathophysiologic

Related to sphincter blockage secondary to:

Strictures
Ureterocele
Bladder neck contractures
Prostatic enlargement
Perineal swelling
Severe pelvic prolapse

Related to impaired afferent pathways or inadequacy secondary to:

Cord injury/tumor/infection
Brain injury/tumor/infection
Cerebrovascular accident
Demyelinating diseases
Multiple sclerosis
Diabetic neuropathy
Alcoholic neuropathy
Tabes dorsalis

Treatment Related

Related to bladder outlet obstruction* or impaired afferent pathways secondary to drug therapy (iatrogenic)

Antihistamines
Theophylline
Epinephrine
Isoproterenol
Decongestants*
Anticholinergics*
Calcium channel blockers*

Situational (Personal, Environmental)

Related to bladder outlet obstruction secondary to:

Fecal impaction*

Related to detrusor hypocontractility* secondary to:

Deconditioned voiding
Association with stress or discomfort

[54]Previously called *Urinary Retention*.

Key Concepts

- Three entities can cause overflow incontinence: bladder outlet obstruction, detrusor inadequacy, and impaired afferent pathways.
- Detrusor inadequacy is characterized by the pressure of uninhibited detrusor contractions sufficient to cause urinary incontinence. One cause of detrusor inadequacy is deconditioned voiding reflexes characterized by anxiety or discomfort associated with voiding. Another cause is central nervous system diseases.
- Impaired afferent pathways occur when both the sensory and motor branches of the simple reflex arc are damaged. Therefore, there are no sensations to tell the individual the bladder is full and no motor impulses for emptying the bladder. Thus, the individual develops a neurogenic bladder (autonomous). With this type of neurogenic bladder, the individual is likely to dribble urine when pressure in the bladder rises because of the bladder filling beyond its normal capacity or because of coughing, straining, or exercising.

Focus Assessment Criteria

Refer to *Impaired Urinary Elimination.*

Goals

NOC

Refer to *Functional Urinary Incontinence.*

The individual will achieve a state of dryness that meets personal satisfaction, as evidenced by the following indicators:

- Empties the bladder using Credé's or Valsalva maneuver with a residual urine of less than 50 mL if indicated
- Voids voluntarily

Interventions

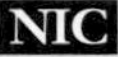

See also *Functional Urinary Incontinence,* Overflow Retention Care, Urinary Bladder Training.

- Refer to Related Factors.

Explain Rationale for Treatment

Develop a Bladder-Retraining or Reconditioning Program

- See *Continuous Incontinence.*

Instruct About Methods to Empty Bladder

- Assist to a sitting position.
- Teach abdominal strain and Valsalva maneuver; instruct individual to
  - Lean forward on thighs
  - Contract abdominal muscles, if possible, and strain or "bear down"; hold breath while straining (Valsalva maneuver—if not contraindicated)
  - Hold strain or breath until urine flow stops; wait 1 minute, and strain again as long as possible
  - Continue until no more urine is expelled

R: *Valsalva maneuver contracts the abdominal muscles, which manually compresses the bladder.*

- Teach Credé's maneuver; instruct to
  - Place hands flat (or place fist) just below umbilical area.
  - Place one hand on top of the other.
  - Press firmly down and in toward the pelvic arch.
  - Repeat six or seven times until no more urine can be expelled.
  - Wait a few minutes and repeat to ensure complete emptying.

R: *In many individuals, Credé's maneuver can help empty the bladder. This maneuver is inappropriate, however, if the urinary sphincters are chronically contracted. In this case, pressing the bladder can force urine up the ureters as well as through the urethra. Reflux of urine into the renal pelvis may result in renal infection.*

Indicate on the Intake and Output Record Which Technique Was Used to Induce Voiding

Obtain Postvoid Residuals After Attempts at Emptying Bladder; If Residual Urine Volumes Are Greater Than 100 mL, Schedule Intermittent Catheterization Program (See *Continuous Incontinence*)

R: *Clean intermittent self-catheterization (CISC) prevents overdistention, helps maintain detrusor muscle tone, and ensures complete bladder emptying. CISC may be used initially to determine residual urine after Credé's maneuver or tapping. As residual urine decreases, catheterization may be tapered. CISC may recondition the voiding reflex in some individuals.*

Initiate Health Teaching

- Teach bladder reconditioning program (refer to *Continuous Incontinence*).
- Teach intermittent catheterization (refer to *Continuous Incontinence*).
- Instruct individual about prevention of urinary tract infections (refer to *Continuous Incontinence*).

R: *If bladder emptying techniques are unsuccessful, other methods of managing incontinence are necessary.*

RISK FOR VASCULAR TRAUMA

Risk for Vascular Trauma

Related to Infusion of Vesicant Medications

NANDA-I Definition

Vulnerable to damage to a vein and its surrounding tissues related to the presence of a catheter and/or infused solutions, which may compromise health

Risk Factors*

Treatment Related

Catheter type[55]
Catheter width[55]
Impaired ability to visualize the insertion site
Inadequate catheter fixation[55]
Infusion rate[55]
Insertions site[55]
Length of insertion time
Nature of solution (e.g., concentration, chemical irritant, temperature, pH)

Author's Note

This NANDA-I diagnosis represents a risk for all individuals with intravenous catheters. Procedure manuals in the clinical unit should contain the correct placement, fixation, and monitoring of all intravenous sites. Nurses needing these guidelines should refer to the procedure manual. Practicing nurses do not need to have this diagnosis on the care plan. Students should refer to their fundamentals of nursing text for specific techniques to start, secure, and monitor intravenous therapy. Consult with your faculty to determine if this should be written on your assigned individual's care plan.

Clinically, certain intravenous medications (e.g., chemotherapy, vesicant medications) are extremely toxic and therefore require specific interventions to prevent occurrence and tissue necrosis. Interventions and goals for preventing and responding to extravasation of the intravenous vesicant medications will be outlined for this diagnosis. These interventions are usually also found in a procedure manual.

Errors in Diagnostic Statements

Risk for Vascular Trauma related to inadequate catheter fixation

This diagnostic statement contains a related factor that is legally problematic. If the catheter was inadequately secured, then this should be corrected. This is not a nursing diagnosis issue. It is a clinician problem that needs to be addressed and corrected.

[55]May indicate poor clinical practice.

Review the preceding Risk Factors; the author has placed a footnote (|) next to all those listed that may indicate poor clinical practice. These situations should not be listed as related factors for this diagnosis; instead, they require immediate correction.

Key Concepts (Payne & Savares, 2015)

- Administration of prescribed intravenous antineoplastic agents requires the nurse to review and know dosage (ranges), solution restrictions when dosage reductions are indicated, administration precautions (time, storage), side effects, and adverse effects.
- Intravenous drugs are categorized as an irritant, nonirritant, or vesicant.
- A local reaction to chemotherapy (e.g., doxorubicin) is a venous flare. It is characterized by a localized erythema, venous streaking, and pruritus along the injected vein. There is no pain or edema and there is a blood return.
- Another local reaction is from an agent carmustine (irritant) that causes pain, venous irritation, and chemical phlebitis. These agents do not cause ulceration if infiltrated.
- A vesicant is a drug that infiltrates (extravasation) and causes pain, ulceration, necrosis, and sloughing of damaged tissue. Prolonged extravasation can cause loss of joint or tendon mobility, vascularity, or tendon function.
- Vesicants can be non-antineoplastic drugs (e.g., Levophed, Dilantin). Many antineoplastic drugs are vesicants.
- The physical and emotional impact of an extensive extravasation injury may prompt legal action.
- The best defenses against claims of negligence related to extravasation are the following:
  - To prevent them if possible
  - To detect them quickly
  - To intervene promptly
- Individuals receiving vesicants intravenously need close monitoring and should be instructed of the signs and symptoms to report.

Focus Assessment Criteria

Objective Data

Assess the Insertion Site Prior to Infusion for

Leaks
Redness
Edema
Blood return

Assess the Site During Infusion for

Redness
Swelling (bled at injection site)
Blood return

Ask the Individual If There Is Any Burning or Pain at the Injection Site

Advise the individual to Report Any Sensations That Occur at the Site During Infusion

Risk for Vascular Trauma • Related to Infusion of Vesicant Medications

Goals

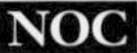
NOC
Knowledge Treatment Procedure, Risk Control

The individual will report or be monitored for early signs and symptoms of extravasation, as evidenced by the following indicators:

- Swelling
- Stinging, burning, or pain at the injection site
- Redness
- Lack of blood return

Interventions

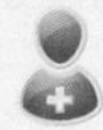

NIC

Intravenous Insertion, Medication Administration: Intravenous, Surveillance, Teaching: Procedure/Treatment, Venous Access Device (VAD) Maintenance, Chemotherapy Management

> **Clinical Alert** The full effect of the extravasation injury is not usually immediately apparent but may evolve over days or weeks. Early local symptoms of a vesicant extravasation resemble those of an irritant extravasation: local pain, erythema, burning, pruritus, or swelling. Over the course of the reaction, however, as tissue necrosis evolves and becomes clinically apparent, progressive erythema, discoloration, blistering, or desquamation may develop. The severity of the local reaction may vary both upon the agent extravasated and upon the total dose of extravasated material (Al-Benna, O'Boyle, & Holley, 2013).

Prior to Administration of a Prescribed Vesicant Medication, Review the Agency Protocol for Hazardous Drug Handling, Physician Order, and Information About the Medication

R: *The institutional policy is written to help prevent extravasation and to direct management if it occurs.*

If Inexperienced in This Procedure, Consult an Experienced Nurse for Assistance

R: *Serious injury from extravasation can be prevented.*

Identify Individuals at Increased Risk for Extravasation (Elderly, Debilitated, Confused, Unable to Communicate, Diabetics, Fragile Veins, Have Received Irritating Drugs in the Past, or Those With General Vascular Disease) and Monitor Them Continuously During Infusion

R: *Individuals who cannot identify and communicate stinging, burning, or pain at the injection site cannot be relied on for early detection of extravasation (Al-Benna et al., 2013; Hayden & Goodman, 2005).*

Avoid Infusing Vesicant Drugs

- Over joints, bony prominences, tendons, neurovascular bundles, or the antecubital fossa
- When venous or lymphatic circulation is poor (e.g., operative side after mastectomy)
- At sites that have been irritated previously

R: *These precautions can prevent movement of the catheter and extravasation.*

Never Give Vesicants Intramuscularly or Subcutaneously; the Drug Is Toxic to Tissues Prior to Infusion

- Gently check for brisk blood return and easy flow of fluids by gravity.
- Check all needle or catheter site for leaks, evidence of swelling, or venous thrombosis.

R: *Excessive pressure on the vein can be prevented with gentle movements. Displacement, damage, or a blockage can be detected before infusion.*

Use the Correct Equipment (Intravenous, Port, Huber-Point Needle); Infuse Solutions Slowly, in a Steady, Even Flow; Check for Blood Return Every 3 to 5 mL According to Policy

R: *Early identification of extravasation can prevent serious tissue damage.*

Assess the Individual Every 3 to 5 mL or Per Institution's Policy for (Wilkes, 2011)

- Swelling (most common)
- Stinging, burning, or pain at the injection site (not always present)
- Redness (not often seen initially)
- Lack of blood return (if this is the only symptom, reevaluate the intravenous line)

R: *Extravasation can occur with or without symptoms and signs.*

If the Aforementioned Signs or Symptoms Occur, Stop Infusion and Contact an Experienced Nurse, Physician, or Nurse Practitioner Immediately

R: *The situation requires a rapid diagnosis and action.*

If Extravasation Occurs, Follow Institutional Policy for Discontinuation, Antidote Administration, Diluents, Site Care, Ice Applications, and Elevation of the Extremity

R: *The institutional policy and extravasation kit should be available for use.*

Document the Extravasation Event, Including (Wilkes, 2011)

- Name of drug
- Dilution

- Estimated volume infused in the infusion method
- Type of device
- Size of catheter and quality of blood return if infusion pump used
- Subjective complaints (discomfort with movement)
- Objective observations (measuring, photographing)
- Range of motion
- Actions taken with a timeline

R: *The best defense against claims of negligence related to extravasation injuries is to prevent them to the extent possible, to detect them quickly, and to intervene properly.*

RISK FOR OTHER-DIRECTED VIOLENCE

Definition

At risk for behaviors in which an individual demonstrates that he or she can be physically, emotionally, and/or sexually harmful to others (NANDA-I)

State in which an individual has been, or is at risk to be, assaultive toward others or the environment[56]

Risk Factors

Presence of risk factors (see Related Factors)

Related Factors

Pathophysiologic

Related to history of aggressive acts and perception of environment as threatening secondary to:

or

Related to history of aggressive acts and delusional thinking secondary to:

or

Related to history of aggressive acts and manic excitement secondary to:

or

Related to history of aggressive acts and inability to verbalize feelings secondary to:

or

Related to history of aggressive acts and psychic overload secondary to:

Temporal lobe epilepsy
Head injury
Progressive central nervous system deterioration (brain tumor)
Hormonal imbalance
Viral encephalopathy
Mental retardation
Minimal brain dysfunction

Related to toxic response to alcohol or drugs

Related to organic brain syndrome

Treatment Related

Related to toxic reaction to medication

[56]This statement added by Lynda Juall Carpenito for clarity and usefulness.

Situational (Personal, Environmental)

Related to history of overt aggressive acts

Related to increase in stressors within a short period

Related to acute agitation

Related to suspiciousness

Related to persecutory delusions

Related to verbal threats of physical assault

Related to low frustration tolerance

Related to poor impulse control

Related to fear of the unknown

Related to response to catastrophic event

Related to response to dysfunctional family throughout developmental stages

Related to dysfunctional communication patterns

Related to drug or alcohol abuse

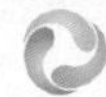

Author's Note

The diagnosis *Risk for Other-Directed Violence* describes an individual who has been assaultive, or because of certain factors (e.g., toxic response to alcohol or drugs, hallucinations or delusions, brain dysfunction) is at high risk for assaulting others. In such a situation, the nursing focus is on decreasing violent episodes and protecting the individual and others.

The nurse should not use this diagnosis to address underlying problems such as anxiety or poor self-esteem, but instead should refer to the diagnoses *Anxiety*, *Ineffective Coping*, or both to focus on the sources of the violence (spouse, child, older adult). When domestic violence is present or suspected, the nurse should explore the diagnosis *Disabled Family Coping*. An individual at risk for suicide would warrant the diagnosis *Risk for Suicide*.

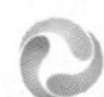

Errors in Diagnostic Statements

Risk for Other-Directed Violence related to reports of abuse by wife

"Reports of abuse by a spouse" represents family dysfunction, which *Risk for Other-Directed Violence* does not cover. Spousal abuse is a complex situation necessitating individual and family therapy. The nursing diagnoses *Disabled Family Coping* and *Ineffective Coping* for the abuser and the victim would be more clinically useful.

Risk for Other-Directed Violence related to poor management or agitation by staff

This diagnostic statement is legally problematic and does not offer constructive strategies. When staff management of an agitated individual is inappropriate, the nurse must treat this as a staff management problem, not an individual problem. If staff members increased the individual's agitation because of lack of knowledge, the nurse must outline specific do's and don'ts in the nursing care plan. In addition, an in-service program about identifying precursors to violence and agitation reduction strategies should be held for staff. For the individual, the nurse could rewrite the diagnosis as *Risk for Other-Directed Violence* related to mental dysfunction and persecutory delusions.

Key Concepts

General Considerations

- There is a reluctance of nurses to report workplace violence and a high incidence of hospitals not reporting violence to authorities (Roche, Diers, Duffield, & Catling-Paull, 2010).
- Roche et al. (2010) reported that 30% of nurses on medical-surgical units reported emotional abuse and 50% reported threats or actual assault.
- A central theme among violent people is helplessness. Assaultive behavior is a defense against passivity and helplessness.

- Aggressive behavior is a defense against anxiety. This coping mechanism is reinforced because it reduces anxiety by increasing the individual's sense of power and control. (Refer to Key Concepts, *Anxiety*, for further discussion of anger.) Interventions that encourage "acting out of anger" reinforce assault behavior and thus are to be avoided.
- Violence is usually preceded by a predictable sequence of events (e.g., a stressor or a series of stressors).
- When brain dysfunction is a prime or contributing factor to violent behavior, social and environmental variables should still be evaluated. Organic impairment may interfere with an individual's ability to handle certain stresses. Exposure to or ingestion of toxic chemicals, such as lead and pesticides, can alter an individual's normal behavior. Examples of violent behavior in brain dysfunction are biting, scratching, temper outbursts, and mood lability.
- Fear and anxiety can distort perceptions of the environment. Suspicious, delusional people often misinterpret stimuli. Alcohol and drugs also impair judgment and decrease internal controls over behavior.
- People who have a history of emotional deprivation in childhood are particularly vulnerable to attacks on their self-esteem.
- Although the individual may identify the person with whom he or she is angry, this may not be the real object of aggression. People often cannot allow themselves to express anger toward a person on whom they are dependent.
- Staff members frequently respond to violent individuals with actual fear or overreactions. This can lead to punitive sanctions such as heavier medication, seclusion, or attempts to cope by avoidance and withdrawal from the individual. Staff must identify their own reactions to violent individuals so they can manage the situation more effectively. Staff should trust an intuition that the individual is potentially violent (Farrell, Harmon, & Hastings, 1998).
- In studies of individuals' perception of seclusion, sense of powerlessness seemed to be the worst feeling, followed by fear, humiliation, loneliness, and shame (*Norris & Kennedy, 1992).
- Physical aggression in long-term care, such as swearing, biting, kicking, spitting, and grabbing, may be in response to a loss of control over life. The more importance the individual attaches to freedom and choice, the more forcefully he or she is likely to respond.

Pediatric Considerations

- In 2015, 13,396 persons were killed by firearm violence (Gun Violence Archive, 2015).
- Homicide is the 16th cause of death in the United States. Homicide is the second cause of death in children ages 5 to 14 years and the second cause of death in children ages 15 to 24 years (Centers for Disease Control and Prevention, 2013).
- The homicide rate among African American victims is 18.71 per 100,000 as compared to the national homicide rate of 4.86 for Hispanics and 2.97 per 100,000 for Caucasians.
- Violent shaking of children, especially those younger than 6 months, can cause fatal intracranial trauma without signs of external head injury (Hockenberry & Wilson, 2015).
- Children who are exposed to community violence experience more depression, anxiety, fear, and aggressive acting-out behaviors than children not exposed (*Veenema, 2006).
- During 2013 the United States, 679,000 children experienced or were at risk for child abuse. Physical abuse of children often results from unreasonable severe corporal punishment or unjustifiable punishment (e.g., hitting an infant for crying; Child Trends Data Bank, 2015).

Focus Assessment Criteria

Refer also to Focus Assessment Criteria for *Ineffective Coping*, *Disabled Family Coping*, *Confusion*, and *Anxiety*.

Subjective Data

Assess for Risk Factors

Medical History
Hormonal imbalance
Head injury
Brain disease
Drug abuse (amphetamines, phencyclidine hydrochloride, marijuana, alcohol, cocaine)

Psychiatric History
Previous hospitalizations
Outpatient therapy

History of Emotional Difficulties in Individual, Family, or Both
Mental retardation
Parental brutality
Cruelty to animals
Pyromania

Interaction Patterns (Note Changes)
Family
Coworkers
Friends
Others

Coping Patterns (Past and Present)

Sources of Stress in Current Environment

Work/School History
How does individual function?
Fights in school?
Understress?
Stable employment
Level of education attained
Frequency of job changes
Learning disabilities
Periods of unemployment

Legal History
Arrests and convictions for violent crimes
Juvenile offenses for violent behavior

History of Violence
Assess recency, severity, and frequency.
"What is the most violent thing you have ever done?"
"What is the closest you have ever come to striking someone?"
"In what kinds of situations have you hit someone or destroyed property?"
"When was the last time this happened?"
"How often does this occur?"
"Were you using drugs or alcohol during these episodes?"

Present Thoughts About Violence
Identify possible victim and weapon.
"How do you feel after an incident?"
"Are you currently having thoughts about harming someone?"
"Is there anyone in particular you think about harming?" (Identify the victim and the individual's access to the victim.)
"Do you have a specific plan for how you might accomplish this?" (Identify the plan, type of weapon, and availability of weapon.)

Thought Content
Helplessness
Suspiciousness or hostility
Perceived intention (e.g., "He meant to hit me" in response to a slight bump)
Fear of loss of control
Persecutory delusions
Disorientation

Child–Adolescent

Conflict Management—Impulse Control
How does the child respond to conflict?
History of fights
History of being a victim of bullying

Relationships
Has he or she experienced pushing, hitting, being afraid, being hurt, or being forced to have sexual contact?

Safety
"Do you feel safe?"
"Are you afraid of someone you know?"
"Have you talked with an adult about this situation?"
If abuse is suspected, refer to *Disabled Family Coping*.

Objective Data

Assess for Risk Factors

Body Language
Posture (relaxed, rigid)
Hands (relaxed, rigid, clenched)
Facial expression (calm, annoyed, tense)

Motor Activity
Within normal limits
Pacing
Immobile
Agitation
Increased

Affect
Within normal limits
Flat
Labile
Inappropriate
Controlled

Goals

NOC
Abuse Cessation, Abusive Behavior Self-Restraint, Aggression Self-Control, Impulse Self-Control

The individual will refrain from abusive behaviors (in all forms) toward others, as evidenced by the following indicators (Varcarolis, 2011):

- Seeks assistance when emotions are escalating
- Refrains from threatening, loud language toward others
- Responds to external controls when at high risk for loss of control
- Identifies factors contributing to abusive behaviors
- Identifies calming strategies
- Uses appropriate methods to express anger

Interventions

NIC
Abuse Protection Support, Anger Control Assistance, Environmental Management: Violence Prevention, Impulse Control Training, Crisis Intervention, Seclusion, Physical Restraint

The nursing interventions for *Risk for Other-Directed Violence* apply to any individual who is potentially violent, regardless of related factors.

Promote Interactions That Increase the Individual's Sense of Trust

- Acknowledge the individual's feelings (e.g., "You are having a rough time").
  - Be genuine and empathetic.
  - Tell the individual that you will help him or her to control behavior and not do anything destructive.
  - Be direct and frank ("I can see you are angry").
  - Be consistent and firm.
- Set limits when the individual poses a risk to others. Refer to *Anxiety* for further interventions for setting limits.
- Offer choices and options. At times, it is necessary to give in to some demands to avoid a power struggle.

R: *Setting limits clarifies rules, guidelines, and standards of acceptable behavior and establishes the consequences of violating the rules.*

- Encourage the individual to express anger and hostility verbally instead of "acting out."
- Encourage walking or exercise as activities that may diffuse aggression.

R: *Physical activity can help reduce muscle tension.*

- Maintain individual's personal space:
  - Do not touch the individual.
  - Avoid feelings of physical entrapment of individual or staff.
- Be aware of your own feelings and reactions.
  - Do not take verbal abuse personally.
  - Remain calm if you are becoming upset; leave the situation to others, if possible.
  - After a threatening situation, discuss your feelings with other staff.

R: *Staff activities may be counterproductive to managing aggressive behavior. Recognition and replacement of attitudes such as "I must be calm and relaxed at all times" with "No matter how anxious I feel, I will keep thinking and decide on the best approach" often prevent escalation of aggression.*

- Observe for cues of increasing anger (Boyd, 2012).
  - Reports of numbness, nausea, and vertigo
  - Choking sensation, chills, and prickly sensations
  - Increased muscle tone, clenched fists, set jaw, and eyebrows lower and drawn together
  - Lips pressed together to form a thin line
  - Flushing or paleness
  - "Goose bumps"
  - Twitching
  - Sweating

R: *Violence can have a pattern. Early detection can prevent escalation (Varcarolis, 2011).*

Initiate Immediate Management of the High-Risk Individual

- Allow the individual with acute agitation a space that is five times greater than that for an individual who is in control. Do not touch the individual unless you have a trusting relationship.
- Avoid physical entrapment of individual or staff.
- Convey empathy by acknowledging the individual's feelings. Let the individual know you will not let him or her lose control. Remind the individual of previous successes with self-control.
- Do not approach a violent individual alone. Often, the presence of three or four staff members is enough to reassure the individual that you will not let him or her lose control. Use a positive tone; do not demand or cajole.

R: *Always place staff safety first. The presence of four or five staff members reassures the individual that you will not let him or her lose control. The focus is respect, concern, and safety.*

R: *Assaultive behavior tends to occur when conditions are crowded, are without structure, and involve activity "demanded" by staff (Farrell et al., 1998).*

- Give the individual control by offering alternatives (e.g., walking, talking).
- Set limits on actions, not feelings. Use concise, easily understood statements.

R: *Minimization of anger and ineffective coping are the most frequent factors contributing to escalation of violence (Varcarolis, 2011).*

- Maintain eye contact, but do not stare. Stand at a friendly angle (45°); keep an open posture if the individual is standing, and sit when the individual sits.

R: *Maintain the same physical level (e.g., both people either sitting or standing prevents feelings of intimidation). The least aggressive stance is at a 45° angle to the individual, rather than face to face.*

- Do not make promises you cannot keep.
- Avoid using "always" and "never."

R: *Although people may verbalize hostile threats and take a defensive stance, most fear losing control and want assistance to maintain their control (Halter, 2014).*

- When interpersonal and pharmacologic interventions fail to control the angry, aggressive individual, physical interventions (restraints, seclusion) are the final resort. Always follow hospital protocols (Varcarolis, 2011).

R: *Hospital protocols should be clear regarding how, when, and for what time period an individual can be restrained or secluded the associated nursing care needed (Varcarolis, 2011).*

Establish an Environment That Reduces Agitation (Farrell et al., 1998)

- Decrease noise level.
- Give short, concise explanations.
- Control the number of persons present at one time.
- Provide a single or semiprivate room.
- Allow the individual to arrange personal possessions.
- Be aware that darkness can increase disorientation and enhance suspiciousness.
- Decrease situations in which the individual is frustrated.
- Provide music if the individual is receptive.

R: *The individual is in an agitated/mentally compromised state. Environmental stimuli that unnecessarily increase this state can increase aggression.*

Assist the Individual to Maintain Control Over His or Her Behavior

- Establish the expectation that the individual can control behavior, and continue to reinforce the expectation. Explain exactly which behavior is inappropriate and why.
- Give three options: offer two choices, whereas the third is the consequence of violent behavior.
- Allow time for the individual to make a choice.
- Provide positive feedback when the individual is able to exercise restraint.
- Enforce consequences when indicated.
- Reassure the individual that you will provide control if he or she cannot. ("I am concerned about you. I will get [more staff, medications] to keep you from doing anything impulsive.")
- Set firm, clear limits when an individual presents a danger to self or others. ("Put the chair down.")
- Call the individual by name in a calm, quiet, respectful manner.
- Avoid threats; refer to yourself, not policies, rules, or supervisors.
- Allow appropriate verbal expressions of anger. Give positive feedback.
- Set limits on verbal abuse. Do not take insults personally. Support others (individuals, staff) who may be targets of abuse.
- Do not give attention to the individual who is being verbally abusive. Tell the individual what you are doing and why.
- Assist with external controls, as necessary.
  - Maintain observation every 15 to 30 minutes.
  - Remove items that the individual could use as weapons (e.g., glass, sharp objects).
  - Assess the individual's ability to tolerate off-unit procedures.
  - If the individual is acutely agitated, be cautious with items such as hot coffee.

R: *Crisis management techniques can help prevent escalation of aggression and help the individual achieve self-control. The least restrictive safe and effective measure should be used (Alvarey, 1998).*

R: *The nurse and the individual should collaborate to find solutions and alternatives to aggression (Boyd, 2005).*

Plan for Unpredictable Violence

- Monitor for cues to potential aggression (Halter, 2014).

Verbal

- Morose silence
- Loud, demanding remarks
- Illogical responses
- Negative response to requests
- Demeaning remarks
- Overt hostility
- Threats
- Sarcasm
- Mistrust

Nonverbal Facial Expression

- Tense jaw
- Staring
- Clenched teeth

- Dilated pupils
- Lip biting
- Pulsing carotid

Nonverbal Body Language

- Hand twisting objects
- Stony withdrawal
- Aggression
- Confrontational stance
- Fist clenching, unclenching (slamming doors)
- Pounding, kicking
- Pacing
- Ensure availability of staff before potential violent behavior (never try to assist the individual alone when physical restraint is necessary).
- Determine who will be in charge of directing personnel to intervene in violent behavior if it occurs.
- Ensure protection for self (door nearby for withdrawal, pillow to protect face).

R: *Crisis management techniques can help prevent escalation of aggression and help the individual achieve self-control. The least restrictive safe and effective measure should be used (Halter, 2014).*

Use Seclusion and/or Restraint, If Indicated

- Remove individual from situation if environment is contributing to aggressive behavior, using the least amount of control needed (e.g., ask others to leave, and take individual to quiet room).
- Reinforce that you are going to help the individual control himself or herself.
- Repeatedly tell the individual what is going to happen before external control begins.
- Ensure that sufficient personnel (five) are present.
- Protect individual from injuring self or others through use of restraints or seclusion.[57]
- When using seclusion, institutional policy provides specifics. The following are general measures:
  - Observe the individual at least every 15 minutes.
  - Search the individual before secluding to remove harmful objects.
  - Check seclusion room to see that safety is maintained.
  - Offer fluids and food periodically (in nonbreakable containers).
  - When approaching an individual to be secluded, have sufficient staff present.
  - Explain concisely what is going to happen ("You will be placed in a room by yourself until you can better control your behavior"); give the individual a chance to cooperate.
  - Assist with toileting and personal hygiene (assess the individual's ability to be out of seclusion; a urinal or commode may need to be used).
  - If the individual is taken out of seclusion, someone must be present continually.
  - Maintain verbal interaction during seclusion (provides information necessary to assess the individual's degree of control).
  - When the individual is allowed out of seclusion, a staff member needs to be in constant attendance to determine whether the individual can handle additional stimulation.
- When using restraint, institutional policy provides specifics. The following are general measures:
  - An individual in a four-point or two-point restraint must be in seclusion or with one-on-one nursing care for protection. Seclusion guidelines should be followed.
  - Restraints must be loosened every hour (one limb at a time).
  - Waist restraints must allow enough arm movement to enable eating/smoking and self-protection against falling.
  - Restraints should be padded.
  - Restraints never should be attached to side rails, but rather to the bed frame.
- Provide an opportunity to clarify the rationale for seclusion and to discuss the individual's reactions after the seclusion period is over.

R: *Seclusion and restraint are options for an individual exhibiting serious, persistent aggression. The nurse must protect the individual's safety at all times. Use of the least restrictive measures allows the individual the most opportunity to regain self-control (Farrell et al., 1998).*

[57] May require a primary care professional's order.

Convene a Group Discussion After a Violent Episode in an Inpatient Unit

- Include all those who witnessed the episode (individual, staff).
- Include individual(s) exhibiting the violent behavior, if possible.
- Discuss what happened, the consequences, and the feelings of the community.

R: *After a violent act, leading a group discussion of the event, outcome, and feelings can decrease anxiety, increase understanding of violence, and address preventable problems that occurred.*

Assist the Individual in Developing Alternative Coping Strategies When the Crisis Has Passed and Learning Can Occur

- Explore what precipitates the individual's loss of control ("What was happening before you felt like hitting her?").
- Assist the individual to recall the physical symptoms associated with anger.
- Teach to use deep breaths and relaxation breathing.

R: *Studies have shown that relaxation therapy is an effective intervention for individuals in an angry state (*Del Vecchio & O'Leary, 2004).*

- Help the individual to evaluate where in the chain of events change was possible.
  - Use role-playing to practice communication techniques.
  - Discuss how issues of control interfere with communication.
  - Help the individual recognize negative thinking patterns associated with low self-esteem.
- Help the individual to practice negotiation skills with family and people in authority.
- Encourage increased recreational activities.
- Use group therapy to decrease sense of aloneness and increase communication skills.
- Instruct about or refer for assertiveness training.
- Instruct about or refer for negotiation skills development.

R: *Discussions after a crisis can help to foster new and more effective approaches to management of aggressive individuals (Halter, 2014).*

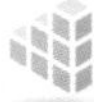

Pediatric Interventions

- Discuss with parents the methods of disciplining the child: Are they realistic? Appropriate? Effective?

To Manage Disruptive Behavior in Children (Varcarolis, 2011)

- Use a preset gesture or signal to remind child/adolescent to use self-control

R: *This can prevent escalation.*

- Move closer to child, put arm around child gently.

R: *This can provide a calming effect.*

- Redirect attention to another activity.
- Use humor or kidding.

R: *This can prevent escalation and frustration.*

- Remove child from situation.
- Initiate therapeutic holding.

R: *This can interrupt the disruptive cycle.*

- Use promises and reward carefully.
- Use threats and punishment carefully.

R: *This may encourage the child to bargain for a reward. Threats and punishment must be realistic and follow-through is critical for it to be effective.*

- Discuss the risks of firearms in the home. Explore the storage of firearms and protective devices (e.g., lockboxes, trigger locks).
- Explore various sources of media violence (e.g., television, video games, music, movies).
- Explain strategies to prevent adverse effects of media (e.g., violence, commercials [Hockenberry & Wilson, 2015; *Willis & Strasburger, 1998]).

- Watch television and videos with children: Limit to 2 hours or less a day
- If possible, avoid programs that emphasize violence.
- Creatively illustrate when violent acts are punished.
- Explore alternatives to violence (e.g., "What could the man have done besides shooting?")
- When selecting programs, consider the following questions:
  - Are good characters violent?
  - Is the violence justified?
  - Are there negative consequences of violence?
- Consider the child's age when selecting television programs and movies.

R: *Discussions that correlate with the actual viewing of violent behavior are more meaningful (*Davies & Flannery, 1998).*

- Discuss programs and commercial content with child to emphasize (Hockenberry & Wilson, 2015):
  - You are smarter than what you see on TV.
  - TV world is not real.
  - Somebody is making money trying to sell you something.
  - TV shows that some people are more important than others.
- Engage the child and peers in a nonthreatening manner to discuss age-related violence (e.g., hitting, bullying, throwing objects, date rape).

R: *Violence is a learned behavior. If it is learned, then prosocial behavior can be taught as an alternative (*Davies & Flannery, 1998).*

- Role-play high-risk situations, such as
  - Finding a gun in a friend's house
  - Bullying a victim
  - Refusing sexual advances

R: *Parents can model appropriate problem-solving strategies. Environments (families, schools, communities) that provide care and support have high expectations and provide opportunities for children to participate in discussions that can increase children's hardiness and invulnerability to violence (*Edari & McManus, 1998).*

RISK FOR SELF-DIRECTED VIOLENCE

NANDA-I Definition

At risk for behaviors in which an individual demonstrates that he or she can be physically, emotionally, and/or sexually harmful to self

Risk Factors*

Age 15 to 19
Age 45 or older
Engagement in autoerotic sexual acts

Author's Note

The remaining risk factors are risk factors for suicide (e.g., suicidal ideation or history of multiple suicide attempts). *Risk for Self-Directed Violence* should be replaced with *Risk for Suicide.* Refer to this diagnosis for additional content.

WANDERING

NANDA-I Definition

Meandering, aimless, or repetitive locomotion that exposes the individual to harm; frequently incongruent with boundaries

Defining Characteristics*

Continuous movement from place to place
Getting lost
Fretful locomotion
Frequent movement from place to place
Haphazard locomotion
Hyperactivity
Inability to locate significant landmarks in a familiar setting
Locomotion resulting in unintended leaving of a premise
Periods of locomotion interspersed with periods of nonlocomotion (e.g., sitting, standing, sleeping)
Pacing
Trespassing
Scanning behaviors
Searching behaviors
Locomotion that cannot be easily dissuaded
Shadowing a caregiver's locomotion
Locomotion into unauthorized or private spaces
Long periods of locomotion without an apparent destination
Persistent locomotion in search of something

Related Factors

Pathophysiologic

Related to impaired cerebral function* secondary to:

Cerebrovascular accident
Mental retardation
Alzheimer's dementia or other dementia

Related to physiologic state or needs (e.g., hunger, thirst, pain, urination, constipation)*

Situational (Personal, Environmental)

Related to emotional state (e.g., frustration, anxiety, boredom, depression, or agitation)*

Related to overstimulating*/understimulating environment

Related to separation from familiar environment* (e.g., people, objects)

Maturational

Older Adult

Related to faulty judgments secondary to:

Medications (e.g., sedation,* hyperactivity)
Alzheimer's dementia or other dementia

Related to separation from familiar environment* (e.g., people, objects)

Children

Related to faulty judgments secondary to (specify) (e.g., Autism, Asperger's syndrome)

Author's Note

This nursing diagnosis is more useful than *Risk for Injury*, which was previously used. *Risk for Injury* focuses on strategies to protect an individual from injury. *Wandering* directs interventions to protect an individual from injury in addition to addressing the reasons for the wandering behavior, if possible.

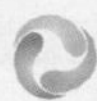

Errors in Diagnostic Statements

Wandering related to repetitive episodes of "being lost" in neighborhood

This diagnosis as written does not have related factors. These related factors are signs of *Wandering*. If the contributing factors to *Wandering* are not known, the nurse can write the diagnosis as *Wandering* related to unknown etiology, as evidenced by repetitive episodes of "being lost" in the neighborhood.

Key Concepts

- There are 5.5 million people with Alzheimer's disease in the United States, and about 70% of those wander away at least once in a year, totaling almost 3 million people. Some are never found (Alzheimer's Association, 2015).
- It is estimated up to 31% of nursing home residents wander away at least once in a year (Lai & Arthur, 2003).
- "In addition to cognitive impairment, risk factors for wandering include older age, male sex, poor sleep patterns, agitation, aggression, and a more socially active and outgoing premorbid lifestyle" (Lester, Garite, & Kohen, 2012).
- Negative consequences of wandering for individuals include elopement, falls, other injuries, and even death (Alzheimer's Association, 2015).

Focus Assessment Criteria

Subjective Data

Assess for Related Factors

Emotional coping patterns
Refer to *Ineffective Coping*.

Objective Data

Assess for Defining Characteristics

Reported episodes of
- Trespassing
- Persistent locomotion
- Getting lost
- Following caregiver
- Hyperactivity
- Pacing
- Locomotion with no apparent destination

Goals

NOC
Risk Control, Elopement Propensity Risk, Safe Wandering, Family Functioning

The individual will not elope or get lost, as evidenced by the following indicators for individual and family:

- Ambulates safely
- Caretakers will identify factors that contribute to wandering behaviors.
- Caretakers will anticipate wandering behaviors.

Interventions

Clinical Alert Wandering, as it is applied to individuals who are disoriented or cognitively impaired, is generally characterized by excessive ambulation that has a tendency to lead to safety concerns or nuisance issues. It is a purposeful behavior triggered by a desire to fulfill a need. Although the nature of the need varies, it may relate to physical discomfort, such as the urge to urinate, or to emotional discomfort, such as the need for more or less stimulation (Lester et al., 2012).

NIC
Surveillance: Safety, Environmental Management: Safety, Referral, Risk Identification, Security Enhancement

Assess for Contributing Factors

- Anxiety
- Confusion
- Frustration
- Boredom
- Agitation
- Separation from familiar people and places
- Faulty judgments
- Physiologic urge (hunger, thirst, pain, urination, constipation)
- Sleep disturbances (Refer to *Disturbed Sleep Pattern.*)

Reduce or Eliminate Contributing Factors, If Possible

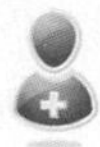

Clinical Alert "Physical handicaps and a lack of prior wandering or elopement attempts are no guarantee against elopement. As our case illustrates, even nonambulatory residents with cognitive impairment may be at high risk of wandering, especially if they are able to self-propel in wheelchairs" (Lester et al., 2012).

Anxiety/Agitation

- If feasible, fence in an area with safety locks.

R: *This can encourage moving around in fresh air, which can reduce anxiety, agitation, and restlessness.*

- Try to take the person for a walk before or after dinner.
- Provide a safe route for walking.
- Encourage activities that involve exercise (e.g., sweeping, raking).

R: *Safe paths within or on the outside of a unit can provide a release for the need to wander.*

Unfamiliar Environment

- Do not leave someone with dementia unsupervised in new surroundings.
- Select a familiar picture to exhibit on the individual's door.
- Redirect the individual if he or she is lost.
- Create nature scenes in the hallways (Cohen-Mansfield, 1998).
- Mark exit door with big signs.
- Place horizontal stripes on the exit door or use a cloth panel across the width of the door.

R: *Safe paths within or on the outside of a unit can provide a release for the need to wander (Logsdon et al. 1998).*

R: *When an environment is enhanced with murals, pictures, and so forth, people with dementia trespass and exit less (Cohen-Mansfield, 1998).*

Physiologic Urges

- Anticipate need for toileting with a schedule.
- Schedule times for fluids and food.
- Evaluate for any pain.
- Ensure the individual is comfortable.

R: *Unmet needs and environmental factors can also contribute to wandering risk. It is well known that people with dementia have a lower threshold for stress, and their ability to cope with internal and environmental stress continues to erode as the disease progresses.*

Promote a Safe Environment. Secure Your Home

- Install locks on doors and windows.
- Install electronic devices with buzzers on doors and property boundaries.
- Use pressure-sensitive alarms (doormats, bed sensor, chair sensor).
- Provide regular opportunities for the individual to walk with a companion or in a safe area.

R: *Modifying the environment rather than using restraints can decrease stress and agitation (Logsdon et al., 1998).*

R: *People with cognitive impairments need external controls for protection.*

Notify Others (Neighbors, Police, Others in Residence, Staff, Community Resources) About the Person's Wandering Behaviors

- Dress your loved one in bright clothing.

R: *Bright clothes are easier to see in crowds, etc.*

- Explain the use of electronic devices.
- Make sure the person always wears ID bracelet or anklet, not only a wallet with ID.
- Instruct others to notify the provider if they see the individual wandering.
- Supply others with a recent photograph and current identification information (age, height, weight, hair color, description of clothes, identifying characteristics) of the individual.
- For Wandering and Elopement Resources refer to online resources like the National Council of Certified Dementia Practitioners (search *wandering*) and the "Safety Center" at the Alzheimer's Association website.

R: *Community residents, personnel, and police need to be alerted to the risk of wandering and injury.*

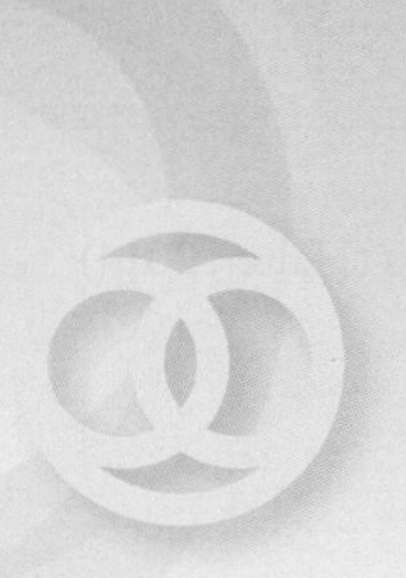

Part 2

Family/Home Nursing Diagnoses

This section focuses on family and home nursing diagnoses. These diagnoses can be used in any setting such as a hospital, skilled care, or a home. Community wellness and health maintenance diagnoses related to the family can be found in Part 4. Key concepts related to the family will be relevant to all types of family and home nursing diagnoses.

Key Concepts

General Considerations

- A family is a set of interacting individuals related by blood, marriage, cohabitation, or adoption, who interdependently perform relevant functions by fulfilling expected roles (Edelman, Kudzma, & Mandle, 2014).
- Pillitteri (2014) reports family types as:
  - Dyad—two people living together (e.g., married, unmarried, gay, lesbian)
  - Nuclear—traditional family of a husband, wife, and children
  - Multigenerational—a nuclear family with other family members such as grandparents, cousins, grandchildren
  - Cohabitation—unmarried couples with children living together
  - Polygamous—although illegal in the United States, a family of one man with several wives may immigrate to the United States
  - Blended—remarriage or reconstituted family with children (e.g., divorced, widowed)
  - Single parent—51% of families are single parent (Vespa, Lewis, & Kreider, 2009)
  - Communal—groups of people who chose to live together
  - Same gender—About one in five families have same-gender parents.
- Healthy families (Edelman et al., 2014; Kaakinen Coehlo, Steele, Tabacco, Hanson, 2015):
  - Are resilient
  - Are adaptable
  - Spend time together
  - Are cohesive
  - Have a sense of spiritual well-being
  - Have a sense of well-being
  - Are able to deal with stress
  - Are committed
  - Exhibit positive communication
  - Show appreciation and affection for one another
  - Each family member influences the entire family unit. Thus, the health of an individual influences the health of the family. Family equilibrium depends on a balance of roles in the family and reciprocation (*Duvall, 1977; Edelman et al., 2014).

Stress/Crisis

- Constructive or functional coping mechanisms of families facing a stress crisis are as follows (Halter, 2014):
  - Greater reliance on one another
  - Maintenance of a sense of humor
  - Increased sharing of feeling and thoughts
  - Promotion of each member's individuality
  - Accurate appraisal of the meaning of the problem
  - Search for knowledge and resources about the problem
  - Use of support systems

- Destructive or dysfunctional coping mechanisms of families facing a crisis are as follows (Halter, 2014):
  - Denial of the problem
  - Exploitation of one or more members (threats, violence, neglect, scapegoating)
  - Separation (hospitalization, institutionalization, divorce, abandonment)
  - Authoritarianism (no negotiation)
  - Preoccupation of family members (who lack affection) with appearing close
- Characteristics of families prone to crisis include the following (Varcarolis, 2011):
  - Apathy (resignation to state in life)
  - Poor self-concept
  - Low income
  - Inability to manage money
  - Unrealistic preferences (materialistic)
  - Lack of skills and education
  - Unstable work history
  - Frequent relocations
  - History of repeated inadequate problem solving
  - Lack of adequate role models
  - Lack of participation in religious or community activities
  - Environmental isolation (no telephone, inadequate public transportation)
- The National Coalition for the Homeless Report (2015):
  - In the United States, more than 3.5 million people experience homelessness each year.
  - 35% of the homeless population are families with children, which is the fastest growing segment of the homeless population.
  - 23% are U.S. military veterans.
  - 25% are children under the age of 18 years.
  - 30% have experienced domestic violence.
  - 20% to 25% suffer from mental illness.
  - In urban communities, people experience homelessness for an average of 8 months.

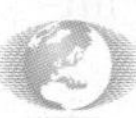

Transcultural Considerations

- The dominant U.S. culture values two goals for families: (1) encouragement and nurturance of each individual and (2) cultivation of healthy, autonomous children. Marital partners are expected to be supportive and share a sense of meaning. Each partner has the freedom for personality development. Children are encouraged to develop their own identity and life directions (Giger, 2013).
- Families in oppressed groups: In Latin families, the needs of the family are more important than those of the individual. The father is the provider, head of the household, and decision maker (Andrews & Boyle, 2012).
- Campinha-Bacote (2011) designed a model for becoming culturally competent as an ongoing, changing process, which includes the following:
  - Awareness of one's own beliefs and biases
  - Acquiring knowledge about worldwide cultures
  - Acquiring skills to conduct a cultural assessment
  - Motivated to understand, know, and work with diverse individuals and groups to avoid cultural conflicts
- Arab-American families are supposed to be supportive. A family is often criticized as a failure if a member is sent to the hospital for psychiatric care. Arab-American families may appear overindulgent and interfering to compensate for criticism (Giger, 2013).
- Japanese Americans identify themselves by the generation in which they are born. First- and second-generation Japanese Americans see the family as one of the most important factors in their lives. They manage problems within the family structure. The father and other male members are in the top positions. Achievement or failure of one member reflects on the entire family. Caring for elderly parents, usually by the oldest son or unmarried child, is expected. Adult children freely provide their parents with goods, money, and assistance (Andrews & Boyle, 2012).
- The nuclear family and the greater Jewish community are the center of Jewish culture. Families are close knit and child oriented. The commandments dictate expected behavior toward parents and within the community (Giger, 2013).
- For the Vietnamese, family has been the chief source of cohesion and continuity for hundreds of years. Immediate family includes parents, unmarried children, and sometimes the husband's parents and sons

with their wives and children. Individual behavior reflects on the whole family. A member is expected to give up personal wishes or ambitions if they disrupt family harmony. Family loyalty is "filial piety," which commands children to obey and honor their parents even after death (Giger, 2013).

Abuse in Families

- The World Health Organization defines violence as "the intentional use of physical force or power, threatened or actual, against oneself, against another person, or against a group or community, which either results in or has a high likelihood of resulting in injury, death, psychological harm, maldevelopment, or deprivation."
- Vagianos (2014) reported[1] the following:
  - Seventy percent of women worldwide experience physical and/or sexual abuse by an intimate partner during their lifetimes.
  - Three women are murdered every day by a current or former male partner in the United States.
  - In the United States, the number of women who experience physical violence by an intimate partner every year is 4,774,000.
  - The percentage of gay or bisexual men who will experience intimate partner violence in their lifetimes is 40.1 %.
  - Fifty percent of lesbian women experience domestic violence (not necessarily intimate partner violence) in their lifetimes.
  - Financial abuse is present ninety-eight percent (98%) of the time in all domestic violence cases. The number one reason domestic violence survivors stay or return to the abusive relationship is because the abuser controls their money supply, leaving them with no financial resources to break free.
  - The incidence of the likelihood a woman will be murdered in the few weeks after leaving her abusive partner is 70% higher than at any other time in the relationship.
- "More significant, however, are the skewed contexts in which media present violence". "In media portrayals, 75 percent of violent acts are committed without remorse, criticism, or penalty; 41 percent are associated with humor; 38 percent are committed by attractive perpetrators; and 58 percent involve victims who show no pain" (American Academy of Family Physicians, 2015).
- Family violence is "the intentional intimidation, abuse or neglect of children, adults or elders by a family member, intimate partner or caretaker in order to gain power and control over the victim" (American Academy of Family Physicians, 2015).
- People involved in family violence have higher levels of depression, suicidal feelings, self-contempt, inability to trust, and inability to develop intimate relationships in later life (*Carson & Smith-DiJulio, 2006).
- Children who witness abuse in their homes after 5 or 6 years of age begin to identify with the aggressor and lose respect for the victim (*Carson & Smith-DiJulio, 2006).

Spousal Abuse

Department of Justice (2014) defines domestic violence as a pattern of abusive behavior in any relationship that is used by one partner to gain or maintain power and control over another intimate partner. Domestic violence can be physical, sexual, emotional, economic, or psychological actions or threats of actions that influence another person. This includes any behaviors that intimidate, manipulate, humiliate, isolate, frighten, terrorize, coerce, threaten, blame, hurt, injure, or wound someone.

Domestic violence is the third leading cause of homelessness among families.

- The battered wife syndrome has three major concepts: cycle of violence (Fig. II.8), learned helplessness, and anticipatory fear (*Blair, 1986).
- Carlson-Catalano (*1998) found that of the battered women in her study, all reported they left to protect another loved one (child or pet). None of the women reported that she left because of her own safety or discomfort.
- Factors contributing to a battered woman's remaining in the relationship include the following:
  - Belief that children need a two-parent family
  - Lack of financial support

[1] To access the references for each of the above statistics refer to the article "30 Shocking Domestic Violence Statistics That Remind Us It's An Epidemic" at the Huffington Post website.

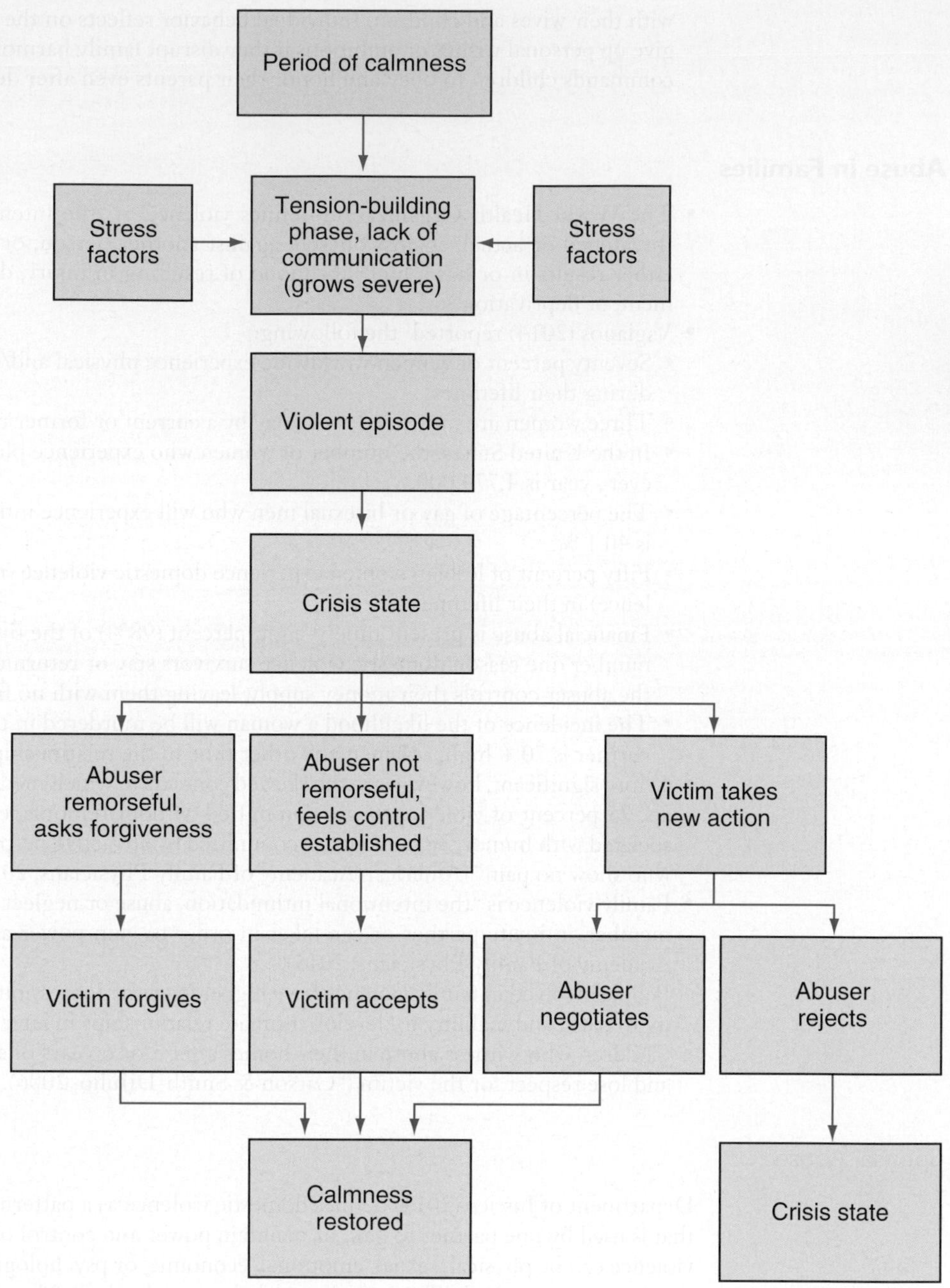

FIGURE II.8 Escalation of violence.

  - Lack of a place to go
  - Belief that the abuse will stop
  - Fear for her life or her children's lives
  - Fear of unknown future
- Personal characteristics of the abuser (Halter, 2014; *Smith-DiJulio & Holzapfel, 1998) include the following:
  - History of a family devoid of love, affection, and security
  - Unfulfilled, overwhelming need for love and security
  - Unrealistic expectations about others (usually spouse or child) as being able to fill void from childhood, resulting in feelings of rejection, anger, and abuse
  - Blaming outside factors for everything that goes wrong; blaming wife for causing him to get angry
  - Denial of the violence or minimizing its severity

- Impulsiveness
- Excessive dependence on and jealousy of spouse (usually the only significant relationship he has)
- Fear of losing spouse or significant other, which can contribute to suicide, homicide, depression, or anger
- Belief in male supremacy

- Personal characteristics of the battered woman (Halter, 2014) include the following:
  - Low self-esteem, defining self in terms of partner
  - Unrealistic hopes for change
  - Belief that she has incited her husband to beat her and is to blame
  - Raised in a family that restricted emotional expression (e.g., anger, hugging)
  - Subscribing to the feminine sex-role stereotype
  - History of marrying to escape restrictive, confining family
  - Extreme resourcefulness and self-sufficiency to survive
  - Usually not abused as a child and did not witness abuse
  - View of herself as a victim with no option but to appease her spouse
  - Gradually increased social isolation
  - Belief that partner "can't help it"
- The likelihood of a woman seeking and using assistance for abuse increases if (*Sammons, 1981)
  - She has been in the relationship less than 5 years.
  - She is employed.
  - She has friends or relatives who live nearby (within a few miles).
  - She has discussed the abuse with others.
  - The abuse is frequent (daily, weekly), severe (requires medical treatment/hospitalization), or increasing in frequency.

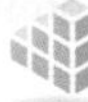

Pediatric Considerations

- The Department of Health and Human Services: Administration for Children & Families (2013) reported:
  - An estimated 679,000 children were victims of abuse and neglect (unique instances).
  - Forty seven states reported approximately 3.1 million children received preventative services from child protective services agencies in the United States.
  - Children in the first year of their life had the highest rate of victimization of 23.1 per 1,000 children in the national population of the same age.
  - Of the children who experienced maltreatment or abuse, nearly 80% suffered neglect; 18% suffered physical abuse; and 9% suffered sexual abuse.
  - Less than 80% of reported child fatalities as a result of abuse and neglect were caused by one or more of the child victim's parents.
  - There were 678,932 victims of child abuse and neglect reported to child protective services in 2013.
  - The youngest children are the most vulnerable with about 27% of reported victims being under the age of 3.
- Child maltreatment includes intentional physical abuse or neglect, emotional abuse or neglect, and sexual abuse of children by adults (Hockenberry & Wilson, 2015).
- "Child neglect is defined as the failure of the child's parents or caretaker to provide the child with the basic necessities of life, when financially able to do so or when offered reasonable means to do so" (*Cowen, 1999). Basic necessities are shelter, nutrition, health care, supervision, education, affection, and protection (*Cowen, 1999). It is the most common form of child maltreatment (Hockenberry & Wilson, 2015).
- Family interactions in neglectful families are "more chaotic, less able to resolve conflict, less cohesive, less verbally expressive and less warm and empathetic" (*Cowen, 1999).
- In one study, 85% of cases of neglected children had a parent who was indifferent, intolerant, or overanxious (*Browne, 1989).
- Abused by someone they know: parent, babysitter, relative, or friend of the family.
- Factors that contribute to child abuse (Hockenberry & Wilson, 2015) include the following:
  - Living in poverty or near poverty (high risk)
  - Lack or unavailability of extended family
  - Lack of role model as a child
  - High-risk children (e.g., unwanted, undesired sex or appearance, physically or mentally handicapped, hyperactive, terminally ill)
  - High-risk parents (e.g., single, adolescent, emotionally disturbed, alcoholic, drug addicted, physically ill)

- Characteristic personal patterns of abusers (*Kaufman & Straus, 1987) include the following:
  - History of abuse by and lack of warmth and affection from parents
  - Social isolation (few friends or outlets for tensions)
  - Marked lack of self-esteem, with low tolerance for criticism
  - Emotional immaturity and dependency
  - Distrust of others
  - Inability to admit the need for help
  - Unrealistic expectations for/of child
  - Desire for the child to give them pleasure

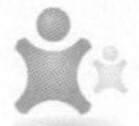

Maternal Considerations

- Intimate partner violence is the leading cause of female homicide and injury-related deaths during pregnancy (American Psychological Association [APA], 2015b).
- According to the Centers for Disease Control and Prevention (2013), at least 4% to 8% of pregnant women—that is over 300,000 per year—report suffering abuse during pregnancy.

Prematurity as a Risk for Child Maltreatment

- Separation of the infant from its parents, as in the case of prematurity, can reduce the attachment and nurturing behaviors of the mother toward her child. A disproportionate number of abused children were premature or ill at birth (Kauffman et al., 1986).
- Maternal characteristics that predict increased risk of both poor pregnancy outcomes and child abuse may contribute to infant/child maltreatment (*Spencer Wallace, Sundrum, Bacchus, & Logan, 2006).
- Spencer et al. (*2006) in a large retrospective whole population birth cohort reported that "lower levels of fetal growth and shorter gestational duration are associated with increased likelihood of child protection registration in all categories including sexual abuse independent of maternal age or socioeconomic status."
- Needell and Barth (*1998) reported that "infants admitted into foster care as a result of maltreatment were more than twice as likely as those not in care to have been born low birth weight after adjustment for single parenthood, family size, and ethnicity" (*Spencer et al., 2006).

Geriatric Considerations

- Elder abuse is the infliction of physical, emotional/psychological, sexual, or financial harm on an older adult. Elder abuse can also take the form of intentional or unintentional neglect of an older adult by the caregiver (APA, 2015a). The following are types of elder abuse or neglect:
  - Physical abuse
  - Sexual Abuse
  - Financial abuse and exploitation
  - Verbal, emotional, or psychological abuse
  - Caregiver neglect
- Caregiver neglect can range from caregiving strategies that withhold appropriate attention from the individual to intentionally failing to meet the physical, social, or emotional needs of the older person. Neglect can include failure to provide food, water, clothing, medications, and assistance with activities of daily living or help with personal hygiene. If the caregiver is responsible for paying bills for the older person, neglect can also include failure to pay the bills or to manage the older person's money responsibly. Family caregivers may inadvertently neglect their older relatives because of their own lack of knowledge, resources, or maturity, although this is a less frequent form of abuse.
- Older adults are increasingly vulnerable to mistreatment as they become economically, physically, socially, and emotionally more dependent and the resources of caretakers are limited (Miller, 2015).
- Acierno et al. (2010) reported that it is estimated that more than two million elders are abused or mistreated each year (APA, 2003). Theories of causation include intrafamily violence, learned behavior (cycle of family violence), psychopathology of the abuser, dependency of the elder, dependency of the caregiver, lack of social support, caregiver burden, poor health of the elder or caregiver, and substance abuse.
- According to Miller (2015), mandatory reporting laws do not require reporters to know that abuse or neglect has occurred, but merely to report it if they suspect it.

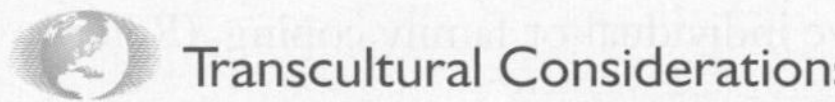

Transcultural Considerations

- Domestic violence is cross-cultural. It exists in every culture and is a sign of individual and family dysfunction.
- Traditional Native American life did not include spousal or child abuse. Unfortunately, domestic violence has evolved and is frequently alcohol related. In the United States, 54% of Hispanic women born in the United States reported abuse compared with 22% of Hispanic women born in Mexico (Harris, Firestone, & Vega, 2005).
- Montalvo-Liendo Koci, McFarlane, Nava, Gilroy, and Maddoux (2013) found that women of Mexican descent, who did not report abuse, were influenced by "familism" and gender role orientations. Other reported factors were protecting their partners, avoidance of worrying their mothers or nonsupportive mothers, fear of losing their children, and their immigration status (Montalvo-Liendo et al., 2013).

Children With Special Needs

- Parental tasks for successful adaptation to children with special needs are as follows:
  - Realistically perceive infant's condition and caregiver's needs.
  - Adapt to hospital environment.
  - Assume primary caregiver role.
  - Progress to total responsibility for care at discharge.
- Parenting behaviors are learned through role modeling, role rehearsal, and reference group interaction. External factors, both developmental (birth of a child) and situational (illness and/or hospitalization of a child), require the acquisition of new behaviors or the modification of existing behaviors. Difficulty mastering the behaviors required for the role transition leads to role strain. Uncertainty about what behaviors the new role requires leads to lack of role clarity. Incompatibility between the new role expectation and already existing expectations leads to role conflict.
- Parents experiencing their child's illness in an acute or a chronic situation face the challenge of role transition to continue effective parenting on either a temporary or permanent basis. The parent must give up the role of parenting a well child and acquire the role of parenting a sick child.
- Role conflicts can develop easily when a child receives home care from a parent or a combination of parents and health-care professionals. Role confusion caused by the intrusion of treatments, providers, or both into the home is a source of stress for the entire family and requires careful role negotiation (*Melnyk, Feinstein, Moldenhouer, & Small, 2001).
- Unhealthy outcomes resulting from maladaptation to family crisis are as follows:
  - Disturbed parent–child relationship
  - Failure to thrive
  - Vulnerable child syndrome
  - Disturbed marital and family equilibrium
  - Child abuse or neglect
- Clements, Copeland, and Loftus (*1990) reported in a study of 30 families with chronically ill children that parenting is more difficult at certain critical times: initial diagnosis; increase in physical symptoms; relocation of the child, such as rehospitalization; developmental changes for the child, such as entrance into school; and physical or emotional absence of one parent (e.g., illness, pregnancy).
- Caring for a child with special needs places high demands on parents' energy, time, and financial resources.
- Fathers of children with special needs are challenged with a situation that they could not protect their family from or control. They have more difficulty adjusting to a son with special needs because of the loss of future joint recreation.
- In a study of 45 mothers of acutely ill children, Schepp (*1991) found that predictability of events and anxiety influenced the mother's coping effort. Mothers who knew what to expect were less anxious.
- Strong families appreciate and encourage all members. There is a commitment toward each member and the family unit. There is a clear set of family rules, values, and beliefs.
- Families acquire children through birth, adoption, and remarriage. Sometimes grandparents assume the parenting role for grandchildren because of the loss of parents, substance abuse, or a history of ineffective parenting (*Clemen-Stone, Eigasti, & McGuire 2001).
- Although many parents anticipate the birth of their child with pleasure, most are unprepared for the accompanying changes. After a child is born, parental self-concepts develop. For a woman, her role as parent often overshadows her role as wife and individual. For a man, parenthood strengthens his role as husband and worker. Parenting often becomes a dominant role for women and a secondary role for men (*Clemens-Stone et al., 2001).

- Situations that contribute to abuse are often related to ineffective individual or family coping. (Refer to Disabled Family Coping, as evidenced by child abuse.)

Parent–Infant Bonding

- Bonding cannot be determined "by particular behaviors, but from patterns of behavior" (*Goulet Bell, & Tribble 1998). Parent–infant bonding is interactional. Attachment requires proximity, reciprocity, and commitment (*Goulet et al., 1998).
- "Children who are cared for in a relatively consistent and predictable way develop confidence in their ability to have a positive influence on their environment and are more likely to express their need for love and security" (*Goulet et al., 1998).
- The mother–child relationship begins before conception: planning, confirming, and accepting the pregnancy; feeling fetal movement, accepting the fetus as an individual; giving birth; hearing and seeing the baby; touching and holding the baby; and caring for the baby.
- Participation of the father in caregiving activities has increased in the United States. Fathers who choose a traditional role (allowing the mother to be totally responsible for caretaking activities) must be accessed in their sociocultural context.
- Mercer and Ferketich (*1990) studied parental attachment of 121 high-risk women, 61 partners of high-risk women, 182 low-risk women, and 117 partners of low-risk women. They found that the major predictor of parental attachment for all four groups was parental competence.

Focus Assessment Criteria

Elder Abuse/Neglect

Assess for Perpetrator Risk Factors

Mental illness
Alcoholism, drug abuse
Hostility
Financial dependency on the victim

Assess for Elder Victim Risk Factors

Dementia
Problem behaviors
Disability

Assess for Perpetrator/Victim Environmental Risk Factors

Shared living arrangements
Social isolation or lack of social support

General Assessment

Family composition (who resides in home)
Literacy (ability to read and/or write, English as a second language)
Family strengths
Decisions (shared, autocratic)
Rules/discipline
Family member responsibilities
Financial status
Participation in community activities
Presence of extended family
Use of alcohol, drugs, tobacco (parents, relatives, children)
Family lifestyle (activities, leisure [individual, family], work, TV/Internet time)
Family rituals
Health care (insurance, access, cost)

Communication Patterns of Each Family Member

Express feelings openly
Expression of feelings are sanctioned

Clear messages
Little or no open dialogue

Emotional/Supportive Pattern
Constructive
- Optimistic
- Rely on each other

Destructive
- Isolated
- Deny problems
- Exploit members (threats, violence, neglect, scapegoating, authoritative)

Assess for Recent Changes

Addition of New Family Member
Birth
Adoption
Marriage
Elderly relative

Loss of Family Member
Relocation
Change in Family Roles
- Financial crisis
- Disaster

Assess Parental Behavior (Prenatal, After Delivery)

Prenatal
Verbalize anticipation.
Seek prenatal care.
Plan room, clothes.

Intrapartum
Participate in decision and birthing process.
Verbalize positive feelings.
Attempt to see infant as soon as delivered.
Respond positively (happy) or negatively (sad, apathetic, disappointed, angry, ambivalent).
Hold and talk to infant.
Use baby's name.

Postpartum
Verbalize positive feelings.
Seek proximity by holding infant closely; touch and hug.
Smile and gaze at infant; seek eye contact.
Refer to infant by name and sex.
Express interest in learning infant care.
Perform nurturing behavior (i.e., feeding, changing).

Assess for Domestic Violence

Have you ever been emotionally or physically abused by your partner or someone important to you?
In the last year, have you been hit, slapped, kicked, or otherwise physically hurt by someone?
Are you or have you ever been pregnant? If yes, have you been hit, slapped, kicked, or otherwise physically hurt by someone? If yes, by whom? How many times?
Within the last year, has anyone forced you to have sexual activities? If yes, who? Number of times?
Are you afraid of your partner or anyone else?
Has your partner:
- Threatened to try suicide?
- Threatened to kill you?

Does your partner:
- Drink to excess?
- Control all the money?
- Use drugs?
- Destroy possessions?
- Try to control your daily activities?
- Try to control who your friends are?
- Exhibit violent jealousy?
- Have a gun?

Assess for Suspicion of Child Abuse

Trauma (fractures, lacerations, bruises, welts, burns, dislocations)
Unexplained or unwitnessed injuries
Nature and extent of injury not consistent with explanation
Injuries in various stages of healing
Injuries to face
Abdominal injuries
Multiple bruises (trunk, buttocks, wrists, ankles, ears, neck, around mouth)
Fractures (rib, metaphyseal, scapular, distal clavicle, all humerus fractures [except supracondylar] in children younger than 3 years, vertebral fractures or subluxations, midshaft ulnar fractures, bilateral fractures)
Bruises of varied colors:
- Red, black, or blue: immediate to 5 days
- Green: 5 to 7 days
- Yellow: 7 to 10 days
- Brown: 10 to 14 days

Physical indicators of sexual abuse
- Vaginal or penile discharges
- Sexually transmitted disease
- Genital or anal injuries or swelling
- Pain or itching in genital area
- Caregiver–sibling interaction

COMPROMISED FAMILY COPING

NANDA-I Definition

A usually supportive primary person (family member, significant other, or close friend) provides insufficient, ineffective, or compromised support, comfort, assistance, or encouragement that may be needed by the individual to manage or master adaptive tasks related to his or her health challenge.

Defining Characteristics*

Subjective

Individual reports a concern about significant person's response to health problem.
Significant person reports preoccupation with personal reaction (e.g., fear, anticipatory grief, guilt, anxiety) to individual's need.
Significant person reports inadequate understanding, which interferes with effective supportive behaviors.

Objective

Significant person attempts assistive or supportive behaviors with unsatisfactory results.
Significant person enters into limited personal communication with the individual.
Significant person displays protective behavior disproportionate to individual's need for autonomy.

Related Factors

Refer to *Interrupted Family Processes.*

Author's Note

This nursing diagnosis describes situations similar to the diagnosis *Interrupted Family Processes or Risk for Interrupted Family Processes.* Until clinical research differentiates this diagnosis from the aforementioned diagnosis, use *Interrupted Family Processes.*

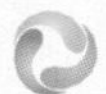

Author's Note

Compromised Family Coping describes a family that reports usual constructive function but is experiencing an alteration from a current stress-related challenge. The family is viewed as a system, with interdependence among members. Thus, life challenges for individual members also challenge the family system. Certain situations may negatively influence family functioning; examples include illness, an older relative moving in, relocation, separation, and divorce. Risk for *Interrupted Family Processes* can represent such a situation.

Compromised Family Coping differs from *Caregiver Role Strain*. Certain situations require one or more family members to assume a caregiver role for a relative. Caregiver role responsibilities can vary from ensuring an older parent has three balanced meals daily to providing for all hygiene and self-care activities for an adult or child. *Caregiver Role Strain* describes the mental and physical burden that the caregiver role places on individuals, which influences all their concurrent relationships and role responsibilities. It focuses specifically on the individual or individuals with multiple direct caregiver responsibilities.

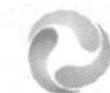

Errors in Diagnostic Statements

***Compromised Family Coping* related to family not discussing the situation**

A family's failure to discuss a situation does not represent a related factor, but a possible validation of the problem. If a failure to support one another represents a response to a stressor affecting the family system, *Compromised Family Coping* related to (specify stressor), as evidenced by report of family not discussing the situation, may be appropriate.

Goals

NOC

Family Coping, Family Environment: Internal, Family Normalization, Parenting

The family will maintain functional system of mutual support for one another, as evidenced by the following indicators:

- Frequently verbalizes feelings to professional nurse and one another
- Identifies appropriate external resources available

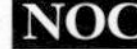

Interventions

NIC

Family Involvement Promotion, Coping Enhancement, Family Integrity Promotion, Family Therapy, Counseling, Referral

Assess Causative and Contributing Factors

Illness-Related Factors

- Sudden, unexpected nature of illness
- Burdensome, chronic problems
- Potentially disabling nature of illness
- Symptoms creating disfiguring change in physical appearance
- Social stigma associated with illness
- Financial burden

Factors Related to Behavior of Ill Family Member

- Refuses to cooperate with necessary interventions
- Engages in socially deviant behavior associated with illness (e.g., suicide attempts, violence, substance abuse)
- Isolates self from family
- Acts out or is verbally abusive to health professionals and family members

Factors related to overall family functioning

- Unresolved guilt, blame, hostility, jealousy
- Inability to solve problems
- Ineffective communication patterns among members
- Changes in role expectations and resulting tension
- Unclear role boundaries

Factors Related to Illness in Family (See Also ***Caregiver Role Strain***)

Factors Related to the Community

- Lack of support from spiritual resources (philosophical, religious, or both)
- Lack of relevant health education resources
- Lack of supportive friends
- Lack of adequate community health-care resources (e.g., long-term follow-up, hospice, respite)

R: *Common sources of family stress are as follows (*Carson & Smith-DiJulio, 2006):*

- External sources of stress (e.g., job or school related) one member is experiencing
- External sources of stress (e.g., finances, relocation) influencing the family unit
- Developmental stressors (e.g., childbearing, new baby, childrearing, adolescence, arrival of older grandparent, marriage of single parents, loss of spouse)
- Situational stressors (e.g., illness, hospitalization, separation, caregiving responsibilities)

Promote cohesiveness.

- Approach the family with warmth, respect, and support.
- Keep family members abreast of changes in ill family member's condition when appropriate.
- Avoid discussing what caused the problem or blaming.
- Encourage verbalization of guilt, anger, blame, and hostility and subsequent recognition of own feelings in family members.

R: *No family is 100% functional; however, healthy families are concerned with each other's needs and encourage expression of feelings (Halter, 2014).*

- Explain the importance of functional communications, which uses verbal and nonverbal communication to teach behavior, share feelings and values, and evolve decisions about family health practices (Kaakinen et al., 2015).

R: *Effective communication is necessary in families to adapt to stressors and develop cohesiveness (Kaakinen et al., 2015).*

Assist Family to Appraise the Situation

- What is at stake? Encourage family to have a realistic perspective by providing accurate information and answers to questions. Ensure all family members have input.
- What are the choices? Assist family to reorganize roles at home and set priorities to maintain family integrity and reduce stress.
- Initiate discussions regarding stressors of home care (physical, emotional, environmental, and financial).
- "Family-oriented approaches that include helping a family gain insight and make behavioral changes are most successful" (Halter, 2014).
- Promote clear boundaries between individuals in family.
- Ensure that all family members share their concerns.
- Elicit the responsibilities of each member.
- Acknowledge the differences.

R: *An individual's emotional, social, and physical functioning is directly related to how clear his or her role is differentiated in the family (Halter, 2014).*

Initiate Health Teaching and Referrals, as Necessary

- Include family members in group education sessions.
- Refer families to lay support and self-help groups:
  - Al-Anon
  - Lupus Foundation of America

- Syn-Anon
- Arthritis Foundation
- Alcoholics Anonymous
- National Multiple Sclerosis Society
- Sharing and Caring
- American Cancer Society
- American Hospital Association
- American Heart Association
- American Diabetes Association
- Ostomy Association
- American Lung Association
- Reach for Recovery
- Alzheimer's Disease and Related Disorders Association

- Facilitate family involvement with social supports.
- Assist family members to identify reliable friends (e.g., clergy, significant others); encourage seeking help (emotional, technical) when appropriate.
- Enlist help of other professionals (social work, therapist, psychiatrist, school nurse).

R: *Families in stress will need extra encouragement to participate in self-help or other community agencies (Hockenberry & Wilson, 2015).*

DISABLED FAMILY COPING

Disabled Family Coping

Related to (Specify), as Evidenced by Partner Violence
Related to (Specify), as Evidenced by Child Abuse/Neglect
Related to Multiple Stressors Associated with Elder Care

Definition

Behavior of primary person (family member, significant other, or close friend) that disables his or her capacities and the individual's capacities to effectively address tasks essential to either person's adaption to the health challenge (NANDA-I)

The state in which a family demonstrates, or is at risk to demonstrate, destructive behavior in response to an inability to manage internal or external stressors due to inadequate resources (physical, psychological, cognitive, financial)[2]

Defining Characteristics

Decisions/actions that are detrimental to family well-being*
Neglectful care of individual in regard to basic human needs*
Neglectful care of individual in regard to illness treatment*
Neglectful relationships with other family members*
Family behaviors that are detrimental to well-being*
Distortion of reality regarding the individual's health problem*
Rejection*
Agitation*
Aggression*
Impaired restructuring of a family unit
Intolerance*
Abandonment*
Depression*
Hostility*

[2] This definition and characteristic have been added by the author for clarity and usefulness.

Related Factors

Pathophysiologic

Related to impaired ability to fulfill role responsibilities secondary to:

Any acute or chronic illness

Situational (Personal, Environmental)

Related to impaired ability to constructively manage stressors secondary to:

Substance abuse (e.g., alcoholism)
Negative role modeling
History of ineffective relationship with own parents
History of abusive relationship with parents

Related to unrealistic expectations of child by parent

Related to unrealistic expectations of parent by child

Related to unmet psychosocial needs of child by parent

Related to unmet psychosocial needs of parent by child

Related to marital stressors secondary to:

Financial difficulties
Separation
Infidelities
Problematic children
Problematic relatives

Maturational

Children
Related to impaired ability to constructively manage stressors secondary to:

Premature infant
Disabled child

Older Adults
Related to impaired ability to constructively manage multipole stressors associated with elder care

Author's Note

Disabled Family Coping describes a family with a history of overt or covert destructive behavior or responses to stressors. This diagnosis necessitates long-term care from a nurse therapist with advanced specialization in family systems and abuse.

The use of this diagnosis in this book focuses on nursing interventions appropriate for a nurse generalist in a short-term relationship (e.g., emergency unit, nonpsychiatric in-house unit) and for any nurse in the position to prevent *Disabled Family Coping* through teaching, counseling, or referrals.

Errors in Diagnostic Statements

Disabled Family Coping related to reports of beatings by alcoholic husband

This diagnostic statement is formulated incorrectly and legally inadvisable for a nurse to write. Reported beating by a husband with alcoholism is not the contributing factor, but rather a diagnostic cue. This diagnosis should be written as *Disabled Family Coping* related to unknown etiology, as evidenced by wife reporting "My husband is an alcoholic and beats me frequently." The quoted statement represents the data as reported by the wife, rather than the nurse's judgment.

Goals

NOC

Caregiver Emotional Health, Caregiver Stressors, Family Coping, Family Normalization

Each family member will respond to the crisis with increased coping skills, emotional growth, and resources that prepare her or him for future stressors as evidenced by the following indicators:

- Appraises unhealthy coping behaviors of family members
- Relates expectations for self and family
- Sets realistic short- and long-term goals
- Relates community resources available

Interventions

NIC

Caregiver Support, Referral, Emotional Support, Family Therapy, Family Involvement Promotion

Identify With Each Family Member Their Strengths

R: *Identification of strengths provides "the family with information regarding the strengths, supporting their coping and functioning capabilities and encouraging movement to health through family education" (Kaakinen et al., 2015).*

Identify With Each Family Member Their Stressors

R: *Identification of stressors begins the process to help family members find and use appropriate treatment and crisis intervention if needed (Kaakinen et al., 2015).*

Assist Members to Appraise Family Behaviors (Effective, Ineffective, Destructive)

Discuss the Effects of Behaviors on Individuals and Family Unit (e.g., interactions, supportive, destructive)

R: *Families with a dysfunctional member (e.g., an alcoholic) are assisted to see that the entire family is dysfunctional, not just the individual.*

Assist Family to Set Short-Term and Long-Term Goals

R: *The family responding to the crisis returns to precrisis functioning, develops improved functioning (adaptation), or develops destructive functioning (maladaptation). Short-term goals focus on stabilizing the family as much as possible. Long-term goals focus on changes needed in functioning and establishing patterns to foster lasting changes.*

Promote Family Resilience

- Ask each family member to identify one activity he or she would like to add to their family.

Promote Adaption to Stressors and Crises (Kaakinen et al., 2015)

- Identify stressors that can be reduced or eliminated.

R: *Stressors are normative or nonnormative.*

- Engage the family members to discuss the situation.
- Allow each member to share their thoughts and suggestions for improving the situation.
- Negotiate necessary changes.
- Identify available resources.

R: *The family's resilience, unity, and resources will affect how they cope with stressors and crises (Kaakinen et al., 2015).*

- Ask each family member to identify one behavior he or she could control. Begin to help members to work through resentments of the past.

R: *Each family member is provided an opportunity to share feelings about the present and past (*Smith-DiJulio & Holzapfel, 2006). Interventions focus on helping the family renegotiate roles and patterns of interactive and functioning.*

Improve Family Cohesiveness

- Determine family recreational activities that include all members and are enjoyable.

R: *Family recreational activities foster family cohesion with positive experiences.*

Provide Anticipatory Guidance (Kaakinen et al., 2015)

- Identify relevant life changes that will occur in this family (e.g., birth of child, relocation, empty nest). Discuss necessary adjustments in the family routines.
- Identify family member's responsibilities. Evaluate the balance of responsibilities.

R: *The nurse can prepare the family for changes and stressors before they become a crisis (Kaakinen et al., 2015).*

Initiate Referrals, as Needed (e.g., support)

- Support groups, family therapy, economic support

R: *Dysfunctional families have a history of isolation. Interventions focus on increasing their socialization and use of community resources.*

Disabled Family Coping • Related to (Specify), as Evidenced by Partner Violence

Definition

Domestic abuse is defined as any action by an individual intended to harm another individual (physical, emotional, financial, social, and sexual) in a shared household.

Goals

NOC

Family Coping, Family Normalization, Family Functioning, Abuse Protection, Abuse Cessation

The individual will seek assistance for abusive behaviors, as evidenced by the following indicators:

- Discusses the physical assaults and fears
- Identifies the characteristics of abusers
- Describes a safety plan
- Seeks assistance for abusive behavior, legally and emotionally
- Relates community resources available when help is desired

Interventions

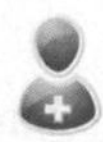

Clinical Alert As clinicians, you can serve an important role as advocates for change in an abused person's life by offering information, compassion, and support. The act of screening itself may be a key intervention that can help an individual begin to improve the quality of her or his life (Centers for Disease Control and Prevention [CDC], 2013).

Interventions to address the complexity and magnitude of the problems inherent in domestic violence are usually beyond the scope of a nurse generalist. Those provided here are to assist the nurse who has a short-term interaction with an individual and family.

NIC

Caregiver Support, Emotional Support, Referral, Counseling, Decision-Making Support, Support Group, Anger Control Assistance, Abuse Protection Support: Domestic Partner, Conflict Mediation

Develop Rapport

- Interview in private. Be empathic.
  - If a partner insists on being present all the time
    - Ask the individual to go with you to provide a urine specimen. Ask the person if someone is hurting her or him.
- Don't assume you know what the person needs.
- Ask, "How can I help you?"
- Avoid displaying shock or surprise at the details.
- If contact is made by telephone, find out how to get in touch with the victim.

R: *The victim is tense and afraid, feels helpless, accepts blame, and is hoping for change in the partner (*Carson & Smith-DiJulio, 2006).*

Evaluate Potential Danger to Victim and Others

Assess Actual Physical Abuse

- Current and past physical/sexual abuse
- Are children hurt?
- When did it happen last?

- Is there danger to children?
- Are you hurt now?

Assess Support System

- Does she have a safe place to go?
- Does she want police called?
- Does she need an ambulance?

Assess Drug and Alcohol Use

- Is victim using drugs/alcohol?
- Is abuser using drugs/alcohol?

R: *Nursing interventions should focus on the level of danger, safety, and protection. Consequences of rash decisions can be fatal.*

Assess for Factors That Inhibit Victims From Seeking Aid

Individual Beliefs

- Fear for safety of self or children
- Fear of embarrassment
- Low self-esteem
- Guilt (punishment justified)
- Myths ("It is normal" or "It will stop")

R: *The nurse must openly dispel myths that offer explanations and tolerance for battering and wrongly give an illusion of control and rationality (*Carson & Smith-DiJulio, 2006).*

Lack of Financial Independence or Support System

R: *Financial abuse is present ninety-eight percent (98%) of the time in all domestic violence cases. The number one reason domestic violence survivors stay or return to the abusive relationship is because the abuser controls.*

Lack of Knowledge of

- The severity of the problem
- Community resources
- Legal rights

R: *When stressed, individuals solve problems poorly and do not seek outside assistance.*

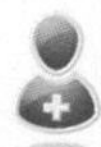

CLINICAL ALERT Myths also held by health-care professionals are abused individual could leave if they really wanted to, violence only occurs in heterosexual couples, alcohol or drug use is responsible, family violence is most prevalent in poor, uneducated couples.

Gently Discuss the Effects of Violence on Children

R: *Carlson-Catalano (*1998) found that of the battered women in her study, all reported they left to protect another loved one (child or pet). None of the women reported that she left because of her own safety or discomfort.*

- Elicit the individual's impression of effects on children.
- Greater lifelong risks for behavioral and emotional problems
- After age 5 to 6, children lose respect for the victim and identify with the aggressor.

R: *"Family violence is common in histories of juvenile criminals, runaways, violent criminals, prostitutes, and those who in turn are violent to others" (*Carson & Smith-DiJulio, 2006).*

Encourage Decision Making

- Provide an opportunity to validate abuse, and talk about feelings and the myths. Be direct and nonjudgmental:
  - How do you handle stress?
  - How does your partner handle stress?
  - How do you and your partner argue?
  - Are you afraid of your partner?
  - Have you ever been hit, pushed, or injured by your partner?

- Provide options but allow the individual to make a decision at her own pace.
- Encourage a realistic appraisal of the situation; dispel guilt and myths.
  - Violence is not normal for most families.
  - Violence may stop, but it usually becomes increasingly worse.
  - The victim is not responsible for the violence.

R: *Nurses must be cautious not to pressure the victim into a premature decision. Victims of abuse are "brainwashed by terror." They use denial and rationalization when they remain in the abusive relationship (*Blair, 1986; Halter, 2014).*

Establish a Safety and/or Escape Plan (Refer to Abuse Specialists/Hotlines)

- Enlist help of coworkers, family, neighbors, school clientele.
- If staying in home, increase safety measures (e.g., new locks, security systems)
- Alert neighbors to call police if they hear or see the problem individual.

R: *A safety plan is a specific plan for a fast escape if the victim identifies "now is the time to leave."*

Provide Legal and Referral Information

- Discreetly inform of community agencies available to victim and abuser (emergency and long-term).
  - Hotlines
  - Legal services
  - Shelters
  - Counseling agencies
- Discuss mandatory reporting.
- Discuss the availability of the social service department for assistance.
- Consult with legal resources in the community and familiarize the victim with state laws regarding
  - Abuse
  - Eviction of abuser
  - Counseling
  - Temporary support
  - Protection orders
  - Criminal law
  - Types of police interventions
- Document findings and dialogue, take pictures of injuries (*Carson & Smith-DiJulio, 2006).

R: *Some states and cities have laws that allow the police to press charges against the abuser when physical evidence of battering exists. This reduces the pressure on the victim filing charges.*

- Refer for individual, group, or couples counseling.
- Explore strategies to reduce stress and more constructively manage stressors (e.g., relaxation exercises, walking, and assertiveness training).

R: *Battering interventions must take place in the context of a coordinated community and criminal justice response to battering.*

Initiate Health Teaching, If Indicated

- Teach the community (e.g., parent–school organizations, women's clubs, and programs for schoolchildren) about the problem of spousal/elder abuse.
- Instruct caregivers about how properly to manage an elderly individual at home (e.g., transferring to chair, modified appliances, how to maintain orientation).
- Refer for financial assistance and transportation arrangements.
- Refer for assertiveness training.
- Refer the abuser to the appropriate community service (only refer men who have asked for assistance or admitted their abuse because revealing the wife's confidential disclosure may trigger more abuse). To secure additional information, contact National Clearinghouse on Domestic Violence through their website.

R: *Information and referrals are provided to encourage decision making when stressed individuals have difficulty accessing outside support (*Carson & Smith-DiJulio, 2006).*

Disabled Family Coping • Related to (Specify), as Evidenced by Child Abuse/Neglect

Definition

Child maltreatment includes intentional physical abuse, or neglect, emotional abuse or neglect, and sexual abuse of children by adults (Hockenberry & Wilson, 2015). "Child neglect is defined as the failure of the child's parents or caretaker to provide the child with the basic necessities of life, when financially able to do so or when offered reasonable means to do so" (*Cowen, 1999). Basic necessities are shelter, nutrition, health care, supervision, education, affection, and protection (*Cowen, 1999). It is the most common form of child maltreatment (Hockenberry & Wilson, 2015).

Goals

NOC

Family Coping, Family Normalization, Family Functioning, Abuse Protection, Abuse Cessation

The child will be free from injury or neglect, as evidenced by the following indicators:

- Receives comfort from another caretaker
- The parent will receive assistance for abusive behavior.
- Acknowledges abusive behaviors

Interventions

NIC

Caregiver Support, Emotional Support, Counseling, Decision-Making Support, Support Group, Anger Control Assistance, Abuse Protection Support: Child, Conflict Mediation, Referral

Identify Families at Risk for Child Abuse

- Poor differentiation of individual within the family
- Lack of autonomy
- Social isolation
- Desperate competition for affection and nurturance among members
- Feelings of helplessness and hopelessness
- Abuse/violence learned as a way to reduce tension
- Low tolerance for frustration; poor impulse control
- Closeness and caring confused with abuse and violence
- Mixed- and double-message communication patterns
- High level of conflict surrounding family tasks
- Nonexistent parental coalition

Intervene With Families at Risk

- Establish a relationship with parents that encourages them to share difficulties ("Being a parent is sure difficult [frustrating] work, isn't it?").
  - Relay your understanding of stresses, but do not condone abuse.
  - Focus on the parent's needs; avoid an authoritative approach.
  - Take opportunities to demonstrate constructive methods for working with children (give the child choices; listen carefully to the child).
- Stress the importance of support systems (e.g., encourage parents to exchange experiences with other parents).
- Encourage parents to allow time for their own needs (e.g., exercise three times a week).
- Discuss with parents how they respond to parental frustrations (share feelings with other parents), and instruct them not to discipline children when angry.
- Explore other methods of discipline aside from physical punishment.

R: *Successful interactions with abusive parents must be provided in the context of acceptance and approval to compensate for their low self-esteem and fear of rejection (Halter, 2014): Programs that teach parents to interpret and understand their children's behaviors and to give appropriate responses can reduce child maltreatment.*

Identify Suspected Cases of Child Abuse

- Assess for and evaluate
  - Evidence of maltreatment
  - History of incident or injury
    - Conflicting stories
    - Story improbable for child's age
    - Story not consistent with injury

- Parental behaviors
  - Seeks care for a minor complaint (e.g., cold) when other injuries are visible
  - Shows exaggerated or no emotional response to the injury
  - Is unavailable for questioning
  - Fails to show empathy for child
  - Expresses anger or criticism of child for being injured
  - Demands to take child home if pressured for answers
- Child behaviors
  - Does not expect to be comforted
  - Adjusts inappropriately to hospitalization
  - Defends parents
  - Blames self for inciting parents to rage

R: *Identification of child abuse depends on recognizing the physical signs, specific parent behavior, specific child behavior, inconsistencies in injury history, and contributing factors) (Hockenberry & Wilson, 2015)*

R: *The first priority of care for the abused child is preventing further injury (Hockenberry & Wilson, 2015).*

Report Suspected Cases of Child Abuse

R: *All states and providences in North America have laws for mandatory reporting of child maltreatment. The nurse reports suspected cases for further investigation (Hockenberry & Wilson, 2015).*

- Know the procedures for reporting child abuse (e.g., Bureau of Child Welfare, Department of Social Services, and Child Protective Services).
- Maintain an objective record:
  - Health history, including accidental or environmental injuries
  - Detailed description of physical examination (nutritional status, hygiene, growth and development, cognitive and functional status)
  - Environmental assessment of home (if in community)
  - Description of injuries, photos of injuries
  - Verbal conversations with parents and child in quotes
  - Description of behaviors, not interpretation (e.g., avoid "angry father," instead, "Father screamed at child, 'If you weren't so bad this wouldn't have happened.'")
  - Description of parent–child interactions (e.g., "shies away from mother's touch")

R: *The nurse should consult the legislation mandating the reporting of child abuse for the specifics of legal definition, penalties for failure to report, reporting procedure, and legal immunity for reporting.*

Promote a Therapeutic Environment

Provide the Child With Acceptance and Affection

- Show child attention without reinforcing inappropriate behavior.
- Use play therapy to allow child self-expression.
- Provide consistent caregivers and reasonable limits on behavior; avoid pity.
- Avoid asking too many questions and criticizing parent's actions.
- Explain in detail all routines and procedures in age-appropriate language.

R: *These strategies can reduce the child's stress and model appropriate behavior for the parent(s).*

Assist Child With Grieving If Placement in Foster Home Is Necessary

- Acknowledge that child will not want to leave parents despite severity of abuse.
- Allow opportunities for child to express feelings.
- Explain reasons for not allowing child to return home; dispel belief it is a punishment.
- Encourage foster parents to visit child in hospital.

R: *Children are attached to their parents despite the abuse (Hockenberry & Wilson, 2015).*

Provide Interventions That Promote Parent's Self-Esteem and Sense of Trust

- Tell them it was good that they brought the child to the hospital.
- Welcome parents to the unit and orient them to activities.
- Promote their confidence by presenting a warm, helpful attitude and acknowledging any competent parenting activities.
- Provide opportunities for parents to participate in child's care (e.g., feeding, bathing).

R: *Strong negative feelings can interfere with the nurse's judgment and effectiveness and alienate the family (*Carson & Smith-DiJulio, 2006).*

Promote Comfort and Reduce Fear for Child (*Carson & Smith-DiJulio, 2006)

- Do not display anger, horror, or shock.
- Do not blame abuser.
- Reassure child that he or she was not "bad" or at fault.
- Do not pressure child to give answers.
- Do not force child to undress.

R: *Children, being egocentric, assume they are responsible for the maltreatment.*

Initiate Health Teaching and Referrals, as Indicated

Provide Anticipatory Guidance for Families at Risk

- Assist individuals to recognize stress and to practice management techniques (e.g., plan for time alone away from child).
- Discuss the need for realistic expectations of the child's capabilities.
- Teach about child development and constructive methods for handling developmental problems (enuresis, toilet training, temper tantrums).
- Discuss methods of discipline other than physical (e.g., deprive the child of favorite pastime: "You may not ride your bike for a whole day"; "You may not play your stereo"; "No cell phone use for 1 day").
- Emphasize rewarding positive behavior.

R: *Unrealistic expectations for the age of the child and severe punishment techniques increase episodes of violence.*

Disseminate Information to the Community About Child Abuse (e.g., Parent–School Organizations, Radio, Television, Newspaper)

- Relay your understanding of stresses, but do not condone abuse.
- Focus on the parent's needs; avoid an authoritative approach.
- Take opportunities to demonstrate constructive methods for working with children (give the child choices; listen carefully to the child).

R: *Primary prevention (public awareness, community education, parenting classes, nutrition programs) is directed at the general population. Secondary prevention is directed at high-risk groups. Home-based and center-based programs have had positive outcomes (e.g., home visitation programs, substance abuse/mental health referrals, crisis intervention) (*Cowen, 1999).*

- Refer at-risk families to a home health nursing agency to assess the following:
  - Interaction of family members
  - Type of physical contact (e.g., comforting, detached, angry)
  - Parenteral attitudes/conflicts about parenting
  - Parenteral history of abuse
  - Environmental conditions (sleep areas, play areas, home management)
  - Financial status
  - Need for immediate services (economic, child care, counseling, protection services)

R: *The best environment in which to assess any family functioning is in their home.*

Disabled Family Coping • Related to Multiple Stressors Associated with Elder Care

Goals

NOC

Family Coping, Family Normalization, Family Functioning, Abuse Protection, Abuse Cessation

The caregiver will acknowledge the need for assistance with abusive or neglectful behavior, as evidenced by the following indicators:

- Discusses the stressors of elder care
- Relates strategies to reduce stressors
- Identifies community resources available

The older adult will be free of abusive behavior.

- Describes methods to increase socialization beyond caregiver
- Identifies resources available for assistance

Interventions

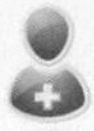

CLINICAL ALERT "Abuse comes in many forms, but the net effect is the same. Abuse creates potentially dangerous situations and feelings of worthlessness, and it isolates the older person from people who can help" (American Psychological Association, 2015a). "Studies show the causes of elder abuse to be wide-ranging—and not necessarily an outcome of caregiver stress. Seeing caregiver stress as a primary cause of abuse has unintended and detrimental consequences that affect the efforts to end this widespread problem" (Brandl & Raymond, 2012).

NIC

Caregiver Support, Emotional Support, Counseling, Support Group, Decision-Making Support, Anger Control Assistance, Abuse Protection Support: Elder, Conflict Mediation, Referral

Identify Individuals (Caregiver, Older Adult) at High Risk for Abuse or Neglect

R: *Risk factors for elder abuse/neglect are the invisibility of the problem, vulnerability of older adults, and psychosocial and caregiver risk factors (Miller, 2015).*

Caregiver

- Social isolation
- Dependency on elder (financial, emotional); coresidency
- Health problems (physical, mental)
- Substance abuse
- Poor relationship history with elder
- Financial problems
- Transgenerational violence
- Relationship problems

Ramsey-Klawsnik (*2000) postulated five types of offenders: (1) the overwhelmed, (2) the impaired, (3) the narcissistic, (4) the domineering, or bullying, and (5) the sadistic (Brandl & Raymond, 2012).

Older Adult

- Dependent on others for activities of daily living
- Isolation
- Financial insecurity
- Impaired cognitive functioning
- Depressive mentality
- History of abuse to caregiver
- Incontinence

R: *Perpetrator who initiates violence or neglect considers their own needs to be more important than others' needs. An elder who is dependent for activities of daily living is most vulnerable (*Carson & Smith-DiJulio, 2006).*

- Establish a relationship with caregivers that encourages them to share difficulties.
- Encourage caregivers to share experiences with others in the same situation.
- Evaluate caregiver's ability to provide long-term, in-home care.
- Explore sources of help (e.g., housekeeping, meals delivered to home, day care, respite care, transportation assistance).
- Encourage caregiver to discuss sharing responsibilities with other family members.
- Discuss alternative sources of care (e.g., nursing home, senior housing).
- Discuss how caregiver can allow time for individual's needs.
- Discuss community resources available for help (e.g., crisis hotline, social services, voluntary emergency caregivers). Refer to *Caregiver Role Strain.*

Assist Caregivers to Reduce Stressors

R: *"Individuals vary in their ability to remain resilient and effectively cope when demands exceed capabilities" (Brandl & Raymond, 2012).*

R: *Interventions focus on assisting caregivers to reduce stress and select constructive coping responses (Miller, 2015).*

Assist Older Adults to Reduce Risks of Abuse

- Encourage contact with old friends and neighbors if living with relative.
- Encourage to plan a weekly contact with a friend, neighbor.
- Encourage to participate in community activities as much as possible.
- Encourage to have his or her own telephone.
- Assist to acquire legal advice.

R: *Strategies to reduce isolation can protect the individual from undetected abuse. Legal advice may be needed to protect accents.*

- Ensure that the individual is not accepting care in exchange for transfer of assets or property without legal advice.
- Ensure that the person is not living with someone who has a history of violence or substance abuse.

R: *Strategies for high-risk elders include access and assessment, intervention, follow-up, and prevention.*

Identify Suspected Cases of Elder Abuse (Miller, 2015)

R: *Signs of elder abuse may be missed by professionals working with older Americans because of lack of training on detecting abuse. The elderly may be reluctant to report abuse themselves because of fear of retaliation, lack of physical and/or cognitive ability to report, or because they don't want to get the abuser (90% of whom are family members) in trouble (National Center for Elder Abuse, 2015).*

- Signs include
  - Failure to adhere to therapeutic regimens, which can pose threats to life (e.g., insulin administration, ulcerated conditions)
  - Evidence of malnutrition, dehydration, elimination problems
  - Bruises, swelling, lacerations, burns, bites
  - Pressure ulcers
  - Caregiver not allowing nurse to be alone with elder
- Consult with home health nurse to plan a home visit for assessment of signs of abuse or neglect (*Smith-DiJulio & Holzapfel, 1998):
  - House in poor repair
  - Inadequate heat, lighting, furniture, or cooking utensils
  - Unpleasant odors
  - Inaccessible food
  - Old food
  - Older adult lying on soiled materials (e.g., urine, food)
  - Medication not being taken
  - Garbage

R: *Abused elders usually do not report abuse because of fear of reprisal or abandonment.*

Report Suspected Cases

R: *The nurse does not have to prove abuse before reporting; a high suspicion should be investigated*

- Consult with manager for procedures for reporting suspected cases of abuse.
- Maintain an objective record, including
  - Description of injuries
  - Conversations with elder and caregiver(s)
  - Description of behaviors
  - Nutritional, hydration status
- Consider the elder's right to choose to live at risk of harm, providing he or she is capable of making that choice.
- Do not initiate an action that could increase the elder's risk of harm or antagonize the abuser.
- Respect the elder's right to secrecy and the right for self-determination.

R: *Each state has specific guidelines for reporting suspected cases of elder abuse.*

Initiate Health Teaching and Referrals, as Indicated

- Refer high-risk families to a home health nursing agency to assess the following (*Carson & Smith-DiJulio, 2006; Miller, 2015):

Environmental Conditions

- Inadequate heat, lighting
- Presence of garbage, old food in kitchen, unpleasant odors
- Blocked stairways, locks on refrigerator

Caretaker

- Attitude, conflict, anger, depression
- Interaction with elder

- Insufficient finances
- Alcohol/drug abuse

Elder's Condition

- Unclean body, unclean clothes and linens
- Medications not taken properly
- Lack of assistive devices
- Inadequate follow-up with primary provider
- Need for immediate services (economic, day care, respite, protection services, counseling)
- Refer elder for counseling to explore choices. Reassure him or her that they did nothing wrong to deserve maltreatment (Varcarolis, 2011).

R: *Educational programs serve to advocate for elders and to raise the consciousness of the community.*

READINESS FOR ENHANCED FAMILY COPING

NANDA-I Definition

A pattern of management of adaptive tasks by primary person (family member, significant other, or close friend) involved with the individual's health change, which can be strengthened.

Defining Characteristics*

Significant person attempts to describe growth impact of crisis.
Significant person moves in direction of enriching lifestyle.
Significant person moves in direction of health promotion.
Significant person chooses experiences that optimize wellness*.
Individual expresses interest in making contact with others who have experienced a similar situation.

Related Factors

Refer to *Compromised Family Coping.*

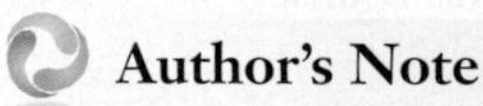

Author's Note

This nursing diagnosis describes components found in *Compromised Family Coping*. Until clinical research differentiates the category from the aforementioned categories, use *Compromised Family Coping*, depending on the data presented.

INTERRUPTED FAMILY PROCESSES

Definition

Change in family relationships and/or functioning (NANDA-I)
State in which a usually supportive family experiences, or is at risk to experience, a stressor that challenges its previously effective functioning[3]

Defining Characteristics

Major (Must Be Present)

Family system cannot or does not:

Adapt constructively to crisis
Communicate openly and effectively between family members

[3] This definition has been added by the author for clarity and usefulness.

Minor (May Be Present)

Family system cannot or does not:

Meet physical needs of all its members
Meet emotional needs of all its members
Meet spiritual needs of all its members
Express or accept a wide range of feelings
Seek or accept help appropriately

Related Factors

Any factor can contribute to *Interrupted Family Processes*. Common factors are listed below.

Treatment Related

Related to:

Disruption of family routines because of time-consuming treatments (e.g., home dialysis)
Physical changes because of treatments of ill family member
Emotional changes in all family members because of treatments of ill family member
Financial burden of treatments for ill family member
Hospitalization of ill family member

Situational (Personal, Environmental)

Related to loss of family member:

Death
Incarceration
Going away to school
Desertion
Separation
Hospitalization
Divorce

Related to addition of new family member:

Birth
Marriage
Adoption
Elderly relative

Related to losses associated with:

Poverty
Economic crisis
Change in family roles (e.g., retirement)
Birth of child with defect
Relocation
Disaster

Related to conflict (moral, goal, cultural)

Related to breach of trust between members

Related to social deviance by family member (e.g., crime)

Author's Note

This nursing diagnosis describes situations similar to the diagnosis *Compromised Family Coping*. Until clinical research differentiates this diagnosis from the aforementioned diagnosis, use *Compromised Family Coping*.

DYSFUNCTIONAL FAMILY PROCESSES • Related to Effects of Alcohol Abuse

NANDA-I Definition

Psychosocial, spiritual, and physiologic functions of the family unit are chronically disorganized, which lead to conflict, denial of problems, resistance to change, ineffective problem solving, and a series of self-perpetuating crises

Defining Characteristics[4]

Major (Must Be Present)

Behaviors

Inappropriate expression of anger*
Inadequate understanding or knowledge of alcoholism
Manipulation*
Denial of problems*
Dependency*
Loss of control of drinking
Refusal to get help*
Impaired communication*
Alcohol abuse
Rationalization*
Enabling behaviors
Blaming*
Ineffective problem solving*
Inability to meet emotional needs
Broken promises*
Criticizing*

Feelings*

Hopelessness
Anger
Guilt
Powerlessness
Loneliness
Responsible for alcoholic's behavior
Embarrassment
Emotional isolation
Worthlessness
Vulnerability
Suppressed rage
Repressed emotions
Anxiety
Shame
Mistrust

Roles and Relationships

Deteriorated family relationships
Inconsistent parenting
Disturbed family dynamics
Closed communication systems
Family denial
Marital problems
Ineffective spouse communication
Intimacy dysfunction
Disruption of family roles

Minor (May Be Present)

Behaviors

Inability to accept a wide range of feelings*
Inability to get or receive help appropriately*
Orientation toward tension relief rather than goal achievement*
Ineffective decision making
Failure to deal with conflict
Contradictory, paradoxical communication*
Family's special occasions are alcohol centered*
Harsh self-judgment*
Escalating conflict*
Isolation
Lying*
Failure to send clear messages
Difficulty having fun*
Immaturity*
Disturbances in concentration*
Chaos*
Inability to adapt to change*
Power struggles*
Substance abuse other than alcohol
Difficulty with life cycle transitions*
Verbal abuse of spouse or parent*
Stress-related physical illnesses*
Failure to accomplish current or past developmental tasks*
Lack of reliability*
Disturbances in academic performance in children*

Feelings

Being different from other people*
Lack of identity*
Moodiness*
Confused love and pity

[4] Lindeman, Hokanson, and Bartek (*1994).

Unresolved grief
Feelings misunderstood
Loss*
Depression*
Fear*
Hostility*
Abandonment*
Emotional control by others*
Dissatisfaction*
Confusion*
Failure*
Being unloved*
Self-blaming

Roles and Relationships

Triangulating family relationships*
Inability to meet spiritual needs of members
Reduced ability to relate to one another for mutual growth and maturation*
Lack of skills necessary for relationships*
Lack of cohesiveness*
Disrupted family rituals or no family rituals*
Inability to meet security needs of members
Does not demonstrate respect for individuality of its members
Decreased sexual communication and individuality of its members
Low perception of parental support*
Pattern of rejection
Neglected obligations*

Related Factors

Related to inadequate coping skills and/or inadequate problem-solving skills secondary to:

Alcohol abuse
Substance abuse*
Mental illness
Compromised cognitive function

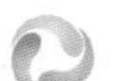

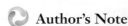

Author's Note

Disabled Family Coping can represent the consequences of the disturbed family dynamics related to chronic mental illness, progressive cognitive decline, substance abuse, and alcohol abuse by a family member. Alcoholism is a family disease. This nursing diagnosis can represent the effects of alcohol abuse on each family member. In addition, the individual with substance abuse will also have a specific nursing diagnosis of *Ineffective Coping* or *Ineffective Denial*.

Key Concepts

The Alcoholic Family

- Problem drinking that becomes severe is given the medical diagnosis of "alcohol use disorder" or AUD. Approximately 7.2% or 17 million adults in the United States aged 18 and older had an AUD in 2012. This includes 11.2 million men and 5.7 million women. Adolescents can be diagnosed with an AUD as well, and in 2012, an estimated 855,000 adolescents aged 12 to 17 had an AUD (National Institute of Alcohol Abuse and Addiction [NIAAA], 2013).
- Excessive alcohol consumption is the third leading preventable cause of death in the United States. More than 85,000 deaths a year in the United States are directly attributed to alcohol use, including resulting medical illness, traffic fatalities, drowning, and suicide (Tetrault & O'Connor, 2015).
- Approximately one in four children is exposed to family alcohol abuse or alcohol dependence.
- Alcoholism, or alcohol dependence, is a disease that causes
  - Craving—a strong need to drink
  - Loss of control—not being able to stop drinking once you've started
  - Physical dependence—withdrawal symptoms
  - Tolerance—the need to drink more alcohol to feel the same effect
- The American Academy of Pediatrics warns binge drinking is a common problem in adolescence and is associated with some of the leading causes of death and serious injury in this age group, including motor vehicle accidents, homicide, and suicide. The report says 21% of students have had more than a small

taste of alcohol by the time they are 13 years old… 79% by the time they hit 12th grade. Furthermore, 28% to 60% of high-school students report binge drinking… and 72% of 18- to 20-year-old drinkers, drink heavily (Siqueira, Smith, & Committee on Substance Abuse, 2015).

- Alcoholism and its denial dominate alcoholic families. When alcohol is the center of the family, developmental tasks are thwarted or ignored. "To keep the family unit intact, each member must change his or her cognitive perceptions to fit into the family's scheme of enabling the drinking to continue, while at the same time denying that it is a problem" (*Starling & Martin, 1990).
- Alcoholics initially use denial about alcohol to relieve stress. After dependence sets in, they use denial to conceal from the self and others how important alcohol is to functioning (Halter, 2014; *Smith -Di Julio & Holzapfel, 1998; Varcarolis, 2011).
- As destructive interactions continue, family members and the alcoholic move away from each other. The alcoholic turns to liquor, while the family finds other means of escape (*Collins, Leonard, & Searles, 1990).
- "Meaningful sobriety is characterized by more than just the abstinence of the alcoholic person. It necessitates an ongoing growth process for all family members to work together toward the goal of a well-functioning family" (*Grisham & Estes, 1982).
- Wegscheider-Cruse & Cruse (2012) described six roles typical in families affected by alcoholism:
  - Alcoholic
  - Chief enabler—often the spouse; super-responsible, takes on alcoholic's duties
  - Family hero—high achiever to provide family with some pride to cover up failures
  - Scapegoat—defiant, angry, diverts family focus from alcoholism
  - Lost child—helpless, powerless
  - Mascot—clowning, joking; a form of tension relief to mask underlying terror
- Wing (*1995) describes a four-stage theory of alcoholism, recovery, and goal setting:
  - *Stage I*: Denial—Alcoholics are coerced into treatment; their goals are to avoid punishment, with no sincere desire to stop drinking.
  - *Stage II*: Dependence—Alcoholics admit that they have a drinking problem and seek treatment to maintain job or a relationship.
  - *Stage III*: Behavior change—Alcoholics attempt to replace unhealthy behaviors with healthy behaviors.
  - *Stage IV*: Life planning—alcoholics integrate family, career, and educational goals with sobriety.
- Men entering treatment services perceive alcohol as the cause of their problems. Women reported that they drank because of their problems (*Kelly, Day, & Streissguth, 2000).
- From the literature, Kalmakis (2010) reported the following:
  - Alcohol was a factor in half of all sexual assaults.
  - Seventy-two percent of college women who were raped were under the influence of alcohol.
  - Alcohol consumption is associated with an increased risk of sexual assault.
- Ullman & Brecklin (*2003) describes a bidirectional model of sexual assault and alcohol use as follows:
  - Drinking may precede sexual assault.
  - Victims of sexual assault may drink excessively.
  - Sexual assault and drinking may influence each other over time.

Pediatric Considerations

- Children learn definitions of love, intimacy, and trust from their families of origin. The environment in the alcoholic family is chaotic and unpredictable. Roles are unclear. Sometimes, children become the parents and the alcoholic member becomes an outsider in the family.
- Children report being more disturbed by parents arguing rather than one parent's drinking. Children can respond in varied ways (e.g., peacemaker, aggression at school).
- Behavioral problems in children need to be assessed in the context of their purpose for the family.
- Children of alcoholics are accustomed to extra and inappropriate responsibilities (*Smith-DiJulio, 1998; Varcarolis, 2011).

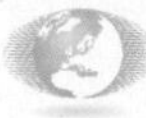

Transcultural Considerations

- Alcoholism is the number one health problem in the African-American community, reducing longevity with high incidences of acute and chronic alcohol-related diseases. Unemployment has been identified as the primary factor. Treatment programs must be accessible within the community or by public transportation. Black churches serve a dual role as a site for therapy meetings and as a referral service (Giger, 2013).

- For Mexican Americans, alcohol consumption is a way to celebrate life. Alcohol contributes to increased incidents and violence. Family pride protects the alcoholic man as long as he provides for the family (Giger, 2013).
- Alcoholism is found among Native Americans in high percentages. Alcohol abuse is responsible for violence, suicides, and fetal alcohol syndrome in this ethnic population.

Focus Assessment Criteria

Assess for Alcohol Abuse

Denial of Problem

Responses of Family Members
Alcohol use influences decisions
Afraid
Embarrassed
Worried
Effects on each member
Overall feelings
Behavior problems (children)
Guilt feelings

Characteristics of Alcoholic Person
Has friends who drink heavily
Justifies alcohol use
Promises to quit or reduce
Is verbally/physically abusive
Drives under the influence
Fails to remember events
Avoids conversations about alcohol
Has periods of remorse

Family/Social Functions
Unsatisfactory, tense
Always include alcohol
Financial, legal problems
Negative comments of others about drinking behavior

Goals

NOC

Family Coping, Family Functioning, Substance Addiction Consequences

The family will acknowledge alcoholism in the family and will set short- and long-term goals, as evidenced by the following indicators:

- Relates the effects of alcoholism on the family unit and individuals
- Identifies destructive response patterns
- Describes resources available for individual and family therapy

Interventions

NIC

Coping Enhancements, Referral, Family Process Maintenance, Substance Use Treatment, Family Integrity Promotion, Limit Setting, Support Group

Establish a Trusting Relationship

- Be consistent; keep promises.
- Be accepting and noncritical.
- Do not pass judgment on what is revealed.
- Focus on family members' responses.

Allow Family Members as Individuals and a Group to Share Pent-Up Feelings

- Validate feelings as normal.
- Correct inaccurate beliefs.

R: *Alcoholism disturbs family communication. Sharing feelings is uncommon because of a history of disappointment. Alcoholism involves shame and stigma, which promotes secrets and silence. Diminished sharing and silence* *can maintain disturbed families for long periods. Communication focuses mainly on family members trying to control the other member's drinking behavior (*Grisham & Estes, 1982).*

Emphasize That Family Members Are Not Responsible for the Person's Drinking (*Carson & Smith-DiJulio, 2006; Starling & Martin, 1990)

- Explain that emotional difficulties are relationship based rather than "psychiatric."
- Instruct that their feelings and experiences are associated frequently with family alcoholism.

R: *"The potential value of reaching the alcoholic individual by first assisting family members should not be underestimated" (*Grisham & Estes, 1982). The family and health-care professional must accept that no certain outcome can be promised for the alcoholic, even when the family gets help.*

Discuss Addiction With the Children of Addicted Parents (*National Association for Children of Alcoholics [NACoA], 2001)

- Alcoholism/drug dependency is a sickness.
- You can't make it better.
- You deserve help for yourself.
- You are not alone.
- There are safe people and places that can help.
- There is hope.

R: *Children of addicted parents are the highest risk group of children to become alcohol and drug abusers due to both genetic and family environment factors.*

Engage the Child/Adolescent in Discussing Their Feeling

- Explain that talking about worries at home is not being mean to your family.
- Sharing your feelings can help you feel less alone.
- Advise not to ride in a car when the driver has been drinking if you can avoid it.
- When you live with addicted parents, feeling love and hate at the same time is common.

Teaching the Seven Cs (*NACoA, 2001)

- I didn't CAUSE it.
- I can't CURE it.
- I can't CONTROL it.
- I can help take CARE of myself by
  - COMMUNICATING my feelings
  - Making healthy CHOICES
  - CELEBRATING me

R: *Children need to know that it is not their fault when their parents drink too much or abuse drugs, and that they cannot control their parents' behavior (NIH, 2012).*

Explain Those at High Risk for Alcohol Abuse (Aronson, 2015)

- Having another mental health problem, such as severe anxiety, depression, or a personality disorder
- Is most common among those aged 18 to 25

R: *"Alcohol use disorder runs in families, and certain genes make people more vulnerable to drinking problems". "In fact, people who have a sibling, parent, or child who abuses alcohol have three to four times the average risk of developing a drinking problem" (Aronson, 2015).*

Explore the Family's Beliefs About Situation and Goals

- Discuss characteristics of alcoholism; review a screening test (e.g., MAST, CAGE) that outlines characteristics of alcoholism.
- Discuss causes and correct misinformation.
- Assist to establish short- and long-term goals.

R: *Wing (*1995) proposes that relapses occur for different reasons in each stage. In stage I, relapse accompanies removal of the threat of punishment. Relapse in stage II occurs when the object of dependence (e.g., marriage, job) is secured or lost. Relapses in stages III and IV are less frequent and triggered by unexpected, stressful events. Nursing interactions for people in stages I and II focus on confronting denial and helping them become more* *internally focused. People in stages III and IV need assistance to learn how to cope with unexpected, stressful events (*Wing, 1995).*

Assist the Family to Gain Insight Into Behavior; Discuss Ineffective Methods Families Use

- Hiding alcohol or car keys
- Anger, silence, threats, crying
- Making excuses for work, family, or friends
- Bailing the individual out of jail
- Does not stop drinking
- Increases family anger
- Removes the responsibility for drinking from the individual
- Prevents the individual from suffering the consequences of his or her drinking behavior

R: *Interventions focus on assisting the family to change their ineffective communication and response patterns (*Carson & Smith-DiJulio, 2006).*

Emphasize to Family That Helping the Alcoholic Means First Helping Themselves

- Focus on changing their response.
- Allow the individual to be responsible for his or her drinking behavior.
- Describe activities that will improve their lives, as individuals and a family.
- Initiate one stress management technique (e.g., aerobic exercise, assertiveness course, meditation).
- Plan time as a family together outside the home (e.g., museum, zoos, and picnic). If the alcoholic is included, he or she must contract not to drink during the activity and agree on a consequence if he or she does.

R: *Family members use denial to avoid admitting the problem and dealing with their contribution to it, in the hope that the problem will disappear if not disclosed (*Collins et al., 1990).*

Discuss With Family That Recovery Will Dramatically Change Usual Family Dynamics

- The alcoholic is removed from the center of attention.
- All family roles will be challenged.
- Family members will have to focus on themselves instead of the alcoholic individual.
- Family members will have to assume responsibility for their behavior, rather than blaming others.
- Behavioral problems of children serve a purpose for the family.

R: *Ending the drinking behavior threatens the family integrity because the family functioning is centered around alcoholism (*Carson & Smith-DiJulio, 2006).*

Discuss Possibility of and Contributing Factors to Relapse

R: *Wing (*1995) proposes that relapses occur for different reasons in each stage. In stage I, relapse accompanies removal of the threat of punishment. Relapse in stage II occurs when the object of dependence (e.g., marriage, job) is secured or lost. Relapses in stages III and IV are less frequent and triggered by unexpected, stressful events. Nursing interactions for people in stages I and II focus on confronting denial and helping them become more internally focused. People in stages III and IV need assistance to learn how to cope with unexpected, stressful events.*

If Additional Family or Individual Nursing Diagnoses Exist, Refer to Specific Diagnosis (e.g., Child Abuse, Domestic Violence)

Initiate Health Teaching Regarding Community Resources and Referrals, as Indicated

- Al-Anon
- Alcoholics Anonymous family therapy
- Individual therapy
- Self-help groups
- Association for Children of Alcoholics (NACoA)

R: *The family is the unit of treatment when one member is an alcoholic. Referrals are needed for long-term therapy.*

Hospitalization of ill family member

READINESS FOR ENHANCED FAMILY PROCESSES

NANDA-I Definition

A pattern of family functioning that is sufficient to support the well-being of family members, which can be strengthened.

Defining Characteristics*

Expresses willingness to enhance family dynamics
Family functioning meets needs of family members.
Activities support the safety and growth of family members
Communication is adequate.
Relationships are generally positive; interdependent with community; family tasks are accomplished.
Family roles are flexible and appropriate for developmental stages.
Respect for family members is evident.
Family adapts to change.
Boundaries of family members are maintained.
Energy level of family supports activities of daily living.
Family resilience is evident.
Balance exists between autonomy and cohesiveness.

Goal

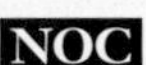

Family Environment: Internal

The family will express willingness to enhance family dynamics and growth.

Interventions

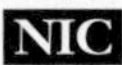

Family Involvement Promotion, Family Integrity Promotion

Discuss Elements That Influence Health Promotion in a Family (Edelman, Kudzma, & Mandle, 2014; Kaakinen et al., 2015)

- Family culture
- Lifestyles patterns/role models
- Family nutrition
- Religion/spirituality
- Family processes

R: *These elements interact with each other and need to be addressed for successful family health promotion interventions. Suggestions for health promotion that conflict with the family's culture, religion, or spirituality will be rejected (Kaakinen et al., 2015).*

- Encourage the family to examine their patterns of communication (verbal, nonverbal) and family interactions (Kaakinen et al., 2015).
  - Are they effective?
  - Are all members involved in feeling sharing and decision making?
  - Is there positive, reinforcing interactions?
  - Are parent's role-modeling positive family processes?

R: *Effective, positive interactions enhance family lifestyle and adaption to transitions/stressors. They promote cohesiveness and healthier family lifestyles (Kaakinen et al., 2015).*

- Convey that the family has the capacity to achieve a higher level of health and has the right to health information to make informed decisions.

R: *A caring, culturally competent nurse can convey that the family has potential for health promotion (Giger, 2013).*

- Elicit from family areas for growth and change. Assure the commitment of all family members (e.g., improved nutrition, exercising, family meals, group relaxation activities, family time). (Edelman et al., 2014).

R: *This collaboration promotes family empowerment to make healthier choices.*

- Determine one area for improvement and write a family self-care contract (*Bomar, 2005; Kaarkinen et al., 2015).
- Set a goal and time frame for initiating and frequency.
- Develop a plan.
- Assign responsibilities.
- Evaluate outcomes.
- Modify, renegotiate, or terminate.

R: *A written self-care contract represents negotiation and commitment of all members (Kaarkinen et al., 2010).*

- Direct family to seek resources independently (e.g., community resources, Web sites).

R: *Families desire information about developmental issues and health promotion, and seeking information is empowering (Edelman et al., 2014; Kaarkinen et al., 2015).*

- Refer to *Interrupted Family Processes* for additional intervention for strengthening family functioning, promoting family integrity, mutual support, and positive functioning.

IMPAIRED HOME MAINTENANCE

NANDA-I Definition

Inability to independently maintain a safe growth-promoting immediate environment.

Defining Characteristics

Major (Must Be Present, One or More)

Expressions or observations of:

Difficulty maintaining home hygiene
Difficulty maintaining a safe home
Inability to keep up home
Lack of sufficient finances

Minor (May Be Present)

Repeated infections
Infestations
Accumulated wastes
Unwashed utensils
Offensive odors
Overcrowding

Related Factors

Pathophysiologic

Related to impaired functional ability* secondary to chronic debilitating disease*

Diabetes mellitus
Arthritis
Chronic obstructive pulmonary disease (COPD)
Multiple sclerosis
Congestive heart failure
Cerebrovascular accident
Parkinson's disease
Muscular dystrophy
Cancer

Situational (Personal, Environmental)

Related to change in functional ability of (specify family member) secondary to:

Injury* (fractured limb, spinal cord injury)
Surgery (amputation, ostomy)
Impaired mental status (memory lapses, depression, anxiety–severe panic)
Substance abuse (alcohol, drugs)

Related to inadequate support system*

Related to loss of family member

Related to deficient knowledge

Related to insufficient finances*

Related to unfamiliarity with neighborhood resources*

Maturational

Infant
Related to multiple care requirements secondary to:

High-risk newborn

Older Adult
Related to multiple care requirements secondary to:

Family member with deficits (cognitive, motor, sensory)

Author's Note

With rising life expectancy and declining mortality rates, the number of older adults is steadily increasing, with many living alone at home. Eighty-five percent of people 65 years or older report one or more chronic diseases. Of adults 65 to 74 years of age, 20% report activity limitations, and 15% cannot perform at least one activity of daily living (ADL) independently (Miller, 2015). The shift from health care primarily in hospitals to reduced lengths of stay has resulted in the discharge of many functionally compromised people to their homes. Often a false assumption is that someone will assume the management of household responsibilities until the individual has recovered.

Impaired Home Maintenance describes situations in which an individual or family needs teaching, supervision, or assistance to manage the household. Usually, a community health nurse is the best professional to complete an assessment of the home and the individual's functioning there. Nurses in acute settings can make referrals for home visits for assessment.

A nurse who diagnoses a need for teaching to prevent household problems may use *Risk for Impaired Home Maintenance* related to insufficient knowledge of (specify).

Errors in Diagnostic Statements

Impaired Home Maintenance related to caregiver burnout

Caregiver burnout is not a sign of or related factor for *Impaired Home Maintenance*. It is associated with *Caregiver Role Strain*. *Impaired Home Maintenance* may be present if multiple responsibilities overwhelm the caregiver. In this situation, both diagnoses are needed because the interventions for them differ.

Key Concepts

- Refer to Chapter 7: Transitional Individual/Family Centered-Care for principles and clinical strategies.

Pediatric Considerations

- Children depend on family members to manage home care.
- Trends in the treatment of children with chronic illness or disability include home care, early discharge, focus on developmental age, and assessment of strengths and uniqueness. Interventions are geared toward the entire family rather than just the ill child (Hockenberry & Wilson, 2015).

- High-risk graduates of neonatal intensive care units require technically complex home care. Transition is planned as early as possible to contain cost and to help reduce adverse effects of hospitalization on the family system.

Geriatric Considerations

- Older people have greater incidence of chronic disease, impaired function, and diminished economic resources and a smaller social network than do younger people (Miller, 2015).
- Functional ability includes ADLs and instrumental ADLs (IADLs) for those skills needed to live independently (e.g., procuring food, cooking, using the telephone, housekeeping, handling finances). IADLs are connected integrally to physical and cognitive abilities. The older adult who lives alone is at great risk of being institutionalized if he or she cannot perform IADLs. The possibility is great that no social network can meet these deficits (Miller, 2015).
- Along with diminished cognitive or physical ability, the older individual frequently has diminished financial resources, sporadic kin, or few neighborhood social supports. He or she also may live in substandard housing or housing that does not allow simple adaptation to meet individual physical or cognitive deficits (Miller, 2015).
- In some cultures and family structures, older adults can seek assistance in some areas of home management and still retain a sense of independence. These people have determined that by choosing selective resources to meet their needs, they will be able to maintain independent living for a longer time (Miller, 2015).

Goals

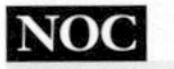
NOC
Family Functioning

The individual or caretaker will express satisfaction with home situation, as evidenced by the following indicators:

- Identifies factors that restrict self-care and home management
- Demonstrates ability to perform skills necessary for care of the home

Interventions

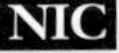
NIC
Home Maintenance Assistance, Environmental Management: Safety, Environmental Management

The following interventions apply to many with impaired home maintenance, regardless of etiology.

Assess for Causative or Contributing Factors

- Lack of knowledge
- Insufficient funds
- Lack of necessary equipment or aids
- Inability (illness, sensory deficits, motor deficits) to perform household activities
- Impaired cognitive functioning
- Impaired emotional functioning

Reduce or Eliminate Causative or Contributing Factors, If Possible

Lack of Knowledge

- Determine the information they need to learn:
  - Monitoring skills (pulse, circulation, urine)
  - Medication administration (procedure, side effects, precautions)
  - Treatment/procedures
  - Equipment use/maintenance
  - Safety issues (e.g., environmental)
  - Community resources
  - Follow-up care
  - Anticipatory guidance (e.g., emotional and social needs, alternatives to home care)
  - Initiate teaching; give detailed written instruction.

Insufficient Funds

- Consult with social service department for assistance.
- Consult with service organizations (e.g., American Heart Association, The Lung Association, American Cancer Society) for assistance.

Lack of Necessary Equipment or Aids

- Determine type of equipment needed, considering availability, cost, and durability.
- Seek assistance from agencies that rent or sanction loans.
- Teach care and maintenance of supplies to increase length of use.
- Consider adapting equipment to reduce cost.

Inability to Perform Household Activities

- Determine the type of assistance needed (e.g., meals, housework, transportation); assist individual to obtain it.

Meals

- Discuss with relatives the possibility of freezing complete meals that require only heating (e.g., small containers of soup, stews, casseroles).
- Determine the availability of meal services for ill people (e.g., Meals on Wheels, church groups).
- Teach people about nutritious foods that are easily prepared (e.g., hard-boiled eggs, tuna fish, peanut butter).

Housework

- Encourage individual to contract with an adolescent for light housekeeping.
- Refer individual to community agency for assistance.

Transportation

- Determine the availability of transportation for shopping and health care.
- Suggest individual request rides with neighbors to places they drive routinely.

Impaired Cognitive Functioning

- Assess individual's ability to maintain a safe household.
- Refer to *Risk for Injury* related to lack of awareness of hazards.
- Initiate appropriate referrals.

Impaired Emotional Functioning

- Assess severity of the dysfunction.
- Refer to *Ineffective Coping* for additional assessment and interventions.

R: *When determining an individual's ability to perform self-care at home, the nurse must assess his or her ability to function and protect self. The nurse considers motor and sensory deficits and mental status (Miller, 2015).*

Initiate Health Teaching and Referrals, as Indicated

- Refer to community nursing agency for a home visit.

R: *A home visit is essential to assess and evaluate what services are needed (Edelman, Kudzma, & Mandle, 2014). The home environment must be assessed for safety before discharge: location of bathroom, access to water, cooking facilities, and environmental barriers (stairs, narrow doorways).*

- Provide information about how to make the home environment safe and clean (Edelman et al., 2014). Refer to community agencies (e.g., visitors, meal programs, homemakers, adult day care).
- Refer to support groups (e.g., local Alzheimer's Association, American Cancer Society).

R: *Transition planning begins at admission, with the nurse determining anticipated needs after discharge: self-care ability, availability of support, homemaker services, equipment, community nursing services, therapy (physical, speech, occupational) (Barnsteiner, Disch, & Walton, 2014; National Transitions of Care Coalition, 2009).*

IMPAIRED PARENTING

Impaired Parenting

Risk for Impaired Parent–Infant Attachment.

NANDA-I Definition

Inability of the primary caregiver to create, maintain, or regain an environment that promotes the optimum growth and development of the child.

Defining Characteristics

The home environment must be assessed for safety before discharge: location of bathroom, access to water, cooking facilities, and environmental barriers (e.g., stairs, narrow doorways).
Inappropriate and/or nonnurturing parenting behaviors
Lack of behavior, indicating parental attachment
Inconsistent behavior management
Inconsistent care
Frequent verbalization of dissatisfaction or disappointment with infant/child
Verbalization of frustration with role
Verbalization of perceived or actual inadequacy
Diminished or inappropriate visual, tactile, or auditory stimulation of infant
Evidence of abuse or neglect of child
Growth and development challenges in infant/child

Related Factors

Individuals or families who may be at risk for developing or experiencing parenting difficulties

Parent(s)

Financial resources
Single
Addicted to drugs
Adolescent
Terminally ill
Abusive
Acutely disabled
Psychiatric disorder
Accident victim
Alcoholic

Child

Of unwanted pregnancy
With undesired characteristics
Terminally ill
With hyperactive characteristics
Mentally handicapped
Of undesired gender
Physically handicapped

Situational (Personal/Environmental)

Related to interruption of bonding process secondary to

Illness (child/parent)
Relocation/change in cultural environment
Incarceration

Related to separation from nuclear family

Related to lack of knowledge

Related to inconsistent caregivers or techniques

Related to relationship problems (specify):

Marital discord
Stepparents
Divorce
Live-in partner
Separation
Relocation

Related to little external support and/or socially isolated family

Related to lack of available role model

Related to ineffective adaptation to stressors associated with

Illness
Economic problems
New baby
Substance abuse
Elder care

Maturational

Adolescent Parent

Related to the conflict of meeting own needs over child's

Related to history of ineffective relationships with own parents

Related to parental history of abusive relationship with parents

Related to unrealistic expectations of child by parent

Related to unrealistic expectations of self by parent

Related to unrealistic expectations of parent by child

Related to unmet psychosocial needs of child by parent

Author's Note

The family environment should provide the basic needs for a child's physical growth and development: stimulation of the child's emotional, social, and cognitive potential; consistent, stable reinforcement to learn impulse control. It is the role of parents to provide such an environment. Most parenting difficulties stem from lack of knowledge or inability to manage stressors constructively. The ability to parent effectively is at high risk when the child or parent has a condition that increases stress on the family unit (e.g., illness, financial problems) (Gage, Everett, & Bullock, 2006).

Impaired Parenting describes a parent experiencing difficulty creating or continuing a nurturing environment for a child. *Parental Role Conflict* describes a parent or parents whose previously effective functioning is challenged by external factors. In certain situations, such as illness, divorce, or remarriage, role confusion and conflict are expected; thus *Risk for Impaired Parenting* would be useful. At present, *Risk for Impaired Parenting* is not an approved NANDA-I nursing diagnosis.

Errors in Diagnostic Statements

Impaired Parenting related to child abuse

Child abuse is a sign of family dysfunction. Usually, each situation involves an abusing adult and a knowing nonabusing adult; the treatment plan must include both. Thus, the diagnosis *Disabled Family Coping* would be more descriptive. *Impaired Parenting* is most appropriate when an external factor challenges the parents. External factors do not cause child abuse; rather, emotional disturbances and ineffective coping do.

Key Concepts

Refer to Key Concepts at the beginning of Part 2 Family/Home Nursing Diagnoses.

Focus Assessment Criteria

Refer to the Focus Assessment Criteria at the beginning of Part 2 Family/Home Nursing Diagnoses.

Goals

NOC

Parenting Performance; Parenting Performance: Specify age, e.g., adolescent, toddler; Child Development; Abuse Cessation; Abuse Recovery

The parent/primary caregiver demonstrates two effective skills to increase parenting effectiveness, as evidenced by the following indicators:

- Will acknowledge an issue with parenting skills
- Identifies resources available for assistance with improvement of parenting skills that are culturally considerate

Interventions

NIC

Anticipatory Guidance; Counseling; Developmental Enhancement; Family Support; Family Therapy; Parenting Promotion; Family Integrity: Promotion

Encourage Parents to Express Frustrations Regarding Role Responsibilities, Parenting, or Both

- Convey empathy.
- Reserve judgment.
- Covey/offer educational information based on assessment.
- Help foster realistic expectations.
- Encourage discussion of feelings regarding unmet expectations.
- Discuss individualized, achievable, and culturally considerate strategies (e.g., discussing with partner, child; setting personal goals).

R: *Several aspects of the parent go into their ability to parent an infant/child. These aspects can include their parental personality, mental well-being, and support systems. These factors can influence the parent's success in their parenting role. By understanding and assessing each aspect, the need for further intervention may become apparent (Hockenberry & Wilson, 2015).*

R: *The Calgary Family Assessment Model may be used to help attain and assess family data (Ball, Bindler, & Cowen, 2015).*

Educate Parents about Normal Growth and Development and Age-Related Expected Behaviors (Refer to *Delayed Growth and Development*)

R: *The Duvall Developmental Theory can be useful in describing the family as something that grows throughout its life span. It is suggested that as the infant grows into a child, and then into an adolescent, the family as a whole grows into new stages of development. Thinking in this way can help parents/caregivers grow along with their children as milestones are met (Hockenberry & Wilson, 2015).*

Explore with Parents the Child's Problem Behavior

- Frequency, duration, context (when, where, triggers)
- Consequences (parental attention, discipline, inconsistencies in response)
- Behavior desired by parents

R: *The parents'/caregiver's parenting style should be assessed and then interventions can be considered for discipline and limit-setting techniques. Parenting styles include authoritarian, permissive, authoritative, and indifferent (Ball et al., 2015).*

Discuss Guidelines for Promoting Acceptable Behavior in Children (Hockenberry & Wilson, 2015)

- Convey to the child that he or she is loved.
- Positive reinforcement is an effective and recommended discipline technique for all ages.
- Redirecting is effective for infants and school-age children, whereas verbal instruction/explanation is most effective for school-age children and adolescents.
- Set realistic expectations for behavior based on child's level of understanding and developmental stage.
- When reprimanding child, focus on the bad behavior or action, not insinuating that the child is bad.
- Watch for potential scenarios where child might be likely to misbehave, such as the child being overtired or overexcited. Change conditions when able to or have strategies in place to minimize bad behavior.
- Help child develop self-control techniques.
- Demonstrate and discuss acceptable and expected social behaviors.
- Minimize bad behavior by ignoring minor transgressions which will eventually stop the act or behavior (Ball et al., 2015).
- Make promises only when they can be kept (Ball et al., 2015).

R: *Keep in mind the parent/caregiver's parenting style when considering ways to encourage good behavior in children (Hockenberry & Wilson, 2015).*

Explain the Discipline Technique of "Time-Out" (Ball et al., 2015)

- "Time-out," refers to a discipline technique that places child in a designated, isolated area. This area does not include toys or games and serves a consequence of undesirable behavior. Typically the length of time recommended is 1 minute/year of age.
- Time-out provides a cooling-off period for both child and parent.
- Explain to the child what to expect from the time-out as well as why they have found themselves in it.
- Start the timer only when child is quiet, and reset the timer for acting out that occurs while in time-out.

- Make sure to minimize any distractions while child is in time-out (e.g., turn off television or make sure television cannot be seen or heard).

R: *Discipline techniques should be implemented at the time of the infraction to increase their effectiveness (Hockenberry & Wilson, 2015).*

R: *Consistency is important in developing patterns of good behavior (Hockenberry & Wilson, 2015).*

Acknowledge Cultural Impacts on Parent/Caregiver's Disciplinary Methods (Ball et al., 2015)

- Expected behaviors emerge from the family's preexisting cultural values and beliefs.
- The child learns cultural values and expected roles and behaviors as they grow.
- Immigrant families may face challenges as they work toward raising their child in their inherent culture but also adapting to the culture of which they have immigrated to.
- Different cultures place varying levels of importance on different aspects of childrearing (e.g., grandparents as active caregivers, families with large numbers of children, responsibilities expected of the child).

Acknowledge and Encourage Parent/Caregiver's Strengths in Their Parenting Role (Ball et al., 2015)

- Focus on family competence.
- Validate family member's emotions.
- Help family member recognize that they can bring prior positive life experiences to their current situation in coping with a child's health-care concern.

Provide General Parenting Guidelines (Hockenberry & Wilson, 2015)

- Be consistent with disciplinary techniques in terms of type of punishment for type of infraction.
- Be adaptable and flexible when it comes to child's behavior and setting.
- As child gets older, provide privacy to administer punishment to avoid public shaming.
- Avoid repeated lecturing or bring up of infraction once punishment for a specific incident is completed and addressed.
- Show unity among parents/caregivers when it comes to discipline and expected behavior.
- Follow through with punishments and the initial details set forth. Avoid becoming distracted.
- Praise children for acceptable or desired behavior.
- Serve as a role model in acting in a way that you wish your child to act.
- Address misbehavior upon its discovery.
- Set and explain clear and expected rules for behavior with consideration to child's age and level of understanding.

Initiate Appropriate Referrals as Indicated

Risk for Impaired Parent–Infant Attachment

NANDA-I Definition

Disruption of the interactive process between parent/significant other and child/infant that fosters the development of a protective and nurturing reciprocal relationship.

Risk Factors

Pathophysiologic

Related to interruption of attachment process secondary to

Parental illness
Infant illness

Treatment Related

Related to barriers to attachment secondary to

Lack of privacy
Intensive care monitoring
Ill child
Structured visitation
Equipment-restricted visitation
Physical barriers
Separation
Premature infant

Situational (Personal/Environmental)

Related to unrealistic expectations (e.g., of child or self)

Related to unplanned/unwanted pregnancy

Related to disappointment with infant (e.g., gender, appearance)

Related to ineffective coping associated with new baby and other responsibilities to

Health issues
Substance abuse
Mental illness
Relationship difficulties
Economic difficulties

Related to lack of knowledge and/or available role model for parental role

Related to physical disabilities of parent (e.g., blindness, paralysis, deafness)

Related to being emotionally unprepared due to premature delivery to infant

Maturational

Adolescent Parent
Related to difficulty delaying own gratification for the gratification of the infant

Author's Note

This diagnosis describes a parent or caregiver at risk for attachment difficulties with his or her infant. Barriers to attachment can be the environment, knowledge, anxiety, and health of parent or infant. This diagnosis is appropriate as a risk or high-risk diagnosis. If the nurse diagnoses a problem in infant–parent attachment, the diagnosis *Risk for Impaired Parenting* related to difficulties in parent–child attachment would be more useful so that the nurse could focus on improving attachment and preventing destructive parenting patterns.

Errors in Diagnostic Statements

***Risk for Impaired Parent–Infant Attachment* related to husband not being the biologic father**

The related factor is certainly a risk factor associated with attachment problems; however, this information is confidential and requires caution to protect its disclosure. If a family shares this information during an assessment or interaction, the nurse should record it exactly in quotes in the progress notes. The nurse can write the nursing diagnosis as *Risk for Impaired Parent–Infant Attachment* related to possible rejection of infant by father.

Key Concepts

- Refer to Key Concepts at the beginning of Part 2 Family/Home Nursing Diagnoses.

Focus Assessment Criteria

Refer to the Focus Assessment Criteria at the beginning of Part 2 Family/Home Nursing Diagnoses.

Goals

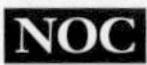

NOC
Refer to Impaired Parenting

The parent will demonstrate increased attachment behaviors, such as holding infant close, smiling and talking to infant, and seeking eye contact with infant, as evidenced by the following indicators:

- Be supported in his or her need to be involved in infant's care
- Begins to verbalize positive feelings regarding infant
- Engages in infant/child care

Interventions

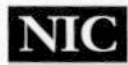

NIC
Refer to Impaired Parenting

Assess Causative or Contributing Factors

Maternal
- Unwanted pregnancy
- Prolonged or difficult labor and delivery
- Postpartum pain or fatigue
- Lack of positive support system (mother, spouse, friends)
- Lack of positive role model (mother, relative, friends/neighbors)
- Inability to prepare emotionally (e.g., an unexpected delivery)

Inadequate Coping Patterns (One or Both Parents)
- Financial/economic stress
- Alcoholism
- Drug addiction
- Marital difficulties (separation, divorce, violence/abuse)
- Change in lifestyle related to new role
- Adolescent parent
- Career change (e.g., working woman or mother)
- Illness in family

Infant
- Premature birth, congenital anomalies, illness
- Multiple births

Eliminate or Reduce Contributing Factors, If Possible

Illness/Fatigue
- Establish with parent/caregiver what infant care activities are feasible.
- Provide parent/caregiver with uninterrupted sleep periods of at least 2 hours during the day and 4 hours at night. Provide relief for discomfort.

Lack of Experience or Positive Parenting Role Model
- Explore parenting feelings and attitudes concerning their own parents.
- Assist parents/caregivers to identify someone who is a positive parent; encourage parent/caregiver to seek that person's aid/advise.
- Outline the teaching program available during hospitalization.
- Determine who will assist parent at home initially.
- Identify community programs and reference material that can increase parental learning about child care after discharge (e.g., support groups, mother/baby group activities).

R: *A person will fulfill many roles in their lifetime (e.g., son/daughter, grandchild, brother/sister, wife/husband, parent). The person has to learn the expectations and responsibilities of each role as they grow by observing others of those same roles around them. By identifying those role models and how effective/positive they are, the new parent/caregiver can transition into their newest role (Durham & Chapman, 2014).*

Lack of Positive Support System (Ball et al., 2015)
- Identify parent's support system; assess its strengths and weaknesses.
- Assess the need for counseling.
- Encourage parents to express feelings about the experience and about the future.
- Be an active listener to the parents.
- Observe the parents interacting with the infant.
- Assess for resources (financial, emotional, and cultural) already available to the family.

- Be aware of resources available both within the hospital and in the community.
- Refer to hospital or community services/specialists.

Barriers to Practicing Cultural Beliefs That May Affect the Family Unit during Hospitalization

- Support mother–infant–family beliefs.
- Integrate culture and traditions into routine care when possible.
- Identify community resources.

R: *Nurses should be aware of the cultural diversity among their client population and know how to attain information and resources concerning culture beliefs or practices that he/she is not familiar with (Kyle & Carman, 2013).*

Elimination of Institutional Barriers That Inhibit Individualization of Care

- Sensitize staff to practicing family-centered care.
- Use families to review practice and policies.
- Encourage cultural sensitization of staff.

R: *Nurses need to be able to assess for and integrate culturally appropriate interventions into the child's care to provide culturally appropriate, family-centered care. By doing this the nurse can effectively care for a culturally diverse population of children (Kyle & Carman, 2013).*

Provide Opportunities for the Process of Mutual Interaction

Promote Bonding Immediately After Delivery and During the Postpartum Phase (Durham & Chapman, 2014)

- Encourage mother to hold infant after birth (mother may need short recovery period).
- Provide/encourage skin-to-skin contact.
- Praise the mother/father for care provided to the infant.
- Provide mother with an opportunity to breastfeed immediately after delivery if possible.
- Give family as much time as they wish together with minimum interruptions from staff.
- Encourage father to hold infant.
- Provide cultural appropriate support to the family.
- Check mother regularly for signs of fatigue, especially if she received anesthesia.
- Offer flexible rooming-in to the mother; establish with her the care she will assume initially and support her requests for assistance.

Provide Support to the Parents (Durham & Chapman, 2014)

- Listen to the mother's replay of her labor and delivery experience and evaluate for possible red-flags or concerning statements.
- Allow for verbalization of feelings.
- Indicate acceptance of feelings.
- Point out the infant's strengths and individual characteristics to the parents/caregivers.
- Demonstrate the infant's responses to the parents/caregivers.
- Have a system of follow-up after discharge, especially for families considered high risk (e.g., telephone call or home visit by community health/home health nurse).
- Be aware of resources and support groups available within the hospital and community; refer the family as needed.
- Provide culturally appropriate care as requested by family.

Assess the Need to Support the Parents/Caregivers' Emerging Confidence in Child Care (Durham & Chapman, 2014)

- Observe the parents/caregivers interacting with the infant.
- Support each parent/caregiver's strengths.
- Help parents understand infant's cues and temperament.
- Assist each parent in those areas in which he or she is uncomfortable (role modeling).
- Assess for level of knowledge in growth and development; provide information as needed.
- Provide handouts, audiovisual aids, and appropriate internet resources for parent/family at their level of understanding and language.

Provide Bonding/Attachment Experiences as Soon as Possible When Immediate Separation Between Parent and Child is Necessary Secondary to Prematurity or Illness (Durham & Chapman, 2014)

- Invite parents to see and touch infant as soon as possible.
- Encourage parents to spend prolonged periods of time with infant.

- Support activities such as skin-to-skin bonding/holding and basic caregiving needs.
- If infant is transported to another facility and is separated from mother,
  - Have staff make frequent calls to mother.
  - Encourage family to spend time in neonatal intensive care unit; bring back verbal reports and pictures of infant to mother.
  - Explore family and community resources to provide means of rejoining mother and infant as soon as possible.

For Adoptive Parents

- Counsel adoptive parents that many emotions are normal on first interaction with their children.
- Counsel adoptive parents about the possibility of postadoption depression.
- Encourage adoptive parents to seek parenting classes before receiving their infant.

R: *Adoptive parents do not always have the same opportunities to prepare for the child's arrival as their biologic parent counterparts do. There aren't always as many resources available to them. The nurse can help connect the adoptive parents with available resources in their area (Hockenberry & Wilson, 2015).*

R: *The sooner the adoptive child is able to be placed into the care of their adoptive parents, the better. This encourages optimal child-adoptive parent bonding (Hockenberry & Wilson, 2015).*

Initiate Referrals as Needed/Appropriate

- Consult with community agencies for follow-up visits if indicated.
- Refer parents to pertinent organizations/specialists in their area.

PARENTAL ROLE CONFLICT

Parental Role Conflict

Related to Effects of Illness and/or Hospitalization of a Child.

Definition

Parental experience of role confusion and conflict in response to crisis (NANDA-I).

State in which a parent or primary caregiver experiences or perceives a change in role in response to external factors (e.g., illness, hospitalization, divorce, separation, birth of child with special needs).

Defining Characteristics

Major (Must Be Present, One or More)

Parent/Caregiver expresses concerns about changes in parental role.
Demonstrated disruption in care and/or caretaking routines.

Minor (May Be Present)

Parent/Caregiver expresses concerns/feelings of inadequacy to provide for child's physical and emotional needs during hospitalization or in the home.
Parent/Caregiver expresses concerns about effect of child's illness on other children.
Parent/Caregiver expresses concerns about care of siblings at home.
Parent/Caregiver expresses concerns about perceived loss of control over decisions relating to the child.

Related Factors

Related to separation from child secondary to

Birth of a child with a congenital defect, chronic illness, or both

Hospitalization of a child with an acute or chronic illness
Change in acuity, prognosis, or environment of care (e.g., transfer to or from intensive care unit)

Related to intimidation with invasive or restrictive treatment modalities (e.g., isolation, intubation)

Related to interruption of family life secondary to

Home care of a child with special needs (e.g., apnea monitoring, tracheostomy, gastrostomy, or all three)
Frequent visits to the hospital
Addition of new family member (aging relative, newborn)

Related to change in ability to parent secondary to

Illness of parent
Remarriage
Travel requirements
Dating
Work responsibilities
Death
Divorce
Change in marital status

Author's Note

This diagnosis differs from *Impaired Parenting*, which describes parenting practices that do not promote optimal growth and development. *Parental Role Conflict* describes an effective parent, whose role has been challenged or changed by external factors.

Errors in Diagnostic Statements

Parental Role Conflict Related to Hospitalization of Their Child

This diagnosis does not describe why hospitalization has caused *Parental Role Conflict.* Further assessments are indicated. If the parent(s) is/are not engaged in caring for their child, the nurse needs to determine why. For example, *Parental Role Conflict* related to fear of interfering with care and making a mistake. As evident by declining to feed child and help with bathing.

Key Concepts

- Refer to Key Concepts at the beginning of Part 2 Family/Home Nursing Diagnoses.

Focus Assessment Criteria

Refer to the Focus Assessment Criteria at the beginning of Part 2 Family/Home Nursing Diagnoses.

Goals

NOC
Refer to Impaired Parenting.

The parent/caregiver and child will demonstrate control over decision making, as evidenced by the following indicators:

- Express feelings regarding the situation
- Identify sources of support

Interventions

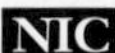
Refer to Impaired Parenting.

Assess the Present Situation

- Parents/Caregivers' and children's perception of and responses to situation
- Parental understanding of the effects of the situation on children and their typical responses
- Changes in parenting practices and daily routines (employment or change in the child care arrangements)
- Other related stressors (financial, job-related)

- Level of conflict between parents/caregivers
- Social support for both parents/caregivers

R: *Childbirth brings on many changes to the lives of the current family member's lives with each family member needing to adjust to a new role or added responsibilities. The ability of the family to adjust should be assessed (Durham & Chapman, 2014).*

Encourage the Involvement of Father in Care (Durham & Chapman, 2014)

- Foster his strengths.
- Provide an appropriate place for discussion of any issues and concerns.
- Encourage the sharing of feelings and concerns as culturally appropriate.
- Include the father in child's care.

Help Parents/Caregivers with Setting Limits with the Child (Hockenberry & Wilson, 2015)

- Explain the boundaries of acceptable behavior.
- Offer age-appropriate choices (e.g., "Which medicine do you want to take first?").
- Expect the child to perform age-appropriate self-care activities when possible.
- Assign age-appropriate chores.
- Channel undesirable feelings into constructive activity.

Encourage Parents/Caregivers to Address Siblings' Responses (Durham & Chapman, 2014)

- Help parents talk to siblings about the child's condition.
- Encourage parents/caregivers to spend special time with siblings, acknowledge siblings' feelings, and allow sibling some participation in child's care as appropriate.
- Allow siblings a life outside of caregiving.

Assist Family to Increase Decision-Making Abilities

- Emphasize parental responsibility for meeting needs and solving problems.
- Emphasize building on parental strengths.
- Provide active and reflective listening.
- Offer normative help that is congruent with parental appraisal of need.
- Ensure appropriate cultural and linguistic support through verbal and written resources.
- Promote acquisition of competencies.
- Use parent–professional collaboration as the mechanism for meeting needs.
- Allow locus of control to reside with the parent.
- Accept and support parental decisions.

R: *The parents/caregivers should be supported and encouraged as they adapt to their new parental roles and make adjustments to their current lives. They may require assistance in identifying causes of difficulties and resources to help alleviate them (Durham & Chapman, 2014).*

Facilitate Parent/Caregiver–Nurse Partnership

- Acknowledge the parents/caregivers' overall competence and their unique expertise.
- Explain everything related to care. Engage parents in team meetings.
- Negotiate differences, be flexible, and offer respite.
- Nurses should be nonjudgmental and accepting of differences that occur within families of what they may perceive as a nontraditional family unit (e.g., LGBT families, polygamous families, communal families, blended families). Showing disapproval of such family situations can have a negative effect on the parent/caregiver–nurse relationship and be detrimental to family-centered care (Hockenberry & Wilson, 2015).

Initiate Teaching and Referrals, as Needed

- Ensure that primary health-care provider, specialty services, and school nurse are aware of care needs.
- Initiate referrals, as needed (e.g., specialty teaching for care at home, day care, respite care).
- Identify local and national disease-oriented organizations as appropriate for child/family.

Parental Role Conflict • Related to Effects of Illness and/or Hospitalization of a Child

Goals

The parent will demonstrate control over decision making concerning the child and collaborate with health professionals to make decisions about the care of the child, as evidenced by the following indicators:

- Relates information about the child's health status and treatment plan
- Participates in caring for the child in the home/hospital setting to the degree desired
- Verbalizes feelings about the child's illness and the hospitalization
- Identifies and use available support systems that allow parent time and energy to cope with ill child's needs

Interventions

Help Adapt Parenting Role During Illness/Hospitalization (Hockenberry & Wilson, 2015)

- Family-centered care is of utmost importance in caring for the family with a child that has a chronic condition or is hospitalized.
- Acknowledge strengths of the family.
- Foster family's competence in caring for the child.
- Empower the family to advocate for the child and their needs as a family.
- Involve parents/caregivers in decision-making process.
- Share information about condition and resources available to them and the child.
- In the parent/caregiver's absence from hospital, the nurse try to maintain the child's home/family routine as much as possible in terms of the child's care.

Allow Parents to Participate in the Care of Their Child to the Degree They Desire (Ball, Bindler, & Cowen, 2015)

- Allow rooming-in, that is to allow parent/caregiver to stay with the child in their hospital room.
- Encourage parents to help in preparing the child for a procedure or planned hospitalization in the form of age-appropriate explanations, reading books about subject, or play involving demonstrating what may happen with a doll.
- Allow the parent to be present as much as possible during child's hospitalization, including preparations for procedures (e.g., allowing the parent to be with child and help with distraction while staff places peripheral IV or performs a laceration repair).
- Encourage parents/caregivers to perform feedings, diaper changes, bathing, and assist with other helpful, daily activities.

Support Parental Ability to Normalize the Hospital/Home Environment (Hockenberry & Wilson, 2015)

- Assess the child's daily routine and try to incorporate as much as possible during hospitalization.
- Help child/family focus on the "normal" aspects of their appearance in the children with physical deformities or anomalies that they may be self-conscious about. Assist in promoting positive self-image. Provide opportunities to make appearance as near-normal as desired through use of wigs, prosthesis, or cosmetics to cover a scar.
- The parent/caregiver's behavior and response to child's condition can be either detrimental or positive in the child's learning to cope with their condition. Assist and encourage the parent/caregiver to have a healthy and beneficial attitude toward their child's condition.

R: *A major contributing factor in the child/family coping with feeling different because of illness or hospitalization can be trying to maximize normalization as much as possible in child/family's life (Hockenberry & Wilson, 2015).*

Provide Physical and Emotional Support for Parents/Caregivers (Hockenberry & Wilson, 2015)

- Help the parents manage their possible feelings of grief over the loss of the "perfect child," and cope with the strain of demands of caregiving.
- Caregiver strain is real possibility as they try to balance the demands of the household and possibly caring for other children while meeting the challenges of caring for their child with a chronic condition or that is hospitalized.

- Assist the family in managing their feelings and stress while adapting to the situation and provide resources as needed (counseling, support groups, education, community agencies).
- Encourage parents/caregivers to remember to take care of themselves (e.g., get enough rest, eat well, maintain their physical health needs).
- Help them develop coping strategies for ongoing stress related to hospitalization or care of their child as well as sudden causes of stress that may arise.
- Assess for a support system and if one is not available or in place, assist parents/caregivers in developing one.

Initiate Referrals as Indicated

- Chaplain, social services, community agencies (respite care), parent self-help groups
- Provide information to parents for self-referral.

Related to lack of available role model

Related to ineffective adaptation to stressors associated with

Illness
Economic problems
New baby
Substance abuse

READINESS FOR ENHANCED PARENTING

NANDA-I Definition

A pattern of providing an environment for children or other dependent client(s)/person(s) that is sufficient to nurture growth and development, and can be strengthened.

Defining Characteristics*

Expresses willingness to enhance parenting.
Children or other dependent individual(s) express satisfaction with home environment.
Emotional support of children or dependent individual(s)/person(s)
Needs of children/dependent client(s) are met (e.g., physical and emotional).
Exhibits realistic expectations of children/dependent person.

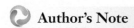

Author's Note

Refer to *Impaired Parenting* for strategies to support effective parenting.

Part 3

Community Nursing Diagnoses

This part includes all the NANDA-I approved community diagnoses and other NANDA-I approved diagnoses with community application. In Part 1, many diagnoses are focused on the individual but would be useful in the community; for example, *Imbalanced Nutrition* related to frequent intake of high-fat and salty foods as evidenced by reports of an average intake of fast foods of more than 10 to 15 meals a week works as an individual as well as community diagnosis. Likewise, if a community is forced to relocate, the diagnosis *Anticipatory Grieving* related to sale of apartment and forced relocation of tenants as manifested by anger, crying, and fear might apply as an individual diagnosis.

The function of community nursing provides an important component in the current evolving healthcare arena called population health. Under the Affordable Care Act of 2012, population health is a major focus of health reform. Community nurses play a key role in population health by applying the community nursing processes and nursing diagnoses within their communities where they work.

Community nursing can be introduced to students by focusing on a small geographic population such as a neighborhood, assisted-living residents, or a group of women in a shelter. Students may also address some common-interest communities such as a senior citizen center, church community, or local chapter of Women Against Rape.

Key Concepts

- Community health care differs from home health care (Allender, Rector, & Warner, 2014).
  - Community health care: continuous
    - Targets populations
    - Focuses on groups that do not seek care
    - Emphasizes wellness and primary prevention
  - Home health care: episodic
    - Targets individuals and families
    - Focuses on individuals who seek care
    - Emphasizes restoring health after an acute episode
- Community competence describes the healthy functioning of the total community unit. A competent community has four important characteristics (Allender et al., 2014):
  - It collaborates effectively to identify community needs and problems.
  - It achieves a working consensus on goals and priorities.
  - It agrees on ways and means to implement the agreed-on goals.
  - It collaborates effectively in the required actions.
- The essential conditions for community competence and health (Allender et al., 2014) are as follows:
  - A high degree of awareness that "we are community"
  - Use of natural resources while taking steps to conserve them for future generations
  - Open recognition of subgroups and encouragement of their participation in community affairs
  - Readiness to meet crises
  - Problem solving: Community identifies, analyzes, and organizes to meet its own needs.
  - Open channels of communication that allow information to flow among all subgroups of citizens in all directions.
  - Desire to make each resource available to all members of the community
  - Legitimate and effective ways to settle disputes
  - Encouragement of maximum citizen participation in decision making
  - Promotion of high-level wellness among all its members

- Community refers "to a collection of people who interact with one another and whose common interests or characteristics form a basis for a sense of unity or belonging" (Allender et al., 2014).
- There are three types of communities (Allender et al., 2014):
  - *Common interest* is a collection of people locally or widespread with a shared interest or goal.
  - *Geographic* is defined as a group in a certain geographic boundary.
  - *Community of solution* is a group of people who come together to address a problem that affects all of them.
- Examples of each type of community:
  - Geographic community
    - City
    - Town
    - Neighborhood
    - County, state
    - Country, world
    - Prison, jail
  - Common-interest community
    - Faith communities
    - Disabled individuals
    - Pregnant teens
    - Women Against Rape
    - Mothers Against Drunk Driving (MADD)
    - Homeless
    - Nurse practitioners
  - Community of solutions
    - County water department
    - City/County health department
    - Disaster team
    - Environmental Protection Agency
    - Ambulance service
    - Health center
- Communities have five common components (Allender et al., 2014; *Clemen-Stone et al., 2001):
  - *People:* People are the most important resource or core of the community. Functional, cohesive communities have shared values.
  - *Goals and needs:* Goals and needs of individuals and groups in the community reflect the community goals and needs. As in Maslow's hierarchy, a community must have its needs of physiology, safety, and social affiliation fulfilled before meeting higher needs of esteem and self-actualization.
  - *Community environment:* The environment (climate, natural resources, buildings, food, water supply, flora, animals, insects, economics, health and welfare services, leadership, social networks, recreation, and religion) has major effects on health.
  - *Service systems:* These are a network of agencies and organizations in the community that help to meet the basic needs (social welfare, education, economic) and the health needs of the community.
  - *Boundaries:* These define communities. Some boundaries are concrete, such as a geographic or political entity (e.g., cities, states) or a situation (e.g., home, school, work). Interests define conceptual boundaries (e.g., book clubs).
- Healthy People 2020 focuses on five determinants of health: policy making, social factors, health services, individual behavior, and biology and genetics. These determinants are based on a range of personal, social, economic, and environmental factors that influence health status. "It is the interrelationships among these that determine individual and population health. Because of this, interventions that target multiple determinants of health are most likely to be effective." (http://healthypeople.gov/2020/about/DOHAbout.aspx, retrieved August 17, 2015). Refer to Box II.7 for a list of the 12 health indicators for the health determinants.
- Communities (local, state) can use Healthy People 2020's new approach to address the overarching goals to:
  - Attain higher quality, longer lives free of preventable disease, disability, injury, and premature death
  - Achieve health equity, eliminate disparities, and improve the health of all groups
  - Create social and physical environments that promote good health for all
  - Promote quality of life, healthy development, and health behaviors across all life stages (http://healthypeople.gov/2020/about/DOHAbout.aspx, retrieved March 20, 2011 and August 17, 2015).

Box II.7 THE LEADING HEALTH INDICATORS THAT REFLECT THE MAJOR PUBLIC HEALTH CONCERNS IN THE UNITED STATES

Access to health services
Clinical preventive services
Environmental quality
Injury and violence
Maternal, infant, and child health
Mental health
Nutrition, physical activity, and obesity
Oral health
Reproductive and sexual health
Social determinants
Substance abuse
Tobacco

- Rural communities have fewer than 2,500 residents. Rural people are more self-reliant and reluctant to seek assistance from others. Researchers have found that "rural residents define health as being able to do what they want to do; it is a way of life and a state of mind; there is a goal of maintaining balance in all aspect of their lives" (Lee & McDonagh, 2006, p. 314, as cited in Winters & Lee, 2009, p. 27).

  "Older rural residents and those with ties to extractive industries are more likely to define health in a functional manner—to work, to be productive, and to do usual tasks" (Lee & McDonagh, 2006, as cited in Winters & Lee, 2009).
- Rural communities often resist outsiders' ideas and prefer health-care providers who live in their community. Although people all know one another, they are reluctant to ask for help or share problems for fear their neighbors will find out (*Bushy, 1990).
- Population health:
  - Kindig and Stoddart (*2003) define population health as "the health outcomes of a group of individuals, including the distribution of such outcomes with the group."
  - Populations are defined groups of individuals with a focus on the health and well-being of these groups. There are five common health segments: (1) health independents, (2) at-risk individuals, (3) early-stage chronic, (4) individuals with complex conditions, and (5) late-stage/polychronics (Clark & Bujnowski, 2014).

Community Assessment (Allender et al., 2014)

The community assessment can be used in its entirety or in segments if a focused assessment is desired. This assessment will direct the collection of data to determine the presence of effective functioning or ineffective functioning. The assessment should also account for the Healthy People 2020 health determinants.

Sources of Data

Individuals
Groups, subgroups (e.g., adolescents, homeless, elders)
Maps
Chamber of commerce
Public library
Health planning boards
Farm labor boards
Social service programs
Health department (local, county, and state health)
U.S. Department of Health and Human Services
Local government
Educational programs
Local hospital community benefit departments
Websites (www.followed by two-letter abbreviation for state.gov; e.g., www.ca.gov)
World Health Organization (WHO)
National Institutes of Health (NIH)
U.S. Public Health Services
U.S. Bureau of Census
Centers for Disease Control and Prevention
Community commons
County health rankings
Non-profit Hospital Community Health Needs Assessment (CHNA)
County Health Needs Assessment

Behavioral Risk Factor Surveillance System
Youth Behavioral Risk Factor Surveillance System

Methods of Data Collection

Windshield survey
Community resident interviews (Key Informants)
Participant observations
Descriptive epidemiologic studies
Focus groups
Asset mapping

Geographic

Location: neighborhood, city, county, state
Physical environment: site of natural disaster (floods, earthquakes, volcano, hurricanes, tornadoes)
Recreational opportunities
Climate: extreme heat or cold, rain or snow
Flora and fauna: poisonous plants, diseased animals, venomous animals, insects
Human-made environment: housing, dams, water supply, chemical waste, air pollution, industrial pollutants, air quality
Food Deserts

Population Demographics

Size
Density: high/low
Composition
- Gender ratio
- Age distribution
- Ethnic origins
- Race distributions
- Other (e.g., married, single, gay)

Characteristics
- Mobility
- Socioeconomic status
- Unemployment rates
- Educational level
- Types of employment
- Migrants, transients (e.g., snow birds, homeless)
- Rate of growth or decline
- Cultural diversity

Data Analysis Questions
What are the population size and age distributions?
What is the distribution of gender, race, and marital status?
What is the distribution of educational level, occupation, and income?

Functional Health Patterns

This section provides a comprehensive assessment of a community using the functional health patterns (*Gordon, 1994). It is designed to allow a focus assessment on only one functional health pattern, such as nutrition of a community. Data analysis questions follow each pattern for assistance in determining if there is effective functioning, a problem, or a risk for a problem.

Health Perception–Health Maintenance Pattern

Mortality rates (age-related, maternal, and neonatal)
Ten leading causes of death
Morbidity rates of cancer, coronary heart disease, alcoholism, substance abuse, communicable diseases (tuberculosis, sexually transmitted diseases, HIV)
Mental illness
Crime rates and types
Motor vehicle accidents, alcohol/drug related

Environmental Hazards

Natural disasters, extreme climates, toxins, venomous insects, reptiles, animals, and poisonous plants

Health-Care Services

Hospital services, nursing homes, assisted-living facilities, ambulatory services
Occupational school health, health department, community services, health centers, home services

Protective Services

Police, fire, disaster response plan, ambulance services
Environmental protection services

Support Available

Financial, food, housing, clothing, and counseling

Data Analysis Questions
What are the major health problems?
How has the community responded to the major health problems?
Are they satisfied with the results?
What health promotion programs are available? Are they affordable?
Is there a group (cultural, ethnic, poor, transients) whose health needs are not addressed?
How do the unemployed and uninsured access health care?
What is the incidence of alcohol- and drug-related crimes and accidents?
What is the community's perception of safety?
What are the climate hazards?
How does the community reduce risks of injury in extreme weather?
What are the flora and fauna hazards?
How does the community reduce risks of injury?

Nutritional–Metabolic Pattern

Access to food (community food banks)
Food insecurity; cost of food
Availability of healthy foods (community gardens, farmers markets)
Sources of food stores, markets, fast food, nutritional services (e.g., WIC, Meals on Wheels)
Incidence of malnourished, overweight, or obesity
Water supply (source, testing results)

Data Analysis Questions
How does the cost of food compare with other communities?
How often is fast food consumed?
Are there food programs for children, elderly, and poor?
What types of foods are in the school (cafeteria, vending machines)?

Elimination Pattern

Sanitation (water supply, sewage disposal, trash and garbage disposal, animal control, rodent and vermin control)
Ecologic concerns (recycling, types of hazardous waste)

Data Analysis Questions
Are hazardous wastes under control?
Are dumps or disposables a risk to water contamination?
Are the disaster plans current?
What is the air pollution index?

Activity–Exercise Pattern

Transportation (options, costs, access)
Recreation facilities (types, costs, access)
Frequency of walking, bike riding, play areas (access, condition, safety)
Housing (availability, quality, cost)

Data Analysis Questions
How adequate is the transportation system?
Are recreation facilities used?
Are there barriers to using these facilities (cost, access, handicap friendly)?
Are there safe play areas for children?
Is housing adequate, safe, and affordable?

Cognitive–Perception Pattern

Educational levels
Language
Process of community decisions
Decision makers (community, business, faith-based)
Educational facilities (public, private, adult education, higher education, health education programs, and quality, availability, and cost of each)
Communication (publications, radio and TV stations, informal network)

Data Analysis Questions
How are the schools rated (county, state, national)?
What is the dropout rate?
What are the reasons for dropouts?
Is adult education available?
What educational programs are available for residents with English as a second language skill?
Do health-related agencies work together?

Role–Relationship Pattern

Community-sponsored events (faith based, senior centers, parenting classes, children's activities)
Community engagement
Socioeconomic groups
Ethnic/racial groups
Communications methods (newspapers, flyers, bulletins, radio, TV)

Data Analysis Questions
How is information communicated to the residents?
Are there public meetings?
Do residents interact with each other?
Is there a friendly atmosphere?
What are the roles of domestic violence, violence, child abuse, and elder abuse?
What is the divorce rate?

Sleep–Rest Pattern

Noise sources (cars, airplanes, industrial)
Work/school routine
Environment conducive to rest/sleep (light, TV, traffic)
Data Analysis Questions
How is the noise level controlled?
Do children get 8 or more hours of sleep?
What are scheduled sleep routines?

Coping–Stress Tolerance Pattern

Assistance programs (local, faith based, state, federal)
Crisis intervention programs (mental health services, crisis centers, telephone help lines)
History of unresolved conflict (racial, gangs)
Crimes (types, drug related)

Data Analysis Questions
Are assistance programs accessible for all residents?
Is there a problem with prostitution or pornography?

What are the crime statistics?
Are residents satisfied with assistance programs?
What is the community response to crisis? Anger? Indifference? Isolation? Helpless? Overwhelmed?
What are the barriers to effective coping?

Sexuality–Reproductive Pattern

Average size of family
Reproduction (birth rate, teen pregnancies, prenatal care, abortion facilities)
Birth control resources
Educational programs (sex education, childbirth education classes, parenting classes)

Data Analysis Questions
Are family planning services available to all residents?
Is there family counseling available and affordable?
Is sex education supported in schools and community?

Value–Belief Pattern

Community origins
Community traditions
Religions in community

Data Analysis Questions
What are the community's priorities?
Do most residents feel they are valued in the community?
Are all ethnic groups accepted?
Are all religious groups accepted?

CONTAMINATION: COMMUNITY

Contamination: Community

Risk for Contamination: Community

NANDA-I Definition

Exposure to environmental contaminants in doses sufficient to cause adverse health effects

Defining Characteristics

Clusters of clients seeking care for similar signs or symptoms
Signs and symptoms are dependent on the causative agent, which include pesticides, chemicals, biologics, waste, radiation, and pollution.
Large numbers of clients with rapidly fatal illnesses
Sick, dying, or dead animals or fish; absence of insects
Measurement of contaminants exceeding acceptable levels
Refer to *Contamination: Individual* for specific contaminant-related health effects.

Related Factors

Pathophysiologic

Presence of bacteria, viruses, toxins

Treatment Related

Insufficient or absent use of decontamination protocol
Inappropriate or no use of protective clothing

Situational

Acts of bioterrorism
Flooding, earthquakes, natural disasters
Sewer line leaks
Industrial plant emissions; intentional or accidental discharge of contaminants by industries or businesses
Physical factors (climatic conditions such as temperature, wind; geographic area)
Social factors (crowding, sanitation, poverty, lack of access to health care)
Biologic factors (presence of vectors such as mosquitoes, ticks, rodents)

Environmental

Contamination of aquifers by septic tanks
Intentional/accidental contamination of food and water supply
Exposure to heavy metals or chemicals, atmospheric pollutants, radiation, bioterrorism, disaster; concomitant or previous exposure

Maturational

Community dynamics (participation, power and decision-making structure, collaborative efforts)

Key Concepts

- More than 70,000 individual industrial chemicals are registered with the Environmental Protection Agency for commercial use, and an average of 2,300 new chemicals are introduced each year. All humans are now exposed to synthetic pollutants in drinking water, air, and food supply, as well as in consumer products and home pesticides (*Thornton, McCally, & Houlihan, 2002).
- Refer to *Contamination: Individual* for additional Key Concepts.

Focus Assessment Criteria

Subjective Data

Assess for Defining Characteristics

Clusters of community members report the following:
- Respiratory/cardiac (e.g., difficulty breathing, cough, flu symptoms, irregular heart beat)
- Gastrointestinal (e.g., stomach ache, diarrhea, cramping, nausea, vomiting)
- Neurologic (e.g., muscle weaknesses, joint and muscle aches, visual changes)
- Dermatologic (e.g., skin lesions, pustules, skin irritation, itching, blistering, burns)
- Exposure to radiation
- Pregnancies resulting in birth defects
- Unusual liquids, sprays, or vapors at work or home
- Dead or dying animals in area
- Explosions or bombs
- Employment or home located near industrial, agricultural, or commercial businesses

Objective Data

Clusters of community members with the following:
- Neurologic (e.g., hallucinations, confusion, seizures, decreased level of consciousness, pupil changes, and blurred vision)
- Pulmonary (e.g., labored breathing, cyanosis)
- Cardiac (e.g., cardiac dysrhythmia, hypertension, hypotension)
- Integumentary (e.g., skin lesions, pustules, scabs, blisters, ulcerations, burns, erythema, dry or moist desquamation, jaundice)
- Fever
- Cancers (thyroid, skin, leukemia)
- Birth defects
- Radiation sickness (weakness, hair loss, changes in blood chemistries, hemorrhage, diminished organ function)

Assess for Related Factors

Refer to Related Factors.

Goals

- Community will use health surveillance data system to monitor for contamination incidents.
- Community will participate in mass casualty and disaster readiness drills.
- Community will use disaster plan to evacuate and triage affected members.
- Community exposure to contaminants will be minimized.
- Community health effects associated with contamination will be minimized.

Interventions

General Interventions

Monitor for Contamination Incidents Using Health Surveillance Data

R: *Early surveillance and detection are critical components of preparation for potential biologic attacks (*Veenema, 2003).*

Provide Accurate Information About Risks Involved, Preventive Measures, and Use of Antibiotics and Vaccines

- Encourage community members to talk to others about their fears.
- Provide general supportive measures (food, water, shelter).

R: *Interventions aimed at supporting and coping help the community deal with feelings of fear, helplessness, and loss of control that are normal reactions in a crisis situation.*

R: *Treatment of contamination before and after exposure will decrease symptoms and reduce mortality. Success of response is related to ability to effectively decontaminate patients, protection of health-care providers, communication, efficient transportation, and competent treatment (Agency for Toxic Substances and Disease Registry [ATSDR], 2014).*

Specific Interventions

Prevention

- Identify community risk factors and develop programs to prevent disasters from occurring.

Preparedness

- Plan for communication, evacuation, rescue, and victim care.
- Schedule mass casualty and disaster readiness drills.

Response

- Identify contaminants in the environment.
- Educate community about the environmental contaminant.
- Collaborate with other agencies (local health department, emergency medical services, state and federal agencies).
- Rescue, triage, stabilize, transport, and treat affected community members.

Recovery

- Mental health services should assist in psychological recovery and should emphasize principles of a sense of safety, calm, a sense of being able to solve problems, connectedness to social support, and hope.

Decontamination Procedure

- Primary decontamination of exposed personnel is agent specific.
- Remove contaminated clothing.
- Use copious amounts of water and soap or diluted (0.5%) sodium hypochlorite.
- Secondary decontamination from clothing or equipment of those exposed; use proper physical protection.

R: *Decontamination procedures prevent exposure of additional community members and health-care workers.*

- Employ appropriate isolation precautions (universal, airborne, droplet, and contact isolation).

R: *Precautions prevent cross-contamination by agent.*

Risk for Contamination: Community

NANDA-I Definition

At risk for exposure to environmental contaminants in doses sufficient to cause adverse health effects

Risk Factors

Refer to Related Factors under *Contamination: Community*.

Key Concepts

Refer to Key Concepts under *Contamination: Community*.

Focus Assessment Criteria

Assess for Related Factors

Refer to Related Factors under *Contamination: Community*.

Goals

- Community will use health surveillance data system to monitor for contamination incidents.
- Community will participate in mass casualty and disaster readiness drills.
- Community will remain free of contamination-related health effects.

Interventions

Monitor for Contamination Incidents Using Health Surveillance Data

R: *Early detection of environmental contamination will decrease the risk of actual contamination occurring.*

Provide Accurate Information About Risks Involved and Preventive Measures

- Encourage community members to talk to others about their fears.

R: *Interventions aimed at supporting and coping help the community deal with feelings of fear, helplessness, and loss of control that are normal reactions in a crisis situation.*

Identify Community Risk Factors and Develop Programs to Prevent Disasters From Occurring

- Notify agencies authorized to protect the environment from contaminants in the area.
- Modify the environment to minimize risk.

R: *Modification of the environment will decrease the risk of actual contamination occurring.*

READINESS FOR ENHANCED COMMUNITY COPING

NANDA-I Definition

A pattern of community's activities for adaptation and problem solving for meeting the demands or needs of the community, which can be strengthened

Defining Characteristics*

Expresses desire to enhance
- Availability of community recreation programs
- Availability of community relaxation programs
- Communication among community members
- Communication between aggregates and larger community
- Community planning for predictable stressors
- Community resources for managing stressors
- Community responsibility for stress management
- Problem solving for identified issue

Seeks social support
Uses broad range of emotion-oriented strategies
Uses a broad range of problem-oriented strategies
Uses spiritual resources

Related Factors

Not applicable.

Author's Note

This diagnosis can be used to describe a community that wishes to improve an already effective pattern of coping. For a community to be assisted to a higher level of functioning, its basic needs for food, shelter, safety, a clean environment, and a supportive network must first be addressed. When these needs are met, programs can focus on higher functioning, such as wellness and self-actualization. Community programs can be designed after a community assessment and because of community requests. They can focus on enhancing health promotion with topics related to optimal nutrition, weight control, regular exercise programs, constructive stress management, social support, role responsibilities, and preparing for and coping with life events such as retirement, parenting, and pregnancy.

Goals

NOC

Community Competence, Community Health Status, Community Risk Control

The community (specify type of community, e.g., the town of Mullica Hill, the southeast neighborhood of South Tucson) will provide programs to improve (specify type of focus, e.g., nutrition), as evidenced by the following indicators:

- Identifies health-promotion needs as (specify: e.g., daily decrease in high-fat foods, increase in fruits and vegetables)
- Accesses resources needed (specify: e.g., local experts, nutritionist, college students)
- Develops programs (specify: health fair, school cafeteria, printed material) based on needs assessment
- Implements policies for health (e.g., American Diabetes Association policy for healthy meals)

Interventions

NIC

Program Development, Risk Identification, Community Health Development, Environmental Risk Protection

Conduct Focus Groups to Discuss Programs to Assist Residents With Positive Coping With Developmental Tasks

- Arrange focus groups according to age, including diverse groups.

R: *Focus groups assessments are advantageous because of their efficiency and low cost (Allender, Rector, & Warner, 2014).*

Plan Programs Targeted for a Specific Population

Adolescents (13 to 18 Years)

- Career planning
- Stress management
- Substance abuse
- Topics associated with sexual activity

Young Adults (18 to 35 Years)

- Career selection
- Constructive relationships
- Balancing one's life
- Parenting issues

Middle Age (35 to 65 Years)

- Launching children
- Parenting issues
- Reciprocal relationships
- Aging parents
- Quality leisure time

Older Adults (65 Years and Older)

- Retirement issues
- Balancing one's life
- Anticipated losses
- Facts and myths of aging
- Exercise options (in home, at a center)

All Ages

- Civic planning
- Meeting needs of all community members
- Crisis intervention
- Grieving
- Community involvement

R: *Life-cycle events are predictable developmental tasks of young adults, middle adults, and older adults (refer to Key Concepts for specifics). Programs in the community can be planned to assist individuals with adapting successfully to life events (*Clemen-Stone et al., 2001; Edelman, Kudzma, & Mandle, 2014).*

Discuss Programs That Promote High-Level Wellness

- Optimal nutrition
- Weight control
- Age-relevant exercise programs
- Socialization programs
- Effective problem solving
- Injury prevention
- Environmental quality

Define the Target Health-Promotion Needs

- Analyze assessment of community.
- Prioritize the needs:
  - Organize the focus group responses.
  - Probability of success
  - Cost:benefit ratio (e.g., resources available)
  - Potential for policy development

Select a Health-Promotion Program

- Identify target population (e.g., entire community, older adults, adolescents).
- Delineate a timetable for the planning and implementation stages.

R: *Focus groups can identify residents' assessment of health needs and promote their involvement in community programming (Allender et al., 2014).*

Meet With Community Groups (Health Centers, Faith-Based Groups, Government Agencies) to Review Findings of Focus Groups and to Discuss Collaborative Programming

R: *Community building can develop new and existing leadership and strengthen community organizations and interorganizational collaboration.*

Plan the Program

- Develop detailed program objectives and the evaluation framework to be used.
  - Content
  - Time needed
  - Ideal teaching method for targeting group
  - Teaching aids (e.g., large-print materials)
- Establish resources needed and sources.
  - Space
  - Transportation facilities
  - Optimal day of the week
  - Optimal time of the year
  - Supplies, audiovisual equipment
  - Financial (budgeted, donations)
- Market the program.
  - Media (e.g., newspaper, TV, radio)
  - Posters (food market, train station)
  - Flyers (distribute via school to home)
  - Word of mouth (religious organizations, community clubs, schools)
  - Guest speaker (community clubs, schools)

R: *As an advocate and community liaison, the community health nurse collaborates with other disciplines and agencies to match resources with community-identified needs for program success (Edelman et al., 2014).*

Provide Program and Evaluate Whether Desired Results (Objectives) Were Achieved

- Number of participants
- Negative feedback
- Objectives achieved
- Actual expenditures versus budgeted
- Statistics (e.g., bicycle accidents)
- Participant evaluations
- Adequate planning
- Revisions for future planning
- Shared responsibility

R: *Evaluation will determine if the program was completely effective, partly effective, or ineffective in achieving the program objectives (Edelman et al., 2014).*

Determine the Strengths and Limitations of the Program and Plan a New Approach if Indicated.

R: *Community health-promotion programs must demonstrate effectiveness to earn continued community and economic support (Edelman et al., 2014).*

INEFFECTIVE COMMUNITY COPING

NANDA-I Definition

Pattern of community activities for adaptation and problem solving that is unsatisfactory for meeting the demands or needs of the community

Defining Characteristics*

Community does not meet its own expectations
Deficits in community participation
Excessive community conflicts
Reports of community powerlessness
Reports of community vulnerability
High rates of illness
Increased social problems (e.g., homicides, vandalism, arson, terrorism, robbery, infanticide, abuse, divorce, unemployment, poverty, militancy, mental illness)
Stressors perceived as excessive

Risk Factors

Presence of risk factors (See Related Factors.)

Related Factors

Situational

Related to ineffective or nonexistent community systems (e.g., lack of emergency medical system, transportation system, disaster planning system)[1]

Related to lack of knowledge of resources

Related to inadequate communication patterns

Related to inadequate community cohesiveness

Related to inadequate resources for problem solving[1]

Related to natural disasters[1] ***secondary to:***

Flood
Hurricane
Earthquake
Epidemic
Avalanche

Related to traumatic effects of[1]***:***

Airplane crash
Industrial disaster
Large fire
Environmental accident
Earthquake

Related to threat to community safety (e.g., murder, rape, kidnapping, robberies)[1]

Related to sudden rise in community unemployment

[1] These represent risk factors for *Risk for Ineffective Community Coping*. Refer to Author's Note for additional clarification.

Maturational

Related to inadequate resources for:

Children
Working parents
Adolescents
Older adults

 **Author's Note**

Ineffective Community Coping is a diagnosis of a community that does not have a constructive system in place to cope with events or changes that occur. The focus of interventions is to improve community dialogue, planning, and resource identification.

When a community has experienced a natural disaster (e.g., hurricane, flood), a threat to safety (e.g., murder, violence, rape), or a man-made disaster (e.g., airplane crash, large fire), the focus should be on preventive strategies. The diagnosis *Risk for Ineffective Community Coping* is more appropriate when the community has been a victim of a disaster or a violent crime.

Goals

NOC

Community Competence, Community Health Status, Community Risk Control

The community will engage in effective problem solving, as evidenced by the following indicators:

- Identifies problem
- Accesses information to improve coping
- Uses communication channels to access assistance

Interventions

NIC

Community Health Development, Environmental Risk Protection, Program Development, Risk Identification

Assess for Causative or Contributing Factors

- Refer to Related Factors.

Provide Opportunities for Community Members (e.g., Schools, Churches, Synagogues, Town Hall) to Meet and Discuss the Situation

- Demonstrate acceptance of community members' anger, withdrawal, or denial.
- Correct misinformation as needed.
- Discourage blaming.

R: *Certain behaviors or beliefs (e.g., anxiety, fear, value conflicts) can interfere with problem solving. They should be explored in discussions (*Clemen-Stone et al., 2001).*

Provide for Effective Communication (Allender, Rector, & Warner, 2014)

- Allow for and address questions.
- Convey the facts.
- Convey seriousness.
- Be clear, simple, and repetitive.
- Present solutions and suggestions.
- Address real and perceived needs.

R: *For communication to elicit effective action, it must be believable, current, clear, authoritative, and predictive of the probability of future events (Allender et al., 2014).*

Promote Community Competence in Coping

- Focus on community goals, not individuals' goals.
- Engage subgroups in group discussions and planning.
- Ensure access to resources for all members (e.g., flexible hours for working members).
- Devise a method for formal disagreements.
- Evaluate each decision's impact on all community members.

R: *For a community to cope effectively, it must function collectively, not as individuals (Allender et al., 2014).*

Establish a Community Information Center at the Local Library to Access Information and Support (e.g., Telephone, Online)

R: *"The public library has the resources and expertise to address the need for prompt, reliable, and relevant information in any conflict or crisis situation at no cost."*

Identify the Collaborative Resources That Can Be Accessed in the Health Department, Faith-Based Organization, Social Services, and Health-Care Provider Agencies

R: *Interorganizational collaboration draws upon each other's strengths and increases community participation.*

Use the Community Information Center (e.g., Local Library) to Inform Residents of Ongoing Activities and Progress

R: *Open channels of communication can reduce speculation, anger, and apathy (Allender et al., 2014).*

DEFICIENT COMMUNITY HEALTH

NANDA-I Definition*

Presence of one or more health problems or factors that deter wellness or increase the risk of health problems experienced by an aggregate

Defining Characteristics*

Incidence of risks relating to hospitalization experienced by aggregates or populations
Incidence of risks relating to physiologic states experienced by aggregates or populations
Incidence of risks relating to psychological states experienced by aggregates or populations
Incidence of health problems experienced by aggregates or populations
No program available to enhance wellness for aggregates or populations[2]
No program available to prevent one or more health problems for aggregates or populations[2]
No program available to reduce one or more health problems for aggregates or populations[2]
No program available to eliminate one or more health problems for aggregates or populations[2]

Related Factors*

Lack of access to public health-care providers
Lack of community experts
Limited resources
Program has inadequate budget.
Program has inadequate community support.
Program has inadequate consumer satisfaction.
Program has inadequate evaluation.
Program has inadequate outcome data.
Program partly addresses health problem.

Author's Note

This NANDA-I nursing diagnosis describes a community that has health problems that need assessment and program development. The programs must be accessible, affordable, available, and realistic for optimal outcomes to be achieved.

This diagnosis, although different from *Ineffective Health Management*, shares the same focus of community assessment and program development. Refer to the Key Concepts and Community Assessment at the beginning of Part 3, Community Nursing Diagnoses.

---

[2]These four defining characteristics do not define community health but instead are related factors that contribute to *Deficient Community Health*.

Goals

NOC
Refer to *Ineffective Community Health Management.*

Refer to *Ineffective Community Health Management.*

Interventions

NIC
Refer to *Ineffective Community Health Management.*

Refer to *Ineffective Community Health Management.*

INEFFECTIVE COMMUNITY HEALTH MANAGEMENT[3]

Definition

Pattern of regulating and integrating into community processes programs for treatment of illness and the sequelae of illness that are unsatisfactory for meeting health-related goals

Defining Characteristics

Verbalized difficulty meeting health needs in communities
Acceleration (expected or unexpected) of illness(es)
Morbidity, mortality rates above norm

Related Factors

Situational (Environmental)

Related to unavailability of community programs for (specify):

Prevention of diseases
Immunizations
Accident prevention
Smoking cessation
Alcohol abuse
Screening for diseases
Dental care
Fire safety
Substance abuse
Child abuse

Related to problem accessing program secondary to:

Inadequate communication
Lack of transportation
Limited hours
Insufficient funds

Related to complexity of population's needs

Related to lack of awareness of availability

Related to multiple needs of vulnerable groups (specify):

Homeless
Below poverty level
Pregnant teenagers
Home-bound individuals

Related to unavailable or insufficient health-care agencies

[3]This diagnosis is not presently on the NANDA-I list but has been added for clarity and usefulness.

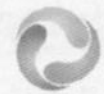

Author's Note

This diagnosis describes a community that is experiencing unsatisfactory management of its health problems. This diagnosis can also describe a community with evidence that a population is underserved because of the lack of availability of, access to, or knowledge of health-care resources. Using the results of community assessments, community nurses can identify at-risk groups and overall community needs. In addition, they assess health systems, transportation, social services, and access.

Goals

NOC

Participation: Health Care Decisions, Risk Control, Risk Detection

This community will achieve the following goals:

- Identifies needed community resources
- Promotes the use of community resources for health problems

Interventions

NIC

Decision-Making Support, Health System Guidance, Risk Identification, Community Health Development, Risk Identification

Use Health Department Data (Local, County, State, National) to Identify Major Health Problems and Associated Risks; for Example:

- Obesity
- Heart disease
- Asthma
- Automobile accidents

R: *These data will provide accurate statistics (Allender, Rector, & Warner, 2010).*

Organize Focus Groups to Assess Health Needs and Assets; Include Different Age Groups, Ethnic/Racial Groups, and Residents With Varied Lengths of Residence

- Initiate discussion with questions (Clark, 2009) such as the following:
  - What is it like to live in this community?
  - What could make life in this community better?
  - What kinds of things could improve the health of people who live in this community?
  - What could the health department do to improve the health of people who live in this community?
  - What could you, or people you know, do to improve life in this community?

R: *"Focus groups specifically targeted to all segments of the population proved to be an effective mechanism to elicit broad community input regarding health needs and assets" (Clark, 2009).*

Meet With Community Groups (Health Centers, Faith-Based Groups, Government Agencies) to Review Findings of Focus Groups and to Discuss Collaborative Planning

R: *Community building can develop new and existing leadership and strengthen community organizations and interorganizational collaboration (*McLeroy Norton, Kegler, Burdine, & Sumaya, 2003).*

Organize Response Data

- Rank-order entire sample.
- Group responses of selected groups (e.g., age, gender, income level, disabled).

R: *The cost of health-related programs and limited resources make priority identification imperative (Edelman et al., 2014).*

Analyze the Findings

- What overall health problems are reported?
- What are the health concerns of
  - Older population
  - Households with children up to 20 years of age
  - Single-parent households
  - Respondents younger than 45 years
  - People living below poverty level
  - Uninsured

- Adolescents
- New immigrants

R: *Health-care program planning provides an orderly structure for organizing large quantities of data to achieve community health goals successfully (*Clemen-Stone et al., 2001).*

Evaluate Community Resources

- What resources are available for the health problems identified?
- Are there utilization or access problems with the services?
- How does the population learn about services?
- Identify problems that do not have community services available.

R: *Evaluation of resources available is needed to match activities planned and to determine if funding is needed for additional resources (Edelman et al., 2014).*

If Services Are Unavailable, Pursue Program Development

Examine and Evaluate Similar Programs in Other Communities

- Basic information
- Purpose, goals
- Services available
- Funding
- Cost to participants
- Accessibility of services

Meet With Appropriate People to Discuss Findings (Survey, On-Site Visits); Address the Following

- Presence of community support
- Available expertise and technology in community
- Financial support

Identify Appropriate Community Sources of Assistance

- Hospital departments
- Health departments
- Faith-based organizations
- Chamber of commerce
- Health-care professionals
- Industry
- Private foundations
- Public assistance agencies
- Professional societies

Collaborate With University Faculty for Collaborative Grant Writing

R: *Grants are a reality in public health efforts (Allender et al., 2010).*

Plan the Program (Refer to Readiness for Enhanced Community Coping for Interventions for Community Planning)

If Services Are Available But Are Underutilized, Assess for (Bamberger et al., 2000)

System Barriers

- Hours of operation (inconvenient)
- Location of services (access, aesthetics, distance)
- Efficiency and atmosphere
- Cost
- Complicated appointment system
- Unfriendly

Personal Barriers
- Mistrust
- Competing life priorities
- Powerlessness
- Illiteracy
- Lacking resources (e.g., telephone, transportation, child care, finances)
- Unpredictable work schedule
- Language other than English

R: *Unless the barriers to accessing health-care services are identified and eliminated, these services will continue to be underused (Bamberger et al., 2000).*

Evaluate Vulnerable Population's Access to Health Care and Knowledge of Risk Factors

- Rural families, elderly
- Migrant workers
- New immigrants
- Homeless
- Those living below poverty level

R: *Access to care is both a distributive and social justice issue (Allender et al., 2010).*

Make a Priority of Ensuring That Basic Needs (Food, Shelter, Clothing, and Safety) Are Met Before Attempting to Address Higher Health Needs

R: *Physiologic needs must be met before a person can focus on meeting higher needs for personal well-being (*Maslow, 1971).*

Provide Information Regarding Illness Prevention, Health Promotion, and Health Services to Vulnerable Populations (e.g., Federally Funded Community Health Centers)

- Be sure reading material is appropriate for targeted group (e.g., reading level, language, pictures).
- Use posters, flyers.
- Select locations that the targeted populating uses regularly:
  - Grocery, convenience stores
  - Day care centers
  - School activities
  - Religious services
  - Laundromats
  - Community fairs
  - Meetings
  - Sporting events

R: *Vulnerable populations (poor, uninsured, ethnic minorities) report no regular source of care, no ambulatory visits within the preceding 12 months, and fair or poor health status (Agency for Healthcare Research and Quality, 2014). Vulnerable groups wait longer to obtain appointments to see a clinician, and they perceive the communication with their clinicians as less than desirable (Agency for Healthcare Research and Quality, 2014). They have higher premature death rates, high morbidities, low functional status, and low quality of life (Agency for Healthcare Research and Quality, 2014).*

Part 4

Health Promotion/Nursing Diagnoses

This section organizes all the health promotion/wellness diagnoses for individuals. *Readiness for Enhanced Self-Health Management* is a broad nursing diagnosis that can be useful, if a specific wellness diagnosis does not address the targeted health topic.

Health Promotion Diagnosis is "a clinical judgment concerning motivation and desire to increase well-being and to actualize human health potential. Health promotion may exist in individual, family group, or community" (Herdman & Kamitsura, 2014). A valid wellness nursing diagnosis has two requirements: (1) An individual has a desire for increased wellness in a particular area and (2) is currently functioning effectively in a particular area.

Wellness nursing diagnoses are one-part statements with no related factors. The goals established by the individual or group will direct their actions to enhance their health.

There is still confusion about the clinical usefulness of this type of diagnosis. This author does support that some of these diagnoses can be strengthened and are clinically useful, such as *Readiness for Enhanced Parenting* or *Readiness for Enhanced Community Coping*; whereas others, such as *Readiness for Enhanced Power*, *Readiness for Enhanced Urinary Elimination*, and other similar diagnoses, are questionable relative to clinical usefulness. Under each diagnosis, Author's Notes will elaborate on the clinical usefulness of the diagnosis.

Clinically, data that represent strengths can be important for nurses to know. These strengths can assist the nurse in selecting interventions to reduce or prevent a problem in another health pattern. Assessment of strengths is discussed in Chapter 6. If nurses want to designate strength, it should be documented as strength on the assessment form or care plan. If the individual desires assistance in promoting a higher level of function, *Readiness for Enhanced (specify)* would be useful in certain settings, such as schools, community centers, and assisted living facilities. Interested clinicians can use these health promotion/wellness diagnoses and are invited to share their work with NANDA as well as this author.

Key Concepts

- Healthy People 2020 has two major goals (http://healthypeople.gov/):
  - Increase quality and years of healthy life
  - Eliminate health disparities
- Health promotion addresses strategies to assist people to live at the highest level of well-being possible (Edelman, Kudzma, & Mandle, 2014).
- All individuals can be assisted to a healthier lifestyle, if motivated and informed. If an individual has deficits in his or her lifestyle, other nursing diagnoses apply, such as *Risk-Prone Health Behavior* or *Imbalanced Nutrition.*
- Some individuals regularly engage in healthy choices. These individuals may desire to increase the strength of these choices to be even healthier in one or more areas, such as decision making or nutrition.
- The nurse is an advocate for healthier lifestyles and personal behavior. Refer to Appendix C: Strategies to Promote Engagement of Individual/families for Healthier Outcomes.
- The nurse must be careful not to judge the overall health practices of the individual/family as barriers to increase wellness in a specific area. For example, a woman may smoke and consume a balanced, low-fat, low-carbohydrate diet; if she desires, she could improve her already nutritious diet. Her smoking habit can be addressed under *Risk-Prone Health Behavior.*

Health Promotion/Wellness Assessment (Carpenito-Moyet, 2007; Edelman, Kudzma, & Mandle, 2014; *Gordon, 2002)

Subjective Data

Health Perception–Health Management Pattern

Ask the individual to place one check next to the category in which they usually practice; place two checks for those they practice daily (*Breslow & Hron, 2004):

- Three meals a day at regular times and no snacking
- Breakfast every day
- Moderate exercise two or three times a week
- 7 to 8 hours of sleep, not more or less
- No smoking
- Moderate weight
- No alcohol or in moderation

What Is His or Her Perception of Their Overall Health?

- What personal practices maintain their health?
- What sources is accessed to maintain or improve their healthy lifestyle?
- How could he or she be healthier?

Nutrition–Metabolic Pattern

- What is the person's body mass index?
- Typical daily fluid intake—What? How much?
- Supplements (vitamins, types of snacks)
- Daily intake of whole grain or enriched breads, legumes, cereals, rice, or pasta
- Three servings of fruit/fruit juice daily
- Unlimited raw, or five to eight servings of cooked nonstarch, vegetables daily
- Skim or low-fat dairy products
- Meats and poultry trimmed of fat and skin
- Caffeine intake
- No fried foods/snacks
- No or limited (fewer than two) sugar drinks (e.g., soda, ice tea, juices)
- Do you see a relationship among stress and tension, emotional upsets, and your eating habits?

Elimination Pattern

- Bowel elimination pattern? (Describe.)
  - Frequency (every 2 to 3 days), character (soft, bulky)
- Urinary elimination pattern? (Describe.)
  - Character (amber, yellow, straw-colored)

Activity–Exercise Pattern

- Exercise pattern? (Type, frequency)
- Leisure activities? (Frequency)
- Energy level? (High, moderate, adequate, low)
- Are there barriers to exercising?
- What are the five things that you do to play?
- What things do you do that make you feel good?

Sleep–Rest Pattern

- Satisfied and rested?
- Average hours of sleep per night
- Relaxation periods? (How often? How long?)

Cognitive–Perceptual Pattern

- Satisfied with
  - Decision making?
  - Memory?
  - Ability to learn?
- Describe briefly your educational background.

Self-Perception–Self-Concept Pattern

- Describe how you feel about
  - Yourself?
  - Your body? Changes?
- Do you have trouble expressing anger, sadness, happiness, love, and/or sexuality?
- What are your major strengths or personal qualities?
- What are your weaknesses or negative aspects?
- In your life right now, what is your most meaningful activity?
- How many more years do you expect to live, and how do you think you will die?
- How do you imagine your future?
- What would you like to accomplish in your future? Are there changes you need to make to accomplish this?

List the Most Important Events, Crises, Transitions, and/or Changes (Positive or Negative) in Your Life

- Take time to reflect on how they affected you. Place an asterisk in front of one or two that were especially important.

Roles–Relationships Pattern

- Satisfied with job? Need a change?
- Satisfied with role responsibilities?
- Describe your relationship with your family/partner.
- Describe your friendships (close, casual).
- List the most important people in your life right now and why they are important.

Sexuality–Reproductive Pattern

- Is sex an important aspect of your life?
- Are you currently in a sexual relationship?
- What would you want to change about your current sexual relationship?

Coping–Stress Tolerance Pattern

- List the most regular sources of stress in your life. How could you make them less stressful?
- How do you usually respond to stressful situations (get angry, withdraw, take it out on others, get sick, drink, eat)?
- What situations make you feel calm or relaxed?
- What situations make you feel anxious or upset? What can you do to make yourself feel better?

Values–Beliefs Pattern

- Write 10 things you most value in life.
- Would you describe yourself as a religious or spiritual person?
- How do your beliefs help you?

READINESS FOR ENHANCED BREASTFEEDING*

NANDA-I Definition

A pattern of providing milk to an infant or young child directly from the breasts, which can be strengthened

Defining Characteristics

Major (Must Be Present)

Mother's ability to position infant at breast to promote a successful latch-on response
Infant content after feeding
Regular and sustained suckling/swallowing at the breast
Infant weight patterns appropriate for age
Effective mother–infant communication patterns* (infant cues, maternal interpretation, and response)

Minor (May Be Present)

Signs or symptoms of oxytocin release are present* (let-down or milk ejection reflex).
Adequate infant elimination patterns for age*
Eagerness of infant to nurse*
Maternal verbalization of satisfaction with breastfeeding

Key Concepts

Refer to *Ineffective Breastfeeding*.

Focus Assessment Criteria

Refer to *Ineffective Breastfeeding*.

Goal

NOC
Knowledge: Breastfeeding

The mother will report an increase in confidence and satisfaction with breastfeeding, as evidenced by the following indicator:

- Identifies two new strategies (specify) to enhance breastfeeding

Interventions

- Refer to the Internet for sites for resources and information on breastfeeding.
- Refer to *Ineffective Breastfeeding* for interventions to enhanced breastfeeding.

READINESS FOR ENHANCED CHILDBEARING PROCESS

NANDA-I Definition

A pattern of preparing for and maintaining a healthy pregnancy, childbirth process, and care of the newborn that is sufficient for ensuring well-being and can be strengthened

Defining Characteristics*

During Pregnancy

Reports appropriate prenatal lifestyle (e.g., nutrition, elimination, sleep, body movement, exercise, personal hygiene)
Reports appropriate physical preparations
Reports managing unpleasant symptoms in pregnancy
Demonstrates respect for unborn baby
Reports a realistic birth plan
Prepares and seeks necessary newborn care items
Seeks necessary knowledge (e.g., of labor and delivery, newborn care)
Reports availability of support systems
Has regular prenatal health visits

During Labor and Delivery

Reports lifestyle (e.g., diet, elimination, sleep, body movement, personal hygiene) that is appropriate for the stage of labor
Responds appropriately to the onset of labor
Is proactive during labor and delivery
Uses relaxation techniques appropriate for the stage of labor
Demonstrates attachment behavior to the newborn baby
Uses support systems appropriately

After Birth

Demonstrates appropriate baby-feeding techniques
Demonstrates appropriate breast care
Demonstrates attachment behavior to the baby
Demonstrates basic baby care techniques
Provides safe environment for the baby
Reports appropriate postpartum lifestyle (e.g., diet, elimination, sleep, body movement, exercise, personal hygiene)
Utilizes support system appropriately

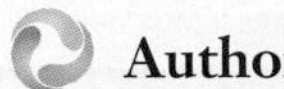

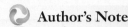

Author's Note

This NANDA-I nursing diagnosis represents the comprehensive care that is needed to promote the following: healthy pregnancy, childbirth and the postpartum process, enhanced relationships (mother, father, infant, and siblings), and optimal care of the newborn. This care is beyond the scope possible in this text. Refer to a text about maternal-child health for the specific interventions for this diagnosis.

READINESS FOR ENHANCED COMFORT

NANDA-I Definition

A pattern of ease, relief, and transcendence in physical, psychospiritual, environmental, and/or social dimensions that is sufficient for well-being and can be strengthened

Defining Characteristics*

Expresses desire to enhance comfort
Expresses desire to enhance feeling of contentment
Expresses desire to enhance relaxation
Expresses desire to enhance resolution of complaints

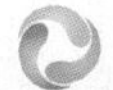

Author's Note

This diagnosis is general and therefore does not direct specific interventions. It encompasses physical, psychological, spiritual, environmental, and social dimensions. It would be more clinically useful to focus on a particular dimension, such as *Readiness for Enhanced Spiritual Well-Being*.

READINESS FOR ENHANCED COMMUNICATION

NANDA-I Definition

A pattern of exchanging information and ideas with others that is sufficient for meeting one's needs and life's goals, and can be strengthened

Defining Characteristics*

Able to speak and/or write a language
Expresses feelings
Expresses satisfaction with ability to share ideas with others
Expresses satisfaction with ability to share information with others
Expresses willingness to enhance communication
Forms phrases

Forms sentences
Forms words
Interprets nonverbal cures appropriately
Uses nonverbal cues appropriately

Author's Note

This diagnosis represents an individual with good communications skills. Interventions to enhance communication skills can be found in Section 2 Part 1 in *Impaired Communication* and *Impaired Verbal Communication*.

READINESS FOR ENHANCED COPING

NANDA-I Definition

A pattern of cognitive and behavioral efforts to manage demands that are sufficient for well-being and can be strengthened

Defining Characteristics*

Acknowledges power
Aware of possible environmental changes
Defines stressors as manageable
Seeks knowledge of new strategies
Seeks social support
Uses a broad range of emotion-oriented strategies
Uses a broad range of problem-oriented strategies
Uses spiritual resources

Key Concepts

Refer to *Stress Overload* for principles of effective coping.

Focus Assessment Criteria

Refer to Health Promotion/Wellness Assessment under Self-Perception–Self-Concept Pattern.

Goal

NOC
Acceptance: Health Status, Self-Awareness. Coping, Social Interaction Skills

The individual will report increased satisfaction with coping with stressors, as evidenced by the following indicator:

- Identifies two new strategies (specify) to enhance coping with stressors

Interventions

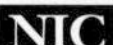

NIC
Coping Enhancement, Anticipatory Guidance, Self-Efficacy Enhancement

If Anxiety Diminishes One's Effective Coping, Teach

- Abdominal relaxation breathing
- Abdominal breathing while imagining a peaceful scene (e.g., ocean, woods, mountains)
- To imagine the feel of the warm sand on your feet, the sun on your face, and the sound of water

R: *Relaxation techniques provide an opportunity to regroup prior to reacting.*

Explain Reframing (Halter, 2014)

- Reassess the situation; ask yourself:
  - What positive thing can come out of the situation?
  - What did I learn?
  - What would I do differently next time?
  - What might be going on with my (boss, partner, sister, friend) that would cause him or her to say or do that?
  - Is she or he stressed out or having problems?

R: *Reframing provides one with the opportunity to analyze and consider reasons for behavior and alternative options.*

Acknowledge Stress-Reducing Tips for Living (Halter, 2014)

- Exercise regularly, at least three times weekly
- Reduce caffeine intake
- Engage in meaningful, satisfying work
- Do not let work dominate your life
- Guard your personal freedom
- Choose your friends; associate with gentle people
- Live with and love whom you choose
- Structure your time as you see fit
- Set your own life goals

R: *The stressors of life are heightened when others decide how one should live his or her life.*

- Refer to the Internet for sites for resources and information about stress reduction techniques.

READINESS FOR ENHANCED DECISION MAKING

NANDA-I Definition

A pattern of choosing a course of action that is sufficient for meeting short- and long-term health-related goals and can be strengthened

Defining Characteristics*

Expresses desire to enhance decision making
Expresses desire to enhance congruency of decisions with personal and/or sociocultural values and goals
Expresses desire to enhance risk–benefit analysis of decisions
Expresses desire to enhance understanding of choices and the meaning of the choices
Expresses desire to enhance use of reliable evidence for decisions

Key Concepts

Refer to *Decisional Conflict* for principles of effective decision making.

Focus Assessment Criteria

Refer to Health Promotion/Wellness Assessment under Cognitive–Perceptual Pattern.

Goal

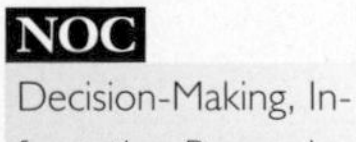

Decision-Making, Information Processing

The individual/group will report increased satisfaction with decision making, as evidenced by the following indicator:

- Identifies two new strategies (specify) to enhance decision making

Interventions

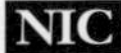
Decision-Making Support, Mutual Goal Setting

- Refer to Interventions for *Decisional Conflict.*
- Refer to the Internet for sites for resources and information about decision making.

READINESS FOR ENHANCED EMANCIPATED DECISION MAKING

Definition

A process of choosing a health-care decision that includes personal knowledge and/or consideration of social norms, which can be strengthened

Defining Characteristics

Expresses desire to enhance ability to choose health-care options that best fit current lifestyle
Expresses desire to enhance ability to enact chosen health-care option
Expresses desire to enhance ability to understand all available health-care options
Expresses desire to enhance ability to verbalize own opinion without constraint
Expresses desire to enhance comfort to verbalize health-care options in the presence of others
Expresses desire to enhance confidence in decision making
Expresses desire to enhance confidence to discuss health-care options openly
Expresses desire to enhance decision making
Expresses desire to enhance privacy to discuss health-care options

Key Concepts

An individual is ready to make an emancipated decision making when she recognizes the social norms placed on health-care options and uses her personal knowledge in a flexible environment to arrive at a health-care option.

Focus Assessment Criteria

Refer to *Impaired Emancipated Decision Making.*

Goals

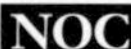
Refer to *Impaired Emancipated Decision Making.*

The individual will report making an emancipated decision about a health-care issue, as evidenced by the following indicators:

- Is satisfied with the decision
- Used her personal knowledge to assist her to arrive at the decision
- Was able to arrive at the decision in a flexible environment without oppressive forces from others
- Chosen fits in best with the individual's lifestyle
- Uninhibited when telling others about the option he or she chose
- Satisfied with the chosen option
- Carries through with the option that was chosen

Interventions

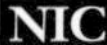
Refer to *Impaired Emancipated Decision Making.*

- Refer to *Impaired Emancipated Decision Making.*

READINESS FOR ENHANCED FLUID BALANCE

NANDA-I Definition

A pattern of equilibrium between the fluid volume and the chemical composition of body fluids that is sufficient for meeting physical needs and can be strengthened

Defining Characteristics

Expresses willingness to enhance fluid balance

Stable weight
Moist mucous membranes
Food and fluid intake adequate for daily needs
Straw-colored urine with specific gravity within normal limits
Good tissue turgor
No excessive thirst
Urine output appropriate for intake
No evidence of edema or dehydration

Author's Note

If an individual has a pattern of equilibrium between the fluid volume and the chemical composition of body fluids that is sufficient for meeting physical needs, how can this be strengthened? Would it be more useful to focus on education under the diagnosis *Risk for Deficient Fluid Volume*?

Key Concepts

Refer to *Imbalanced Nutrition* and *Deficient Fluid Volume* for key concepts of balanced nutrition and fluid volume.

Goal

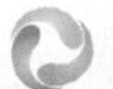

Fluid Balance, Hydration, Electrolyte Balance

The individual will report increased satisfaction with fluid balance, as evidenced by the following indicator:

- Identifies two new strategies (specify) to enhance fluid balance

Interventions

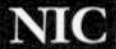

Fluid/Electrolyte Management

- Refer to Interventions for *Deficient Fluid Balance.*
- Refer to the Internet for sites for resources and information about nutrition.

READINESS FOR ENHANCED HEALTH MANAGEMENT

Definition

A pattern of regulating and integrating into daily living a therapeutic regimen for the treatment of illness and its sequelae, which can be strengthened

Defining Characteristics

Expresses desire to enhance

Choices of daily living for meeting goals
Management of illness

Management of prescribed regimens
Management of risk factors
Management of symptoms
Immunization/vaccination status

Key Concepts

Refer to *Ineffective Health Management* for principles of Health Management.

Focus Assessment Criteria

Refer to Health Promotion/Wellness Assessment under Health Perception–Health Management Pattern.

Goal

NOC
Refer to *Ineffective Health Management.*

The individual will report increased hope, as evidenced by the following indicator:

- Identifies two new strategies (specify) to manage their condition

Interventions

NIC
Refer to *Ineffective Health Management.*

- Refer to *Ineffective Health Management* for interventions to promote enhanced management of the condition.

READINESS FOR ENHANCED HOPE

NANDA-I Definition

A pattern of expectations and desires for mobilizing energy on one's own behalf that is sufficient for well-being and can be strengthened

Defining Characteristics*

Expresses desire to enhance congruency of expectations with desires
Expresses desire to enhance ability to set achievable goals
Expresses desire to enhance problem solving to meet goals
Expresses desire to enhance belief in possibilities
Expresses desire to enhance spirituality and sense of meaning to life
Expresses desire to enhance interconnectedness with others
Expresses desire to enhance hope

Key Concepts

Refer to *Hopelessness* for principles of hope.

Focus Assessment Criteria

Refer to Health Promotion/Wellness Assessment under Self-Perception–Self-Concept Pattern.

Goal

NOC
Refer to *Hopelessness.*

The individual will report increased hope, as evidenced by the following indicator:

- Identifies two new strategies (specify) to enhance hope

Interventions

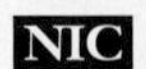

Refer to Hopelessness.

- Refer to *Hopelessness* for interventions to promote hope.

READINESS FOR ENHANCED ORGANIZED INFANT BEHAVIOR

NANDA-I Definition

A pattern of modulation of the physiologic and behavioral systems of functioning (i.e., autonomic, motor, state-organization, self-regulatory, and attention-interactional systems) in an infant that is sufficient for well-being and can be strengthened

Defining Characteristics (Blackburn & Vandenberg, 1993)

Autonomic System

Regulated color and respiration
Reduced visceral signals (e.g., smooth)
Reduces tremors, twitches
Digestive functioning, feeding tolerance

Motor System

Smooth, well-modulated posture and tone
Synchronous smooth movements with
  Hand/foot clasping
  Suck/suck searching
  Grasping
  Hand holding
  Hand-to-mouth activity
  Tucking

State System

Well-differentiated range of states
Clear, robust sleep states
Focused, shiny-eyed alertness with intent or animated facial expressions
Active self-quieting/consoling "ooh" face
Attentional smiling
Cooing

Author's Note

This diagnosis describes an infant who is responding to the environment with stable and predictable autonomic, motor, and state cues. The focus of interventions is to promote continued stable development and to reduce excess environmental stimuli that may stress the infant. Because this is a wellness diagnosis, the use of related factors is not needed. The nurse can write the diagnostic statement as *Readiness for Enhanced Organized Infant Behavior* as evidenced by ability to regulate autonomic, motor, and state systems to environmental stimuli.

Key Concepts

Refer to *Disorganized Infant Behavior*.

Focus Assessment Criteria

Objective Data

Refer to Defining Characteristics.

Reciprocal Interactions

Eye contact

Exploratory behavior
Mutual gazing
Easy consolation
Reaching toward
Attending to social stimuli

Goals

NOC

Newborn Adaptation, Neurologic Status, Preterm Infant Organization, Sleep, Comfort Level, Parent–Infant Attachment

The infant will continue age-appropriate growth and development and not experience excessive environmental stimuli. The parent(s) will demonstrate handling that promotes stability, as evidenced by the following indicators:

- Describes developmental needs of infant
- Describes early signs of stress of exhaustion
- Demonstrates
  - Gentle, soothing touch
  - Melodic tone of voice, coos
  - Mutual gazing
  - Rhythmic movements
  - Acknowledgment of all baby's vocalizations
  - Recognition of soothing qualities of actions

Interventions

NIC

Environmental Management: Comfort Neurologic Monitoring, Sleep Enhancement, Newborn Care, Parent Education: Newborn Positioning, Pain Management

Explain to Parents the Effects of Excess Environmental Stress on the Infant

Provide a List of Signs of Stress for Their Infant; Refer to *Disorganized Infant Behavior* for a List of Signs

Teach Parents to Terminate Stimulation If Infant Shows Signs of Stress

R: *Premature infants must adapt to the extrauterine environment with underdeveloped body systems (*Vandenberg, 1990). These infants can tolerate only one activity at a time (*Blackburn, 1993).*

Model Developmental Interventions

- Offer only when the infant is alert (if possible, show parents examples of alert and not alert).
- Begin with one stimulus at a time (touch, voice).
- Provide intervention for a short time.
- Increase interventions according to infant's cues.
- Provide frequent, short interventions instead of infrequent, long-term ones.
- Stimulation (visual, auditory, vestibular, tactile, olfactory, gustatory)
- Periods of alertness
- Sleep requirements

R: *Parents need to understand that they must pace the type, amount, intensity, and timing of stimulation. Behavioral cues from the infant should guide these decisions (Lawhon, 2002).*

Explain, Model, and Observe Parents Engaging in Developmental Interventions

Visual
- Eye contact
- Face-to-face experiences
- High-contrast colors, geometric shapes (e.g., black and white shapes on paper mobile); up to 4 weeks, simple mobiles of four dessert-size paper plates with stripes, four-square checkerboards, a black dot, and a simple bull's eye hung 10 to 13 inches from baby's eyes.

Auditory
- Use high-pitched vocalizations.
- Play classical music softly.
- Use a variety of voice inflections.

- Avoid loud talking.
- Call infant by name.
- Avoid monotone speech patterns.

Vestibular (Movement)
- Rock baby in chair.
- Place infant in sling and rock.
- Close infant's fist around a soft toy.
- Slowly change position during handling.
- Provide head support.

Tactile
- Use firm, gentle touch as initial approach.
- Use skin-to-skin contact in a warm room.
- Provide alternative textures (e.g., sheepskin, velvet, satin).
- Avoid stroking if responses are disorganized.

Olfactory
- Wear a light perfume.

Gustatory
- Allow nonnutritive sucking (e.g., pacifier, hand in mouth).

R: *Individualized developmental care can improve developmental outcomes, weight gain, sleep, motor function, pain tolerance, and feeding. Parents are helped to understand the infant's needs, which will improve attachment and reduce fears (Pillitteri, 2014).*

Promote Adjustment and Stability in Caregiving Activities (Blackburn & Vandenberg, 1993; *Merenstein & Gardner, 1998)

Waking
- Enter room slowly.
- Turn on light and open curtains slowly.
- Avoid waking baby if he or she is asleep.

Changing
- Keep room warm.
- Gently change position; contain limbs during movement.
- Stop changing if infant is irritable.

Feeding
- Time feedings with alert states.
- Hold infant close and, if needed, swaddle in a blanket.

Bathing
- Ventral openness may be stressful. Cover body parts not being bathed.
- Proceed slowly; allow for rest.
- Offer pacifier or hand to suck.
- Eliminate unnecessary noise.
- Use a soft, soothing voice.

R: *To minimize stress and conserve energy, patterns of routine care should be adhered to (Blackburn & Vandenberg, 1993).*

Explain the Need to Reduce Environmental Stimuli When Taking the Infant Outside

- Shelter eyes from light.
- Swaddle the infant so his or her hands can reach the mouth. Protect from loud noises.

R: *To minimize stress and conserve energy, patterns of routine care should be adhered to (Blackburn & Vandenberg, 1993).*

Praise Parent(s) for Interaction Patterns; Point out Infant's Engaging Responses

R: *Parental confidence can be increased and thus enhance bonding and nurturing behavior at home (Pillitteri, 2014).*

Initiate Health Teaching and Referrals, as Needed

- Explain that developmental interventions will change with maturity. Refer to *Delayed Growth and Development* for specific age-related developmental needs.
- Provide parent(s) with resources for assistance at home (e.g., community resources).
- Refer to the Internet for sites for resources and information about preterm newborns.

R: *Families of preterm infants need continued support and anticipatory guidance to improve the transition from the neonatal intensive care unit to home (Pillitteri, 2014).*

READINESS FOR ENHANCED KNOWLEDGE (SPECIFY)

NANDA-I Definition

A pattern of cognitive information related to a specific topic, or its acquisition, that is sufficient for meeting health-related goals and can be strengthened

Defining Characteristics*

Expresses an interest in learning
Explains knowledge of the topic
Behaviors congruent with expressed knowledge
Describes previous experiences pertaining to the topic

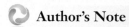

Author's Note

Readiness for Enhanced Knowledge is broad. All nursing diagnoses—actual, risk, and wellness—seek to enhance knowledge. Once the specific area of enhanced knowledge is identified, refer to that specific diagnosis, for example, *Readiness for Enhanced Nutrition, Grieving, Risk for Ineffective Parenting, Deficient Health Behavior*, or *Ineffective Therapeutic Regimen Management*. *Readiness for Enhanced Knowledge* is not needed because it lacks the reason for the desired or needed knowledge.

READINESS FOR ENHANCED NUTRITION

NANDA-I Definition

A pattern of nutrient intake that is sufficient for meeting metabolic needs and can be strengthened

Defining Characteristics*

Expresses willingness to enhance nutrition
Eats regularly
Consumes adequate food and fluid
Expresses knowledge of healthy food and fluid choices
Follows an appropriate standard for intake (e.g., MyPlate or American Diabetic Association guidelines)
Safe preparation and storage of food and fluids
Attitude toward eating and drinking is congruent with health goals

Key Concepts

Refer to *Imbalanced Nutrition* for principles of balanced nutrition.

Focus Assessment Criteria

Refer to Health Promotion/Wellness Assessment under Nutrition–Metabolic Pattern.

Goal

NOC
Nutritional Status, Teaching Nutrition

The individual/group will report an increase in balanced nutrition, as evidenced by the following indicator:

- Identifies two new strategies (specify) to enhance nutrition

Interventions

- Refer to Internet for sites for resources and information about nutrition:
  - www.myplate.gov
  - www.health.gov/dietaryguidelines
  - www.lifestyleadvantage.org

READINESS FOR ENHANCED POWER

NANDA-I Definition

A pattern of participating knowingly in change that is sufficient for well-being and can be strengthened

Defining Characteristics*

Expresses readiness to enhance awareness of possible changes to be made
Expresses readiness to enhance freedom to perform actions for change
Expresses readiness to enhance identification of choices that can be made for change
Expresses readiness to enhance involvement in creating change
Expresses readiness to enhance knowledge for participation in change
Expresses readiness to enhance participation in choices for daily living and health
Expresses readiness to enhance power

Key Concepts

Refer to *Powerlessness* for principles of power and locus of control.

Focus Assessment Criteria

Refer to *Powerlessness*.

Goal

NOC
Health Beliefs: Perceived Control, Participation: Health Care Decisions

The individual/group will report increased power, as evidenced by the following indicator:

- Identifies two new strategies (specify) to enhance power

Interventions

NIC
Decision-making Support, Self-responsibility Facilitation, Teaching: Individual

- Refer to *Powerlessness* for strategies to increase power.

READINESS FOR ENHANCED RELATIONSHIP

NANDA-I Definition

A pattern of mutual partnership that is sufficient to provide each other's needs and can be strengthened

Defining Characteristics*

Reports desire to enhance communication between partners
Reports satisfaction with sharing of information and ideas between partners
Reports satisfaction with fulfilling physical and emotional needs by one's partner
Demonstrates mutual respect between partners
Meets developmental goals appropriate for family life stage
Demonstrates well-balanced autonomy and collaboration between partners
Demonstrates mutual support in daily activities between partners; partners identify each other as a key person
Demonstrates understanding of partner's insufficiencies (physical, social)
Express satisfaction with complementary relation between partners

Goal

The individual will report increased satisfaction with partnership, as evidenced by the following indicator:

- Identifies two new strategies (specify) to enhance partnership

Interventions

Teach to (*Murray, Zentner, & Yakimo, 2009)

- Talk daily about feelings
- Elicit feelings of partner
- Explore "what if . . ." conversations

R: *Regular sharing of feelings provides opportunities to solve small problems before they escalate.*

Vary Family Responsibilities, Schedule, Chores, and Roles

R: *This can prepare the family to adapt during times of crises.*

Engage Partner to Discuss Individual Problems and Validate Solutions or Ask for Partner's Opinion About the Problem

R: *This sharing promotes mutual respect.*

Establish a Support System That Can Help When Needed; Provide Such Support to Other Families or Individuals in Need

R: *Outside support is needed during crises.*

During Times of High Stress or Crises, Share Feelings of Guilt, Anger, or Helplessness

R: *Discussion of feelings about the situation clarifies that the stress is situation related not about the partner.*

Engage in Activities Together as Partners, Family

R: *Isolating behaviors can increase fears and anger.*

Refer to the Internet for Sites and Resources for Coping With Difficult Family Situations (e.g., Death of Member, Ill Family Member)

READINESS FOR ENHANCED RELIGIOSITY

NANDA-I Definition

A pattern of reliance on religious beliefs and/or participation in rituals of a particular faith tradition that is sufficient for well-being and can be strengthened

Defining Characteristics

Expresses a desire to strengthen religious belief patterns
- Comfort or religion in the past
- Questions harmful belief patterns
- Rejects belief patterns that are harmful
- Requests assistance in expanding religious options
- Requests assistance to increase participation in prescribed religious beliefs
- Requests forgiveness
- Requests reconciliation
- Requests meeting with religious leaders/facilitators
- Requests religious materials, experiences, or both

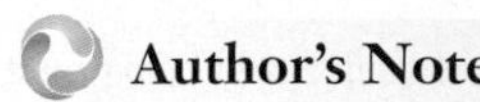

Author's Note

This diagnosis represents a variety of foci. Request for forgiveness may be related to an actual nursing diagnosis such as *Grieving*, *Ineffective Individual Coping*, or *Compromised Family Coping*. Further assessment is needed for interventions. Refer to *Impaired Religiosity* in Section 2, Part 1, for additional information.

READINESS FOR ENHANCED RESILIENCE

NANDA-I Definition

A pattern of positive responses to an adverse situation or crisis that is sufficient for optimizing human potential and can be strengthened

Defining Characteristics*

- Access to resources
- Effective use of conflict-management strategies
- Expresses desire to enhance resilience
- Identifies support systems
- Involvement in activities
- Presence of a crisis
- Sets goals
- Uses effective communication skills
- Verbalizes self-control
- Demonstrates positive outlook
- Enhances personal coping skills
- Identifies available resources
- Increases positive relationships with others
- Makes progress toward goals
- Maintains safe environment
- Takes responsibilities for actions
- Verbalizes an enhanced sense of control

Related Factors

Demographics that increase the chance of maladjustment
- Drug used
- Gender
- Inconsistent parenting
- Low intelligence
- Low maternal education
- Large family size
- Minority status

Parental mental illness
Poor impulse control
Poverty
Psychological disorders
Condition
Violence

Vulnerability factors that encompass indices that exacerbate the negative reflects of the risk

Author's Note

This NANDA-I diagnosis focuses on the concept of resilience. Resilience is a strength that allows one to persevere and overcome difficulties. When faced with a crisis or problem, resilient people respond constructively with solutions or effective adaptation. Resilience is not a nursing diagnosis. It is an important and vital characteristic that can be nurtured and taught to children to assist them to cope with problematic life events.

The Defining Characteristics describe enhanced or effective coping. In contrast, the Related Factors are contributing factors for ineffective coping.

This author recommends

- Using *Risk for Infective Coping* related to the Related Factors listed earlier to assist someone to prevent ineffective coping
- Using *Ineffective Coping* related to the above Related Factors if Defining Characteristics of *Ineffective Coping* exist. (Refer to Section 2 under *Ineffective Coping* for specific defining characteristics.)
- Referring to the interventions for promoting resiliency in children and adults. (Refer to Index under resiliency for specific pages.)

READINESS FOR ENHANCED SELF-CARE

NANDA-I Definition

A pattern of performing activities for oneself that helps to meet health-related goals and can be strengthened

Defining Characteristics*

Expresses a desire to enhance independence in maintaining life
Expresses desire to enhance independence in maintaining health
Expresses desire to enhance knowledge of strategies of self-care
Expresses a desire to enhance responsibility for self-care
Expresses desire to enhance self-care

Author's Note

This diagnosis focuses more on improving self-care activities. Refer to *Self-Care Deficits* for interventions to improve self-care.

READINESS FOR ENHANCED SELF-CONCEPT

NANDA-I Definition

A pattern of perceptions or ideas about the self that is sufficient for well-being and can be strengthened

DefiningCharacteristics*

Expresses willingness to enhance self-concept
Expresses satisfaction with thoughts about self, sense of worthiness, role performance, body image, and personal identity

Actions are congruent with expressed feelings and thoughts
Expresses confidence in abilities
Accepts strengths and limitations

Key Concepts

Refer to *Disturbed Self-Concept* for principles related to self-concept.

Focus Assessment Criteria

Refer to Health Promotion/Wellness Assessment under Self-Perception–Self-Concept Pattern.

Goal

NOC
Quality of Life, Self-Esteem, Coping

The individual will report increased self-concept in (specify situation), as evidenced by the following indicator:

- Identifies two new strategies (specify) to enhance self-concept

Interventions

NIC
Hope Instillation, Values Clarification, Coping Enhancement

- Refer to *Disturbed Self-Concept* for interventions to improve self-concept.

READINESS FOR ENHANCED HEALTH MANAGEMENT

NANDA-I Definition

A pattern of regulating and integrating into daily living a therapeutic regimen for the treatment of illness and its sequelae that is sufficient for meeting health-related goals and can be strengthened

Defining Characteristics*

Expresses desire to manage the illness (e.g., treatment and prevention of sequelae)
Choices of daily living are appropriate for meeting goals (e.g., treatment, prevention)
Expresses little difficulty with prescribed regimens
Describes reduction of risk factors
No unexpected acceleration of illness symptoms

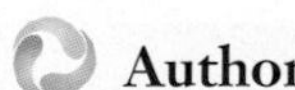

Author's Note

This diagnosis can be used to focus on a personal or lifestyle change in a specific area that is effective and can be enhanced to increase management of an illness.

Key Concepts

Refer to *Ineffective Health Management*.

Focus Assessment Criteria

Subjective and Objective Data

Assess for Defining Characteristics

Is knowledgeable about
Illness/condition (severity, susceptibility to complications, prognosis, ability to cure it or control its progression)

Treatment/diagnostic studies
Preventive measures
Has a pattern of adherence to recommended health behaviors or regimen
Expresses a desire to increase the ability to manage condition (progression, sequelae)
Reports that symptoms of condition are stable or diminished

Goal

NOC
Adherence Behavior, Health Beliefs, Health Promoting Behaviors, Well-Being, Knowledge: specify

The individual will express a desire to move from wellness to a higher level of wellness in management of a disease for condition (specify) (e.g., nutrition, decision making), as evidenced by the following indicator:

- Identifies two new strategies (specify) to enhance management of a disease/condition

Interventions

NIC
Health Education, Risk Identification, Values Classification, Behavior Modification, Coping Enhancement, Knowledge: Health Resources

The following interventions are appropriate for any health promotion/wellness nursing diagnosis that focuses on lifestyle changes and choices, for example, *Readiness for Enhanced Nutrition*, *Parenting*, *Sleep*, *Breastfeeding*, *Family Coping*, and *Family Processes.* These areas of wellness and health promotion can be found readily in the self-help literature and on the Internet. Some of the interventions for the wellness diagnoses, such as *Readiness for Enhanced Grieving*, *Readiness for Enhanced Coping*, or *Readiness for Enhanced Decision Making* can be found in Section 2, Part 1, under the individual nursing diagnoses. For example, in *Decisional Conflict*, there are interventions that can promote better decision making even for someone already making good decisions.

Complete Assessment of One or More or All Functional Health Patterns as the Individual Desires

R: *This structured assessment provides the individual with an opportunity to focus on segments of their health behavior and/or lifestyle to judge their satisfaction or desire for enhancement.*

Renew Data With the Individual or Group

- Does the individual/group report good or excellent health?
- Does the individual desire to learn a behavior to maximize health in a specific pattern?

R: *Every day individuals decide what they are going to eat, whether they will exercise, and other lifestyle choices (*Bodenheimer, MacGregor, & Sharifi, 2005).*

Refer to Appendix C: Strategies to Promote Engagement of Individual/Families for Healthier Outcomes for interventions to Promote Health Literacy and Engagement

Encourage Select Only One Wellness Focus at a Time (e.g., Exercise, Decrease Intake of Carbohydrates, Increase Intake of Water)

R: *Addressing multiple behavioral changes at once is time consuming, which may discourage the change (*Bodenheimer et al., 2005).*

Refer to Educational Resources About a Particular Focus (Print, Online)

- Examples of generic databases/websites include the following:
  - www.seekwellness.com/wellness/
  - www.cdc.gov—Centers for Disease Control and Prevention
  - www.agingblueprint.org—focuses on aging well
  - www.nhlbi.nih.gov—US Department of Health and Human Services
  - www.ahrq.gov—US Preventive Services Task Force
  - www.health.gov—various health topics
  - www.nih.gov—National Institutes of Health
  - www.fda.gov—Food and Drug Administration
  - www.mbmi.org—Mind-Body Medical Institute
  - www.ahha.org—American Holistic Health Association

R: *Self-management tools for autonomous or highly motivated individuals are assistive technologies, such as smart treadmills, online education, and support groups, and self-help books that are used independently (Edelman, Kudzma, & Mandle, 2014).*

Advise to Contact the Nurse to Discuss the Outcome of Resource Review via Telephone or E-Mail

R: *Motivated, autonomous individuals can be supported via the telephone or e-mail, which is efficient and cost-effective for them (*Piette, 2005).*

Discuss the Strategies or Targeted Behavioral Changes; Have the Individual Record Realistic Goals and Time Frames That Are Highly Specific; Avoid Recommendations of "Exercise More" or "Eat Less"

- For example: Goal—I will reduce my daily intake of carbohydrates.
- Indicators—Reduce cookie intake from five to two each day.
- Change pasta to multigrain pasta.
- Reduce potato intake by 50% and replace with 50% root vegetables.

R: *To increase self-efficacy, the individual must be successful. Success is more predictable if goals and indicators are concrete and achievable (*Bodenheimer et al., 2005). Vague recommendations are subjective and ineffective (Waryasz & McDermott, 2010).*

In Primary Care, Ask the If You Can Contact Him or Her at Designated Intervals (Every Month, at 4 to 6 Months, at 1 Year); Call or E-Mail to Discuss Progress.

R: *All types of individuals, motivated or not, can benefit from the support from their health-care professional.*

Advise That This Process Can Be Repeated as They Desire in Other Functional Health Patterns

R: *Enhanced wellness can be a continuous, lifelong journey with the individual as navigator and the health-care professional as the travel agent.*

READINESS FOR ENHANCED SLEEP

NANDA-I Definition

A pattern of natural, periodic suspension of consciousness that provides adequate rest, sustains a desired lifestyle, and can be strengthened

Defining Characteristics*

Amount of sleep is congruent with developmental needs
Reports being rested after sleep
Expresses willingness to enhance sleep
Follows sleep routines that promote sleep habits
Uses medications to induce sleep on occasion

Key Concepts

Refer to Health Promotion/Wellness Assessment under Elimination Pattern.

Focus Assessment Criteria

Refer to *Disturbed Sleep Pattern*.

Goal

The individual will report satisfactory sleep pattern, as evidenced by the following indicator:

- Identifies two new strategies (specify) to enhance sleep

Interventions

Refer to *Disturbed Sleep Patterns* for strategies to promote sleep.

READINESS FOR ENHANCED SPIRITUAL WELL-BEING

NANDA-I Definition

A pattern of experiencing and integrating meaning and purpose in life through connectedness with self, others, art, music, literature, nature, and/or a power greater than oneself that is sufficient for well-being and can be strengthened.

Defining Characteristics (*Carson, 1998)

Inner strength that nurtures:
- Sense of awareness
- Inner peace
- Sacred source
- Unifying force
- Trust relationships

Intangible motivation and commitment directed toward ultimate values of love, meaning, hope, beauty, and truth

Trusts relations with or in the transcendent that provide bases for meaning and hope in life's experiences and love in one's relationships

Has meaning and purpose to existence

Key Concepts

- Growth in spirituality is a dynamic process in which an individual becomes increasingly aware of the meaning of, purpose of, and values in life (*Carson, 1999). Spiritual growth is a two-directional process: horizontal and vertical. The horizontal process increases the individual's awareness of the transcendent values inherent in all relationships and activities of life (*Carson, 1999). The vertical process moves the individual into a closer relationship with a higher being, as conceived by him or her. Carson illustrates that it is possible to develop spirituality through the horizontal process and not the vertical. For example, an individual can define his or her spirituality in terms of relationships, art, or music without a relationship with a higher being, just as an individual can focus his or her spirituality on a higher being and may not express spirituality through other avenues.
- Faith is necessary for spiritual growth, particularly for a relationship to a higher being. Hope is also critical for spiritual development and is integral to the horizontal and vertical processes (*Carson, 1999).
- Research suggests that HIV-positive individuals who are spiritually well and who find meaning and purpose in life are also hardier (*Carson & Green, 1992).
- Regardless of an individual's religion or lack of belief, the process of spiritual growth is similar. The religious foundations that guide the growth are different. When people are together on the level of spirituality, they meet on the level of the heart. On this level, all people are one. When the experiences are reframed into religious dogma, that is when disagreements begin (*Carson, 1999).
- Spirituality has been found especially important to caregivers of victims of chronic illness. Older individuals with strong spiritual connections adapt to losses associated with aging better than those who do not report these connections (Underwood, 2012).

Focus Assessment Criteria

Refer to Health Promotion/Wellness Assessment under Values–Beliefs Pattern.

Goals

NOC
Hope, Spiritual Well-Being

The individual will express enhanced spiritual harmony and wholeness, as evidenced by the following indicators:

- Maintains previous relationship with higher being
- Continues spiritual practices not detrimental to health

Interventions

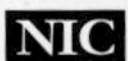

Spiritual Growth Facilitation, Spiritual Support, Hope

- Refer to the Internet for resources and information about spiritual health.

READINESS FOR ENHANCED URINARY ELIMINATION

NANDA-I Definition

A pattern of urinary functions that is sufficient for meeting eliminatory needs and can be strengthened

Defining Characteristics*

Expresses willingness to enhance urinary elimination.
Urine is straw colored with no odor.
Specific gravity is within normal limits.
Amount of output is within normal limits for age and other factors.
Positions self for emptying of bladder.
Fluid intake is adequate for daily needs.

Key Concepts

Refer to Health Promotion/Wellness Assessment under Elimination Pattern.

Focus Assessment Criteria

Refer to *Impaired Urinary Elimination*.

Goals

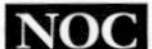

Fluid Balance, Hydration, Electrolyte Balance

The individual will report an increased balance in urinary elimination, as evidenced by the following indicator:

- Identifies two new strategies (specify) to enhance urinary elimination

Interventions

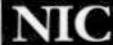

Education: Fluid/Electrolyte

- Refer to the Internet for sites for resources and information about fluid balance:

Section 3

Manual of Collaborative Problems

INTRODUCTION

This Manual of Collaborative Problems presents 55 specific collaborative problems grouped under nine generic collaborative problem categories. Previously, collaborative problems have been labeled as *Potential Complication: (specify)* or *PC (specify)*. The terminology for collaborative problems was revised in the 13th edition. These problems have been selected because of their high incidence or morbidity. Information on each generic collaborative problem is presented under the following subheads:

- Definition
- Author's Note: Discussion of the problem to clarify its clinical use
- Significant Laboratory/Diagnostic Assessment Criteria: Laboratory findings useful in monitoring

Discussions of the specific collaborative problems cover the following information:

- Definition
- High-Risk Populations
- Collaborative Goals: A statement specifying the nursing accountability for monitoring, for physiologic instability, and for providing interventions (nursing and medical) to maintain or restore stability. Indicators of physiologic stability have been added to evaluate the individual's condition.
- General Interventions and Rationales: These specifically direct the nurse to
  - Monitor for onset or early changes in status.
  - Initiate physician- or advanced practice nurse-prescribed interventions as indicated.
  - Initiate nurse-prescribed interventions as indicated.
  - Evaluate the effectiveness of these interventions.

Clinical Alerts

Clinical Alerts are found in the intervention section to advise the student nurse or nurse to take an immediate action because of a serious event or a change in the individual's physiologic status. For example, Notify Rapid Response Team.

Rationale

A rationale statement noted with an "**R**" and italics explains why a sign or symptom is present or gives the scientific explanation for why an intervention produces the desired response.

Carp's Cues

This feature provides additional information to challenge the reader to consider other options or to emphasize the severity of an event.

Keep in mind that for many of the collaborative problems in Section 3, associated nursing diagnoses also can be predicted to be present. For example, an individual with diabetes mellitus would receive care under the collaborative problem *Risk for Complications of Hypo/Hyperglycemia* along with the nursing diagnosis *Risk for Ineffective Health Maintenance related to insufficient knowledge of (specify)*; an individual with renal calculi would be under the collaborative problem *Risk for Complications of Renal Calculi* and also the nursing diagnosis *Risk for Ineffective Self-Health Management related to insufficient knowledge of prevention of recurrence, dietary restrictions, and fluid requirements.*

RISK FOR COMPLICATIONS OF CARDIAC/VASCULAR DYSFUNCTION

Risk for Complications of Cardiac/Vascular Dysfunction

Risk for Complications of Bleeding
Risk for Complications of Decreased Cardiac Output
Risk for Complications of Arrhythmias
Risk for Complications of Pulmonary Edema
Risk for Complications of Deep Vein Thrombosis/Pulmonary Embolism
Risk for Complications of Hypovolemia
Risk for Complications of Compartment Syndrome
Risk for Complications of Intra-Abdominal Hypertension

Definition

Describes a person experiencing or at high risk to experience various cardiac and/or vascular dysfunctions

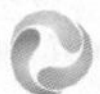

Author's Note

The nurse can use this generic collaborative problem to describe a person at risk for several types of cardiovascular problems. For example, all individuals in a critical care unit are vulnerable to cardiovascular dysfunction, using *Risk for Complications of Cardiac/Vascular Dysfunction* would direct nurses to monitor cardiovascular status for various problems, based on focus assessment findings. Nursing interventions for this individual would focus on detecting abnormal functioning and providing the appropriate response or interventions.

For an individual with a specific cardiovascular complication, the nurse would add the applicable collaborative problem to the individual's problem list, along with specific nursing interventions for that problem. For example, a Standard of Care for an individual after myocardial infarction could contain the collaborative problem *Risk for Complications of Cardiac/Vascular Dysfunction,* directing nurses to monitor cardiovascular status. If this individual later experienced a dysrhythmia, the nurse would add *Risk for Complications of Dysrhythmia* to the problem list, along with specific nursing management information (e.g., *Risk for Complications of Dysrhythmia related to myocardial infarction*). When the risk factors or etiology is not directly related to the primary medical diagnosis, the nurse still should add them, if known (e.g., *Risk for Complications of Hypo/Hyperglycemia related to diabetes mellitus* in an individual who has sustained myocardial infarction).

Significant Laboratory/Diagnostic Assessment Criteria

- Deep vein thrombosis diagnostic work-up:
  - D-Dimer—D-dimer is a substance in the blood that is often increased in people with deep vein thrombosis or PE
  - Compression ultrasonography—Compression ultrasonography uses sound waves to generate pictures of the structures inside the leg
  - Contrast venography
  - Magnetic resonance imaging (MRI)—Screening for risk of cardiovascular disease (Labs on Line, 2014)
- Lipid profile (LDL-C, HDL-C, cholesterol, triglycerides)
- High-sensitivity CRP—detects low concentrations of C-reactive protein, a marker of inflammation that is associated with atherosclerosis, among other conditions
- Lipoprotein (a)—an additional lipid test that may be used to identify an elevated level of lipoprotein (a), a modification to LDL-C that increases risk of atherosclerosis
- Cardiac biomarkers (Labs on Line, 2014)
  - Troponin—(elevated within a few hours of heart damage and remain elevated for up to 2 weeks)
  - CK-MB—(elevated when there is damage to the heart muscle cells)
  - BNP or NT-proBNP—(released by the body as a natural response to heart failure; increased levels of BNP, while not diagnostic for a heart attack, indicate an increased risk of cardiac complications in persons with acute coronary syndrome.)
- Serum potassium (fluctuates with diuretic therapy, parenteral fluid replacement)

- Serum calcium, magnesium, phosphate
- White blood cell count (elevated with inflammation)
- Erythrocyte sedimentation rate (elevated with inflammation, tissue injury)
- Arterial blood gas (ABG) values (lowered SaO_2 indicates hypoxemia; elevated pH, alkalosis; lowered pH, acidosis)
- Coagulation studies (elevated with anticoagulant and/or thrombolytic therapy or coagulopathies)
- Hemoglobin and hematocrit (elevated with polycythemia, lowered with anemia)
- Electrocardiograph with or without stress test
- Doppler ultrasonic flow meter
- Cardiac catheterization
- Intravascular ultrasonography (IVU)
- Electrophysiology studies
- Computed tomography (CT), ultrafast CT
- Magnetic resonance imaging
- Signal-averaged electrocardiography
- Echocardiography with or without stress test
- Phonocardiography
- Exercise (physical or chemical) electrocardiography (ECG)
- Perfusion imaging
- Infarct imaging
- Angiocardiography
- Holter monitoring
- Inflatable loop monitor

Risk for Complications of Bleeding

Definition

Describes a person experiencing or at high risk to experience a decrease in blood volume

High-Risk Populations

- Intraoperative status
- Postoperative status

Postprocedural cannulation of any arterial vessel, but particularly those at risk for retro-peritoneal bleed due to cannulation of femoral vessel

- Anaphylactic shock
- Trauma
- A history of bleeding disease or dysfunction
- Anticoagulant use, including over-the-counter use of aspirin or NSAIDs (nonsteroidal anti-inflammatory drugs)
- Chronic steroid use
- Acetaminophen use with associated liver dysfunction
- Anemia
- Liver disease
- Disseminated intravascular coagulation (DIC)
- Rupture of esophageal varices
- Dissecting aneurysms
- Trauma in pregnancy
- Pregnancy-related complications (Placenta previa, molar pregnancy, abruption placenta)
- Thrombolytic therapy

Collaborative Outcomes

The individual will be monitored for early signs and symptoms of bleeding and will receive collaborative interventions if indicated to restore physiologic stability.

Indicators of Physiologic Stability

- Alert, oriented, calm
- Urine output >0.5 mL/kg/hr
- Neutrophils 60% to 70%
- Red blood cells
  - Male: 4.6 to 5.9 million/mm^3
  - Female: 4.2 to 5.4 million/mm^3
- Platelets 150,000 to 400,000/mm^3
- No petechiae or purpura
- No gum or nasal bleeding
- Regular menses
- No headache
- Clear vision
- Intact coordination, facial symmetry, and muscle strength
- No splenomegaly
- Identify risk factors that can be reduced
- Relate early signs and symptoms of infection
  - Oxygen saturation >95%
  - Normal sinus rhythm
  - No chest pain
  - No life-threatening dysrhythmias
  - Skin warm and dry, usual skin color (appropriate for race)
  - Pulse: regular rhythm, rate 60 to 100 beats/min
  - Respirations 16 to 20 breaths/min
  - Blood pressure >90/60, <140/90 mm Hg, MAP >70, or CVP >11
  - Urine output >0.5 mL/kg/hr
  - Serum pH 7.35 to 7.45
  - Serum RCO$_2$ 35 to 45 mm Hg
  - Spo$_2$ goals >95% for those without history of lung disease
  - Breath sounds without evidence of new, abnormal sounds (rales)
  - No presence of distended neck veins (JVD)

Interventions and Rationales

Note that indicates provided measures to prevent thrombosis.

Monitor fluid status; evaluate

- Intake (parenteral and oral)
- Output and other losses (urine, drainage, and vomiting), nasogastric tube
- Increase monitoring of urine output to hourly.

R: *Decreased blood volume reduces blood to kidneys, which decreases the glomerular filtration rate (GFR) causing a decrease urine output. When blood flow to the kidneys is less than 20% to 25% of normal, ischemic damage occurs (Grossman & Porth, 2014). Decreased urine output is an early sign of bleeding/hypovolemia*

Monitor for signs and symptoms of bleeding dependent on site

- Integumentary system:
  - Petechiae
  - Ecchymoses
  - Hematomas
  - Oozing from venipuncture sites
  - Cyanotic patches on arms/legs
- Increase in bleeding from surgical wound
- Eyes and ears:
  - Visual disturbances
  - Periorbital edema
  - Subconjunctival hemorrhage
  - Ear pain

- Nose, mouth, and throat:
  - Petechiae
  - Epistaxis
  - Tender or bleeding gums
- Cardiopulmonary system:
  - Crackles and wheezes
  - Stridor and dyspnea
  - Tachypnea and cyanosis
  - Hemoptysis
- Gastrointestinal system:
  - Pain
  - Blood streaks in stool/emesis
  - Bleeding around rectum
  - Occult blood in stools
  - Dark stools
- Genitourinary system:
  - Increased menses
  - Decreased urine output
- Musculoskeletal system:
  - Painful joints
- Central nervous system:
  - Mental status changes
  - Vertigo
  - Seizures
  - Restlessness

Monitor for signs and symptoms of shock

- Increased pulse rate with normal or slightly decreased blood pressure, narrowing pulse pressure, decrease in mean or mean arterial pressure (MAP)
- Urine output <5 mL/kg/hr
- Restlessness, agitation, decreased mentation
- Increased respiratory rate, thirst
- Diminished peripheral pulses
- Cool, pale, moist, or cyanotic skin
- Decreased oxygenation saturation (SaO_2, SvO_2); pulmonary artery pressures, right atrial pressure, wedge/occlusion pressure, cardiac output/index
- Decreased hemoglobin/hematocrit
- Decreased central venous pressure
- Capillary refill >3 seconds (indicates poor tissue perfusion)

R: *The compensatory response to decreased circulatory volume aims to increase oxygen delivery through increased heart and respiratory rates and decreased peripheral circulation (manifested by diminished peripheral pulses and cool skin). Decreased oxygen to the brain alters mentation. Decreased circulation to the kidneys leads to decreased urine output. Hemoglobin and hematocrit values decline if bleeding is significant (Grossman & Porth, 2014).*

If shock occurs, place the individual in the supine position unless contraindicated (e.g., head injury)

R: *This position increases blood return (preload) to the heart.*

Insert an IV line; use a large-bore catheter if blood or large volume fluid replacement is anticipated. Initiate appropriate protocols for shock (e.g., vasopressor therapy). Refer also to *Risk for Complications of Acidosis* or *Risk for Complications of Alkalosis*, if indicated, for more information

R: *Protocols aim to increase peripheral resistance and elevate blood pressure.*

Contact physician, PA, or advanced practice nurse with assessment data that may indicate bleeding and to replace fluid losses at a rate sufficient to maintain urine output >0.5 mL/kg/hr (e.g., saline or Ringer's lactate)

R: *This measure promotes optimal renal tissue perfusion.*

Monitor the surgical site for bleeding, dehiscence, and evisceration

R: *Careful monitoring allows early detection of complications.*

Teach the individual to splint the surgical wound with a pillow when coughing, sneezing, or vomiting

R: *Splinting reduces stress on suture line by equalizing pressure across the wound.*

If anticoagulant or thrombolytic therapy, monitor for

- Bruises, nosebleeds
- Bleeding gums
- Hematuria
- Severe headaches
- Red or black stools

R: *The prolonged clotting time of anticoagulants by anticoagulant therapy can cause spontaneous bleeding anywhere in the body. Hematuria is a common early sign.*

Monitor for signs of bleeding from venous access devices (e.g., IVs, long-term venous access devices)

- Hematoma at site
- Bleeding at site

R: *Bleeding can occur several hours after insertion after blood pressure returns to normal and puts increased pressure on newly formed clot at the insertion site. It can also develop later, secondary to vascular erosion due to infection*

Monitor for bleeding during pregnancy and postpartum (Refer to specific collaborative problems as *Risk for Complications of Placenta Previa*)

Minimize individual's movement and activity

R: *This helps decrease tissue demands for oxygen.*

Provide reassurance, simple explanations, and emotional support to help reduce anxiety

R: *High anxiety increases metabolic demands for oxygen.*

Administer oxygen as ordered

R: *Diminished blood volume causes decreased circulating oxygen levels.*

Risk for Complications of Decreased Cardiac Output

Definition

Describes a person experiencing or at high risk to experience inadequate blood supply for tissue and organ needs because of insufficient blood pumping by the heart.

Decreased Cardiac Output is a phenomenon that is not restricted to individuals or environments that specifically focus on cardiovascular care. It is not only prevalent in cardiovascular care units, but also in post-anesthesia units and noncardiac care units among individuals with noncardiogenic disorders. A significant decrease in cardiac output is a life-threatening situation, demonstrating the need for developing a risk nursing diagnosis for early intervention (Pereira de Melo et al., 2011).

High-Risk Populations

- Acute coronary syndrome (ACS)
- Congestive heart failure
- Cardiogenic shock
- Hypertension
- Valvular heart disease
- Cardiomyopathy

- Cardiac tamponade
- Hypothermia
- Anaphylaxis
- Dilated cardiomyopathy
- Streptococcal toxic shock syndrome
- Severe diarrhea
- Systemic inflammatory response syndrome (SIRS)
- Coarctation of the aorta
- Chronic obstructive pulmonary disease (COPD)
- Pheochromocytoma
- Chronic renal failure
- Adult respiratory distress syndrome
- Hypotension/hypovolemia (e.g., postsurgery, severe bleeding or burns)
- Bradycardia
- Tachycardia

Collaborative Outcomes

The individual will be monitored for early signs and symptoms of *Decreased Cardiac Output* and will receive collaborative interventions if indicated to restore physiologic stability.

Indicators of Physiologic Stability

- Calm, alert, oriented
- Oxygen saturation >95%
- Normal sinus rhythm
- No chest pain
- No life-threatening dysrhythmias
- Skin warm and dry
- Usual skin color (appropriate for race)
- Pulse: regular rhythm, rate 60 to 100 beats/min
- Respirations 16 to 20 breaths/min
- Blood pressure >90/60, <140/90 mm Hg, MAP >70, or CVP >11
- Urine output >0.5 mL/kg/hr

Interventions and Rationales

Monitor for signs and symptoms of decreased cardiac output/index

- Increased, decreased, and/or irregular pulse rate
- Increased respiratory rate
- Decreased blood pressure, increased blood pressure
- Abnormal heart sounds
- Abnormal lung sounds (crackles, rales)
- Decreased urine output (<5 mL/kg/hr)
- Changes in mentation
- Cool, moist, cyanotic, mottled skin
- Delayed capillary refill time
- Neck vein distention
- Weak peripheral pulses
- Abnormal pulmonary artery pressures
- Abnormal renal artery pressures
- Decreased mixed venous oxygen saturation
- Electrocardiogram (ECG) changes
- Dysrhythmias
- Decreased SaO_2
- Decreased $ScvO_2$

R: *Decreased cardiac output/index leads to insufficient oxygenated blood to meet the metabolic needs of tissues. Decreased circulating volume can result in hypoperfusion of the kidneys and decreased tissue perfusion with a* *compensatory response of decreased circulation to extremities and increased pulse and respiratory rates (Grossman & Porth, 2014). Changes in mentation may result from cerebral hypoperfusion. Vasoconstriction and venous congestion in dependent areas (e.g., limbs) produce changes in skin and pulses.*

Closely monitor urine output hourly

R: *Decreased blood volume reduces blood to kidneys, which decreases the glomerular filtration rate (GFR) causing a decrease urine output. When blood flow to the kidneys is less than 20% to 25% of normal, ischemic damage occurs (Grossman & Porth, 2014). Decreased urine output is an early sign of bleeding/hypovolemia.*

Initiate appropriate protocols or standing orders, depending on the underlying etiology of the problem affecting ventricular function

R: *Nursing management differs based on etiology (e.g., measures to help increase preload for hypovolemia and to decrease preload for impaired ventricular contractility).*

Position with the legs elevated, unless ventricular function is impaired

R: *This position can help increase preload and enhance cardiac output.*

Assist with measures to conserve strength, such as resting before and after activities (e.g., meals, baths)

R: *Adequate rest reduces oxygen consumption and decreases the risk of hypoxia.*

With impaired ventricular function, cautiously administer IV fluids. Be sure to include any additional IV fluids (e.g., antibiotics) when calculating fluid allocation. Consult with pharmacist to concentrate IVs and medications when necessary

R: *An individual with poorly functioning ventricles may not tolerate increased blood volumes.*

If decreased cardiac output results from hypovolemia, septic shock, or dysrhythmia, refer to the specific collaborative problem in this section

Risk for Complications of Arrhythmias

Definition

Describes a person experiencing or at high risk to experience a disorder of the heart's conduction system that results in an abnormal heart rate, abnormal rhythm, or a combination of both

High-Risk Populations

- A-type coronary artery disease (CAD):
  - Angina
  - Myocardial infarction (acute coronary syndrome [ACS])
  - Congestive heart failure
- Significant Hypoglycemia (Chow et al., 2014)
- Accidental Hypothermia
  - Mild hypothermia > tachycardia
  - Moderate hypothermia > atrial fibrillation, junctional bradycardia
  - Severe hypothermia > bradycardia, ventricular arrhythmias (including ventricular fibrillation, and asystole Zafren & Mechem, 2014)
- Sepsis
- Increased intracranial pressure
- Electrolyte imbalance (calcium, potassium, magnesium, phosphorus)
- Atherosclerotic heart disease
- Medication side effects (e.g., aminophylline, dopamine, stimulants, digoxin, beta-blockers, calcium-channel blockers, dobutamine, lidocaine, procainamide, quinidine, diuretics, class 1C antiarrhythmic drugs, anticonvulsants such as phenytoin, tricyclic antidepressants, and some agents used to treat neuropathic pain and immunomodulators) (Heist & Ruskin, 2010)

- COPD
- Cardiomyopathy, valvular heart disease
- Anemia
- Postoperative cardiac surgery
- Postoperative after any major anesthesia
- Trauma
- Sleep apnea
- Hypoxia

Collaborative Outcomes

The individual will be monitored for early signs and symptoms of d arrhythmias and decreased cardiac output and will receive collaborative interventions if indicated to restore physiologic stability.

Indicators of Physiologic Stability

- Normal sinus rhythm
- Refer also to *Decreased Cardiac Output* indicators of physiologic stability.

Interventions and Rationales

Monitor for signs and symptoms of arrhythmias

- Abnormal rate, rhythm
- Palpitations, chest pain, syncope, fatigue
- Decreased SaO_2
- Hypotension
- Change in level of consciousness

R: *Ischemic tissue is electrically unstable, causing arrhythmias. Certain congenital cardiac conditions fibrosis or scar tissue of conduction system, inflammatory disease, cardiac surgery, infection, cancer, electrolyte imbalances, and medications also can cause disturbances in cardiac conduction.*

Monitor ECG patterns and changes as

- Acute coronary syndrome (ST-segment elevation, prolongation of Q wave, inversion of T wave)

R: *The above ECG changes may not be present immediately. The first ECG change seen clinically is usually ST-segment elevation, which indicates myocardial injury in tissue underlying the electrodes. ECG changes of infarction include ST elevation (indicating injury), Q waves (indicating necrosis), and T-wave inversion (indicating ischemia and evolution of the infarction). These signs of ischemia can be isolated to ECG leads overlying the involved myocardium and indicating localized ischemia. If they are present in many ECG leads, more widespread ischemia is suspected (Grossman & Porth, 2014).*

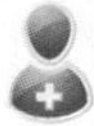

Clinical Alert If the initial ECG is normal or inconclusive, additional recordings should be obtained if the individual develops symptoms. These should be compared with recordings obtained in an asymptomatic state. The standard ECG at rest does not adequately reflect the dynamic nature of coronary thrombosis and myocardial ischemia. Almost two-thirds of all ischemic episodes in the phase of instability are clinically silent, and hence are unlikely to be detected by a conventional ECG. Accordingly, online continuous computer-assisted 12-lead ST-segment monitoring is also a valuable diagnostic tool.

Notify physician, PA, or nurse practitioner of ST elevation and of other serious EKG changes

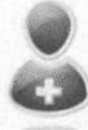

Clinical Alert This is termed ST-elevation ACS (STE-ACS) and generally reflects an acute total coronary occlusion. Most of these individuals will ultimately develop an ST-elevation MI (STEMI). The therapeutic objective is to achieve rapid, complete, and sustained reperfusion by primary angioplasty or fibrinolytic therapy.

- Sinus node arrhythmias (sinus tachycardia, sinus bradycardia, sinus block, sinus pause or arrest, sick sinus syndrome)

R: *Alterations in SA node function leads to changes in rate or rhythm of the heartbeat (Grossman & Porth, 2014)*

- Atrial origin arrhythmias (premature atrial contractions (PAC), multifocal/focal atrial tachycardia, atrial flutter, atrial fibrillation, paroxysmal supraventricular tachycardia)

R: *PAC's and tachycardia can be caused by stress, caffeine, alcohol, tobacco, cardiac ischemia, digitalis toxicity, hypokalemia, hypomagnesemia, and hypoxia. Atrial flutter rarely occurs in healthy persons and is usually seen in children and young adults, who have had surgery for complex congenital heart disease (Grossman & Porth, 2014).*

- Junctional arrhythmias (bradycardia, nonparoxysmal, junctional tachycardia)
- Ventricular arrhythmias (premature ventricular contractions, ventricular tachycardia, ventricular flutter, ventricular fibrillation)

R: *Ventricular arrhythmias are considered more serious than those in the atria because the pumping action of the heart can be impaired causing decrease cardiac output (Grossman & Porth, 2014).*

- Disorders of atrioventricular conduction (first-degree AV Block, second-degree block, third-degree AV Block)

R: *Heart block is caused by abnormal impulse conduction. It may be normal, physiologic (vagal tone), or pathologic. Causes can be scar tissue, certain medications, electrolyte imbalances, acute MI, inflammatory diseases, or cardiac surgery (Grossman & Porth, 2014).*

Initiate appropriate protocols depending on the type of arrhythmia

- Administer supplemental oxygen

R: *It increases circulating oxygen levels and decreases cardiac workload.*

- Monitor oxygen saturation (SaO_2) with pulse oximetry and ABGs as necessary.
- Monitor serum electrolyte levels (e.g., sodium, potassium, calcium, magnesium).

R: *High or low electrolyte levels may exacerbate a dysrhythmia.*

Risk for Complications of Pulmonary Edema

Definition

Cardiogenic pulmonary edema (CPE) is defined as pulmonary edema due to increased capillary hydrostatic pressure secondary to elevated pulmonary venous pressure. CPE reflects the accumulation of fluid with a low-protein content in the lung interstitium and alveoli as a result of cardiac dysfunction usually heart failure

Non-Heart-Related (Noncardiogenic) Pulmonary Edema

Pulmonary edema that is not caused by increased pressures in the heart is called noncardiogenic pulmonary edema (Givertz, 2015).

- **High Altitude Pulmonary Edema.** The exact cause is not completely understood. It seems to develop as a result of increased pressure from constriction of the pulmonary capillaries.
- **Nervous system conditions.** A type of pulmonary edema called neurogenic pulmonary edema can occur after some nervous system conditions or procedures—such as after a head injury, seizure, or subarachnoid hemorrhage—or after brain surgery.

High-Risk Populations

Pulmonary edema can be caused by cardiac related or noncardiac-related causes

Cardiac Causes

This condition usually occurs when the diseased, compromised or overworked left ventricle, or heart valves are not able to pump out enough of the blood it receives though the pulmonary artery. The increased pressure extends into the left atrium and then to the pulmonary veins, causing fluid to accumulate in the lungs (Givertz, 2015).

- Hypertension (untreated or uncontrolled)
- Dysrhythmias
- Myocardial infarction
- Acute cardiac syndrome
- Angina
- Congestive heart failure
- Cardiomyopathy
- Failed pacemaker, lead wires, and/or generator
- Coronary artery disease
- Aortic or mitral cardiac valve disease
- Congenital heart defects

Noncardiac Causes

In this condition, fluid may leak from the capillaries in your lungs' air sacs because the capillaries themselves become more permeable or leaky, even without the buildup of back pressure from your heart. the integrity of the alveoli become compromised as a result of underlying inflammatory response, and this leads to leaky alveoli that can fill up with fluid from the blood vessels (Givertz, 2015).

- Acute respiratory distress syndrome (ARDS)
- Diabetes mellitus (episodic severe hyperglycemia, underlying cause of CAD)
- Inhalation of toxins (ammonia and chlorine)
- Drug overdose (pathophysiology unknown, e.g., heroin, cocaine, methadone, aspirin; Givertz, 2015)
- Smoke inhalation
- Neurologic trauma/surgery
- Volume overload (in the presence of compromised cardiac function)
- Renal failure (inability to excrete fluid from the body can cause fluid buildup in the blood vessels)
- Pulmonary embolism ("PE can cause pulmonary edema by injuring the pulmonary and adjacent pleural systemic circulations, elevating hydrostatic pressures in pulmonary and/or systemic veins, and perhaps by lowering pleural pressure due to atelectasis"; Givertz, 2015.)
- Pneumothorax (pulmonary edema can occur with rapid expansion of the lung post collapse)
- Viral infections (rapidly progressive noncardiogenic pulmonary edema associated with profound hypotension and a high case fatality rate with, e.g., hantavirus infection, dengue hemorrhagic fever, coronavirus infection, H1N1 influenza A; Givertz, 2015)
- Near drowning
- High altitudes (an abnormally pronounced degree of hypoxic pulmonary vasoconstriction at a given altitude appears to underlie the pathogenesis of this disorder; Givertz, 2015)
- Hypothermia (When core temperature reaches 32° C, metabolism, ventilation, and cardiac output begin to decline causing decreased cardiac output, which can lead to pulmonary edema, oliguria, areflexia, coma, hypotension, bradycardia, ventricular arrhythmias [including ventricular fibrillation], and asystole.) (Mechem & Zafren, 2014)
- Circulating toxins (e.g., snake venom, alpha-naphthyl thiourea [rat poison inhaled])
- Systemic inflammatory response syndrome (SIRS)
- Sepsis causes low cardiac output, low peripheral vascular pressure, and high pulmonary vascular resistance due to vasoconstriction, causing increased pulmonary congestion.

Collaborative Outcomes

The individual will be monitored for early signs and symptoms of pulmonary edema and will receive collaborative interventions if indicated to restore physiologic stability.

Indicators of Physiologic Stability

- Alert, calm, oriented
- Symmetrical easy, rhythmic respirations

- Warm, dry skin
- Full breath sounds all lobes
- No crackles and wheezing
- Usual color (for race)
- Refer to *Risk for Complications of Decreased Cardiac Output* for additional indicators

Interventions and Rationales

Address the overwhelming terrifying experience of sudden, critical breathlessness

R: *Individuals report breathlessness in terms of the feelings associated with bad episodes of breathlessness as distress, anxiety, panic, and fear of dying (Gysels & Higginson, 2011; Schneidman, Reinke, Donesky, & Carrieri-Kohlman. 2014)*

- Validate how frighten he or she must be.
- Reassure the person and do not leave them alone.

R: *These strategies attempt to reduce anxiety/fear.*

Elevate the head of the bed or use extra pillows under the head and shoulders

R: *This position will decrease resistance to inspiration.*

If possible, increase air flow around person, for example, fan, open window

R: *Increasing circulating cooler air can decrease breathlessness.*

Monitor for signs and symptoms of pulmonary edema

- Dry, hacking cough, especially when lying down
- Confusion, sleepiness, and disorientation may occur in older people
- Dizziness, fainting, fatigue, or weakness
- Fluid buildup, especially in the legs, ankles, and feet
- Increased urination at night (peripheral edema during the day returns to circulation when legs are elevated, resulting in nocturia)
- Nausea, abdominal swelling, tenderness, or pain (may result from the buildup of fluid in the body and the backup of blood in the liver)
- Weight gain (fluid accumulation increases weight)
- Weight loss (nausea causes a loss of appetite)
- Rapid breathing, bluish skin, and feelings of restlessness, anxiety, and suffocation
- Shortness of breath and lung congestion

R: *Symptoms are caused by congestion in lungs from fluid accumulation.*

- Tiring easily
- Wheezing and spasms of the airways similar to asthma
- Jugular vein distention (JVD)
  - Persistent cough
  - Productive cough with frothy sputum
  - Cyanosis
  - Diaphoresis

R: *Impaired pumping of left ventricle accompanied by decreased cardiac output and increased pulmonary artery pressure produce pulmonary edema. Circulatory overload can result from the reduced size of the pulmonary vascular bed. Hypoxia causes increased capillary permeability that, in turn, causes fluid to enter pulmonary tissue. Venous pressure and pulmonary lungs become so congested with fluid that it affects the exchange of oxygen, which is considered pulmonary edema (Grossman & Porth, 2014).*

Weigh individual daily

- Ensure accuracy by weighing at the same time every day on the same scale and with the individual wearing the same amount of clothing.

R: *Daily weights and strict input and output (I&O) are vital in determining the effects of treatment and for early detections of fluid retention or worsening of condition.*

Closely monitor urine output hourly

R: *Decreased blood volume reduces blood to kidneys, which decreases the glomerular filtration rate (GFR) causing a decrease urine output. When blood flow to the kidneys is less than 20% to 25% of normal, ischemic damage occurs (Grossman & Porth, 2014). Decreased urine output is an early sign of bleeding or hypovolemia.*

Monitor with pulse oximetry

R: *This will provide for continuous monitoring of oxygen saturation.*

Take steps to maintain adequate hydration while avoiding overhydration

R: *Adequate hydration helps liquefy pulmonary secretions; overhydration can increase preload and worsen pulmonary edema.*

Cautiously administer intravenous (IV) fluids

- Consult with the physician/NP if the ordered rate plus the PO intake exceeds 2 to 2.5 L/24 hr. Be sure to include additional IV fluids (e.g., antibiotics) when calculating the hourly allocation. Oral fluid intake must also be monitored and, if indicated, possibly restricted.

R: *Failure to regulate IV and oral fluids carefully can cause circulatory overload with worsening of the condition.*

If indicated, administer oxygen as prescribed

R: *Hypoxia produces increased capillary pressure, causing fluid to enter pulmonary tissue and triggering signs and symptoms of pulmonary edema.*

Initiate appropriate treatments according to protocol, which may include

- Diuretics

R: *To decrease preload.*

- Vasodilators

R: *To decrease preload & afterload.*

- Positive inotropic agents (e.g., digitalis).

R: *To enhance ventricular contractions.*

- Morphine

R: *To decrease anxiety, preload and afterload, and metabolic demands.*

Risk for Complications of Deep Vein Thrombosis

Definition

Describes a person experiencing venous clot formation because of blood stasis, vessel wall injury, or altered coagulation and/or experiencing or at high risk to experience obstruction of one or more pulmonary arteries from a blood clot, air or fat embolus

High-Risk Populations

(Barbar et al., 2010; Lip & Hull, 2014)

- Active cancer (3)
- History of deep vein thrombosis (DVT) or pulmonary embolism (3)
- Reduced mobility >72 hours (3)
- Known thrombophilic condition (3) (e.g., polycythemia, blood dyscrasias)
- High levels of factor VIII in white people (Payne, Miller, Hooper, Lally, & Austin, 2014)
- High levels of factor VIII and Von Willebrand factor in black people (Payne et al., 2014)
- Recent trauma/surgery (2)
- Over 70 years old (1)

- Obesity >30 BMI (1)
- Acute coronary or ischemic stroke (1)
- Acute infection and/or rheumatologic disorder (1)
- Ongoing hormonal therapy (1)
- Heart/respiratory failure (1)
- Age (risk rises steadily from age 40)
- Fractures (especially hip, pelvis, and leg)
- Chemical irritation of vein
- All major surgeries that involve general anesthesia and immobility (over 30 minutes) in the operative course (preop, periop, and postop combined), especially surgeries involving abdomen, pelvis, and lower extremities
- Orthopedic (hips/knees), urologic, or gynecologic surgery
- History of venous insufficiency
- Varicose veins
- Inflammatory bowel disease
- Pregnancy
- Surgery greater than 30 minutes (2)
- Over 40 years of age
- Valve malfunction
- Systemic lupus erythematosus
- Central venous catheters
- Nephrotic syndrome

These risk factors have been identified in the Padua Prediction risk assessment for venous thrombolytic events. A score of ≥4 is a high-risk individual (Barbar et al., 2010).

- Air Embolism
  - Central line insertion or removal, sheath central line tubing changes, manipulation, or disconnection
- Fat Embolism (Eriksson, Schultz, Cohle, & Post, 2011)
  - Fractures—closed fractures produce more emboli than open fractures. Long bones, pelvis and ribs cause more emboli. Sternum and clavicle furnish less. Multiple fractures produce more emboli.
  - Orthopedic procedures—most commonly, intramedullary nailing of the long bones, hip, or knee replacements [6]
  - Massive soft tissue injury
  - CPR is associated with a high incidence of PFE regardless of cause of death (Eriksson, 2011).
  - Severe burns
  - Bone marrow biopsy
  - Nontraumatic settings occasionally lead to fat embolism. These include conditions associated with:
    - Liposuction
    - Fatty liver
    - Prolonged corticosteroid therapy
    - Acute pancreatitis
    - Osteomyelitis
    - Conditions causing bone infarcts, especially sickle cell disease

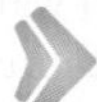

Carp's Cues

In more than 90% of cases of PE, the thrombosis originates in the deep veins of the legs. Deep vein thrombosis (DVT) is a distressing but often avoidable condition that leads to long-term complications such as the post-phlebitic syndrome and chronic leg ulcers in a large proportion of individuals who have proximal vein thrombosis. Pulmonary embolism remains the most common preventable cause of death in hospital (Lip & Hull, 2014)

- The incidence of fat embolism syndrome (FES) varies from 1% to 29%. Fat emboli occur in all individuals with long-bone fractures, but only few patients develop systemic dysfunction, particularly the triad of skin, brain, and lung dysfunction, known as FES (Eriksson, 2011).

Collaborative Outcomes

The individual will be monitored for early signs and symptoms of (a) deep vein thrombosis and (b) pulmonary embolism and the individual will receive collaborative interventions if indicated to restore physiologic stability.

Indicators of Physiologic Stability

- No leg pain (a)
- No leg edema (a)
- No change in skin temperature or color (a, b)
- No acute dyspnea, restlessness, decreased mental status, or anxiety (b)
- No acute, sharp chest pain (b)
- Pulse: regular rhythm, rate 60 to 100 beats/min (b)
- Respirations 16 to 20 breaths/min (b)
- Blood pressure >90/60, <140/90 mm Hg, MAP >70, or CVP >11
- Breath sounds without evidence of new, abnormal sounds (rales, crackles) (b)
- No presence of distended neck veins (JVD) (b)

Interventions and Rationales

Screen for prevention and institute prophylaxis per protocol

Consult with physician or advanced practice nurse for low-dose heparin/anticoagulant therapy for a high-risk individual (see Anticoagulant Therapy in *Risk for Complications* of Medication Therapy Adverse Effects)

R: *Heparin therapy decreases platelet adhesiveness, reducing the risk of embolism. In the presence of thrombosis, treatment goals are preventing the clot from becoming larger, preventing new blood clots from forming,*

Monitor for onset or status of venous thrombosis, noting

- Diminished or absent peripheral pulses

R: *Insufficient circulation causes pain and diminished peripheral pulses.*

- Unusual warmth and redness or coolness and cyanosis, increased leg swelling

R: *Unusual warmth and redness point to inflammation; coolness and cyanosis indicate vascular obstruction.*

- Increasing leg pain

R: *Leg pain results from tissue hypoxia.*

- A rapid heart rate and/or a feeling of passing out
- New chest pain with difficulty breathing

R: *These findings may indicate mobilization of thrombi to the lungs (pulmonary embolism)*

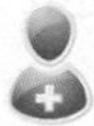

Clinical Alert Stay with person and call for Rapid Response Team.

- Fit with inflatable compression devices for high-risk individuals.
- Continue use of elastic graduated compression stockings (GCS) if prescribed.

R: *These devices apply gentle pressure to improve circulation and help prevent clots. They should be used prior to surgery and before anticoagulant therapy (Lip & Hull, 2014).*

All individuals should receive VTE risk assessment on admission (Institute for Clinical System Improvement [ICSI], 2008; Partnership for Patient Care, 2007)

R: *In all individuals, the decision to anticoagulate should be individualized and the benefits of venous thromboembolism (VTE) prevention carefully weighed against the risk of bleeding.*

Assess for contraindications to anticoagulation (Lip & Hull, 2014)

- Absolute contraindications:
  - Active bleeding, severe bleeding diathesis
  - Platelet count <50,000/µL
  - Recent, planned, or emergent surgery/procedure
  - Major trauma
  - A history of intracranial hemorrhage
- Relative contraindications:
  - Recurrent bleeding from multiple gastrointestinal telangiectasias
  - Intracranial or spinal tumors

- Platelet count <150,000/μL
- Large abdominal aortic aneurysm with concurrent severe hypertension, and stable aortic dissection
- Additional relative contraindications in older patients (e.g., >65 years)
- Include a history of multiple falls and the presence of more than one factor that elevates the bleeding risk

R: *"Such patients are at high risk of bleeding or have a high risk of a catastrophic result should a bleed occur. Consequently, the decision to anticoagulate in this population should be even more cautious to allow the benefits of VTE prevention to be carefully weighed against the risk of bleeding" (Lip & Hull, 2014).*

Monitor for signs and symptoms of pulmonary embolism

- Acute, sharp chest pain
- Dyspnea, restlessness, cyanosis, decreased mental status, or anxiety
- Decreased oxygen saturation (SaO_2, SvO_2)
- Tachycardia
- Tachypnea (Shaughnessy, 2007)
- Neck vein distention
- Hypotension
- Acute right ventricular dilation without parenchymal disease (on chest X-ray)
- Confusion
- Cardiac dysrhythmias (can be lethal)
- Low-grade fever
- Productive cough with blood-tinged sputum
- Pleural friction rub or new murmur (Shaughnessy, 2007)
- Crackles

R: *Occlusion of pulmonary arteries impedes blood flow to the distal lung, producing a hypoxic state.*

If these manifestations occur, promptly initiate protocols for shock

- Establish an IV line (for medication and fluid administration).
- Administer fluid replacement therapy according to protocol.
- Insert indwelling urinary (Foley) catheter (to monitor circulatory volume through urine output).
- Initiate ECG monitoring and invasive hemodynamic monitoring (to detect dysrhythmias and guide therapy).
- Initiate unit protocols.
- Refer to *Risk for Complications of Hypovolemic Shock* for additional interventions.
- Prepare for angiography and/or perfusion lung scans (to confirm diagnosis and detect the extent of atelectasis).

R: *Because death from massive pulmonary embolism commonly occurs in the first 2 hours after onset, prompt intervention is crucial.*

Initiate oxygen therapy; monitor oxygen saturation

R: *This measure rapidly increases circulating oxygen levels.*

Monitor serum electrolyte levels, ABG values, blood urea nitrogen, and complete blood count results

R: *These laboratory tests help determine perfusion and volume status. Monitor D-Dimer & chest X-ray aids in diagnosis (Shaughnessy, 2007).*

- Evaluate hydration status based on urine specific gravity, intake/output, weights, and serum osmolality. Take steps to ensure adequate hydration.

R: *Increased blood viscosity and coagulability and decreased cardiac output may contribute to thrombus formation.*

- Encourage individual to perform isotonic leg exercises, flexing knees, and ankles hourly.

R: *They promote venous return.*

- Ambulate as soon as possible with at least 5 minutes of walking each waking hour. Avoid prolonged chair sitting with legs dependent.

R: *Walking contracts leg muscles, stimulates the venous pump, and reduces stasis (ICSI, 2008).*

- Elevate the affected extremity above the level of the heart.

R: *This positioning can help reduce interstitial swelling by promoting venous return.*

- Discourage smoking.

R: *Nicotine can cause vasospasms.*

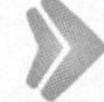

Carp's Cues

In 2002, the National Quality Forum created and endorsed a list of Serious Reportable Events (SREs), which was updated in 2006. There are 28 events that have been labeled as SREs; also called never events. "The 28 events on the list are largely preventable, grave errors and events that are of concern to the public and healthcare providers and that warrant careful investigation and should be targeted for mandatory public reporting" (National Quality Forum, 2011). One of the 28 events is patient death or serious disability associated with intravascular air embolism that occurs while being cared for in a healthcare facility.

For Prevention of Air Emboli (Weinhouse, 2016)

Explain to the individual what was going to happen and why it is important to follow the specific instructions

R: *Positioning during central line removal is a critical intervention to prevent air embolism*

Perform hand hygiene and put on clean gloves. Remove the dressing carefully and discard it with your gloves. Repeat hand hygiene and put on sterile gloves

Assess the catheter insertion site for evidence of complications such as redness, swelling, or drainage. Notify the physician if you see any of these signs; she may order a culture. Clean the site according to facility policy, preferably with chlorhexidine

- Never using scissors near the venous access device, as this could result in accidental severing of the catheter.
- Remove the catheter-securing device.

Before central line catheter insertion and tubing changes, place person in supine or Trendelenburg's position and instruct him or her to perform Valsalva maneuver during the procedure. Instruct to take a deep breath and bear down simulating applying downward pressure as if having a bowel movement. Have person demonstrate it. Remove the catheter as the person bears down.[1]

If the individual is unable to cooperate with procedure, perform during positive pressure portion of respiratory cycle (Luettel, 2011; *Lynn-McHale Wiegand, & Carlson, 2005)

- Spontaneous breathing—during exhalation.
- Mechanical ventilation—during inhalation.

R: *These measures increase intrathoracic pressure and help prevent air from entering the catheter.*

After you have removed the catheter, tell the person to breathe normally. Apply pressure with the sterile gauze until bleeding stops (O'Dowd & Kelle, 2015)

Apply a sterile air-occlusive dressing over the insertion site to prevent a delayed air embolism

Assess the length and integrity of the catheter and visually inspect the tip for smoothness. Remove your gloves and perform hand hygiene (O'Dowd & Kelle, 2015)

- Instruct individual to remain supine for 30 minutes after removal (O'Dowd & Kelle, 2015)

Document the date and time of CVC removal, noting the CVC's length and integrity, the site assessment, patient response, and nursing interventions (O'Dowd & Kelle, 2015)

Do not pull harder if resistance is met while removing a CVC (O'Dowd & Kelle, 2015)

Do not remove it when the person is inhaling (O'Dowd & Kelle, 2015)

Do not apply any dressing that is not air-occlusive, this would increase the risk of a delayed air embolism (O'Dowd & Kelle, 2015)

[1] Follow protocol to remove central line catheter

R: *These measures help prevent air entry and infection at insertion site.*

Monitor for signs and symptoms of air embolism during dressing and IV tubing changes and after any accidental separation of IV connections

- Sucking sound on insertion
- Dyspnea
- Tachypnea
- Wheezing
- Substernal chest pain
- Anxiety

R: *Air embolism can occur with IV tubing changes, with accidental tubing separation, and during catheter insertion, removal, and disconnection (e.g., an individual can aspirate as much as 200 mL of air from a deep breath during subclavian line disconnection). Entry of air into the pulmonary arterial system can obstruct blood flow, causing bronchoconstriction of the affected lung area. Use lure lock connections to help prevent accidental disconnection.*

If air embolism is suspected call the Rapid response team or call 911, do not leave the person

Administer 100% oxygen

R: *This promotes diffusion of nitrogen, which compresses an air embolism in about 80% of cases*

Place person flat or in Trendelenburg position and turn on to left side

R: *This position displaces air away from pulmonary valve and traps it in the ventricle for radiological aspiration.*

Initiate protocols for respiratory or cardiac arrest if indicated

For Risk for Complications of Fat Embolism

Carp's Cues

Fat emboli occur in all patients with long-bone fractures, but only few individuals develop systemic dysfunction of the skin, brain, and lung dysfunction, known as fat embolism syndrome (FES). FES typically manifests 24 to 72 hours after the initial insult, but may rarely occur as early as 12 hours or as late as 2 weeks after the inciting event. Affected patients develop a classic triad—hypoxemia, neurologic abnormalities, and a petechial rash (Weinhouse, 2016).

Monitor for signs and symptoms of fat embolism

R: *FES typically manifests 24 to 72 hours after the initial insult, but may rarely occur as early as 12 hours or as late as 2 weeks after the inciting event. Affected patients develop a classic triad—hypoxemia, neurologic abnormalities, and a petechial rash.*

- Hypoxemia, dyspnea, and tachypnea are the most frequent early findings. A syndrome indistinguishable from acute lung injury (ALI) or acute respiratory distress syndrome (ARDS) may develop. Approximately one-half of patients with FES caused by long-bone fractures develop severe hypoxemia and require mechanical ventilation.
- The onset is then sudden, with:
  - Breathlessness ± vague pains in the chest—Depending on severity this can progress to respiratory failure with tachypnea, increasing breathlessness and hypoxia.
  - Fever—often in excess of 38.3° C with a disproportionately high pulse rate.
  - Petechial rash—commonly over the upper anterior part of the trunk, arm and neck, buccal mucosa, and conjunctivae. The rash may be transient, disappearing after 24 hours.
  - Central nervous system symptoms, varying from a mild headache to significant cerebral dysfunction (restlessness, disorientation, confusion, seizures, stupor, or coma).
  - Renal—oliguria, hematuria, anuria.
- Tachypnea more than 30 per minute
- Sudden onset of chest pain or dyspnea
- Restlessness, apprehension
- Confusion

R: *Drowsiness with diminished urine output (oliguria) is almost diagnostic. Neurologic abnormalities develop in the majority of patients with FES. They typically occur after the development of respiratory distress, with affected patients developing a confusional state followed by an altered level of consciousness (Weinhouse, 2016)*

- Elevated temperature above 103° F
- Increased pulse rate more than 140 per minute
- Petechial skin rash (12 to 96 hours postoperative)

R: *These changes are the result of hypoxemia. Fatty acids attack red blood cells and platelets to form microaggregates, which impair circulation to vital organs, such as the brain. Fatty globules passing through the pulmonary vasculature cause a chemical reaction that decreases lung compliance and ventilation/perfusion ratio and raises body temperature. Rash results from capillary fragility. Common sites are conjunctiva, axilla, chest, and neck; (Weinhouse, 2016).*

Minimize movement of a fractured extremity for the first 3 days after the injury.

R: *Immobilization minimizes further tissue trauma and reduces the risk of embolism dislodgement (Weinhouse, 2016).*

Consider prophylactic corticosteroids if long-bone or pelvic fractures to prevent Fat Embolism Syndrome (Weinhouse, 2016)

Ensure adequate hydration.

R: *Optimal hydration dilutes the irritating fatty acids through the system (Weinhouse, 2016).*

Monitor intake/output, urine color, and specific gravity.

R: *These data reflect hydration status.*

Risk for Complications of Hypovolemia

Definition

Describes a person experiencing or at high risk to experience inadequate cellular oxygenation and inability to excrete waste products of metabolism secondary to decreased fluid volume (e.g., from bleeding, plasma loss, prolonged vomiting, or diarrhea)

Hypovolemic shock refers to rapid fluid loss results in multiple organ failure due to inadequate circulating volume and subsequent inadequate perfusion. Most often caused by rapid blood loss due to a medical or surgical condition. Refer to *Risk for Complications of Bleeding* if indicated.

High-Risk Populations

(Grossman & Porth, 2014)

- Intraoperative status
- Postoperative status
- Postprocedural cannulation of any arterial vessel, but particularly those at risk for retro-peritoneal bleed due to cannulation of femoral vessel
- Anaphylactic shock
- Trauma
- Bleeding (e.g., external [laceration, gunshot wound] or internal [gastrointestinal, surgical site])
- Diabetic ketoacidosis (DKA) or hyperosmolar hyperglycemic state (HHS)
- Excessive GI fluid losses (vomiting, diarrhea, gastrointestinal suctioning, draining GI fistula)
- Excessive renal losses (diuretic therapy, osmotic diuresis related to hyperglycemia)
- Excessive skin losses (fever, exposure to hot environment, loss of skin due to burns, wounds)
- Infants, children, older persons
- Acute pancreatitis
- Major burns
- Disseminated intravascular coagulation (DIC)
- Diabetes insipidus
- Ascites

- Peritonitis
- Intestinal obstruction
- Systemic inflammatory response syndrome (SIRS)/Sepsis
- Hyponatremia

Collaborative Outcomes

The individual will be monitored for early signs and symptoms of hypovolemia and will receive collaborative interventions if indicated to restore physiologic stability.

Indicators of Physiologic Stability

Refer to *Risk for Complications of Decreased Cardiac.*

Interventions and Rationales

Monitor fluid status hourly if indicated; evaluate

- Intake (parenteral and oral)
- Output and other losses (urine, drainage, and vomiting), nasogastric tube

R: *Decreased blood volume reduces blood to kidneys, which decreases the glomerular filtration rate (GFR) causing a decrease urine output. When blood flow to the kidneys is less than 20% to 25% of normal, ischemic damage occurs (Grossman & Porth, 2014). Decreased urine output is an early sign of bleeding/hypovolemia.*

Monitor the surgical site for bleeding, dehiscence, and evisceration

R: *Careful monitoring allows early detection of complications.*

Teach individual to splint the surgical wound with a pillow when coughing, sneezing, or vomiting

R: *Splinting reduces stress on suture line by equalizing pressure across the wound.*

Monitor for signs and symptoms of shock

- Increased pulse rate with normal or slightly decreased blood pressure, narrowing pulse pressure, decrease in mean or mean arterial pressure (MAP)
- Urine output <5 mL/kg/hr (early sign)
- Restlessness, agitation, decreased mentation
- Increased respiratory rate, thirst
- Diminished peripheral pulses
- Cool, pale, moist, or cyanotic skin
- Decreased oxygenation saturation (SaO_2, SvO_2), pulmonary artery pressures, cardiac output/index, right atrial pressure, wedge/occlusion pressure
- Decreased hemoglobin/hematocrit, decreased cardiac output/index
- Decreased central venous pressure

R: *The compensatory response to decreased circulatory volume aims to increase oxygen delivery through increased heart and respiratory rates and decreased peripheral circulation (manifested by diminished peripheral pulses and cool skin). Decreased oxygen to the brain alters mentation. Decreased circulation to the kidneys leads to decreased urine output. Hemoglobin and hematocrit values decline if bleeding is significant (Grossman & Porth, 2014).*

If shock occurs, place individual in the supine position unless contraindicated (e.g., head injury)

R: *This position increases blood return (preload) to the heart.*

Insert an IV line; use a large-bore catheter if blood or large volume fluid replacement is anticipated. Initiate appropriate protocols for shock (e.g., vasopressor therapy). Refer also to *Risk for Complications of Acidosis* or *Risk for Complications of Alkalosis*, if indicated, for more information

R: *Protocols aim to increase peripheral resistance and elevate blood pressure.*

Collaborate with physician, physician assistant, or advanced practice nurse to replace fluid losses at a rate sufficient to maintain urine output >0.5 mL/kg/hr (e.g., saline or Ringer's lactate)

R: *This measure promotes optimal renal tissue perfusion.*

Restrict individual's movement and activity

R: *This helps decrease tissue demands for oxygen.*

Provide reassurance, simple explanations, and emotional support to help reduce anxiety

R: *High anxiety increases metabolic demands for oxygen.*

Administer oxygen as ordered

R: *This will increase the circulating oxygen available for tissue use.*

Risk for Complications of Compartment Syndrome

Definition

Describes a person experiencing increased pressure in a limited space, such as a fascial envelope, which compromises circulation and function, usually in the forearm or leg. Acute compartment syndrome is a surgical emergency. Compartment syndrome can also occur in the abdomen, when there is a sustained or repeated elevation of 12 mm Hg or greater (Stracciolini & Hammerberg, 2014). Refer to *Risk for Complications of Intra-Abdominal Hypertension*

High-Risk Populations

A prerequisite for the development of increased compartment pressure is a fascial structure that prevents adequate expansion of tissue volume to compensate for an increase in fluid.

Internal Factors

- Fractures
- Musculoskeletal surgery
- Injuries (crush, electrical, vascular)
- Allergic response (snake, insect bites)
- Excessive edema
- Thermal injuries
- Vascular obstruction
- Intramuscular bleeding
- Extremely vigorous exercise, especially eccentric movements (extension under pressure)
- Anabolic steroids

External Factors

- Extravasation of IV fluids
- Procedural cannulation of vessel for diagnostic or interventional reasons:
  - Casts
  - Prolonged use of tourniquet
  - Tight dressings
  - Tight closure of fascial defects
  - Positioning during surgery
  - Lying on limb for extended periods
- Drug abuse (arterial injection; Stracciolini & Hammerberg, 2014)

Collaborative Outcomes

The individual will be monitored for early signs and symptoms of compartment syndrome and will receive collaborative interventions if indicated to restore physiologic stability.

Indicators of Physiologic Stability

- Pedal pulses 2+, equal
- Capillary refill <3 seconds
- Warm extremities
- No complaints of paresthesia (numbness), tingling
- Minimal swelling
- Ability to move toes or fingers

Interventions and Rationales

Explain to individual/family the reason for the specific questions and examinations

R: *Diagnosing changes in neurovascular function in individuals with trauma is difficult, thus cooperation of involved persons can be useful.*

Assess for specific signs of compartment syndrome (Shadgan et al., 2010; Stracciolini & Hammerberg, 2014)

- Complaints of tingling or burning sensations > numbness

R: *Sensory deficits typically precede motor deficits and manifest distal to the involved compartment.*

- Pain is out of proportion to the injury, unrelieved by narcotics
- Pain with passive stretch of muscles in the affected compartment or hyperextension of digits (toes or fingers) (early finding).

R: *Passive stretching of muscles decreases muscle compartment, thus increasing pain. Pain in response to passive stretching of muscles within the affected compartment is widely described as a sensitive early sign of ACS (Stracciolini, & Hammerberg, 2014).*

- A new and persistent deep ache in an arm or leg
- Electricity-like pain in the limb

R: *Pain and paresthesia indicate compression of nerves and increasing pressure within muscle compartment.*

- Increases with the elevation of the extremity

R: *This increases the pressure in the compartment.*

- Involved compartment or limb will feel tense and warm on palpation.
- Skin is tight and shiny.
- Late signs/symptoms
- Diminished or absent pulse
- Pallor, cool skin
- Pale, grayish, or whitish tone to skin

R: *Arterial occlusion produces these late signs*

- Prolonged capillary refill (>3 seconds)

R: *Delayed capillary refill or pale, mottled, or cyanotic skin indicates obstructed capillary blood flow.*

- Care of weakness when moving affected limb
- Progresses to inability to move joint or fingers/toes
- Pulselessness

R: *Decreased arterial perfusion results in pulselessness.*

Examine laboratory findings of compartment syndrome

- Elevated WBC (white blood cell count) and ESR (erythrocyte sedimentation rate)

R: *These elevations are a result of the severe inflammatory response.*

- Lowered serum pH

R: *This reflects tissue damage with acidosis.*

- Elevated temperature

R: *This is due to necrosis of tissue.*

- Elevated serum potassium

R: *Cellular damage releases potassium.*

Assess neurovascular function at least every hour for first 24 hours

R: *A delay in diagnosis is the most important determinant of a poor individual outcome.*

Instruct to report unusual, new, or different sensations (e.g., tingling, numbness, and/or decreased ability to move toes or fingers)

R: *Early detection of compromise can prevent serious.*

When the individual is unconscious or heavily sedated and unable to complain or report sensations, intensive assessment is required

R: *Permanent nerve injury can occur 12 to 24 hours of nerve compression.*

If pain medications become ineffective, consider compartmental syndrome

R: *Opioids are ineffective for neurovascular pain (Pasero & McCaffery, 2011).*

If signs of compartment syndrome occur

- Discontinue excessive elevation and ice applications.
- Keep the body part below the level of the heart.

R: *This will to improve blood flow into the compartment*

- Remove restrictive dressings, splints

R: *Elevation and external devices will impede perfusion.*

Initiate nasal oxygen

R: *This will improve oxygenation to compromised tissue.*

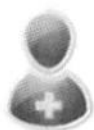

Clinical Alert Immediately, advise physician, physician assistant/NP of the need for the evaluation of the neurovascular changes assessed or reported by the individual (Stracciolini & Hammerberg, 2014).

R: *Immediate medical assessment will determine what specific interventions are needed (e.g., measurement of compartment pressures, emergency surgery [fasciotomy], removal of cast, splints). Measurement of compartment pressures can be done with a handheld manometer (e.g., Stryker device), a simple needle manometer system, or the wick or slit catheter technique.*

Monitor and document compartment pressures according to protocol. Report elevated pressures promptly

R: *"The normal pressure of a tissue compartment falls between 0 and 8 mmHg. Clinical findings associated with ACS generally correlate with the degree to which tissue pressure within the affected compartment approaches systemic blood pressures. Capillary blood flow becomes compromised when tissue pressure increases to within 25 to 30 mmHg of mean arterial pressure" (Stracciolini & Hammerberg, 2014).*

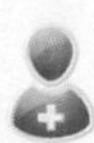

Clinical Alert Many surgeons involved in trauma care use a threshold based upon the difference between systemic blood pressures and compartment pressures to confirm the presence of ACS. These authors concur with this approach and suggest that a difference between the diastolic blood pressure and the compartment pressure (delta pressure) of 30 mm Hg or less be used as the threshold for diagnosing ACS. The delta pressure is found by subtracting the compartment pressure from the diastolic pressure. Many clinicians use the delta pressure of 30 mm Hg to determine the need for fasciotomy, while others use a difference of 20 mm Hg (Stracciolini & Hammerberg, 2014).

Carefully maintain hydration with at least 0.5 mL/kg[2]

R: *Muscle necrosis or rhabdomyolysis may lead to the accumulation of myoglobin in the kidneys, causing acute renal failure in up to 50% of individuals with rhabdomyolysis (Mabvuure, Malahias, Hindocha, Khan, & Juma, 2012).*

R: *Eight liters of fluid can extravasate into a limb, causing hypovolemia, decreased renal function, and shock.*

Risk for Complications of Intra-Abdominal Hypertension

Definition

Describes a person experiencing or at high risk to experience sustained or repeated pathologic elevation of intra-abdominal pressure (IAP) of 12 mm Hg or greater (WSACS, 2013). Abdominal compartment syndrome refers to organ dysfunction caused by intra-abdominal hypertension (Gestring, 2015).

High-Risk Populations

(Gestring, 2015; Lee, 2012)

- Causes of primary (i.e., acute) intra-abdominal hypertension include the following:
  - Penetrating trauma
  - Intraperitoneal hemorrhage
  - Pancreatitis
  - External compressing forces, such as debris from a motor vehicle collision or after a large structure explosion
  - Pelvic fracture
  - Rupture of abdominal aortic aneurysm
  - Perforated peptic ulcer
- Secondary intra-abdominal hypertension may occur in individuals without an intra-abdominal injury, when fluid accumulates in volumes sufficient to cause intra-abdominal hypertension. Causes include the following:
  - Large-volume resuscitation: The literature shows significantly increased risk with infusions greater than 3 L, for example, trauma
  - Large areas of full-thickness burns (>30% total body surface area)
  - Penetrating or blunt trauma without identifiable injury
  - Abdominal surgery
  - Packing and primary fascial closure, which increases incidence
  - Sepsis
  - Liver transplantation
- Causes of chronic intra-abdominal hypertension include the following:
  - Peritoneal dialysis
  - Morbid obesity
  - Cirrhosis
  - Chronic alcohol abuse
  - Pancreatitis
  - Meigs syndrome
  - Intra-abdominal mass
  - Massive ascites
  - Bowel distention

Collaborative Outcomes

The individual will be monitored for early signs and symptoms of intra-abdominal hypertension; will receive collaborative interventions if indicated to restore physiologic stability.

[2] Continue to monitor cardiovascular and renal status: pulse, respiration, blood pressure, and urine output.

Indicators of Physiologic Stability

- Intra-abdominal pressure 0 to 5 mm Hg
- No increase in abdominal girth
- Urine output > 0.5 mL/kg/hr
- No melena

Interventions and Rationales

Monitor for intra-abdominal hypertension (IAH)

R: *Organ dysfunction with intra-abdominal hypertension is a product of the effects of IAH on multiple organ systems.*

- Increase in abdominal girth

R: *The effect of IAH on the GI system leads to diminished perfusion, which results in ischemia, acidosis, capillary leak, intestinal edema, and release of GI flora into the lymph and vascular systems (Lee, 2012).*

- Wheezes, rales, increased respiratory rate, cyanosis
- Limited respiratory excursion

R: *As the abdomen distends, the diaphragm is pushed upward, preventing the lungs from full expansion and increasing intrathoracic pressure (Lee, 2012).*

- Decreased urine output

R: *Increasing abdominal distention compresses renal parenchyma and decreased renal perfusion (Lee, 2012).*

- Wan appearance, syncope, headache, confusion

R: *Increasing intrathoracic pressure causes back pressure on the jugular veins and impedes drainage of cerebrospinal fluid, producing increased intracranial pressure (Lee, 2012).*

- Intra-abdominal hypertension (IAH) that increases to 20 mm Hg or greater and is associated with new organ dysfunction or failure is abdominal compartmental syndrome. Abdominal compartmental syndrome has a mortality rate of over 50%. Medical treatment focuses on attempting to reduce IAP with mechanical drainage and diuretics. If these methods are not effective, a decompressive laparotomy must be performed (Lee, 2012).

To manage individuals with IAH appropriately, nurses must perform IAP measurements

The gold standard of indirect measurement is measurement via a urinary bladder catheter

R: *Hands-on assessments of the abdomen and serial measurements of abdominal girth are not sensitive as direct and indirect measurements of IAP (Lee, 2012).*

Monitor intra-abdominal pressure in high-risk individuals who

- Are intubated with high peak and plateau pressures
- Have GI bleeding or pancreatitis, who are nonresponsive to intravenous (IV) fluids, blood products, and pressors
- Have severe burns or sepsis, who are not responding to IV fluids and pressors
- Have contradictory Swann-Ganz readings, when compared to clinical condition

Institute interventions to prevent or reduce abdominal distention

R: *Preventing abdominal compartment syndrome is much more effective than treating it.*

Prevent constipation and fecal impactions

R: *These conditions will increase abdominal distention.*

Maintain patency of nasogastric tube and monitor for increased residuals with enteral feedings

R: *Increased residual feedings or retained GI fluids will further increase distention.*

Ensure that individuals who are eating; avoid all gas-producing food

R: *These gases can further aggravate abdominal distention.*

Avoid the prone position and elevating the head of bed more than 20°

R: *The prone position and elevations over 20° will increase intra-abdominal pressure.*

Remove heavy blankets, constrictive abdominal dressings

R: *Any external pressure on the abdomen will increase pressure (must be avoided to prevent).*

Aggressively manage fluid balance to keep the individual in negative or equal state

R: *Excessive fluid administration will increase abdominal hypertension. Careful attention needs to be paid to the amount of fluid being administered and closely monitoring individuals for early signs/symptoms of ACS (Gestring, 2015).*

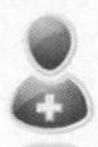

CLINICAL ALERT One trial randomly assigned 71 patients with severe acute pancreatitis to rapid fluid expansion or controlled fluid expansion. The rapid expansion group received significantly greater volumes of crystalloid (4,028 vs. 2,472 mL) and colloid (1,336 vs. 970 mL) on the day of admission with no differences after 4 days. The incidence of abdominal compartment syndrome was higher in the rapid expansion group (72% vs. 38%) (Gestring, 2015).

RISK FOR COMPLICATIONS OF RESPIRATORY DYSFUNCTION

Risk for Complications of Respiratory Dysfunction

Risk for Complications of Atelectasis, Pneumonia
Risk for Complications of Hypoxemia

Definition

Describes a person experiencing or at high risk to experience various respiratory problems

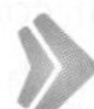

Carp's Cues

The nurse uses the generic collaborative problem *Risk for Complications of Respiratory Dysfunction* to describe a person at risk for several types of respiratory problems and to identify the nursing focus—monitoring respiratory status for detection and diagnosis of abnormal functioning. Nursing management of a specific respiratory complication is then described under the appropriate collaborative problem for that complication. For example, a nurse using *Risk for Complications of Respiratory Dysfunction* for an individual in whom hypoxemia later develops would then add *Risk for Complications of Hypoxemia* to the individual's problem list. If the risk factors or etiology was not related directly to the primary medical diagnosis, the nurse would add this information to the diagnostic statement (e.g., *Risk for Complications of Hypoxemia* related to COPD in an individual with chronic obstructive pulmonary disease [COPD] who experiences respiratory problems after gastric surgery).

For a person vulnerable to respiratory problems because of immobility or excessive tenacious secretions, the nurse should apply the nursing diagnosis *Risk for Ineffective Respiratory Function* related to immobility rather than *Risk for Complications of Respiratory Dysfunction*.

Significant Laboratory/Diagnostic Assessment Criteria

- Blood pH (elevated in alkalosis, lowered in acidosis)
- Arterial blood gas (ABG) values:
  - pH (elevated in alkalemia, lowered in acidemia) (more commonly referred to as alkalosis and or acidosis)
  - PCO_2 (elevated in pulmonary disease, lowered in hyperventilation)
  - PO_2 (lowered in pulmonary disease)
  - CO_2 content (elevated in COPD, lowered in hyperventilation)
- Sputum stain and culture
- Chest X-ray
- Pulmonary angiography
- Bronchoscopy
- Thoracentesis
- Pulmonary function tests

- Ventilation/perfusion scanning
- Pulse oximetry
- End-tidal carbon monitoring ($ETCO_2$)

Risk for Complications of Atelectasis, Pneumonia

Definition

Describes a person experiencing impaired respiratory functioning because of a complete or partial collapse of a lung or lobe of a lung, which can result in pneumonia[3]

High-Risk Populations

- Mechanical ventilation
- Pulmonary edema
- Impaired swallowing (increased risk for aspiration)
- Shallow breathing (due to abdominal pain or rib fracture)
- Postoperative status (especially abdominal or thoracic surgery)
- Immobilization
- Decreased level of consciousness
- Nasogastric feedings
- Chronic lung disease (COPD, bronchiectasis, cystic fibrosis)
- Chronic heart, liver or renal disease
- Diabetes mellitus
- Alcoholism
- Cancer
- Asplenia
- Immunosuppressed conditions or on immunosuppressing medications (within previous 3 months)
- Debilitation
- Decreased surfactant production
- Compression of lung tissue (e.g., from cancer, abdominal distention, obesity, pneumothorax)
- Airway obstruction
- Impaired ability to cough (e.g., poor cough reflex, too weak, or in pain from recent surgery or an accident), to cough vigorously

Presence of comorbidities such as chronic heart, lung, liver, or renal disease; diabetes mellitus; alcoholism; malignancies; asplenia; immunosuppressing conditions or use of immunosuppressing drugs; or use of antimicrobials within the previous 3 months (in which case an alternative from a different class should be selected).

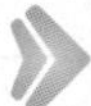

Carp's Cues

Pneumonia can be classified as community-acquired or hospital-acquired. The following scoring helps to determine which individuals should be treated at home or admitted to the hospital.

CURB-65 uses five prognostic variables (Lim et al., 2003):

- Confusion (based upon a specific mental test or disorientation to person, place, or time)
- Urea (blood urea nitrogen in the United States) >7 mmol/L (20 mg/dL)
- Respiratory rate ≥30 breaths/min
- Blood pressure (BP) (systolic <90 mm Hg or diastolic ≤60 mm Hg)
- Age ≥65 years

"The authors (Lim et al., 2003) of the original CURB-65 report suggested that patients with a CURB-65 score of 0 to 1, who comprised 45 percent of the original cohort and 61 percent of the later cohort, were at low risk and could probably be treated as outpatients. Those with a score of 2 should be admitted to the hospital, and those with a score of 3 or more should be assessed for care in the intensive care unit (ICU), particularly if the score was 4 or 5" (Bartlett, 2014).

[3]The nurse should use the nursing diagnosis *Risk for Ineffective Respiratory Function* for people at high risk for atelectasis and pneumonia, to focus on prevention. The collaborative problem *Risk for Complications of Atelectasis, Pneumonia* is applicable only if the condition occurs.

Collaborative Outcomes

In the following section, () indicates *closely monitor individuals over 65 years of age*

The individual will be monitored for early signs and symptoms of atelectasis and/or pneumonia and the individual will receive collaborative interventions if indicated to restore physiologic stability.

Indicators of Physiologic Stability

- Alert, calm, oriented (baseline for individual)
- Respiratory rate 16 to 20 breaths/min
- Respirations easy, rhythmic
- Temperature 98° F to 99.5° F
- No change in usual skin color
- Pulse oximetry >95%

Interventions and Rationales

Evaluate the individual's risk for mortality using the CURB-65 scale (Bartlett, 2014; Lim et al., 2003)

- One point is given for the presence of each of the following (Lim et al., 2003):
  - **C**onfusion—altered mental status
  - **U**remia—blood urea nitrogen (BUN) level greater than 20 mg/dL
  - **R**espiratory rate—30 breaths or more per minute
  - **B**lood pressure—systolic pressure less than 90 mm Hg or diastolic pressure less than 60 mm Hg
  - Age older than 65 years

Current guidelines suggest that individuals may be treated in an outpatient setting or may require hospitalization according to their CURB-65 score, as follows

- Score of 0 to 1—outpatient treatment
- Score of 2—admission to medical unit
- Score of 3 or higher—admission to intensive care unit (ICU)

Ensure blood culture is done prior to the start of any antibiotic

- Culture any suspected infection sites (urine, sputum, invasive lines).

R: *Poor outcomes are associated with inadequate or inappropriate antimicrobial therapy (i.e., treatment with antibiotics to which the pathogen was later shown to be resistant in vitro). They are also associated with delays in initiating antimicrobial therapy, even short delays (e.g., an hour) (Schmidt & Mandel, 2012).*

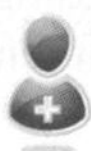

CLINICAL ALERT Blood culture obtained after the initiation of antibiotic therapy can be inaccurate. Research on individuals with septic shock demonstrated that the time to initiation of appropriate antimicrobial therapy was the strongest predictor of mortality (Schmidt & Mandel, 2012).

Monitor for signs and symptoms of pneumonia, atelectasis

- Increased respiratory rate >24 breaths/min (tachypnea) 45% to 70% frequency
- Fever (80% frequency) and chills (50%) (sudden or insidious)*
- Productive cough with Mucopurulent sputum*
- Diminished or absent breath sounds
- Rales, or crackles, (30% frequency)*
- Pleuritic chest pain (30% frequency)
- Marked dyspnea*

R: *Bacteria can act as a pyrogen by raising the hypothalamic thermostat through the production of endogenous pyrogens, which may mediate through prostaglandins. Chills can occur when the temperature setpoint of the hypothalamus changes rapidly. High fever increases metabolic needs and oxygen consumption. The impaired respiratory system cannot compensate, and tissue hypoxia results (Grosssman & Porth, 2014). In older adults, tachypnea ≥26 respirations/min is one of the earliest signs of pneumonia and often occurs 3 to 4 days before a confirmed diagnosis.*

- Lethargy, change in mental status

R: *Delirium or mental status changes are often seen early in pneumonia in older individuals. Decreased blood flow to brain, heart, and kidneys triggers baroreceptors, and release of catecholamines increases heart rate/cardiac output, further increasing vasoconstriction (Grossman & Porth, 2014).*

- Gastrointestinal symptoms (e.g., nausea, vomiting, diarrhea)

Monitor laboratory and other diagnostic tests

- White blood cells

R: *"The major blood test abnormality is leukocytosis (typically between 15,000 and 30,000 per mm³) with a leftward shift. Leukopenia can occur and generally connotes a poor prognosis" (Bartlett, 2014).*

- Chest X-ray

R: *"The presence of an infiltrate on plain chest radiograph is considered the gold standard for diagnosing pneumonia when clinical and microbiologic features are supportive" (Bartlett, 2014).*

R: *Tracheobronchial inflammation, impaired alveolar capillary membrane function, edema, fever, and increased sputum production disrupt respiratory function and compromise the blood's oxygen-carrying capacity. Reduced chest wall compliance in older adults affects the quality of respiratory effort. In older adults, tachypnea (≥26 respirations/min) is an early sign of pneumonia, often occurring 3 to 4 days before a confirmed diagnosis. Delirium or mental status changes are often seen early in pneumonia in older adults (Grossman & Porth, 2014).*

Evaluate the effectiveness of cough suppressants and expectorants

R: *A dry, hacking cough interferes with sleep and affects energy. Cough suppressants should be used judiciously, however, because complete depression of the cough reflex can lead to atelectasis by hindering movement of tracheobronchial secretions.*

Monitor for signs and symptoms of septic shock

R: *Bacterial infections are the most common cause of sepsis. The infection can begin anywhere bacteria or other infectious agents can enter the body. Sepsis can be caused by skin laceration, appendicitis, pneumonia, or a urinary tract infection (Grossman & Porth, 2014).*

- Altered body temperature (>38° C or <36° C)
- Hypotension (140/90, >90/60 mm Hg; MAP [mean arterial pressure] >70; CVP >11)
- Decreased level of consciousness
- Weak, rapid pulse
- Rapid, shallow respirations or CO_2 <32

R: *Diminishing oxygen saturation as seen by pulse oxime*

- Cold, clammy skin
- Oliguria (urine output <0.5 mL/kg/hr)

R: *Septic shock is a systemic inflammatory response syndrome (SIRS) associated with infection because of microorganisms resulting in hypotension and perfusion abnormalities despite fluid resuscitation or vasopressors.*

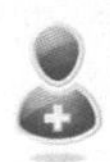

Clinical Alert Immediate action is needed, call Rapid Response Team.

- Refer to *Risk for Complications of Systemic Inflammatory Response Syndrome (SIRS)/Sepsis*
- Evaluate if individual has had the influenza vaccine and if indicated Pneumovax and Prevnar 13 immunizations. When the individual is stable, the vaccines can be given in the hospital per protocols.

R: *This increased the likelihood of vaccination.*

Risk for Complications of Hypoxemia

Definition

Describes a person experiencing or at high risk to experience insufficient plasma oxygen saturation (PO_2 less than normal for age) because of alveolar hypoventilation, pulmonary shunting, or ventilation–perfusion inequality

High-Risk Populations

- COPD
- Asthma
- Acute lung injury
- Sepsis
- Pneumothorax
- Pleural effusion
- Pneumonia
- Atelectasis
- Pulmonary edema
- Adult respiratory distress syndrome
- Central nervous system depression
- Medulla or spinal cord disorders
- Guillain–Barré syndrome
- Myasthenia gravis
- Muscular dystrophy
- Obesity
- Compromised chest wall movement (e.g., trauma)
- Drug overdose
- Head injury
- Near-drowning
- Multiple trauma
- Anemia and/or hypovolemia
- Pulmonary embolism

Collaborative Outcomes

The individual will be monitored for early signs and symptoms of hypoxemia and the individual will receive collaborative interventions if indicated to restore physiologic stability.

Indicators of Physiologic Stability

- Serum pH 7.35 to 7.45
- $PaCO_2$ 35 to 45
- PaO_2 80 to 100
- Pulse: regular rhythm, rate 60 to 100 beats/min
- Respirations 16 to 20 breaths/min
- Blood pressure <140/90, >90/60 mm Hg (MAP >70; CVP >11)
- Urine output >30 mL/hr (use of a standardized volume that is weight-based, e.g., >0.5 mL/kg/hr)

Interventions and Rationales

Monitor for signs of acid–base imbalance

- ABG analysis: pH <7.35, $PaCO_2$ >48 mm Hg

R: *ABG analysis helps evaluate gas exchange in the lungs. In mild to moderate COPD, the individual may have a normal $PaCO_2$ level as chemoreceptors in the medulla respond to increased $PaCO_2$ by increasing ventilation. In severe COPD, however, the individual cannot sustain this increased ventilation, and the $PaCO_2$ value gradually increases (Grossman & Porth, 2014).*

- Increased and irregular pulse, and increased respiratory rate initially, followed by decreased rate

R: *Respiratory acidosis develops as a result of excessive CO_2 retention. An individual with respiratory acidosis from chronic disease at first experiences increased heart rate and respirations in an attempt to compensate for decreased oxygenation. After a while, the individual breathes more slowly and with prolonged expiration. Eventually, the respiratory center may stop responding to the higher CO_2 levels, and breathing may stop abruptly (Grossman & Porth, 2014).*

- Changes in mentation (somnolence, confusion, irritability, anxiety)

R: *Changes in mentation result from cerebral tissue hypoxia.*

- Decreased urine output (<0.5 mL/hr); cool, pale, or cyanotic skin

R: *The compensatory response to decreased circulatory oxygen aims to increase blood oxygen by increasing heart and respiratory rates and to decrease circulation to the kidneys and extremities (marked by decreased pulses and skin changes) (Grossman & Porth, 2014).*

Administer low-flow (2 L/min) oxygen as needed through nasal cannula; if indicated, titrate up to keep pulse oximetry between 90% and 92%

R: *Oxygen therapy increases circulating oxygen levels. Using a cannula rather than a mask may help reduce the individual's fears of suffocation.*

Limit O_2 flow to 1 to 2 L/min in individuals with COPD

R: *High concentrations of oxygen decrease the respiratory drive causing hypoventilation with increase in carbon dioxide ($PaCO_2$).*

Evaluate the effects of positioning on oxygenation, using ABG values as a guide

- Change individual's position every 2 hours, avoiding positions that compromise oxygenation.

R: *This measure promotes optimal ventilation*

Ensure adequate hydration

- Teach individual to avoid dehydrating beverages (e.g., caffeinated drinks, grapefruit juice).

R: *Optimal hydration helps liquefy secretions. Avoid milk-based products.*

Ensure adequate nutrition

- Teach individual to eat small frequent meals.

R: *Small frequent meals will be more comfortable and allow greater dietary intake. Individuals often are short of breath and fatigue while eating.*

Monitor for signs of right-sided heart failure

- Elevated diastolic pressure
- Distended neck veins
- Edema
- Elevated central venous pressure

R: *The causes of right-sided heart failure are conditions that impede blood flow into the lungs. The heart must work harder to pump oxygen-rich blood throughout your body. The combination of arterial hypoxemia and respiratory acidosis acts locally as a strong vasoconstrictor of pulmonary vessels. This leads to pulmonary arterial hypertension, increased right ventricular systolic pressure, and, eventually, right ventricular hypertrophy and failure (Grossman & Porth, 2014).*

- Refer to the nursing diagnosis *Activity Intolerance* in Section 1 for specific adaptive techniques to teach an individual with chronic pulmonary insufficiency.

RISK FOR COMPLICATIONS OF METABOLIC/IMMUNE/ HEMATOPOIETIC DYSFUNCTION

Risk for Complications of Metabolic/Immune/Hematopoietic Dysfunction

Risk for Complications of Hypo/Hyperglycemia
Risk for Complications of Negative Nitrogen Balance
Risk for Complications of Electrolyte Imbalances
Risk for Complications of Systemic Inflammatory Response Syndrome (SIRS)/Sepsis
Risk for Complications of Acidosis (Metabolic, Respiratory)
Risk for Complications of Alkalosis (Metabolic, Respiratory)
Risk for Complications of Allergic Reaction
Risk for Complications of Thrombocytopenia
Risk for Complications of Opportunistic Infections
Risk for Complications of Vaso-Occlusive/Sickling Crisis

Definition

Describes a person experiencing or at high risk to experience various endocrine, immune, or metabolic dysfunctions

Author's Note

The nurse can use this generic collaborative problem to describe a person at risk for several types of metabolic and immune system problems. For example, for an individual with pituitary dysfunction who is at risk for various metabolic problems, using *Risk for Complications of Metabolic Dysfunction* directs nurses to monitor endocrine system function for specific problems, based on focus assessment findings. Under this collaborative problem, nursing interventions would focus on monitoring metabolic status to detect and diagnose abnormal functioning.

If the individual develops a specific complication, the nurse would add the appropriate specific collaborative problem, along with nursing management information, to the individual's problem list. For an individual with diabetes mellitus, the nurse would add the diagnostic statement *Risk for Complications of Hypo/Hyperglycemia.* For an individual receiving chemotherapy, the nurse would use *Risk for Complications of Immunodeficiency,* a collaborative problem that encompasses leukopenia, thrombocytopenia, and erythrocytopenia. If thrombocytopenia were an isolated problem, it would warrant a separate diagnostic statement (i.e., *Risk for Complications of Thrombocytopenia*).

For an individual with a condition or undergoing a treatment that produces immunosuppression (e.g., AIDS, graft-versus-host disease, immunosuppressant therapy), the collaborative problem *Risk for Complications of Immunosuppression* would be appropriate. When conditions have or possibly could have affected coagulation (e.g., chronic renal failure, alcohol abuse, anticoagulant therapy), a collaborative problem such as *Risk for Complications of Hemolysis* or *Risk for Complications of Erythrocytopenia* would be indicated. If the risk factors or etiology were not directly related to the primary medical diagnosis, they could be added (e.g., *Risk for Complications of Immunosuppression related to chronic corticosteroid therapy* in an individual who has sustained a myocardial infarction).

Significant Laboratory/Diagnostic Assessment Criteria

- Serum amylase (elevated in acute pancreatitis, lowered in chronic pancreatitis)
- Serum albumin (lowered in malnutrition)
- Lymphocyte count (lowered in malnutrition)
- Serum calcium (elevated in hyperparathyroidism, certain cancers, and acute pancreatitis, lowered in hypoparathyroidism)
- Blood pH (elevated in alkalosis, lowered in acidosis)
- Serum glucose (elevated in diabetes mellitus and pancreatic insufficiency, lowered in pancreatic islet cell tumors)
- Cystatin C to screen for and monitor kidney dysfunction in those with known or suspected kidney disease
- Serum antidiuretic hormone (ADH) (elevated levels indicate syndrome of inappropriate antidiuretic hormone excretion [SIADH]), reduced levels indicate central diabetes insipidus)
- Urine specific gravity (reflects the kidneys' ability to concentrate and dilute urine)
- Serum osmolarity (represents concentration of particles in blood)
- Urine osmolarity (measures urine concentration—increased in Addison's disease, SIADH, dehydration renal disease; decreased in diabetes insipidus, psychogenic water drinking)
- Serum glycosylated hemoglobin (Hgb A1c) (reflects mean glucose levels for preceding 2 to 3 months)
- Urine acetone, urine glucose (present in diabetes mellitus)
- Urine ketone bodies (present in uncontrolled diabetes)
- Platelets (elevated in polycythemia and chronic granulocytic leukemia, lowered in anemia and acute leukemia)
- Immunoglobulins (elevated in autoimmune disease)
- Coagulation tests (elevated in thrombocytopenia, purpura, and hemophilia)
- Prothrombin time (elevated in anticoagulant therapy, cirrhosis, and hepatitis)
- Red blood cell (RBC) count (lowered in anemia, leukemia, and renal failure)
- CT, MRI of targeted organ
- Bone marrow aspirate with diagnostic pathology
- Spinal tap with appropriate analysis, culture, and sensitivity

Risk for Complications of Hypo/Hyperglycemia

Definition

Describes a person experiencing or at high risk to experience a blood glucose level that is too low or too high for metabolic function.[4]

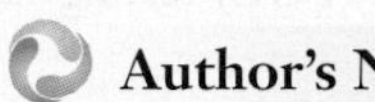

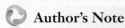

Author's Note

In 2006, NANDA approved the nursing diagnosis, *Risk for Unstable Blood Sugar.* This author defines this condition as a collaborative problem. The nurse can choose which terminology is preferred. The student should consult with the instructor for direction.

High-Risk Populations

- Diabetes mellitus
- Parenteral nutrition
- Systemic inflammatory response syndrome (SIRS)/sepsis
- Enteral feedings
- Medications
- Hyperglycemia—corticosteroid therapy, acute response to stimulants as amphetamine, some psychotropic medications such as olanzapine (Zyprexa) and duloxetine (Cymbalta)
- Hypoglycemia—chronic use of stimulants
- Hypoglycemia
  - Excess alcohol intake
  - Pancreatic tumor—insulinoma
  - Lack (deficiency) of a hormone, such as cortisol or thyroid hormone
  - Severe heart, kidney, or liver failure or a body-wide infection
  - Some types of weight-loss surgery
- Pancreatitis (hyperglycemia), cancer of pancreas
- Addison's disease (hypoglycemia)
- Adrenal gland hyperfunction
- Liver disease (hypoglycemia)

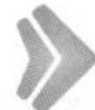

Carp's Cues

Over twenty-nine million (29.1 million) people or 9.3% of the US population have diabetes—diagnosed 21.0 million people; undiagnosed 8.1 million people (27.8% of people with diabetes are undiagnosed) (National Diabetes Statistics Report, 2014).

Collaborative Outcomes

The individual will be monitored for early signs and symptoms of hyperglycemia and/or hypoglycemia and will receive collaborative interventions if indicated to restore physiologic stability.

Indicators of Physiologic Stability

- pH 7.35 to 7.45 and HCO_3 18 to 22 mmol/L
- Fasting blood glucose 70 to 130 mg/dL No ketones in urine
- Serum sodium 135 to 145 mmol/L Serum osmolality, >295 mOsm/kg
- BP <130/80 clear, oriented
- Pulse (60 to 100 beats/min)
- Respiration 16 to 20 breaths/min
- Peripheral pulses, equal and full, capillary refill <3 seconds
- Warm, dry skin
- No vision changes
- Bowel sounds, present

[4] If the person is not at risk for both, the diagnosis should specify the problem (e.g., *Risk for Complications of Hyperglycemia related to corticosteroid therapy*).

- White blood cells 4,000 to 10,800 mm
- Urine, protein-negative
- Creatinine 0.8 to 1.3 mg/dL
- Blood urea nitrogen 5 to 25 mg/dL

Interventions and Rationales

Many labs and institutions require a repeat of or a second method of validation for treatment of "Critical Lab Values." The organizations define them and require them even for Point of Care (POC) testing for blood glucose values.

Monitor for signs and symptoms of diabetic ketoacidosis (DKA) with type 1 diabetes

- Recent illness/infection
- Blood glucose >300 mg/dL
- Malaise and generalized weakness
- Moderate/large ketones
- Dehydration
- Anorexia, nausea, vomiting, abdominal pain
- Kussmaul's respirations (shallow, rapid)
- Fruity acetone odor of the breath
- pH <7.30 and HCO_3 <15 mEq
- Decreased sodium, potassium, phosphates

R: *When insulin is not available, blood glucose (BG) levels rise and the body metabolizes fat for energy; the byproduct of this fat metabolism is ketones. Excessive ketone bodies results in ketoacidosis and a drop in pH and bicarbonate serum levels. This acidosis causes headaches, nausea, vomiting, and abdominal pain. Increased respiratory rate helps CO_2 excretion in effort to reduce acidosis. Elevated glucose levels inhibit water reabsorption in the renal glomerulus, leading to osmotic diuresis with loss of water, sodium, potassium, and phosphates, leading to severe dehydration and electrolyte imbalance (Grossman & Porth, 2014).*

Monitor for signs and symptoms of hyperosmolar hyperglycemic state (HHS) type 2

- Blood glucose >600 mg/dL
- pH >7.30 and HCO_3 >15 mEq/L
- Severe dehydration
- Serum osmolality >320 mOsm/kg
- Hypotension, tachycardia
- Altered sensorium, lethargy
- Nausea, vomiting
- Urine ketones negative or <2+

R: *Hyperosmolar hyperglycemic state is marked by profound dehydration and hyperglycemia without ketoacidosis. Decreased renal clearance and utilization of glucose result in an osmotic dieresis and osmotic shift of fluid to the intravascular space, resulting in intracellular dehydration and loss of electrolytes. Cerebral impairment is due to this intracellular dehydration (Grossman & Porth, 2014).*

Monitor for signs and symptoms of hypoglycemia

- Blood glucose <70 mg/dL
- Pale, moist, cool skin
- Tachycardia, diaphoresis
- Jitteriness, irritability
- Confusion
- Drowsiness
- Hypoglycemia unawareness

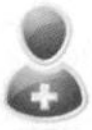

Clinical Alert Hypoglycemia is defined as any BG <70 mg/dL and may be caused by too much insulin, too little food, or too much physical activity. Hypoglycemia symptoms are related to sympathetic system stimulation and brain dysfunction related to decreased levels of glucose. Sympathoadrenal activation and release of adrenaline causes diaphoresis, cool skin, tachycardia, anxiety, and jitteriness. Reduction in cerebral glucose will result in confusion, difficulty with concentration, focal impairments, and if severe, can cause seizures and eventually coma and death (Hamdy, 2012).

Treatment of hypoglycemia is considered emergent.

R: *Hypoglycemia unawareness is a defect in the body's defense system that impairs the ability to experience the warning symptoms usually associated with hypoglycemia. The individual may rapidly progress from being alert to unconsciousness.*

Institute "Rule of 15" with a goal to achieve BG >100 mg/dL

- If the individual is alert and cooperative, give 15 g of carbohydrate orally and monitor for 15 minutes; repeat BG—if above 100 mg/dL may give light snack if not time for a meal. If not above 70 mg/dL, repeat treatment with 15 g of carbohydrate—monitor and recheck BG in 15 minutes and may repeat until at goal.
- Nonalert individual: Call for help—if IV access, give 24 g dextrose (1 amp D50); if none, give 1 mg glucagon IM, monitor for 15 minutes, and repeat BG; may repeat treatment q15–30 minutes depending on response.
- If hypoglycemia is severe (BG <40), recurrent, or caused by sulfonylurea or long-acting insulin, follow D50 treatment with D5 or D10 drip.
- Continued follow-up is mandatory until individual is stable. Cause of the hypoglycemia should always be investigated (Inzucchi et al., 2012).

Continue to monitor hydration status every 30 minutes; assess skin moisture and turgor, urine output and specific gravity, and fluid intake

R: *Accurate assessments are needed during the acute stage (first 10 to 12 hours) to prevent overhydration or underhydration.*

Continue to monitor blood glucose levels according to protocol

R: *Careful monitoring enables early detection of medication-induced hypoglycemia or continued hyperglycemia.*

Monitor serum potassium, sodium, and phosphate levels

R: *Acidosis causes hyperkalemia and hyponatremia. Insulin therapy promotes potassium and phosphate return to the cells, causing serum hypokalemia and hypophosphatemia.*

Monitor neurologic status every hour

R: *Fluctuating glucose levels, acidosis, and fluid shifts can affect neurologic functioning.*

Carefully protect individual's skin from microorganism invasion, injury, and shearing force; reposition every 1 to 2 hours

R: *Dehydration and tissue hypoxia increase the skin's vulnerability to injury.*

Do not allow a recovering individual to drink large quantities of water

- Give a conscious individual ice chips to quench thirst.

R: *Excessive fluid intake can cause abdominal distention and vomiting*

Monitor cardiac function and circulatory status; evaluate

- Rate, rhythm (cardiac, respiratory)
- Skin color
- Capillary refill time, central venous pressure
- Peripheral pulses
- Serum potassium

R: *Severe dehydration can cause reduced cardiac output and compensatory vasoconstriction. Cardiac dysrhythmias can result from potassium imbalances.*

Follow protocols for ketoacidosis, as indicated

Investigate for causes of ketoacidosis or hypoglycemia, and teach prevention and early management, using the nursing diagnosis *Risk for Ineffective Self-Health Management related to insufficient knowledge of (specify)* (see Section 2)

Risk for Complications of Negative Nitrogen Balance

Definition

Describes a person experiencing or at risk to experience catabolism, when more nitrogen is excreted from tissue breakdown than is replaced by intake.

High-Risk Populations

- Severe malnutrition
- Prolonged NPO state
- Elderly with chronic disease
- Uncontrolled diabetes
- Digestive disorders
- Prolonged use of glucose or saline IV therapy
- Inadequate enteral replacement
- Excessive catabolism (e.g., due to cancer, infection, burns, surgery, excess stress)
- Anorexia nervosa, bulimia
- Critical illness
- Chemotherapy
- Sepsis

Indicators

- Temperature 98° F to 99.5° F
- White blood count 4,300 to 10,800 mm^3
- No extremity edema
- Serum prealbumin 20 to 50 g/dL
- Serum albumin 3.5 to 5 g/dL

Interventions and Rationale

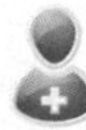

CLINICAL ALERT "After a variety of insults (shock, trauma, burns, sepsis, pancreatitis, etc.), patients develop a systemic inflammatory response that is presumably beneficial and resolves as the patient recovers. However, if the systemic inflammatory response is exaggerated or perpetuated, severe disturbances in protein metabolism may arise. The resulting hypermetabolism and catabolism can cause acute protein malnutrition, with impairment in immune function and subclinical multiple organ dysfunction, including acute renal failure" (Beretta, Rocchetti, & Braga, 2010).

Establish the individual's optimum weight for height

R: *This establishes baseline goals.*

When possible, weigh individual daily at same time, wearing same amount of clothes, same scale, and same bedding

R: *Monitoring weight helps detect excessive catabolism.*

Ensure a consult with nutritionist regarding optimal source of nutrients is obtained

R: *"The current guidelines on nutritional intervention in critically ill patients recommend the utilization of enteral nutrition (EN) in all ICU patients who are not expected to take a full oral diet within 3 days. EN should begin during the first 24 h, using a standard high-protein formula" (Beretta et al., 2010). The early initiation of goal-directed enteral nutrition support improves wound healing, decreases intensive care unit (ICU) and hospital length of stay, and might improve survival following critical illness or injury (Singer et al., 2009).*

Monitor for signs of negative nitrogen balance

- Weight loss
- 24-hour urine nitrogen balance below zero

R: *Impaired carbohydrate metabolism causes increased metabolism of fats and protein, which—especially with metabolic acidosis—can lead to negative nitrogen balance and weight loss. Sustained periods of negative energy balance decrease body mass due to losses of both fat and skeletal muscle mass. Decreases in skeletal muscle mass are associated with a myriad of negative consequences, including suppressed basal metabolic rate, decreased protein turnover, decreased physical performance, and increased risk of injury. Decreases in skeletal muscle mass in response to negative energy balance are due to imbalanced rates of muscle protein synthesis and degradation.*

Monitor for signs and symptoms of hypoalbuminemia, which can have a rapid or insidious onset

- Emotional depression, fatigue

R: *These effects result from decreased energy supplies.*

- Muscle wasting

R: *This results from insufficient protein available for tissue repair.*

- Poorly healing wounds

R: *This results from insufficient protein available for tissue repair.*

- Edema

R: *Edema results from a plasma-to-interstitial fluid shift because of insufficient vascular osmotic pressure.*

Monitor laboratory values

- Serum prealbumin and transferring

R: *These values evaluate visceral protein. Prealbumin is a precursor to albumin and a much more sensitive measure of visceral protein.*

- BUN

R: *This value measures kidney clearance ability.*

- 24-hour urine nitrogen

R: *Because the glomerulus reabsorbs 99% of what is filtered, measurement of urea nitrogen, a waste product of protein metabolism, gives data to calculate the nitrogen balance.*

- Electrolytes, osmolality

R: *These values help assess kidney function.*

- Total lymphocyte count

R: *Lymphocyte production requires protein.*

- Continually reevaluate the individual's energy/protein requirements. Consult with a nutritionist for evaluation (e.g., indirect calorimetry test, anthropometric measures).

R: *Increasing dietary protein intake, and perhaps leucine, to more than the RDA has been demonstrated to spare muscle mass (Carbone, McClung, & Pasiakos, 2012).*

- Administer total parenteral solutions, intralipid fat emulsions, and/or enteral formulas as prescribed by the physician, physician assistant, or advanced practice nurse and in accordance with appropriate procedures and protocols.

R: *This individual's increased caloric requirements for tissue repair cannot be met with routine IV therapy. Refer to Carpenito-Moyet (2014) for care related to Total Parenteral Therapy*

For specific nursing interventions to increase oral nutrient intake

- Refer to the nursing diagnosis *Imbalanced Nutrition: Less Than Body Requirements* (see Section 2).

Risk for Complications of Electrolyte Imbalances[5]

Risk for Complications of Hypokalemia
Risk for Complications of Hyperkalemia
Risk for Complications of Hyponatremia
Risk for Complications of Hypernatremia
Risk for Complications of Hypocalcemia
Risk for Complications of Hypercalcemia

[5] For a person experiencing or at high risk to experience a deficit or excess in a single electrolyte, the diagnostic statement should specify the problem (e.g., *Risk for Complications of Hypokalemia related to diuretic therapy*).

Risk for Complications of Hypophosphatemia
Risk for Complications of Hyperphosphatemia
Risk for Complications of Hypomagnesemia
Risk for Complications of Hypermagnesemia
Risk for Complications of Hypochloremia
Risk for Complications of Hyperchloremia

Definition

Describes a person experiencing or at risk to experience a deficit or excess of one or more electrolytes

High-Risk Populations
(Grossman & Porth, 2014)

For Hypokalemia

Inadequate Intake
- Decreased potassium intake
- Inability to eat
- Potassium-free parenteral solution
- Crash dieting

Excessive Renal Losses
- Diuretic therapy
- Diuretic phase of renal failure
- Increased mineralocorticoid levels (steroid use, hyperaldosteronism)
- Excessive Gastrointestinal Losses
- Excessive nasogastric suctioning
- Vomiting
- Diarrhea
- Draining gastrointestinal fistula
- Laxative misuse

Transcompartmental Shift
- Metabolic or respiratory alkalosis
- Administration of insulin for treatment diabetic ketoacidosis
- Administration of Beta-adrenergic agonist (e.g., albuterol)

Miscellaneous
- Excessive intake of licorice
- Estrogen use
- Malabsorption
- Salt depletion
- Severe magnesium depletion

For Hyperkalemia

Excessive intake
- Excessive or rapid infusion of potassium-containing parenteral fluids
- Treatment with oral potassium supplements
- Excessive intake of potassium-rich foods

Release from Intracellular Compartment
- Cell damage (e.g., from burns, trauma, surgery)
- Extreme exercising
- Seizures
- Acidosis

Inadequate Elimination by kidneys
- Renal failure
- Adrenal insufficiency
- Potassium-sparing diuretic use
- ACE inhibitors or ARBs

For Hyponatremia

Hypotonic hypernatremia (shift of water from intracellular fluids to extracellular fluids)

- Excessively diluted infant formula
- Sodium-free parenteral solutions
- Vomiting, diarrhea
- Excessive diaphoresis (sweating)
- Irrigation with nonsaline solutions (GI tubes, enemas, prostate post-op irrigations)
- Potent diuretic use
- Gastric suctioning
- Burns
- Excessive wound drainage

Euvolemic (decreased serum with normal extracellular fluids)

- Increased antidiuretic hormone levels
- Trauma, stress, pain
- Syndrome of inappropriate antidiuretic hormone (SIADH) (resulting from central nervous system [CNS] disorders, major trauma, malignancies, or endocrine disorders)
- Medications that increase ADH (e.g., vasopressin and its analogues, thiazide and thiazide-like diuretics, chlorpropamide, carbamazepine, antipsychotics, antidepressants nonsteroidal anti-inflammatory drugs, barbiturates, desipramine, morphine, nicotine, amitriptyline) (Pillai, Unnikrishnan, & Pavithran, 2011)
- Diuretic use
- Glucocorticoid deficiency
- Hypothyroidism
- Psychogenic polydipsia
- Endurance exercise
- MDMA ("ecstasy") abuse

Hypovolemic (Decreased Serum Sodium with Increased ECF volume)

- Renal failure without nephrosis
- Decompensated heart failure
- Advance liver disease
- Hypertonic Hyponatremia (Osmotic Shift of Water from ICF to the ECF Compartment)

For Hypernatremia

Excessive Water Losses

- Watery diarrhea
- Hypertonic tube feeding
- Severe insensible fluid loss (e.g., through hyperventilation or sweating)
- Excessive sodium intake (oral, IV, medications)
- Hypertonic tube feeding
- Diabetes insipidus

Decreased Water Intake

- Elderly, infants
- Unconscious or inability to express thirst
- Unavailability of water
- Oral trauma or inability to sallow
- Impaired thirst sensation

Excessive Sodium Intake

- Rapid or Excessive sodium intake (oral, IV, medications)
- Near drowning in salt water

For Hypocalcemia

Impaired ability to mobilize Calcium from Bone

- Hypoparathyroidism
- Resistance to action of parathyroid hormone
- Hypermagnesemia

Decreased Intake or Absorption
- Malabsorption
- Vitamin D deficiency
- Failure to Activate
- Liver disease
- Kidney disease
- Medications that impair activation of vitamin D, for example, antiepileptic drugs, antineoplastic drugs, antibiotics (clotrimazole, rifampicin), anti-inflammatory agents (dexamethasone), antihypertensives (nifedipine, spironolactone), antiretroviral drugs (ritonavir, saquinavir), endocrine drugs (cyproterone acetate), herbal medicines (Kava kava), hyperforin (St. John's wort) (Grober & Kister, 2012)

Abnormal Renal Losses
- Renal failure and increased phosphorus

Increased Protein Binding or Chelation
- Increased pH
- Increased Fatty Acids
- Rapid transfusion of citrated blood

Increased Sequestration
- Acute Pancreatitis

For Hypercalcemia

Increased Intestinal Absorption
- Excessive vitamin D intake
- Milk-alkali syndrome
- Excessive calcium intake (dietary, calcium-containing antacids)

Increased Bone Reabsorption
- Parathyroid hormone-secreting tumors (e.g., lung, kidney)
- Cancers (Hodgkin's disease, myeloma, leukemia, neoplastic bone disease)
- Prolonged immobilization
- Multiple fractures

Decreased Elimination
- Thiazide diuretics
- Lithium therapy

For Hypophosphatemia

Decreased Intestinal Absorption
- Antacids(aluminum and calcium)
- Steatorrhea and chronic diarrhea
- Lack of vitamin D
- Post Parathyroidectomy

Increased Bone Reabsorption
- Alkalosis
- Hypoparathyroidism
- Diabetic ketoacidosis
- Renal tubular absorption deficit (wasting of phosphorus)

Increased Urinary Excretion
- Vitamin D deficiency or resistance
- Primary renal phosphate wasting
- Primary and secondary hyperparathyroidism
- Thiazide diuretics

Malnutrition and Intracellular Shifts
- Alcoholism
- Total parenteral hyperalimentation
- Recovery from malnutrition
- Administration of insulin during treatment for diabetic ketoacidosis

For Hyperphosphatemia

Acute Phosphate Overload
- Laxatives and enemas containing phosphorus
- Excessive IV or PO phosphate

Intracellular-to-Extracellular Shift
- Massive trauma
- Heat Stroke
- Seizures
- Rhabdomyolysis
- Tumor lysis syndrome
- Potassium deficiency

Impaired Elimination
- Renal failure
- Hypoparathyroidism

For Hypomagnesemia (Yu, 2013)

Impaired Intake or Absorption
- Malnutrition
- Malabsorption
- Alcoholism
- Small bowel surgery
- Prolonged IV therapy without magnesium
- High calcium intake without concomitant amounts of magnesium

Increased Losses
- Gastrointestinal losses (chronic use of proton pump inhibitors; e.g., omeprazole usually for more than 1 year)
- Renal loses
  - Volume expansion
  - Alcohol
  - Uncontrolled diabetes mellitus
  - Familial hypomagnesemia
  - Magnesium-wasting kidney disease
- Miscellaneous
  - Increased magnesium uptake by renewing bone, following parathyroidectomy, thyroidectomy, or correction of severe metabolic acidosis "hungry bone syndrome"

For Hypermagnesemia

Excessive intake
- Excessive use of oral magnesium-containing antacids, laxatives
- Intravenous administration of magnesium for treatment of preeclampsia

Decreased Excretion
- Kidney disease
  - Glomerulonephritis
  - Tubulointerstitial kidney disease
- Acute renal failure

For Hypochloremia

- Loss of GI fluids (e.g., through vomiting, diarrhea, suctioning)
- Loss of fluids through skin (e.g., burns, diaphoresis, high fever)
- Metabolic alkalosis
- Diabetic acidosis
- Prolonged use of IV dextrose
- Cystic Fibrosis
- Drugs such as: androgens, corticosteroids, estrogens, and certain diuretics.

For Hyperchloremia Acidosis

- Underlying GI or autoimmune conditions
- Loss of bicarbonate stores through diarrhea or renal tubular wasting
- Renal failure, ketoacidosis, lactic acidosis, and ingestion of certain toxins
- Renal failure
- Cushing's syndrome
- Hyperventilation
- Eclampsia
- Anemia
- Cardiac decompensation

Collaborative Outcomes

The individual will be monitored for early signs and symptoms of electrolyte imbalances and will receive collaborative interventions if indicated to restore physiologic stability.

Indicators of Physiologic Stability with Critical Value Alerts[6] (Mayo, 2014; Stanford Medicine, 2009; Williamson & Snyder, 2014)

- Serum or plasma sodium: 135 to 145 mmol/L; alert levels: <120 mmol/L and ≥160 mmol/L
- Serum potassium: 3.6 to 5.4 mmol/L (plasma, 3.6 to 5.0 mmol/L); alert levels: <3.0 mmol/L and ≥6.0 mmol/L
- Serum or plasma chloride: 98 to 108 mmol/L
- Serum or plasma bicarbonate: 18 to 24 mmol/L (as total carbon dioxide, 22 to 26 mmol/L); alert levels: <10 mmol/L and ≥40 mmol/L
- Serum calcium: 8.5 to 10.5 mg/dL (2.0 to 2.5 mmol/L); alert levels: <6.5 mg/dL and ≥13.0 mg/dL
- Ionized calcium: 1.0 to 1.3 mmol/L
- Serum phosphates 125 to 300 mg/dL
- Serum magnesium: 1.8 to 3.0 mg/dL (1.2 to 2.0 mEq/L or 0.5 to 1.0 mmol/L); alert levels ≤1.0 mg/dL and ≥9.0 mg/dL
- Osmolality (calculated) 280 to 300 mOsm/kg; alert levels ≤190 mOsm/kg and ≥39 mOsm/kg

Interventions and Rationales

Identify the electrolyte imbalance(s) for which the individual is vulnerable, and intervene as follows. (Refer to High-Risk Populations under the specific imbalance.)

Risk for Complications of Hypo/Hyperkalemia

Monitor for signs and symptoms of hyperkalemia

- Serum potassium >6 mmol/L (mEq/L)
  - Weakness to flaccid paralysis
  - Muscle irritability
  - Paresthesias
  - Nausea, abdominal cramping, or diarrhea
  - Oliguria
  - Electrocardiogram (ECG) changes (deJong, 2014):
    - P-waves are widened and of low amplitude due to slowing of conduction
    - Prolonged PR interval
    - Bradycardia
    - QRS complex:
      - QRS widening
      - Fusion of QRS-T
      - Loss of the ST segment
      - Tall tented T waves
      - At concentrations >7.5 mmol/L, atrial and ventricular fibrillation can occur.

[6] Critical values are defined as values that are outside the normal range to a degree that may constitute an immediate health risk to the individual or require immediate action (Stanford Medicine, 2009).

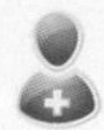

Clinical Alert Early changes in EKG need reporting to physician, physician assistant, or nurse practitioner. Call Rapid Response Team for critical EKG changes.

R: *Hyperkalemia can result from the kidney's decreased ability to excrete potassium or from excessive potassium intake. Acidosis increases the release of potassium from cells. Fluctuations in potassium level affect nerve and muscle transmission, producing cardiac arrhythmias, and reducing action of GI smooth muscle. There is an increase in cardiac irritability and cardiac monitoring may show early changes as premature ventricular beats (Grossman & Porth, 2014).*

For an individual with hyperkalemia

- Restrict potassium-rich foods, fluids, and IV solutions with potassium.

R: *High potassium levels necessitate a reduction in potassium intake.*

- Provide passive range-of-motion (ROM) exercises to extremities.

R: *ROM improves muscle tone and reduces cramps.*

- Per orders or protocols, give medications to reduce serum potassium levels, such as IV calcium.

R: *To block effects on the heart muscle temporarily*

- Give sodium bicarbonate, glucose, insulin.

R: *To force potassium back into cells*

- Give cation-exchange resins (e.g., Kayexalate, hemodialysis)

R: *To force excretion of potassium*

Monitor for signs and symptoms of hypokalemia

- Serum potassium <3.0 mmol/L (mEq/L)
- Nausea, vomiting, anorexia
- Weakness or flaccid paralysis
- Decreased or absent deep tendon reflexes
- Hypoventilation, change in consciousness
- Polyuria
- Hypotension
- Paralytic ileus
- ECG changes (deJong, 2014):
  - ST depression and flattening of the T-wave
  - Negative T waves
  - A U-wave may be visible

R: *Hypokalemia results from losses associated with vomiting, diarrhea, or diuretic therapy, or from insufficient potassium intake. Hypokalemia impairs neuromuscular transmission and reduces the efficiency of respiratory muscles. Kidneys are less sensitive to antidiuretic hormone and thus excrete large quantities of dilute urine. GI smooth muscle action also is reduced. Abnormally low potassium levels also impair electrical conduction of the heart (Grossman & Porth, 2014).*

For a individuals with hypokalemia

- Encourage increased intake of potassium-rich foods.

R: *An increase in dietary potassium intake helps ensure potassium replacement.*

If parenteral potassium replacement (always diluted) is instituted, do not exceed 10 mEq/hr in adults. Monitor serum potassium levels during replacement

R: *Rapid infusion can cause cardiac dysrhythmias.*

- Monitor for discomfort at peripheral infusion site. Observe the IV site for infiltration.

R: *Potassium is very caustic to tissues.*

Risk for Complications of Hypo/Hypernatremia (Grossman & Porth, 2014)

Monitor for signs and symptoms of hyponatremia

- Serum sodium levels below135 mEq/L (mmol/L)
- Apprehension weakness, muscle cramps
- Headache, diarrhea
- Abdominal cramps
- Muscle twitching or convulsions
- Anorexia, nausea, vomiting, diarrhea
- CNS effects ranging from lethargy to coma

R: *Hyponatremia results from sodium loss through vomiting, diarrhea, or diuretic therapy; excessive fluid intake; or insufficient dietary sodium intake. Cellular edema, caused by osmosis, produces cerebral edema, weakness, and muscle cramps.*

For an individual with hyponatremia, initiate IV sodium chloride solutions and discontinue diuretic therapy, as ordered

R: *These interventions prevent further sodium losses.*

Monitor for signs and symptoms of hypernatremia with fluid overload (Grossman & Porth, 2013)

- Serum sodium levels >145mEq/L (mmol/L)
- Increased hematocrit, and BUN
- Elevated serum osmolality
- Thirst, decreased urine output, high urine specific gravity
- CNS effects ranging from decreased reflexes, headache, agitation to seizures, coma
- Tachycardia. Decreased blood pressure

R: *Hypernatremia results from excessive sodium intake or increased aldosterone output. Water is pulled from the cells, causing cellular dehydration and producing CNS symptoms. Thirst is a compensatory response to dilute sodium.*

For an individual with hypernatremia

- Initiate fluid replacement in response to serum osmolality levels, as ordered.

R: *Rapid reduction in serum osmolality can cause cerebral edema and seizures.*

- Monitor for changes in sensorium, decreased reflexes, seizures.

R: *Sodium excess causes cerebral edema.*

- Monitor intake and output.

R: *This evaluates fluid balance.*

Risk for Complications of Hypo/Hypercalcemia

Monitor for signs and symptoms of hypocalcemia

- Serum calcium <6.5 mg/dL
- Altered mental status
- Numbness or tingling in fingers and toes
- Muscle cramps
- Seizures
- ECG changes (deJong, 2014):
  - Narrowing of the QRS complex
  - Reduced PR interval
  - T wave flattening and inversion
  - Prolongation of the QT-interval
  - Prominent U-wave
  - Prolonged ST and ST-depression
- Chvostek's or Trousseau's sign for neuromuscular excitability (tapping the face on the point located 0.5 to 1 cm below the zygomatic process of the temporal bone, 2 cm anterior to the ear lobe causes a spasm of face, lip, or nose, indicating tetany from hypocalcemia]
- Tetany (spasms of the hands and feet, cramps, spasm of the voice box (larynx)

R: *Hypocalcemia can result from the kidney's inability to metabolize vitamin D (needed for calcium absorption). Retention of phosphorus causes a reciprocal drop in serum calcium level. A low serum calcium level produces increased neural excitability, resulting in muscle spasms tetany (cardiac, facial, extremities) and CNS irritability (seizures). It also causes cardiac muscle hyperactivity, as evidenced by ECG changes.*

For an individual with hypocalcemia, follow protocols (Goltzman, 2014)

- For those with milder symptoms of neuromuscular irritability (paresthesias) and corrected calcium concentrations greater than 7.5 mg/dL, oral calcium supplementation can be initiated.
- Intravenous calcium for symptomatic individuals (carpopedal spasm, tetany, seizures), with a prolonged QT-interval, and for asymptomatic patients with an acute decrease in serum corrected calcium to ≤7.5 mg/dL (1.9 mmol/L).

Assess for hyperphosphatemia or hypomagnesemia

R: *Hyperphosphatemia inhibits calcium absorption; in hypomagnesemia, the kidneys excrete calcium to retain magnesium (Goltzman, 2014).*

Monitor for ECG changes: prolonged QT-interval, irritable dysrhythmias, and atrioventricular conduction defects

R: *Calcium imbalances can cause cardiac muscle hyperactivity.*

Monitor for signs and symptoms of hypercalcemia

- Serum calcium ≥13.0 mg/dL
- Altered mental status
- Anorexia, nausea, vomiting, constipation
- Numbness or tingling in fingers and toes
- Muscle cramps, hypotoxicity
- Deep bone pain
- AV blocks (ECG)

R: *Insufficient calcium level reduces neuromuscular excitability, resulting in decreased muscle tone, numbness, anorexia, and mental lethargy.*

For an individual with hypercalcemia

- Initiate normal saline IV therapy and loop diuretics, as ordered; avoid thiazide diuretics.

R: *IV fluids dilute serum calcium. Loop diuretics enhance calcium excretion; thiazide diuretics inhibit calcium excretion.*

- Per order, administer phosphorus preparations and mithramycin (contraindicated in individuals with renal failure).

R: *These increase bone deposition of calcium.*

- Monitor for renal calculi (see *Risk for Complications of Renal Calculi*).

Risk for Complications of Hypo/Hyperphosphatemia

Monitor for signs and symptoms of hypophosphatemia

- Muscle weakness, pain
- Bleeding

Depressed white cell function

- Confusion
- Anorexia

R: *Phosphorus deficiency impairs cellular energy resources and oxygen delivery to tissues and also causes decreased platelet aggregation.*

For an individual with hypophosphatemia, per order, replace phosphorus stores slowly by oral supplements, and discontinue phosphate binders

R: *This helps prevent precipitation with calcium.*

Monitor for signs and symptoms of hyperphosphatemia

- Tetany
- Numbness or tingling in fingers and toes

- Soft tissue calcification
- Chvostek's and Trousseau's signs
- Coarse, dry skin

R: *Hyperphosphatemia can result from the kidneys' decreased ability to excrete phosphorus. Elevated phosphorus does not cause symptoms in and of itself, but contributes to tetany and other neuromuscular symptoms in the short term and to soft tissue calcification in the long term.*

For an individual with hyperphosphatemia, administer phosphorus-binding antacids, calcium supplements, or vitamin D, and restrict phosphorus-rich foods

R: *Supplements are needed to overcome vitamin D deficiency and to compensate for a calcium-poor diet. High phosphate decreases calcium, which increases parathyroid hormone (PTH). PTH is ineffective in removing phosphates due to renal failure, but causes calcium reabsorption from bone and decreases tubular reabsorption of phosphate.*

Risk for Complications of Hypo/Hypermagnesemia

Monitor for hypomagnesemia

- Serum magnesium ≤1.0
- Dysphagia, nausea, anorexia
- Muscle weakness
- Facial tics
- Athetoid movements (slow, involuntary twisting movements)
- Cardiac dysrhythmias, flat or inverted T waves, prolonged QT intervals, tachycardia, depressed ST segment. Torsades, a specific type of ventricular dysrhythmia, is associated with hypomagnesemia.
- Confusion

R: *Magnesium deficit causes neuromuscular changes and hyperexcitability.*

For an individual with hypomagnesemia, initiate magnesium sulfate replacement (dietary for mild deficiency, parenteral for severe deficiency), as ordered

Initiate seizure precautions

R: *This protects from injury.*

Monitor for hypermagnesemia

- Serum magnesium ≥9.0
- Decreased blood pressure, bradycardia, decreased respirations
- Flushing
- Lethargy, muscle weakness
- Peaked T waves

R: *Magnesium excess causes depression of central and peripheral neuromuscular function, producing vasodilation (Grossman & Porth, 2014).*

Risk for Complications of Hypo/Hyperchloremia

Carp's Cues

The serum chloride value, like the serum sodium value, is a *concentration* measurement (e.g., the amount of chloride/liter of plasma water). Therefore, the serum chloride concentration can be elevated above the normal range—hyperchloremia—either by the addition of excess chloride to the ECF compartment or by the loss of water from this compartment, and vice versa. The serum chloride concentration can be reduced below the normal range—hypochloremia—by the loss of chloride from the ECF or the addition of water to this compartment. This means that one cannot evaluate total body chloride stores from the serum chloride concentration. Clinical parameters must be used in conjunction with serum chloride values to assess the significance of hypochloremia or hyperchloremia.

Interventions/Rationale

Monitor electrolytes of individuals, who are vomiting closely

R: *Severe vomiting may lead to the most disproportionate loss of chloride compared to sodium since gastric chloride content is greater than 100 mEq/L and gastric sodium content is relatively low (20 to 30 mEq/L). In individuals with* *protracted vomiting or nasogastric suction, the serum sodium concentration may be only mildly depressed (130 mEq/L), whereas the serum chloride concentration is usually markedly lowered (80 to 90 mEq/L) (Grossman & Porth, 2014).*

Monitor for hypochloremia

- Hyperirritability
- Slow respirations
- Decreased blood pressure

R: *Hypochloremia occurs with metabolic alkalosis, resulting in loss of calcium and potassium, which produces the symptoms.*

For an individual with hypochloremia, see *Risk for Complications of Metabolic Alkalosis* for interventions

Monitor for hyperchloremia

- With acute onset or high levels—headache, lack of energy, nausea, and vomiting
- Weakness
- Lethargy
- Deep, rapid breathing
- Persistent tachycardia

R: *Metabolic acidosis causes loss of chloride ions.*

For an individual with hyperchloremia

- See *Risk for Complications of Metabolic Acidosis* for interventions.

Risk for Complications of Systemic Inflammatory Response Syndrome (SIRS)/Sepsis

Definition of Risk for Complications of Systemic Inflammatory Response Syndrome (SIRS)

Describes a person experiencing or at high risk to experience a life-threatening condition related to dysregulated systemic inflammation, organ dysfunction, and organ failure in response to both infectious processes (sepsis) and noninfectious insults, such as an autoimmune disorder, pancreatitis, vasculitis, thromboembolism. The microorganisms may or may not be present in the bloodstream. SIRS has replaced the terminology *septic syndrome*. Sepsis is one contributing factor to SIRS (Neviere, 2015).

Definition of Risk for Complications of Sepsis

Describes a person experiencing or at risk for experiencing a loss of circulatory volume (hypovolemia) and impaired perfusion caused by an infectious agent (bacterial, viral) resulting in compromised tissue perfusion and cellular dysfunction (Neviere, 2015).

High-Risk Populations

Individuals with

- Bacterial infection (urinary, respiratory, wound)
- Viral infection
- Complication of surgery (GI, thoracic)
- Drug overdose
- Burns, multiple trauma
- Immunosuppression, AIDS
- Invasive lines (urinary, arterial, endotracheal, or central venous catheter)
- Pressure ulcers
- Extensive slow-healing wounds
- Immunocompromised (transplants, cancer, chemotherapy, AIDS, cirrhosis, pancreatitis)
- Diabetes mellitus
- Extreme age (<1 year and >65 years)

Collaborative Outcomes

The individual will be monitored for early signs and symptoms of septic shock and will receive collaborative interventions if indicated to restore physiologic stability.

Indicators of Physiologic Stability (Neviere, 2015)

- Alert
- No edema
- Temperature 98° F to 99.5° F
- Pulse 60 to 100 beats/min
- Capillary refill <2 seconds
- Urine output >0.5/mL/kg/hr
- Urine specific gravity 1.005 to 1.030
- White blood count greater than 4,000 cells/mm^3 or less than 12,000 cells/mm^3
- Less than 10% immature neutrophils (band forms)
- Activated protein C (APC) 65 to 135 International Units/dL
- Platelets 150 to 400
- Prothrombin time 11 to 13.5 seconds
- INR 1.5 to 2.5
- Partial thromboplastin time (PTT) 30 to 45 seconds
- Serum potassium 3.5 to 5.0 mEq/L
- Serum sodium 135 to 145 mEq/L
- Blood glucose (fasting) <100 mg/dL
- Serum lactate levels 1.0 to 2.5 mmol/L
- Plasma C-reactive protein—<0.8 mg/L
- Plasma procalcitonin— the normal value

Interventions and Rationales

Monitor for septic shock and systemic inflammatory response syndrome (SIRS) (Halloran, 2009; Neviere, 2015)

- Urine output <0.5 mL/kg/hr

R: *Urine output is decreased when sodium shifts into the cells, which pulls water into cells. Decreased circulation to kidneys reduces their ability to detoxify the toxins that result from anaerobic metabolism (Grossman & Porth, 2014).*

- Body temperature greater than 38° C or less than 36° C
- Heart rate greater than 90 per minute

R: *High heart rate decreases blood flow to brain, heart, and kidneys.*

- Triggers baroreceptors and release of catecholamines, increasing heart rate/cardiac output and further increasing vasoconstriction
- Hyperkalemia

R: *Potassium moves into the cell with the sodium, impairing nervous, cardiovascular, and muscle cell function.*

- Decreasing blood pressure

R: *Movement of water into the cell causes hypovolemia.*

- Respiratory rate greater than 20 per minute

R: *Anaerobic metabolism decreases circulating oxygen. The body attempts to increase oxygenation by increasing respiratory rate.*

- Hyperglycemia

R: *The liver and kidneys produce more glucose in response to the release of epinephrine, norepinephrine, cortisol, and glucagon. Anaerobic metabolism reduces the effects of insulin. Insulin resistance contributes to multiple organ failure, nosocomial infection, and renal injury (Ball et al., 2007).*

- White blood cell count greater than 12,000 per microliter or less than 4,000 per microliter or presence of 10% immature neutrophils

R: *Increased white cells indicate an infectious process.*

- Plasma C-reactive protein more than two standard deviations above the normal value
- Plasma procalcitonin more than two standard deviations above the normal value

R: *CRP is increased by inflammatory disease as well as infection and is therefore not a good indicator of infection in patients with severe SIRS. PCT level is useful for diagnosis of sepsis and as an indicator of severity of organ failure in patients with SIRS (Kibel, Adams, & Barlow, 2011).*

Ensure that blood culture is done prior to the start of any antibiotic. Culture any suspected infection sites (e.g., urine, sputum, invasive lines)

R: *"Poor outcomes are associated with inadequate or inappropriate antimicrobial therapy (i.e., treatment with antibiotics to which the pathogen was later shown to be resistant in vitro. They are also associated with delays in initiating antimicrobial therapy, even short delays (e.g., an hour)" (Schmidt & Mandel, 2012).*

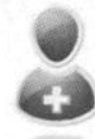

Clinical Alert Blood culture obtained after the initiation of antibiotic therapy can be inaccurate. Research on individuals with septic shock demonstrated that the time to initiation of appropriate antimicrobial therapy was the strongest predictor of mortality (Schmidt & Mandel, 2012).

Assess fluid status

- Monitor central venous pressure and follow protocol for fluid replacement. Early goal-directed therapy (EGDT) with fluid replacement improves cardiac output, tissue perfusion, and oxygen delivery, improving mortality and morbidity.

R: *Sepsis causes vasodilation and capillary leak, resulting in hypovolemia.*

Monitor blood pressure

- Administer replacement fluids and vasopressors (especially norepinephrine) to maintain mean arterial pressure (MAP) >65.

R: *In EGDT, maintaining MAP >65 improves tissue perfusion and outcomes (Neviere, 2015).*

Assess for evidence of adequate tissue perfusion: heart rate, respirations, urine output, mentation, $ScvO_2/SvO_2$

Monitor older adults for changes in mentation; weakness, malaise; normothermia or hypothermia; and anorexia

R: *These individuals do not exhibit the typical signs of infection. Usual presenting findings—fever, chills, tachypnea, tachycardia, and leukocytosis—frequently are absent in older adults with significant infection (Neviere, 2015).*

Risk for Complications of Metabolic or Respiratory Acidosis

Definition

Metabolic acidosis is defined as a pathologic process that, if unopposed, results in a reduction of the serum bicarbonate concentration (normal is 24 mEq/L, with a normal range of 22 to 28 mEq/L) and a low arterial pH (normal 7.4, with a normal range of 7.35 to 7.45). Acidemia (as opposed to acidosis) is defined as a low arterial pH (<7.35), which can result from a metabolic acidosis, respiratory acidosis, or both.

Carp's Cues

Differential Diagnosis (Emmett, 2013)

- Metabolic acidosis is characterized by a low serum HCO_3 and a low arterial pH; the serum anion gap may be increased or normal.
- Metabolic alkalosis is characterized by an elevated serum HCO_3 and an elevated arterial pH.
- Respiratory acidosis is characterized by an elevated arterial PCO_2 and a low arterial pH.
- Respiratory alkalosis is characterized by low arterial PCO_2 and an elevated arterial pH.

- "Mixed acid–base disorders" has a normal arterial pH in the presence of substantial changes in both serum HCO_3 and arterial PCO_2 is usually indicative of a mixed acid–base disorder (which could include an iatrogenic acute respiratory alkalosis if discomfort from the arterial puncture causes the patient to hyperventilate).

High-Risk Populations

For Respiratory Acidosis

Acute result from depression of the central respiratory center by one or another of the following:

- CNS disease or drug-induced respiratory depression
- Inability to ventilate adequately, due to a neuromuscular disease or paralysis (e.g., myasthenia gravis, amyotrophic lateral sclerosis [ALS], Guillain–Barré syndrome, muscular dystrophy)
- Airway obstruction, usually related to asthma or chronic obstructive pulmonary disease (COPD)
- Pneumothorax

Chronic respiratory acidosis may be secondary to many disorders, including COPD. Hypoventilation in COPD involves multiple mechanisms, including the following:

- Decreased responsiveness to hypoxia and hypercapnia
- Increased ventilation-perfusion mismatch leading to increased dead space ventilation
- Decreased diaphragmatic function due to fatigue and hyperinflation
- Obesity hypoventilation syndrome, amyotrophic lateral sclerosis, and severe restrictive ventilatory defects are observed in interstitial fibrosis and thoracic skeletal deformities.

For Metabolic Acidosis

Increased acid production with increased anion gap

- Lactic acidosis
- Ketoacidosis
  - Diabetes mellitus
  - Starvation
  - Alcohol-associated
- Ingestions
  - Methanol
  - Ethylene glycol
  - Aspirin
- Toluene (if early or if kidney function is impaired)
- Diethylene glycol
- Propylene glycol
- D-lactic acidosis
- Pyroglutamic acid (5-oxoproline)

Loss of bicarbonate or bicarbonate precursors with normal anion gap

- Diarrhea or other intestinal losses (e.g., tube drainage)
- Type 2 (proximal) renal tubular acidosis (RTA)
- Post treatment of ketoacidosis
- Carbonic anhydrase inhibitors
- Ureteral diversion (e.g., ileal loop)

Decreased renal acid excretion with increased anion gap

- Chronic kidney disease

Decreased renal acid excretion with normal anion gap

- Chronic kidney disease and tubular dysfunction (but relatively preserved glomerular filtration rate)
- Distal renal tubular acidosis (dRTA) or Type 1 Renal tubular acidosis (RTA)
- Type 4 RTA (hypoaldosteronism)

Collaborative Outcomes

The individual will be monitored for early signs and symptoms of metabolic or respiratory acidosis and will receive collaborative interventions if indicated to restore physiologic stability.

Indicators of Physiologic Stability

- Refer to *Electrolyte Imbalances* for Indicators
- Blood urea nitrogen 10 to 20 mg/dL
- Creatinine 0.2 to 0.8 mg/dL
- Alkaline phosphate 30 to 150 International Units/mL
- Serum prealbumin 1 to 3 g/dL
- No muscle cramps

Interventions and Rationales

For Metabolic Acidosis

Monitor for signs and symptoms of metabolic acidosis

- Rapid, shallow respirations
- Headache, lethargy, coma
- Nausea and vomiting
- Low plasma bicarbonate and pH of arterial blood
- Behavior changes, drowsiness
- Increased serum potassium
- Increased serum chloride
- PCO_2 <35 to 40 mm Hg
- Decreased HCO_3

R: *Metabolic acidosis results from the kidney's inability to excrete hydrogen ions, phosphates, sulfates, and ketone bodies. Bicarbonate loss results when the kidney reduces its resorption. Hyperkalemia, hyperphosphatemia, and decreased bicarbonate levels aggravate metabolic acidosis. Excessive ketone bodies cause headaches, nausea, vomiting, and abdominal pain. Respiratory rate and depth increase to increase CO_2 excretion and reduce acidosis. Acidosis affects the CNS and can increase neuromuscular irritability because of the cellular exchange of hydrogen and potassium.*

For an individual with metabolic acidosis

- Initiate IV fluid replacement as ordered, depending on the underlying etiology.

R: *Dehydration may result from gastric and urinary fluid losses.*

- If the etiology is diabetes mellitus, refer to *Risk for Complications of Hypo/Hyperglycemia* for interventions.
- Assess for signs and symptoms of hypocalcemia, hypokalemia, and alkalosis as acidosis is corrected.

R: *Rapid correction of acidosis may cause rapid excretion of calcium and potassium and rebound alkalosis.*

- Correct, per orders, any electrolyte imbalances. Refer to *Risk for Complications of Electrolyte Imbalances* for specific interventions for each type of electrolyte imbalance.
- Monitor arterial blood gas (ABG) values, urine pH.

R: *These values help evaluate the effectiveness of therapy.*

For Respiratory Acidosis

Monitor for signs and symptoms of respiratory acidosis (Manifestations vary, depending on the severity of the disorder and on the rate of development of hypercapnia.)

- Early:
  - Anxious, complaints of dyspnea
  - Disturbed sleep, daytime hypersomnolence
  - Decreased respiratory rate
- Later as the partial arterial pressure of carbon dioxide ($PaCO_2$) increases:
  - Increased anxiety
  - Tachycardia, dysrhythmias, bounding pulses
  - Increased respiratory effort
  - Diaphoresis
  - Nausea and/or vomiting
  - Neurological changes (blurred vision, decreased reflexes decreased level of consciousness, restlessness, headaches)
  - Diagnostic (increased PCO, normal or decreased PO_2, increased serum calcium, decreased sodium chloride)

R: *Respiratory acidosis can occur when an impaired respiratory system cannot remove CO_2, or when compensatory mechanisms that stimulate increased cardiac and respiratory efforts to remove excess CO_2 are overtaxed. Elevated $PaCO_2$ is the chief criterion (Grossman & Porth, 2014).*

For an individual with respiratory acidosis

- Improve ventilation by positioning with head of bed up

R: *This will promote diaphragmatic descent*

- Coaching in deep breathing with prolonged expiration

R: *This will increase exhalation of CO_2*

- Aiding expectoration of mucus followed by suctioning, if needed.

R: *This will improve ventilation–perfusion*

Promote optimal hydration

R: *This helps liquefy secretions and prevent mucous plugs.*

Limit use of sedatives and tranquilizers

R: *Both can cause respiratory depression.*

Refer to metabolic acidosis earlier in this section and initiate the first five interventions to correct metabolic acidosis

Risk for Complications of Metabolic or Respiratory Alkalosis[7]

Definition

Describes a person experiencing or at high risk for experiencing an acid–base imbalance due to excessive bicarbonate or loss of hydrogen ions

High-Risk Populations

For Respiratory Alkalosis (Byrd, 2014)

CNS related causes:

- Pain
- Hyperventilation syndrome
- Anxiety, Panic disorders, Psychosis
- Cerebrovascular accident
- Meningitis
- Encephalitis
- Tumor, Trauma

Hypoxia-related causes are as follows:

- High altitude
- Right-to-left shunts
- Severe anemia
- Heart Failure
- Pulmonary edema
- Pulmonary embolism
- Interstitial lung disease
- Asthma
- Emphysema
- Chronic bronchitis

---

[7] When indicated, the nurse should specify the diagnosis as either *Risk for Complications of Metabolic Acidosis* or *Risk for Complications of Respiratory Acidosis.*

Drug-related causes are as follows:

- Progesterone
- Methylxanthine toxicity
- Salicylate toxicity
- Catecholamines
- Nicotine

Endocrine-related causes are as follows:

- Pregnancy
- Hyperthyroidism

Miscellaneous causes are as follows:

- Sepsis
- Severe anemia
- Hepatic failure
- Mechanical ventilation
- Heat exhaustion
- Recovery phase of metabolic acidosis
- Congestive heart failure

For Metabolic Alkalosis (Emmett, 2014)

Increased acids from ketoacidosis, excessive renal hydrogen loss from

- Uncontrolled diabetes
- Starvation or fasting
- Alcohol abuse
- Lactic acidosis
- Ingestion of toxins such as ethylene glycol (antifreeze) or cyanide
- Certain medications and other substances, such as excessive amounts of aspirin, iron, loop or thiazide diuretics or paraldehyde

Loss of HCO_3 (bicarbonate); gastrointestinal hydrogen loss:

- Prolonged vomiting
- Diarrhea
- Gastric tubes or ileostomies
- Type 2 (proximal) renal tubular acidosis

Decreased acid excretion from intracellular shift of hydrogen:

- Hypokalemia
- Renal failure or Type 1 (distal) renal tubular acidosis

Decreased production of HCO_3 (bicarbonate)

- Renal, hepatic, or pancreatic failure.
- Alkali administration:
  - Administration of large quantities of citrate salts (e.g., multiple blood transfusions)
  - Use of citrate salts as an anticoagulant in hemodialysis
  - Freebase and crack cocaine, when renal function is very compromised

Collaborative Outcomes

The individual will be monitored for early signs and symptoms of metabolic or respiratory alkalosis and will receive collaborative interventions if indicated to restore physiologic stability.

Indicators

See *Risk for Complications of Metabolic or Respiratory Acidosis* for indicators.

Interventions and Rationales

For Metabolic Alkalosis

Monitor for signs and symptoms of metabolic alkalosis

- Weakness, myalgia, polyuria, and cardiac arrhythmias
- Hypoventilation develops because of inhibition of the respiratory center in the medulla. Symptoms of hypocalcemia (e.g., jitteriness, perioral tingling, muscle spasms) may be present.
- Tingling of fingers, dizziness, tremors
- Hypoventilation
- Polyuria, polydipsia
- Jitteriness
- Hypoventilation
- Cardiac dysrhythmias

R: *Symptoms of metabolic alkalosis are not specific. Hypokalemia is usually present which can cause weakness, myalgia, polyuria, and cardiac arrhythmias. Hypoventilation develops because of inhibition of the respiratory center in the medulla. Hypocalcemia causes complaints of jitteriness, perioral tingling, muscle spasms (Emmeritt, 2014).*

For an individual with metabolic alkalosis

- Initiate order for parenteral fluids.

R: *To correct sodium, water, chloride deficits*

- Monitor carefully the administration of ammonium chloride if ordered.

R: *Ammonium chloride increases circulating hydrogen ions, which results in decreased pH. Treatment can cause too-rapid decrease in pH and hemolysis of RBCs.*

- Evaluate renal and hepatic function before administration of ammonium chloride.

R: *Impaired renal or hepatic function cannot accommodate increased hemolysis.*

- Administer sedatives and tranquilizers cautiously, if ordered.

R: *Both depress respiratory function.*

- Monitor ABG values, urine pH, serum electrolyte levels, and BUN.

R: *These values help evaluate response to treatment and detect rebound metabolic acidosis resulting from too-rapid correction.*

For Respiratory Alkalosis

Monitor for respiratory alkalosis

- Early
  - Paresthesias
  - Numbness/tingling around mouth
  - Tingling of fingers, dizziness

R: *A decrease in ionized calcium produces the early symptoms.*

- Later
  - Chest pain or tightness
  - Dyspnea
  - Tetany, mental confusion
  - Seizures
  - Decreased serum chloride, serum potassium, serum calcium

R: *Acute onset of hypocapnia (decrease in $PaCO_2$) reduces cerebral blood flow and can cause neurologic symptoms.*

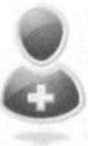

CLINICAL ALERT "The treatment of respiratory alkalosis is primarily directed at correcting the underlying disorder. Respiratory alkalosis itself is rarely life-threatening. Therefore, emergent treatment is usually not indicated unless the pH level is greater than 7.5" (Bryd, 2014).

For an individual hyperventilating with respiratory alkalosis

- Provide reassurance

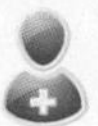

Clinical Alert "In individuals presenting with hyperventilation, a systematic approach should be used to rule out potentially life-threatening, organic causes first before considering less serious disorders" (Bryd, 2014).

- Determine the cause of hyperventilation.

R: *Different etiologies warrant different interventions (e.g., anxiety versus incorrect mechanical ventilation).*

- Calm the anxious person by maintaining eye contact and remaining with him or her.

R: *Anxiety increases respiratory rate and CO_2 retention.*

- Coach the person to breathe slowly with you and to rebreathe into a paper bag.

R: *This increases CO_2 retention.*

- Alternatively, have the anxious person breathe into a paper bag and rebreathe from the bag.

R: *This increases $PaCO_2$ as the person rebreathes his or her own exhaled CO_2.*

- If anxiety is causative, refer to the nursing diagnoses *Anxiety* and *Ineffective Breathing Patterns* in Section 2 for additional interventions.

Encourage to explore treatment for underlying stress

- Consult with physician, physician assistant, or advanced practice nurse for use of sedation as necessary.

R: *Sedation can help reduce respiratory rate and anxiety.*

- Monitor ABG values and electrolyte levels (e.g., potassium, calcium).

R: *Monitoring these values helps evaluate the individual's response to treatment.*

- As necessary, refer to *Risk for Complications of Electrolyte Imbalances* for specific management of electrolyte imbalance.

Risk for Complications of Allergic Reaction

Definition

Describes a person experiencing or at high risk to experience hypersensitivity and release of mediators to specific substances (antigens) and anaphylaxis. Idiopathic anaphylaxis (IA) is a well-described syndrome of anaphylaxis without any recognized external trigger. IA is one of the most common causes of anaphylaxis, accounting for approximately one-third of cases in one retrospective study (Greenberger, Lessard, Chen, & Farruggia, 2008).

High-Risk Populations

- History of allergies
- Asthma
- Immunotherapy
- Hereditary angioedema
- IA is more common (65%) in women (Greenberger, Lessard, Chen, & Farruggia, 2008)
- Individuals exposed to high-risk antigens:
  - Insect stings (e.g., bee, wasp, hornet, ant)
  - Animal bites/stings (e.g., stingray, snake, jellyfish)
  - Radiologic iodinated contrast media (e.g., used in arteriography, intravenous pyelography)
- Transfusion of blood and blood products
- High-risk individuals exposed to:
  - High-risk medications (e.g., aspirin, antibiotics, opiates, local anesthetics, animal insulin, chymopapain)
  - High-risk foods (e.g., peanuts, chocolate, eggs, seafood, shellfish, strawberries, milk)
  - Chemicals (e.g., floor waxes, paint, soaps, perfume, new carpets)

Collaborative Outcomes

The individual will be monitored for early signs and symptoms of allergic response and will receive collaborative interventions if indicated to restore physiologic stability.

Indicators of Physiologic Stability

- Calm, alert, oriented
- No complaints of urticaria or pruritus
- No complaints of tightness in throat
- No complaints of shortness of breath or wheezing

Interventions and Rationales

Review allergy profile prior to administrating any medications

Carefully assess for history of allergic responses (e.g., rashes, difficulty breathing)

R: *Identifying a high-risk individual allows precautions to prevent anaphylaxis.*

Screen individual/family for hereditary angioedema (HAE)

R: *"Hereditary angioedema (HAE) is a rare disorder characterized by recurrent episodes of well-demarcated angioedema without urticaria, which most often affect the skin or mucosal tissues of the upper respiratory and gastrointestinal tracts. Although swelling resolves spontaneously in two to four days in the absence of treatment, laryngeal edema may cause fatal asphyxiation, and the pain of gastrointestinal attacks may be incapacitating" (Atkinson, Cicardi, & Zuraw, 2014).*

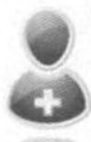

Clinical Alert It is critical to determine that an allergic reaction is HAE, since the treatment needed targets specifically HAE. Plasma-derived C1INH is the best studied first-line therapy for acute episodes of angioedema in patients with HAE (Atkinson et al., 2014).

Assess for sensitivities/allergies to

- Food

R: *Most common food allergens are milk, eggs, peanuts, tree nuts, fish, shellfish, soy, and wheat, which account for over 90% of all food allergies. Foods commonly mistaken for IA include mustard and other spices (Auckland Allergy Clinic, 2012).*

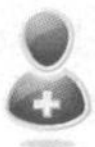

Clinical Alert "Unfortunately, approximately 20% to 30% of the population reports having an FA, yet reliable estimates of FA prevalence are between 3% and 4%." Food allergies are the commonest cause of anaphylaxis and occur in 1% to 2% of the population. Symptoms usually start 5 to 30 minutes after ingestion, occasionally after 1 to 2 hours, but rarely any longer. Consider an alternative diagnosis if symptoms began many hours after ingestion or if the individual has since eaten the suspected food without any reaction (Auckland Allergy Clinic, 2012).

- Medications/drugs are another common cause of anaphylaxis.
- It is important to focus on drugs/supplements/herbal preparation (bee pollen, echinacea) and other over-the-counter formulations (especially aspirin and NSAIDs) in the history taking.

If the individual has a history of allergic response, inform physician, physician assistant, or advanced practice nurse

R: *Skin testing can confirm hypersensitivity.*

Monitor for signs and symptoms of localized allergic reaction

- Wheals, flares (due to histamine release)
- Itching
- Nontraumatic edema (perioral, periorbital)

R: *The antigen–antibody reaction causes vasodilatation with pooling of blood (edema), histamine release (wheals, itching), and diminished perfusion to tissues followed by vascular and circulatory vasoconstriction. Patients may experience fevers, chills, rigors, flushing, and diaphoresis (sweating) as temperature regulation is disrupted by circulating cytokines*

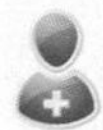

CLINICAL ALERT At first sign of hypersensitivity, promptly initiate emergency protocol for anaphylaxis and access the rapid response team stat page physician or advanced practice nurse.

R: *Progression from hives and itching to life-threatening symptoms of wheeze, loss of consciousness, and laryngeal edema may occur in 10 minutes to hours after onset.*

Monitor for systemic allergic reaction and anaphylaxis

- Light-headedness, skin flushing, angioedema, and slight hypotension (resulting from histamine-induced vasodilation)
- Throat or palate tightness, wheezing, hoarseness, dyspnea, and chest tightness (from smooth muscle contraction from prostaglandin release)
- Irregular, increased pulse and decreased blood pressure (from leukotriene release, which constricts airways and coronary vessels)
- Decreased level of consciousness, respiratory distress, and shock (resulting from severe hypotension, respiratory insufficiency, and tissue hypoxia)
- If an allergic reaction is suspected to infusion, discontinue infusion but maintain IV access.

Follow Protocol

- Establish IV access, administer epinephrine IV or endotracheally.

R: *Establishing venous access prior to vasoconstriction is optimal for rapid medication administration, Epinephrine produces peripheral vasoconstriction, which raises blood pressure and acts as a β agonist to promote bronchial smooth muscle relaxation, and to enhance inotropic and chronotropic cardiac activity (Garzon, Kempker, & Piel, 2011).*

- Administer oxygen; establish a patent airway if indicated. Have suction available. Oropharyngeal intubation may be required.

R: *Laryngeal edema interferes with breathing.*

- Administer other medications, as ordered, which may include:
  - Corticosteroids

R: *Corticosteroids inhibit enzyme and WBC response to reduce bronchoconstriction.*

  - Aminophylline

R: *Aminophylline produces bronchodilation.*

  - Vasopressors

R: *Vasopressors counter profound hypotension.*

  - Diphenhydramine

R: *Diphenhydramine prevents further antigen–antibody reaction.*

  - H_1 antihistamines and epinephrine

R: *H_1 antihistamines and epinephrine mediate GI*

Continue to monitor to evaluate response to therapy

R: *Within minutes, such reactions can progress to severe hypotension, decreased level of consciousness, and respiratory distress (Garzon et al., 2011).*

- Vital signs
- Level of consciousness
- Lung sounds, peak flows
- Cardiac function
- Intake and output
- ABG values

R: *Careful monitoring is necessary to detect complications of shock and identify the need for additional interventions.*

For those history of or significant risk for anaphylaxis

- Discuss with the individual and family preventive measures for anaphylaxis:
  - Stress the need to carry an anaphylaxis kit, which contains injectable epinephrine and oral antihistamines for use in self-treating allergic reaction and to seek emergency treatment.
  - Have individual and family member practice with a nonactive demo autoinjector.
  - Advice that serious reaction may require two injections.

R: *Demonstration of demo auto injectors explains the force needed to activate the auto injector and for the loud sound occurring with needle ejection, is particularly helpful as many patients do not realize the force required to activate an auto injector, and are usually unaware and startled by the loud sound made as the needle ejects (Garzon et al., 2011).*

Risk for Complications of Thrombocytopenia

Definition

Describes a person experiencing or at high risk to experience insufficient circulating platelets (less than 150,000). This decrease can be caused by a reduction in platelet production, a change in platelet distribution, platelet destruction, or vascular dilution.

High-Risk Populations

(Gauer & Braun, 2012)

- Decreased platelet production
- Bone marrow failure (e.g., aplastic anemia, paroxysmal nocturnal hemoglobinuria, Shwachman-Diamond syndrome)
- Bone marrow suppression (e.g., from medication, chemotherapy, or irradiation)
- Chronic alcohol abuse
- Congenital macrothrombocytopenias (e.g., Alport syndrome, Bernard-Soulier syndrome, Fanconi anemia, platelet-type or pseudo–Von Willebrand disease, Wiskott-Aldrich syndrome)
- Infection (e.g., cytomegalovirus, Epstein-Barr virus, hepatitis C virus, HIV, mumps, parvovirus B19, rickettsia, rubella, varicella-zoster virus)
- Myelodysplastic syndrome
- Neoplastic marrow infiltration
- Nutritional deficiencies (vitamin B_{12} and folate)
- Increased platelet consumption
- Alloimmune destruction (e.g., posttransfusion, neonatal, posttransplantation)
- Autoimmune syndromes (e.g., antiphospholipid syndrome, systemic lupus erythematosus, sarcoidosis)
- Disseminated intravascular coagulation/severe sepsis
- Drug-induced thrombocytopenia e.g. sulfa, aspirin, interferon, anticonvulsants, digoxin)
- Heparin-induced thrombocytopenia
- Immune thrombocytopenic purpura
- Infection (e.g., cytomegalovirus, Epstein-Barr virus, hepatitis C virus, HIV, mumps, parvovirus B19, rickettsia, rubella, varicella-zoster virus)
- Mechanical destruction (e.g., aortic valve, mechanical valve, extracorporeal bypass)
- Preeclampsia/HELLP syndrome
- Thrombotic thrombocytopenic purpura/hemolytic uremic syndrome
- Sequestration/other
- Chronic alcohol abuse
- Dilutional thrombocytopenia (e.g., hemorrhage, excessive crystalloid infusion)
- Gestational Incidental thrombocytopenia (mild, 5% incidence)
- Hypersplenism (e.g., distributional thrombocytopenia)
- Liver disease (e.g., cirrhosis, fibrosis, portal hypertension)
- Pseudothrombocytopenia
- Pulmonary emboli
- Pulmonary hypertension

Collaborative Outcomes

The individual will be monitored for early signs and symptoms of thrombocytopenia and will receive collaborative interventions if indicated to restore physiologic stability.

Indicators of Physiologic Stability

- Platelet count >150,000 per mm^3

Interventions and Rationales

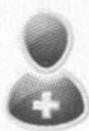

Clinical Alert Thrombocytopenia may be associated with a variety of conditions, with associated risks that may range from life-threatening to no risk at all (George & Arnold, 2014).

The concept of a "safe" platelet count is imprecise, lacks evidence-based recommendations, and depends on the disorder and on the individual (even with the same disorder) (George & Arnold, 2014). The following may be used as guides, but should not substitute for clinical judgment based on individual patient and disease factors:

- Surgical bleeding generally may be a concern with platelet counts <50,000 per microliter (<100,000 per microliter for some high-risk procedures such as neurosurgery or major cardiac or orthopedic surgery).
- Severe spontaneous bleeding is most likely with platelet counts <10,000 per microliter.

Monitor complete blood count (CBC), hemoglobin, coagulation tests, and platelet counts

R: *These values help evaluate response to treatment and risk for bleeding. Platelet count <20,000 per mm^3 indicates a high risk for intracranial bleeding.*

Assess for other factors that may lower platelet count in addition to the primary cause

- Abnormal hepatic/splenetic function
- Infection, fever
- Anticoagulant use
- Alcohol use
- Aspirin use
- Administration of several units of nonplatelet-containing fluids (e.g., packed RBCs)

R: *Assessment may identify factors that could be controllable.*

Monitor for signs and symptoms of spontaneous or excessive bleeding

- Spontaneous petechiae, ecchymoses, hematomas
- Bleeding from nose or gums
- Prolonged bleeding from invasive procedures such as venipunctures or bone marrow aspiration
- Hematemesis or coffee-ground emesis
- Hemoptysis
- Hematuria
- Unusual Vaginal bleeding
- Rectal bleeding
- Black, tarry stools
- Gross blood in stools

R: *Constant monitoring is needed to ensure early detection of bleeding.*

Assess for systemic signs of bleeding and hypovolemia

- Increased pulse, increased respirations, decreased blood pressure
- Changes in neurologic status (e.g., subtle mental status changes, blurred vision, headache, disorientation)

R: *Changes in circulatory oxygen levels produce changes in cardiac, vascular, and neurologic functioning.*

If hemorrhage is suspected, refer to *Risk for Complications of Hypovolemic Shock* for specific interventions

Anticipate platelet transfusion

Apply direct pressure for 5 to 10 minutes, then a pressure dressing, to all venipuncture sites. Monitor carefully for 24 hours

R: *These measures promote clotting and reduce blood loss.*

Treat nausea aggressively to prevent vomiting

R: *Severe vomiting can cause GI bleeding.*

Using the nursing diagnosis *Risk for Injury related to bleeding tendency* (see Section 2), implement nursing interventions and teaching to reduce the risk of trauma

Teach individual/family signs/symptoms to report to primary care provider or specialist

- Frequent nosebleeds
- Bleeding gums after brushing teeth
- Long bleeding times after a minor cut or scratch
- Easy bruising

Risk for Complications of Opportunistic Infections

Definition

Describes a person with a compromised immune system experiencing or at high risk to experience a condition and/or infection caused by an organism (bacterial, protozoa, fungus, viral)

High-Risk Populations

- Immunosuppressive therapy (chemotherapy, antiviral)
- Antibiotic therapy (disruption of physiologic balance of microorganisms
- Malignancy (HPV-related, sarcoidosis)
- Sepsis
- AIDS
- Nutritional deficits
- Skin damage (burns, extensive pressure ulcers)
- Recurrent infections
- Leukopenia
- Trauma
- Extensive pressure ulcers
- Pregnancy
- Radiation therapy (long bones, skull, sternum)
- Elderly with chronic illness
- Drug/alcohol addiction

Collaborative Outcomes

The individual will be monitored for early signs and symptoms of opportunistic infections and will receive collaborative interventions if indicated to restore physiologic stability.

Indicators of Physiologic Stability

- Temperature 98° F to 99.5° F
- Respirations 16 to 20 breaths/min
- No cough
- Alert, oriented
- No seizures, no headache
- Regular, formed stools
- No herpetic or zoster lesions
- No swallowing complaints
- No change in vision
- No weight loss
- No new lesions; for example, mouth
- No lymphadenopathy

Interventions and Rationales

Monitor CBC, WBC differential (neutrophils, lymphocytes), and absolute neutrophil count (WBC and neutrophil)

R: *These values help evaluate response to treatment.*

Monitor for signs and symptoms of primary or secondary infection

- Slightly increased temperature
- Chills
- Dysphagia
- Adventitious breath sounds
- Cloudy or foul-smelling urine
- Complaints of urinary frequency, urgency, or dysuria
- WBCs and bacteria in urine
- Redness, change in skin temperature, swelling, or unusual drainage in any area of disrupted skin integrity, including previous and current puncture sites
- Irritation or ulceration of oral mucous membrane
- Complaints of perineal or rectal pain and any unusual vaginal or rectal discharge
- Increased hemorrhoidal pain, redness, or bleeding
- Painful, pruritic skin lesions (herpes zoster), particularly in cervical or thoracic area
- Change in WBC count, especially increased immature neutrophils

R: *In an individual with severe neutropenia, usual inflammatory responses may be decreased or absent.*

Obtain culture specimens (e.g., urine, vaginal, rectal, mouth, sputum, stool, blood, skin lesions, indwelling lines) as ordered

R: *Testing determines the type of causative organism and guides treatment.*

Monitor for signs and symptoms of sepsis

R: *Gram-positive and gram-negative organisms can invade open wounds, causing septicemia. A debilitated individual is at increased risk. Sepsis produces massive vasodilation, resulting in hypovolemia and subsequent tissue hypoxia. Hypoxia leads to decreased renal function and cardiac output, triggering a compensatory response of increased respirations and heart rate in an attempt to correct hypoxia and acidosis. Bacteria in urine or blood indicate infection (Neviere, 2015).*

Explain the human Papilloma virus (HPV) and the risks of cancer

- The difference between low-risk and high-risk HPV.
- Some types of HPV, typically HPV 6 and HPV 11, cause genital warts. The warts are rarely associated with cervical cancers. They are considered "low-risk" HPV.

R: *There are more than 100 types of HPV. About 30 or so types can cause genital infections. Most of the time, HPV goes away by itself within 2 years and does not cause health problems. It is thought that the immune system fights off HPV naturally. It is only when certain types of HPV do not go away over years that it can cause these cancers.*

- Certain HPV types are classified as "high-risk" because they lead to abnormal cell changes and can cause genital cancers: cervical cancer as some vaginal, vulvar, penile, and oropharyngeal cancers.

R: *High-risk HPVs cause virtually all cervical cancers. They also cause most anal cancers and the most common of the high-risk strains of HPV are types 16 and 18, which cause about 70% of all cervical cancers.*

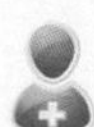

Clinical Alert National Cancer Institute (2012)

- Cervical cancer: The most common HPV cancer. More than 99% of cervical cancer is caused by HPV.
- Vulvar cancer: About 69% are linked to HPV.
- Vaginal cancer: About 75% are linked to HPV.
- Penile cancer: About 63% are linked to HPV.
- Anal cancer: About 91% are linked to HPV.
- Oropharyngeal cancers (cancers of the back of the throat, including the base of the tongue and tonsils): About 72% are linked to HPV. (Note: Many of these cancers may be related to tobacco and alcohol use.)

Teach measures that can prevent or provide early detection

- Vaccination with Gardasil or Cervarix between ages 11 to 26 (series of three vaccinations)
- Cervical cancer screening with the HPV test and the Pap test in women aged 30 and older
- For men, monitor abnormalities on your penis, scrotum, or around the anus and seek medical evaluation if you find warts, blisters, sores, ulcers, white patches, or other abnormal areas on your penis—even if they do not hurt.
- Avoid smoking, multiple partners.
- The risk for cervical cancer is increased in multiple pregnancies and long-term use of oral contraceptives.

Monitor for signs and symptoms of opportunistic protozoal infections (Centers for Disease Control and Prevention [CDC], 2014)

- *Pneumocystis carinii* pneumonia: dry, nonproductive cough, low-grade fever, gradual to severe dyspnea
- *Toxoplasma gondii* encephalitis: headache, lethargy, seizures
- *Cryptosporidium* enteritis: watery diarrhea, nausea, abdominal cramps, malaise

R: *Individuals with immunodeficiency are at risk for secondary diseases of opportunistic infections; protozoal infections are the most common and serious*

Monitor for signs and symptoms of opportunistic viral infections conditions (CDC, 2014)

- Herpes simplex oral, genital: blisters, severe pain
- Perirectal abscesses: bleeding, rectal discharge
- Cytomegalovirus retinitis, colitis, pneumonitis, encephalitis, or other organ disease
- Progressive multifocal leukoencephalopathy: headache, decreased mentation
- Varicella-zoster, disseminated (shingles)
- *Streptococcus pneumoniae* (pneumococcus): loss of muscle control, speech problems, blindness, altered mental state
- HPV with no signs and symptoms can progress to lesions, cancer of cervix, penis, anus, oropharynx.
- Kaposi's sarcoma (human herpes virus 8, HHV 8) can occur anywhere, with pink/purple spots on skin, lymphomas in lungs, lymph nodes, intestines.

Monitor for signs and symptoms of opportunistic fungal infections (CDC, 2014)

- *Candida albicans* stomatitis and esophagitis: exudate, complaints of unusual taste in mouth
- *Cryptococcus neoformans* meningitis: fever, headaches, blurred vision, stiff neck, confusion
- *Pneumocystis carinii*: difficulty breathing, high fever, dry cough

Monitor for signs and symptoms of opportunistic bacterial infections, which commonly affect the pulmonary system

- *Mycobacterium avium* (intracellular disseminated)
- *Mycobacterium tuberculosis* (extrapulmonary and pulmonary)
- Salmonella: diarrhea, nausea, vomiting

Teach individuals and significant others how specific infections are acquired and prevention strategies (CDC, 2014)

- Vaccines for pneumonia (Pneumovax, Prevnar 13)
- Zostavax vaccine if indicated

R: *This is given after age 65 unless one is immune compromised.*

- Diligent hand-washing
- Emphasize the need to report symptoms promptly.

R: *Early treatment of adverse manifestations often can prevent serious complications (e.g., septicemia) and also increases the likelihood of a favorable response to treatment.*

- Explain the need to balance activity and rest and to consume a nutritious diet.

R: *Rest and a nutritious diet give energy for healing and enhancement of the body's defense system.*

- Use safe food handling: for example, keep cold foods cold; hot foods hot. Avoid undercooked foods, handle raw food properly in preparation, avoid cross contamination.

R: *Salmonella enters the body with ingestion of contaminated food or water.*

- Explain the importance of adhering to medication regimen (prophylaxis and antiviral).
- Explain that it is acceptable to expect health-care providers to use hand hygiene before providing care.
- Refer to *Risk for Infection* in Section 2 for additional preventive measures.

Risk for Complications of Vaso-occlusive/Sickling Crisis

Definition

Describes a person with sickle cell disease experiencing vascular occlusion by the sickled cells, which damages cells and tissue and causes hemolytic anemia, massive splenomegaly, and hypovolemic shock, acute chest syndrome, cerebrovascular accidents (See Table III.1.)

High-Risk Populations

Individuals with sickle cell disease with precipitating factors, such as the following:

- High altitude (>7,000 feet above sea level)
- Unpressurized aircraft
- Dehydration (e.g., diaphoresis, diarrhea, vomiting)
- Strenuous physical activity
- Cold temperatures (e.g., iced liquids)
- Infection (e.g., respiratory, urinary, vaginal) parvovirus
- Ingestion of alcohol
- Cigarette smoking

Collaborative Outcomes

The individual will be monitored for early signs and symptoms of vasoocclusion crisis and will receive collaborative interventions if indicated to restore physiologic stability.

Indicators of Physiologic Stability

- BP <130/80
- Clear, oriented
- Pulse 60 to 100 beats/min
- Respiration 16 to 20 breaths/min
- Peripheral pulses, equal and full, capillary refill <3 seconds
- Pain control to a pre-established acceptable level
- Oxygen saturation >95%
- No or minimal bone, abdominal, or chest pain
- No or minimal fatigue or headache
- Urine output >5 mL/kg/hr

Interventions and Rationales

Monitor for signs and symptoms of anemia

- Lethargy
- Weakness
- Fatigue
- Increased pallor
- Dyspnea on exertion

Table III.1 COMPARISON OF NORMAL RED CELLS TO SICKLE CELLS

	Red Blood cells	Sickle Cells
Shape	Disc-shaped	Sickle or crescent shape
Character	Smooth	Stiff and sticky
Circulation	Move easily	Blocks blood flow
Lifespan	120 days	10–20 days
RBC production	Optimal for tissue needs	Insufficient for tissue needs

R: *As illustrated in Table III.1, the short life span of sickle cells (hemoglobin S) compromise the bone marrow's ability to produce red blood cells necessary for tissue needs. Anemia is common with sickle cell (Vishinsky, 2014). Because anemia is common with most of these individuals and low hemoglobins are relatively tolerated, changes should be described in reference to person's baseline or acute symptoms (Field, Vichinsky, & DeBaun, 2011).*

Monitor laboratory values, including CBC with reticulocyte count

R: *Reticulocyte (normal level about 1%) elevation represents active erythropoiesis. Lack of elevation with anemia may represent a problem*

Evaluate pain

R: *Acute pain is the first symptom of disease in more than 25% of individuals. It is the most frequent symptom after the age of 2 years. The frequency of pain peaks between the ages of 19 and 39; more frequent pain is associated with a higher mortality rate in individuals over age (Vishinsky, 2014).*

Have individual rate their pain using age appropriate scales

R: *The pain severity can range from trivial to excruciating. Approximately one-third of the individuals had acute or chronic pain approximately 95% of the time.*

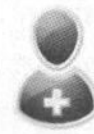

Clinical Alert The literature reports:

- 86% of physicians in academic teaching hospital do not believe that self-report is the most reliable indicator of pain among individuals with sickle cell disease (SCD) (Labbé, Herbert, & Haynes, 2005).
- In a survey of the nurses who treat individuals with SCD, 63% believed that addiction was prevalent, and 30% were reluctant to provide high-dose morphine. Approximately, 33% believed that a common barrier in the management of sickle cell pain was clinicians' reluctance to prescribe opioids (33%), and the belief that most individuals with SCD were drug addicts (32%) (*Pack-Mabien, Labbe, Herbert, & Haynes, 2001).
- The percentage of adults with SCD who exhibit behavior consistent with substance abuse is similar to that seen in the general population. Large academic centers in Cincinnati, Philadelphia, and London have estimated the percentage of adults with SCD abusing opioids to be in the range of zero to 9%. In comparison, in similar communities, the prevalence of substance abuse in the general population is 6% to 9%.
- SCD patients with high ED use were found to be more severely ill, have more pain, more distress, and lower quality of life compared to low utilizers (Aisiku et al., 2009).
- Shapiro, Benjamin, Payne, and Heidrich (*1997) study found that 53% of ED physicians and 23% of hematologists thought that more than 20% of patients were addicted.

Explore your own perceptions of individuals with STD and c/o of pain

R: *Many health-care providers perceive that individuals with SCD are addicted to opioids and exhibit drug-seeking behavior.*

- What is the difference between addiction, dependence, and tolerance?
- Consider that SCD is inherited, chronic, and frequently incurable.
- Acknowledge the differences in the sociocultural background between individuals and health-care providers.
- How would you care change if you considered treating sickle cell pain like cancer pain?
- When individuals seek pain relief in the emergency room, is it because there is no credible pain management plan at home?

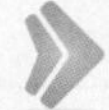

Carp's Cues

For over 20 years I have practiced as a Family Nurse Practitioner in a community with high rate of crime, much related to drug abuse. On a weekly basis, I am evaluating a request for opioids. Is it credible? Can another medication be substituted? I carefully evaluate the situation (e.g., clinical examination, urine drug screen, previous prescriptions) and make my decision. I can report several incidences when I was prescribed the controlled substance, only to find out I was fooled. However, I can report no incidences when I declined a prescription for someone, who needed it. I prefer to live with this second outcome.

Implement the acute pain management plan

- Fixed schedule of parenteral opioids with rescue doses (DeBaun & Vishinsky, 2014; Solomon, 2010)

R: *Pain therapy during the first 2 to 3 days of hospitalization should be aggressive. Analgesia should be given parentally on a fixed schedule (usually every 2 hours) and not on an "as needed" basis.*

- Engage in ongoing assessments of pain intensity and titration of the dose of opioid analgesics to achieve pain relief. The pain should be assessed every 30 to 60 minutes and the dose of the opioid titrated with rescue injection equal to 25% to 50% of the initial dose. If three or more rescue doses are needed within 24 hours or less to achieve adequate pain relief, the initial dose should be increased by 25% to 50% and the process repeated until adequate pain relief is achieved.
- Sedation and vital signs should be monitored as described above.

Explain (DeBaun & Vichinsky, 2014)

- Addiction, in contrast to tolerance and physical dependence, is a psychological disorder.
- Tolerance refers to increasing dose requirements because of changes in drug metabolism.
- Physical dependence characterized by withdrawal symptoms is a normal occurrence after 7 days of opioid exposure.

R: *Confusion in there terms can increase fears in individuals and families and biased responses from health-care providers*

Management of pain in the frequent utilizers cf care facilities (difficult or "problem" patients)

R: *"Every adult with sickle cell disease (SCD) should have an established pain plan tailored to his/her individual needs. This plan should instruct the individual how to appropriately manage mild, moderate, and severe pain, with a pre-defined threshold for the use of opioids and when to contact health care providers" (DeBaun & Vichinsky, 2014).*

- Consider possible reasons:
  - Under treatment as outpatients
  - Secondary gain (social, financial, or psychological problems)
  - Convenience of emergency department
  - Drug seeking
- Complete a pain management contract with

R: *Treatment contracts designed to set limits are perhaps the best method to deal with these individuals and family.*

- Involvement of individual and family/support system to include behavioral modification techniques to improve their coping with a chronic pain syndrome and to clarify expectations for treatment of pain in the emergency department and during hospitalizations
- Encouragement to become involved in sickle cell and other community programs
- One primary care provider or specialist assumes the primary responsibility for the person's continuity of care both in and out of the hospital. Only this provider should write prescriptions for opioids to control pain and only one pharmacy should be utilized to fill these prescriptions to ensure an accurate assessment of opioid use by the individual. Random urine drug screens are also in the contract and the consequences of failure to comply with contract

Provide comfort measures

- Bed rest
- Fluids and foods high in folic acid
- Warm compresses to areas of pain
- Refer to the nursing diagnosis *Acute Pain* (see Section 2, Part 1) for interventions to manage the pain associated with a sickling crisis.

Monitor for signs and symptoms of acute chest syndrome (Field & DeBaun, 2014)

- Temperature ≥38.5° C
- >2% decrease in SpO_2 (O_2 saturation) from a documented steady-state value on room air (FiO_2 = 0.21)
- PaO_2 <60 mm Hg
- Tachypnea (per age-adjusted normal)
- Intercostal retractions, nasal flaring, or use of accessory muscles of respiration

- Acute chest pain
- Cough
- Wheezing
- Rales

R: *Acute chest syndrome (ACS) is a leading cause of death for patients with SCD. Vasoocclusion within the pulmonary microvasculature is the basis for ACS pathophysiology. Etiologies for ACS either trigger vasoocclusion (e.g., infection, asthma, hypoventilation) or are a result of vasoocclusion (e.g., bone marrow and fat emboli). These etiologies can occur together; once intrapulmonary vasoocclusion is initiated, it is propagated by hypoxia, inflammation, and acidosis. ACS with intrapulmonary vasoocclusion and respiratory failure due to fat emboli*

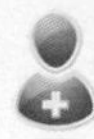

CLINICAL ALERT Access Rapid Response Team, in event of sudden onset of symptoms.

Access a chest X-ray

R: *Radiographic evidence of consolidation: a new segmental (involving at least one complete segment) radiographic pulmonary infiltrate with signs/symptoms of acute onset confirms acute chest syndrome (Field & DeBaun, 2014).*

Monitor for signs and symptoms of infection

- Fever
- Pain
- Chills
- Increased WBCs

R: *Bacterial infection is a major cause of morbidity and mortality. Decreased spleen function (asplenia) results from sickle cell anemia. The loss of the spleen's ability to filter and destroy various infectious organisms increases the risk of infection (Grossman & Porth, 2014).*

Monitor for changes in neurologic function

- Speech disturbances
- Sudden headache
- Numbness, tingling

R: *Cerebral infarction and intracranial hemorrhage are complications of SCD. Occlusion of nutrient arteries to major cerebral arteries causes progressive wall damage and eventual occlusion of the major vessel. Intracerebral hemorrhage may be secondary to hypoxic necrosis of vessel walls (Vichinsky, 2014).*

Monitor for splenic sequestration crisis

- Sudden onset of lassitude
- Very pale, listless
- Rapid pulse
- Shallow respirations
- Low blood pressure

R: *Increased obstruction of blood from the spleen together with rapid sickling can cause sudden pooling of blood into the spleen. This causes intravascular hypovolemia and hypoxia, progressing to shock (Vichinsky, 2014).*

Instruct individual to report the following

- Any acute illness
- Severe joint or bone pain
- Chest pain
- Abdominal pain
- Headaches, dizziness
- Gastric distress
- Priapism
- Recurrent vomiting

R: *These symptoms may indicate vasoocclusion in varied sites as a result of sickling. Some illnesses may predispose the individual to dehydration (Vichinsky, 2014).*

Initiate therapy per physician, physician assistant, or nurse practitioner prescription (e.g., antisickling agents, analgesics, transfusions)

- Provide
  - Bed rest
  - Fluids and foods high in folic acid
  - Warm compresses to areas of pain
  - Refer to the nursing diagnosis *Acute Pain* (see Section 2, Part 1) for interventions to manage the pain associated with a sickling crisis.

RISK FOR COMPLICATIONS OF RENAL/URINARY DYSFUNCTION

Risk for Complications of Renal/Urinary Dysfunction

Risk for Complications of Acute Urinary Retention
Risk for Complications of Renal Calculi
Risk for Complications of Renal Insufficiency

Definition

Describes a person experiencing or at high risk to experience various renal or urinary tract dysfunctions

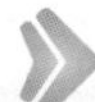

Carp's Cues

The nurse can use this generic collaborative problem to describe a person at risk for several types of renal or urinary problems. For such an individual (e.g., an individual in a critical care unit, who is vulnerable to various renal/urinary problems), using *Risk for Complications of Renal/Urinary Dysfunction* directs nurses to monitor renal and urinary status, based on the focus assessment, to detect and diagnose abnormal functioning. Nursing management of a specific renal or urinary complication would be addressed under the collaborative problem applying to the specific complication. For example, a standard of care for an individual recovering from coronary bypass surgery could contain the collaborative problem *Risk for Complications of Renal/Urinary Dysfunction*, directing the nurse to monitor renal and urinary status. If urinary retention is developed in this individual, the nurse would add *Risk for Complications of Urinary Retention* to the problem list, along with specific nursing interventions to manage this problem. If the risk factors or etiology was not directly related to the primary medical diagnosis, the nurse still would specify them in the diagnostic statement (e.g., *Risk for Complications of Renal Insufficiency* related to chronic renal failure in an individual who has sustained a myocardial infarction).

Keep in mind that the nurse must differentiate those problems in bladder function that nurses can treat primarily as nursing diagnoses (e.g., incontinence, chronic urinary retention) from those that nurses manage using both nurse-prescribed and physician-prescribed interventions (e.g., acute urinary retention).

Significant Laboratory/Diagnostic Assessment Criteria

(Methven, MacGregor, Traynor, O'Reilly, & Deighan, 2010)

- Serum chemistries
- Albumin, prealbumin, and serum (lowered in renal disease)
- Amylase (elevated with renal insufficiency)
- Blood urea nitrogen (BUN) (elevated in acute or chronic renal failure)
- Calcium (lowered in uremic acidosis)
- Chloride (elevated with renal tubular acidosis)
- Creatinine (elevated with kidney disease)
- Magnesium (lowered in chronic nephritis)
- pH, base excess, bicarbonate (lowered in metabolic acidosis, elevated in metabolic alkalosis)
- Phosphorus (elevated with chronic glomerular disease, lowered with renal tubular acidosis)
- Potassium (elevated in renal failure, lowered with chronic diuretic therapy, renal tubular acidosis)
- Proteins (total, albumin, globulin) (lowered in nephritic syndrome)

- Sodium (elevated with nephritis, lowered with chronic renal insufficiency)
- Uric acid (elevated with chronic renal failure)
- Complete blood count
- Hemoglobin (lowered in chronic renal disorders)
- MCHC—normal or lowered with accompanying iron deficiency anemia
- MCV—normal or lowered with accompanying iron deficiency anemia
- White blood cell (WBC) count (elevated with acute infection)
- Urine
- Blood
  - Acute—present with hemorrhagic cystitis, renal calculi, renal, bladder tumors
  - Chronic—glomerular damage
- WBC count (elevated with infection, obstruction). Obtain clean catch sample.
- Creatinine (elevated in acute/chronic glomerulonephritis, nephritis, lowered in advanced degeneration of kidneys)
- pH (decreased with metabolic acidosis, increased with metabolic alkalosis)
- Specific gravity (elevated with dehydration, lowered with overhydration, renal tubular disease)
- Myoglobin—present in muscle injury (medications, trauma)
- Protein to creatinine ratio (>200 mg/g is positive) or albumin to creatinine ratio (>30 mg/g is positive). Obtain random urine sample.
- Urine sodium and osmolarity (level depends on type—acute/chronic and site of kidney injury—prerenal or intrarenal)
- Culture and sensitivity—positive in infection
- 24-hour urine creatinine clearance—used in unstable clinical situations or to confirm clearance
- Imaging studies:
  - Helical noncontrast computerized tomography or ultrasonography
  - Renal ultrasound—normal renal size 9 to 10 cm
  - Magnetic resonance imaging for evaluating mass or cyst
  - Kidneys, ureters, bladder X-ray—evaluating for overall size and obstructions
  - Renal biopsy—diagnoses specific kidney disease to determine treatment options
  - Renal angiography—evaluates for stenosis

Risk for Complications of Acute Urinary Retention

Definition

Describes a person experiencing or at high risk to experience an acute abnormal accumulation of urine in the bladder and the inability to void due to a temporary situation (e.g., postoperative status) or to a condition reversible with surgery (e.g., prostatectomy) or medications

High-Risk Populations

(Barrisford & Steele, 2014; Selius & Subedi, 2008)

Acute urinary retention is most often secondary to obstruction, but may also be related to trauma, medication, neurologic disease, infection, and occasionally psychological issues

- Postoperative status (e.g., surgery of the perineal area, lower abdomen)
- Postpartum status
- Benign masses (e.g., fibroids)
- Malignant tumors of the pelvis, urethra, or vagina
- Postpartum vulvar edema
- Anxiety
- Prostate enlargement, prostatitis, prostate cancer
- Medication side effects (e.g., atropine, antidepressants, antihistamines)
- Postarteriography status
- Bladder outlet obstruction (infection, tumor, calculi/stone, constipation, urethral stricture, perianal abscess)
  - Impaired detrusor contractility (spinal cord injuries, progressive neurologic diseases, diabetic neuropathy, cerebrovascular accidents)

- Malignancy—bladder neoplasm, other tumors causing spinal cord compression
- Other infections—genital herpes, varicella zoster, infected foreign bodies

Collaborative Outcomes

The individual will be monitored for early signs and symptoms of acute urinary retention and receive collaborative intervention to restore physiologic stability.

Indicators of Physiologic Stability

- Urinary output >1,500 mL/24 hr
- Can verbalize bladder fullness
- No complaints of lower abdominal pressure

Interventions and Rationales

Monitor a postoperative individual for urinary retention

R: *Trauma to the detrusor muscle and injury to the pelvic nerves during surgery can inhibit bladder function. Anxiety and pain can cause spasms of the reflex sphincters. Bladder neck edema can cause retention. Sedatives and narcotics can affect the CNS and effectiveness of smooth muscles (Grossman & Porth, 2014; Urinary Retention, 2012).*

Monitor for urinary retention by palpating and percussing the suprapubic area for signs of bladder distention (overdistention, etc.)

- Instruct individual to report bladder discomfort or inability to void.

R: *These problems may be early signs of urinary retention.*

If individual does not void within 8 to 10 hours after surgery or complains of bladder discomfort, take the following steps

- Warm the bedpan.
- Encourage the individual to get out of bed to use the bathroom, if possible.
- Instruct a man to stand when urinating, if possible. If unable to stand, even sitting at the side of the bed helps.
- Run water in the sink as individual attempts to void.
- Pour warm water over individual's perineum.

R: *These measures help promote relaxation of the urinary sphincter and facilitate voiding.*

After the first voiding postsurgery, continue to monitor and to encourage individual to void again in 1 hour or so

R: *The first voiding usually does not empty the bladder completely.*

If the individual still cannot void after 10 hours, follow protocols for straight catheterization, as ordered by physician, physician assistant, advanced practice nurse

- Consider bladder scanning to determine if the amount of urine in the bladder necessitates catheterization.

R: *Straight catheterization is preferable to indwelling catheterization because it carries less risk of urinary tract infection from ascending pathogens. Bladder scanning is not a risk for infection.*

If person is voiding small amounts, use straight catheterization; if postvoid residual is >200 mL, leave catheter indwelling. Notify physician or advanced practice nurse

Risk for Complications of Renal Calculi

Definition

Describes a person with or at high risk for development of a solid concentration of mineral salts in the urinary tract

High-Risk Populations

(Curhan, Aronson, & Preminger, 2014)

- Leads to the formation of uric acid stones, as acidic urine is seen in bicarbonate loss [28, 31–35]. In addition to having acidic urine, patients with gout and these other metabolic defects may have increased uric acid excretion, although they are typically so-called "underexcretors of uric acid." (See "Uric acid nephrolithiasis".)
- Classic symptoms of nephrolithiasis are uncommon. The diagnosis is suggested in a patient with recurrent urinary tract infections, mild flank pain, or hematuria, who has a persistently alkaline urine pH (>7.0), often with multiple magnesium ammonium phosphate crystals in the urine sediment.
- History of renal calculi
- Family history of renal calculi
- Urinary infection
- Urinary stasis, obstruction
- Immobility
- Hypercalcemia (dietary)
- Enhanced enteric oxalate absorption (e.g., gastric bypass procedures, bariatric surgery, short bowel syndrome)
- Medications that may crystallize in the urine such as indinavir, acyclovir, sulfadiazine, and triamterene
- Low fluid intake is associated with increased stone risk
- A persistently acidic urine promotes uric acid precipitation (e.g., chronic diarrheal states, volume depletion lead to a concentrated acid urine, or with other metabolic defects, including gout, diabetes, insulin resistance, and obesity).
- Struvite stones form with an upper urinary tract infection due to a urease-producing organism such as *Proteus* or *Klebsiella*.
- Conditions that cause hypercalcemia
  - Hyperparathyroidism
  - Renal tubular acidosis (decreased serum bicarbonate)
  - Myeloproliferative disease (leukemia, polycythemia vera, multiple myeloma)
  - Excessive excretion of uric acid
  - Inflammatory bowel disease
  - Gout
  - Dehydration

Collaborative Outcomes

The individual will be monitored for early signs and symptoms of renal calculi and the individual will receive collaborative interventions as indicated to restore physiologic stability.

Indicators of Physiologic Stability

- Temperature 98° F to 99.5° F
- Urine output >1,500 mL/24 hr
- Urine specific gravity 1.005 to 1.030
- BUN 5 to 25 mg/dL
- Clear urine
- No flank pain

Interventions and Rationales

Monitor for signs and symptoms of calculi

- Increased or decreased urine output
- Sediment in urine
- Flank or loin pain
- Hematuria (with symptomatic nephrolithiasis and also often present in asymptomatic individuals)
- Abdominal pain, distention, nausea, vomiting, diarrhea
- Flank pain or tenderness, ipsilateral testicle or labium
- Dysuria, and urgency (when the stone is located in the distal ureter)

R: *Upper ureteral or renal pelvic obstruction lead to flank pain or tenderness, whereas lower ureteral obstruction causes pain that may radiate to the ipsilateral (same side as calculi) testicle or labium. Calculi-stimulating* *renointestinal reflexes can cause GI symptoms (Curhan et al., 2014). Stones in the urinary tract can cause obstruction, infection, and edema, manifested by loin/flank pain, hematuria, and dysuria. Stones in the renal pelvis may raise urine production.*

Send urine for culture and sensitivity

- Send 24-hour urine for calcium, oxalate, phosphorus, and uric acid. Urinary potassium, citrate, ammonium, sulfate, and magnesium may be ordered. Corresponding serum chemistries (e.g., bicarbonate and calcium will be simultaneously sent to lab).

Prepare person for KUB X-ray, excretory urography, magnetic resonance (if pregnant) renal ultrasound, helical noncontrast computerized tomography or ultrasonography is indicated

R: *Tests are needed to determine type of stone and infection (Zisman, Worcester, & Coe, 2012).*

Strain urine to obtain a stone sample; send samples to the laboratory for analysis

R: *Acquiring a stone sample confirms stone formation and enables analysis of stone constituents.*

If the individual complains of pain, consult with the physician or advanced practice nurse for aggressive therapy (e.g., narcotics, antispasmodics)

R: *Calculi can produce severe pain from spasms and proximity of the nerve plexus.*

Track the pain by documenting location, any radiation, duration, and intensity (using a rating scale of 0 to 10)

R: *This measure helps evaluate movement of calculi.*

Instruct the individual to increase fluid intake, if not contraindicated

R: *Increased fluid intake promotes increased urination, which can help facilitate stone passage and flush bacteria and blood from the urinary tract.*

Monitor for signs and symptoms of pyelonephritis

- Fever, chills
- Costovertebral angle pain (a dull, constant backache below the 12th rib)
- Leukocytosis
- Bacteria, blood, and pus in urine
- Dysuria, frequency

R: *Urinary stasis or irritation of tissue by calculi can cause urinary tract infections. Signs and symptoms reflect various mechanisms. Bacteria can act as pyrogens by raising the hypothalamic thermostat through the production of endogenous pyrogen, which may be mediated through prostaglandins. Chills can occur when the temperature set-point of the hypothalamus changes rapidly. Costovertebral angle pain results from distention of the renal capsule. Leukocytosis reflects increased leukocytes to fight infection through phagocytosis. Bacteria and pus in urine indicate a urinary tract infection. Bacteria can irritate bladder tissue, causing spasms and frequency (Grossman & Porth, 2014).*

Monitor for early signs and symptoms of renal insufficiency

- Refer to *Risk for Complications of Renal Insufficiency.*

Explain importance of following instructions for current care and prevention or minimization of risk for future stone formation

- Provide educational materials (e.g., Kidney stones: Client Fact Sheet http://www.suna.org/members/kidney_stones.pdf).

Risk for Complications of Renal Insufficiency/Failure

Definition

Renal insufficiency is an early sign of poor function of the kidneys that may be due to a reduction in blood flow to the kidneys caused by renal artery disease. Proper kidney function may be disrupted, however, when the arteries that provide the kidneys with blood become narrowed, a condition called renal artery stenosis.

Some patients with renal insufficiency experience no symptoms or only mild symptoms. Others develop dangerously high blood pressure, poor kidney function, or kidney failure that requires dialysis (Kovesdy, Kopple, & Kalantar-Zadeh, 2015).

Stages of Renal Failure (Kovesdy et al., 2015)

Stage 1

Glomerular Filtration Rate (GFR) *>90+*
Normal kidney function but urine findings or structural abnormalities or genetic trait point to kidney disease. Observation, control of blood pressure.

Stage 2

GFR >60 to 89
Mildly reduced kidney function, and other findings (as for stage 1) point to kidney disease. Observation, control of blood pressure and risk factors.

GFR > 45 to 59

Stage 3B

Stage 3A

GFR > 30 to 44
Moderately reduced kidney function. Observation, control of blood pressure and risk factors.

Stage 4

GFR>15 to 29
Severely reduced kidney function. Planning for endstage renal failure. More on management of Stages 4 and 5 CKD.

Stage 5

GFR <15 or on dialysis
Very severe, or endstage kidney failure (sometimes call established renal failure)

High-Risk Populations

(Grossman & Porth, 2014; Kovesdy et al., 2015)

- Older age
- Gender
- Family history
- Race or ethnicity
- Genetic factors
- Hyperlipidemia (elevated fats in the blood)
- Hypertension (high blood pressure)
- Smoking
- Diabetes
- Obesity
- High-risk individuals
  - Older persons
  - Postsurgical
  - Major trauma
  - Underlying chronic kidney disease
- Renal tubular necrosis from ischemic causes
  - Excessive diuretic use
  - Pulmonary embolism
  - Burns
  - Intrarenal thrombosis
  - Rhabdomyolysis
  - Renal infections
  - Renal artery stenosis/thrombosis
  - Peritonitis

    - Sepsis
    - Hypovolemia
    - Hypotension
    - Congestive heart failure
    - Myocardial infarction
    - Aneurysm
    - Aneurysm repair
- Renal tubular necrosis from toxicity
- Nonsteroidal anti-inflammatory drugs
    - Gout (hyperuricemia)
    - Hypercalcemia
    - Certain street drugs (e.g., PCP)
    - Gram-negative infection
    - Radiocontrast media
    - Aminoglycoside antibiotics
    - Antineoplastic agents
    - Methanol, carbon tetrachloride
    - Snake venom, poison mushroom
    - Phenacetin-type analgesics
    - Heavy metals
    - Insecticides, fungicides
    - Diabetes mellitus
    - Malignant hypertension
    - Hemolysis (e.g., from transfusion reaction)

Collaborative Outcomes

The individual will be monitored for early signs and symptoms of renal insufficiency with a goal of preventing or minimizing chronic damage. The individual will receive collaborative interventions as indicated to restore and/or maintain physiologic stability.

Indicators of Physiologic Stability

- Blood pressure less than 120 over less than 80
- Urine specific gravity 1.005 to 1.030
- Urine output >0.5 mL/hr
- Urine sodium 40 to 220 mEq/L/24 hr (varies by dietary intake, medications)
- BUN 10 to 20 mg/dL
- Serum potassium 3.8 to 5 mEq/L
- Serum sodium 135 to 145 mEq/L
- Serum phosphorus 2.5 to 4.5 mg/dL
- Serum creatinine clearance 100 to 150 mL/min (varies by age, gender, and race)
- Glomerular filtration rate of 90-120 mL/min

Interventions and Rationales

Monitor for hematuria and proteinuria (The Renal Association, 2013)

Visible (macroscopic) hematuria (usually referred immediately to urology or to nephrology if acute renal pathology is suspected)

Invisible (microscopic) hematuria without proteinuria, GFR >60 mL/min/1.73 m^2

- Age >40, usually refer to urology (recommended age may vary locally)
- Age <40, or >40 with negative urological investigations, refer to nephology

Microscopic hematuria with protein/creatinine ratio >50 mg/mmol

- Refer to nephrology if urological investigations negative
- Refer nephrology

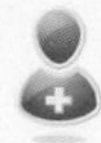

Clinical Alert Glomerular Filtration Rate, usually based on serum Creatinine level, age, sex, and race. For Afro-Caribbean black individuals, eGFR was 21% higher for any given creatinine.

Most laboratory reports indicate a normal range for white and blank individual (The Renal Association, 2013).

Monitor for signs and symptoms of increasing renal failure

Glomerular filtration rate over 90

- Sustained elevated urine specific gravity, elevated urine sodium levels
- Sustained insufficient urine output (<30 mL/hr), elevated blood pressure
- Elevated BUN, serum creatinine, potassium, phosphorus, and decreased bicarbonate (CO_2); decreased creatinine clearance
- Dependent edema (periorbital, pedal, pretibial, sacral)
- Nocturia
- Lethargy
- Itching
- Nausea/vomiting

R: *Hypovolemia and hypotension activate the renin–angiotensin system, which causes peripheral vasoconstriction and decreases glomerular filtration rate (blood flow.) The result is increased sodium and water reabsorption with decreased urine output. BUN is also reabsorbed. If this adaptive mechanism is inadequate, acute kidney injury from ischemia develops. Urine output remains low or diminishes and blood pressure is elevated (Fazia, Lin, & Staros, 2012). Decreased excretion of urea and creatinine in the urine elevates BUN and creatinine levels. Dependent edema results from increased plasma hydrostatic pressure, salt, and water retention, and/or decreased colloid osmotic pressure from plasma protein losses (Grossman & Porth, 2014).*

Notify physician, physician assistant/NP of changes in condition or laboratory results, which reflect increasing renal insufficiency/failure

Weigh the individual daily at a minimum

- Ensure accurate findings by weighing at the same time each day, on the same scale, and with the individual wearing the same amount of clothing.

R: *Daily weights and intake and output records help evaluate fluid balance and guide fluid intake recommendations.*

Maintain strict intake and output records

Explain prescribed fluid management goals to individual and family

R: *Individual and family understanding may enhance cooperation.*

Distribute fluid intake fairly evenly throughout the entire day and night

- It may be necessary to match fluid intake with loss every 8 hours or even every hour if the individual is critically imbalanced.

R: *Maintaining a constant fluid balance, without major fluctuations, is essential. Allowing toxins to accumulate because of poor hydration can cause complications such as nausea and sensorium changes.*

Encourage individual to express feelings, give positive feedback

R: *Fluid and diet restrictions can be extremely frustrating. Emotional support can help reduce anxiety and may improve compliance with the treatment regimen.*

Consult with a dietitian regarding the fluid and diet plan

R: *Important considerations in fluid management, requiring a specialist's attention, include the fluid content of nonliquid food, appropriate amount and type of liquids, liquid preferences, and sodium content.*

Administer oral medications with meals whenever possible

- If medications must be administered between meals, give with the smallest amount of fluid necessary.

R: *This measure avoids using parts of the fluid allowance unnecessarily.*

Avoid continuous IV fluid infusion whenever possible

- Dilute all necessary IV drugs in the smallest amount of fluid that is safe for IV administration.
- Use small IV bags and an IV controller or pump, if possible, to prevent accidental infusion of a large volume of fluid.

R: *Extremely accurate fluid infusion is necessary to prevent fluid overload.*

Monitor for signs and symptoms of metabolic acidosis

- Rapid, shallow respirations
- Headaches
- Nausea and vomiting
- Low plasma pH
- Behavioral changes, drowsiness, lethargy

R: *Acidosis results from the kidney's inability to excrete hydrogen ions, phosphates, sulfates, and ketone bodies. Bicarbonate loss results from decreased renal resorption. Hyperkalemia, hyperphosphatemia, and decreased bicarbonate levels aggravate metabolic acidosis. Excessive ketone bodies cause headaches, nausea, vomiting, and abdominal pain. Respiratory rate and depth increase in an attempt to increase CO_2 excretion and thus reduce acidosis. Acidosis affects the CNS and can increase neuromuscular irritability because of the cellular exchange of hydrogen and potassium (Grossman & Porth, 2014).*

For an individual with metabolic acidosis, ensure adequate caloric intake while limiting fat and protein intake

- Consult with a dietitian for an appropriate diet.

R: *Restricting fats and protein helps prevent accumulation of acidic end products.*

Assess for signs and symptoms of hypocalcemia, hypokalemia, and alkalosis as acidosis is corrected

R: *Rapid correction of acidosis may cause rapid excretion of calcium and potassium and result in rebound alkalosis.*

Dialysis may be necessary to correct metabolic acidosis

R: *Bicarbonate in the dialysate is a higher concentration than the serum. The bicarbonate is delivered during dialysis to help correct the acidosis. Bicarbonate solutions can be tailored to meet individual needs (The Renal Association, 2013).*

Notify physician/PA/NP of s/s of metabolic acidosis

Monitor for signs and symptoms of hypernatremia with fluid overload

- Extreme thirst
- CNS effects ranging from agitation to convulsion

R: *Hypernatremia results from excessive sodium intake or increased aldosterone output. Water is pulled from the cells, causing cellular dehydration and producing CNS symptoms. Thirst is a compensatory response aimed at diluting sodium.*

Maintain prescribed sodium restrictions

R: *Hypernatremia must be corrected slowly to minimize CNS deterioration.*

Monitor for electrolyte imbalances

- Potassium
- Calcium
- Phosphorus
- Sodium
- Magnesium

R: *Refer to Risk for Complications of Electrolyte Imbalances for specific signs and symptoms and interventions. Renal dysfunction can cause hyperkalemia, hypernatremia, hypocalcemia, hypermagnesemia, or hyperphosphatemia. Diuretic therapy can cause hypokalemia or hyponatremia.*

Monitor for gastrointestinal (GI) bleeding

R: *The poor platelet aggregation and capillary fragility associated with high serum levels of nitrogenous wastes may aggravate bleeding. Heparinization required during dialysis in cases of gastric ulcer disease also may precipitate GI bleeding.*

- Refer to *Risk for Complications of GI Bleeding* for specific interventions.

Monitor for manifestations of anemia

- Dyspnea
- Fatigue
- Tachycardia, palpitations

- Cold intolerance
- Pallor of nail beds and mucous membranes
- Low hemoglobin and hematocrit levels
- Easy bruising

R: *Chronic renal failure results in decreased red blood cell production because of decreased erythropoietin production and decreased survival time because of elevated uremic toxins.*

Instruct individual to use a soft toothbrush and to avoid vigorous nose blowing, constipation, and contact sports

R: *Trauma prevention reduces the risk of bleeding and infection.*

Demonstrate the pressure method to control bleeding should it occur

R: *Applying direct, constant pressure on a bleeding site can help prevent excessive blood loss.*

Monitor for manifestations of hypoalbuminemia (Deegens &Wetzels, 2011)

- Serum albumin level <3.5 g/dL; proteinuria (>150 mg/24 hr)
- Edema formation: pedal, facial, sacral
- Hypovolemia (more common in very low <1 m/dL serum albumin levels)
- Decreased hematocrit and hemoglobin levels in advancing disease
- Hyperlipidemia

R: *Refer to Risk for Complications of Negative Nitrogen Balance for more information and interventions. When albumin leaks into the urine because of changes in the glomerular electrostatic barrier or because of peritoneal dialysis, the liver responds by increasing production of plasma proteins. When the loss is great, the liver cannot compensate, and hypoalbuminemia results.*

Monitor for hypervolemia

- Evaluate daily:
  - Weight
  - Fluid intake and output records
  - Rales in lungs
  - Circumference of the edematous parts
  - Laboratory data: hematocrit, serum sodium, and plasma protein in specific serum albumin

R: *As glomerular filtration rate decreases and the functioning nephron mass continues to diminish, the kidneys lose the ability to concentrate urine and to excrete sodium and water, resulting in hypervolemia.*

Monitor for signs and symptoms of congestive heart failure and decreased cardiac output

- Gradual increase in heart rate
- Increasing dyspnea
- Diminished breath sounds, rales
- Decreased systolic blood pressure
- Presence of or increase in S_3 and/or S_4 heart sounds
- Gallop rhythm
- Peripheral edema
- Distended neck veins

R: *Congestive heart failure can result from increased cardiac output, hypervolemia, dysrhythmias, and hypertension, reducing the ability of the left ventricle to eject blood, with subsequent decreased cardiac output and increased pulmonary vascular congestion.*

Encourage adherence to strict fluid restrictions: 800 to 1,000 mL/24 hr, or 24-hour urine output plus 500 mL

R: *Fluid restrictions are based on urine output. In an anuric individual, restriction usually is 800 mL/day, which accounts for insensible losses from metabolism, the GI tract, perspiration, and respiration.*

Collaborate with physician, advanced practice nurse, or dietitian to plan an appropriate diet. Encourage adherence to a low-sodium diet (2 to 4 g/day)

R: *Sodium restrictions should be adjusted based on urine sodium excretion.*

If hemodialysis or peritoneal dialysis is initiated, follow institutional protocols

RISK FOR COMPLICATIONS OF NEUROLOGIC/SENSORY DYSFUNCTION

Risk for Complications of Neurologic/Sensory Dysfunction

Risk for Complications of Alcohol Withdrawal
Risk for Complications of Increased Intracranial Pressure
Risk for Complications of Seizures

Definition

Describes a person experiencing or at high risk to experience various neurologic or sensory dysfunctions

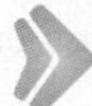

Carp's Cues

The nurse can use this generic collaborative problem to describe a person at risk for several types of neurologic or sensory problems (e.g., an individual recovering from cranial surgery or who has sustained multiple traumas). For such a person, using *Risk for Complications of Neurologic/Sensory Dysfunction* directs nurses to monitor neurologic and sensory function based on focus assessment findings. Should a complication occur, the nurse would add the applicable specific collaborative problem (e.g., *Risk for Complications of Increased Intracranial Pressure*) to the individual's problem list to describe the nursing management of the complication. If the risk factors or etiology were not related directly to the primary medical diagnosis or treatment, the nurse could add this information to the diagnostic statement. For example, for an individual with a seizure disorder admitted for abdominal surgery, the nurse would add *Risk for Complications of Seizures related to epilepsy* to the problem list.

For information on Focus Assessment Criteria, visit thePoint.

Significant Laboratory/Diagnostic Assessment Criteria

Cerebrospinal Fluid

Cloudy Presentation (Indicative of an Infection)

- Protein (increased in meningitis)
- White blood cell (WBC) count (increased in meningitis)
- Albumin (elevated with brain tumors)
- Glucose (decreased with bacterial meningitis)

Blood

- WBC count (elevated with bacterial infection, decreased in viral infection)
- Creatine phosphokinase (CPK)
- Cortisol
- Lactate dehydrogenase
- pCO_2
- Ammonia
- Neuron-specific enolase
- Alcohol level
- Glucose calcium
- Mercury and lead levels if indicated

Radiologic/Imaging

- Skull and spine X-rays
- Computed tomography (CT)
- Magnetic resonance imaging (MRI)
- Cerebral angiography
- Position emission tomography (PET) (measures physiologic and biochemical process in the nervous system; can detect tumors, vascular diseases, and behavioral disturbances such as dementia or schizophrenia)
- Myelography

Other
- Doppler
- Lumbar puncture
- Electroencephalography (EEG)
- Continuous bedside cerebral blood flow monitoring

Risk for Complications of Alcohol Withdrawal

Definition

Describes a person experiencing or at high risk to experience the complications of alcohol withdrawal (e.g., delirium tremens, autonomic hyperactivity, seizures, alcohol hallucinosis, and hypertension)

Carp's Cues

There are about 8 million alcohol-dependent people in the United States. Approximately 500,000 episodes of withdrawal severe enough to require pharmacologic treatment occur each year (Hoffman & Weinhouse, 2015).

Delirium tremens (DT) is associated with a mortality rate of up to 5%. Death usually is due to arrhythmia, complicating illnesses such as pneumonia, or failure to identify an underlying problem that led to the cessation of alcohol use, such as pancreatitis, hepatitis, or central nervous system injury or infection. Older age, preexisting pulmonary disease, core body temperature greater than 40° C (104° F), and coexisting liver disease are associated with a greater risk of mortality (Hoffman & Weinhouse, 2015).

High-Risk Populations

(Hoffman & Weinhouse, 2015)

- A history of sustained drinking
- A history of previous DT
- Age greater than 30
- The presence of a concurrent illness
- The presence of significant alcohol withdrawal in the presence of an elevated ethanol level
- A longer period (more than 2 days) between the last drink and the onset of withdrawal

Collaborative Outcomes

The individual will be monitored for early signs and symptoms of alcohol withdrawal and will receive collaborative interventions if indicated to restore physiologic stability.

Indicators of Physiologic Stability

- No seizure activity
- Calm, oriented
- Temperature 98° F to 99.5° F
- Pulse 60 to 100 beats/min
- BP >90/60, <140/90 mm Hg
- No reports of hallucinations
- No tremors

Interventions and Rationales

Carefully attempt to determine if the individual abuses alcohol

- Consult with the family regarding their perception of alcohol consumption. Explain why accurate information is necessary.

R: *It is critical to identify high-risk people so potentially fatal withdrawal symptoms can be prevented.*

If alcohol abuse is confirmed, obtain history of previous withdrawals

- Delirium tremens
- Seizures

Maintain the IV running continuously

R: *This may be necessary for fluid replacement and dextrose, thiamine bolus, benzodiazepine, and magnesium sulfate administration. Chlordiazepoxide and diazepam should not be given IM because of unpredictable absorption.*

Monitor vital signs at least every 2 hours

R: *Individuals in withdrawal have elevated heart rate, respirations, and fever. Those experiencing DT can be expected to have a low-grade fever. Rectal temperature greater than 37.7° C (99.9° F) is a clue to possible infection.*

Observe for minor withdrawal symptoms (Hoffman & Weinhouse, 2015)

- Insomnia
- Tremulousness
- Mild anxiety
- Gastrointestinal upset; anorexia
- Headache
- Diaphoresis
- Palpitations

R: *Minor withdrawal symptoms are due to central nervous system hyperactivity. Withdrawal occurs 6 to 96 hours after drinking ends. Withdrawal can occur in people who are considered "social drinkers" (6 oz of alcohol daily for a period of 3 to 4 weeks). Withdrawal patterns may resemble those of previous episodes. Seizure patterns unlike previous episodes may indicate another underlying pathology (Hoffman & Weinhouse, 2015).*

When alcohol abuse is suspected and/or minor withdrawal symptoms are assessed, notify the physician/NP for initiation of benzodiazepine therapy, with dosage determined by assessment findings

R: *Benzodiazepine requirements in alcohol withdrawal are highly variable and specific to the individual. Fixed schedules may oversedate or undersedate.*

Obtain a complete history of prescription and nonprescription drugs taken

R: *Benzodiazepine or barbiturate withdrawal may mimic alcohol withdrawal and complicate the picture (Hoffman & Weinhouse, 2015).*

Observe for the desired effects of benzodiazepine therapy

- Relief from withdrawal symptoms
- Peaceful sleep but arousable

R: *Long-acting benzodiazepines are the drugs of choice in controlling withdrawal symptoms except with hepatic dysfunction. With hepatic dysfunction, the shorter half-life of lorazepam and the absence of active metabolites with oxazepam may prevent prolonged effects if oversedation occurs.*

Monitor for withdrawal seizures

- Refer also to *Risk for Complications of Seizures.*

R: *Withdrawal seizures can occur 6 to 96 hours after drinking ends. They are usually nonfocal and grand mal, last minutes or less, and occur singularly or in clusters of two to six.*

Monitor for and intervene promptly in cases of status epilepticus. Follow institution's emergency protocol

R: *Status epilepticus is life-threatening if not controlled immediately with IV diazepam. Monitor and determine onset of alcohol hallucinosis. Hallucinations are usually visual, although auditory and tactile phenomena may also occur. The person senses that the hallucinations are not real and is aware of surroundings.*

R: *Alcoholic hallucinosis is the same as DT. "Alcoholic hallucinosis refers to hallucinations that develop within 12 to 24 hours of abstinence and resolve within 24 to 48 hours (which is the earliest point at which delirium tremens typically develops). In contrast to delirium tremens, alcoholic hallucinosis is not associated with global* *clouding of the sensorium, but with specific hallucinations, and vital signs are usually normal" (Hoffman & Weinhouse, 2015).*

Monitor for delirium tremens

- Delirium component (vivid hallucinations, confusion, extreme disorientation, and fluctuating levels of awareness)

Extreme hyperadrenergic stimulation (tachycardia, hypertension or hypotension, extreme tremor, agitation, diaphoresis, and fever)

R: *DT appears on days 3 to 5 after cessation of drinking and can persist for up to 7 days (Hoffman & Weinhouse, 2015).*

Monitor fluid and electrolyte status

R: *Severe alcohol withdrawal can severely impact fluid and electrolyte status (Hoffman & Weinhouse, 2015).*

- Hypovolemia

R: *This results from hyperthermia, vomiting, and tachypnea.*

- Hypokalemia

R: *This results from renal and extrarenal losses.*

- Hypomagnesemia

R: *Etiology is unknown but may predispose to dysrhythmia and seizures.*

- Hypophosphatemia

R: *This may be due to malnutrition; if severe, may contribute to bleeding.*

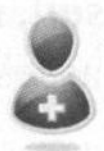

CLINICAL ALERT Prior to providing care, advise ancillary staff/student to report the following to the professional nurse assigned to the individual:

- Insomnia
- Observed tremors
- Mild anxiety
- Complaints of gastrointestinal upset; decreased appetite
- Headache
- Diaphoresis

Risk for Complications of Increased Intracranial Pressure

Definition

Describes a person experiencing or at high risk to experience increased cranial pressure (>20 mm Hg) exerted by cerebrospinal fluid (CSF) within the brain's ventricles or the subarachnoid space

High-Risk Populations

(Rangel-Castillo, Gopinath, & Robertson, 2008; Smith & Amin-Hanjani, 2013)

Intracranial (Primary)

- Brain tumor
- Cerebral edema (such as in acute hypoxic ischemic encephalopathy, large cerebral infarction, severe traumatic brain injury)
- Nontraumatic intracerebral hemorrhage (aneurysm rupture and subarachnoid hemorrhage, hypertensive brain hemorrhage, intraventricular hemorrhage)
- Ischemic stroke
- Hydrocephalus

- Idiopathic or benign intracranial hypertension
- Idiopathic intracranial hypertension (pseudotumor cerebri)
- Other (e.g., pneumocephalus, abscesses, cysts)
- Meningitis, encephalitis
- Status epilepticus

Extracranial (Secondary)

- Airway obstruction
- Hypoxia or hypercarbia (hypoventilation)
- Hypertension (pain/cough) or hypotension (hypovolemia/sedation)
- Posture (head rotation)
- Obstruction of venous outflow (e.g., venous sinus thrombosis, jugular vein compression, neck surgery)
- Hyperpyrexia
- Seizures
- Drug and metabolic (e.g., tetracycline, rofecoxib, divalproex sodium, lead intoxication)
- High altitude
- Hepatic failure (mass lesion [hematoma] edema)
- Increased cerebral blood volume (vasodilation)
- Decreased CSF absorption (e.g., arachnoid granulation adhesions after bacterial meningitis)
- Increased CSF production (e.g., choroid plexus papilloma)

Collaborative Outcomes

The individual will be monitored for early signs and symptoms of increased intracranial pressure (ICP) and will receive collaborative interventions if indicated to restore physiologic stability.

Indicators of Physiologic Stability

- Adult ICP 5 to 15 mm Hg (7.5 to 20 cm H_2O)
- ICP monitoring device (e.g., ventriculostomy)
- Pupils equal; reactive to light and accommodation
- Intact extraocular movements
- Pulse 60 to 100 beats/min
- Respirations 16 to 20 breaths/min
- BP >90/60, <140/90 mm Hg
- Stable pulse pressure (difference between diastolic and systolic readings)
- No nausea/vomiting

If Conscious:

- Alert, oriented, calm, or no change in usual cognitive status
- Appropriate speech
- Mild to no headache

General Interventions and Rationales

Maintain ICP monitoring per protocol

- If using an ICP monitoring device (e.g., ventriculostomy), refer to the procedure manual for guidelines.

R: *Ventriculostomy is utilized to monitor ICP and as an access to drain CSF to reduce ICP.*

Monitor the system for proper functioning at least every 2 to 4 hours, and any time there is a change in the ICP, neurologic examination, and CSF output

R: *The functioning of the monitoring system should be evaluated when malfunctioning is suspected.*

Report immediately an increase in ICP

R: *"ICP values greater than 20 to 25 mm Hg require treatment in most circumstances. Sustained ICP values of greater than 40 mm Hg indicate severe, life-threatening intracranial hypertension"* (Rangel-Castillo et al. 2008).

Differentiate between cerebral perfusion pressure (CPP) and increased ICP

R: *Impaired cerebral perfusion results in decreased cerebral blood flow and a rise in ICP. CPP can be impaired by an increase in ICP, a decrease in blood pressure, or a combination of both factors. With normal autoregulation, the brain is able to maintain a normal cerebral blood flow (CBF). After injury, the ability of the brain to pressure autoregulate may be absent or diminished (Rangel-Castillo et al., 2008).*

Maintain oxygenation and ventilation to keep PaO_2 >100, $PaCO_2$ 30 to 35

R: *This will increase the oxygenation of cerebral tissue.*

Monitor for signs and symptoms of increased ICP

Assess the following (Glasgow Coma Scale [GCS]) (Hickey, 2014):

- Best eye-opening response: spontaneously, to auditory stimuli, to painful stimuli, or no response
- Best motor response: obeys verbal commands, localizes pain, flexion–withdrawal, flexion–decorticate, extension–decerebrate, or no response
- Best verbal response: oriented to person, place, and time; confused conversation; inappropriate speech; incomprehensible sounds; or no response

R: *Deficiencies of cerebral blood supply resulting from hemorrhage, hematoma, cerebral edema, thrombus, or emboli compromise cerebral tissue. These responses evaluate the individual's ability to integrate commands with conscious and involuntary movement. The nurse can assess cortical function by evaluating eye-opening and motor response. No response may indicate damage to the midbrain.*

Assess for changes in vital signs

- Pulse changes: slowing rate to 60 beats/min or lower, or increasing rate to 100 beats/min or higher

R: *Bradycardia is a late sign of brain stem ischemia. Tachycardia may indicate hypothalamic ischemia and sympathetic discharge.*

- Respiratory irregularities: slowing rate with lengthening apneic periods

R: *Respiratory patterns vary depending on the site of impairment. Cheyne–Stokes breathing (a gradual increase followed by a gradual decrease, then a period of apnea) points to damage in cerebral hemispheres, midbrain, and upper pons. Central neurogenic hyperventilation occurs with midbrain and upper pontine lesions. Ataxic breathing (irregular with random sequence of deep and shallow breaths) indicates pontine dysfunction. Hypoventilation and apnea occur with medullary lesions (Hickey, 2014).*

- Rising blood pressure and/or widening pulse pressure
- Bradycardia, increased systolic blood pressure, and increased pulse pressure

R: *These are late signs (known as Cushing response) of brain stem ischemia, leading to cerebral herniation (Hickey, 2014).*

Assess pupillary responses

R: *Changes indicate pressure on oculomotor or optic nerves.*

- Inspect the pupils with a bright pinpoint light to evaluate size, configuration, and reaction to light. Compare both eyes for similarities and differences.

R: *The oculomotor nerve (cranial nerve III) in the brain stem regulates pupil reactions.*

- Evaluate gaze to determine whether it is conjugate (paired, working together) or if eye movements are abnormal.

R: *Conjugate eye movements are regulated from parts of the cortex and brain stem.*

- Evaluate the ability of the eyes to adduct and abduct.

R: *Cranial nerve VI, or the abducens nerve, regulates abduction and adduction of the eyes. Cranial nerve IV, or the trochlear nerve, also regulates eye movement.*

- Note any other signs and symptoms.
  - Vomiting

R: *Vomiting results from pressure on the medulla, which stimulates the brain's vomiting center.*

- Headache: constant, increasing in intensity, or aggravated by movement
- Straining

R: *Compression of neural tissue increases ICP and causes pain.*

- Subtle changes (e.g., lethargy, restlessness, forced breathing, purposeless movements, changes in mentation)

R: *These signs may be the earliest indicators of cranial pressure changes.*

Elevate the head of the bed 20° to 30° unless contraindicated (e.g., hypovolemia)

R: *Slight elevation of the head of the bed to 30° improves jugular venous outflow, reduces cerebrovascular congestion, and lowers ICP. In individuals who are hypovolemic, this may be associated with a fall in blood pressure and an overall fall in CPP. Care must therefore initially be taken to exclude hypovolemia. Positioning is very dependent on the type of surgery done and the approach used and should always be clarified before repositioning (Hickey, 2014).*

Maintain negative fluid balance

- Carefully monitor hydration status; evaluate fluid intake and output, serum osmolality, urine specific gravity, and osmolality.

R: *Significant departures from the normal intravascular volume can adversely affect ICP and/or cerebral perfusion. Increased intravascular volume will increase cranial pressure; decreased intravascular volume will decrease cardiac output and cerebral tissue perfusion (Hickey, 2014).*

Monitor intravenous (IV) fluid therapy (hypertonic saline, mannitol); carefully administer IV fluids with an infusion pump

R: *Careful IV fluid administration is necessary to prevent overhydration, which increases ICP, and dehydration, which decreases cerebral tissue perfusion.*

Monitor for diabetes insipidus (Hickey, 2014)

- More than 200 mL/hr of urine output for 2 consecutive hours

R: *Cerebral edema can damage the pituitary gland or hypothalamus where antidiuretic hormone (ADH) is produced. This results in decreased ADH and the development of central diabetes insipidus in individuals with traumatic brain injury (Hickey, 2014).*

Dehydration can occur rapidly and further compromise cerebral vascular perfusion. Immediate action is required

Monitor temperature. As indicated, initiate antipyretics and cooling blankets per orders/institutional protocols

R: *A fever increases metabolic rate by 10% to 13% per degree Celsius and is a potent vasodilator. Fever-induced dilation of cerebral vessels can increase CBF and may increase ICP. Fever should be avoided as it increases ICP, being an independent predictor of poor outcome after severe head injury (Rangel-Castillo et al., 2008).*

For individuals with posttraumatic brain injury, consult with physician/NP for seizure prophylaxis (phenytoin)

R: *The risk of seizures after trauma is related to the severity of the brain injury; seizures occur in 15% to 20% of individuals with severe head injury. Seizures increase cerebral metabolic rate and ICP. Seizure prophylaxis is recommended for the first 7 days after severe brain injury (Rangel-Castillo et al., 2008).*

Avoid the following situations or maneuvers, which can increase ICP (Hickey, 2014; Smith & Amin-Hanjani, 2013)

- Carotid massage

R: *This slows the heart rate and reduces systemic circulation, which is followed by a sudden increase in circulation.*

- Neck flexion or extreme rotation; if intubated, do not use securing device with circumferential wrapping

R: *This inhibits jugular venous drainage, which increases cerebrovascular congestion and ICP.*

- Digital anal stimulation, breath-holding, straining

R: *These can initiate the Valsalva maneuver, which impairs venous return by constricting the jugular veins, thus increasing ICP.*

- Extreme flexion of the hips and knees

R: *Flexion increases intrathoracic pressure, which inhibits jugular venous drainage, increasing cerebrovascular congestion and, thus, ICP.*

- Rapid position changes

Teach to exhale during position changes

R: *This helps prevent the Valsalva maneuver.*

Consult with the physician or nurse practitioner for stool softeners, if needed

R: *Stool softeners prevent constipation and straining during defecation, which can trigger the Valsalva maneuver.*

Maintain a quiet, calm, softly lit environment. Schedule several lengthy periods of uninterrupted rest daily. Cluster necessary procedures and activities to minimize interruptions

R: *These measures promote rest and decrease stimulation, both of which can help decrease ICP.*

Avoid sequential performance of activities that increase ICP (e.g., coughing, suctioning, repositioning, bathing)

R: *Research has validated that such sequential activities can cause a cumulative increase in ICP (Hickey, 2014).*

Limit suctioning time to 10 seconds at a time; hyperoxygenate individual both before and after suctioning

R: *These measures help prevent hypercapnia, which can increase cerebral vasodilation and raise ICP, and prevent hypoxia, which may increase cerebral ischemia.*

Consult with physician or advanced practice nurse about administering prophylactic lidocaine before suctioning

R: *This measure may help prevent acute intracranial hypertension.*

CLINICAL ALERT Prior to providing care, advise ancillary staff/student to report the following to the professional nurse assigned to the individual:

- Change in orientation
- Complaints of new or worsening headaches
- Slowed responses (speech, movements)
- Vomiting

Risk for Complications of Seizures

Definition

Describes a person experiencing or at high risk to experience paroxysmal episodes of involuntary muscular contraction (tonus) and relaxation (clonus)

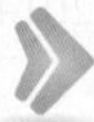

Carp's Cues

Alcohol abuse is one of the most common causes of adolescent- and adult-onset seizures. Seizures, nearly always generalized tonic–clonic, occur in about 10% of adults during withdrawal. Multiple seizures happen in about 60% of these individuals. The first seizure occurs 7 hours to 2 days after the last drink, and the time between the first and last seizures is usually 6 hours or less (Hoffman & Weinhouse, 2015). Less than one-half of epilepsy cases have an identifiable cause (Schachter, 2015).

High-Risk Populations

Carp's Cues

"Less than one-half of epilepsy cases have an identifiable cause" (Schachter, 2015).

"It is presumed that epilepsy in most of these other individuals is genetically determined" (Schachter, 2015). Some seizures are provoked, that is, they occur in the setting of metabolic derangement, drug or alcohol withdrawal, and acute neurologic disorders such as stroke or encephalitis. Such patients are not considered to have epilepsy, because the presumption is that these seizures would not recur in the absence of the provocation (Fisher et al., 2014).

- Family history of seizure disorder
- Congenital brain malformations
- Inborn errors of metabolism
- Cerebral cortex lesions
- Head injury
- Infectious disorder (e.g., meningitis)
- Cerebral circulatory disturbance (e.g., cerebral palsy, stroke)
- Brain tumor
- Alcohol overdose or withdrawal; refer to *Risk for Complications of Alcohol Withdrawal*
- Drug overdose (e.g., cocaine)
- Poststroke
- Sudden withdrawal from certain anti-anxiety or antidepressant drugs such as benzodiazepines, barbiturates, and tricyclic antidepressants
- Medications (overdose, abrupt withdrawal) such as theophylline, meperidine, tricyclic antidepressants, phenothiazines, lidocaine, quinolones, penicillins, selective serotonin reuptake inhibitors, isoniazid, antihistamines, cyclosporine, interferons, lithium
- Electrolyte imbalances (e.g., hypocalcemia, pyridoxine deficiency)
- Hypoglycemia as a complication of diabetes mellitus
- High fever
- Eclampsia
- Metabolic abnormalities (e.g., renal, hepatic, electrolyte)
- Alzheimer's or other degenerative brain diseases in older persons
- Poisoning (e.g., mercury, lead, carbon monoxide)

Collaborative Outcomes

The individual will be monitored for early signs and symptoms of seizure activity and will receive collaborative interventions, if indicated, to restore physiologic stability.

Indicators of Physiologic Stability

- No seizure activity

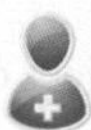

Clinical Alert "Seizures and epilepsy are not the same. An epileptic seizure is a transient occurrence of signs and/or symptoms due to abnormal excessive or synchronous neuronal activity in the brain. Epilepsy is a disease characterized by an enduring predisposition to generate epileptic seizures and by the neurobiological, cognitive, psychological, and social consequences of this condition. Translation: a seizure is an event and epilepsy is the disease involving recurrent unprovoked seizures" (Fisher et al., 2014).

Interventions and Rationales

Determine whether the individual senses an aura before onset of seizure activity. If so, advise him or her to immediately report to nursing staff and, if standing, to sit or lie down

R: *This can prevent injuries from falling or hitting head on an object.*

If seizure activity occurs, observe or acquire details from those who witnessed it and document the following (Hickey, 2014)

R: *An accurate, comprehensive description of a seizure can assist the physician/NP/PA with appropriate anticonvulsant and optimal seizure management (Hickey, 2014).*

Behavior Prior to Seizure

- Site of onset of seizure
- Progression and sequencing of activity

R: *Site of onset and order of progression are important in diagnosing causation.*

- Type of movements: clonic (jerking), tonic (stiffening)
- Twitching, head turning, dystonia (muscle spasms and twisting of limbs)
- Parts of body involved (symmetric, unilateral, bilateral)
- Changes in pupil size or position (open, rolling, deviation)
- Skin changes (color, temperature, perspiration)
- Urinary or bowel incontinence
- Duration
- Unconsciousness (duration)
- Behavior after seizure
- Weakness, paralysis after seizure
- Sleep after seizure (postictal period)

R: *Progression of seizure activity may assist in identifying its anatomic focus.*

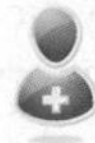

CLINICAL ALERT A high proportion (25%) of new seizures occur in persons over the age of 65 years, and nearly 25% of all people with epilepsy are elderly (Lawn et al., 2013). The causes and clinical manifestations of seizures and epilepsy differ in this age group and affect the diagnostic approach (Boggs, 2015). Lawn et al. found that older adults with new-onset seizures had remote symptomatic etiologies such as head injury, epileptogenic lesions, or focal EEG abnormalities, and that age was not an independent factor.

In older adults, assess for presence of partial or focal seizures (Boggs, 2015)

- May or may not lose consciousness
- Strange feelings, staring
- Minor behavioral changes, memory lapses
- Unaccountable loss of time
- Transient confusion
- Abrupt jerking muscle movements in an arm or leg
- Chewing or other mouth or tongue movements, or pulling or fumbling with clothing without a purpose
- A blank stare with no apparent awareness of one's surroundings
- A sudden feeling of fear, joy, or rage that comes without reason
- Repeating a phrase or word
- A change in vision or a hallucination (seeing something that is not real)
- A sensation of smell or taste, usually unpleasant, that does not come from a real object or food
- Sudden loss of balance or dizziness
- After a seizure, a person may be disoriented for a few minutes.

R: *Age-related changes in the brain produce seizures that present differently in older adults. Only 25% of older adults with epilepsy present with tonic–clonic seizures (Boggs, 2015).*

Provide privacy during and after seizure activity

R: *Privacy protects the individual from embarrassment.*

During seizure activity, take measures to ensure adequate ventilation (e.g., loosen clothing). Do not try to force an airway or tongue blade through clenched teeth

R: *Strong clonic–tonic movements can cause airway occlusion. Forced airway insertion can cause injury.*

During seizure activity, gently guide movements to prevent injury. Do not attempt to restrict movements

R: *Physical restraint could result in musculoskeletal injury.*

If the individual is sitting when seizure activity occurs, ease to the floor if needed and place something soft under his or her head

R: *These measures help prevent injury.*

After seizure activity subsides, position individual on the side

R: *This position helps prevent aspiration of secretions.*

Allow person to sleep after seizure activity; reorient on awakening

R: *The person may experience amnesia; reorientation can help him or her regain a sense of control and can help reduce anxiety.*

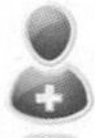

CLINICAL ALERT "Status epilepticus is a condition resulting either from the failure of the mechanisms responsible for seizure termination or from the initiation of mechanisms, which lead to abnormally prolonged seizures (after time point t1). It is a condition, which can have long-term consequences (after time point t2), including neuronal death, neuronal injury, and alteration of neuronal networks, depending on the type and duration of seizures" (Trinka et al., 2015).

Call rapid response team if seizure continues more than 2 consecutive minutes or the individual experiences two or more generalized seizures without full recovery of consciousness between seizures

- Initiate protocol:
  - Establish airway.
  - Suction PRN.
  - Administer oxygen through nasal catheter.
  - Initiate an IV line.

R: *Status epilepticus is a medical emergency with a 10% mortality rate. Impaired respiration can cause systemic and cerebral hypoxia. IV administration of a rapid-acting anticonvulsant (e.g., diazepam) is indicated (Hickey, 2014).*

Keep the bed in a low position with the side rails up, and pad the side rails with blankets

R: *These precautions help prevent injury from fall or trauma.*

If appropriate, question individual when stable about

- Any strange feelings, smells, movements that precede a seizure, time of day; reports of fatigue and confusion.

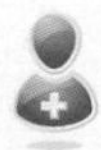

CLINICAL ALERT Prior to providing care, advise ancillary staff/student to report the following to the professional nurse assigned to the individual:

- Any signs of seizure activity
- Intermittent nonresponsive, blank stares

RISK FOR COMPLICATIONS OF GASTROINTESTINAL/HEPATIC/ BILIARY DYSFUNCTION

Risk for Complications of Gastrointestinal/Hepatic/Biliary Dysfunction

Risk for Complications of Paralytic Ileus
Risk for Complications of GI Bleeding
Risk for Complications of Hepatic Dysfunction
Risk for Complications of Hyperbilirubinemia

Definition

Describes a person experiencing or at high risk for experiencing compromised function in the gastrointestinal (GI), hepatic, or biliary systems. (*Note:* These three systems are grouped together for classification purposes. In a clinical situation, the nurse would use either *Risk for Complications of Gastrointestinal Dysfunctional*, *Risk for Complications of Hepatic Dysfunction*, *Risk for Complications of GI Bleeding*, or *Risk for Complications of Biliary Dysfunction* to specify the applicable system.)

Carp's Cues

The nurse can use these generic collaborative problems to describe a person at risk for various problems affecting the GI, hepatic, or biliary system. Doing so focuses nursing interventions on monitoring GI, hepatic, or biliary status to detect and diagnose abnormal functioning. Should a complication develop, the nurse would add the applicable specific collaborative problem (e.g., *Risk for Complications of GI Bleeding*, *Risk for Complications of Hepatic Dysfunction*) to the problem list, specifying appropriate nursing management.

In most cases, along with these collaborative problems, the nurse treats other associated responses, using nursing diagnoses (e.g., *Impaired Comfort related to accumulation of bilirubin pigment and bile salts*).

Significant Laboratory/Diagnostic Assessment Criteria

- Urinalysis (to detect low amylase levels, which indicate pancreatic insufficiency)
- Serum *Helicobacter pylori (H. pylori)* (positive as a risk factor for peptic ulcer disease)
- Serum albumin (lowered in chronic liver disease)
- Serum amylase (elevated in biliary tract disease)
- Serum lipase (elevated in pancreatitis)
- Serum calcium (high total calcium levels in cancer of liver, pancreas, and other organs)
- Stool specimen (can be analyzed for blood, parasites, fat)
- Bilirubin (elevated in hepatic disease, newborn hyperbilirubinemia)
- Potassium (lowered in liver disease with ascites, vomiting, diarrhea)
- Blood urea nitrogen (BUN; increased in hepatic failure)
- Prothrombin time (elevated in cirrhosis, hepatitis)
- Hemoglobin, hematocrit (decreased with bleeding)
- Sodium (decreased with dehydration)
- Platelets (decreased with liver disease or bleeding)
- Serum ammonia level elevated in liver dysfunction
- Hepatitis panel for primary differential diagnosis of diseases of the liver
- Abdominal X-ray
- Ultrasound (to detect masses, obstruction, gallstones)
- CT scan, MRI (to evaluate soft tissue for abscesses, tumors, sources of bleeding)
- Colonoscopy, barium enema, sigmoidoscopy
- Endoscopy, upper GI series, endoscopic retrograde cholangiopancreatography (ERCP) (visual examination of the inside of the stomach and duodenum, with the injection of radiographic contrast into the ducts in the biliary tree and pancreas for visualization on X-rays)
- Balloon assistive enteroscopy (visual examination of the small bowel using an instrument called an endoscope with a balloon, which allows the scope to pass further into the small bowel)
- Esophagogastroduodenoscopy (EGD) (to examine the lining of the esophagus, stomach, and first part of the small intestine)

Risk for Complications of Paralytic Ileus

The stages of hepatic failure will impact the functioning of the individual and family. When indicated in this section by, refer to Individual Nursing Diagnoses in Section 2—Part 1 as *Fatigue, Risk for Injury, Confusion, Risk for Pressure Ulcers, Compromised Family Coping.*

Definition

Describes a person experiencing or at high risk for experiencing neurogenic or functional bowel obstruction

High-Risk Populations

- Bacteria or viruses that cause intestinal infections (gastroenteritis)
- Thrombosis or embolus to mesenteric vessels
- Any major surgery with use of general anesthesia and subsequent limitation of mobility, as well as minor surgery of the abdomen
- Postoperative status (bowel, retroperitoneal, or spinal cord surgery)
- Kidney or lung disease
- Use of certain medications, especially narcotics
- Decreased blood supply to the intestines (mesenteric ischemia)
- Postshock status
- Hypovolemia
- Infections inside the abdomen, such as appendicitis
- Chemical, electrolyte, mineral imbalances (e.g., hypokalemia)
- Posttrauma (e.g., spinal cord injury)
- Uremia
- Spinal cord lesion
- Mechanical causes of intestinal obstruction may include (Bordeianou & Yeh, 2015):
  - Adhesions or scar tissue that forms after surgery
  - Foreign bodies that block the intestines
  - Gallstones (rare)
  - Hernias
  - Impacted stool
  - Intussusception (telescoping of one segment of bowel into another)
  - Tumors blocking the intestines
  - Volvulus (twisted intestine)

Collaborative Outcomes

The individual will be monitored for early signs and symptoms of paralytic ileus and will receive collaborative interventions, if indicated, to restore physiologic stability.

Indicators of Physiologic Stability

- Bowel sounds present
- No nausea and vomiting
- No abdominal distention
- No change in bowel function
- Evidence of flatus

Interventions and Rationales

Auscultate each of the four abdominal quadrants to evaluate the specific function of large (colon) and small intestines

- The right upper quadrant contains the lower margin of the liver, the gallbladder, part of the large intestine, a few loops of the small intestine.

- The right lower quadrant contains the appendix, the connection between the large and small intestines, loops of bowel.
- The left upper quadrant contains the lower margin of the spleen, part of the pancreas, some of the stomach and duodenum.
- The left lower quadrant contains bowel loops and the descending colon.

R: *Knowing the structures under the stethoscope will help to determine the nature of the bowel sounds. Large intestine's (colon) function can be auscultated at the outer (distal) aspects of each quadrant. Small intestine's function can be auscultated in the inner aspect of each quadrant (refer to Fig. III.1).*

In a postoperative individual, monitor bowel function, looking for

- Bowel sounds in small intestines can return within 24 to 48 hours of surgery.
- Bowel sounds in large intestines can return within 3 to 5 days of surgery.
- Flatus and defecation resuming by the second or third postoperative day.

R: *Resolution of normal bowel function starts in the proximal or right colon and progresses to the distal or left colon. Normally, the small bowel regains function within hours, whereas it may take 3 to 5 days for the colon to regain function. Bowel sounds should be auscultated to help differentiate paralytic ileus from a mechanical ileus. Continued absence of bowel sounds suggests paralytic ileus, whereas hyperactive bowel sounds may indicate a mechanical ileus (McCutcheon, 2013).*

Monitor for signs and symptoms of paralytic ileus (McCutcheon, 2013)

- Mild abdominal pain and bloating
- Nausea, vomiting, poor appetite
- Distended and tympanic abdomen
- Constipation, obstipation
- Absent or hypoactive bowel sounds
- Passing flatus or stool

R: *Intraoperative manipulation of abdominal organs and the depressive effects of narcotics and anesthetics on peristalsis reduce bowel motility. The physiologic postoperative ileus that usually follows surgery has a benign and self-limited course. However, when ileus is prolonged, it leads to increasing discomfort and must be differentiated from other potential complications, for example, bowel obstruction, intra-abdominal abscess (McCutcheon, 2013).*

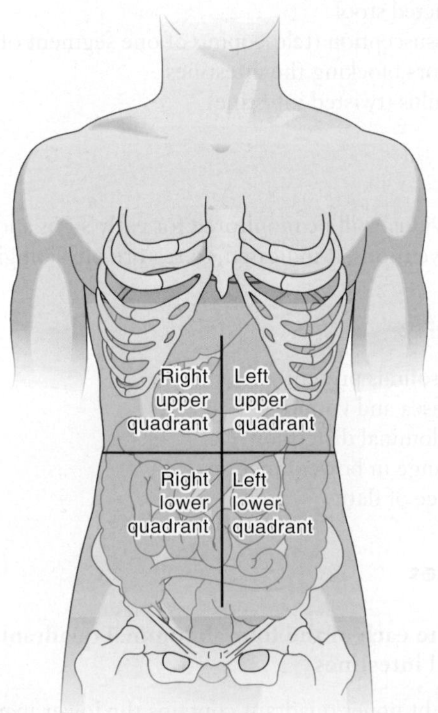

FIGURE III.1 Diagram of the location of small and large intestines in quadrants for auscultation.

Differentiate between paralytic ileus and mechanical bowel obstruction

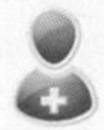

Clinical Alert It is useful to note that nearly all individuals with early postoperative bowel obstruction have an initial return of bowel function and oral intake, which is then followed by nausea, vomiting, abdominal pain, and distention, whereas patients with ileus generally do not experience return of bowel function (Bordeianou & Yeh, 2015).

- Abdominal distention, vomiting, obstipation—may be present with both
- Bowel sounds: Paralytic ileus—usually quiet or absent
  - Bowel obstruction—may be high-pitched or may be absent
- Pain: Paralytic ileus—mild and diffuse
  - Bowel obstruction—moderate to severe, colicky
- Fever, tachycardia: paralytic ileus—absent
  - Bowel obstruction—should raise suspicion

R: *Localized tenderness, fever, tachycardia, and peritoneal signs suggest bowel ischemia or perforation, which indicate the need for emergent surgical intervention.*

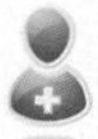

Clinical Alert Notify physician/NP of new onset or increasing signs and symptoms of paralytic ileus. If the obstruction blocks the blood supply to the intestine, it may cause infection and tissue death (gangrene). The duration of the blockage and its cause are risk factors for tissue death. Hernias, volvulus, and intussusception carry a higher gangrene risk (Bordeianou & Yeh, 2015).

When bowel obstruction is suspected, a plain abdominal X-ray or computed tomographic (CT) scan with contrast is indicated

R: *Small bowel obstruction can be diagnosed on X-ray if the more proximal small bowel is dilated and the more distal small bowel is not dilated. The stomach may also be dilated. However, if there remains any suspicion for small bowel obstruction or another diagnosis, we suggest computed tomography (CT) of the abdomen (Bordeianou & Yeh, 2015).*

Restrict fluids until bowel sounds are present. When indicated, begin with small amounts of clear liquids only

- Monitor individual's response to resumption of fluid and food intake, and note the nature and amount of any emesis or stools

R: *The individual will not tolerate fluids until bowel sounds resume.*

Risk for Complications of GI Bleeding

Definition

Describes a person experiencing or at high risk for experiencing GI bleeding

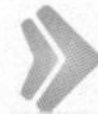

Carp's Cues

The three nonsurgical modalities used to diagnose lower gastrointestinal bleeding (LGIB) are colonoscopy, radionuclide scans, and angiography. Apart from colonoscopy, endoscopic procedures such as esophagogastroduodenoscopy (EGD), wireless capsule endoscopy (WCE), push enteroscopy, and double-balloon enteroscopy are used, depending on the clinical circumstance. The sequence of using various modalities depends on such factors as rate of bleeding, hemodynamic status of the individual, and inability to localize bleeding with the initial modality.

High-Risk Populations

Upper GI Bleeding

- Miscellaneous causes
  - Older persons
  - Daily use of aspirin or nonsteroidal anti-inflammatory drugs (NSAIDs)

- Antiplatelet therapy and proton pump inhibitor (PPI) cotherapy
- Selective serotonin reuptake inhibitors or serotonin-specific reuptake inhibitor (SSRIs)
- Prolonged mechanical ventilation >48 hours
- Recent stress (e.g., trauma, sepsis)
- Platelet deficiency
- Coagulopathy
- Shock, hypotension
- Major surgery (>3 hours)
- Head injury
- Severe vascular disease
- Disorders of GI, hepatic, and biliary systems
- Transfusion of 5 units (or more) of blood
- Burns (>35% of body)
- Hematobilia, or bleeding from the biliary tree
- Hemosuccus pancreaticus, or bleeding from the pancreatic duct
- Severe superior mesenteric artery syndrome

- Esophageal causes
  - Esophageal varices
  - Esophagitis
  - Esophageal cancer
  - Esophageal ulcers
  - Mallory–Weiss tear
- Gastric causes
  - Gastric ulcer
  - Gastric cancer
  - Gastritis
  - Gastric varices
  - Gastric antral vascular ectasia
  - Dieulafoy's lesions
- Duodenal causes
  - Duodenal ulcer
  - Vascular malformation
  - Antithrombolytic therapy

Lower Gastrointestinal Bleeding in Adults/Percentage

- Diverticular disease (60%)
  - Diverticulosis/diverticulitis of small intestine
  - Diverticulosis/diverticulitis of colon
- Inflammatory bowel disease (13%)
  - Crohn's disease of small bowel, colon, or both
  - Ulcerative colitis
  - Noninfectious gastroenteritis and colitis
- Benign anorectal diseases (11%)
  - Hemorrhoids
  - Anal fissure
  - Fistula-in-ano
- Neoplasia (9%)
  - Malignant neoplasia of small intestine
  - Malignant neoplasia of colon, rectum, and anus
- Coagulopathy (4%)
- Arteriovenous malformations (AVMs) (3%)

Collaborative Outcomes

The individual will be monitored for early signs and symptoms of GI bleeding and will receive collaborative interventions, if indicated, to restore physiologic stability.

Indicators of Physiologic Stability

- Negative stool occult blood
- Calm, oriented
- Hemodynamic stability (BP, pulse, urine output)
- Refer to *Risk for Complications of Hypovolemia*

Interventions and Rationales

Initiate prophylaxis stress ulcers protocol for persons on mechanical ventilation, for example, oral PPI or intravenous histamine-2 receptor antagonist (H_2 blocker) or intravenous PPI (Weinhouse, 2016)

R: *Researchers have reported an incidence of 46.7% of GI bleeding in individuals on mechanical ventilation (Chu et al., 2010, p. 34).Critically ill individuals experience a decrease in the protective mucous layer in the stomach, hypersecretion of acid because of excessive gastrin stimulation, and inadequate perfusion to stomach secondary to shock, infection, or trauma (Weinhouse, 2016).*

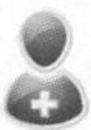

Clinical Alert Acute respiratory failure requiring mechanical ventilation (MV) for >48 hours has been shown to be one of the two strongest *independent risk factors for clinically important GI bleeding in the ICU* (Chu et al., 2010).

Monitor for complications associated with MV, such as stress ulcer and GI hypomotility

- Diarrhea
- Decreased bowel sounds
- High gastric residuals
- Constipation
- Ileus

R: *MV, with increased positive end expiratory pressure (PEEP), increases intrathoracic pressure. This decreases perfusion to the GI tract.*

Monitor for signs and symptoms of acute upper GI bleeding

- Hematemesis (vomiting blood)
- Melena (dark stool)
- Dysphasia, dyspepsia
- Epigastric pain
- Heartburn
- Diffuse abdominal pain
- Weight loss
- Presyncope, syncope

R: *Clinical manifestations depend on the amount and duration of upper GI bleeding. Early detection enables prompt intervention to minimize complications.*

Monitor for lower GI bleeding

- Maroon-colored stools
- Bright-red blood

R: *LGIB ranges from trivial hematochezia (blood in stool) to massive hemorrhage with shock, and accounts for up to 24% of all cases of GI bleeding. This condition is associated with significant morbidity and mortality (10% to 20%). LGIB is one of the most common gastrointestinal indications for hospital admission, particularly in older persons. Diverticulitis accounts for up to 50% of cases, followed by ischemic colitis and anorectal lesions.*

Monitor for occult blood in gastric aspirates and bowel movements

R: *An individual can lose 100 mL of blood in stool and may have normal-appearing stools. Testing stool for occult blood is more accurate.*

- Test nasogastric aspirate with Gastroccult.

R: *The Hemoccult test's sensitivity is reduced by the acidic environment, and the Gastroccult test is the most accurate.*

- Test stool for occult blood with the fecal occult blood test (FOBT)

R: *The Gastroccult test is not recommended for use with fecal samples.*

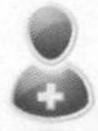

CLINICAL ALERT Massive LGIB is a life-threatening condition; although this condition manifests as maroon stools or bright-red blood from the rectum, individuals with massive upper gastrointestinal bleeding (UGIB) may also present with similar findings. Regardless of the level of the bleeding, one of the most important elements of the management of individuals with massive UGIB or LGIB is restoring hemodynamic stability.

Institute protocols for volume replacement (e.g., 2 large-bore intravenous [IV] catheters and isotonic crystalloid infusions)

R: *Orthostatic hypotension (i.e., a blood pressure fall of >10 mm Hg) is usually indicative of blood loss of more than 1,000 mL.*

Prepare for transfusion per physician/PA/advanced practice nurse orders and protocol

R: *The goal is to increase blood volume and treat or prevent hypovolemic shock.*

Monitor hemoglobin, hematocrit, red blood cell count, platelets, prothrombin time, partial thromboplastin time, type blood and crossmatch, and BUN values

R: *These values reflect the effectiveness of therapy.*

- If hypovolemia occurs, refer to *Risk for Complications of Hypovolemia* for more information and specific interventions.

Risk for Complications of Hepatic Dysfunction

Definition

Describes a person experiencing or at high risk for experiencing progressive liver dysfunction

High-Risk Populations

- Infections
  - Hepatitis A, B, C, D, E, non-A, non-B, non-C
  - Herpes simplex virus (types 1 and 2)
  - Epstein–Barr virus
  - Varicella zoster
  - Dengue fever virus
  - Rift Valley fever virus
- Drugs/toxins
  - Industrial substances (vinyl chloride, chlorinated hydrocarbons, phosphorus, carbon tetrachloride)
  - *Amanita phalloides* (mushrooms)
  - Aflatoxin (herb)
  - Medications (isoniazid, rifampin, halothane, methyldopa, tetracycline, valproic acid, monoamine oxidase inhibitors, phenytoin, nicotinic acid, tricyclic antidepressants, isoflurane, ketoconazole, cotrimethoprim, sulfasalazine, pyrimethamine, octreotide, antivirals)
  - Acetaminophen toxicity
  - Cocaine
  - Alcohol
- Hypoperfusion (shock liver)
  - Venous obstructions
  - Budd–Chiari's syndrome
  - Veno-occlusive disease
  - Ischemia

- Metabolic disorders
  - Hyperbilirubinemia
  - Hereditary (Wilson's disease, hemochromatosis)
  - Tyrosinemia
  - Heat stroke
  - Galactosemia
  - Nutritional deficiencies
- Surgery
  - Traumatized liver
  - Jejunoileal bypass
  - Partial hepatectomy
  - Liver transplant failure
- Other
  - Reye's syndrome
  - Acute fatty liver of pregnancy
  - Massive malignant infiltration
  - Autoimmune hepatitis
  - Rh incompatibility
  - Ingestion of raw contaminated fish
  - Thalassemia

Collaborative Outcomes

The individual will be monitored for early signs and symptoms of hepatic dysfunction and will receive collaborative interventions, if indicated, to restore physiologic stability.

Indicators of Physiologic Stability

- Prothrombin time (PT) 9.5 to 13.8 seconds
- Partial prothrombin time (PTT) 25 to 35 seconds
- Aspartate aminotransferase (AST) male 8 to 48 units/L, female 6 to 18 units/L
- Alanine aminotransferase (ALT) 7 to 55 units/L
- Alkaline phosphatase 45 to 115 units/L
- Serum barbiturates 2 to 21 μmol/L
- Serum electrolytes within normal range

Interventions and Rationales

Monitor for signs and symptoms of hepatic dysfunction

- Anorexia, indigestion

R: *GI effects result from circulating toxins.*

- Jaundice

R: *Yellowed skin and sclera result from excessive bilirubin production.*

- Petechiae, ecchymoses

R: *These skin changes reflect impaired synthesis of clotting factors.*

- Clay-colored stools

R: *This can result from decreased bile in stools.*

- Elevated liver function tests (e.g., serum bilirubin, serum transaminase)

R: *Elevated values indicate extensive liver damage.*

- Bleeding, prolonged prothrombin time

R: *This reflects reduced production of clotting factors.*

- Edema, ascites

R: *Decreased synthesis of protein results in hypoalbuminemia and fluid shifts into extravascular space.*

With hepatic dysfunction, monitor for hemorrhage

R: *The liver has a central role in hemostasis. Decreased platelet count results from impaired production of new platelets from the bone marrow. Decreased clearance of old platelets by the reticuloendothelial system also results. In addition, synthesis of coagulation factors (II, V, VII, IX, and X) is impaired, resulting in bleeding. The most frequent site is the upper GI tract. Other sites include the nasopharynx, lungs, retroperitoneum, kidneys, and intracranial and skin puncture sites (Grossman & Porth, 2014).*

Teach individual to report any unusual bleeding (e.g., in the mouth after brushing teeth)

R: *Mucous membranes are prone to injury because of their high surface vascularity.*

Monitor for hepatic encephalopathy by assessing orientation, cognition, speech patterns (Goldberg & Chopra, 2015)

- *Grade I*: Changes in behavior, mild confusion, slurred speech, disordered sleep
- *Grade II*: Lethargy, moderate confusion
- *Grade III*: Marked confusion (stupor), incoherent speech, sleeping but wakes with stimulation
- *Grade IV*: Coma, unresponsive to pain

R: *Profound liver failure results in accumulation of ammonia and other toxic metabolites in the blood. The blood–brain barrier permeability increases, and both toxins and plasma proteins leak from capillaries to the extracellular space, causing cerebral edema (Goldberg & Chopra, 2015).*

Create a quiet environment

- Explain to family the reason
- Post a sign to remind staff, for example, "Maintain a quiet environment"
- Decrease audible stimuli, for example, alarms, loud voices
- Reduce harsh lights

R: *Stimulation can contribute to increased intracranial pressure and should be minimized (Goldberg & Chopra, 2015).*

Monitor for signs and symptoms of (refer to the index under each electrolyte for specific signs and symptoms)

- Hypoglycemia

R: *Hypoglycemia is caused by loss of glycogen stores in the liver from damaged cells and decreased serum concentrations of glucose, insulin, and growth hormones.*

- Hypokalemia

R: *Potassium losses occur from vomiting, NG suctioning, diuretics, or excessive renal losses.*

- Hypophosphatemia

R: *The loss of potassium ions causes the proportional loss of magnesium ions. Increased phosphate loss, transcellular shifts, and decreased phosphate intake contribute to hypophosphatemia.*

- Acid–base disturbances

R: *Hepatocellular necrosis can result in accumulation of organic anions, resulting in metabolic acidosis. People with ascites often have metabolic alkalosis from increased bicarbonate levels resulting from increased sodium/hydrogen exchange in the distal tubule.*

Assess for side effects of medications. Avoid administering narcotics, sedatives, and tranquilizers and exposing the individual to ammonia products

R: *Liver dysfunction results in decreased metabolism of certain medications (e.g., opiates, sedatives, tranquilizers), increasing the risk of toxicity from high drug blood levels. Ammonia products should be avoided because of the individual's already high serum ammonia level.*

Monitor for signs and symptoms of renal failure (refer to Risk for Complications of Renal Failure for more information)

R: *Obstructed hepatic blood flow results in decreased blood flow to the kidneys, impairing glomerular filtration and leading to fluid retention and decreased urinary output.*

Teach individual and family to report signs and symptoms of complications, such as

- Increased abdominal girth

R: *Increased abdominal girth may indicate worsening portal hypertension.*

- Rapid weight loss or gain

R: *Weight loss points to negative nitrogen balance; weight gain points to fluid retention.*

- Bleeding

R: *Unusual bleeding indicates decreased prothrombin time and clotting factors.*

- Tremors

R: *Tremors can result from impaired neurotransmission because of failure of the liver to detoxify enzymes that act as false neurotransmitters.*

- Increasing confusion and/or somnolence

R: *Cognitive impairments will worsen as cerebral hypoxia increases, caused by continuing increases in serum ammonia levels resulting from the liver's impaired ability to convert ammonia to urea.*

Risk for Complications of Hyperbilirubinemia

Definition

(Blackburn, 2013)

Describes a newborn with or at high risk for development of an abnormally high concentration (given the age in hours of the infant) of the bile pigment bilirubin in the blood. Hyperbilirubinemia affects at least 60% of all term newborns and up to 80% of preterm infants. It is usually benign and self-limiting and the majority of infants do not experience any problems.

Severe hyperbilirubinemia occurs when the concentration and rates of bilirubin accumulation have progressed or are progressing to levels where there is risk for neurotoxicity and neurologic sequelae are severe. Although still rare, bilirubin encephalopathy and kernicterus continue to occur with breastfed and late-preterm infants at higher risk.

There is not a specific bilirubin level that can be considered safe or dangerous. Multiple factors, including postnatal age, gestational age, comorbidity, and other factors influence how well each infant can metabolize and excrete the bilirubin he or she produces (Association of Women's Health, Obstetric and Neonatal Nurses [AWHONN], 2006; Blackburn, 2013).

Significant Laboratory/Diagnostic Assessment Criteria

(American Academy of Pediatrics [AAP], 2004)

- Prenatal maternal ABO and Rh(D) typing
- Blood type and Rh(D) and direct antibody test (Coombs) from cord blood when mother is blood type O
- Transcutaneous bilirubin meter (TcB) levels
- Total serum bilirubin (TSB) and direct bilirubin levels
- Indirect bilirubin
- Serum albumin
- Perinatal sepsis workup
  - Urinalysis and cultures
  - Complete blood cell (CBC) count with differential and smear for red cell morphology
  - Reticulocyte count
  - Blood culture
  - Lumbar puncture
- Glucose-6-phospate dehydrogenase (G6PD) deficiency (if suggested by ethnic or geographic origin or if poor response to phototherapy)

High-Risk Populations

(AAP, 2004; AWHONN, 2006; Blackburn, 2013; Smith & Carley, 2014)

Newborn

- Birthweight <1,500 g
- Preterm delivery

- Gestational age 35 to 38 weeks
- Blood group incompatibilities (ABO or Rh)
- Male sex
- Hypothermia
- Hypoxia, acidosis, asphyxia
- Hypoglycemia
- Bruising or extravascular hemolysis (cephalohematoma, intracranial hemorrhage, swallowing blood)
- Hypoalbuminemia
- Sepsis
- Meningitis
- Delayed cord clamping
- Polycythemia (Hct >65%)
- Delayed meconium passage
- Previous sibling with jaundice and phototherapy
- Infant from ethnic group originating from South and Eastern Asia, African coasts, the Mediterranean, parts of the Middle East, and Native Americans
- Congenital red blood cell disorders, for example, G6PD deficiency
- Congenital conditions that can cause hepatic obstruction (biliary atresia, cystic fibrosis)
- Intestinal obstruction
- Congenital hypothyroidism
- Poor feeding
- Exclusive breastfeeding, particularly if nursing is not going well and weight loss is excessive
- Inborn errors of metabolism

Maternal

- Macrosomic infant of a diabetic mother
- Medications that affect albumin binding, for example, bupivacaine, sulfonamides, salicylate, ibuprofen
- Forceps or vacuum delivery
- From ethnic group originating from South and Eastern Asia, African coasts, the Mediterranean, parts of the Middle East, and Native American
- Gestational hypertension
- Family history of newborn jaundice
- Family history of jaundice, liver disease, anemia, or splenectomy

Collaborative Outcomes

The newborn will be monitored for early signs of hyperbilirubinemia, and the newborn will receive collaborative interventions if indicated to restore physiologic stability.

Indicators of Physiologic Stability

TSB level interpreted according to newborn's age in hours using the Hour-Specific Bilirubin Nomogram (AAP, 2004) (Figure III.2)

Interventions and Rationales

(AAP, 2004; AWHONN, 2006; McGrath & Hardy, 2011; Smith & Carley, 2014)

Assess maternal history for

- Blood type and Rh, positive antibody titer (Coombs) test

R: *Mother's blood type can cause intravascular hemolysis via an antigen–antibody reaction. Infants with ABO or Rh incompatibilities may develop severe hyperbilirubinemia within the first 24 hours after birth. Increased hemolysis results from maternal antibodies reacting with fetal and neonatal antigens (AWHONN, 2006; McGrath & Hardy, 2011).*

- Diabetes mellitus

R: *Infants born to women with maternal diabetes are at increased risk, especially if the newborn is macrosomic. The newborn may have an increased RBC mass at birth, which can lead to the breakdown of a*

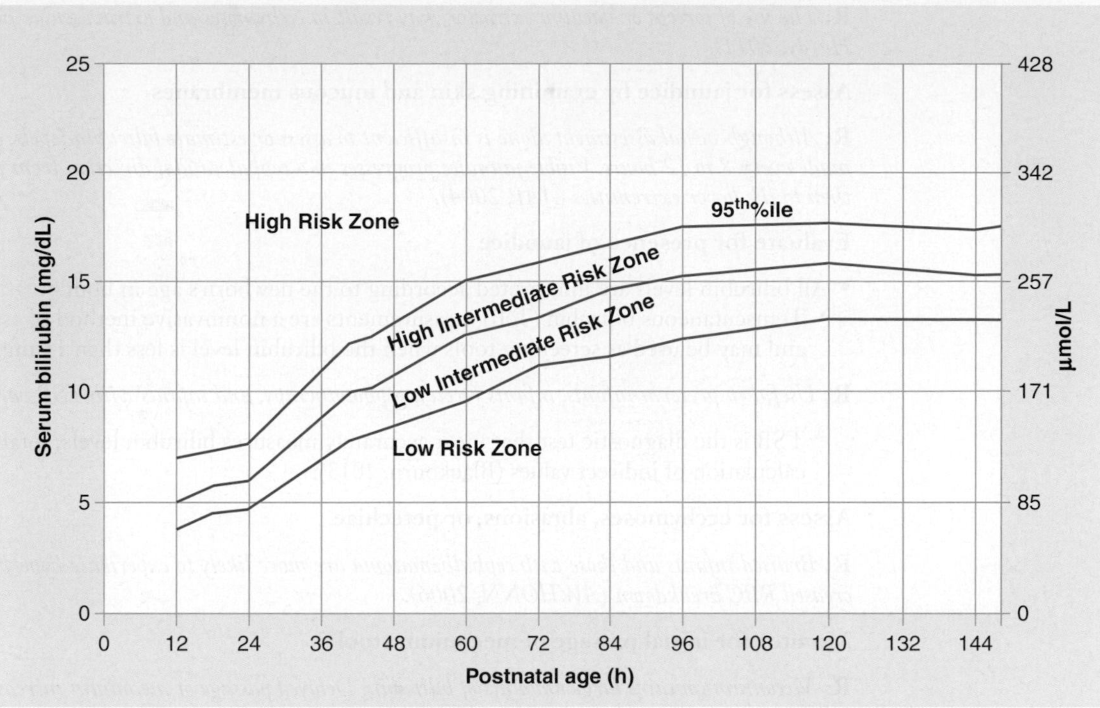

FIGURE III.2 Nomogram for designation of risk of developing hyperbilirubinemia (*Bhutani, Johnson, & Sivievri, 1999).

high number of aged RBCs, resulting in excessive amounts of bilirubin in the newborn (AAP, 2004; McGrath & Hardy, 2011).

- Maternal and paternal ethnicity

R: *Ethnic group originating from South and Eastern Asia, African coasts, the Mediterranean, and parts of the Middle East has higher rates of hyperbilirubinemia (AWHONN, 2006).*

- Maternal drugs used during the last 3 months of pregnancy, that is, sulfonamides, salicylates, ibuprofen

R: *These drugs interfere with the binding of bilirubin to albumin in neonates (McGrath & Hardy, 2011).*

- History of sibling with hyperbilirubinemia

R: *Infants with siblings who had jaundice are at risk, perhaps because those infants share genetic polymorphisms that influence bilirubin metabolism (AWHONN, 2006).*

Assess labor and delivery history for

- Perinatal complications

R: *Infants with perinatal sepsis and asphyxia are more vulnerable to bilirubin toxicity and neuronal susceptibility at lower concentrations of bilirubin (AWHONN, 2006)*

- Gestational age at birth between 35 and 37-6/7 weeks gestation

R: *Near-term/late-preterm newborns are at risk for bilirubin neurotoxicity and severe hyperbilirubinemia (AAP, 2004). Elevated bilirubin levels are primarily due to immature liver function and diminished capacity for bilirubin conjugation (Smith & Carley, 2014).*

- Delayed cord clamping

R: *Allows excessive amount of blood to be transfused from the placenta to the neonate, which increases the quantity of RBCs which can lead to excessive amounts of bilirubin from the breakdown of aged RBCs (McGrath & Hardy, 2011).*

- Use of bupivacaine (synthetic oxytocin) during labor.

R: *Associated with higher incidence of neonatal jaundice (McGrath & Hardy, 2011)*

- Operative delivery

R: *The use of forceps or vacuum extractor may result in ecchymoses and extravascular hemolysis (McGrath & Hardy, 2011).*

Assess for jaundice by examining skin and mucous membranes

R: *Although visual assessment alone is insufficient to assess or estimate bilirubin levels, assessments should be made every 8 to 12 hours. Visible jaundice progresses in a cephalocaudal direction from the face to the trunk and then to the lower extremities (AAP, 2004).*

Evaluate for presence of jaundice

- All bilirubin levels are interpreted according to the newborn's age in hours:
  - Transcutaneous bilirubin (TcB) measurements are a noninvasive method of assessing bilirubin levels and may be used as screening tools when the bilirubin level is less than 15 mg/dL.

R: *Useful in preterm infants, infants receiving phototherapy, and infants with TSB values >15 mg/dL*

- TSB is the diagnostic test that most accurately measures bilirubin levels, total and direct bilirubin and calculation of indirect values (Blackburn, 2013).

Assess for ecchymoses, abrasions, or petechiae

R: *Bruised infants and those with cephalhematoma are more likely to experience hyperbilirubinemia due to increased RBC breakdown (AWHONN, 2006).*

Monitor for initial passage of meconium stool

R: *Meconium contains large amounts of bilirubin. Delayed passage of meconium increases the potential for bilirubin in the small intestine to be deconjugated and be recirculated via enterohepatic circulation (Blackburn, 2013; Smith & Carley, 2014).*

Prevent cold stress

R: *Hypothermia stimulates the release of free fatty acids which compete for albumin-binding sites (McGrath & Hardy, 2011).*

Ensure adequate hydration and caloric intake by supporting adequate breastfeeding and decreasing the likelihood of subsequent signs of significant hyperbilirubinemia

R: *Poor caloric intake and/or dehydration associated with inadequate breastfeeding may contribute to the development of hyperbilirubinemia (AAP, 2004).*

Differentiate physiologic jaundice from pathologic jaundice

- *Physiologic jaundice*: normal process in the first few days after birth due to physiologic adaptation
  - Bilirubin level increase first appears after 24 hours of age in term neonates and after 48 hours of age in preterm neonates.
  - It reaches peak at day 3 or 4 and returns to a normal level by the end of day 7 in term neonates.
  - It reaches peak at day 5 or 6 and returns to a normal level by the end of day 9 or 10 in preterm neonates.
  - Pattern for breastfed infants is slightly different: peak level often occurs on day 4 and the decline may be slower.
- *Pathologic jaundice*: associated with pathologic factors such as Rh or ABO incompatibility. Elevated bilirubin level
  - Appears within the first 24 hours of life
  - Persists beyond the age for return to a normal level in term and preterm neonates
  - No specific serum level can be used for diagnosis (Blackburn, 2013; McGrath & Hardy, 2011).

Monitor for severe hyperbilirubinemia

- Severe hyperbilirubinemia can result in acute bilirubin encephalopathy (ABE). ABE describes the acute clinical characteristics of bilirubin toxicity and includes a broad continuum of neurologic signs ranging from subtle behavioral changes to seizures. ABE may progress to kernicterus (the chronic form of bilirubin encephalopathy) or death.

R: *Severe hyperbilirubinemia and the resultant bilirubin toxicity can induce injury to specific parts of the neonatal brain: the basal ganglia, brainstem nuclei, and parts of the pons, the brainstem, and cerebellum. A spectrum of deficits may appear (AWHONN, 2006).*

- Early signs of ABE include the following:
  - Extreme jaundice

- Alterations in level of consciousness (lethargy)
- Hypotonia, then later hypertonia
- Abnormal movement (opisthotonos, retrocollis)
- Poor feeding
- Shrill, high-pitched cry

- Initiate phototherapy according to protocol/policy, if indicated.

R: *The goal of phototherapy is to decrease the level of unconjugated bilirubin. Phototherapy accomplishes this by*

- Absorption of light by the bilirubin molecule
- Photoconversion of bilirubin by photochemical reaction, restructuring the molecule into an isomer
- Excretion of bilirubin through urine and bile, bypassing the conjugation process (Smith & Carley, 2014)
- The efficacy of phototherapy depends on several factors:
  - Spectrum of light delivered by the phototherapy unit, which is determined by the type of light source and the wavelength range
  - Light intensity
  - Surface area of the infant exposed to phototherapy (AAP, 2011)
- Explain procedure for phototherapy to parents. Reassure parents that no serious long-term side effects have been reported (Smith & Carley, 2014).

Monitor for short-term side effects of phototherapy (Szucs & Rosenman, 2013; AWHONN, 2006)

- Increased insensible water loss through the skin from increased metabolic rate is caused by phototherapy lights, hyperthermia, and increase in water content of stools (McGrath & Hardy, 2011).
- Loose watery stools with potential for loss of nutrients are an unavoidable side effect of phototherapy and can also result in increased insensible water loss and dehydration.

R: *May be related to increased bile flow, which stimulates gastrointestinal activity (Blackburn, 2013).*

- Skin rashes—a generalized macular rash frequently develops and resolves spontaneously when phototherapy is discontinued (Smith & Carley, 2014).

R: *Due to injury of mast cells with release of histamine; erythema from violet light (Blackburn, 2013)*

- Hyperthermia or hypothermia: Hyperthermia increases the newborn's metabolic rate and can result in tachycardia and increased insensible water loss and dehydration (Smith & Carley, 2014). Hypothermia stimulates the release of free fatty acids, which compete for albumin-binding sites (McGrath & Hardy, 2011).
- Decreased maternal–infant interaction due to separation of newborn from its parents
- Lack of visual sensory input from eye patches
- Can cause alteration in state organization and neurobehavioral organization; may interfere with parent–infant interaction and increase parental stress (Blackburn, 2013)
- Thermal injury due to devices used in the environment with high humidity, and oxygen must meet fire hazard safety standards (AAP, 2011).
- Electrical hazards due to devices used in the environment with high humidity, and oxygen must meet electrical safety standards (AAP, 2011).
- The focus of nursing care is to prevent or minimize side effects.

Skin care

- Expose as much skin surface as possible. The newborn is placed naked under the phototherapy light and repositioned at least every 2 hours to ensure adequate light exposure to all areas (Smith & Carley, 2014).
- Meticulous skin care is necessary to prevent skin breakdown resulting from loose stools (Smith & Carley, 2014).
- Lotions, balms, and ointments are avoided because they may increase the risk of burns (AWHONN, 2006).
- Hydration:
  - Intake, output, and urine specific gravity are measured accurately and documented.
  - Usually supplementation with expressed breast milk or formula will improve hydration and urine output, and the increased gastrointestinal motility could inhibit the enterohepatic circulation of bilirubin. Providing supplements of water or dextrose water does not lower bilirubin levels in jaundiced, healthy, breastfeeding infants. Routine supplementation during phototherapy is not indicated (AAP, 2004).

R: *Because bilirubin by-products from phototherapy are excreted in the urine, maintaining adequate hydration and good urine output can improve the efficacy of phototherapy (AWHONN, 2006).*

Eye care

- Protect infant's eyes from potential retinal damage during phototherapy treatment using an opaque mask to prevent exposure to the light. The eye shield should be properly sized and positioned to cover the eyes completely, but prevent any occlusion of the nares. The infant's eyelids are closed before the mask is applied.

R: *Corneal injury can result from eye patches that apply excessive pressure to the eyes or are loose enough to allow eye opening under the patch (Smith & Carley, 2014).*

- Eye patches should be removed during feedings or at least every 4 hours to observe for drainage and to promote social stimulation and visual development (Smith & Carley, 2014).

Thermoregulation

- Maintain thermal homeostasis while newborn is under phototherapy lights by using a servo-control mechanism such as an Isolette or radiant warmer.

R: *Hypothermia stimulates release of free fatty acids, which compete for albumin-binding sites. Hyperthermia increases the newborn's metabolic rate (McGrath & Hardy, 2011).*

- Monitor axillary temperature at least every 2 to 4 hours to assess for hyperthermia and hypothermia (Smith & Carley, 2014).

Maternal–infant separation

- If the mother has been discharged, the parents may require a great deal of emotional support during the temporary separation from their infant. Scheduling the infant's feeding times during parent visits allows the parents more time with their newborn.
- Parents need accurate and useful information about their newborn's condition.
- The breastfeeding mother should receive individualized lactation counseling whenever possible. Education regarding expression and storage of breast milk and information about electric breast pump rental should be offered (AWHONN, 2006).

Monitor clinical improvement or progression of jaundice including signs of early bilirubin encephalopathy

- Changes in sleeping patterns
- Deterioration of feeding pattern
- Inability to be consoled while crying

Provide family support

- Provide parents with written and verbal information about newborn jaundice (Smith & Carley, 2014).
- Prepare parents for home phototherapy if indicated.
- Perform systematic assessment on all newborns before discharge for the risk of severe hyperbilirubinemia (AAP, 2004; Smith & Carley 2014).
- Teach warning signs of neurotoxicity (provide written instructions):
  - Extreme jaundice
  - Alterations in level of consciousness (lethargy)
  - Hypotonia, then later hypertonia
  - Abnormal movement (opisthotonos, retrocollis)
  - Poor feeding
  - Shrill, high-pitched cry

Provide appropriate follow-up based on the time of discharge and risk assessment (Smith & Carley, 2014)

- Follow-up for all newborns within 48 hours after discharge by a physician or trained health-care provider who is experienced in the care of newborns to provide follow-up physical assessment (McGrath & Hardy, 2011)
- Ongoing lactation support to ensure adequacy of intake for breastfed infants (McGrath & Hardy, 2011)
- Arrange for daily home health nurse visits, if indicated.

RISK FOR COMPLICATIONS OF MUSCULAR/SKELETAL DYSFUNCTION

Risk for Complications of Muscular/Skeletal Dysfunction

Risk for Complications of Pathologic Fractures
Risk for Complications of Joint Dislocation

Definition

Describes a person experiencing or at high risk to experience various musculoskeletal problems

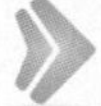

Carp's Cues

The nurse can use this generic collaborative problem to describe people at risk for several types of musculoskeletal problems (e.g., all individuals who have sustained multiple traumas). This collaborative problem focuses nursing management on assessing musculoskeletal status to detect and to diagnose abnormalities.

For an individual exhibiting a specific musculoskeletal problem, the nurse would add the applicable collaborative problem (e.g., *Risk for Complications of Pathologic Fractures)* to the problem list. If the risk factors or etiology were not related directly to the primary medical diagnoses, the nurse would add this information to the diagnostic statement (e.g., *Risk for Complications of Pathologic Fractures related to osteoporosis*).

Because musculoskeletal problems typically affect daily functioning, the nurse must assess the individual's functional patterns for evidence of impairment. Findings may have significant implications—for instance, a casted leg that prevents a woman from assuming her favorite sleeping position and impairs her ability to perform housework. After identifying any such problems, the nurse should use nursing diagnoses to address specific responses of actual or potential altered functioning.

Significant Laboratory/Diagnostic Assessment Criteria

- Laboratory
  - Serum calcium (decreased in osteoporosis)
  - Serum phosphorus (decreased in osteoporosis)
  - Sedimentation rate (increased in inflammatory disorders)
- Diagnostic
  - X-ray
  - Bone scan (uses a radioactive material to evaluate bone tissue, such as fractures, tumors, areas of inflammation (arthritis)
  - Bone density test—Dexa Scan, DXA (measures and calculates the relative density of that bone, primarily to diagnose osteopenia or osteoporosis)
  - Computed tomography (CT) scan (exams bone for bone detail and cortical destruction)
  - Magnetic resonance imaging (MRI)
  - Arthrography (multiple X-rays of a joint using a fluoroscope to examine ligaments, cartilage, tendons, or the joint capsule, e.g., hip, shoulder)
  - Discography (uses injection of contrast medium into one or more spinal discs to determine source of back pain)

Risk for Complications of Pathologic Fractures

Definition

A pathologic fracture occurs when a bone breaks without adequate trauma in an area that is weakened by another disease process. Causes of weakened bone include tumors (metastatic cancer), infection, and certain inherited bone disorders (osteoporosis, Paget's disease)

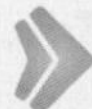

Carp's Cues

Pathologic fractures can be caused by any type of bone tumor, but the overwhelming majority of pathologic fractures in older persons are secondary to metastatic carcinomas. Multiple myeloma is also common in older persons and has a high incidence of pathologic fractures.

High-Risk Populations

- Tumors
  - Primary
  - Benign (fibroxanthoma)
  - Secondary (metastatic) (most common) (e.g., fibrous dysplasia, osteosarcoma, Ewing's, malignant fibrous histiocytoma, fibrosarcoma)
- Metabolic
  - Osteoporosis (most common)
  - Paget's disease
  - Hyperparathyroidism (Brown tumors)
  - Renal failure
- Cushing's syndrome
- Malnutrition
- Long-term corticosteroid therapy
- Osteogenesis imperfecta
- Prolonged immobility
- Radiation osteonecrosis (Ewing's, Lyme's disease)
- Rickets
- Osteomalacia
- Multiple myeloma
- Lymphatic leukemia
- Unicameral bone cyst
- Infection

Collaborative Outcomes

The individual will be monitored for early signs and symptoms of pathologic fractures and will receive collaborative interventions, if indicated, to restore physiologic stability.

Indicators of Physiologic Stability

- No new onset of pain
- No changes in range of motion

General Interventions and Rationales

In individuals with cancer, identify those at high risk for pathologic fractures. Primary site with % of frequency of metastasis to bone (Balach & Peabody, 2011)

- Breast 50 to 85
- Kidneys 30 to 50
- Thyroid 40
- Lung 30 to 50
- Melanoma 30 to 40
- Prostate 50 to 70
- Bladder 12 to 25
- Hodgkin's 50 to 70

R: *The majority of bone metastases originate from cancers of the breast, lung, and prostate, followed by the thyroid and kidney. The most common sites of spread in the skeleton include the spine, pelvis, ribs, skull, upper arm, and leg long bones. These sites correspond to areas of bone marrow that demonstrate high levels of red blood cell production, the cells responsible for carrying oxygen to tissues in the body (Balach & Peabody, 2011; Monczewski, 2013).*

Monitor for signs and symptoms of pathologic fractures

- Hip pain (61% of all pathologic fractures occur in the femur)
- Thoracic or lumbar spine pain that typically presents with sitting or standing.
- Localized pain that is continuous and unrelenting (back, neck, or extremities)
- Visible bone deformity
- Crepitation on movement
- Loss of movement or use
- Localized soft tissue edema
- Skin discoloration/bruising

R: *Detection of pathologic fractures enables prompt intervention to prevent or minimize further complications.*

If a fracture is suspected, maintain proper alignment and immobilize the site using pillows or a splint; notify the physician or advanced practice nurse promptly[8]

R: *Timely, appropriate intervention can prevent or minimize soft tissue damage.*

R: *In individuals with tumors destroying >50% of the diameter of bone or with lesions >2.5 cm, prophylactic internal fixation will be needed because of the increased risk to fracture.*

For postoperative radiation therapy following surgery, individual will be referred to radiation oncology to (O'Donnell, 2012)[9]

- Decrease pain
- Slow progression
- Treat remaining tumor burden not removed at surgery

R: *Radiation alone can provide complete pain relief in 50% of individuals and partial pain relief in 35%.*

In an individual with osteoporosis, teach them the signs and symptoms of vertebral, hip, and wrist fractures, such as

- Pain in the lower back, neck, or wrist
- Localized tenderness
- Pain radiating to abdomen and flank
- Spasm of paravertebral muscles

R: *Progressive osteoporosis more readily affects bones with high amounts of trabecular tissue (e.g., hip, vertebrae, wrist).*

Risk for Complications of Joint Dislocation

Definition

Describes a person experiencing or at high risk to experience displacement of a bone from its position in a joint

High-Risk Populations

- Total hip replacement
- Total knee replacement
- Fractured hip, knee, shoulder

For Infants/Children

- Birth trauma (e.g., breech, firstborn)
- Sports
- Cerebral palsy (hip)

Collaborative Outcomes

The individual will be monitored for early signs and symptoms of pathologic fractures and will receive collaborative interventions, if indicated, to restore physiologic stability.

---

[8] For some individuals with pathological fractures, surgical fixation is indicated.
[9] In individuals with fracture, radiation therapy may be indicated.

Indicators of Physiologic Stability

- Hip in abduction or neutral position
- Aligned affected extremity

Interventions and Rationales

Maintain correct positioning (Martin, Thornhill, & Katz, 2015)

- *Hip*: Maintain the hip in abduction, neutral rotation, or slight external rotation.
- *Hip*: Avoid hip flexion over 60°.
- *Knee*: Slightly elevated from hip; avoid using bed knee Gatch or placing pillows under the knee (to prevent flexion contractures). Place pillows under the calf.

R: *Specific positions are used to prevent prosthesis dislocation.*

Assess for signs of joint (hip, knee) dislocation

- Hip
  - Acute groin pain in operative hip
  - Shortening of leg with external rotation
- Hip, Knee, Shoulder
  - "Popping" sound heard by individual
  - Bulge at surgical site
  - Inability to move
  - Pain with mobility

R: *Until the surrounding muscles and joint capsule heal, joint dislocation may occur if positioning exceeds the limits of the prosthesis, as in flexing or hyperextending the knee or abducting the hip >45°.*

The individual may be turned toward either side unless contraindicated. Always maintain an abduction pillow when turning; limit the use of Fowler's position

R: *If proper positioning is maintained, including the abduction pillow, individuals may safely be turned toward the operative and nonoperative side. This promotes circulation and decreases the potential for pressure ulcer formation as a result of immobility. A prolonged Fowler's position can dislocate the prosthesis.*

Monitor for shoulder joint dislocation/subluxation

R: *Total shoulder arthroplasty has a higher risk of joint dislocation/subluxation because the shoulder is capable of movement in three planes (flexion/extension, abduction/adduction, internal/external rotation).*

Provide instruction regarding precautions needed at home to prevent joint dislocation

Posthip Replacement

- Do not drive until cleared by surgeon at office visit.
- When getting in or out of a car, it is important to keep your leg straight and out to the side.
- Care must be taken to not lean forward when getting into or out of the chair.
- Keep your legs and knees apart, and avoid excessive flexion at the hip joint.
- Use chairs with arms to assist you in getting into and out of the chair.
- An elevated toilet seat will be required for at least 6 weeks after surgery.
- Can shower or sponge bath at home. A shower seat may also be useful.
- When dressing, use the devices provided by the occupational therapist (sock donner, long shoe horn, reacher) for at least 6 weeks. These assistive devices are helpful in dressing and will help you maintain your hip precautions.

Postshoulder Replacement

- Keep sling or immobilizer splint on until instructed otherwise
- Minimize or prevent swelling
- Elevate the arm
- Perform exercises to the other joints of the arm
- Avoid any stressful or sudden movements of the arm
- Do not lift, push, or pull until instructed otherwise (e.g., do not push yourself up in bed or push up from a chair with the new shoulder arm)
- Do not drive until cleared by surgeon at office visit

RISK FOR COMPLICATIONS OF MEDICATION THERAPY ADVERSE EFFECTS[10]

Risk for Complications of Medication Therapy Adverse Effects

Risk for Complications of Anticoagulant Therapy Adverse Effects
Risk for Complications of Antianxiety Therapy Adverse Effects
Risk for Complications of Adrenocorticosteroid Therapy Adverse Effects
Risk for Complications of Antineoplastic Therapy Adverse Effects
Risk for Complications of Anticonvulsant Therapy Adverse Effects
Risk for Complications of Antidepressant Therapy Adverse Effects
Risk for Complications of Antiarrhythmic Therapy Adverse Effects
Risk for Complications of Antipsychotic Therapy Adverse Effects
Risk for Complications of Antihypertensive Therapy Adverse Effects
Risk for Complications of β-Adrenergic Blocker Therapy Adverse Effects
Risk for Complications of Calcium Channel Blocker Therapy Adverse Effects
Risk for Complications of Angiotensin-Converting Enzyme Inhibitor and Angiotensin Receptor Blocker Therapy Adverse Effects
Risk for Complications of Diuretic Therapy Adverse Effects

Definition

Describes a client experiencing or at high risk to experience potentially serious effects or reactions related to medication therapy

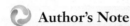

Author's Note

The nurse can use these collaborative problems to describe an individual who has experienced or who is at risk for adverse effects of medication therapy. In contrast to side effects, which are troublesome and annoying but rarely serious, adverse effects are unusual, unexpected, and potentially serious reactions. Adverse drug reactions are drug-induced toxic reactions. Examples of adverse effects include dysrhythmias, gastric ulcers, blood dyscrasias, and anaphylactic reactions; examples of side effects include drowsiness, dry mouth, nausea, and weakness. Side effects usually can be managed by changing the dose, form, route of administration, or diet, or by using preventive measures with continuation of the medication. Adverse effects usually require discontinuation of the medication. A care plan will not contain a collaborative problem for every medication that the individual is taking. Nurses routinely teach individuals about side effects of medications and monitor for side effects as part of the standard of care for every individual. These collaborative problems are indicated for individuals who are at high risk for adverse effects or reactions because of the duration of the therapy, high predictability of their occurrence, the potential seriousness if they occur, and previous history of an adverse response. Students may add these collaborative problems to care plans.

High-Risk Populations

- Prolonged medication therapy
- History of hypersensitivity
- History of adverse reactions
- High single or daily doses
- Changes in daily doses
- Newly prescribed medications
- Multiple medication therapy
- Physical disabilities
- Mental instability
- Hepatic insufficiency

[10] This section is intended as an overview of the nursing accountability for adverse effects of medication therapy. It is not intended to provide the reader with complete information on individual drugs, which can be found in pharmacology texts or manuals.

- Renal insufficiency
- Disease or condition that increases the risk of a specific adverse response (e.g., history of gastric ulcer)

Risk for Complications of Anticoagulant Therapy Adverse Effects

High-Risk Populations for Adverse Effects

- Diabetes mellitus
- Hypothyroidism
- Gastrointestinal (GI) bleeding
- Bleeding tendency, comply with
- Hyperlipidemia
- Elderly women
- Compromised cognitive function
- History of noncompliance (e.g., missed appointments, failure to comply with lab test monitoring)
- Vitamin K deficiency
- Debilitation
- Congestive heart failure
- Children
- Mild hepatic or renal dysfunction
- Tuberculosis
- Pregnancy
- Immediately postpartum

Collaborative Outcomes

The individual will be monitored for early signs and symptoms of adverse effects of anticoagulant therapy and will receive collaborative interventions if indicated to restore physiologic stability

Indicators

Individual/family can report signs and symptoms that need immediate reporting:

- Hypersensitivity
- Dark, tarry colored stools
- Chest pain
- Edema
- Dizziness

Interventions and Rationales

(Arcangelo & Peterson, 2016)

Refer also to a pharmacology text for specific information on the individual drug

Assess for contraindications to anticoagulant therapy

- History of hypersensitivity
- Wounds
- Presence of active bleeding
- Blood dyscrasias
- Anticipated or recent surgery
- GI ulcers
- Subacute bacterial endocarditis
- Pericarditis
- Severe hypertension
- Impaired renal function
- Impaired hepatic function
- Hemorrhagic cerebrovascular accident
- Use of drugs that affect platelet formation (e.g., salicylates, dipyridamole, NSAIDs)
- Presence of drainage tubes
- Eclampsia
- Hemorrhagic tendencies

- Threatened abortion
- Ascorbic acid deficiency
- Spinal puncture
- Regional anesthesia
- Pregnancy (Coumadin)
- Inadequate lab facilities
- Compliance risk
- Spinal puncture

Explain possible adverse effects

- Systemic
  - Hypersensitivity (fever, chills, runny nose, headache, nausea, vomiting, rash, itching, tearing)
  - Bleeding, hemorrhage
    - Fatigue/malaise/lethargy
    - Alopecia
    - Rash
    - Fever
    - Cold intolerance
    - Anemia
- Gastrointestinal
  - Vomiting
  - Diarrhea
  - Dark, tarry colored stools
  - Abdominal cramps
  - Hepatitis
  - Flatulence/bloating
- Cardiovascular
  - Hypertension
  - Chest pain
  - Edema
  - Vasculitis
- Renal
  - Impaired renal function
- Neurologic
  - Dizziness
  - Paresthesias

Monitor for and reduce the severity of adverse effects

- For warfarin (Coumadin) and heparin, monitor laboratory results of activated partial thromboplastin time (APTT) for heparin therapy and prothrombin time (PT) and international normalized ratio (INR) for oral therapy. Report values over target for therapeutic range.

R: *The therapeutic range for APTT on heparin therapy is 1.5 to 2.5 times normal. For dalteparin (Fragmin), enoxaparin (Lovenox) no APTT monitoring is necessary. The therapeutic range for PT is INR of 2.0 to 3.0.*

- For dabigatran (Paradoxa), fondaparinux (Arixtra), apixaban (Eliquis), clopidogrel (Plavix) rivaroxaban (Xarelto), no PT/INR monitoring is needed.
- Monitor for signs of bleeding (e.g., bleeding gums, skin bruises, dark stools, hematuria, epistaxis).
- For an individual recciving heparin therapy, have protamine sulfate available during administration. For warfarin, the antidote is vitamin K.

R: *Protamine sulfate is the antidote to reverse the effects of heparin.*

- Carefully monitor older adult individuals.

R: *They are more sensitive to the effects of anticoagulants.*

- Consult with the pharmacist about medications that can potentiate (e.g., antibiotics, cimetidine, salicylates, phenytoin, acetaminophen, antifungals, NSAIDs, bismuth) or inhibit (e.g., barbiturates, dicloxacillin, carbamazepine, nafcillin, bile acid binding agents, griseofulvins) anticoagulant action.
- Monitor for signs and symptoms of heparin-induced thrombocytopenia (fever, weakness, difficulty speaking, seizures, yellowing of skin/eyes, dark or bloody urine, petechiae).

R: *Antibodies directed against platelet membrane are produced in the presence of heparin, causing increased platelet consumption.*

- Reduce hematomas and bleeding at injection sites.
- Use small-gauge needles.
- Do not massage sites.
- Rotate sites.
- Use subcutaneous route.
- Apply steady pressure for 1 to 2 minutes.

R: *These techniques reduce the trauma to tissues and avoid highly vascular areas (e.g., muscles).*

- Instruct individual to avoid use of razors or to use electric razors.
- Instruct individual to avoid pregnancy while on therapy.

R: *Warfarin is toxic to fetuses.*

Teach individual and family how to prevent or reduce the severity of adverse effects

- Instruct them to monitor for and report signs of bleeding.
- Tell them to inform physicians, dentists, and other health care providers of anticoagulant therapy before invasive procedures.

R: *Precautions may be needed to prevent bleeding.*

- Instruct them to contact physician or advanced practice nurse immediately after the onset of a fever or rash.

R: *These can indicate an infection or allergic response.*

- Tell them that it takes 2 to 10 days for PT levels to return to normal after warfarin (Coumadin) is stopped.
- Explain that certain medications can inhibit or potentiate anticoagulant effect, and advise them to consult with a pharmacist before taking any prescribed or over-the-counter drug (e.g., aspirin, antibiotics, ibuprofen, diuretics).
- Teach persons on Coumadin to avoid or learn how to incorporate foods high in vitamin K if desired; such foods include turnip greens, asparagus, broccoli, watercress, cabbage, beef liver, lettuce, and green tea.

R: *Vitamin K decreases anticoagulant action. If desired, plan to consume foods high in potassium in portions that are consistent daily. Keeping the portion consistent daily will establish their Coumadin dose to maintain an INR within range for effective anticoagulation. Other anticoagulant medications have no dietary restrictions.*

- Teach individual to avoid alcohol, which potentates the effects of the anticoagulant if hepatic disease is also present.
- Instruct individual to wear Medic-Alert identification.
- Stress the importance of regular follow-up care and regular monitoring of blood levels.
- Instruct the individual and family to report the following:
  - Bleeding
  - Dark stools
  - Fever
  - Chills
  - Sore throat, difficulty speaking
  - Itching
  - Dark urine
  - Yellowing of skin or eyes
  - Mouth sores
  - Severe headache
  - New rash
  - Persistent abdominal pain
  - Episode of fainting

Risk for Complications of Antianxiety Therapy Adverse Effects

High-Risk Populations for Adverse Effects

- Children
- Older adults
- Impaired liver or kidney function

- Psychosis
- Depression
- Pregnancy or breast-feeding
- Severe muscle weakness
- Limited pulmonary reserves

Collaborative Outcomes

The individual will be monitored for early signs and symptoms of adverse effects of antianxiety therapy and will receive collaborative interventions if indicated to restore physiologic stability

Indicators

Individual/family can report signs and symptoms that need immediate reporting:

- Dyspnea
- Impaired judgment
- Paradoxical excitement
- Tremors
- Slurred speech
- Confusion

Interventions and Rationales

(Arcangelo & Peterson, 2016)

Refer also to a pharmacology text for specific information on the individual drug

Assess for contraindications to antianxiety therapy

- Hypersensitivity
- Impaired consciousness
- Compromised respiratory function
- Shock
- Porphyria
- History of drug or alcohol (for benzodiazepines) abuse
- Undiagnosed neurologic disorders
- Glaucoma, paralytic ileus, prostatic hypertrophy (for benzodiazepines)
- Pregnancy or breast-feeding
- Alcohol use
- Severe, uncontrolled pain
- Narrow-angle glaucoma
- CNS depression

Explain possible adverse effects

- Systemic
  - Hypersensitivity (pruritus, rash, hypotension)
  - Hair loss
  - Drug dependency
  - Sleep disturbances
  - Drowsiness
  - Dry mouth
  - Blurred vision
  - Altered libido
  - Appetite change
  - Weight change
- Cardiovascular
  - Decreased heart rate, blood pressure
  - Transient tachycardia, bradycardia
  - Edema
- Central nervous system
  - Impaired judgment
  - Paradoxical excitement

- Excessive drowsiness
- Tremors
- Dizziness
- Slurred speech
- Confusion
- Dysphagia
- Headache
- Ataxia
- Amnesia
- Respiratory
- Respiratory depression
- Hematologic
  - Leukopenia
- Ophthalmic
  - Blurred vision
- Genitourinary
  - Urine retention
- Hepatic
  - Jaundice

Monitor for and reduce the severity of adverse effects

- Monitor for history of drug dependency.
- Evaluate the individual's mental status before drug administration. Consult the physician or advanced practice nurse if the individual exhibits confusion or excessive drowsiness.
- Evaluate the individual's risk for injury; see *Risk for Injury* for more information.
- Monitor for signs of overdose (e.g., slurred speech, continued somnolence, respiratory depression, confusion).
- Monitor for signs of tolerance (e.g., increased anxiety, wakefulness).

Teach individual and family how to prevent or reduce the severity of adverse effects

- Instruct individual never to discontinue taking the medication abruptly after long-term use.

R: *Abrupt cessation can cause vomiting, tremors, and convulsions.*

- Teach family or significant others the signs of overdose (e.g., slurred speech, continued somnolence, respiratory depression, confusion).
- Remind individual and family that alcohol and other sedatives potentiate the action of the medication.
- Instruct individual to avoid driving and other hazardous activities when drowsy.
- Discuss the possibility of drug tolerance and dependence with long-term use.

Instruct the individual and family to report the following signs or symptoms

- Slurred speech
- Continued somnolence
- Confusion
- Respiratory insufficiency
- Hostility, rage
- Muscle spasms
- Vivid dreams
- Euphoria
- Hallucinations
- Sore throat
- Fever
- Mouth ulcers

Risk for Complications of Adrenocorticosteroid Therapy Adverse Effects

High-Risk Populations for Adverse Effects

- AIDS
- Thrombophlebitis
- Congestive heart failure
- Diabetes mellitus
- Hypothyroidism
- Glaucoma
- Osteoporosis

- Myasthenia gravis
- Bleeding ulcers
- Seizure disorders or mental illness
- Older adults
- Pregnancy or breast-feeding
- Severe stress, trauma, or illness systemic fungal infection

Collaborative Outcomes

The individual will be monitored for early signs and symptoms of adverse effects of adrenocorticosteroid therapy and will receive collaborative interventions if indicated to restore physiologic stability

Indicators

Individual/family can identify signs and symptoms that need immediate reporting:

- Delayed wound healing
- Hallucinations
- Mood swings
- Psychosis
- Bleeding

Interventions and Rationales

(Arcangelo & Peterson, 2016)

Refer also to a pharmacology text for specific information on the individual drug

Assess for contraindications to steroid therapy

- History of:
  - Hypertension
  - Hypersensitivity
  - Active peptic ulcer disease
  - Active tuberculosis
  - Active fungus infection
  - Herpes
  - Cardiac disease

Explain possible adverse effects

- Systemic
  - Hypersensitivity (rash, hives, hypotension, respiratory distress, anaphylaxis)
  - Increased susceptibility to infection
  - Acute adrenal insufficiency (response to abrupt cessation after 2 weeks of therapy)
  - Hypokalemia
  - Delayed wound healing
  - Hypertriglyceridemia
  - Acne
  - Insomnia
  - Ecchymosis
  - Hyperglycemia
  - Appetite change
- Central nervous system
  - Hallucinations
  - Headaches
  - Mood swings
  - Depression
  - Psychosis
  - Papilledema
  - Anxiety
- Ophthalmic
  - Glaucoma
  - Cataracts

- Cardiovascular
  - Thrombophlebitis
  - Hypertension
  - Embolism
  - Edema
  - Dysrhythmias
- Gastrointestinal
  - Bleeding
  - Pancreatitis (especially children)
  - Ulcers
  - Nausea/vomiting
  - Dyspepsia
- Musculoskeletal
  - Osteoporosis
  - Growth retardation in children
  - Muscle wasting
  - Buffalo hump

Monitor for adverse effects

- Establish baseline assessment data.
  - Weight
  - Serum potassium
  - Complete blood count (CBC)
  - Blood glucose
  - Serum sodium
  - Blood pressure
- Monitor:
  - Weight
  - CBC
  - Blood pressure
  - Serum potassium
  - Blood glucose
  - Serum sodium
  - Stool for guaiac
- Report changes in monitored data.

Teach the individual and family how to prevent or reduce the severity of adverse effects

- Instruct to take the medication with food or milk.

R: *This reduces gastric distress.*

- Advise to weigh self daily at the same time and wearing the same clothes each time.

R: *Weight gain may indicate fluid retention.*

- Instruct to avoid people with infections.

R: *The individual's compromised immune system increases his or her vulnerability to infection.*

- Advise to consult with a physician, advanced practice nurse, or pharmacist before taking any over-the-counter drugs.

R: *Serious drug interactions can occur.*

- Instruct to inform physicians, advanced practice nurse, dentists, and other health care providers of therapy before any invasive procedure.

R: *Precautions should be taken to prevent bleeding.*

- Instruct to contact the physician or advanced practice nurse if signs of infection occur.
- Teach to take medication in the morning.

R: *This can help reduce adrenal suppression and decrease insomnia.*

- Instruct to wear Medic-Alert identification.

R: *He or she may need more medication in an emergency.*

- Warn never to discontinue the medication without consulting the physician or advanced practice nurse about side effects.

R: *The medication needs to be weaned because adrenal function needs a gradual return time.*

- Limit sodium intake to 6 g/day.

R: *Excess sodium will increase fluid retention.*

- Discuss the possible problems of weight gain and sodium retention (Refer to *Imbalanced Nutrition: More Than Body Requirements* and *Excess Fluid Volume* for more information).
- Explain possible drug-induced appearance changes (e.g., moon face, hirsutism, abnormal fat distribution).
- Explain the possible effects on mood and emotions (e.g., euphoria, mood swings, hyperactivity)
- Encourage individual to establish a system to prevent dosage omission or double dosage (e.g., check sheet, prefilled daily dose containers, or place with toothbrush).
- Explain the risk for hyperglycemia.

R: *Steroids interfere with glucose metabolism.*

Instruct the individual and family to report the following signs and symptoms

- Gastric pain
- Darkened stool color
- Unusual weight gain
- Vomiting
- Sore throat, fever
- Adrenal insufficiency (fatigue, anorexia, palpitations, nausea, vomiting, diarrhea, weight loss, mood swings)
- Menstrual irregularities
- Change in vision, eye pain
- Persistent, severe headache
- Leg pain, cramps
- Excessive thirst, hunger, urination
- Diarrhea
- Change in mental status
- Dizziness
- Palpitations
- Fatigue, weakness

Risk for Complications of Antineoplastic Therapy Adverse Effects

High-Risk Populations for Adverse Effects

- Debilitation
- Bone marrow depression
- Malignant infiltration of kidney
- Malignant infiltration of bone marrow
- Liver dysfunction
- Renal insufficiency
- Older adult
- Children

Collaborative Outcomes

The individual will be monitored for early signs and symptoms of adverse effects of antineoplastic therapy and will receive collaborative interventions if indicated to restore physiologic stability

Indicators

Individual/family can identify signs and symptoms that need immediate reporting:

- Rash
- Fever
- Confusion

- Headaches
- Pain/swelling at IV site
- Weakness
- Dizziness
- Bleeding

Interventions and Rationales
(Arcangelo & Peterson, 2016)

Refer also to a pharmacology text for specific information on the individual drug

Assess for contraindications to antineoplastic therapy

- Hypersensitivity to the drug
- Radiation therapy within the previous 4 weeks
- Severe bone marrow depression
- Breast-feeding
- First trimester of pregnancy

Explain possible adverse effects

- Systemic
  - Hypersensitivity (pruritus, rash, chills, fever, difficulty breathing, anaphylaxis)
  - Immunosuppression
  - Alopecia
  - Fever
  - Rash
  - Infection
  - Thrombocytopenia
  - SIADH
- Cardiovascular
  - Congestive heart failure
  - Dysrhythmias
- Respiratory
  - Pulmonary fibrosis
- Central nervous system
  - Confusion
  - Headaches
  - Weakness
  - Depression
  - Dizziness
  - Neurotoxicity
- Hematologic
  - Leukopenia
  - Bleeding
  - Thrombocytopenia
  - Agranulocytosis
  - Anemia
  - Hyperuricemia
  - Electrolyte imbalances
- Gastrointestinal
  - Diarrhea
  - Anorexia
  - Vomiting
  - Mucositis
  - Enteritis
  - Intestinal ulcers
  - Paralytic ulcer
- Hepatic
  - Hepatotoxicity
- Genitourinary/Reproductive
  - Renal failure

- Amenorrhea
- Sterility
- Decreased sperm count
- Hemorrhagic cystitis
- Renal calculi

Take steps to reduce extravasation of vesicant medications (agents that cause severe necrosis if they leak from blood vessels into tissue)

- Refer to *Risk for Vascular Trauma related to Infusion of Vesicant Medications* for specific interventions.

Monitor for and reduce the severity of adverse effects

- Document a baseline assessment of vital signs, cardiac rhythm, and weight. Monitor daily.

R: *This facilitates subsequent assessments for adverse reactions.*

- Ensure that baseline electrolyte, blood chemistry, bone marrow, and renal and hepatic function studies are done before administering the first dose.

R: *This enables monitoring for adverse reactions.*

- Ensure adequate hydration, at least 2 L/day.

R: *Good hydration can help prevent kidney damage from rapid destruction of cells.*

- Monitor for early signs of infection.

R: *Bone marrow suppression increases the risk of infection.*

- Monitor for sodium, potassium, magnesium, phosphate, and calcium imbalances.

R: *Electrolyte imbalances are commonly precipitated by renal injury, vomiting, and diarrhea.*

- Monitor for renal insufficiency: insufficient urine output, elevated specific gravity, elevated urine sodium levels.

R: *Certain antineoplastics have toxic effects on renal glomeruli and tubules.*

- Monitor for renal calculi: flank pain, nausea, vomiting, abdominal pain; refer to *Risk for Complications of Renal Calculi* if it occurs.

R: *Rapid lysis of tumor cells can produce hyperuricemia.*

- Monitor for neurotoxicity: paresthesias, gait disturbance, disorientation, confusion, foot drop or wrist drop, fine motor activity disturbances.

R: *Some antineoplastics impair neural conduction.*

Teach the individual and family how to prevent or reduce the severity of adverse effects

- Stress the importance of follow-up assessments and laboratory tests.

R: *This can help detect adverse effects early.*

- Instruct to avoid crowds and people with infectious diseases.

R: *An individual receiving antineoplastic therapy is very susceptible to infectious diseases.*

- Teach to monitor weight and intake and output daily.

R: *Regular monitoring can detect adverse effects early.*

- Instruct to consult with primary health care provider before taking any over-the-counter drugs.

R: *Serious drug interactions can occur.*

- Advise to avoid live vaccines. (e.g., varicella, flu mist, etc.)

R: *A compromised immune system increases the risk for onset of disease.*

- Refer to appropriate nursing diagnoses for selected responses (e.g., *Imbalanced Nutrition, Impaired Oral Mucous Membranes).*

Instruct the individual and family to report the following signs and symptoms

- Fever (>100° F)
- Chills, sweating
- Diarrhea
- Severe cough
- Sore throat
- Unusual bleeding
- Burning on urination
- Muscle cramps
- Flulike symptoms
- Pain, swelling at IV site
- Abdominal pain
- Confusion, dizziness
- Decreased urine output

Risk for Complications of Anticonvulsant Therapy Adverse Effects

High-Risk Populations for Adverse Effects

- Hepatic insufficiency
- Renal insufficiency
- Coagulation problems
- Hyperthyroidism
- Diabetes mellitus
- Older adults
- Cognitive impairments
- Debilitation
- Cardiac dysfunction
- Glaucoma
- Myocardial insufficiency
- MAOI use within 14 days

Collaborative Problems

The individual will be monitored for early signs and symptoms of adverse effects of anticonvulsant therapy and will receive collaborative interventions if indicated to restore physiologic stability

Indicators

Individual/family can identify signs and symptoms that need immediate reporting:

- Suicidality
- Depression
- Personality changes
- Tremors
- Ataxia
- Cognitive impairment
- Seizures
- Urine retention

Interventions and Rationales

(Arcangelo & Peterson, 2016)

Refer also to a pharmacology text for specific information on the individual drug

Assess for contraindications to anticonvulsant therapy

- Hypersensitivity
- Bone marrow depression
- Heart block, sinus bradycardia (Dilantin)

- Pregnancy
- Hepatic insufficiency (Depakote)
- Blood dyscrasias
- Respiratory obstruction

Explain possible adverse effects

- Systemic
  - Hypersensitivity
  - Lupus-like reactions (excessive side effects, rashes)
  - Folate deficiency
  - SIADH
  - Hyponatremia
  - Fatigue/weakness
  - Suicidality
- Central nervous system
  - Depression
  - Personality changes
  - Irritability
  - Tremors
  - Ataxia
  - Cognitive impairment
  - Blurred vision
  - Nystagmus
  - Dizziness
  - Withdrawal seizures
- Cardiovascular
  - A-V block
- Hematologic
  - Leukopenia
  - Anemias
  - Thrombocytopenia
  - Agranulocytosis
  - Bone marrow suppression
- Gastrointestinal
  - Gingival hyperplasia (with hydantoin)
  - Pancreatitis
- Hepatic
  - Hepatitis
  - Elevated liver enzymes
- Genitourinary
  - Albuminuria
  - Impotence
  - Urine retention
  - Renal calculi

Monitor for and reduce the severity of adverse effects

- Document baseline information on seizures: type, frequency, usual time, presence of aura, precipitating factors.
- Administer medication at regular intervals.

R: *Regular administration helps prevent fluctuating serum drug levels.*

- Keep a flow record of serum drug levels; report levels outside the therapeutic range.

R: *Seizures can occur with lower levels; higher levels can cause toxicity.*

- Monitor hepatic and blood count studies.

R: *These studies can detect blood dyscrasias and hepatic dysfunction.*

- Monitor for sore throat, persistent fatigue, fever, and infections.

R: *These signs and symptoms can indicate blood dyscrasias.*

- Take vital signs before and after parenteral drug administration.

R: *Vital signs demonstrate the drug's effect on cardiac function.*

- When administering the drug IV, monitor vital signs closely and give the drug slowly.

R: *Close monitoring can enable early detection of bradycardia, hypotension, and respiratory depression.*

Teach the individual and family how to prevent or reduce the severity of adverse effects

- Stress not to alter the dosage or abruptly discontinue the medication.

R: *Changing the regimen can precipitate severe seizures.*

- Emphasize the importance of taking the medication on time, around-the-clock if needed.

R: *Regular administration helps maintain therapeutic drug levels.*

- Instruct to consult with a pharmacist before taking any medications (e.g., aspirin, oral contraceptives, folic acid).

R: *Certain medications reduce the effects of anticonvulsants.*

- Stress the importance of maintaining a proper diet; encourage to consult with a physician or advanced practice nurse to determine the need for supplements.

R: *Some anticonvulsants interfere with vitamin and mineral absorption.*

- Advise the need for regular dental examinations.

R: *Long-term phenytoin (Dilantin) therapy can cause gingival hyperplasia*

- Avoid azoles, MAO inhibitors, protease inhibitors, acetaminophen, *Ginkgo biloba*, and macrolide antibiotics while on medication.
- Medications that can decrease the effect of the medications include cimetidine, warfarin, and tramadol. Grapefruit can interfere with absorption of the medication.

Instruct the individual and family to report the following signs and symptoms

- Systemic
  - Hypersensitivity
  - Suicidality
  - Depression
  - Personality changes
  - Irritability
  - Tremors
  - Ataxia
  - Cognitive impairment
  - Blurred vision
  - Dizziness
  - Urine retention
    - Gingival hyperplasia
    - Abdominal pain
    - Yellowing of sclera
    - Kidney stones

Risk for Complications of Antidepressant Therapy Adverse Effects

High-Risk Populations for Adverse Effects

- Increased ocular pressure
- Impaired renal function
- Impaired hepatic function
- Urine retention
- Diabetes mellitus
- Seizure disorder

- Hyperthyroidism
- Parkinson's disease
- Pregnancy or breast-feeding
- Electroconvulsive therapy
- Cardiovascular disease
- Schizophrenia, psychosis
- Older adults
- Individuals younger than 25 years
- Diuretic users

Collaborative Outcomes

The individual will be monitored for early signs and symptoms of adverse effects of antidepressant therapy and will receive collaborative interventions if indicated to restore physiologic stability

Indicators

Individual/family can identify signs and symptoms that need immediate reporting:

- Suicidal ideation
- Delusions
- Seizures
- Extrapyramidal symptoms
- Confusion
- Mania
- Hallucinations
- Tachycardia

Interventions and Rationales

(Arcangelo & Peterson, 2016)

Refer also to a pharmacology text for specific information on the individual drug

Assess for contraindications to antidepressant therapy

- Hypersensitivity
- Narrow-angle glaucoma
- Acute recovery phase after myocardial infarction
- Severe renal impairment
- Severe hepatic impairment
- Prostatic hypertrophy
- Cerebrovascular disease
- Cardiovascular disease
- Schizophrenia (for monoamine oxidase [MAO] inhibitors)
- Anesthesia administration within the past 1 to 2 weeks (for MAO inhibitors)
- Hypertension (for MAO inhibitors)
- Concomitant use of MAO inhibitors and tricyclics
- Seizure disorder (for tricyclics)
- Ingestion of foods containing tyramine (for MAO inhibitors)
- Concomitant use of MAO inhibitors, sympathomimetics, narcotics, sedatives, hypnotics, barbiturates, phenothiazines, alcohol, street drugs, and antihypertensives

Explain possible adverse effects

- Systemic
  - Hypersensitivity (rash, petechiae, urticaria, photosensitivity)
  - Diaphoresis
  - Hyponatremia
  - Suicidal ideation
  - Dry mouth
  - Sweating
  - Anorexia
  - Weight gain

- Central nervous system
  - Nightmares
  - Tremors
  - Ataxia
  - Delusions
  - Seizures
  - Agitation
  - Paresthesias
  - Hypomania
  - Extrapyramidal symptoms
  - Confusion
  - Mania
  - Hallucinations
- Cardiovascular
  - Orthostatic hypotension (MAO inhibitors)
  - Tachycardia
  - Hypertension crisis (MAO inhibitors)
  - Dysrhythmias (MAO inhibitors)
- Hematologic
  - Blood dyscrasias
  - Bone marrow suppression
- Gastrointestinal
  - Paralytic ileus
  - Vomiting
  - Diarrhea/constipation
- Hepatic
  - Hepatotoxicity
- Genitourinary
  - Urine retention
  - Impotence
  - Prostatic hypertrophy
  - Nocturia
  - Acute renal failure
  - Priapism (MAO inhibitors)
  - Ejaculatory dysfunction
- Endocrine
  - Altered blood glucose levels
  - SIADH

Monitor for and reduce the severity of adverse effects

- Consult with a pharmacist regarding potential interactions with the individual's other medications.

R: *MAO inhibitors cause many adverse interactions.*

- Document baseline pulse, cardiac rhythm, and blood pressure.

R: *Antidepressants can seriously affect cardiac function; baseline assessment enables accurate monitoring during drug therapy.*

- Ensure that baseline blood, renal, and hepatic function studies are done.

R: *Baseline values allow monitoring for changes.*

- Record signs and symptoms of depression before initiating therapy.

R: *This information facilitates evaluation of the individual's response to therapy.*

- Monitor weight and intake and output, and assess for edema.

R: *Some antidepressants can cause fluid retention and anorexia.*

Teach the individual and family how to prevent or reduce the severity of adverse effects

- Stress that alcohol potentiates medication effects.

- Instruct the individual to consult a pharmacist before taking any over-the-counter drugs.

R: *Many medications interact with antidepressants.*

- Warn the individual not to adjust dosage or discontinue medication without consulting a physician, nurse practitioner, or nurse. Abrupt discontinuation of some antidepressant medications can cause seizures.
- For an individual taking an MAO inhibitor, stress the importance of avoiding certain foods containing tyramine, such as avocados, bananas, fava beans, raisins, figs, aged cheeses, sour cream, red wines, sherry, beer, yeast, yogurt, pickled herring, chicken liver, aged meats, fermented sausages, chocolate, caffeine, soy sauce, licorice.

R: *These foods have a pressor effect, which may cause a hypertensive reaction.*

- Instruct the individual to continue to avoid hazardous foods and medications for several weeks after the medication is discontinued

R: *MAO enzyme regeneration takes several weeks.*

- Advise family members to watch for and report signs of increased depression, hypomania, or exaggerated symptoms in the individual.
- Explain that MAO inhibitors must be discontinued 1 week before anesthesia administration.

R: *MAO inhibitors can have serious interactions with anesthetics and narcotics.*

- For diaphoresis-related electrolyte depletion associated with selective serotonin reuptake inhibitors, instruct to:
  - Avoid caffeine.
  - Avoid activity in hot weather.
  - When at risk for dehydration, drink enough fluids to keep urine color pale (colorless) unless contraindicated.

Instruct the individual to report the following signs and symptoms

- Hypertensive reaction (headache, neck stiffness, palpitations, sweating, nausea, photophobia)
- Visual disturbances
- Yellowed skin or eyes
- Rash
- Abdominal pain
- Pruritus
- Urinary problems
- Seizures
- Changes in mental status (e.g., increased depression, thoughts of suicide)

Risk for Complications of Antiarrhythmic Therapy Adverse Effects

High-Risk Populations for Adverse Effects

- Hypertension
- Diabetes mellitus
- Children
- Older adults
- Impaired hepatic function
- Impaired renal function
- Cardiomegaly
- Pulmonary pathology
- Thyrotoxicosis
- Peripheral vascular disease
- Atrioventricular conduction abnormalities
- Congestive heart failure
- Hypotension
- Digitalis intoxication
- Potassium imbalance

Collaborative Problems

The individual will be monitored for early signs and symptoms of adverse effects of antiarrhythmic therapy and will receive collaborative interventions if indicated to restore physiologic stability

Indicators

Individual/family can identify signs and symptoms that need immediate reporting:

- Palpitations
- Dizziness
- Apprehension

Interventions and Rationales

(Arcangelo & Peterson, 2016)

Refer also to a pharmacology text for specific information on the individual drug

Assess for contraindications to antiarrhythmic therapy

- Hypersensitivity
- Ventricular fibrillation (digoxin)
- Thrombocytopenia purpura
- Myasthenia gravis
- Cardiac, renal, or hepatic failure
- Heart block (diltiazem, metoprolol, propranolol)
- Ventricular tachycardia (digoxin)

Explain possible adverse effects

- Systemic
  - Hypersensitivity (rash, difficulty breathing, heightened side effects)
  - Lupus-like reaction
- Cardiovascular
  - Worsening or new dysrhythmia
  - Hypotension
  - Cardiotoxicity (widened QRS complex >25%, ventricular extrasystoles, absent P waves)
- Central nervous system
  - Dizziness
  - Apprehension
- Hematologic
  - Agranulocytosis

Monitor for and reduce the severity of adverse effects

- Establish a baseline assessment of blood pressure, heart rate, respiratory rate, peripheral pulses, lung sounds, and intake and output.

R: *Baseline assessment facilitates evaluation for adverse reactions to drug therapy.*

- Report any electrolyte imbalance, acid–base imbalance, or oxygenation problems.

R: *Dysrhythmias are aggravated by these conditions.*

- Withhold the dose and consult the physician or advanced practice nurse if the individual experiences a significant drop in blood pressure, bradycardia, worsening dysrhythmia, or a new dysrhythmia after receiving the medication.

R: *These signs may indicate an adverse reaction.*

- During parenteral administration, have emergency drugs (e.g., vasopressors, cardiac glycosides, diuretics) available and resuscitation equipment on hand; use microdrip infusion equipment to ensure close regulation of IV flow rate.

Teach the individual and family how to prevent or reduce the severity of adverse effects

- Stress the importance of ongoing follow-up with the primary health care provider and/or cardiologist.
- Emphasize the need to take the medication on time and to avoid "doubling up" on doses.

R: *A regular schedule prevents toxic blood levels.*

- Instruct to take the medication with food.

R: *This can help minimize GI distress.*

- Teach to monitor pulse and blood pressure daily.

R: *Careful monitoring can detect early signs of adverse effects.*

- Advise to consult a pharmacist before taking any over-the-counter drugs.

R: *Possible drug interactions may alter cardiac stability.*

Instruct the individual and family to report the following signs and symptoms

- Dizziness, faintness
- Palpitations
- Visual disturbances
- Hallucinations
- Confusion
- Headache
- 1- to 2-lb weight gain
- Coldness and numbness in extremities

Risk for Complications of Antipsychotic Therapy Adverse Effects

High-Risk Populations for Adverse Effects

- Glaucoma
- Prostatic hypertrophy
- Elderly
- Dementia
- Epilepsy
- Diabetes mellitus
- Severe hypertension
- Ulcers
- Cardiovascular disease
- Chronic respiratory disorders
- Hepatic insufficiency
- Pregnancy or breast-feeding
- Exposure to extreme heat, phosphorus insecticides, or pesticides

Collaborative Problems

The individual will be monitored for early signs and symptoms of adverse effects of antipsychotic therapy and will receive collaborative interventions if indicated to restore physiologic stability

Indicators

Individual/family can identify signs and symptoms that need immediate reporting:

- Changes in mental status
- Palpitations
- Orthostatic hypotension
- Dystonia
- Dyspnea

Interventions and Rationales

(Arcangelo & Peterson, 2016)

Refer also to a pharmacology text for specific information on the individual drug

Assess for contraindications to antipsychotic therapy

- Bone marrow suppression
- Blood dyscrasias
- Parkinson's disease
- Hepatic insufficiency
- Renal insufficiency
- Cerebral arteriosclerosis
- Coronary artery disease
- Circulatory collapse
- Mitral insufficiency
- Severe hypotension
- Alcoholism, drug abuse
- Subcortical brain damage
- Comatose states

Explain possible adverse effects

- Systemic
  - Hypersensitivity (rash, abdominal pain, jaundice, blood dyscrasias)
  - Photosensitivity
  - Fever
  - Weight change
- Cardiovascular
  - Hypertension
  - Orthostatic hypotension
  - Palpitations
  - QT prolongation
- Central nervous system
  - Extrapyramidal (acute dystonia, akathisia, pseudoparkinsonism)
  - Hyperreflexia
  - Tardive dyskinesia
  - Cerebral edema
  - Neuroleptic malignant syndrome
  - Sleep disturbances
  - Bizarre dreams
  - Anxiety
  - Drowsiness
- Gastrointestinal
  - Constipation
  - Paralytic ileus
  - Fecal impaction
- Hematologic
  - Agranulocytosis
  - Thrombocytopenia
  - Leukopenia
  - Purpura
  - Leukocytosis
  - Pancytopenia
  - Anemias
- Ophthalmic
  - Ptosis
  - Lens opacities
  - Pigmentary retinopathy
- Respiratory
  - Laryngospasm
  - Dyspnea
  - Bronchospasm

- Genitourinary
  - Urine retention
  - Incontinence
  - Enuresis
  - Impotence
- Endocrine
  - Gynecomastia
  - Glycosuria
  - Altered libido
  - Hyperglycemia
  - Amenorrhea
  - Galactorrhea

Monitor for and reduce the severity of adverse effects

- Document a baseline assessment of blood pressure (sitting, standing, and lying), pulse, and temperature.

R: *Baseline assessment facilitates monitoring for adverse reactions.*

- Ensure that baseline bone marrow, renal, and hepatic function studies are done before administering the first dose.

R: *Results of these studies enable monitoring for changes.*

- After parenteral administration, keep the individual flat and monitor blood pressure.

R: *These measures help reduce hypotensive effects.*

- Monitor blood pressure during initial treatment.

R: *Blood pressure monitoring detects early hypotensive effects. Assess bowel and bladder functioning.*

R: *Anticholinergic and antiadrenergic effects decrease sensory stimulation to the bowel and bladder.*

- Observe for fine, worm-like movements of the tongue.

R: *Early detection of tardive dyskinesia enables prompt intervention and possible reversal of its course.*

- Monitor for acute dystonic reactions, neck spasms, eye rolling, dysphagia, convulsions.

R: *Early detection of these signs may indicate the need for dose reduction.*

- Ensure optimal hydration; evaluate urine specific gravity regularly.

R: *Dehydration increases susceptibility to dystonic reactions.*

- Monitor for signs and symptoms of blood dyscrasias: decreased white cells, platelets, and red cells; sore throat; fever; malaise.

R: *Antipsychotic medication can cause bone marrow suppression. Monitor weight.*

R: *Antipsychotic medication can cause hypothyroidism, commonly marked by weight gain. Monitor for neuroleptic malignant syndrome; refer to Risk for Complications of Neuroleptic Malignant Syndrome for interventions.*

R: *Neuroleptic malignant syndrome is a potentially dangerous adverse effect of antipsychotic drug therapy.*

Teach the individual and family how to prevent or reduce the severity of adverse effects

- Instruct to consult a pharmacist before taking any over-the-counter drugs.

R: *Serious drug interactions can occur with various over-the-counter medications.*

- Stress the need to continue the medication regimen as prescribed and never abruptly stop taking it.

R: *Abrupt cessation can cause vomiting, tremors, and psychotic behavior.*

- Caution the individual to protect himself from sun exposure with clothing, hat, sunglasses, and sunscreen.

R: *Photosensitivity is a common side effect of antipsychotic therapy.*

- Warn against using alcohol, barbiturates, or sedatives.

R: *Their effects are potentiated in combination with antipsychotic medication.*

Instruct the individual and family to report the following signs and symptoms

- Urine retention
- Changes in mental status
- Fine, worm-like tongue movements
- Visual disturbances
- Neck spasms
- Fever
- Dysphagia
- Sore throat
- Eye rolling
- Signs of infection
- Involuntary chewing, puckering
- Tremors
- Puffing movements
- Abdominal pain

Risk for Complications of Antihypertensive Therapy Adverse Effects

- β-Adrenergic Blocker therapy adverse effects
- Calcium channel blocker therapy adverse effects
- Angiotensin-converting enzyme inhibitor and angiotensin receptor blocker therapy adverse effects
- Diuretic therapy adverse effects

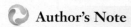

Author's Note

Antihypertensive medications are classified into nine groups: central adrenergic agents, ganglionic blockers, peripherally acting catecholamine depleters, calcium channel blockers, β-adrenergic blockers, vascular smooth muscle relaxants, angiotensin-converting enzymes, and diuretics. Because their sites of action differ greatly, it is not useful to present a generic collaborative problem of *Risk for Complications of Antihypertensive Therapy Adverse Effects*. Instead, three classifications are addressed: β-adrenergic blockers, calcium channel blockers, and angiotensin-converting enzymes. For information on other classifications, consult a pharmacology text.

Risk for Complications of β-Adrenergic Blocker Therapy Adverse Effects

High-Risk Populations for Adverse Effects

- Diabetes mellitus
- Severe liver disease
- Pregnancy or breast-feeding
- Chronic bronchitis, emphysema
  - Asthma/bronchospasm
  - Bradycardia
  - Second- or third-degree heart failure pheochromocytoma
- Peripheral vascular insufficiency
- Allergic rhinitis
- Renal insufficiency
- Hepatic insufficiency
- Myasthenia gravis

Collaborative Outcomes

The individual will be monitored for early signs and symptoms of adverse effects of β-adrenergic blocker therapy and will receive collaborative interventions if indicated to restore physiologic stability

Indicators

Individual/family can identify signs and symptoms that need immediate reporting:

- Difficulty breathing
- Dark urine
- Difficult urination
- Mental changes
- Behavioral changes

Interventions and Rationales

(Arcangelo & Peterson, 2016)

Refer also to a pharmacology text for specific information on the individual drug

Assess for contraindications to β-adrenergic blockers

- Hypersensitivity
- Sinus bradycardia
- Second- or third-degree heart block
- PR interval greater than 0.24 seconds on electrocardiogram (ECG)
- Heart (except carvedilol, metoprolol)
- Cardiogenic shock
- MAO inhibitor or tricyclic antidepressant therapy
- Asthma (for nonselective β-adrenergic blockers)
- Diabetes
- Hyperlipidemia
- Peripheral
- Arterial insufficiency
- Pregnancy—first trimester

Explain possible adverse effects

- Systemic
  - Hypersensitivity (rash, pruritus)
  - Increased triglycerides
  - Decreased high-density lipoproteins (HDL)
  - Feeling of cold
  - Lethargy
  - Leg pain
- Central nervous system
  - Depression
  - Memory loss
  - Paresthesias
  - Bizarre dreams
  - Insomnia
  - Hallucinations
  - Behavior changes
  - Catatonia
  - Vertigo
- Cardiovascular
  - Bradycardia
  - Cerebrovascular accident
  - Edema
  - Tachycardia
  - Hypotension
  - Peripheral arterial insufficiency
  - Arrhythmia
  - Congestive heart failure
  - Raynaud's phenomenon
- Hematologic
  - Agranulocytosis
  - Thrombocytopenia
  - Eosinophilia

- Gastrointestinal
  - Diarrhea
  - Vomiting
  - Ischemic colitis
  - Gastric pain
- Hepatic
  - Hepatomegaly
- Respiratory
  - Bronchospasm
  - Dyspnea
  - Rales
- Endocrine
  - Hypoglycemia or hyperglycemia
- Genitourinary
  - Difficulty urinating
  - Elevated blood urea nitrogen and serum transaminase
- Ophthalmic
  - Blurred vision

Monitor for and reduce the severity of adverse effects

- Establish a baseline assessment of pulse, blood pressure (lying, sitting, standing), lung fields, and peripheral pulses.

R: *Baseline assessment facilitates monitoring for adverse reactions.*

- Ensure that baseline renal, hepatic, glucose, and blood studies are done before drug therapy begins.

R: *Results of these studies enable monitoring for changes.*

- Establish with the provider the parameters (blood pressure, pulse) that call for withholding the medication.

R: *Hypotension and bradycardia can reduce cardiac output.*

- Monitor intake, output, and weight and assess for edema.

R: *Reduced cardiac output can cause fluid accumulation*

- Monitor for congestive heart failure.

R: *β-Adrenergic blockers can compromise cardiac function.*

- Monitor for hypoglycemia in an individual with diabetes.

R: *β-Adrenergic blockers interfere with the conversion of glycogen to glucose by occupying β-adrenergic receptor sites.*

Teach the individual how to prevent or reduce the severity of adverse effects

- Stress the importance of continuing the medication regimen as prescribed, and warn individual never to discontinue the drug abruptly.

R: *Abrupt cessation may precipitate dysrhythmias or angina.*

- Emphasize the need to monitor pulse and blood pressure daily. Explain the pulse and blood pressure values that indicate the need to withhold the medication.
- Instruct to weigh self daily, at the same time each day and wearing the same clothes every time; tell individual to report any weight gain of 1 lb or more.

R: *Weight gain may indicate fluid retention resulting from decreased cardiac output.*

- Instruct to taper slowly because abrupt withdrawal in someone with CAD can cause exacerbation of angina, MI, or arrhythmia.
- Explain the need to protect hands and feet from prolonged exposure to cold.

R: *β-Adrenergic blockers decrease circulation in the skin and extremities.*

- Instruct to consult with primary health care provider before exercising.

R: *The medication impedes the body's adaptive response to stress.*

- Stress the importance of follow-up laboratory tests.

R: *Significant abnormalities in liver or renal function studies and blood count may be seen.*

Instruct the individual and family to report the following signs and symptoms

- 1- to 2-lb weight gain
- Edema
- Difficulty breathing
- Pulse or blood pressure above or below pre-established parameters
- Dark urine
- Difficult urination
- Visual disturbances
- Sore throat
- Fever
- Sleep disturbances
- Memory loss
- Mental changes
- Behavioral changes

Risk for Complications of Calcium Channel Blocker Therapy Adverse Effects

High-Risk Populations for Adverse Effects

- Renal insufficiency
- Hepatic insufficiency
- Hypotension
- Decreased left ventricular function
- Pregnancy or breast-feeding
- Digitalis therapy
- β-Adrenergic blocker therapy
- Congestive heart failure
- Impaired liver/renal function

Collaborative Outcomes

The individual will be monitored for early signs and symptoms of adverse effects of calcium channel blocker therapy and will receive collaborative interventions if indicated to restore physiologic stability

Indicators

Individual/family can identify signs and symptoms that need immediate reporting:

- Hypotension
- Confusion
- Chest pain

Interventions and Rationales

(Arcangelo & Peterson, 2016)

Refer also to a pharmacology text for specific information on the individual drug

Assess for contraindications to calcium channel blocker therapy

- Severe left ventricular dysfunction
- Sick sinus syndrome
- Second- or third-degree heart block
- Cardiogenic shock
- Acute myocardial infarction (with diltiazem)
- IV use of verapamil and β-adrenergic blockers
- Symptomatic hypotension
- Advanced congestive heart failure

Explain possible adverse effects

- Systemic
  - Hypersensitivity (rash, pruritus, extreme hypotension)
  - Hair loss
  - Sweating, chills
- Central nervous system
  - Tremors
  - Insomnia
  - Confusion
  - Headache
  - Mood changes
- Cardiovascular
  - Palpitations
  - Heart failure
  - Myocardial infarction
  - Bradycardia
  - Hypotension
  - Third-degree heart block (with verapamil)
  - Arrhythmias
  - Peripheral edema
- Gastrointestinal
  - Diarrhea
  - Cramping
  - Constipation
  - Dyspepsia
- Hepatic
  - Elevated liver enzymes
- Respiratory
  - Dyspnea
  - Pulmonary edema
  - Wheezing
- Musculoskeletal
  - Muscle cramping
  - Inflammation
  - Joint stiffness
- Genitourinary
  - Impotence
  - Menstrual irregularities

Monitor for and reduce the severity of adverse effects

- Establish a baseline assessment of pulse, blood pressure, cardiac rhythm, and lung fields.

R: *Baseline data facilitate detection of adverse reactions.*

- Ensure that baseline hepatic function studies are performed before starting drug therapy.

R: *Calcium channel blockers can cause liver enzyme elevation.*

- Carefully monitor blood pressure and heart rate during initial stages of therapy.

R: *Bradycardia and hypotension may occur.*

- Monitor for congestive heart failure.

R: *Decreased cardiac output can compromise heart function.*

- Establish with the provider the parameters (blood pressure, pulse) for withholding the medication.

R: *Hypotension and bradycardia can reduce cardiac output.*

- Monitor intake and output and weight, and assess for edema.

R: *Reduced cardiac output can cause fluid accumulation.*

Teach the individual and family how to prevent or reduce the severity of adverse effects.

- Refer to *Risk for Complications of* β*-Adrenergic Blocker Therapy Adverse Effects* for specific interventions.

Instruct the individual and family to report the following signs and symptoms

- 1- to 2-lb weight gain
- Edema
- Difficulty breathing
- Pulse or blood pressure above or below pre-established parameters
- Sleep disturbances
- Mental changes

Instruct not to stop or miss medication doses

R: *Withdrawal hypertension can occur.*

Instruct not to chew, divide, or crush

R: *Medication will be absorbed too quickly.*

Risk for Complications of Angiotensin-Converting Enzyme Inhibitor and Angiotensin Receptor Blocker Therapy Adverse Effects

High-Risk Populations for Adverse Effects

- Severe renal dysfunction
- Systemic lupus-like syndrome
- Reduced white blood cell count
- Valvular stenosis
- Diabetes mellitus
- Pregnancy or breast-feeding
- Congestive heart failure
- Volume depletion
- Hyponatremia
- Hyperkalemia
- Autoimmune disease (for captopril)
- Coronary disease (for captopril)
- Cerebrovascular disease (for captopril)
- Medication therapy that causes leukopenia or agranulocytosis
- Collagen vascular disease (for enalapril)

Collaborative Outcomes

The individual will be monitored for early signs and symptoms of adverse effects of angiotensin-converting enzyme inhibitor and angiotensin receptor blocker therapy and will receive collaborative interventions if indicated to restore physiologic stability

Indicators

Individual/family can identify signs and symptoms that need immediate reporting:

- Fainting
- Tachycardia
- Chest pain
- GI bleeding

Interventions and Rationales

(Arcangelo & Peterson, 2016)

Refer also to a pharmacology text for specific information on the individual drug

Assess for contraindications to angiotensin-converting enzyme inhibitor therapy

- History of adverse effects
- Renal stenosis (bilateral, unilateral)
- Previous hypersensitivity
- Pregnancy

Explain possible adverse effects

- Systemic
  - Hypersensitivity (urticaria; rash; angioedema of face, throat, and extremities; difficulty breathing; stridor)
  - Photosensitivity
  - Alopecia
- Central nervous system
  - Vertigo
  - Insomnia
  - Fainting
  - Headache
- Cardiovascular
  - Tachycardia
  - Angina pectoris
  - Congestive heart failure
  - Chest pain
  - Hypotension
  - Palpitations
  - Pericarditis
  - Flushing
  - Raynaud's disease
- Gastrointestinal
  - Loss of taste
  - Diarrhea
  - Vomiting
  - Peptic ulcer
  - Anorexia
- Hematologic
  - Neutropenia
  - Eosinophilia
  - Agranulocytosis
  - Hyperkalemia
  - Hemolytic anemia
- Musculoskeletal
  - Joint pain
- Genitourinary
  - Proteinuria
  - Urinary frequency
  - Polyuria
  - Renal insufficiency
  - Oliguria
  - Elevated BUN/creatinine
- Respiratory
  - Cough
  - URI symptoms

Monitor for and reduce the severity of adverse effects

- Establish a baseline assessment of pulse, blood pressure (lying, sitting, and standing), cardiac rhythm, and lung fields.

R: *Baseline assessment data are vital to evaluating response to therapy and identifying adverse reactions.*

- Ensure that baseline electrolyte, blood, and renal and hepatic function studies are performed.

R: *The medication can cause liver enzyme elevation and hypokalemia.*

- Repeat BUN/creatinine and electrolytes in 4 to 6 weeks then periodically
- Carefully monitor blood pressure and heart rate during initial stages of therapy.

R: *Bradycardia and hypotension may occur.*

- Monitor for congestive heart failure.

R: *Decreased cardiac output can compromise heart function.*

- Establish with the physician or advanced practice nurse the parameters (blood pressure, pulse) for withholding the medication.

R: *Hypotension and bradycardia can reduce cardiac output.*

- Monitor intake and output and weight, and assess for edema.

R: *Reduced cardiac output can cause fluid accumulation.*

Teach the individual and family how to prevent or reduce the severity of adverse effects

- Refer to *PRC of ß-Adrenergic Blocker Therapy Adverse Effects.*
- Stress the importance of follow-up laboratory tests.

R: *Significant abnormalities in urinary protein and blood counts can occur.*

Instruct the individual and family to report the following signs and symptoms

- 1- to 2-lb weight gain
- Edema
- Difficulty breathing
- Persistent cough
- Pulse or blood pressure above or below pre-established parameters
- Dark urine
- Difficult urination
- Visual disturbances
- Sore throat
- Fever
- Sleep disturbances
- Memory loss
- Mental changes
- Behavioral changes

Risk for Complications of Diuretic Therapy Adverse Effects

High-Risk Populations for Adverse Effects

- Diabetes mellitus
- Acute MI
- Arrhythmias
- Impaired liver function
- History of gout
- History of pancreatitis
- Elderly
- SLE
- Sulfa allergy (with most diuretics except spironolactone and triamterene)

Collaborative Outcomes

The individual will be monitored for early signs and symptoms of adverse effects of diuretic therapy and will receive collaborative interventions if indicated to restore physiologic stability

Indicators

Individual/family can identify signs and symptoms that need immediate reporting:

- Edema
- Shortness of breath
- Visual and hearing disturbances
- Blood pressure below established parameters
- Dark urine

Interventions and Rationales
(Arcangelo & Peterson, 2016)

Refer to a pharmacology text for specific information on the individual drug

Assess for contraindications to diuretic therapy

- History of adverse effects
- Sulfa allergy
- Anuria
- Electrolyte imbalance
- Hepatic coma

Explain possible side effects

- Systemic
  - Hypokalemia
  - Electrolyte imbalance
  - Metabolic alkalosis
  - Dehydration
  - Ototoxicity/tinnitus
  - Blurred vision
  - Hyperuricemia
  - Hypocalcemia
  - Hyperglycemia
  - Hypomagnesemia
  - Leukopenia
  - Muscle cramps
  - Anorexia
  - Rash
  - Pruritus
  - Tinnitus
- Central nervous system
  - Paresthesias
  - Photosensitivity
- Cardiovascular
  - Hypovolemia
  - Anemia
  - Vasculitis
  - Orthostatic hypotension
- Gastrointestinal
  - Abdominal cramps
  - Diarrhea
  - Nausea/vomiting
  - Cholestatic jaundice
  - Pancreatitis
  - Hematologic
  - Thrombosis
  - Thrombocytopenia
  - Leukopenia
- Genitourinary
  - Interstitial nephritis
  - Urinary frequency

Monitor for and reduce the severity of adverse effects

- Identify a base line of pulse and blood pressure (lying, sitting, and standing).
- Monitor lab results, especially electrolytes.
- Establish with the provider the parameters (blood pressure) for withholding the medication.
- Monitor intake and output and weight daily.

Teach the individual and family how to prevent the severity of adverse events

- Stress the importance of follow-up laboratory tests
- Instruct the individual to change position slowly

Instruct the individual and family to report the following signs and symptoms

- 1- to 2-lb weight gain
- Edema
- Shortness of breath
- Visual and hearing disturbances
- Blood pressure below established parameters
- Dark urine
- Muscle cramps
- Increased lethargy
- Abdominal pain

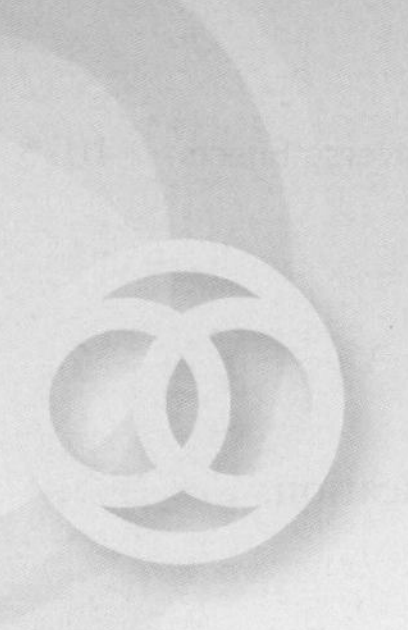

Appendix A

Nursing Diagnoses Grouped by Functional Health Pattern[1]

1. Health Perception–Health Management

Contamination: Community
  Contamination: Community, Risk for
Energy Field, Disturbed
Growth and Development, Delayed
  Failure to Thrive, Adult
  Development, Risk for Delayed
[2]Engagement, Compromised
  [2]Engagement, Risk for Compromised
[2]Elderly Syndrome, Frail
  [2]Elderly Syndrome, Risk for Frail
Health Management, Deficient Community
Health Behavior, Risk-Prone
Health Maintenance, Ineffective
Injury, Risk for
  Aspiration, Risk for
  Falls, Risk for
  [2]Urinary Tract Injury, Risk for
  Perioperative Positioning Injury, Risk for
  Poisoning, Risk for
  Suffocation, Risk for
  Thermal Injury, Risk for
  Trauma, Risk for
Noncompliance
[2]Obesity
  [2]Overweight
  [2]Overweight, Risk for
Health Management, Ineffective
Health Management, Ineffective Community
Health Management, Ineffective Family
Health Management, Readiness for Enhanced
Surgical Recovery, Delayed
  Surgical Recovery, Risk for Delayed

2. Nutritional–Metabolic

Adverse Reaction to Iodinated Contrast Media, Risk for
Allergy Response, Risk for
Blood Glucose Level, Risk for Unstable
Body Temperature, Risk for Imbalanced
  Hyperthermia
  Hypothermia
  Thermoregulation, Ineffective
Breastfeeding, Ineffective
Breastfeeding, Interrupted
Breastfeeding, Readiness for Enhanced
Breast Milk, Insufficient
Electrolyte Imbalance, Risk for
Fluid Balance, Readiness for Enhanced
Fluid Volume, Deficient
Fluid Volume, Excess
Fluid Volume, Risk for Imbalanced
Infection, Risk for
[2]Infection Transmission, Risk for
Intracranial Adaptive Capacity, Decreased
Jaundice, Neonatal
  Jaundice, Risk for Neonatal
Latex Allergy Response
  Latex Allergy Response, Risk for
Liver Function, Risk for Impaired
Nutrition, Imbalanced
  Dentition, Impaired
  Infant Feeding Pattern, Ineffective
  Swallowing, Impaired
Nutrition, Readiness for Enhanced
Protection, Ineffective
  [2]Corneal Injury, Risk for
  Dry Eye, Risk for
  Oral Mucous Membrane, Impaired
  [2]Oral Mucous Membrane, Risk for Impaired
  [2]Pressure Ulcer, Risk for
  Skin Integrity, Impaired
  Skin Integrity, Risk for Impaired
  Tissue Integrity, Impaired
  Tissue Integrity, Risk for Impaired

3. Elimination

Bowel Incontinence
[2]Constipation, Chronic Functional
  Constipation, Perceived
Diarrhea
Gastrointestinal Motility, Dysfunctional
  Gastrointestinal Motility, Risk for Dysfunctional
Urinary Elimination, Impaired
  [2]Incontinence, Continuous Urinary
  Incontinence, Functional Urinary
  Maturational Enuresis
  Incontinence, Overflow Urinary
  Incontinence, Reflex Urinary
  Incontinence, Stress Urinary
  Incontinence, Urge Urinary
Urinary Elimination, Readiness for Enhanced

4. Activity–Exercise

Activity Intolerance
Activity Planning, Ineffective
  Activity Planning, Risk for Ineffective
Bleeding, Risk for
Cardiac Output, Decreased
Disuse Syndrome, Risk for
Diversional Activity, Deficient
Home Maintenance, Impaired
Infant Behavior, Disorganized
  Infant Behavior, Risk for Disorganized
Infant Behavior, Readiness for Enhanced Organized
Intracranial Adaptive Capacity, Decreased
Lifestyle, Sedentary
Liver Function, Risk for Impaired
Mobility, Impaired Physical
  Bed Mobility, Impaired
  [2]Sitting, Impaired
  [2]Standing, Impaired
  Transfer Ability, Impaired
  Walking, Impaired
  Wheelchair Mobility, Impaired
[2]Respiratory Function, Risk for Ineffective
  Airway Clearance, Ineffective
  Breathing Pattern, Ineffective
  Gas Exchange, Impaired
  Spontaneous Ventilation, Impaired

[1] The Functional Health Patterns were identified in Gordon, M. (1994). *Nursing diagnosis: Process and application*. New York: McGraw-Hill, with minor changes by the author.
[2] Indicates the new nursing diagnoses, per NANDA-I Nursing Diagnoses 2015–2017.

Ventilatory Weaning Response, Dysfunctional
[2]Ventilatory Weaning Response, Risk for Dysfunctional
Self-Care, Readiness for Enhanced
[2]Self-Care Deficit Syndrome
Feeding Self-Care Deficit
Bathing Self-Care Deficit
Dressing Self-Care Deficit
[2]Instrumental Self-Care Deficit
Toileting Self-Care Deficit
Shock, Risk for
Sudden Infant Death Syndrome, Risk for
Tissue Perfusion, Ineffective
Cardiac Tissue Perfusion, Risk for Decreased
Cerebral Tissue Perfusion, Risk for Ineffective
Gastrointestinal Tissue Perfusion, Risk for Ineffective
Peripheral Neurovascular Dysfunction, Risk for
Peripheral Tissue Perfusion, Ineffective
Peripheral Tissue Perfusion, Risk for Ineffective
Renal Perfusion, Risk for Ineffective
Vascular Trauma, Risk for
Wandering

5. Sleep–Rest

Sleep, Readiness for Enhanced
Sleep Pattern, Disturbed
Insomnia
Sleep Deprivation

6. Cognitive–Perceptual

Aspiration, Risk for
Comfort, Impaired
Nausea
Pain, Acute
[2]Pain Syndrome, Chronic
Pain, Labor
Comfort, Readiness for Enhanced
Confusion, Acute
Confusion, Chronic
Decisional Conflict
Decision Making, Impaired Emancipated
Decision Making, Risk for Impaired Emancipated
Decision Making, Readiness for Enhanced Emancipated
Decision Making, Readiness for Enhanced
Dysreflexia, Autonomic
Dysreflexia, Risk for Autonomic
Environmental Interpretation Syndrome, Impaired
Knowledge, Deficient
Knowledge (Specify), Readiness for Enhanced
Memory, Impaired
Neglect, Unilateral

7. Self-Perception

Anxiety
Anxiety, Death
Fatigue
Fear
Hope, Readiness for Enhanced
Hopelessness
Human Dignity, Risk for Compromised
[2]Labile Emotional Control
Neglect, Self
Power, Readiness for Enhanced
Powerlessness
Powerlessness, Risk for
[2]Self-Concept, Disturbed
Body Image, Disturbed
Personal Identity, Disturbed
Personal Identity, Risk for Disturbed
Self-Esteem, Chronic Low
Self-Esteem, Risk for Chronic Low
2Self-Esteem, Disturbed
Self-Esteem, Situational Low
Self-Esteem, Risk for Situational Low
Self-Concept, Readiness for Enhanced

8. Role–Relationship

Childbearing Process, Ineffective
Childbearing Process, Risk for Ineffective
[2]Communication, Impaired
Communication, Impaired Verbal
Communication, Readiness for Enhanced
Family Processes, Dysfunctional
Family Processes, Interrupted
Family Processes, Readiness for Enhanced
Grieving
[2]Grieving, Anticipatory
Grieving, Complicated
Loneliness, Risk for
Parental Role Conflict
Parenting, Impaired
Parent–Infant Attachment, Risk for Impaired
Parenting, Readiness for Enhanced
Relationship, Ineffective
Relationship, Ineffective, Risk for
Relationship, Readiness for Enhanced
Role Performance, Ineffective
Social Interaction, Impaired
Social Isolation
Sorrow, Chronic

9. Sexuality–Reproductive

Childbearing Process, Readiness for Enhanced
Sexuality Patterns, Ineffective
Sexual Dysfunction

10. Coping–Stress Tolerance

Caregiver Role Strain
Caregiver Role Strain, Risk for
Coping, Compromised Family
Coping, Disabled Family
Coping, Ineffective
[2]Mood Regulation, Impaired
Coping, Defensive
Coping, Readiness for Enhanced
Denial, Ineffective
Impulse Control, Labile Emotional Control
Coping, Ineffective Community
Coping, Readiness for Enhanced Community
Coping, Readiness for Enhanced Family
Post-Trauma Syndrome
Post-Trauma Syndrome, Risk for
Rape-Trauma Syndrome
Relocation Stress [Syndrome]
Relocation Stress [Syndrome], Risk for
Resilience, Impaired Individual
Resilience, Readiness for Enhanced
Resilience, Risk for Compromised
[2]Self-Harm, Risk for
Self-Mutilation
Self-Mutilation, Risk for
Suicide, Risk for
Stress Overload
Violence, Risk for Other-Directed
Violence, Risk for Self-Directed

11. Value–Belief

Moral Distress
[2]Moral Distress, Risk for
Religiosity, Readiness for Enhanced
Spiritual Distress
Religiosity, Impaired
Religiosity, Risk for Impaired
Spiritual Distress, Risk for
Spiritual Well-Being, Readiness for Enhanced

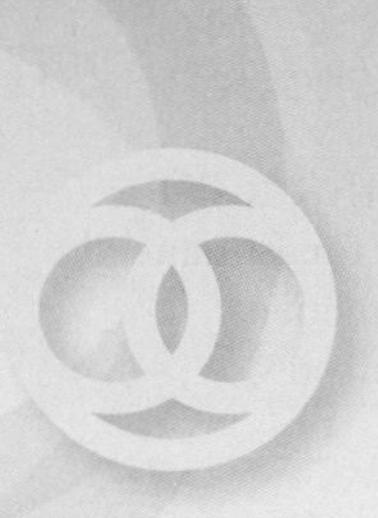

Appendix B

Nursing Admission Baseline Assessment

Nursing Admission Data Base

Date ________ Arrival Time ________ Contact Person ________ Phone ________

ADMITTED FROM: ____ Home alone ____ Home with relative ____ Long-term care facility
____ Homeless ____ Home with ____ (Specify)
____ ER ____ Other ________

MODE OF ARRIVAL: ____ Wheelchair ____ Ambulance ____ Stretcher

REASON FOR HOSPITALIZATION: ____
____
____

LAST HOSPITAL ADMISSION: Date ________________ Reason ________________
____

MEDICAL HISTORY: ____
____

MEDICATION (Prescription/Over-the-Counter)	***DOSAGE***	***LAST DOSE***	***FREQUENCY***

Health Maintenance–Perception Pattern

USE OF:

Tobacco: ____ None ____ Quit (Date) ____ Pipe ____ Cigar ____ <1 pk/day
____ 1–2 pks/day ____ >2 pks/day Pks/year history ________________

Alcohol: ____ Date of last drink ____ Amount/type
____ No. of days in a month when alcohol is consumed ____ In recovery

Other Drugs: ____ No ____ Yes Type ________ Use ________ History ________

Allergies (drugs, food, tape, dyes): ________________ Reaction ________
____

Activity–Exercise Pattern

SELF-CARE ABILITY:

0 = Independent 1 = Assistive device 2 = Assistance from others
3 = Assistance from person and equipment 4 = Dependent/Unable

	0	1	2	3	4
Eating/Drinking					
Bathing					
Dressing/Grooming					
Toileting					
Bed Mobility					
Transferring					
Ambulating					
Stair Climbing					
Shopping					
Cooking					
Home Maintenance					

ASSISTIVE DEVICES: ____ None ____ Crutches ____ Bedside commode ____ Walker
____ Cane ____ Splint/Brace ____ Wheelchair ____ Other

CODE: (1) Not applicable (2) Unable to acquire (3) Not a priority at this time
(4) Other (specify in notes)

Side One

Nutrition–Metabolic Pattern

Special Diet/Supplements: ______

Previous Dietary Instruction: ____ Yes ____ No

Appetite: ____ Normal ____ Increased ____ Decreased ____ Decreased taste sensation
____ Nausea ____ Vomiting

Weight Fluctuations Last 6 Months: ____ None ______ lbs. Gained/Lost

Swallowing difficulty: ____ None ____ Solids ____ Liquids

Dentures: ____ Upper (___ Partial ___ Full) ____ Lower (___ Partial ___ Full)
With Person ____ Yes ____ No

History of Skin/Healing Problems: ____ None ____ Abnormal Healing ____ Rash
____ Dryness ____ Excess Perspiration

Elimination Pattern

Bowel Habits: ____ # BMs q __/day ____Date of last BM ____Within normal limits
____ Constipation ____ Diarrhea ____ Incontinence
____ Ostomy: Type: ____ Appliance ____ Self-care ____ Yes ____ No

Bladder Habits: ____ WNL ____ Frequency ____ Dysuria ____ Nocturia ____ Urgency
____ Hematuria ____ Retention

Incontinency: ____ No ____Yes ____Total ____ Daytime ____ Nighttime
____ Occasional ____ Difficulty delaying voiding ____ Stress
____ Difficulty reaching toilet ____ Difficulty perceiving cues

Assistive Devices: ____ Intermittent catheterization
____ Indwelling catheter ____ External catheter
____ Incontinent briefs

Sleep–Rest Pattern

Habits: ____ hrs/night ____ AM nap ____ PM nap
Feel rested after sleep ____ Yes ____ No

Problems: ____ None ____ Early waking ____Difficulty falling asleeep ____ Nightmares
____ frequent awaking ____ reason

Cognitive–Perceptual Pattern

Mental Status: ____ Alert ____ Receptive aphasia ____ Poor historian
____ Oriented ____ Confused ____ Combative ____ Unresponsive

Speech: ____ Normal ____ Slurred ____ Garbled ____ Expressive aphasia

Language Spoken: ____ English ____ Spanish ____ Other ______ Interpreter ______

Ability to Read English: ____ Yes ____ No ______

Ability to Communicate: ____ Yes ____ No ___Verbally____Written____

Ability to Comprehend: ____ Yes ____ No ______

Level of Anxiety:____Appropriate ____ Mild ____ Moderate ____ Severe ____ Panic

Interactive Skills: ____ Appropriate ____ Other ______

Hearing: ____ WNL ____ Impaired (__ Right __ Left) ____ Deaf (__ Right __ Left)
____ Hearing Aid ______ number ______ with person now

Vision: ____ WNL ____ Eyeglasses ____ Contact lenses
____ Impaired ____ Right ____ Left
____ Blind ____ Right ____ Left
____ Prosthesis ____ Right ____ Left

Vertigo: ____ Yes ____ No Memory intact ____ Yes ____ No

Discomfort/Pain: ____ None ____ Acute ____ Chronic ____ Description ______
______

Onset______Duration______ (Rate 0–no pain to 10–worst pain ever)

Pain Management: Meds, other therapies ______

Coping–Stress Tolerance/Self-Perception/Self-Concept Pattern

Major concerns regarding hospitalization or illness (financial, self-care): ______
______

Major loss/change in past year: ____ No ____ Yes Specify ______
______

Fear of Violence: ____ Yes ____ No From Whom ______

Outlook on Future: ______ (Rate 1–poor to 10–very optimistic)
______

CODE: (1) Not applicable (2) Unable to acquire (3) Not a priority at this time
(4) Other (specify in notes)

Side Two

Sexuality–Reproductive Pattern

LMP: ______________ Post-menopause ______ Gravida ____ Para__________
Birth Control _________________________
Menstrual/Hormonal Problems: ____ Yes ____ No ____
Last Pap Smear: ___________________ Hx of Abnormal PAP ______________________________
Monthly Self-Breast/Testicular Exam: ____ Yes ____ No Last Mammogram: ________________
Sexual Concerns: ____
____

Role–Relationship Pattern

Marital status: ___________ Lives with ___________
Occupation: ____
Employment Status: ____ Employed ____ Short-term disability
____ Long-term disability ____ Unemployed
Support System: ____ Spouse/Partner ____ Neighbors/Friends ____ None
____ Family in same residence ____ Family in separate residence
____ Other ____
Family concerns regarding hospitalization: ____
____

Value–Belief Pattern

Religion: ______________________________
Religious Restrictions: ____ No ____ Yes (Specify) ___________________________________
Request Chaplain Visitation at This Time: ____ Yes ____ No

PHYSICAL ASSESSMENT (Objective)

1. CLINICAL DATA

Age ______ Height ______ Weight ______ BMI ______ Temperature ______
Pulse: ____ Strong ____ Weak ____ Regular ____ Irregular____
Blood Pressure: Right Arm ____ Left Arm ____ Sitting ____ Lying ____

2. RESPIRATORY/CIRCULATORY

Rate:______
Quality: ____ WNL ____ Shallow ____ Rapid ____ Labored ____ Other ___________________
Cough: ____ No ____ Yes
Describe ____
Auscultation:
Upper rt lobes ____ WNL ____ Decreased ____ Absent ____ Abnormal sounds ____
Upper lt lobes ____ WNL ____ Decreased ____ Absent ____ Abnormal sounds ____
Lower rt lobes ____ WNL ____ Decreased ____ Absent ____ Abnormal sounds ____
Lower lt lobes ____ WNL ____ Decreased ____ Absent ____ Abnormal sounds ____
Right Pedal Pulse: ____ Strong ____ Weak ____ Absent
Left Pedal Pulse: ____ Strong ____ Weak ____ Absent

3. METABOLIC–INTEGUMENTARY

SKIN: Take photos per protocol of lesions, injuries
Color: ____ WNL ____ Pale ____ Cyanotic ____ Ashen ____ Jaundice ____ Other ____
Temperature: ____ WNL ____ Warm ____ Cool
Edema: ____ No ____ Yes/Description/location ______________________________________
Lesions: ____ None ____ Yes/Description/location ___________________________________
Bruises: ____ None ____ Yes/Description/location ___________________________________
Reddened: ____ No ____ Yes/Description/location ____________________________________
Pruritus: ____ No ____ Yes/Description/location ____________________________________
MOUTH:
Gums: ____ WNL ____ White plaque ____ Lesions ____ Other ________________________
Teeth: ____ WNL ____ Other ____
ABDOMEN:
Bowel Sounds: ____ Present ____ Absent

Side Three

4. NEURO/SENSORY

Pupils: ____ Equal ____ Unequal describe ____
Reactive to light:
Left: ___ Yes ___ No/Specify ___________
Right: ____ Yes ____ No/Specify ___________
Eyes: ___ Clear ___ Draining ___ Reddened ___ Other ___________

5. MUSCULAR–SKELETAL

Range of Motion: ____ Full ____ Other ___________
Balance and Gait: ____ Steady ____ Unsteady
Hand Grasps: ____ Equal ____ Strong ____ Weakness/Paralysis (__Right __ Left)
Leg Strength: ____ Equal ____ Strong ____ Weakness/Paralysis (__ Right __ Left)

6. OTHER SIGNIFICANT OBSERVATIONS FOR TRANSITION PLANNING

Lives: Alone ____ With ___________ No known residence ___________
Intended Destination Post Discharge: ____ Home ____ Undetermined ____ Other ____
Previous Utilization of Community Resources:
____ Home care/Hospice ____ Adult day care ____ Church groups ____ Other ___________
____ Meals on Wheels ____ Homemaker/Home health aide ____ Community support group
Post-transition Transportation:
____ Car ____ Ambulance ____ Bus/Taxi
____ Unable to determine at this time
Anticipated Financial Assistance Post-discharge?:____ No ____ Yes ___________
Anticipated Problems with Self-care Post-discharge?: ____ No ____ Yes ___________
Assistive Devices Needed Post-discharge?: ____ No ____ Yes ___________
Referrals: (record date)
Transition Coordinator ___________ Home Health ___________
Social Service ___________
Other Comments: ___________
____
SIGNATURE/TITLE ___________ Date ___________

Side Four

Appendix C

Strategies to Promote Engagement of Individual/Families for Healthier Outcomes

Types of Literacy

Functional illiteracy is when someone who has minimal reading and writing skills does not have the capacity for health literacy to manage ordinary everyday needs and requirements of most employments.

Health literacy is the capacity to obtain, process, and understand basic health information and services needed to

- Make appropriate health decisions (*Ratzan, 2001)
- Follow instructions for treatments and medications (*White & Dillow, 2005)
- Sign a consent form
- Make appointments

Carp's Cues

Individuals who are illiterate (who cannot read or write) are easier to identify than those who are functionally illiterate. Do not assume an individual can read and understand health literature even if translated.

R: *The National Assessment of Adult Literacy (NAAL) (*2003) reported that 9 out of 10 English-speaking adults in the United States do not have health literacy (Kutner, Greenberg, Jiny, & Paulson, 2006). A large study on the scope of health literacy at two public hospitals (*Williams et al., 1995) found the following:*

- *Half of English-speaking patients could not read and understand basic health education material.*
- *60% could not understand a routine consent form.*
- *26% could not understand the appointment card.*
- *42% failed to understand directions for taking their medications.*

Assess for the Red Flags of Low Literacy

- Frequently missed appointments
- Incomplete registration forms
- Noncompliance with medication
- Inability to name medications, explain purpose, or describe dosing
- Identification of pills by appearance, not by reading of label
- Inability to give coherent, sequential history
- Few questions asked
- Lack of follow-through on tests or referrals

Strategies to Improve Comprehension

R: *Research shows that individuals remember and understand less than half of what clinicians explain to them (Williams et al., 1995; Roter, Rune, & Comings, 1998). Testing general reading levels does not ensure understanding in the clinical setting (Weiss, 2007).*

- For comprehension to occur, the nurse must accept that there is limited time and that the use of this time is enhanced by
  - Using every contact time to teach something
  - Creating a relaxed encounter

- Using eye contact
- Slowing down—break it down into short statements
- Having limited content—focus on 2 or 3 concepts
- Using plain language
- Engaging individual/family in discussion
- Using graphics
- Explaining what you are doing to the individual/family and why
- Asking them to tell you about what you taught. Tell them to use their own words.

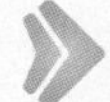

Carp's Cues

Health-care professionals must quiet themselves regarding what they *think* a person or family needs to know. The goal is to find what information the individual wants to know; otherwise even the best teaching techniques will "fall on deaf ears." "Making the suggestion to lose 20 pounds, start going to the gym, and regularly take their hypertension medication to a person who has little understanding that they even have a chronic illness, the nature of that illness, or that they must play a part in managing it, is unlikely to result in the desired outcome" (Hibbard & Greene, 2013).

The Teach–Back Method (DeWalt, Callahan, Hawk et al, 2010)

- This method includes (source: www.teachbacktraining.org/) the following:
  - A way to make sure you—the health-care provider—explained information clearly; it is not a test or quiz of individuals or families.
  - Asking an individual (or family member) to explain—*in their own words*—what they need to know or do, in a caring way.
  - A way to check for understanding and, if needed, re-explain and check again.

Use the Teach-Back Method

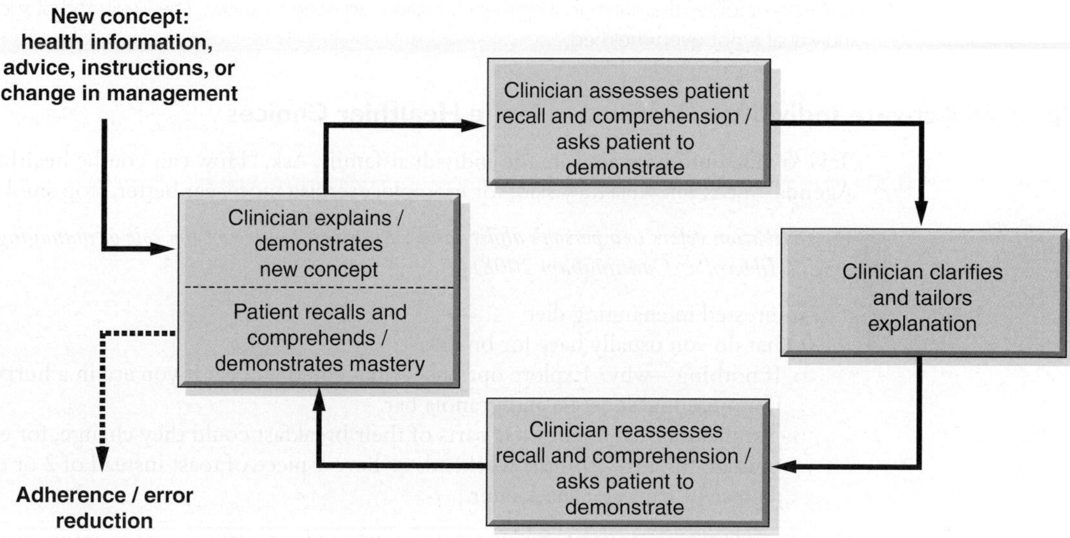

- Explain/demonstrate
  - Explain one concept (e.g., medication, condition, when to call PCP).
  - Demonstrate one procedure (e.g., dressing charge, use of inhaler).
- Assess
  - I want to make sure, I explained ______ clearly, can you tell me ______.
  - Tell me what I told you.
  - Show me how to ______.
  - Avoid asking, "Do you understand?"
- Clarify
  - Add more explanation if you are not satisfied that the person understands or can perform the activity.
  - If the person cannot report the information, don't repeat the same explanation; rephrase it.

Carp's Cues

Be careful the person/family does not think you are testing him or her. Assure them it is important that you help them to understand that the teaching method can help you teach and also diagnose educational needs.

- Teach-back questions (examples):
  - When should you call your PCP?
  - How do you know your incision is healing?
  - What foods should you avoid?
  - How often should you test your blood sugar?
  - What should you do for low blood sugar?
  - What weight gain should you report to your PCP?
  - Which inhaler is your rescue inhaler?
  - Is there something you have been told to do that you do not understand?
  - What should you bring to your PCP office?
  - Is there something you have a question about?

Carp's Cues

Use every opportunity to explain a treatment, a medication, the condition, and/or restrictions. Focus on "need to know" and "need to do."

- For example, as you change a dressing
  - Explain and ask the individual/family member to redress the wound.
  - Point out how the wound is healing and what would indicate signs of infection.

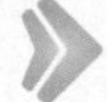

Carp's Cues

When individual/family do not understand what was said or demonstrated, the teach-back needs to be revised in a manner that will improve understanding. Teach-back has the potential to improve health outcomes, because if done correctly, it forces the nurse to limit the information to need to know. The likelihood of success is increased when the individual is not overwhelmed.

Helping to Activate Individuals/Families to Make Healthier Choices

Take opportunities to activate the individual/family. Ask, "How can you be healthier?" regardless of "Your Agenda" focus on what they said, for example, exercise more, eat better, stop smoking.

R: *"Activation refers to a person's ability and willingness to take on the role of managing their health and health care" (Hibbard & Cunningham 2008).*

- If interested in changing diet:
  - What do you usually have for breakfast?
    - If nothing—why? Explore options—what could you eat if you are in a hurry? Wait for an answer—if none, suggest cereal and granola bar.
    - If unhealthy, ask them what parts of their breakfast could they change, for example, save bacon/sausage for a treat on the weekends or have 1 piece of toast instead of 2 or delete the juice and have a piece of fruit as a snack later.

R: *A breakfast increases the body's metabolism early and can reduce excessive eating as the day continues.*

  - What did you have for dinner last night?
    - 10 Fried wings and a large soda.
    - Do you think eating 1 to 2 pieces of chicken is better than 10 wings? They have less fat and more meat than wings.
    - Give them the diagram of MyPlate from www.choosemyplate.gov/. Ask them what they can add to their plate in each section.

R: *Asking the person to select foods from each type of food section will help to teach the person/family what is a starch e.g., corn, peas, (not vegetables) sources of protein, as beans e.g., legumes not green beans, which are a vegetable,*

    - What vegetable could you include in this meal? Carrots, green beans, salad.

Carp's Cues

Have copies of readable educational materials that can be easily accessed (e.g., picture of Choose MyPlate).

- How could you eat healthier?
  - Stress that there are no bad foods but bad amounts. Yes, there are healthier foods/drinks? What are they? Roasted chicken.
  - What do you drink during the day? Could you substitute water or diet drinks for soda or sugar drinks? "The body has to burn calories to process the water you drink, and since water has no calories, it burns other calories in your food."
  - When you eat out, do you think you are given too much food? If yes, how about asking for a take-out box before you start eating? Share a dessert.
- What three changes can you make to eat better?

R: *Keep it simple so the individual sees it as doable.*

- If interested in exercising more, focus on moving more.

R: *The word "exercise" has images of 1/2 to 1 hour sessions, joining a gym.*

- How do you travel to work? School?
  - If you drive, park further away from the building, the store, etc.
  - If you take the train or bus, get off 1 to 2 blocks or stops from your usual stop.
  - Use stairs. If walking upstairs is a problem, walk down only.
  - Walk your dog.
  - Arrange to walk with someone for the company and to increase the commitment.
- If interested in stopping smoking:
  - Set a date.
  - Be realistic, relapses occur.
  - Print out something for the person to take.
    - Go to THE POINT and print out "Getting Started to Quit Smoking?" for individuals with low health literacy.
    - Go to 5 steps to quitting > http://smokefree.gov/steps-on-quit-day for most individuals.
    - Go to www.helpguide.org/articles/addiction/how-to-quit-smoking.htm for more educated individuals.

R: *"Strategies are needed to ensure that individuals/families are supported to become engaged, at the level they desire, instead of teaching what 'we' think they need" (Frosch & Elwyn. 2014).*

- If the individual does not offer what healthier choices they could choose, focus on 1 or 2 consequences of their unhealthy choices as follows:
  - If weight loss would be helpful:
    - Do your legs swell during the day and return to normal when you wake up?
      - "Your weight is compressing the tubes/vessels in your legs which prevent the fluid from returning to your body. At some point the swelling will not go away when you are sleeping. It is permanent! Look at overweight people's feet; many wear slippers as shoes.
    - What could you do if you lost 20 lb that you cannot do now?
      - Pick up 5 pounds of sugar. It is heavy; imagine how your joints or heart would like 5 pounds less of stain. Imagine 2 bags of sugar as 2 pounds of sugar. Focus on 3 pounds at a time as the goal.
  - If the person smokes:
    - How much does smoking cost you each month?
    - If respiratory infections or chronic lung diseases are present, acknowledge that smoking will continue to cause deterioration. Ask them if they ever experienced trouble breathing? Gently explore how frightening it was. Continued smoking will cause progression of the breathing difficulties, with no treatments offering a cure.
    - Do you have leg cramps when you walk? If yes, explain that smoking changes their blood vessels that reduce the blood flow when walking. Eventually the pain will prevent them from walking at all.
    - Smoking interferes with circulation, so your body cannot heal well after an injury or surgery. Smokers also get leg ulcers that never heal.
- If a person is reporting not taking medications as prescribed, explore why. Refer to Medication Reconciliation and Barriers to Adherence later in this section. If the reason is "Don't think I need it," ask, "Do you know anyone with diabetes mellitus, heart disease, had a stroke, or kidney failure?" If yes, say, "Tell me about them."

- Try to make a connection with failure to adhere to treatment plan to the unsatisfactory effect on their daily life or death.
- Does he/she think the poor outcome could have been prevented?

R: *Some individuals report "diabetes (or cardiac disease, or strokes, or renal failure) runs in my family." Discussions can focus on what they do to prevent or reduce this from happening to them.*

- Personalized information (paper and electronic) which
  - Determines person's goal in treatment
  - Serves to identify barriers to adherence and solutions.

R: *"Starting with appropriate goals that fit the person's level of activation, and working toward increasing activation step by step, he/she can experience small successes and steadily build up the confidence and skill for effective self-management" (Hibbard & Greene, 2013).*

R: *The potential for individuals to contribute to their safety by speaking up about their concerns depends heavily on the quality of professional interactions and relationships (Entwistle et al., 2010).*

- Offer praise for honesty about problems with compliance and for sharing reasons. For example (Sofaer & Schumann, 2013, p. 19):
  - "I'm glad you told me that you stopped taking Motrin because it made your stomach hurt. Now I understand why your hands still ache. Let's talk about other ways we can get you some comfort."
  - "It's good that you told me about your stopping the blood pressure pills. That explains your headaches and higher pressure today. Let's discuss how those pills made you feel."

R: *Individuals/Families "will only be successful in taking greater responsibility for their health care decisions and actions if they are well-nurtured in this process, consistently protected from making profoundly negative decisions along the way, and kept safe" (Sofaer & Schumann, 2013, p. 19).*

- Suggest self-monitoring is useful to determine positive and negative influences on compliance.
  - Daily records
  - Charts
  - Diary of progress or symptoms, clinical values (e.g., blood pressure), or dietary intake

R: *"Involving the individual/family in decision-making places some responsibility on him or her to make sure the plan works, promoting engagement with treatment/plan" (Sofaer & Schumann 2013).*

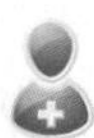

Clinical Alert Many persons who are ready to engage believe that they will engage at their peril and that clinicians and others will react negatively if they ask probing questions, disagree, suggest an alternative approach, ask for a second opinion, question an insurance company decision, or indicate dissatisfaction (Frosch, May, Rendle, Tietbohl, & Elwyn, 2012; Sofaer & Schumann, 2013).

Medication Reconciliation and Barriers to Adherence (Carpenito, 2014)

Medication errors occur 46% of the time during transitions, admission, transfer, or discharge from a clinical unit/hospital. Almost 60% of individuals have at least one discrepancy in their medication history completed on admission. "The most common error (46.4%) was omission of a regularly used medication. Most (61.4%) of the discrepancies were judged to have no potential to cause serious harm. However, 38.6% of the discrepancies had the potential to cause moderate to severe discomfort or clinical deterioration" (Cornish et al., 2005, p. 424).

Medication reconciliation on admission to the health-care facilities often entails the following:

- Name of medication (prescribed, over-the-counter)
- Prescribed dose
- Frequency (daily, bid, tid, as needed)

A list of medications that have been prescribed by a provider does not represent a process of medication reconciliation. A family member recently took an older relative to the ER with chest pain. A typed list of her medications was given to the ER nurse. No discussion occurred about her medication.

Unfortunately, one of two hypertension medications she regularly took was not entered in the electronic health record. Since her blood pressure was elevated on admission and persisted, another antihypertensive medication was ordered. After two days, another medication was added with good results.

The first medication that was added was the medication she was already taking before admission. So essentially, no new medication was added as a result of the error. She spent three unnecessary days in the hospital with increased costs to Medicare and would have definitely rather been home eating her own food and having a good night's sleep in her own bed.

According to the Joint Commission (p. 1), Medication reconciliation is the process of comparing an individual's medication orders to all of the medications that the patient has been taking. This reconciliation is done to avoid medication errors such as omissions, duplications, dosing errors, or drug interactions. It should be done at every transition of care in which new medications are ordered or existing orders are rewritten. Transitions in care include changes in setting, service, practitioner, or level of care. The process comprises five steps: (1) develop a list of current medications; (2) develop a list of medications to be prescribed; (3) compare the medications on the two lists; (4) make clinical decisions based on the comparison; and (5) communicate the new list to appropriate caregivers to the patient.

Critical to acquiring a list of medications are the additional assessment questions, which are the defining elements for medication reconciliation: "*versus a list of medications reported to be taking.*"

For each medication reported, ask the individual/family member the following questions (DeWalt et al., 2010):

- What is the reason you are taking each medication?
- Are you taking the medication as prescribed? Specify once a day, twice a day, etc.
- Are you skipping any doses? Do you sometimes run out of medications?
- How often are you taking the medication prescribed "if needed as a pain medication"?
- Have you stopped taking any of these medications?
- How much does it cost you to take your medications?
- Are you taking anybody else's medication?

Prepare the Individual/Family for Correctly Taking Medications at Home

- Explain what OTC not to take.
- Finish all the medications like antibiotics.
- Do not to take any medications that are at home unless approved by PCP.
- Ask bring all his or her medications to next visit to PCP (e.g., prescribed, OTC, vitamins, herbal medicines).
- As indicated:
  - Create a list of each medication, what used for, times to take, with food or without food.
  - Create a pill card with columns, pictures of pill.
  - For a printable pill card to use with individuals, refer to thePoint.
  - Have individual or family member fill a weekly pill box with sections for bid and tid slots.
  - Warn that if a pill looks different, check with pharmacy.
- Remember, as a nurse:
  - Create a habit of using every contact time to teach something.
  - The more you do it, the better you get.
  - The better you get, the better it is for those you care for.

Appendix D

High-Risk Assessment Tools for Preventable Hospital-Acquired Conditions

This edition has identified the importance of prevention of eight conditions identified by Centers for Medicare and Medicaid Services.

These eight events or conditions are as follows:

- Pressure ulcer stages III and IV
- Falls and trauma
- Surgical site infection after bariatric surgery for obesity, certain orthopedic procedures, and bypass surgery (mediastinitis)
- Vascular catheter-associated infection
- Catheter-associated urinary tract infection
- Administration of incompatible blood
- Air embolism
- Foreign object unintentionally retained after surgery

Using evidence-based guidelines, the following can be accessed:

- Nursing diagnoses that represent prevention of infection, falls, pressure ulcers, and delayed discharge
- Collaborative problems that identify individuals at high risk for air emboli, deep vein thrombosis, and sepsis
- Medical condition, postsurgical care, and treatment plan specifically identify adverse events that are associated with clinical diagnoses or situations (refer to Section 3: Collaborative Problems)
- Standardized risk assessment tools for falls, infection, and pressure ulcers that are incorporated in every care plan. Refer the following for these tools.

For the assessment tools to identify individuals at high risk for one or more of these condition(s), refer to the table of contents for

- Infection—Risk for Infection
- Risk for Delayed Surgical Healing
- Risk for Complications of Deep Vein Thrombosis
- Risk for Complication of Sepsis

Standardized Risk Assessment Tools for Falls, Infection, and Pressure Ulcer

High Risk for Falls

Fall Risk Assessment

Assess for the following risk factors. Record the number of checks in the fall assessment scores in the ( ) as High Risk for Falls (score), or add the risk factors, for example, as High Risk for Falls related to instability, postural hypotension, and IV equipment.

Assess all individuals for risk factors for falls, using the assessment tool in the institution. The following represents one assessment tool:

Variables Score

History of falling

No (score as 0)

Yes (score as 25)

Secondary diagnosis

No (score as 0)

Yes (score as 15)

Ambulatory aid
Bed rest/nurse assistance (score as 0)
Crutches/cane/walker (score as 15)
Furniture (score as 30)

IV or IV access
No (score as 0)
Yes (score as 20)

Gait
Normal/bed rest/immobile (score as 0)
Weak (score as 10)
Impaired (score as 20)

Mental status
Knows own limits (score as 0)
Overestimates or forgets limits (score as 15)

Total Score ________

Risk Level Morse Fall Scale (MFS) Score Action
No risk
0–24 Good basic nursing care
Low to moderate risk
25–45 Implement standard fall prevention interventions
High risk
46+ Implement high-risk fall prevention interventions
Morse Fall Scale (*Morse, 1997). Used with permission.

Timed Up and Go (Podsiadlo & Richardson, 1991)

For individuals who are independent and ambulatory but frail, fatigued, and/or with possible compromised ambulation, assess the person's ability to Timed Up and Go (TUG):

- Have the person wear their usual footwear, and use any assistive device they normally use.
- Have the person sit in the chair with their back to the chair and their arms resting on the arm rests.
- Ask the person to stand up from a standard chair and walk a distance of 10 ft (3 m).
- Have the person turn around, walk back to the chair, and sit down again.
- Timing begins when the person starts to rise from the chair and ends when he or she returns to the chair and sits down.

The person should be given one practice trial and then three actual trials if needed. The times from the three actual trials are averaged.

Predictive Results

Seconds	***Rating***
<10	Freely mobile
10–19	Mostly independent
20–29	Variable mobility
>29	Impaired mobility

Risk Factors for Surgical Site Infection

The risk of surgical site infection is influenced by the amount and virulence of the microorganism and the ability of the individual to resist it (Pear, 2007).

Assess for the following risk factors. Record the number of risk factors in the ( ) as High Risk for Surgical Site Infection (1–10) or add the risk factors, for example, as High Risk for Surgical Site Infection related to obesity, diabetes mellitus, and tobacco use.

Infection colonization of microorganisms (1)
Preexisting remote body site infection (1)
Preoperative contaminated or dirty wound (e.g., posttrauma) (1)
Glucocorticoid steroids (2)
Tobacco use (3)
Malnutrition (4)
Obesity (5)
Perioperative hyperglycemia (6)
Diabetes mellitus (7)
Altered immune response (8)
Chronic alcohol use/acute alcohol intoxication (9)

1. Preoperative nares colonization with *Staphylococcus aureus* noted in 30% of most healthy populations, and especially methicillin-resistant *Staph. aureus* (MRSA), predisposes individuals to have higher risk of surgical site infection (Price et al., 2008).
2. Systemic glucocorticoids, which are frequently used as anti-inflammatory agents, are well-known to inhibit wound repair via global anti-inflammatory effects and suppression of cellular wound responses, including fibroblast proliferation and collagen synthesis. Systemic steroids cause wounds to heal with incomplete granulation tissue and reduced wound contraction (Franz et al., 2007).
3. Smoking has a transient effect on the tissue microenvironment and a prolonged effect on inflammatory and reparative cell functions, leading to delayed healing and complications. Quit smoking four weeks before surgery; restores tissue oxygenation and metabolism rapidly (Sørensen, 2012).
4. Malnourished individuals have been found to have less competent immune response to infection and decreased nutritional stores which will impair wound healing (Speaar, 2008).
5. An obese individual may experience a compromise in wound healing due to poor blood supply to adipose tissue. In addition, antibiotics are not absorbed well by adipose tissue. Despite excessive food intake, many obese individuals have protein malnutrition, which further impedes the healing (Cheadle, 2006).
6. There are two primary mechanisms that place individuals experiencing acute perioperative hyperglycemia at increased risk for surgical site infection. The first mechanism is the decreased vascular circulation, reducing tissue perfusion and impairing cellular-level functions. A clinical study by Akbari et al. (1998) noted that when healthy, nondiabetic subjects ingested a glucose load, the endothelial-dependent vasodilatation in both the micro and macro circulations were impaired similar to that seen in diabetic patients. The second affected mechanism is the reduced activity of the cellular immunity functions of chemotaxis, phagocytosis, and killing of polymorphonuclear cells as well as monocytes/macrophages that have been shown to occur in the acute hyperglycemic state.
7. Postsurgical adverse outcomes related to diabetes mellitus are believed to be related to the preexisting complications of chronic hyperglycemia, which include vascular atherosclerotic disease and peripheral as well as autonomic neuropathies (Geerlings et al., 1999).
8. Suppression of the immune system by disease, medication, or age can delay wound healing (Cheadle, 2006).
9. Chronic alcohol exposure causes impaired wound healing and enhanced host susceptibility to infections. Wounds from trauma in the presence of acute alcohol exposure have a higher rate of postinjury infection due to decreased neutrophil recruitment and phagocytic function (Guo & DiPietro, 2010).

BRADEN SCALE FOR PREDICTING PRESSURE SORE RISK

Patient's Name ______________ Evaluator's Name ______________________ Date of Assessment ________

SENSORY PERCEPTION ability to respond meaningfully to pressure-related discomfort

1. Completely Limited
Unresponsive (does not moan, flinch, or grasp) to painful stimuli, due to diminished level of consciousness or sedation OR limited ability to feel pain over most of body.

2. Very Limited
Responds only to painful stimuli. Cannot communicate discomfort except by moaning or restlessness OR has a sensory impairment which limits the ability to feel pain or discomfort over ½ of body.

3. Slightly Limited
Responds to verbal commands, but cannot always communicate discomfort or the need to be turned OR has some sensory impairment which limits ability to feel pain or discomfort in 1 or 2 extremities.

4. No Impairment
Responds to verbal commands. Has no sensory deficit which would limit ability to feel or voice pain or discomfort.

MOISTURE degree to which skin is exposed to moisture

1. Constantly Moist
Skin is kept moist almost constantly by perspiration, urine, etc. Dampness is detected every time patient is moved or turned.

2. Very Moist
Skin is often, but not always moist. Linen must be changed at least once a shift.

3. Occasionally Moist
Skin is occasionally moist, requiring an extra linen change approximately once a day.

4. Rarely Moist
Skin is usually dry, linen only requires changing at routine intervals.

ACTIVITY degree of physical activity

1. Bedfast
Confined to bed.

2. Chairfast
Ability to walk severely limited or non-existent. Cannot bear own weight and/or must be assisted into chair or wheelchair.

3. Walks Occasionally
Walks occasionally during day, but for very short distances, with or without assistance. Spends majority of each shift in bed or chair.

4. Walks Frequently
Walks outside room at least twice a day and inside room at least once every two hours during waking hours.

MOBILITY ability to change and control body position

1. Completely Immobile
Does not make even slight changes in body or extremity position without assistance.

2. Very Limited
Makes occasional slight changes in body or extremity position but unable to make frequent or significant changes independently.

3. Slightly Limited
Makes frequent though slight changes in body or extremity position independently.

4. No Limitation
Makes major and frequent changes in position without assistance.

NUTRITION usual food intake pattern

1. Very Poor
Never eats a complete meal. Rarely eats more than ⅓ of any food offered. Eats 2 servings or less of protein (meat or dairy products) per day. Takes fluids poorly. Does not take a liquid dietary supplement OR is NPO and/or maintained on clear liquids or IVs for more than 5 days.

2. Probably Inadequate
Rarely eats a complete meal and generally eats only about ½ of any food offered. Protein intake includes only 3 servings of meat or dairy products per day. Occasionally will take a dietary supplement OR receives less than optimum amount of liquid diet or tube feeding.

3. Adequate
Eats over half of most meals. Eats a total of 4 servings of protein (meat, dairy products) per day. Occasionally will refuse a meal, but will usually take a supplement when offered OR is on a tube feeding or TPN regimen which probably meets most of nutritional needs.

4. Excellent
Eats most of every meal. Never refuses a meal. Usually eats a total of 4 or more servings of meat and dairy products. Occasionally eats between meals. Does not require supplementation.

FRICTION & SHEAR

1. Problem
Requires moderate to maximum assistance in moving. Complete lifting without sliding against sheets is impossible. Frequently slides down in bed or chair, requiring frequent repositioning with maximum assistance. Spasticity, contractures or agitation leads to almost constant friction.

2. Potential Problem
Moves feebly or requires minimum assistance. During a move skin probably slides to some extent against sheets, chair, restraints or other devices. Maintains relatively good position in chair or bed most of the time but occasionally slides down.

3. No Apparent Problem
Moves in bed and in chair independently and has sufficient muscle strength to lift up completely during move. Maintains good position in bed or chair.

Total Score ____________

Scoring: The Braden Scale is a summated rating scale made up of six subscales scored from 1-3 or 4, for total scores that range from 6-23. A lower Braden Scale Score indicates a lower level of functioning and, therefore, a higher level of risk for pressure ulcer development. A score of 19 or higher, for instance, would indicate that the patient is at low risk, with no need for treatment at this time. The assessment can also be used to evaluate the course of a particular treatment.

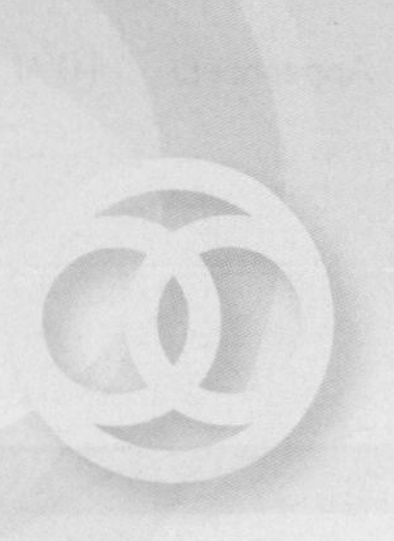

Bibliography

Author's Notes

Classic publications are designated with an asterisk (*)

Citations listed under the general category are used throughout the book

GENERAL REFERENCES

American Nurses Association. (2012). *ANA social policy statement.* Washington, DC: Author.

American Psychiatric Association. (2014). *DSMV: Diagnostic and statistical manual of mental disorders* (4th ed., text revision). Washington, DC: Author.

Alfaro-Lefevre, R. (2014). *Applying nursing process: The foundation for clinical reasoning* (8th ed.). Philadelphia: Wolters Kluwer.

Andrews, M., & Boyle, J. (2012). *Transcultural concepts in nursing* (8th ed.). Philadelphia: Lippincott Williams & Wilkins.

Arcangelo, V. P., & Peterson, A. (2016). *Pharmacotherapeutics for advanced practice* (4th ed.). Philadelphia: Wolters Kluwer.

Barnsteiner, J., Disch, J., & Walton, M. K. (2014). *Person and family-centered care*. Indianapolis, IN: Sigma Theta Tau International.

Boyd, M. A. (2012). *Psychiatric nursing: Contemporary practice* (5th ed.). Philadelphia: Lippincott Williams & Wilkins.

Carpenito, L. J. (1986). *Nursing diagnosis: Application to clinical practice*. Philadelphia: Lippincott Williams & Wilkins.

Carpenito, L. J. (1989). *Nursing diagnosis: Application to clinical practice* (3rd ed.). Philadelphia: Lippincott Williams & Wilkins.

Carpenito, L. J. (1995). *Nurse practitioner and physician discipline specific expertise in primary care*. Unpublished manuscript.

Carpenito, L. J. (1999). *Nursing diagnosis: Application to clinical practice* (5th ed.). Philadelphia: Lippincott Williams & Wilkins.

Carpenito-Moyet, L. J. (2007). *Understanding the nursing process: Concept mapping and care planning for students*. Philadelphia: Lippincott Williams & Wilkins.

Carpenito-Moyet, L. J. (2010a). Teaching nursing diagnosis to increase utilization after graduation. *International Journal of Nursing Terminologies and Classifications, 21*(10), 124–133.

Carpenito-Moyet, L. J. (2014). *Nursing care plans/Transitional patient & family centered care* (6th ed.). Philadelphia: Wolters Kluwer.

Carpenito-Moyet, L. J. (2016). *Handbook of nursing diagnoses* (15th ed.). Philadelphia: Wolters Kluwer.

Centers for Disease Control and Prevention (CDC). (2015a). *Vaccines & immunizations*. Retrieved from www.cdc.gov/vaccines/

CDC. (2015b). *Sexually transmitted diseases* (STDS). Retrived from www.cdc.gov/std/

*Clemen-Stone, E., Eigasti, D. G., & McGuire, S. L. (2001). *Comprehensive family and community health nursing* (6th ed.). St. Louis, MO: Mosby-Year Book.

Coulter, A. (2012). Patient engagement—What works? *Ambulatory Care Manage, 35*(2), 80–89.

*Cunningham, R. S., & Huhmann, M. B. (2011). Nutritional disturbances. In C. H. Yarbro, D. Wujcik, & B. H. Gobel (Eds.), *Cancer nursing: Principles and practice* (7th ed.). Boston: Jones and Bartlett.

DeWalt, D. A., Callahan, L., Hawk, V. H,. Broucksou, K. A., & Hink, A. (2010). *Health literacy universal precautions tool kit* (Prepared by North Carolina Network Consortium, The Cecil G. Sheps Center for Health Services Research, The University of North Carolina at Chapel Hill, under Contract No. HHSA290200710014.) AHRQ Publication No. 10-0046-EF). Rockville, MD: Agency for Healthcare Research and Quality. Retrieved from www.ahrq.gov/professionals/quality-patient-safety/quality-resources/tools/literacy-toolkit/healthliteracytoolkit.pdf

Dudek, S. (2014). *Nutrition essentials for nursing practice* (7th ed.). Philadelphia: Wolters Kluwer.

Edelman, C. L., & Mandle, C. L. (2010). *Health promotion throughout the life span* (7th ed.). St. Louis, MO: Mosby-Year Book.

Giger, J. (2013). *Transcultural nursing: Assessment and intervention* (6th ed.). St. Louis, MO: Mosby-Year Book.

*Gordon, M. (1982). Historical perspective: The National Group for Classification of Nursing Diagnoses. In M. J. Kim & D. A. Moritz (Eds.), *Classification of nursing diagnoses: Proceedings of the fourth national conference.* New York: McGraw-Hill.

Grossman, S., & Porth, C. A. (2014). *Porth's pathophysiology: Concepts of altered health states* (9th ed.). Philadelphia: Wolters Kluwer.

Halter, M. J. (2014). *Varcarolis' foundations of psychiatric mental health nursing* (7th ed.). Philadelphia: W. B. Saunders.

Herdman, H., & Kamitsuru, S. (Eds.). (2014). *Nursing diagnoses/definitions and classification 2015–2017*. Ames, IA: Wiley Blackwell.

Hibbard, J. H., & Greene, J. (2013). What the evidence shows about patient activation: better health outcomes and care experiences; fewer data on costs. *Health Affairs, 32*(2), 207–214.

Hickey, J. (2014). *The clinical practice of neurological and neurosurgical nursing* (5th ed.). Philadelphia: Wolters Kluwer.

Hockenberry, M. J., & Wilson, D. (2015). *Wong's essentials of pediatric nursing* (10th ed.). New York: Elsevier.

Jenny, J. (1987). Knowledge deficit: Not a nursing diagnosis image. *The Journal of Nursing Scholarship, 19*(4), 184–185.

Joint Commission. (2010). *Achieving effective communication, cultural competence, and patient-family-centered care: A roadmap for hospitals*. Oakbrook Terrace, IL: Author.

Labs on Line. (2014). Retrieved from https://labtestsonline.org/

Lutz, C., Mazur, R., & Litch, N. (2015). *Nutrition and diet therapy*. Philadelphia: F.A. Davis.

Lutz, C., & Przytulski, K. (2011). *Nutrition and diet therapy* (5th e d.). Philadelphia: FA Davis.

Miller, C. (2015). *Nursing for wellness in older adults* (7th ed.). Philadelphia: Wolters Kluwer.

Morse, J. M. (1997). *Preventing patient falls*. Thousand Oaks: Sage Broda.

*Murray, R. B., Zentner, J. P., & Yakimo, R. (2009). *Health promotion strategies through the life span* (8th ed.). Upper Saddle River, NJ: Pearson Prentice Hall.

*National Association of Adult Literacy. (2003). *Health literacy of America's adults: Results of the National Assessment of Adult Literacy (NAAL)*. Retrieved from https://nces.ed.gov/naal/

*Norris, J., & Kunes-Connell, M. (1987). Self-esteem disturbance: A clinical validation study. In A. McLane (Ed.), *Classification of nursing diagnoses: Proceedings of the seventh NANDA national conference*. St. Louis, MO: C. V. Mosby.

*North American Nursing Diagnosis Association. (2002). *Nursing diagnosis: Definitions and classification 2001–2002*. Philadelphia: Author.

Pasero, C., Paice, J., & McCaffery, M. (2010). Basic mechanisms underlying the causes and effects of pain. In M. McCaffery & C. Pasero (Eds.), *Clinical pain manual* (pp. 15–34). New York: Mosby.

Pillitteri, A. (2014). *Maternal and child health nursing* (7th ed.). Philadelphia: Wolters Kluwer.

Procter, N., Hamer, H., McGarry, D., Wilson, R., & Froggatt, T. (2014). *Mental health: A person-centered approach*. Sydney: Cambridge Press.

*Ratzan, S. C. (2001). Health literacy: Communication for the public good. *Health Promotion International, 16*(2), 207–214.

Soussignan, R., Jiang, T., Rigaud, D., Royet, J., & Schaal, B. (2010). Subliminal fear priming potentiates negative facial reactions to food pictures in women with anorexia nervosa. *Psychological Medicine, 40*(3), 503–514. Retrieved from ProQuest Health and Medical Complete (Document ID: 1961359321).

Underwood, P. W. (2012). Social support. In V. H. Rice (Ed.), *Handbooks of stress, coping and health* (2nd ed.). Thousand Oaks, CA: SAGE Publications.

Varcarolis, E. M. (2011). *Manual of psychiatric nursing care planning* (4th ed.). St. Louis, MO: Saunders.

Varcarolis, E. M., & Halter, M. J. (2010). *Foundations of psychiatric mental health nursing* (6th ed.). Philadelphia: W. B. Saunders.

Weiss, B. D. (2007). *Health literacy and patient safety: Help patients understand*. Retrieved from http://med.fsu.edu/userFiles/file/ahec_health_clinicians_manual.pdf. American Medical Association.

*White, S., & Dillow, S. (2005). Key concepts and features of the 2003 National Assessment of adult literacy. National Center for Education Statistics. Retrieved from http://nces.ed.gov/NAAL/PDF/2006471.PDF.

Yarbro, C., Wujcik, D., & Gobel, B. (2013). *Cancer nursing: Principles and practice* (17th ed.). Boston: Jones & Bartlett.

SECTION I: THE FOCUS OF NURSING CARE

Agency for Healthcare Research and Quality. (2010). *2009 national healthcare quality report*. AHRQ Publication No. 10-0003. Rockville, MD. Retrieved August 2010, from www.ahrq.gov/qual/nhqr09/nhqr09.pdf

*Bulechek, G., & McCloskey, J. C. (1985). *Nursing interventions: Treatments for nursing diagnoses*. Philadelphia: J. P. Lippincott.

*Bulechek, G., & McCloskey, J. (1989). Nursing interventions: Treatments for nursing diagnoses. In R. M. Carroll-Johnson (Ed.), Classification of nursing diagnoses: Proceedings of the eighth national conference. Philadelphia: J. B. Lippincott.

Buerhaus, P. I., Staiger, D. O., & Auerbach, D. I. (2009). The future of the nursing workforce in the United States: Data, trends and implications. Boston, MA: Jones & Bartlett Publishers.

*Carlson-Catalano, J. (1998). Nursing diagnoses and interventions for post-Acute-phase battered women. *International Journal of Nursing Terminologies and Classifications, 9*(3), 101–110.

Carpenito-Moyet, L. J. (2016). *Handbook of Nursing Diagnoses* (15th ed.). Philadelphia: Wolters Kluwer.

Carpenito-Moyet, L. J. (2017). *Nursing Care Plans: Transitional and Family Centered Care Plans* (7th ed.). Philadelphia: Wolters Kluwer.

Centers for Medical and Medicaid Services (CMS). (2008). *Roadmap for implementing value driven healthcare in the traditional medicare fee for service program*. Retrieved July 25, 2013 from www.cms.gov/QualityInitiativesGenInfo/downloads/VBPRoadmap_QEA_1_16_508.pdf

*Cornish, P. L., Knowles, S. R., Marchesano, R., Tam, V., Shadowitz, S., Juurlink, D. N., & Etchells, E. E. (2005). Unintended medication discrepancies at the time of hospital admission. *Archives of Internal Medicine, 165*(4), 424–429.

Edelman, C. L., Kudzma, E. C., & Mandle, C. L. (2014). *Health promotion throughout the life span* (8th ed.). St. Louis: CV Mosby.

*Henderson, U., & Nite, G. (1960). *Principles and practice of nursing* (5th ed.). New York: Macmillan.

Leonardi, B. C., Faller, M., Siroky, K. (2011). *Preventing never events/evidence-based practice* (White Paper). San Diego, CA: AMN Healthcare. Retrieved July 24, 2013, from http://amnhealthcare.com/uploadedFiles/MainSite/Content/Healthcare_Industry_Insights/Healthcare_News/Never_Events_white_paper_06.16.11.pdf

*McCourt, A. (1991). Syndromes in nursing. In Carroll-Johnson RM (Ed.), *Classification of nursing diagnoses: Proceedings of the ninth NANDA national conference*. Philadelphia: J.B. Lippincott.

National Conference of NANDA International in Miami (November, 2008).

North American Nursing Diagnosis Association. (2009). *Nursing diagnoses: Definitions and Classifications 2009–2010*. Ames, IA: Wiley-Blackwell.

North American Nursing Diagnosis Association. (2012). *Nursing diagnoses: Definitions and Classifications 2012–2014*. Ames, IA: Wiley-Blackwell.

Shreve, J., Van Den Bos, J., Gray, T., Halford, M., Rustagi, K., & Ziemkiewicz, E. (2010). *The economic measurement of medical errors*. Sponsored & Published by Society of Actuaries' Health Section and Sponsored by Milliman, Inc. Retrieved from www.soa.org/files/pdf/research-econ-measurement.pdf

*Wallace, D., & Ivey, J. (1989). The bifocal clinical nursing model: Descriptions and application to patients receiving thrombolytic or anticoagulant therapy. *Journal of Cardiovascular Nursing*, *4*(1), 33–45.

SECTION 2, PART 1: INDIVIDUAL NURSING DIAGNOSES

Activity Intolerance

*Balfour, I. C. (1991). Pediatric cardiac rehabilitation. *American Journal of Diseases of Children*, *145*, 627–630.

Bauldoff, G. S. (2015). When breathing is a burden: How to help patients with COPD. *American Nurse Today*, *10*(2).

*Bauldoff, G., Hoffman, L., Sciurba, F., & Zullo, T. (1996). Home based upper arm exercises training for patients with chronic obstructive pulmonary disease. *Heart and Lung*, *25*(4), 288–294.

*Breslin, E. H. (1992). Dyspnea-limited response in chronic obstructive pulmonary disease: Reduced unsupported arm activities. *Rehabilitation Nursing*, *17*, 12–20.

Centers for Disease Control and Prevention. (2014). *Smoking and COPD*. Atlanta, GA: Author. Retrieved from www.cdc.gov/tobacco/campaign/tips/diseases/copd.html

*Cohen, J., Gorenberg, B., & Schroeder, B. (2000). A study of functional status among elders at two academic nursing centers. *Home Care Provider*, *5*(3), 108–112.

COPD Foundation. (2015). *Breathing techniques*. Washington, DC: Author. Retrieved from www.copdfoundation.org/What-is-COPD/Living-with-COPD/Breathing-Techniques.aspx

*Day, M. J. (1984). 40 years of development in diagnostic imaging. *Physics in Medicine and Biology*, *29*(2), 121–125.

*Fleg, J. L. (1986). Alterations in cardiovascular structure and function with advancing age. *American Journal of Cardiology*, *5*(7), 33C–44C.

*Garrett, K., Lauer, K., & Christopher, B. A. (2004). The effects of obesity on the cardiopulmonary system: Implications for critical care nursing. *Progress in Cardiovascular Nursing*, *19*(4), 155–161.

*Haskell, W. L., Lee, I. M., Pate, R. R., Powell, K. E., Blair, S. N., Franklin, B. A., . . . Bauman, A. (2007). Physical activity and public health: Updated recommendation for adults from the American College of Sports Medicine and the American Heart Association. *Circulation*, *116*(9), 1081.

Hogan, C. L., Mata, J., & Castensen, L. L. (2013). Exercise holds immediate benefits for affect and cognition in younger and older adults. *Psychology of Aging*, *28*(2), 587–594.

La Gerche, A., Robberecht, C., & Kuiperi, C. (2010). Lower than expected desmosomal gene mutation prevalence in endurance athletes with complex ventricular arrhythmias of right ventricular origin. *Heart*, *96*(16), 1268–1274.

Longmuir, P. E., Brothers, J. A., de Ferranti, S. D., Hayman, L. L., Van Hare, G. F., Matherne, G. P., . . .American Heart Association Atherosclerosis, Hypertension and Obesity in Youth Committee of the Council on Cardiovascular Disease in the Young. (2013). Promotion of physical activity for children and adults with congenital heart disease: A scientific statement from the American Heart Association. *Circulation*, *127*, 2147–2159.

McAfee, T., Davis, K. C., Alexander, R. L., Jr., Pechacek, T. F., & Bunnell, R. (2013). Effect of the first federally funded U.S. antismoking national media campaign. *The Lancet*, *9909*, 1857–2038. Retrieved from www.thelancet.com/pdfs/journals/lancet/PIIS0140-6736(13)61686-4.pdf

National Institute of Health and Care Excellence. (2010). *Prevention of cardiovascular disease*. NICE Public Health Guidance 23. Retrieved from www.nice.org.uk/

O'Keefe, J. H., Patil, H. R., Lavie, C. J., Magalski, A., Vogel, R. A., & McCullough, P. A. (2012). Potential adverse cardiovascular effects from excessive endurance exercise. *Mayo Clinical Proceedings*, *87*(6), 587–595.

*Punzal, P. A., Ries, A. L., Kaplan, R. M., & Prewitt, L. M. (1991). Maximum intensity exercise training in patients with chronic obstructive pulmonary disease. *Chest*, *100*, 618–623.

Reilly, J., & Kelly, J. (2011). Long-term impact of overweight and obesity in childhood and adolescence on morbidity and premature mortality in adulthood: Systematic review. *International Journal of Obesity*, *35*, 891–898.

*Sciamanna, C. N., Hoch, J. S., Duke, G. C., Fogle, M. N., & Ford, D. E. (2000). Comparison of five measures of motivation to quit smoking among a sample of hospitalized smokers. *Journal of General Internal Medicine*, *15*(1), 16–23.

*Scott, L. D., Setter-Kline, K., & Britton, A. S. (2004). The effects of nursing interventions to enhance mental health and quality of life among individuals with heart failure. *Applied Nursing Research*, *17*(4), 248–256.

*Stiller, K. (2007). Safety issues that should be considered when mobilizing critically ill patients. *Critical Care Clinics*, *23*(1), 35–53.

Zomorodi, M., Darla Topley, D., & McAnaw, M. (2012). Developing a mobility protocol for early mobilization of patients in a surgical/trauma ICU critical research and practice. Critical *Care Research and Practice*, *2012*. Retrieved from www.hindawi.com/journals/ccrp/2012/964547/

Risk for Adverse Reaction to Iodinated Contrast Media

American College of Radiology Committee on Drugs and Contrast Media. (2013). *ACR manual on contrast media: Version 9*. Reston, VA: American College of Radiology. Retrieved from www.acr.org/quality-%20safety/resources/~/media/37D84428BF1D4E1B9A3A2918DA9E27A3.pdf/

*Maguire, D., Walsh, J. C., & Little, C. L. (2004). The effect of information and behavioral training on endoscopy patient's clinical outcomes. *Patient Education Counsel*, *54*(1), 61–65.

Pasternak, J., & Williamson, E. (2012). Clinical pharmacology, uses, and adverse reactions of iodinated contrast agents: A primer for the non-radiologist. *Mayo Clinical Proceedings*, *87*(4), 390–402. Retrieved from www.ncbi.nlm.nih.gov/pmc/articles/PMC3538464/

Robbins, J. B., & Pozniak, M. A. (2010). *Contrast media tutorial*. Retrieved from www.radiology.wisc.edu/fileShelf/contrastCorner/files/ContrastAgentsTutorial.pdf

Siddiqi, N. (2011). Contrast medium reactions. In *Medscape*. Retrieved from http://emedicine.medscape.com/article/422855-overview

Siddiqi, N. (2015). Contrast medium reactions. In *Medscape*. Retrieved from http://emedicine.medscape.com/article/422855-overview

Singh, J., & Daftary, A. (2008). Iodinated contrast media and their adverse reactions. *Journal of Nuclear Medicine Technology, 36*(2), 69–74.

Risk for Allergy Response

Asthma and Allergy Foundation of America. (2011). *Reducing allergens in the home: A room-by-room guide*. Retrieved from msdh.ms.gov/msdhsite/_static/resources/2111.pdf

Burks, W. (2014). Patient information: Food allergy symptoms and diagnosis (beyond the basics). In *UpToDate*. Retrieved from www.uptodate.com/contents/food-allergy-symptoms-and-diagnosis-beyond-the-basics

Mayo Clinic Staff. (2011). *Allergy-proof your house*. Retrieved from www.mayoclinic.com/health/allergy/HQ01514

Porth, C. M., Gaspard, K. J., & Noble, K. A. (2010). *Essentials of pathophysiology: Concepts of altered health states*. Philadelphia: Lippincott Williamson and Wilkins.

Anxiety

Alici, Y., & Levin, T. T. (2010). Anxiety disorders. In *Psycho-oncology* (2nd ed.). New York: Oxford University Press.

Berger, A. M., Shuster, J. L., & Von Roenn, J. (Eds.). (2013). *Principles and practice of palliative care and supportive oncology* (4th ed.). Philadelphia: Wolters Kluwer.

*Blanchard, C. M., Courneya, K. S., & Laing, D. (2001). Effects of acute exercise on state anxiety in breast cancer survivors. *Oncology Nursing Forum, 28*(10), 1617–1621.

Blay, S. L., & Marinho, V. (2012). Anxiety disorders in old age. *Current Opinion in Psychiatry, 25*(6), 462–467. doi:10.1097/YCO.0b013e3283578cdd

*Brant, J. M. (1998). The art of palliative care: Living with hope, dying with dignity. *Oncology Nursing Forum, 25*(6), 995–1004.

Campbell, T. C. (2008). Communication and palliative care in head and neck cancer. In P. M. Harari, N. P. Connor, & C. Grau, (Eds.), *Functional preservation and quality of life in head and neck radiotherapy* (pp. 299–306). New York: Springer.

Centers for Disease Control and Prevention. (2013). *Adult participation in aerobic and muscle-strengthening physical activities*. Morbidity and Mortality Weekly Report. Retrieved from www.cdc.gov/mmwr/preview/mmwrhtml/mm6217a2.htm

*Clover, A., Browne, J., MsErwin, F., & Vanderberg, B. (2001). Patient approaches to clinical conversations in palliative care. *Journal of Advanced Nursing, 48*(4), 33–41.

Coombs-Lee, B. (2008). Washington "Death with Dignity Act", Initiative 1000. Retrieved from http://endoflifewa.org/wp-content/uploads/2012/11/DOH-FAQ.pdf

*Courts, N. F., Barba, B. E., & Tesh, A. (2001). Family caregivers attitudes towards aging, caregiving, and nursing home placement. *Journal of Gerontological Nursing, 27*(8), 44–52.

*Grainger, R. (1990). Anxiety interrupters. *American Journal of Nursing, 90(2)*, 14–15.

*Grealish, L., Lomasney, A., & Whiteman, B. (2000). Foot massage. A nursing intervention to modify the distressing symptoms of pain and nausea in patients hospitalized with cancer. *Cancer Nursing, 23*, 237–243.

*Hunt, B., & Rosenthal, D. (2000). Rehabilitation counselors' experiences with client death and death anxiety. *Journal of Rehabilitation, 66*(4), 44–50.

*Jones, P. E., & Jakob, D. F. (1984). Anxiety revisited from a practice perspective. In M. J. Kim, G. K. McFarland, & A. M. McLane (Eds.), *Classification of nursing diagnoses: Proceedings of the fifth national conference*. St. Louis, MO: C. V. Mosby.

*Lehrner, J., Marwinski, G., Lehr, S., Johren, P., & Deecke, L. (2005). Ambient odors of orange and lavender reduce anxiety and improve mood in a dental office. *Physiology & Behavior, 86*(1–2), 92–95.

*Lugina, H. I., Christensson, K., Massawe, S., Nystrom, L., & Lindmark, G. (2001). Change in maternal concerns during the 6 weeks postpartum period: A study of primiparous mothers in Dar es Salaam, Tanzania. *Journal of Midwifery and Women's Health, 46*(4), 248–257.

*Lyon, B. L. (2002). Cognitive self-care skills: A model for managing stressful lifestyles. *Nursing Clinics of North America, 37*(2), 285–294.

*Matzo, M., & Sherman, D. W. (2001). Palliative care: Quality care at the end of life. New York: Springer.

*May, R. (1977). *The meaning of anxiety*. New York: W. W. Norton.

*Maynard, C. K. (2004). Assess and manage somatization. *Holistic Nursing Practice, 18*(2), 54–60.

McCann, C. M., Beddoe, E., McCormick, K., Huggard, P., Kedge, S., Adamson, C., & Huggard, J. (2013). Resilience in the health professions: A review of recent literature. *International Journal of Wellbeing, 3*(1), 60–81. doi:10.5502/ijw.v3i1.4

*McCreight, B. S. (2004). A grief ignored: Narratives of pregnancy loss from a male perspective. *Sociology of Health and Illness, 26*(3), 326–350.

*Mok, E., & Woo, C. P. (2004). The effects of slow-stroke back massage on anxiety and shoulder pain in elderly stroke patients. *Complementary Therapy Nurse Midwifery, 10*(4), 209–216.

Peters, L., Cant, R., & Payne, S. (2013). How death anxiety impacts nurses' caring for patients at the end of life: A review of literature. *Open Nursing Journal*, 7, 14–21.

*Singer, L. T., Salvator, A., Guo, S., Collin, M., Lilien, L., & Baley, J. (1999). Maternal psychological distress and parenting stress after the birth of a very low-birth-weight infant. *JAMA, 281*(9), 799–805.

*Stephenson, N. L., Weinrich, S. P., & Tavakoli, A. S. (2000). The effects of foot reflexology on anxiety and pain in patients with breast and lung cancer. *Oncology Nursing Forum, 27*, 67–72.

*Tarsitano, B. P. (1992). Structured preoperative teaching. In G. Bulechek & J. McCloskey (Eds.), *Nursing interventions: Essential nursing interventions*. Philadelphia: W. B. Saunders.

*Taylor-Loughran, A., O'Brien, M., LaChapelle, R., & Rangel, S. (1989). Defining characteristics of the nursing diagnoses fear and anxiety: A validation study. *Applied Nursing Research, 2*, 178–186.

*Tusaie, K., & Dyer, J. (2004). Resilience: A historical review of construct. *Holistic Nursing Practice, 18*(1), 3–8.

Varcarolis, N., Carson, V. B., & Shoemaker, N. (2005). *Foundations of psychiatric mental health nursing: A clinical approach* (4th ed.). Philadelphia: Saunders.

Videbeck, S. L. (2014). *Psychiatric-mental health nursing* (6th ed.). Philadelphia: Wolters Kluwer.

Volker, D. L., & Wu, H. (2011). *Death anxiety* reduction as the result of exposure to a *death* and dying symposium. *Omega: Journal of Death and Dying, 14*, 323–328.

*Whitley, G. (1994). Concept analysis in nursing diagnosis research. In R. Carroll-Johnson & M. Paquette (Eds.), *Classification of nursing diagnosis: Proceedings of the tenth conference.* Philadelphia: J. B. Lippincott.

*Wong, H. L. C., Lopez-Nahas, V., & Molassiotis, A. (2001). Effects of music therapy on anxiety in ventilator dependent patients. *Heart Lung Journal of Acute Critical Care, 30*(5), 376–387.

Yakimo, R. (2008). Mental health promotion of the young and middle-aged adult. In M. A. Boyd (Ed.), *Psychiatric nursing: Contemporary perspectives* (4th ed.). Philadelphia: Lippincott.

*Yilmaz, E., Ozcan, S., Basar, M., Basar, H., Batislam, E., & Ferhat, M. (2003). Music decreases anxiety and provides sedation in extracorporeal shock wave lithotripsy. *Urology, 61*(2), 282–286.

Yochim, B. P., Mueller, A. E., June, A., & Segal, D. L. (2011). Psychometric properties of the geriatric anxiety scale: Comparison to the beck anxiety inventory and geriatric anxiety inventory. *Clinical Gerontologist, 34*, 21–33.

*Yokom, C. J. (1984). The differentiation of fear and anxiety. In M. J. Kim, G. K. McFarland, & A. M. McLane (Eds.), *Classification of nursing diagnoses: Proceedings of the fifth national conference.* St. Louis, MO: C. V. Mosby.

Yun, K., Watanabe, K., & Shimojo, S. (2012). Interpersonal body and neural synchronization as a marker of implicit social interaction. *Scientific Reports, 2*, 959.

Death Anxiety

Ball, J., Bindler, R., & Cowen, K. (2015). *Principles of pediatric nursing: Caring for children* (6th ed.). Upper Saddle River, NJ: Pearson.

*Brant, J. M. (1998). The art of palliative care: Living with hope, dying with dignity. *Oncology Nursing Forum, 25*(6), 995–1004.

Braun, M., Gordon, D., & Uziely, B. (2010). Associations between oncology nurses' attitudes toward death and caring for dying patients. *Oncology Nursing Forum, 37*(1), E43–E49.

Campbell, T. C. (2008). Communication and palliative care in head and neck cancer. In P. M. Harari, N. P. Connor, & C. Grau (Eds.), *Functional preservation and quality of life in head and neck radiotherapy* (pp. 299–306). New York: Springer.

*Clover, A., Browne, J., MsErwin, F., Vanderberg, B. (2001). Patient approaches to clinical conversations in palliative care. *Journal of Advanced Nursing, 48*(4), 33–41.

Corwin, M. J., & McClain, M. (2014). Sudden unexpected infant death including SIDS: Initial management. In *UpToDate*.

Hockenberry, M. J., Wilson, D., & Winkelstein, M. L. (2013). Wong's nursing care of infants and children. New York: Elsevier.

Irwin, S., & Hirst, J. (2014). Overview of anxiety in palliative care. In *UpToDate*. Retrieved from www.uptodate.com/contents/overview-of-anxiety-in-palliative-care

*Matzo, M., & Sherman, D. W. (2001). Palliative care: Quality care at the end of life. New York: Springer.

*Nelson, K. A., Walsh, D., Behrens, C., Zhukovsky, D. S., Lipnickey, V., & Brady, D. (2000). The dying cancer patient. *Seminars in Oncology, 27*(1), 84–89.

*Singer, L. T., Salvator, A., Guo, S., Collin, M., Lilien, L., & Baley, J. (1999). Maternal psychological distress and parenting stress after the birth of a very low-birth-weight infant. *JAMA, 281*(9), 799–805.

Volker, D. L., & Wu, H. (2011). *Death anxiety* reduction as the result of exposure to a *death* and dying symposium. *Omega: Journal of Death and Dying, 14*, 323–328.

*Yakimo, R. (2008). Mental health promotion of the young and middle-aged adult. In M.A. Boyd (Ed.), *Psychiatric nursing: Contemporary perspectives* (4th ed.). Philadelphia: Lippincott Wilkins & Williams.

Yun, K., Watanabe, K., & Shimojo, S. (2012). Interpersonal body and neural synchronization as a marker of implicit social interaction. *Scientific Reports, 2*, 959.

Risk for Imbalanced Body Temperature

Daabiss, M. (2011). Physical status classification. *Indian J Anaesthesia, 55*(2), 111–115. American Society of Anesthesiologists (ASA)(2014) Physical Status (PS) Classification System. Retrieved from www.asahq.org/resources/clinical-

*DeFabio, D. C. (2000). Fluid and nutrient maintenance before, during, and after exercise. *Journal of Sports Chiropractic and Rehabilitation, 14*(2), 21–24, 42–43.

*Edwards, S. L. (1999). Hypothermia. *Professional Nurse, 14*(4), 253.

*Fallis, W. M. (2000). Oral measurement of temperature in orally intubated critical care patients: State-of-the-science review. *American Journal of Critical Care*, 9(5): 334–343.

*Giuliano, K. K., Giuliano, A. J., Scott, S. S., & MacLachlan, E. (2000). Temperature measurement in critically ill adults: A comparison of tympanic and oral methods. *American Journal of Critical Care*, 9(4), 254.

Güneş, Ü. Y., Zaybak, A., & Tamsel, S. (2008). Examining the reliability of the method used for the determination of ventrogluteal. *Cumhuriyet University School of Nursing Journal, 12*(2), 1–8.

*Güneş, U. & Zaybak, A. (2008). Does the body temperature change in older people? *Journal of Clinical Nursing, 17*(17), 2284–2287.

Moran, D. S., & Mendal, L. (2002). Core temperature measurement. *Sports Medicine, 32*(14), 879–885.

National Institutes of Health. (2010). *Hypothermia: A Cold Weather Hazard*. Retrieved from www.nia.nih.gov/health/publication/hypothermia

*Nicoll, L. H. (2002). Heat in motion: Evaluating and managing temperature. *Nursing, 32*, S12.

Noe, R. S., Jin, J. O., & Wolkin, A. F. (2012). Exposure to natural cold and heat: hypothermia and hyperthermia Medicare claims, United States, 2004–2005. *American Journal of Public Health, 102*(4), e11–e18.

*Smith, L. S. (2004). Temperature measurement in critical care adults: A comparison of thermometry and measurement routes. *Biological Research for Nursing, 6*(2), 117–125.

Smitz, S., Van de Winckel, A., & Smitz M. F. (2009). Reliability of infrared ear thermometry in the prediction of rectal temperature in older inpatients. *Journal of Clinical Nursing, 18*(3), 451–456.

Waalen, J., & Buxbaum, J. N. (2011). Is older colder or colder older? The association of age with body temperature in

18,630 individuals. *The Journals of Gerontology Series A: Biological* Sciences *and Medical Sciences*, *66*(5), 487–492.

Ineffective Thermoregulation

*Varda, K. E., & Behnke, R. S. (2000). The effect of timing of initial bath on newborn temperature. *Journal of Obstetric, Gynecologic, and Neonatal Nursing*, *29*(1), 27–32.

Bowel Incontinence

*Bliss, D. Z., Savik, K., Jung, H. J. G., Whitebird, R., & Lowry, A. (2011). Symptoms associated with dietary fiber supplementation over time in individuals with fecal incontinence. *Nursing Research*, *60*(3, Suppl), S58.

*Demata, E. U. (2000). Faecal incontinence. *Journal of Wound Care and Enterostomal Therapy*, 19(4), 6–11.

Markland, D., & Tobin, V. J. (2010). Need support and behavioural regulations for exercise among exercise referral scheme clients: The mediating role of psychological need satisfaction. *Psychology of Sport and Exercise*, *11*(2), 91–99.

Shah, B. J., Chokhavatia, S., & Rose, S. (2012). Fecal incontinence in the elderly: FAQ. *The American Journal of Gastroenterology*, *107*(11), 1635–1646.

Ineffective Breastfeeding

American Academy of Pediatrics (AAP). (2009). *Breastfeeding and the use of human milk*. Retrieved from www2.aap.org/breastfeeding/files/pdf/Breastfeeding2012ExecSum.pdf

American Academy of Pediatrics. (2012). Policy statement: Breastfeeding and the use of human milk. *Pediatrics*, *129*(3), 827–841.

Amir, L. H., & The Academy of Breastfeeding Medicine Protocol Committee. (2014). ABM clinical protocol #4: Mastitis. *Breastfeeding Medicine*, *9*(5), 293–243.

Association of Women's Health, Obstetric and Neonatal Nurses (AWHONN). (2015). *Breastfeeding*. Retrieved from http://onlinelibrary.wiley.com/enhanced/doi/10.1111/1552-6909.12530/

AZDHS. (2012). *Arizona baby steps to breastfeeding success*. Retrieved from www.azdhs.gov/phs/gobreastmilk/BFAzBabySteps.htm

BFAR. (2010). *Breastfeeding after breast and nipple surgeries*. Retrieved from http://bfar.org

Evans, A., Marinelli, K. A., Taylor, J. S., & The Academy of Breastfeeding Medicine. (2014). ABM clinical protocol #2: Guidelines for hospital discharge of the breastfeeding term newborn an mother " The going home protocol" (revised 2014). *Breastfeeding Medicine*, *9*(1), 3–8.

Hale, T. W. (2012). *Medications and mother's milk* (15th ed.). Amarillo, TX: Hale Publications.

Lawrence, R. A., & Lawrence, R. M. (2010). *Breastfeeding – A guide for the medical professional* (7th ed.). Philadelphia: Elsevier Health Services.

Riordian, J., & Wombach, K. (2009). *Breastfeeding and human lactation* (5th ed.). Sudbury, MA: Jones & Bartlett.

*Walker, M. (2006). *Breastfeeding management for the clinician: Using the evidence*. Boston: Jones and Bartlett.

Walker, M. (2013). *Breastfeeding management for the clinician: Using the evidence* (3rd ed.). Sudbury, WA: Jones & Bartlett.

Caregiver Role Strain

American Association of Retired Persons (AARP). (2009). *AARP statement to the 53rd session of the United Nations Commission on the status of women*. Retrieved from www.un.org/womenwatch/daw/ csw/53sess.htm

AARP. (2014). *About Grandfacts*. Retrieved from www.aarp.org/relationships/friends-family/grandfacts-sheets/

*Clipp, E., & George, L. (1990). Caregiver needs and patterns of social support. *Journal of Gerontology*, *45*(3), S102–S111.

Cousino, M., & Hazen, R. (2013). Parenting stress among caregivers of children with chronic illness: A systematic review *Journal of Pediatric Psychology*. Retrieved from www.researchgate.net/publication/248397943_Parenting_Stress_Among_Caregivers_of_Children_With_Chronic_Illness_A_Systematic_Review

*Dilworth-Anderson, P., Williams, I. C., & Gibson, B. E. (2002). Issues of race, ethnicity, and culture in caregiving research: A 20-year review (1980–2000). *The Gerontologist*, *42*(2), 237–272.

*Lindgren, C. (1990). Burnout and social support in family caregivers. *Western Journal of Nursing Research*, *12*, 469–481.

Luo, Y., LaPierre, T. A., Hughes, M. E., & Waite, L. J. (2012). Grandparents providing care to grandchildren a population-based study of continuity and change. *Journal of Family Issues*, *33*(9), 1143–1167.

Namkung, E. H., Greenberg, J. S., & Mailick, M. R. (2016). Well-being of sibling caregivers: Effects of Kinship relationship and race. *The Gerontologist*. Retrieved from http://gerontologist.oxfordjournals.org/content/early/2016/02/15/geront.gnw008.abstract

National Center for Health Statistics. (2015). *Summary of NCHS surveys and data collection systems*. Retrieved from www.cdc.gov/nchs/data/factsheets/factsheet_summary.htm

National Women's Health Information Center. (2011). *Woman's health USA*. Retrievd from www.mchb.hrsa.gov/whusa11/more/downloads/pdf/w11.pdf

*Pearlin, L., Mullan, J., Semple, S., & Skaff, M. (1990). Caregiving and the stress process: An overview of concepts and their measures. *The Gerontologist*, *30*, 583–594.

*Shields, C. (1992). Family interaction and caregivers of Alzheimer's disease patients: Correlates of depression. *Family Process*, *31*(3), 19–32.

Shim, B., Barroso, J., Gilliss, C. L., Davis, L. L. (2013). Finding meaning in caring for a spouse with dementia. *Applied Nursing Research*, *26*(3), 121–126. Accessed at www.ncbi.nlm.nih.gov/pubmed/23827824

Smith, M., & Segal, J. (2015). Caregiving support and help. *Helpguide.org*. Retrieved from www.helpguide.org/articles/caregiving/caregiving-support-and-help.htm

*Smith, G., Smith, M., & Toseland, R. (1991). Problems identified by family caregivers in counseling. *The Gerontologist*, *31*(1), 15–22.

*Winslow, B., & Carter, P. (1999). Patterns of burden in wives who care for husbands with dementia. *Nursing Clinics of North America*, *34*(2), 275–287.

Yahirun, J. J. (2012). Take me home: Return migration among Germany's older immigrants. *International Migration*, *52*(4), 231–254.

Impaired Comfort

American Psychiatric Association. (2014). *DSMV: Diagnostic and statistical manual of mental disorders* (4th ed., text revision). Washington, DC: Author.

American Society of Addiction Medicine. (2015). *Definition of addiction*. Retrieved from www.asam.org/for-the-public/definition-of-addiction

American Speech-Language-Hearing Association (ASH). (2014). *Augmentative and alternative communication*. Retrieved from www.asha.org/slp/clinical/

Arcangelo, V. P., & Peterson, A. (2016). *Pharmacotherapeutics for advanced practice* (4th ed.). Philadelphia: Wolters Kluwer.

Archie, P., Bruera, E., & Cohen, L. (2013). Music-based interventions in palliative cancer care: A review of quantitative studies and neurobiological literature. *Supportive Care in Cancer*, *21*(9), 2609–2624.

*Apfel, C. C., Läärä, E., Koivuranta, M., Greim, C. A., & Roewer, N. (1999). A simplified risk score for predicting postoperative nausea and vomiting conclusions from cross-validations between two centers. *The Journal of the American Society of Anesthesiologists*, *91*(3), 693–700.

Ball, J., Bindler, R., & Cowen, K. (2015). *Principles of pediatric nursing: Caring for Children* (6th ed.). Upper Saddle River, NJ: Pearson.

Barsky, A. J. (2014). Assessing somatic symptoms in clinical practice. *JAMA Internal Medicine*, *174*(3), 407.

Beebe, L. H., & Wyatt, T. H. (2009). Guided imagery and music: Using the Bonny method to evoke emotion and access the unconscious. *Journal of Psychosocial Nursing and Mental Health Services*, *47*(1), 29–33.

Bell, K., & Salmon, A. (2009). Pain, physical dependence and pseudoaddiction: Redefining addiction for 'nice' people? *International Journal of Drug Policy*, *20*(2), 170–178.

Bermas, B. (2014). Rheumatoid arthritis and pregnancy. In *UpToDate*. Retrieved from www.uptodate.com/contents/rheumatoid-arthritis-and-pregnancy

Bernhofer, E., & Sorrell, J. M. (2014). Nurses managing patients' pain may experience moral distress. *Clinical Nursing Research*. doi:10.54773814533124.

Boyd, M. A. (2012). *Psychiatric nursing: Contemporary practice* (5th ed.). Philadelphia: Lippincott Williams & Wilkins.

Brown, S. T., Kirkpatrick, M. K., Swanson, M. S., & McKenzie, I. L. (2011). Pain experience of the elderly. *Pain Management Nursing*, *12*(4), 190–196.

Campbell, C., & Edwards, R. (2012). Ethnic differences in pain and pain management. *Pain Management*, *2*(3), 219–230.

*Chang, J. T., Morton, S. C., Rubenstein, L. Z., Mojica, W. A., Maglione, M., Suttorp, M. J., … & Shekelle, P. G. (2004). Interventions for the prevention of falls in older adults: systematic review and meta-analysis of randomised clinical trials. *BMJ*, *328*(7441), 680.

D'Arcy, Y. (2008). Pain in older adults. *Nurse Practitioner*, *38*(3), 19–25.

Deandrea, S., Lucenteforte, E., Bravi, F., Foschi, R., La Vecchia, C., & Negri, E. (2010). Risk factors for falls in community-dwelling older people: A systematic review and meta-analysis. *Epidemiology*, *21*(5), 658–668.

Denny, D. L., & Guido, G. W. (2012). Undertreatment of pain in older adults: An application of beneficence. *Nursing Ethics*, *19*(6), 800–809.

*Dickson, B. E., Hay Smith, E. J. C., & Dean, S. G. (2009). Demonised diagnosis: The influence of stigma on interdisciplinary rehabilitation of somatoform disorder. *New Zealand Journal of Physiotherapy*, *37*(3), 115–121.

Doran, K., & Halm, M. A. (2010). Integrating acupressure to alleviate postoperative nausea and vomiting. *American Journal of Critical Care*, *19*(6), 553–556.

*Ezzo, J., Streitberger, K., & Schneider, A. (2006). Cochrane systematic reviews examine P6 acupuncture-point stimulation for nausea and vomiting. *Journal of Alternative and Complementary Medicine*, *12*(5), 489–495.

*Ferrell, B. R. (1995). The impact of pain on quality of life. *Nursing Clinics of North America*, *30*, 609–624.

Forouhari, S., Ghaemi, S. Z., Roshandel, A., Moshfegh, Z., Rostambeigy, P., & Mohaghegh, Z. (2014). The effect of acupressure on nausea and vomiting during pregnancy. *Researcher*, *6*(6).

*Fuchs-Lacelle, S., & Hadjistavropoulos, T. (2004). Development and preliminary validation of the pain assessment for seniors with limited ability to communicate (PACSLAC). *Pain Management Nursing*, *5*(10), 37–49.

Galicia-Castillo, M. C., Weiner, D. K. (2014). Treatment of persistent pain in older adults. In *UpToDate*. Retrieved from www.uptodate.com/contents/treatment-of-persistent-pain-in-older-adults

Greco, M. T., Roberto, A., Corli, O., Deandrea, S., Bandieri, E., Cavuto, S., & Apolone, G. (2014). Quality of cancer pain management: An update of a systematic review of undertreatment of patients with cancer. *Journal of Clinical Oncology*, *32*(36):4149–4154.

*Green, C. R. (2002). The unequal burden of pain: Confronting racial and ethnic disparities in pain. *Pain Medicine*, *4*(3), 277–294.

Greenberg, D. B. (2015). Somatization: Treatment and prognosis. In *UpToDate*. Retrieved from www.uptodate.com/contents/somatization-treatment-and-prognosis

Grossman, S., & Porth, C. A. (2014). *Porth's pathophysiology: Concepts of altered health states* (9th ed.). Philadelphia: Wolters Kluwer.

Halter, M. J. (2014). *Varcarolis' foundations of psychiatric mental health nursing* (7th ed.). Philadelphia: W. B. Saunders.

*Hayes, B. J., Craig, K. D., & Wing, P. C. (2002). Diagnostic judgment: Chronic pain syndrome, pain disorder, and malingering. *British Columbia Medical Journal*, *44*(6), 312–316. Retrieved from www.bcmj.org/article/diagnostic-judgment-chronic-pain-syndrome-pain- disorder-and-malingering

Hockenberry, M. J., & Wilson, D. (2015). *Wong's essentials of pediatric nursing* (10th ed.). New York: Elsevier.

Humphreys, J., Cooper, B. A., & Miaskowski, C. (2010). Differences in depression, posttraumatic stress disorder, and lifetime trauma exposure in formerly abused women with mild versus moderate to severe chronic pain. *Journal of Interpersonal Violence*, *25*(12), 2316–2338.

Institute of Medicine. (2011). *Relieving pain in America: A blueprint for transforming prevention, care, education, and research*. Washington, DC: National Academies Press.

Jiyeon, L., & Heeyoung, O. H. (2013). Ginger as an antiemetic modality for chemotherapy-induced nausea and vomiting: A systematic review and meta-analysis. *Oncology Nursing Forum*, *40*(2), 163–170.

Jungquist, C. R., Karan, S., Perlis, & M. L. (2011). Risk factors for opioid-induced excessive respiratory depression. *Pain Management*, *12*(3), 180–187.

*Johnson, R. E., Fudala, P. J., & Payne, R. (2005). Buprenorphine: considerations for pain management. *Journal of pain and symptom management*, *29*(3), 297–326.

*King, T., & Murphy, P. (2009). Evidence-based approaches to managing nausea and vomiting in early pregnancy. *Journal of Midwifery & Women's Health*, *54*(6), 430–444.

Kyle, T., & Carman, S. (2013). *Essentials of pediatric nursing* (2nd ed.). Philadelphia, PA: Wolters Kluwer; Lippincott Williams & Wilkins.

*Lacroix, R., Eason, E., & Melzack, R. (2000). Nausea and vomiting during pregnancy: A prospective study of its frequency, intensity, and patterns of change. *American Journal of Obstetrics and Gynecology*, *182*(4), 931–937.

*Lovering, S. (2006). Cultural attitudes and beliefs about pain. *Journal of Transcultural Nursing*, *17*(4), 389–395.

*Ludwig-Beymer, P. (1989). Transcultural aspects of pain. In M. Andrews & J. Boyle (Eds.), *Transcultural concepts in nursing*. Glenview, IL: Scott, Foresman.

McCaffery, M., & Beebe, A. (1989). *Pain: Clinical manual for nursing practice*. St. Louis: CV Mosby.

*McCaffrey, M., & Portenoy, R. (1999). Acetaminophen and nonsteroidal anti-inflammatory drugs (NSAIDs). In M. McCaffrey & Pasero, C. (Eds.), *Pain: Clinical manual* (2nd ed., pp. 129–160). New York: Mosby.

*McGuire, D., Sheidler, V., & Polomano, R. C. (2000). Pain. In S. Groenwald, M. Frogge, M. Goodman, & C. Yarbo (Eds.), *Cancer nursing: Principles and practice* (5th ed.). Boston: Jones and Bartlett.

McMenamin, E. (2011). Pain management principles. *Current Problems in Cancer*, *35*(6), 317–323.

Miller, C. (2015). *Nursing for wellness in older adults* (7th ed.). Philadelphia: Wolters Kluwer.

Mosset, J. M. (2011). Defining racial and ethnic disparities in pain management. *Clinical Orthopedics and Related Research*, *469*(7), 1859–1870.

Myers-Glower, M. (2013). Preventing complications in patients receiving opioids. *American Nurse Today*, *8*(12).

Narayan, M. C. (2010). Culture's effects on pain assessment and management. *The American Journal of Nursing*, *110*(4), 38–47. Accessed at www.nursingcenter.com/lnc/cearticle?tid=998868#sthash.VV2KzGeo.dpuf

National Cancer Institute. (2011). *Pain for health professionals*. Retrieved from www.cancer.gov/about-cancer/treatment/side-effects/pain/pain-hp-pdq

National Institute of Drug Abuse. (2007). *The neurobiology of drug addiction*. Bethesda, MD: Author. Retrieved from www.drugabuse.gov/publications/teaching-packets/neurobiology-drug-addiction/section-iii-action-heroin-morphine/8-definition-dependence

*Paice, J. A., Noskin, G. A., & Vanagunas, A. (2005). Efficacy and safety of scheduled dosing opioid analgesics: A quality improvement study. *Journal of Pain*, *6*, 639–643.

Pasero, C. (2010). Pain care around-the-clock (ATC) dosing of analgesics. *Journal of PeriAnesthesia Nursing*, *25*(1), 36–39.

Pasero, C., & McCaffery, M. (2011). *Pain assessment and pharmacologic management*. St. Louis: Mosby.

Pillitteri, A. (2014). *Maternal and child health nursing* (7th ed.). Philadelphia: Wolters Kluwer.

Portenoy, R. K., Mehta, Z., & Ahmed, E. (2015). Cancer pain management with opioids: Prevention and management of side effects. In: J. Abrahm (Ed.), *UpToDate*. Retrieved from www.uptodate.com

*Price, D. D. (1999). *Psychological mechanisms of pain and analgesia*. Seattle, WA: IASP Press.

Procter, N., Hamer, H., McGarry, D., Wilson, R.I., Frogget, T. (2014). *Mental health: A person-centered approach*. Sydney: Cambridge.

Rosenquist, E. (2015). Evaluation of chronic pain in adults. In *UpToDate*. Retrieved from www.uptodate.com/contents/evaluation-of-chronic-pain-in-adults?source=see_link§ionName=Older+adults&anchor=H15544523#H15544523

Sauls, D. J. (2004). Adolescents' perception of support during labor. *The Journal of Perinatal Education*, *13*(4), 36–42.

*Savage, S., Covington, E. C., Heit, H. A., Hunt, J., Joranson, D., & Schnoll, S. H. (2001). *Definitions related to the use of opioids for the treatment of pain:* A consensus document from the American Academy of Pain Medicine, the American Pain Society, and the American Society of Addiction Medicine. Glenview, IL: Author.

*Sherman, P.W., & Flaxman, S. M. (2002). Nausea and vomiting of pregnancy in an evolutionary perspective. *American Journal of Obstetrics and Gynecology*, *186*(5) 190–197.

Simkin, P., & Bolding, A. (2004). Update on nonpharmacologic approaches to relieve labor pain and prevent suffering. *Journal of Midwifery & Women's Health*, *49*(6), 489–504.

Singh, M. (2014). Chronic pain syndrome treatment & management. In *Medscape*. Retrieved from http://emedicine.medscape.com/article/310834-treatment

Sloan Kettering Center. (2012). Pain management. Retrieved from www.mskcc.org/cancer-care/treatments/symptom-management/palliative-care

*Sloman, R. (1995). Relaxation and relief of cancer pain. *Nursing Clinics of North America*, *30*, 697–709.

Stevens, B. J., Abbott, L. K., Yamada, J., Harrison, D., Stinson, J., Taddio, A., . . . Finley, G. A. (2011). Epidemiology and management of painful procedures in children in Canadian hospitals. *Canadian Medical Association Journal*, *183*(7), E403–E410.

*Streitberger, K., Witte, S., Mansmann, U., Knauer, C., Krämer, J., Scharf, H. P., & Victor, N. (2004). Efficacy and safety of acupuncture for chronic pain caused by gonarthrosis: a study protocol of an ongoing multi-centre randomised controlled clinical trial [ISRCTN27450856]. *BMC Complementary and Alternative Medicine*, *4*(1), 1.

Tiran, D. (2012). Ginger to reduce nausea and vomiting during pregnancy: evidence of effectiveness is not the same as proof of safety. *Complementary Therapies in Clinical Practice*, *18*(1), 22–25.

*Voda, A. M. & Randall, M. P. (1982). Nausea and vomiting of pregnancy: "Morning sickness". In: C. M. Norris (Ed.), *Concept clarification in nursing* (pp. 133–165). Aspen Systems.

*Von Korff, M., & Simon, G. (1996). The relationship between pain and depression comorbidity of mood. *The British Journal of Psychiatry*, *168*(30), 101–108.

Walter-Nicole, E., Annequin, D., Biran, V., Mitanchez, D., & Tourniaire, B. (2010). Pain management in newborns: From prevention to treatment. *Pediatric Drugs, 12*(6), 353–365.

*Weber, S. E. (1996). Cultural aspects of pain in childbearing women. *Journal of Obstetric, Gynecologic, and Neonatal Nursing, 25*(1), 67–72.

*Weisberg, J. N., & Boatwright, B. A. (2007). Mood, anxiety and personality traits and states in chronic pain. *Pain, 133*(1–3), 1–2.

World Health Organization. (2015). *Dependence syndrome.* Geneva: Author. Retrieved from www.who.int/substance_abuse/terminology/definition1/en

*Zborowski, M. (1952). Cultural components in response to pain. *Journal of Social Issues, 8*, 16–30.

Zeidan, F., Grant, J. A., Brown, C. A., McHaffie, J. G., & Coghill, R. C. (2012). Mindfulness meditation-related pain relief: evidence for unique brain mechanisms in the regulation of pain. *Neuroscience letters, 520*(2), 165–173.

Labor Pain

*Association of Women's Health, Obstetric and Neonatal Nurses (AWHONN). (2008a). *Nursing care and management of the second stage of labor: Evidence-Based Clinical Practice Guideline* (2nd ed.). Washington, DC: Author.

*Association of Women's Health, Obstetric and Neonatal Nurses (AWHONN). (2008b). *Nursing care of the woman receiving regional analgesia/anesthesia in labor: Evidence-based clinical practice guideline* (2nd ed.). Washington, DC: Author.

Association of Women's Health, Obstetric and Neonatal Nurses (AWHONN). (2011). *Nursing support of laboring women*. Position Statement. Washington, DC: Author.

Blackburn, S. T. (2013). *Maternal, fetal & neonatal physiology: A clinical perspective* (3rd ed., pp. 512–515). St. Louis: Saunders Elsevier.

Burke, C. (2014). Pain in labor: Nonpharmacologic and pharmacologic management. In K. R. Simpson & P. Creehan (Eds.), *AWHONN's perinatal nursing* (4th ed., pp. 493–529). Philadelphia: Wolters Kluwer.

Mattson, S. (2011). Ethnocultural considerations in the childbearing period. In S. Mattson & J. E. Smith (Eds), *Core Curriculum for maternal-newborn nursing* (4th ed., pp. 61–79). St. Louis: Saunders Elsevier.

*Montgomery, K. S. (2002). Nursing care for pregnant adolescents. *Journal of Obstetric, Gynecologic and Neonatal Nursing, 32*(2), 49–257.

Simkin, P., & Ancheta, R. (2011). *The labor progress book: Early interventions to prevent and treat dystocia* (3rd ed.). New York: Wiley-Blackwell.

United States Department of Health & Human Services Office of Adolescent Health. (2014). *Trends in teen pregnancy and childbearing*. Retrieved from www.hhs.gov/ash/oah/adolescent-health-topics/reproductive-health/teen-pregnancy/trends.html

Impaired Communication

*American Medical Association Ad Hoc Committee on Health Literacy for the Council on Scientific Affairs. (1999). Health literacy: Report of the concil on scientific affairs. *Journal of the American Medical Association, 281*, 552–557.

American Speech Language Hearing Association. (2014). Retrieved from www.asha.org/

*Bauman, R. A., & Gell, G. (2000). The reality of picture archiving and communication systems (PACS): A survey. *Journal Digit Imaging, 13*(4), 157–169.

Centers for Disease Prevention and Control. (2015). *Cerebrovascular disease or stroke*. Retrieved from www.cdc.gov/nchs/fastats/stroke.htm

Clark, D. (2015). Aphasia: Prognosis and treatment. In *UpToDate*. Retrieved from www.uptodate.com/contents/aphasia-prognosis-and-treatment

Davidson, B., Worrall, L., & Hickson, L. (2008). Exploring the interactional dimension of social communication: A collective case study of older people with aphasia. *Aphasiology, 22*(3), 235–257.

DeWalt, D. A., Callahan, L., Hawk, V. H,. Broucksou, K. A., & Hink, A. (2010). *Health literacy universal precautions tool kit*. Rockville, MD: Agency for Healthcare Research and Quality. Retrieved from www.ahrq.gov/professionals/quality-patient-safety/quality-resources/tools/literacy-toolkit/healthliteracytoolkit.pdf

Grossbach, I., Stranberg, S., & Chlan, L. (2011). Promoting effective communication for patients receiving mechanical ventilation. *Critical Care Nurse, 31*(3), 46–60.

Houle, L. (2010). Language barriers in health care (Unpublished Paper). Retrieved from http://digitalcommons.uri.edu/srhonorsprog/175/

Institute of Medicine (IOM). (2011). *Innovations in health literacy research: Workshop summary*. Washington DC: The National Academies Press.

Joint Committee on Infant Hearing. (2007). Year 2007 Position Statement: Principles and Guidelines for Early Hearing Detection and Intervention Programs. *Pediatrics, 120*(4), 898–921.

Khalaila, R., Zbidat, W., Anwar, K., Bayya, A., Linton, D. M., & Sviri, S. (2011). Communication difficulties and psychoemotional distress in patients receiving mechanical ventilation. *American Journal of Critical Care, 20*(6), 470–479.

*Kutner, M., Greenberg, E., Jin, Y., & Paulsen, C. (2006). *The health literacy of America's adults: Results from the 2003 National Assessment of Adult Literacy.* U.S. Dept. of Education. Washington, DC: National Center for Education Statistics. Retrieved from http://nces.ed.gov/pubs2006/2006483.pdf

Magee, W., & Baker, M. (2009). The use of music therapy in neuro-rehabilitation of people with acquired brain injury. *British Journal of Neuroscience Nursing, 5*(4), 151–156. Retrieved from CINAHL Plus with Full Text database.

McGilton, K. S., Sorin-Peters, R., Sidani, S., Boscart, V., Fox, M., & Rochon, E. (2012). Patient-centred communication intervention study to evaluate nurse-patient interactions in complex continuing care. *BMC Geriatrics, 12*(1), 61.

National Institute on Deafness and Other Communication Disorders. (2013). American sign language. Retrieved from www.nidcd.nih.gov/health/hearing/pages/asl.aspx

Office of Student Disabilities Services, University of Chicago. (2014). *Teaching students with disabilities resources for instructors 2014–2015*. Chicago, IL: Author. Retrieved from https://disabilities.uchicago.edu/sites/disabilities.uchicago.edu/files/uploads/docs/Teaching%20Students%20with%20Disabilities%20201415.pdf

*Ratzan, S. C. (2001). Health literacy: communication for the public good. *Health Promotion International, 16*(2), 207–214.

Roland, P. S., Smith, T. L., Schwartz, S. R., Rosenfeld, R. M., Ballachanda, B., Earll, J. M., . . . Krouse, H. J. (2008). Clinical practice guideline: Cerumen impaction. *Otolaryngology—Head and Neck Surgery*, *139*(3 Suppl, 1), S1–S21.

Schyve, P. M. (2007). Language differences as a barrier to quality and safety in health care: the Joint Commission perspective. *Journal of General Internal Medicine*, *22*(2), 360–361.

Singleton, K., & Krause, E. (2009). Understanding cultural and linguistic barriers to health literacy. *The Online Journal of Issues in Nursing*, *14*(3). Retrieved from www.nursingworld.org/MainMenuCategories/ANAMarketplace/ANAPeriodicals/OJIN/TableofContents/Vol142009/No3Sept09/Cultural-and-Linguistic-Barriers-.html

Speros, C. (2005). Health literacy: concept analysis. *Journal of Advanced Nursing*, *50*(6), 633–640.

*Storbeck, C., & Calvert-Evers, J. (2008). Towards integrated practices in early detection of and intervention for deaf and hard of hearing children. *American Annals of the Deaf*, *153*(3), 314–321. Retrieved from CINAHL Plus with Full Text database.

Stroke Association. (2012). Retrieved from www.stroke.org/we-can-help/healthcare-professionals/improve-your-skills/post-stroke-programs

Summers, D., Leonard, A., Wentworth, D., Saver, J. L., Simpson, J., Spilker, J. A., . . . American Heart Association Council on Cardiovascular Nursing and the Stroke Council. (2009). Comprehensive overview of nursing and interdisciplinary care of the acute ischemic stroke patient: A scientific statement from the American Heart Association. *Stroke*, *40*(8), 2911–2944.

*Williams, M. V., Parker, R. M., Baker, D. W., Parikh, N. S., Pitkin, K., Coates, W. C., & Nurss, J. R. (1995). Inadequate functional health literacy among patients at two public hospitals. *JAMA*, *274*(21), 1677–1682.

White, S. (2008). *Assessing the nation's health literacy: Key concepts and findings of the National Assessment of Adult Literacy (NAAL)*. Chicago, IL: American Medical Association Foundation.

*White, S., & Dillow, S. (2005). Key concepts and features of the 2003 National Assessment of Adult Literacy. National Center for Education Statistics. Retrieved from http://nces.ed.gov/NAAL/PDF/2006471.PDF

Confusion (Acute & Chronic)

Ahlskog, J. E., Geda, Y. E., Graff-Radford, N. R., & Petersen, R. C. (2011). Physical exercise as a preventive or disease-modifying treatment of dementia and brain aging. *Mayo Clinic Proceedings*, *86*(9), 876–884.

Aine, C. J., Sanfratello, L., Adair, J. C., Knoefel, J. E., Caprihan, A., & Stephen, J. M. (2011). Development and decline of memory functions in normal, pathological and healthy successful aging. *Brain Topography*, *24*(3/4), 323–339.

Alzheimer's Association. (2015a). Alzheimer's disease facts and figures—Includes a special report on disclosing a diagnosis of Alzheimer's Disease. *Alzheimer's & Dementia*, *11*(3), 332.

Alzheimer's Association. (2015b). Practical information/statistics. Retrieved from www.alz.org/aaic/

American Geriatrics Society. (2015a). *Clinical practice guideline for postoperative delirium in older adults*. Retrieved from http://geriatricscareonline.org/ProductAbstract/american-geriatrics-society-clinical-practice-guideline-for-postoperative-delirium-in-older-adults/CL018

American Geriatrics Society. (2015b). *Alzheimer's disease*. Retrieved from www.americangeriatrics.org/

Andreessen, L., Wilde, M. H., & Herendeen, P. (2012). Preventing catheter-associated urinary tract infections in acute care: The bundle approach. *Journal of Nursing Care Quality*, *27*(3), 209–217.

*Bamford, C., Lamont, S., Eccles, M., Robinson, L., May, C., & Bond, J. (2004). Disclosing a diagnosis of dementia: A systematic review. *International Journal of Geriatric Psychiatry*, *19*(2), 151–169.

*Bliwise, D. L., & Lee, K. A. (1993). Development of an Agitated Behavior Rating Scale for discrete temporal observations. *Journal of Nursing Measurement*, *1*(2), 115–124.

Bradford, A., Kunik, M. E., Schulz, P., Williams, S. P., & Singh, H. (2009). Missed and delayed diagnosis of dementia in primary care: prevalence and contributing factors. *Alzheimer Disease and Associated Disorders*, *23*(4), 306–314.

Caljouw, M. A., den Elzen, W. P., Cools, H. J., & Gussekloo, J. (2011). Predictive factors of urinary tract infections among the oldest old in the general population. A population-based prospective follow-up study. *BMC Medicine*, *9*(1), 57.

*Carpenter, B., & Dave, J. (2004). Disclosing a dementia diagnosis: A review of opinion and practice, and a proposed research agenda. *The Gerontologist*, *44*(2), 149–158.

Center for Medicare and Medicaid Services. (2012). *Advancing excellence in America's nursing homes*. Retrieved from www.nhqualitycampaign.org

Chatterton, W., Baker, F., & Morgan, K. (2010). The singer or the singing: Who sings individually to persons with dementia and what are the effects? *American Journal of Alzheimer's Disease and Other Dementias*, *25*(8), 641–649.

Clair, A., & Tomaino, C. (2015). *Music*. New York: Alzheimer's Foundation of America. Retrieved from www.alzfdn.org/EducationandCare/musictherapy.html

Clegg, A., Siddiqi, N., Heaven, A., Young, J., & Holt, R. (2014). Interventions for preventing delirium in older people in institutional long-term care. *Cochrane Database Systematic Review*, *1*.

Cohen-Mansfield, J., Marx, M. S., Freedman, L. S., Murad, H., Thein, K., & Dakheel-Ali, M. (2012). What affects pleasure in persons with advanced stage dementia? *Journal of Psychiatric Research*, *46*(3), 402–406.

*Dennis, H. (1984). Remotivation therapy groups. In I. M. Burnside (Ed.), *Working with the elderly group: Process and techniques* (2nd ed.). Monterey, CA: Jones & Bartlett.

Deschodt, M., Braes, T., Flamaing, J., Detroyer, E., Broos, P., Haentjens, P., . . . Milisen, K. (2012). Preventing delirium in older adults with recent hip fracture through multidisciplinary geriatric consultation. *Journal of the American Geriatrics Society*, *60*(4), 733–739.

Farlow, M. R. (2015). *Clinical features and diagnosis of dementia with Lewy bodies*. Retrieved from www.uptodate.com/contents/clinical-features-and-diagnosis-of-dementia-with-lewy-bodies

Francis, J., & Young, B. (2014). Diagnosis of delirium and confusional states. In *UpToDate*. Retrieved from www.uptodate.com/contents/diagnosis-of-delirium-and-confusional-states

*Foreman, M. D., Mion, L. C., Tyrostad, L., & Flitcher, K. (1999). Standard of practice protocol: Acute confusion/delirium. *Geriatric Nursing, 20*(3), 147–152.

*Gerdner, L. (1999). Individualized music intervention protocol. *Journal of Gerontological Nursing, 25*(10), 10–16.

Gibson, A. K., & Anderson, K. A. (2011). Difficult diagnoses: Family caregivers' experiences during and following the diagnostic process for dementia. *American journal of Alzheimer's Disease and Other Dementias, 26*(3):212–217.

Godfrey, M., Smith, J., Green, J., Cheater, F., Inouye, S. K., & Young, J. B. (2013). Developing and implementing an integrated delirium prevention system of care: A theory driven, participatory research study. *BMC Health Services Research, 13*(1), 1.

*Haffmans, P. M., Sival, R. C., Lucius, S. A., Cats, Q., & van Gelder, L. (2001). Bright light therapy and melatonin in motor restless behaviour in dementia: A placebo-controlled study. *International Journal of Geriatric Psychiatry, 16*(1), 106–110.

*Hall, G. R. (1991). Altered thought processes: Dementia. In M. Maas, K. Buckwalter, & M. Hardy (Eds.), *Nursing diagnoses and interventions for the elderly.* Menlo Park, CA: Addison-Wesley.

*Hall, G. R. (1994). Caring for people with Alzheimer's disease using the conceptual model of progressively lowered stress threshold in the clinical setting. *Nursing Clinics of North America, 29,* 129–141.

*Hall, G. R., & Buckwalter, K. C. (1987). Progressively lowered stress threshold: A conceptual model for care of adults with Alzheimer's disease. *Archives of Psychiatric Nursing, 1,* 399–406.

Harvard School of Public Health. (2011). *Value of knowing—Research.* Luxembourg: Alzheimer Europe. Retrieved from www.alzheimer-europe.org/Research/Value-of-knowing

Hattori, H., Hattori, C., Hokao, C., Mizushima, K., & Mase, T. (2011). Controlled study on the cognitive and psychological effect of coloring and drawing in mild Alzheimer's disease patients. *Geriatrics & Gerontology International, 11*(4), 431–437.

Hulme, C., Wright, J., Crocker, T., Oluboyede, Y., & House, A. (2010). Non-pharmacological approaches for dementia that informal carers might try or access: A systematic review. *International Journal of Geriatric Psychiatry, 25*(7), 756–763.

Higgins, P. (2010). Doll therapy in dementia care remains a controversial intervention but it may well provide people with sensory stimulation and purposeful activity. *Nuring Times.* Retrieved from www.nursingtimes.net/using-dolls-to-enhance-the-wellbeing-of-people-with-dementia/5020017.fullarticle

Inouye, S. K., Westendorp, R. G., & Saczynski, J. S. (2014). Delirium in elderly people. *The Lancet, 383*(9920), 911–922.

Khachiyants, N., Trinkle, D., Son, S. J., & Kim, K. Y. (2011). Sundown syndrome in persons with dementia: An update. *Psychiatry investigation, 8*(4), 275–287.

Lecouturier, J., Bamford, C., Hughes, J. C., Francis, J. J., Foy, R., Johnston, M., & Eccles, M. P. (2008). Appropriate disclosure of a diagnosis of dementia: Identifying the key behaviours of 'best practice'. *BMC Health Services Research, 8*(1), 95.

Lykkeslet, E., Gjengedal, E., Skrondal, T., & Storjord, M. B. (2014). Sensory stimulation—A way of creating mutual relations in dementia care. *International journal of qualitative studies on health and well-being, 9.* Retrieved from www.ncbi.nlm.nih.gov/pmc/articles/PMC4090364/

Meddings, J., Rogers, M. A., Krein, S. L., Fakih, M. G., Olmsted, R. N., & Saint, S. (2013). *Reducing unnecessary urinary catheter use and other strategies to prevent catheter-associated urinary tract infection: Brief update review.* Retrieved from www.ncbi.nlm.nih.gov/books/NBK133354/#_NBK133354_pubdet_

Mitchell, G. (2014). Use of doll therapy for people with dementia: an overview. *Nursing Older People, 26*(4), 24–26.

Pezzati, R., Molteni, V., Bani, M., Settanta, C., Di Maggio, M. G., Villa, I., ... & Ardito, R. B. (2014). Can doll therapy preserve or promote attachment in people with cognitive, behavioral, and emotional problems? A pilot study in institutionalized patients with dementia. *Frontiers in Psychology, 21*(5), 342.

Pinner, G., & Bouman, W. P. (2002). To tell or not to tell: On disclosing the diagnosis of dementia. *International Psychogeriatrics, 14*(02), 127–137.

*Rasin, J. (1990). Confusion. *Nursing Clinics of North America, 25,* 909–918.

*Roberts, B. L. (2001). Managing delirium in adult intensive care patients. *Critical Care Nurse, 21*(1), 48–55.

Rompaey, B., Elseviers, M. M., Van Drom, W., Fromont, V., & Jorens, P. G. (2012). The effect of earplugs during the night on the onset of delirium and sleep perception: A randomized controlled trial in intensive care patients. *Critical Care, 16*(3), R73.

Scherder, E. J., Bogen, T., Eggermont, L. H., Hamers, J. P., & Swaab, D. F. (2010). The more physical inactivity, the more agitation in dementia. *International Psychogeriatrics, 22*(08), 1203–1208.

Simmons-Stern, N. R., Budson, A. E., & Ally, B. A. (2010). Music as a memory enhancer in patients with Alzheimer's disease. *Neuropsychologia, 48*(10), 3164–3167.

Stotts, M., & Dyer, J., (2013). *Handbook of remotivation therapy.* New York: Routledge Press.

Wollen, K. A. (2010). Alzheimer's disease: the pros and cons of pharmaceutical, nutritional, botanical, and stimulatory therapies, with a discussion of treatment strategies from the perspective of patients and practitioners. *Alternative Medicine Review, 15*(3), 223–244.

Chronic Functional Constipation

Erichsén, E., Milberg, A., Jaarsma, T., & Friedrichsen, M. (2015). Constipation in specialized palliative care: Prevalence, definition, and patient-perceived symptom distress. *Journal of Palliative Medicine, 18*(7), 585–592.

McCay, S. L., Fravel, M., & Scanlon, C. (2012). Evidence-based practice guideline: Management of constipation. *Journal of Gerontological Nursing, 38*(7), 9–15.

*Shua-Haim, J., Sabo, M., & Ross, J. (1999). Constipation in the elderly: A practical approach. *Clinical Geriatrics,* 7(12), 91–99.

Wald, A. (2015). Patient information: Constipation in adults (Beyond the Basics). In *UpToDate.* Retrieved from www.uptodate.com/contents/constipation-in-adults-beyond-the-basics#H1

*Wisten, A., & Messner, T. (2005). Fruit and fibre (Pajala porridge) in the prevention of constipation. *Scandinavian Journal of Caring Sciences*, *19*(1), 71–76.

Ineffective Coping

*The ADHD Molecular Genetics Network. (2002). Report from the third international meeting of the attention-deficit hyperactivity disorder molecular genetics network. *American Journal of Medical Genetics*, *114*, 272–277.

Ahmed, A., & Simmons, Z. (2013). Pseudobulbar affect: Prevalence and management. *Therapeutics and Clinical Risk Management*, *9*, 483.

American Academy of Pediatrics. (2015). *Attention-deficit/hyperactivity disorder (ADHD)*. Retrieved from www.cdc.gov/ncbddd/adhd/guidelines.html

*Bodenheimer, T., MacGregor, K., & Shariffi, C. (2005). Helping patients manage their chronic conditions. Retrieved from www.chef.org/publications

Centers for Disease Control and Prevention. (2010). Attitudes toward mental illness. *Morbidity and Mortality Weekly Report*, *59*(20), 619–625. Retrieved from www.cdc.gov/mmwr/preview/mmwrhtml/mm5920a3.htm

Clark, M. S., Jansen, K. L., & Cloy, J. A. (2012). Treatment of childhood and adolescent depression. *American Family Physician*, *86*(5), 442–448.

Conwell, Y., Van Orden, K., & Caine, E. D. (2011). Suicide in older adults. *The Psychiatric Clinics of North America*, *34*(2), 451–468.

*Cramer, P. (1998). Coping and defense mechanisms: What's the difference? *Journal of Personality*, *66*(6), 919–946.

Fahim, C., He, Y., Yoon, U., Chen, J., Evans, A., & Perusse, D. (2011). Neuroanatomy of childhood disruptive behavior disorders. *Aggressive Behavior*, *37*(4), 326–337.

*Finkelman, A. W. (2000). Self-management for psychiatric patient at home. *Home Care Provider*, *5*(6), 95–101.

*Flaskerud, J. H. (1984). A comparison of perceptions of problematic behavior by six minority groups and mental health professionals. *Nursing Research*, *33*, 190–197.

*Folkman, S., Lazaraus, R. S., Pimley, S., & Novacek, J. (1987). Age differences in stress and coping processes. *Psychology and Aging*, *2*(2), 171–184.

Garcia, C. (2010). Conceptualization and measurement of coping during adolescence: A review of the literature. *Journal of Nursing Scholarship*, *42*(2): 166–185. Retrieved from www.ncbi.nlm.nih.gov/pmc/articles/PMC2904627

Galor, S., & Hentschel, U. (2012). Problem-solving tendencies, coping styles, and self-efficacy among Israeli veterans diagnosed with PTSD and depression. *Journal of Loss and Trauma*, *17*(6), 522–535.

Giger, J., (2013). *Transcultural nursing: Assessment and intervention* (6th ed.). St. Louis: Mosby-Year Book.

Grant, J. E. (2011). *Gambling and the brain: Why neuroscience research is vital to gambling research*. Beverly, MA: National Center for Responsible Gaming. Retrieved from www.ncrg.org/sites/default/files/uploads/docs/monographs/ncrgmonograph6final.pdf

Hayward, R. D., & Krause, N. (2013). Trajectories of late-life change in god-mediated control. *The Journals of Gerontology Series B: Psychological Sciences and Social Sciences*, *68*(1), 49–58.

Hayward, M., & Strauss, C. (2013). Group person-based cognitive therapy for distressing psychosis. In E. M. J. Morris, L. C. Johns & J. E. Oliver (Eds.), *Acceptance and commitment therapy and mindfulness for psychosis* (pp. 240–255): Hoboken, NJ: Wiley.

*Lazarus, R. (1985). The costs and benefits of denial. In A. Monat & R. Lazarus (Eds.), *Stress and coping: An anthology* (2nd ed.). New York: Columbia.

*Lazarus, R., & Folkman, S. (1984). *Stress, appraisal and coping*. New York: Springer.

Lee, J., & Harley, V. R. (2012). The male fight-flight response: A result of SRY regulation of catecholamines? *Bioessays*, *34*(6): 454–457.

Mitchell, J., Trangle, M., Degnan, B., Gabert, T., Haight, B., Kessler, D., . . . Vincent, S. (2013). *Adult depression in primary care*. Bloomington, MN: Institute for Clinical Systems Improvement.

National Institute on Drug Abuse. (2010). *Drug, brains and behavior: The science of addiction*. Retrieved from www.drugabuse.gov/sites/default/files/sciofaddiction.pdf

*Potenza, M. N. (2006). Should addictive disorders include non-substance-related conditions? *Addiction*, *101*(1), 142–151.

*Prochasaska, J., DiClemente, C. C., & Norcross, J. C. (1982). In search of how people change. *American Psychology*, *47*(8), 1102–1104.

Procter, N., Hamer, H., McGarry, D., Wilson, R.I., Frogget, T. (2014). *Mental health: A person-centered approach*. Sydney: Cambridge.

*Selye, H. (1974). *Stress without distress*. Philadelphia: J. B. Lippincott.

Stawski, R. S., Mogle, J. A., & Sliwinski, M. J. (2013). Daily stressors and self-reported changes in memory in old age: The mediating effects of daily negative affect and cognitive interference. *Aging Mental Health*, *17*(2), 168–172. Retrieved from www.ncbi.nlm.nih.gov/pmc/articles/PMC3652656

Uren, S. A., & Graham, T. M. (2013). Subjective experiences of coping among caregivers in palliative care. *Online journal of issues in nursing*, *18*(1), 88. Retrieved from www.nursingworld.org/MainMenuCategories/ANAMarketplace/ANAPeriodicals/ OJIN/TableofContents/Vol-18-2013/No2-May-2013/Articles-Previous-Topics/Subjective-Experiences-of-Coping-Among-Caregivers-in-Palliative-Care

World Health Organization. (2014). *Mental health: A state of well-being*. Retrieved from www.who.int/features/factfiles/mental_health/en/

Defensive Coping

*Bodenheimer, T., MacGregor, K., & Shariffi, C. (2005). *Helping patients manage their chronic conditions*. Retrieved from www.chef.org/publications

*Ewing, J. A. (1984). Detecting alcoholism: The CAGE questionnaire. *Journal ofthe American Medical Association*, *252*, 1905–1907.

*Kappas-Larson, P., & Lathrop, L. (1993). Early detection and intervention for hazardous ethanol use. *Nurse Practitioner*, *18*(7), 50–55.

Mohr, W. K. (2010). Restraints and the code of ethics: An uneasy fit. *Archives of Psychiatric Nursing*, *24*(1), 3–14.

Substance Abuse

*Bodenheimer, T., MacGregor, K., & Shariffi, C. (2005). *Helping patients manage their chronic conditions*. Retrieved from www.chef.org/publications

*Ewing, J. A. (1984). Detecting alcoholism: The CAGE questionnaire. *Journal ofthe American Medical Association, 252*, 1905–1907.

*Kappas-Larson, P., & Lathrop, L. (1993). Early detection and intervention for hazardous ethanol use. *Nurse Practitioner, 18*(7), 50–55.

Labile Emotional Response

Ahmed, A., & Simmons, Z. (2013). Pseudobulbar affect: Prevalence and management. *Therapeutic Clinical Risk Management, 9*, 483–489.

Beauchaine, T., Gatze-Kopp, L., & Mead, H. (2007). Polyvagal theory and developmental psychopathology: Emotion dysregulation and conduct problems from preschool to adolescence. *Biological Psychology, 74*, 174–184.

Colamonico, J., Formella, A., & Bradley, W. (2012). Pseudobulbar affect: Burden of illness in the USA. *Advances in Therapy, 29*(9), 775–798.

Decisional Conflict

Cicirelli, V. G., MacLean, A. P., Cox, L. S. (2000). Hastening death: A comparison of two end-of-life decisions. *Death Studies, 24*(5), 401–419.

Danis, M., Southerland, L. I., Garrett, J. M., Smith, J. L., Hielema, F., Pickard, C. G., . . . Patrick, D. L. (1991). A prospective study of advance directives for life-sustaining care. *New England Journal of Medicine, 324*(13), 882–888.

*Jezewski, M. A., Scherer, Y., Miller, C., & Battista, E. (1993). Consenting to DNR: Critical care nurses' interactions with patients and family members. *American Journal of Critical Care, 2*(4), 302–309.

*Sims, S. L., Boland, D. L., & O'Neill, C. A. (1992). Decision making in home health care. *Western Journal of Nursing Research, 14*, 186–200.

*Soholt, D. (1990). *A life experience: Making a health care treatment decision* (Unpublished master's thesis). South Dakota State University, Brookings, SD.

Thompson, C., Aitken, L., Doran, D., & Dowding, D. (2013). An agenda for clinical decision making and judgement in nursing research and education. *International Journal of Nursing Studies, 50*(12), 1720–1726.

Impaired Emancipated Decision-making

Allen, K. A. (2014). Parental decision-making for medically complex infants and children: An integrated literature review. *International Journal of Nursing Studies, 51*(9), 1289–1304.

Boykins, D. (2014). Core communication competencies in patient-centered care. *Association of Black Nursing Faculty, 25*(2), 40–45.

Brown, E., Patel, R., Kaur, J. & Coad, J. (2013). The interface between South Asian culture and palliative care for children, young people, and families—A discussion paper. *Issues in Comprehensive Pediatric Nursing, 36*(1/2), 120–143.

Carling-Rowland, A., Black, S., McDonald, L., & Kagan, A. (2014). Increasing access to fair capacity evaluation for discharge decision-making for people with aphasia: A randomised controlled trial. *Aphasiology, 28*(6), 750–765.

*Clark, H. D., O'Connor, A. M., Graham, I. D., & Wells, G. A. (2003). What factors are associated with a woman's decision to take hormone replacement therapy? Evaluated in the context of a decision aid. *Health Expectations, 6*(2), 110–117.

Delany, C. & Galvin, J. (2014). Ethics and shared decision-making in paediatric occupational therapy practice. *Developmental Neurorehabilitation, 17*(5), 347–354.

Ernst, J., Berger, S., Weißflog, G., Schröder, C., Körner, A., Niederwieser, D., . . . Singer, S. (2013). Patient participation in the medical decision-making process in haemato-oncology—A qualitative study. *European Journal of Cancer Care, 22*(5), 684–690.

Goldberg, H. B., & Shorten, A. (2014). Patient and provider perceptions of decision making about use of epidural analgesia during childbirth: A thematic analysis. *The Journal of Perinatal Education, 23*(3), 142–150.

Hain, D. J. & Sandy, D. (2014). Partners in care: Patient empowerment through shared decision-making. *Nephrology Nursing Journal, 40*(2), 153–157.

Hamaker, M. E., Schiphorst, A. H., ten Bokkel Huinink, D., Schaar, C., & van Munster, B. C. (2014). The effect of a geriatric evaluation on treatment decisions for older cancer patients—A systematic review. *Acra Oncologica, 53*(3), 289–296.

Hardin, S. (2012). Geriatric care. Hearing loss in older critical care patients: Participation in decision making. *Critical Care Nurse, 32*(6), 43–50.

Harris, A. L. (2014). "I got caught up in the game": Generational influences on contraceptive decision making in African–American women. *Journal of the American Association of Nurse Practitioners, 25*, 156–165.

Hatfield, L. A. & Pearce, M. M. (2014). Factors influencing parents' decision to donate their healthy infant's DNA for minimal-risk genetic research. *Journal of Nursing Scholarship, 46*(6), 398–407.

Hershberger, P. E., Finnegan, L. Pierce, P. F., & Scoccia, B. (2013). The decision-making process of young adult women with cancer who considered fertility cryopreservation. *Journal of Obstetric, Gynecologic, and Neonatal Nursing (JOGNN), 42*(1), 59–69.

Holland, D. E., Conlon, P. M., Rohlik, G. M., Gillard, K. L., Tomlinson, A. L., Raadt, D. M., . . . Rhudy, L. M. (2014). Developing and testing a discharge planning decision support tool for hospitalized pediatric patients. *Journal for Specialists in Pediatric Nursing, 19*(2), 149–161.

Jacobson, C. H., Zlatnik, M. G., Kennedy, H. P., & Lyndon, A. (2013). Nurses' perspectives on the intersection of safety and informed decision making in maternity care. *Journal of Obstetric, Gynecologic, and Neonatal Nursing (JOGNN), 42*(5), 577–587.

James, J. P., Taft, A., Amir, L. H., & Agius, P. (2014). Does intimate partner violence impact on women's initiation and duration of breastfeeding? *Breastfeeding Review, 22*(2), 11–19.

Légaré, F., Moumjid-Ferdjaoui, N., Drolet, R., Stacey, D., Härter, M., Bastian, H., . . . Desroches, S. (2013). Core competencies for shared decision making training programs: Insights from an international, interdisciplinary working group. *Journal of Continuing Education in Health Professions, 33*(4), 267–273.

Lessa, H. F., Tyrrell, M. A. R., Alves, V. H., & Rodrigues, D. P. (2014). Social relations and the option for planned home birth: An institutional ethnographic study. *Online Brazilian Journal of Nursing, 13*(2), 235–245.

Lewis, K. B., Starzomski, R., & Young, L. (2014). A relational approach to implantable cardioverter-defibrillator generator replacement: An integrative review of the role of nursing in shared decision-making. *Canadian Journal of Cardiovascular Nursing, 24*(3). 6–14.

Lilley, M., Christian, S., Hume, S., Scott, P., Montgomery, M., Semple, L., ... Somerville, M. J. (2010). Newborn screening for cystic fibrosis in Alberta: Two years of experience. *Paediatrics & Child Health, 15*(9), 590.

Mahon, M. (2010). Advanced care decision making: Asking the right people the right questions. *Journal of Psychosocial Nursing & Mental Health Services, 48*(7), 13–19.

Müllersdorf, M., Zander, V., & Eriksson, H. (2011). The magnitude of reciprocity in chronic pain management: Experiences of dispersed ethnic populations of Muslim women. *Scandinavian Journal of Caring Sciences, 25*(4), 637–645.

National Health Service. (2010). *Liberating the NHS: No decision about me, without me*. Retrieved from www.gov.uk/government/uploads/system/uploads/attachment_data/file/216980/Liberating-the-NHS-No-decision-about-me-without-me-Government-

Rivera-Spoljaric, K., Halley, M., & Wilson, S. R. (2014). Shared clinician-patient decision- making about treatment of pediatric asthma: What do we know and how can we use it? *Current Opinion in Allergy & Clinical Immunology, 14*(2), 161–167.

Scaffidi, R. M., Posmontier, B., Bloch, B. R., & Wittmann-Price, R. A. (2014). The relationship between personal knowledge and decision self-efficacy in choosing trial of labor after cesarean. *Journal of Midwifery & Women's Health, 59*(3), 246–253.

Silva, G. P. S., de Jesus, M. C. P., Merighi, M. A. B., Domingos, S. R., & Oliveria, D. M. (2014). The experience of women regarding cesarean section from the perspective of social phenomenology. *Online Brazilian Journal of Nursing, 13*(1), 5–14.

*Sims, S. L., Boland, D. L., & O'Neill, C. A. (1992). Decision making in home health care. *Western Journal of Nursing Research, 14*, 186–200.

*Soholt, D. (1990). *A life experience: Making a health care treatment decision* (Unpublished master's thesis). South Dakota State University, Brookings, SD.

Stepanuk, K. M., Fisher, K. M., Wittmann-Price, R. A., Posmontier, B., & Bhattacharya, A. (2013). Women's decision-making regarding medication use in pregnancy for anxiety and/or depression. *Journal of Advanced Nursing*, (11), 2470–2480.

Suhonen, R., Papastavrou, E., Efstathiou, G., Lemonidou, C., Kalafati, M., da Luz, M. D. A., . . . Kanan, N. (2011). Nurses' perceptions of individualized care: an international comparison. *Journal of advanced nursing, 67*(9), 1895–1907.

Szeto, M.O.P., O'Sullivan, M. J., Body, R. A., & Parrott, J. S. (2014). Registered dietitians' roles in decision-making processes for PEG placement in the elderly. *Canadian Journal of Dietary Practice & Research, 75*(2), 78–83.

Thompson, C., Aitken, L., Doran, D., & Dowding, D. (2013). An agenda for clinical decision making and judgement in nursing research and education. *Nursing Studies, 50*(12), 1720–1726.

*Wittmann-Price, R. A. (2004). Emancipation in decision-making in women's health care. *Journal of Advanced Nursing, 47*, 437–445.

*Wittmann-Price, R. A. (2006). Exploring the subconcepts of the Wittmann-Price theory of emancipated decision-making in women's health care. *Journal of Nursing Scholarship. 38*(4), 377–382.

Wittmann-Price, R. A. & Bhattacharya, A. (2008). Reexploring the subconcepts of the Wittmann-Price theory of emancipated decision-making in women's healthcare. *Advances in Nursing Science, 31*(3), 225–236.

Wittmann-Price, R. A. & Fisher, K. M. (2009). Patient decision aids: Tools for patients and professionals. *American Journal of Nursing, 109*(12), 60–64.

Wittmann-Price, R. A. & Price, S. W. (2014). Development and revision of the Wittmann-Price Emancipated Decision-making Scale. *Journal of Nursing Measurement, 22*(3), 361–367.

Wittmann-Price, R. A., Fliszar, R., Bhattacharya, A. (2011). Elective cesarean births: Are women making emancipated decisions? *Applied Nursing Research, 24*, 147–152.

Diarrhea

Clay, P. G., & Crutchley, R. D. (2014). Noninfectious diarrhea in HIV seropositive individuals: a review of prevalence rates, etiology, and management in the era of combination antiretroviral therapy. *Infectious Diseases and Therapy, 3*(2), 103–122.

Elseviers, M. M., Van Camp, Y., Nayaert, S., Duré, K., Annemans, L., Tanghe, A., & Vermeersch, S. (2015). Prevalence and management of antibiotic associated diarrhea in general hospitals. *BMC Infectious Diseases, 15*(1), 129. Retrieved from www.biomedcentral.com/1471-2334/15/129

Food and Drug Administration. (2014). While you're pregnant—What is foodborne illness? Retrieved from www.fda.gov/Food/ResourcesForYou/HealthEducators/ucm083316.htm

*Goodgame, R. (2006). A Bayesian approach to acute infectious diarrhea in adults. *Gastroenterology Clinics, 35*(2), 249–273.

MacArthur, R. (2014). Understanding noninfectious diarrhea in HIV-infected individuals. *GI Digest*. Retrieved from www.salix.com/healthcare-professionals-resources/gi-digest-newsletter/gi-digest-archive/id/432/understanding-noninfectious-diarrhea-in-hiv-infected-individuals

*Ravry, M. J. (1980). Dietic food diarrhea. *JAMA, 244*(3), 270.

Siegal, K., Schrimshaw, E. W., Brown-Bradley, C. J., & Lekas, H. M. (2010). Sources of emotional distress associated with diarrhea among late middle-age and older HIV-infected adults. *Journal of Pain and Symptom Management, 40*(3), 353–369.

Spies, L. (2009). Diarrhea A to Z: America to Zimbabwe. *Journal of the American Academy of Nurse Practitioners, 21*(6), 307–313.

*Tramarin, A., Parise, N., Campostrini, S., Yin, D. D., Postma, M. J., Lyu, R., . . . Palladio Study Group. (2004). Association between diarrhea and quality of life in HIV-infected patients receiving highly active antiretroviral therapy. *Quality of Life Research, 13*(1), 243–250.

Wanke, C. A. (2016a). Epidemiology and causes of acute diarrhea in resource-rich countries. In *UpToDate*. Retrieved from www.uptodate.com/contents/epidemiology-and-causes-of-acute-diarrhea-in-resource-rich-countries

Wanke, C. A. (2016b). Acute diarrhea in adults (beyond the basics). In *UpToDate*. Retrieved from www.uptodate.com/contents/acute-diarrhea-in-adults-beyond-the-basics

Weller, P. (2015). Patient information: General travel advice (beyond the basics). In *UpToDate*. Retrieved from www.uptodate.com/contents/general-travel-advice-beyond-the-basics?source=see_link

Disuse Syndrome

*Christian, B. J. (1982). Immobilization: Psychosocial aspects. In C. Norris (Ed.), *Concept clarification in nursing*. Rockville, MD: Aspen Publications.

Jiricka, M. K. (2008). Activity tolerance and fatigue pathophysiology: Concepts of altered health states. In: C. M. Porth (Ed.), *Essentials of pathophysiology: Concepts of altered Health States*. Philadelphia: Lippincott Williams & Wilkins.

Kalisch, B. J., Lee, S., Dabney, B. W. (2013). Outcomes of inpatient mobilization: A literature review. *Journal of Clinical Nursing*. Retrieved from www.rgpeo.com/media/61250/jcn%20outcomes.pdf

Lim, R., Lewis, E., Bowles, S., Goenka, N., Joseph, F., & Ewins, D. (2011). *Immobility: A rare cause of hypercalcaemia. Endocrine Abstracts*, 25, 22.

*Maher, A., Salmond, S., & Pellino, T. (2006). *Orthopedic nursing* (3rd ed.). Philadelphia: W. B. Saunders.

*Nigam, Y., Knight, J., Jones, A. (2009). The physiological effects of bed rest and immobility—Part 3. *Nursing Times*, *105*(23), 18–22.

*Stuemple, K. J., & Drury, D. G. (2007). The physiological consequences of bed rest. *JEP Online*, *10*(3), 32–41. Retrieved from http://cupola.gettysberg.edu/cgi/viewcontent.cgi?article=1029&context=healthfac

*Timmerman, R. A. (2007). A mobility protocol for critically ill adults. *Dimensions of Critical Care Nursing*, *26*(5), 175–179.

Zomorodi, M., Topley, D., & McAnaw, M. (2012). Developing a mobility protocol for early mobilization of patients in a surgical/trauma ICU. *Critical Research and Practice*, *2012*, 10. Retrieved from www.hindawi.com/journals/ccrp/2012/964547/

Deficient Diversional Activity

*Barba, B. E., Tesh, A. S., & Courts, N. F. (2002). Promoting thriving in nursing homes. *The Eden Alternative Journal of Gerontological Nursing*, *28*(3), 7.

*Rantz, M. (1991). Diversional activity deficit. In M. Maas, K. Buckwalter, & M. Hardy (Eds.), *Nursing diagnoses and interventions for the elderly*. Redwood City, CA: Addison-Wesley Nursing.

Dysreflexia

Andrade, L. T. D., Araújo, E. G. D., Andrade, K. D. R. P., Souza, D. R. P. D., Garcia, T. R., & Chianca, T. C. M. (2013). Autonomic dysreflexia and nursing interventions for patients with spinal cord injury. *Revista da Escola de Enfermagem da USP*, *47*(1), 93–100.

Bhambhani, Y., Mactavish, J., Warren, S., Thompson, W. R., Webborn, A., Bressan, E., . . . & Van De Vliet, P. (2010). Boosting in athletes with high-level spinal cord injury: knowledge, incidence and attitudes of athletes in paralympic sport. *Disability and Rehabilitation*, *32*(26), 2172–2190.

*McClain, W., Shields, C., & Sixsmith, D. (1999). Autonomic dysreflexia presenting as a severe headache. *American Journal of Emergency Medicine*, *17*(3), 238–240.

Somali, B. K. (2009). Autonomic dysreflexia: A medical emergency with spinal cord injury. *International Journal of Clinical Practice*, *63*(3), 350–352. doi:10.1111/j.1742-1241.2008.01844.x

Stephenson, R. (2014). Autonomic dysreflexia in spinal cord injury. *Medscape*. Retrieved from http://emedicine.medscape.com/article/322809-overview

*Teasell, R., Arnold, J., & Delaney, G. (1996). Sympathetic nervous system dysfunction in high level spinal cord injuries. *Physical Medicine and Rehabilitation*, *10*(1), 37–55.

Energy Field Disturbance

Note: The pioneers in the field of Therapeutic Touch are represented in those citations with an (*) asterisk.

Aghabati, N., Mohammadi, E., & Pour Esmaiel, Z. (2010). The effect of therapeutic touch on pain and fatigue of cancer patients undergoing chemotherapy. *Evidence-Based Complementary and Alternative Medicine*, 7(3), 375–381.

Anderson, J. G., & Taylor, A. G. (2011). Effects of healing touch in clinical practice. *Journal of Holistic Nursing*, *29*(3), 221–228.

*Bradley, D. B. (1987). Energy fields: Implications for nurses. *Journal of Holistic Nursing*, *5*(1), 32–35.

Bulbroook, J. A., & Mentgen, M. J. (2009). *Healing touch: Level 1*. Carrboro, NC: North Carolina Center for Healing Touch.

*Denison, B. (2004). Touch the pain away. *Holistic Nursing Practice*, *18*(3), 142–151.

*Gronowicz, G., McCarthy, M. B., & Jhaveri, A. (2006). Therapeutic Touch inhibits bone formation of human osteosarcoma cells in vitro. In *Transactions of the North American Conference on complementary and integrative*, Edmonton, Canada.

Hart, J. (2008). Complementary therapies for chronic pain management. *Alternative & Complementary Therapies*, *14*(2), 64–68.

*Heidt, P. R. (1990). Openness: A qualitative analysis of nurses' and patients' experiences of therapeutic touch. *Image: The Journal of Nursing Scholarship*, *22*(3), 180–186.

*Kiernan, J. (2002). The experience of therapeutic touch in the lives of five postpartum women. *MCN: The American Journal of Maternal/Child Nursing*, *27*(1), 47–53.

*Krieger, D. (1987). *Living the therapeutic touch: Healing as a lifestyle*. New York: Dodd, Mead.

*Krieger, D. (1997). *Therapeutic touch: Inner workbook*, Santa Fe: Bear & Company.

*Macrae, J. (1988). *Therapeutic touch: A practical guide*. New York: Knopf.

*Meehan, T. C. (1991). Therapeutic touch. In G. Bulechek & J. McCloskey (Eds.), *Nursing interventions: Essential nursing treatments*. Philadelphia: W. B. Saunders.

*Meehan, T. C. (1998). Therapeutic touch as nursing intervention. *Journal of Advanced Nursing*, *28*(1), 117–125.

Mentgen, M. J. (2007). Path of healership: The importance of self care for the healer. *Energy Magazine*, Issue 14.

Monroe, C. M. (2009). The effects of therapeutic touch on pain. *Journal of Holistic Nursing*, *27*(2), 85–92.

*Movaffaghi, Z., Hasanpoor, M., Farsi, M., Hooshmand, P., & Abrishami, F. (2006). Effects of therapeutic touch on blood

hemoglobin and hematocrit. *Journal of Holistic Nursing, 24*(1), 41–48.

*Quinn, J. F. (1989). Therapeutic touch as energy exchange: Replication and extension. *Nursing Science Quarterly, 2*(2), 79–87.

*Quinn, J., & Strelkauskas, A. (1993). Psychoimmunologic effects of therapeutic touch on practitioners and recently bereaved recipients: A pilot study. *Advances in Nursing Science, 15*(4), 13–26.

*Turner, J. G., Clark, A. J., Gauthier, D. K., & Williams, M. (1998). The effect of therapeutic touch on pain and anxiety in burn patients. *Journal of Advanced Nursing, 28*(1), 10–20.

*Umbreit, A. W. (2000). Healing touch: Applications in the acute care setting. *ACCN Clinical Issues of Advanced Practice in Acute Critical Care, 11*(1), 105–119.

Van Aken, R., & Taylor, B. (2010). Emerging from depression: The experiential process of healing touch explored through grounded theory and case study. *Complementary therapies in clinical practice, 16*(3), 132–137. doi:10.1016/j.ctcp.2009.11.001

*Wardell, D. W., & Weymouth, K. F. (2004). Review of studies of healing touch. *Journal of Nursing Scholarship, 36*(2), 147–154.

Wicking, K. (2012). A randomized controlled trial of effects of energy based complimentary therapies of healing touch on functional health status of community-dwelling single older woman (Dissertation). James Cook University. Retrieved from http://researchonline.jcu.edu.au/38394/1/38394-wicking-2012-thesis.pdf

Woods, D. L., Craven, R. F., & Whitney, J. (2005). The effect of therapeutic touch on behavioral symptoms of persons with dementia. *Alternative therapies in health and medicine, 11*(1), 66.

Compromised Engagement

Beverley, M. (2014). Connect patient engagement and cultural competence to drive health management. *Engaging Patients*. Retrieved from www.engagingpatients.org/patient-centered-care-2/connect-patient-engagement-cultural-competence-drive-health-management/

*Cornish, P. L., Knowles, S. R., Marchesano, R., Tam, V., Shadowitz, S., Juurlink, D. N., & Etchells, E. E. (2005). Unintended medication discrepancies at the time of hospital admission. *Archives of Internal Medicine, 165*(4), 424–429.

Entwistle, V. A., McCaughan, D., Watt, I. S., Birks, Y., Hall, J., Peat, M., . . . Wright, J. (2010). Speaking up about safety concerns: multi-setting qualitative study of patients' views and experiences. *Quality and Safety in Health Care, 19*(6), e33–e33.

Frosch, D. L., & Elwyn, G. (2014). Don't blame patients, engage them: Transforming health systems to address health literacy. *Journal of Health Communication, 19*(Suppl 2), 10–14.

Frosch, D. L., May, S. G., Rendle, K. A., Tietbohl, C., & Elwyn, G. (2012). Authoritarian physicians and patients' fear of being labeled 'difficult'among key obstacles to shared decision making. *Health Affairs, 31*(5), 1030–1038.

Gallup Poll. (2015). *Honesty/ethics in professions*. Retrieved from www.gallup.com/poll/1654/honesty-ethics-profession.aspx

Gruman, J. (2011). Engagement does not mean compliance. *Center for Advancing Health*. Retrieved from www.cfah.org/blog/2011/engagement-does-not-mean-compliance

Gruman, J., Holmes-Rovner, M., French, M. E., Jeffress, D., Sofaer, S., Shaller, D., Prager, D. C. (2010). From patient education to patient engagement: Implications for the field of patient education. *Patient Education and Counseling, 78*(3), 350–356. doi:10.1016/j.pec.2010.02.002

*Hibbard, J. H., Stockard, J., Mahoney, E. R., Tusler, M. (2004). Development of the patient activation measure (PAM): Conceptualizing and measuring activation in patients and consumers. *Health Services Research, 39*, 1005–1026.

*Hibbard, J. H., & Cunningham, P. J. (2008). *How engaged are consumers in their health and health care, and why does it matter? Findings from HSC No. 8: Providing insights that contribute to better health policy*. Washington, DC: HSC

Hibbard, J. H., & Greene, J. (2013). What the evidence shows about patient activation: Better health outcomes and care experiences; fewer data on costs. *Health Affairs, 32*(2), 207–214.

Holmes Rovner, M., French, M., Sofaer, S., Shaller, D., Prager, D., & Kanouse, D. (2010). *A new definition of patient engagement: What is engagement and why is it important?* Washington, DC: Center for Advancing Health.

The Joint Commission. (2015). *National patient safety*. Hospital Accreditation Program Retrieved from www.jointcommission.org/topics/hai_standards_and_npsgs.aspx

*Martin, L. R., Williams, S. L., Haskard, K. B., & DiMatteo, M. R. (2005). The challenge of patient adherence. *Therapeutic Clinical Risk Management, 1*(3), 189–199. Retrieved from www.ncbi.nlm.nih.gov/pmc/articles/PMC1661624/

Martin, L. R., Haskard-Zolnierek, K. B., & DiMatteo, M. R. (2010). Health behavior change and treatment adherence evidence-based guidelines for improving healthcare. New York: Oxford University Press.

Merriam-Webster. (2015). Compliance. *Merriam-Webster.* Retrieved from www.merriam-webster.com/thesaurus/compliance

Millenson, M. L., & Macri, J. (2012). *Will the Affordable Care Act move patient-centeredness to center stage?* Retrieved from www.rwjf.org/content/dam/farm/reports/reports/2012/rwjf72412

Pelzang, R. (2010). Time to learn: Understanding patient-centered care. *British Journal of Nursing, 19*(14), 912–917.

Robinson, J. H., Callister, L. C., Berry, J. A., & Dearing, K. A. (2008). Patient-centered care and adherence: definitions and applications to improve outcomes. *Journal of American Academy of Nurse Practioners, 20*, 600–607.

Sofaer, S., & Schumann, M. J. (2013). *Fostering successful patient and family engagement*. This White Paper was prepared for the Nursing Alliance for Quality Care with grant support from the Agency for Healthcare Research and Quality (AHRQ); Approved. Retrieved from www.naqc.org/WhitePaper-PatientEngagement

U.S. Congress. (2010). Patient Protection and Affordable Care Act, H.R. 3590. Public Law 111–148. 111th Cong.

Wong, J. D., Bajear, J. M., Wong, G. G., Alibhai, S. M., Huh, J. H., Cesta, A., ... & Fernandes, O. A. (2008). Medication reconciliation at hospital discharge: evaluating discrepancies. *Annals of Pharmacotherapy, 42*(10), 1373–1379.

Frail Elderly Syndrome

Ahmed, N., Mandel, R., & Fain, M. (2007). Frailty: An emerging geriatric syndrome. *The American Journal of Medicine, 120*, 748–753. doi:10.1016/j.amjmed.2006.10.018

*Blaum, C. S., Xue, Q. L., Michelon, E., Semba, R. D., & Fried, L. P. (2005). The association between obesity and the frailty syndrome in older women: The Women's Health and Aging Studies. *Journal of the American Geriatrics Society, 53*(6), 927–934.

Byard, R. W. (2015). Frailty syndrome—Medicolegal considerations. *Journal of Forensic and Legal Medicine, 30*, 34–38. doi:10.1016/j.jflm.2014.12.016

Clegg, A., Young, J. Y., LLiffe, S., Rikkert, M. O., & Rockwood, K. (2013). Frailty in elderly people. *Lancet, 381*,752–762. doi:10.1016/SO140-6736(12)62167-9.

deVries, N. M., Staal, J. B., vanRavensberg, C. D., Hobbelen, J. S. M., Olde Rikkert, M. G. M., & Nijhuis-van der Sanden, M. W. G. (2011). Outcome instruments to measure frailty: A systematic review. *Ageing Research Reviews, 10*, 104–114. doi:10.1016/j.arr.2010.09.001.

Ensrud, K. E., Blackwell, T. L., Cauley, J. A., Cummings, S. R., Barrett-Connor, E., Dam, T. T. L., . . . Cawthon, P. M. (2011). Circulating 25-hydroxyvitamin D levels and frailty in older men: The osteoporotic fractures in men study. *Journal of the American Geriatrics Society, 59*(1), 101–106.

*Fried, L. P., Tangen, C. M., Walston, J., Newman, A. B., Hirsch, C., Gottdiener, J., . . . McBurnie, M. A. (2001). Frailty in older adults evidence for a phenotype. *The Journals of Gerontology Series A: Biological Sciences and Medical Sciences, 56*(3), M146–M157. Retrieved from www.ncbi.nlm.nih.gov/pubmed/11253156

Janssen, H. C., Samson, M. M., & Verhaar, H. J. (2002). Vitamin D deficiency, muscle function, and falls in elderly people. *The American Journal of Clinical Nutrition*, 75(4), 611–615.

Kennel, K., Drake, M., & Hurley, D. (2010). Vitamin D deficiency in adults: When to test and how to treat. Mayo Clinic Proceedings, 85(8), 752–758. Retrieved from www.mayoclinicproceedings.org/article/S0025-6196(11)60190-0/

Palace, Z. J., & Flood-Sukhdeo, J. (2014). The frailty syndrome. *Today's Geriatric Medicine*, 7(1), 18.

Pijpers, E., Ferreira, I., Stehouwer, C. D., & Kruseman, A. C. N. (2012). The frailty dilemma. Review of the predictive accuracy of major frailty scores. *European Journal of Internal Medicine*, 23(2), 118–123. doi:10.1016/j.ejim.2011.09.003

*Rockwood, K. (2005). Frailty and its definition: A worthy challenge. *Journal of the American Geriatrics Society, 53*(6), 1069–1070.

*Walston, J., Hadley, E. C., Ferrucci, L., Guralnik, J. M., Newman, A. B., Studenski, S. A., . . . Fried, L. P. (2006). Research agenda for frailty in older adults: Towards a better understanding of physiology and etiology. *Journal of the American Geriatrics Society*, 54(6), 991–1001.

Xue, Q. L. (2011). The frailty syndrome: Definition and natural history. *Clinics in Geriatric Medicine*, 27(1), 1–15. Retrieved from www.ncbi.nlm.nih.gov/pmc/articles/PMC3028599/

Fatigue

Bardwell, W. A., & Ancoli-Israel, S. (2008). Breast cancer and fatigue. *Sleep Medicine Clinics, 3*(1), 61–71. Retrieved from www.ncbi.nlm.nih.gov/pmc/articles/PMC2390812/

Corwin, E. J., & Arbour, M. (2007). Postpartum fatigue and evidence-based interventions. *The American Journal of Maternal/Child Nursing, 32*(4), 215–220.

Gambert, S. R. (2013). Why do i always feel tired? Evaluating older patients reporting fatigue. *Consultant*, 53(11), 785–789.

*Gardner, D. L. (1991). Fatigue in postpartum women. *Applied Nursing Research*, 4(2), 57–62.

*Greenberg, D. B., Sawicka, J., Eisenthal, S., & Ross, D. (1992). Fatigue syndrome due to localized radiation. *Journal of Pain and Symptom Management*, 7(1), 38–45.

Haas, M. L. (2011). Radiation therapy: Toxicities and management. In C. H. Yarbro, M. H. Frogge, M. Goodman, & S. L. Groenwald (Eds.), *Cancer nursing/principles and practice* (7th ed.). Boston: Jones & Bartlett.

Hutnik, N., Smith, P., & Koch, T. (2012). What does it feel like to be 100? Socio-emotional aspects of well-being in the stories of 16 centenarians living in the United Kingdom. *Aging Mental Health*, 16(7), 811–818.

Jong, E., Oudhoffc, L. A., & Epskamp, C. (2010). Predictors and treatment strategies of HIV-related fatigue in the combined antiretroviral therapy era. *AIDS*, 24(19), 1387–1405.

*Longino, C. F., & Kart, C. S. (1982). Explicating activity theory: A formal replication. *Journal of Gerontology, 37*, 713–722.

*Nail, L., & Winningham, M. (1997). Fatigue. In S. Groenwald, M. Frogge, M. Goodman, & C. Yarbo (Eds.), *Cancer nursing: Principles and practice* (4th ed.). Boston: Jones and Bartlett.

*Rhoten, D. (1982). Fatigue and the postsurgical patient. In C. Norris (Ed.), *Concept clarification in nursing*. Rockville, MD: Aspen Systems.

*Tilden, V. P., & Weinert, C. (1987). Social support and the chronically ill individual. *Nursing Clinics of North America, 22*, 613–620.

Fear

American Psychiatric Association. (2014). *DSMV: Diagnostic and statistical manual of mental disorders* (4th ed., text revision). Washington, DC: Author.

*Broome, M. E., Bates, T. A., Lillis, P. P., & McGahee, T. W. (1990). Children's medical fears, coping behaviors, and pain perceptions during a lumbar puncture. *Oncology Nursing Forum, 17*, 361–367.

*Cesarone, D. (1991). Fear. In M. Maas, K. Buckwalter, & M. Hardy (Eds.), *Nursing diagnoses and interventions for the elderly*. Redwood City, CA: Addison-Wesley Nursing.

*Crossley, M. L. (2003). 'Let me explain': Narrative emplotment and one patient's experience of oral cancer. *Social Science & Medicine, 56*(3): 439–448.

Kim, S., & So, W.Y. (2013). Prevalence and correlates of fear falling in korean community-dwelling elderly subjects. *Experimental Gerontology, 48*(11), 1323–1328.

Lach, H., & Pasons, J. (2013). Impact of fear of falling in long term care: An integrative review. *Journal of the American Medical Directors Association, 14*(8), 573–577.

Deficient and Excess Fluid Volume

American Academy of Pediatrics. (2011). Policy statement—Climatic heat stress and exercising children and adolescents. Council on Sports Medicine and Fitness and Council on School Health. *Pediatrics*, 128(3), e741–e747.

Cooper, K. (2011). Care of the lower extremities in patients with acute decompensated heart failure. *Critical Care Nurse, 31*(4), 21–28.

*Maughan, R. J., Leiper, J., & Shirreffs, S. M. (1997). Factors influencing the restoration of fluid and electrolyte balance after exercise in the heat. *British Journal of Sports Medicine, 31*(3), 175–182.

Zembruski, C. D. (1997). A three-dimensional approach to hydration of elders: Administration, clinical staff, and in-service education. *Geriatric Nursing, 18*(1), 20–26.

Grieving

Ball, J., Bindler, R., & Cowen, K. (2015). *Principles of pediatric nursing: Caring for children* (6th ed.). Upper Saddle River, NJ: Pearson.

*Bateman, A. L. (1999). Understanding the process of grieving and loss: A critical social thinking perspective. *Journal of American Psychiatric Nurses Association, 5*(5), 139–149.

Block, S. (2013). Grief and bereavement. In *UptoDate*. Retrieved from www.uptodate.com

Bonanno, G. A., & Lilienfeld, S. O. (2008). Let's be realistic: When grief counseling is effective and when it's not. *Professional Psychology: Research and Practice, 39*(3), 377–378.

*Caserta, M. S., Lund, D. A., & Dimond, M. F. (1985). Assessing interviewer effects in a longitudinal study of bereaved elderly adults. *Journal of Gerontology, 40*, 637–640.

Conwell, Y. (2014). Suicide later in life: Challenges and priorities for prevention. *American Journal of Preventive Medicine, 47*(3), S244–S250.

*Cotton, S., Puchalski, C. M., Sherman, S. N., Mrus, J. M., Peterman, A. H., Feinberg, J., . . . Tsevat, J. (2006). Spirituality and religion in patients with HIV/AIDS. *Journal of General Internal Medicine, 21*(Suppl 5), S5–S13.

*Gibson, L. (2003). *Complicated grief: A review of current issues.* White River Junction, VT: Research Education in Disaster Mental Health.

*Hooyman, N. R., & Kramer, B. J. (2006). *Living through loss: Interventions across the life span.* New York: Columbia University Press.

Kain, C. (2016). Teaching tip sheet: Multiple loss and aids-related bereavement. In *American Psychological Association*. Retrieved fom www.apa.org/pi/aids/resources/education/bereavement.aspx

*Lemming, M. R., & Dickinson, G. E. (2010). *Understanding dying, death, and bereavement* (7th ed.). Belmont, CA: Wadsworth.

*Mallinson, R. K. (1999). The lived experience of AIDS-related multiple losses by HIV-negative gay men. *Journal of the Association of Nurses in AIDS Care, 10*(5), 22–31.

*Mina, C. (1985). A program for helping grieving parents. *Maternal-Child Nursing Journal, 10*, 118–121.

*O'Mallon, M. (2009). Vulnerable populations: Exploring a family perspective of grief. *Journal of Hospice & Palliative Nursing, 11*(2), 91–98.

Purnell, L. D. (2013). *Transcultural health care: A culturally competent approach* (4th ed.). Philadelphia: F. A. Davis

*Rando, T. A. (1984). Grief, dying, and death: Clinical interventions for caregivers. Champaign, IL: Research Press.

Smith, M., & Segal, J. (2016). *Coping with grief and loss understanding the grieving process.* Retrieved from www.helpguide.org/articles/grief-loss/coping-with-grief-and-loss.htm

*Vanezis, M., & McGee, A. (1999). Mediating factors in the grieving process of the suddenly bereaved. *British Journal of Nursing, 8*(14), 932–937.

Wright, P. M., & Hogan, N. S. (2008). Grief theories and models: Applications to hospice nursing practice. *Journal of Hospice & Palliative Nursing, 10*(6), 350–355.

Worden, J. W. (2009). *Grief counseling and grief therapy :A handbook for the mental health practitioner* (4th ed.). New York : Springer Publishing.

Growth and Development

Adult Failure to Thrive

Agarwal, K. (2014). Failure to thrive in elderly adults: Management. In *UpToDate*. Retrieved from www.uptodate.com/contents/failure-to-thrive-in-elderly-adults-management

Cornwell, B., Laumann, E., & Schumm, L. P. (2008). The social connectedness of older adults: A national profile. *American Sociological Review, 73*(2), 185–203.

*Gosline, M. B. (2003). Client participation to enhance socialization for frail elders. *Geriatric Nursing, 24*(5), 286–289.

Gregory, C., & Singh, A. (2014). Household food security in the United States in 2013. In Economic Research Report No. 173 (p. 44). Retrieved from www.ers.usda.gov/publications/err-economic-research-report/err173.aspx

*Haight, B. K. (2002). Thriving: A life span theory. *Journal of Gerontological Nursing, 28*(3), 14–22.

Jonas-Simpson, C., McMahon, E., Watson, J., & Andrews, L. (2010). Nurses' experiences of caring for families whose babies were born still or died shortly after birth. *International Journal for Human Caring, 14*(4), 14–21.

*Kimball, M. J., & Williams-Burgess, C. (1995). Failure to thrive: The silent epidemic of the elderly. *Archives of Psychiatric Nursing, 9*(2), 99–105.

*Newbern, V. B., & Krowchuk, H. V. (1994). Failure to thrive in elderly people: A conceptual analysis. *Journal of Advanced Nursing, 19*(5), 840–849.

*Robertson, R.G., & Montagini, M. (2004). Adult failure to thrive. *American Family Physician*, 70(2), 343–350.

*Sarkisian, C. A., & Lachs, M. S. (1996). "Failure to thrive" in older adults. *Annals of Internal Medicine, 124*, 1072.

*Tusaie, K., & Dyer, J. (2004). Resilience: A historical review of construct. *Holistic Nursing Practice, 18*(1), 3–8.

Tuso, P., & Beattle, S. (2015). Nutrition reconciliation and nutrition prophylaxis: Toward total health. *The Permanente Journal*, 19(2), 80–86.

*Wagnil, G., & Young H. M. (1990). Resilience among older women. *Image: Journal of Nursing Scholarship, 22*, 252–255.

Ineffective Health Maintenance

American Lung Association. (2015). *Why kids start.* Chicago, IL: Author. Retrieved from www.lung.org/stop-smoking/about-smoking/preventing-smoking/why-kids-start.html?referrer=https://www.google.com/

Andrews, M., & Boyle, J. (2012). *Transcultural concepts in nursing* (8th ed.). Philadelphia: Lippincott Williams & Wilkins.

Andrews, J. O., Heath, J., Barone, C. P., & Tingen, M. S. (2008). Time to quit? New strategies for tobacco-dependent patients. *The Nurse Practitioner*, *33*(11), 34–42.

Bagaitkar, J., Demuth, D. R., & Scott, D. A. (2008). Tobacco use increases susceptibility to bacterial infection. *Tobacco induced* diseases, *4*(1), 1–10.

Bjartveit, K., & Tverdal, A. (2005). Health consequences of smoking 1–4 cigarettes per day. *Tobacco control*, *14*(5), 315–320.

Bohaty, K., Rocole, H., Wehling, K., & Waltman, N. (2008). Testing the effectiveness of an educational intervention to increase dietary intake of calcium and vitamin D in young adult women. *Journal of the American Academy of Nurse* Practitioners, *20*(2), 93–99.

*Cahill, L., Gorski, L., & Le, K. (2003). Enhanced human memory consolidation with post-learning stress: Interaction with the degree of arousal at encoding. *Learning & Memory*, *10*(4), 270–274.

Centers of Disease Control and Prevention. (2016). Smoking and tobacco use. Retrieved from www.cdc.gov/tobacco/basic_information/index.htm

Cleveland Clinic. (2014). Smoking cessation. Retrieved from https://my.clevelandclinic.org/health/treatments_and_procedures/hic_Quitting_Smoking

Cosman, F., De Beur, S. J., LeBoff, M. S., Lewiecki, E. M., Tanner, B., Randall, S., & Lindsay, R. (2014). Clinician's guide to prevention and treatment of osteoporosis. *Osteoporosis International*, *25*(10), 2359–2381.

*Cutilli, C. C. (2005). Do your patients understand? Determining your patients' health literacy skills. Orthopaedic Nursing, 24(5), 372–377; quiz 378–379.

DeWalt, D. A., Callahan, L. F., Hawk, V. H., Broucksou, K. A., Hink, A, Rudd, R., & Brach, C. (2010). *Health literacy universal precautions tool kit*. Retrieved from www.ahrq.gov/professionals/quality-patient-safety/quality-resources/tools/literacy-toolkit/index.html

Di Leonardi, B. C., Faller, M., & Siroky, K. (2011). *Preventing never events: Evidence based nurse staffing*. San Diego, CA: AMA Healthcare. Retrieved from www.amnhealthcare.com/uploadedFiles/MainSite/Content/Healthcare_Industry_Insights/Industry_Research/Never_Events_white_paper_06.16.11.pdf

Edelman, C. L., & Mandle, C. L. (2010). *Health promotion throughout the life span* (7th ed.). St. Louis, MO: Mosby-Year Book.

Federal Interagency Forum on Aging-Related Statistics.(2012) Older Americans 2012: Key indicators of well-being. *Federal Interagency Forum on Aging-Related Statistics*. Washington, DC: U.S. Government Printing Office. Retrieved from www.agingstats/gov/Main_Site/Data/2012_Documents/Health_status.aspx

Healthy People 2020. (2010). Retrieved from HealthyPeople.gov/2020topoicsobjectives

HHS Poverty Guidelines. (2011). Retrieved from www.ASPE.hhs.gov/poverty

Joint Commmission. (2010). Achieving effective communication, cultural competence, and patient-family-centered care: A roadmap for hospitals. Oakbrook Terrace, IL: The Joint Commission.

Hicks, M., McDermott, L. L., Rouhana, N., Schmidt, M., Seymour, M. W., & Sullivan, T. (2008). Nurses' body size and public confidence in ability to provide health education. *Journal of Nursing Scholarship*, *40*(4), 349–354.

Hockenberry, M. J., & Wilson, D. (2015). *Wong's essentials of pediatric nursing* (10th ed.). New York: Elsevier.

Institute of Medicine. (2009). *Secondhand smoke exposure and cardiovascular effects: Making sense of the evidence*. Retrieved from www.nationalacademies.org/hmd/Reports/2009/Secondhand-Smoke-Exposure-and-Cardiovascular-Effects-Making-Sense-of-the-Evidence.aspx#sthash.pRh3mmNS.dpuf

Institute of Medicine. (2010). *Updates vitamin D recommendations*. Retrieved from http://nof.org/news/79

Kiefer, R. A. (2008). An integrative review of the concept of well-being. *Holistic Nursing Practice*, *22*(5), 244–252.

Leon, L. (2002). Smoking cessation—Developing a workable program. *Nursing Spectrum*, *9*(18), 12–13.

Mayo Foundation for Medical Education and Research. (2013). *Nicotine dependence*. Mayo Clinic.

Mischel, W., & Shoda, Y. (1995). A cognitive-affective system theory of personality: reconceptualizing situations, dispositions, dynamics, and invariance in Personality structure. *Psychological Review*, 102(2), 246–268.

*McLaughlin, L., & Braun, K. (1998). Asian and Pacific Islander cultural values: Considerations for health care decision making. *Health and Social Work*, *23*(2), 116–126.

McMahon, S., & Fleury, J. (2012). Wellness in older adults: A concept analysis. *Nursing Forum*, *47*(1), 39–51.

Miller, C. (2015). *Nursing for wellness in older adults* (7th ed.). Philadelphia: Wolters Kluwer.

*Moore, S. M., & Charvat, J. M. (2002). Using the CHANGE intervention to enhance long-term exercise. *Nursing Clinics of North America*, *37*(2), 273–283.

Morbidity and Mortality Weekly Reports (MMWR). (2016). Retrieved from www.cdc.gov/tobacco/data_statistics/mmwrs/

National Cancer Institute. (2015). *Report offers comprehensive look at global smokeless tobacco use*. Retrieved from www.cancer.gov/news-events/cancer-currents-blog/2015/smokeless-tobacco-report

NIH. (2014). Vitamin D: Moving toward evidence-based decision making in primary care. Retrieved from https://ods.od.nih.gov/Research/VitaminDConference2014.aspx

Nguyen, K., Marshall, L. T., Hu, S., & Neff, L. (2015). State-specific prevalence of current cigarette smoking and smokeless tobacco use among adults aged ≥18 years—United States, 2011–2013. *Morbidity and Mortality Weekly Report*, *64*(19), 532–536.

Parker, R., & Ratzan, S. C. (2010). Health literacy: A second decade of distinction for Americans. *Journal of Health Communication*, *15*(Suppl 2), 20–33.

Pender, N., Murdaugh, C., & Parsons, M. A. (2011). Health promotion in nursing practice (6th ed.). NewYork. Pearson

Progress Update. (2014). *Healthy people 2020 leading health indicators: Progress update*. Retrieved from www.healthypeople.gov/sites/default/files/LHI-ProgressReport-ExecSum_0.pdf

*Ridner, S. H. (2004). Psychological distress: Concept analysis. *Journal of Advanced Nursing*, *45*(5), 536–545.

Shahab, L. (2012). *Smoking and bone health*. National Centre for Smoking Cessation and Training (NCSCT). Retrieved from www.ncst.co.uk/usr/pub/smoking_and_bone_health.pdf

*Sheahan, S. L., & Latimer, M. (1995). Correlates of smoking, stress, and depression among women. *Health Values: The Journal of Health Behavior, Education & Promotion*, *19*, 29–36.

Stead, L. F., Lancaster, T., & Perera, R. (2006). Telephone counselling for smoking cessation. *The Cochrane Library*, *19*(3).

U.S. Bureau of Census. (2011). Census Bureau Releases 2011 American Community Survey estimates. Retrieved from www.census.gov/newsroom/releases/archives/american_community_survey_acs/cb12-175.html

*U.S. Department of Health and Human Services. (2000). *Healthy people 2010*. Washington, DC: U.S. Government Printing Office.

U.S. Department of Health and Human Services. (2015). *Tobacco use and pregnancy*. Washington, DC: U.S. Government Printing Office. Retrieved from http://betobaccofree.hhs.gov/health-effects/pregnancy/

Ineffective Health Management

*Bodenheimer, T., MacGregor, K., & Sharifi, C. (2005). *Helping patients manage their chronic conditions*. Retrieved from www.chef.org/publications

Centers for Medicare and Medicaid Services (CMS). (2008). *Roadmap for implementing value driven healthcare in the traditional medicare fee-for-service-program*. Retrieved from www.cms.gov/Medicare/Quality-Initiatives-Patient-Assessment-Instruments/QualityInitiativesGenInfo/downloads/QualityMeasures

*Cutilli, C. C. (2005). Do your patients understand? Determining your patients' health literacy skills. *Orthopaedic Nursing*, *24*(5), 372–377; quiz 378–379.

Di Leonardi, B.C., Faller, M., & Siroky, K. (2011). Preventing never events: Evidence based nurse staffing. *AMA Healthcare*. Retrieved at www.amnhealthcare.com/uploadedFiles/MainSite/Content/Healthcare_Industry_Insigh ts/Industry_Research/Never_Events_white_paper_06.16.11.pdf

Federal Interagency Forum on Age-Related Statistics. (2012). *Older Americans 2012: Key indicators of well-being*. Retrieved from AgingStats.Gov

Iuga, A. O., & McGuire, M. J. (2014). Adherence and health care costs. *Risk Management and Healthcare Policy*, 7, 35.

*Kalichman, S. C., Cain, D., Fuhel, A., Eaton, L., Di Fonzo, K., & Ertl, T. (2005). Assessing medication adherence self-efficacy among low-literacy patients: Development of a pictographic visual analogue scale. *Health Education Research*, *20*(1), 24–35.

*Kutner, M., Greenberg, E., Jin, Y., & Paulsen, C. (2006). *The Health Literacy of America's Adults: Results from the 2003 National Assessment of Adult Literacy*. U.S. Dept. of Education. Washington, DC. National Center for Education Statistics. Retrieved from http://nces.ed.gov/pubs2006/2006483.pdf

Lee, P. G., Cigolle, C., & Blaum, C. (2009). The co-occurrence of chronic diseases and geriatric syndromes: The health retirement study. *Journal of the American Geriatrics Society*. *57*(3), 511–516.

Parker, R., & Ratzan, S. C. (2010). Health literacy: A second decade of distinction for Americans. *Journal of Health Communication*, *15*(S2), 20–33.

Pelikan, M., Röthlin, F., Ganahl, K., Slonska, Z., Doyle, G., Fullam, J., & Kondilis, B. (2015). *Health literacy in Europe: Comparative results of the European Health Literacy Survey (HLS-EU)*. Oxford: Oxford University Press. Retrieved from http://eurpub.oxfordjournals.org/content/early/2015/04/04/eurpub.ckv043

*Rollnick, S., Mason, P., & Butler, C. (2000). *Health behavior change: A guide for practitioners*. Edinburgh: Churchill Livingstone.

*Roter, D. L., Rune, R. E., & Comings, J. (1998). Patient literacy: A barrier to quality of care. *Journal General Internal Medicine*, *13*(12), 850–851.

Sørensen, K., Van den Broucke, S., Fullam, J., Doyle, G., Pelikan, J., Slonska, Z., & Brand, H. (2012). Health literacy and public health: A systematic review and integration of definitions and models. *BMC Public Health*, *12*(1), 80.

Speros, C. (2009). More than words: Promoting health literacy in older adults. *The Online Journal of Issues in Nursing*, *14*(3). Retrieved from www.nursingworld.org/MainMenuCategories/ANAMarketplace/ANAPeriodicals/OJIN/TableofContents/Vol142009/No3Sept09/Health-Literacy-in-Older-Adults.html

*Williams, M. V., Parker, R. M., Baker, D. W., Parikh, N. S., Pitkin, K., Coates, W. C., & Nurss, J. R. (1995). Inadequate functional health literacy among patients at two public hospitals. *JAMA*, *274*(21), 1677–1682.

Risk Prone Health Behavior

*Bodenheimer, T., MacGregor, K., & Sharifi, C. (2005). *Helping patients manage their chronic conditions*. Retrieved from www.chef.org/publications

Centers for Disease Control and Prevention (CDC). (2014). Youth risk behavior surveillance—United States, 2013. *MMWR: Surveillance Summaries*, *63*(Suppl 4), 1–168.

*Cutilli, C. C. (2005). Health literacy? What you need to know. *Orthopaedic Nursing*, *24*(3), 227–231.

*Kalichman, S. C., Cain, D., Fuhrel, A., Eaton, L., Di Fonzo, K., & Ertl, T. (2005). Assessing medication adherence self-efficacy among low-literacy patients: Development of a pictographic visual analogue scale. *Health Education Research*, *20*(1), 24–35.

*Murphy, P. W., Davis, T. C., Long, S. W., Jackson, R. H., & Decker, B. C. (1993). Rapid estimate of adult literacy in medicine (REALM): A quick reading test for patients. *Journal of Reading*, 124–130.

*Piette, J. D. (2005). *Using telephone support to manage chronic disease*. Oakland, CA: California Healthcare Foundation. Retrieved from www.chef.org/topics/chronicdisease/index.cfm

*Rollnick, S., Mason, P., & Butler, C. (2000). *Health behavior change: A guide for practitioners*. Edinburgh: Churchill Livingstone.

Tyler, D. O., & Horner, S. D. (2008). Family-centered collaborative negotiation: A model for facilitating behavior change in primary care. *Journal of the American Academy of Nurse Practitioners*, *20*(4), 194–203.

Hopelessness

Bayat, M., Erdem, E., & Kuzucu, E. G. (2008). Depression, anxiety, hopelessness, and social support levels of parents of children with cancer. *Journal of Pediatric Oncology Nursing*, *25*(5), 247–253.

*Benzein, E. G., & Berg, A. C. (2005). The level of a relation between hope, hopelessness, and fatigue in patients and

family members in palliative care. *Palliative Medicine, 19*(3), 234–240.

Brothers, B.M. & Anderson, B.L. (2009). Hopelessness as a predictor of depressive symptoms for breast cancer patients coping with recurrence. *Psycho-Oncology, 18*, 267–275. doi: 10.1002/pon.1394

*Engel, G. (1989). A life setting conducive to illness: The giving up-given up complex. *Annals of Internal Medicine, 69*, 293–300.

Govender, R. D., & Schlebusch, L. (2012). Hopelessness, depression and suicidal ideation in HIV-positive persons. *South African Journal of Psychiatry*, 18(1), 16–21.

*Herth, K. (1993). Hope in the family caregiver of terminally ill people. *Journal of Advanced Nursing, 18*, 538–547.

*Hinds, P., Martin, J., & Vogel, R. (1987). Nursing strategies to influence adolescent hopefulness during oncologic illness. *Journal of the Association of Pediatric Oncology Nurses, 4*(1/2), 14–23.

*Jennings, P. (1997). The aging spirit. Faith and hope—therapeutic tools for case managers. *Aging Today, 18*(2), 17.

*Korner, I. N. (1970). Hope as a method of coping. *Journal of Consultation and Clinical Psychology, 34*, 134–139.

*Kübler-Ross, E. (1975). *Death: The final stage of growth*. Englewood Cliffs, NJ: Prentice-Hall.

*Leininger, M. (1978). *Transcultural nursing: Concepts, theories, and practices*. New York: Wiley.

*Lin, H. R., & Bauer-Wu, S.M. (2003). Psychospiritual well-being in patients with advanced cancer: An integrative review of the literature. *Journal of Advanced Nursing, 44*(1), 69–80.

Liu, R. T., & Mustanski, B. (2012). Suicidal ideation and self-harm in lesbian, gay, bisexual, and transgender youth. *American Journal of Preventive Medicine, 42*(3), 221–228. doi:10.1016/j.amepre.2011.10.023

Mair, C., Kaplan, G. A., & Everson-Rose, S. A. (2012). Are there hopeless neighborhoods? An exploration of environmental associations between individual-level feelings of hopelessness and neighborhood characteristics. *Health & Place, 18*(2), 434–439. doi:10.1016/j.healthplace.2011.12.012

Mihaljević, S., Aukst-Margetić, B., Vuksan-Ćusa, B., Koić, E., & Milošević, M. (2012). Hopelessness, suicidality and religious coping in Croatian war veterans with PTSD. *Psychiatria Danubina, 24*(3), 292–297.

*Miller, J. F. (1989). Hope inspiring strategies of the critically ill. *Applied Nursing Research, 2*(1), 23–29.

*Notewotney, M. L. (1989). Assessment of hope in patients with cancer: Development of an instrument. *Oncology Nursing Forum, 16*, 57–61.

Öztunj, G., Yeşil, P., Paydaş, S., & Erdoğan, S. (2013). Social support and hopelessness in patients with breast cancer. *Asian Pacific Journal of Cancer Prevention, 14*(1), 571–578. doi:10.7314/APJCP.2013.14.1.571

*Parse, R. R. (1990). Parse's research methodology within an illustration of the lived experience of hope. *Nursing Science Quarterly, 3*(3), 9–17.

Polanco-Roman, L., & Miranda, R. (2013). Culturally related stress, hopelessness, and vulnerability to depressive symptoms and suicidal ideation in emerging adulthood. *Behavior Therapy, 44*(1), 75–87.doi:10.1016/j.beth.2012.07.002

Robinson, J. D., Hoover, D. R., Venetis, M. K., Kearney, T. J., & Street, R. L. (2012). Consultations between patients with breast cancer and surgeons: A pathway from patient-centered communication to reduced hopelessness. *Journal of Clinical Oncology*. doi:10.1200/JCO.2012.44.2699

Sar, A. H., & Sayar, B. (2013). Relationship between hopelessness and submissive behaviours and humor styles of university students. *International Journal of Human Sciences, 9*(2), 1702–1718.

Sirey, J. A., Bruce, M. L., & Alexopoulos, G. S. (2014). The Treatment Initiation Program: An intervention to improve depression outcomes in older adults. *American Journal of Psychiatry*. doi:10.1176/appi.ajp.162.1.184

*Stotland, E. (1969). *The psychology of hope*. San Francisco: Jossey-Bass.

*Watson, J. (1979). *Nursing: The philosophy and science of caring*. Boston: Little, Brown.

Ye, S. C., & Yeh, H. F. (2007). Using complementary therapy with a hemodialysis patient with colon cancer and a sense of hopelessness. *Hu Li Za Zhi (Chinese), 54*(5): 93–98.

Risk for Compromised Human Dignity

*Angus, D. C., Barnato, A. E., Linde-Zwirble, W. T., Weissfeld, L. A., Watson, R. S., Rickert, T., . . . Robert Wood Johnson Foundation ICU End-Of-Life Peer Group. (2004). Use of intensive care at the end of life in the United States: an epidemiologic study. *Critical Care Medicine, 32*(3), 638–643.

*American Medical Association. (2001). *The principles of medical ethics*. Retrieved 23 March, 2016 from www.ama-assn.org/ama/pub/physician-resources/medical-ethics/code-medical-ethics/principles-medical-ethics.page.

American Nurses Association. (2012). *ANA social policy statement*. Washington, DC: Author.

Ditillo, B. A. (2002). Should there be a choice for cardiopulmonary resuscitation when death is expected? Revisiting an old idea whose time is yet to come. *Journal of Palliative Medicine, 5*(1), 107–116.

*Elpern, E., Covert, B., & Kleinpell, R. (2005). Moral distress of staff nurses in a medical intensive care unit. *American Journal of Critical Care, 14*(6), 523–530.

European Commission. (2016). EU charter of fundamental rights. Retrieved from http://fra.europa.eu/en/charterpedia/article/1-human-dignity

*Haddock, J. (1994). Towards further clarification of the concept "dignity." *Journal of Advanced Nursing, 24*(5), 924–931.

*Halcomb, E., Daly, J., Jackson, D., & Davidson, P. (2004). An insight into Australian Nurses' experience of withdrawal/withholding of treatment in the ICU. *Intensive & Critical Care Nursing, 20*(4), 214–222.

Hamric, A. B., Borchers, C. T., & Epstein, E. G. (2012). Development and testing of an instrument to measure moral distress in healthcare professionals. *AJOB Primary Research, 3*(2), 1–9.

LaSala, C. A., & Bjarnason, D. (2010). Creating workplace environments that support moral courage. *The Online Journal of Issues in Nursing*, 15(3), 1–11.

*Mairis, E. (1994). Concept clarification of professional practice—Dignity. *Journal of Advanced Nursing, 19*(5), 947–953.

*Reed, P., Smith, P., Fletcher, M., & Bradding, A. (2003). Promoting the dignity of the child in hospital. *Nursing Ethics, 10*(1), 67–78.

*Söderberg, S., Lundman, B., & Norberg, A. (1999). Struggling for dignity: The meaning of women's experiences of living with fibromyalgia. *Qualitative Health Research, 9*(5), 575–587.

*Walsh, K., & Kowanko, I. (2002). Nurses' and patients' perceptions of dignity. *International Journal of Nursing Practice, 8*(3), 143–151.

*Zomorodi, M., & Lynn, M. R. (2010). Instrument development measuring critical care nurses' attitudes and behaviors with end-of-life care. *Nursing Research, 59*(4), 234–240.

*Zuzelo, P. R. (2007). Exploring the moral distress of registered nurses. *Nursing Ethics, 14*(3), 344–359.

Disorganized Infant Behavior

*Aita, M. & Snider, L. (2003). The art of developmental care in NICU: A concept analysis. *Journal of Advanced Nursing, 41*(3), 223.

*Als, H. (1986). A synactive model of neonatal behavioral organization: Framework for the assessment of neurobehavioral development in the premature infant and for the support of infants and parents in the neonatal intensive care environment. *Physical and Occupational Therapy in Pediatrics, 6*, 3–53.

*Als, H., Gilkerson, L., Duffy, F. H., McAnulty, G. B., Buehler, D. M., Vandenberg, K., . . . Jones, K. J. (2003). A three-center, randomized, controlled trial of individualized developmental care for very low birth weight preterm infants: Medical, neurodevelopmental, parenting, and caregiving effects. *Journal of Developmental and Behavioral Pediatrics, 24*(6), 399–408.

*American Academy of Pediatrics (AAP), Committee on Environmental Health. (1997). Noise: A hazard for the fetus and newborn. *Pediatrics, 100*(4), 724–727.

*American Academy of Pediatrics (AAP) Committee on Fetus and Newborn, American Academy of Pediatrics Section on Surgery, Canadian Paediatric Society Fetus and Newborn Committee. (2006). Prevention and management of pain in the neonate: An update. *Pediatrics, 118*(5), 2231–2241.

Askin, D., & Wilson, D. (2007). The high risk newborn and family. In M. J. Hockenberry & D. Wilson (Eds.), *Wong's nursing care of infants and children* (8th ed.). St. Louis: Mosby Elsevier.

*Blackburn, S. (1993). Assessment and management of neurologic dysfunction. In C. Kenner, A. Brueggemeyer, & L. Gunderson (Eds.), *Comprehensive neonatal nursing.* Philadelphia: W. B. Saunders.

Blackburn, S. T. (Eds.). (2007). *Maternal, fetal, & neonatal physiology: A clinical perspective* (pp. 560–591). St. Louis, MO: Saunders.

*Blackburn, S., & Vandenberg, K. (1993). Assessment and management of neonatal neurobehavioral development. In C. Kenner, A. Brueggemeyer, & L. Gunderson (Eds.), *Comprehensive neonatal nursing.* Philadelphia: W. B. Saunders.

Blackburn, S., & Ditzenberger, G. (2007). Neurologic system. In C. Kenner & J. W. Lott (Eds.), *Comprehensive neonatal care: An interdisciplinary approach* (4th ed.), pp. 267–299. St. Louis: Saunders Elsevier.

*Bozzette, M. (1993). Observations of pain behavior in the NICU: An exploratory study. *Journal of Perinatal and Neonatal Nursing, 7*(1), 76–87.

*Harrison, L., Olivet, L., Cunningham, K., Bodin, M. B., & Hicks, C. (1996). Effects of gentle human touch on preterm infants: pilot study results. *Neonatal Network, 15*(2), 35–42.

Holditch-Davis, D., & Blackburn, S. (2007). Neurobehavioral development. In C. Kenner & J. W. Lott (Eds.), *Comprehensive neonatal care: An interdisciplinary approach* (4th ed., pp. 448–479). St. Louis: Saunders Elsevier.

Kenner, C., & McGrath, J.M. (Eds.) (2010). Developmental care of newborns and infants, *The Neonatal Intensive Care Unit Environment* (pp.63–74). Glenview, IL: NANN.

*Merenstein, G. B., & Gardner, S. L. (1998). *Handbook of neonatal intensive care* (4th ed.). St. Louis: Mosby-Year Book.

*Merenstein, G. B. & Gardner, S. L. (Eds.). (2002). The neonate and the environment: Impact on development. In *Handbook of neonatal intensive care* (pp. 219–282). St. Louis, MO: Mosby.

Padrón, E., Carlson, E. A., Sroufe, L. A. (2014). Frightened versus not frightened disorganized infant attachment: Newborn characteristics and maternal caregiving. *American Journal of Orthopsychiatry, 84*(2), 201–208.

*Thomas, K. A. (1989). How the NICU environment sounds to a preterm infant. *MCN: American Journal of Maternal-Child Nursing, 14*, 249–251.

*Vandenberg, K. (1990). The management of oral nippling in the sick neonate, the disorganized feeder. *Neonatal Network, 9*(1), 9–16.

VandenBerg, K. (2007). State systems development in high-risk newborns in the neonatal intensive care unit: Identification and management of sleep, alertness, and crying. *Journal Perinatal & Neonatal Nursing, 21*(2), 130–139.

*Williamson, P. S., & Williamson, M. L. (1983). Physiologic stress reduction by local anesthetic during newborn circumcision. *Pediatrics*, 7, 36–40.

*Yecco, G. J. (1993). Neurobehavioral development and developmental support of premature infants. *Journal of Perinatal and Neonatal Nursing*, 7(1), 56–65.

Risk for Infection

*Akbar, S. K., Fazle, M., & Onji, M. (1998). Hepatitis B virus (HBV)-transgenic mice as an investigative tool to study immunopathology during HBV infection. *International Journal of Experimental Pathology, 79*(5), 279–291.

American Academy of Otolaryngology. (2014). Ear infection and vaccines: Patient health information. Received 23 March, 2016, from www.entnet.org/content/ear-infection-and-vaccines.

Anderson, D. J., & Sexton, D. J. (2015). Epidemiology of surgical site infection in adults. In *UpToDate*. Retrieved from www.uptodate.com/contents/epidemiology-of-surgical-site-infection-in-adults.

Armstrong, D. G., & Mayr, A. (2014). Wound healing and risk factors for non-healing. In *UpToDate*. Retrieved from www.uptodate.com/contents/wound-healing-and-risk-factors-for-non-healing.

Centers for Disease Control and Prevention (CDC). (2013a). *Guidance for the selection and use of personal protective equipment (PPE) in healthcare settings.* CDC. Retrieved from www.google.com/webhp?sourceid=chrome-instant&ion=1&espv=2&1e=UTF-

CDC. (2013b). *Diagnoses of HIV infection among adults aged 50 years and older in the United States and dependent areas, 2007–2010.* Retrieved from www.cdc.gov/hiv/pdf/statistics_2010_hiv_surveillance_report_vol_18_no_3.pdf

CDC. (2015a). *HIV in the United States: At a glance.* Retrieved from www.cdc.gov/hiv/statistics/basics/ataglance.html

CDC. (2015b). *Reported STDs in the United States 2014 National Data for Chlamydia, Gonorrhea, and Syphilis.* Retirieved from / www.cdc.gov/std/stats14/std-trends-508.pdf)?

CDC. (2015c). *Hand hygiene in healthcare settings.* CDC. Retrieved from www.cdc.gov/handhygiene/.

CDC. (2015d). *Surgical site infection (SSI) event.* Retrieved from www.cdc.gov/nhsn/PDFs/pscManual/9pscSSIcurrent.pdf

CDC. (2015e). *Youth risk behavior surveillance system (YRBSS).* Retrieved from www.cdc.gov/healthyyouth/data/yrbs/index .tm

CDC. (2015f). *Catheter-associated urinary tract infections (CAUTI).* Retrieved from www.cdc.gov/HAI/ca_uti/uti.html

CDC. (2016). *Urinary tract infection (UTI) event for long-term care facilities.* Retrieved from www.cdc.gov/nhsn/pdfs/ltc/ ltcf-uti-protocol-current.pdf

Diaz, V., & Newman, J. (2015). Surgical site infection and prevention guidelines: A primer for certified registered nurse anesthetists. *AANA Journal, 83*(1), 63.

Fekete, T. (2015). Catheter-associated urinary tract infection in adults. In *UpToDate*. Retrieved from www.uptodate.com/contents/catheter-associated-urinary-tract-infection-in-adults.

Franz, M. G., Robson, M. C., Steed, D. L., Barbul, A., Brem, H., Cooper, D. M., . . . Wiersema-Bryant, L. (2008). Guidelines to aid healing of acute wounds by decreasing impediments of healing. *Wound Repair and Regeneration, 16*(6), 723–748.

*Geerlings, M. I., Deeg, D. J. H., Penninx, B. W. J. H., Schmand, B., Jonker, C., Bouter, L. M., & Van Tilburg, W. (1999). Cognitive reserve and mortality in dementia: the role of cognition, functional ability and depression. *Psychological Medicine, 29*(5), 1219–1226.

Gouin, J. P., & Kiecolt-Glaser, J. K. (2010). The impact of psychological stress on would healing: Methods and mechanisms. *Immunology and Allergy Clinics of North America, 31*(1): 81–93.

Gould, C. V., Umscheid, C. A., Agarwal, R. K., Kuntz, G., Pegues, D. A., & The Healthcare Infection Control Practices Advisory Committee (HICPAC). (2009). *Guideline for prevention of catheter associated urinary tract infections.* Retrieved from www.cdc.gov/hicpac/pdf/CAUTI/CAUTIguideline-2009final.pdf.

Guo, S., & DiPietro, L. A. (2010). Factors affecting wound healing. *Journal of Dental Research, 89*(3), 219–229.

High, K. (2015). Evaluation of infection in the older adult. In *UptoDate*. Retrieved from www.uptodate.com/contents/evaluation-of-infection-in-the-older-adult?source=search_result&search=infection+in+elderly&selectedTitle=1~150

Hockenberry, M. J., Wilson, D., & Winkelstein, M. L. (2013). Wong's nursing care of infants and children. New York: Elsevier.

*Kovach, T. (1990). Nip it in the bud: Controlling wound infection with preoperative shaving. *Today's O.R. Nurse, 9,* 23–26.

Kwon, S., Thompson, R., & Dellinger, P. (2013). Importance of perioperative glycemic control in general surgery. Surgical care and outcomes assessment program. *Annals of Surgery, 257*(1), 8.

Magill, S. S., Edwards, J. R., Bamberg, W., Beldavs, Z. G., Dumyati, G., Kainer, M. A., . . . Ray, S. M. (2014). Multistate point-prevalence survey of health care-associated infections. *New England Journal of Medicine, 370*(13),: 1198–1208.

Miller, C. (2015). *Nursing for wellness in older adults* (7th ed.). Philadelphia: Wolters Kluwer.

Newman, D. K. (2015). Using the bladder scan for bladder volume assessment. In *SeekWellness*. Retrieved from www.seekwellness.com/incontinence/using_the_bladderscan.htm.

O'Grady, N. P., Alexander, M., Burns, L. A., Dellinger, P. E., Garland, J., Heard, S. O., . . . The Healthcare Infection Control Practices Advisory Committee (HICPAC). (2011). *Guidelines for the prevention of intravascular catheter-related infections.* Atlanta, GA: Centers for Disease Control and Prevention. Retrieved from www.cdc.gov/hicpac/pdf/guidelines/bsi-guidelines-2011.pdf

Pear, S. M. (2007). *Managing infection control: Patients risk factors and best practices for surgical site infection prevention* (pp. 56–63). Tucson, AZ: University of Arizona.

Price, C. S., Williams, A., Philips, G., Dayton, M., Smith, W., & Morgan, S. (2008). Staphylococcus aureus nasal colonization in preoperative orthopaedic outpatients. *Clinical Orthopaedics and Related Research, 466*(11), 2842–2847.

Schaeffer, A. J. (2015). Placement and management of urinary bladder catheters. In: *UpToDate*. Retrieved from www.uptodate.com/contents/placement-and-management-of-urinary-bladder-catheters?source=search_result&search=Placement+and+management+of+urinary+bladder+catheters&selectedTitle=1~150

Sessler, D. I. (2006). Non-pharmacologic prevention of surgical wound infection. *Anesthesiology Clinics of North America, 24*(2), 279–297.

*Siegel, J. D., Rhinehart, E., Jackson, M., Chiarello, L., & The Healthcare Infection Control Practices Advisory Committee. (2007, June). *2007 guideline for isolation precautions: Preventing transmission of infectious agents in healthcare settings.* Retrieved August 12, 2008, from www.cdc.gov/ncidod/dhqp/pdf/isolation2007.pdf

Sørensen, L. T. (2012). Wound healing and infection in surgery: The pathophysiological impact of smoking, smoking cessation, and nicotine replacement therapy: A systematic review. *Annals of Surgery, 255*(6), 1069–1079. Retrieved from http://archsurg.jamanetwork.com/article.aspx?articleid=1151013

Speaar, M. (2008). Wound care management: Risk factors for surgical site infections. *Plastic Surgical Nursing, 28*(4), 201–204.

Tanner, J., Norrie, P., & Melen, K. (2011). Preoperative hair removal to reduce surgical site infection. *Cochrane Database System Review, 9,* 11.

The Joanna Briggs Institute. (2007). Pre-operative hair removal to reduce surgical site infection. *Best Practice, 11*(4). Retrieved from http://connect.jbiconnectplus.org/ViewSourceFile.aspx?0=4347

Risk for Infection Transmission

Centers for Disease Control and Prevention. (2015). *HIV in the United States: At a glance.* Retrieved from www.cdc.gov/hiv/statistics/basics/ataglance.html.

Cohen, M. S., Hoffman, I. F., Royce, R. A., Kazembe, P., Dyer, J. R., Daly, C. C., . . . Eron, J. J. (1997). Reduction of concentration of HIV-1 in semen after treatment of urethritis:

Implications for prevention of sexual transmission of HIV-1. *The Lancet*, *349*(9069), 1868–1873.

Grant, R. M., Lama, J. R., Anderson, P. L., McMahan, V., Liu, A. Y., Vargas, L., . . . Montoya-Herrera, O. (2010). Preexposure chemoprophylaxis for HIV prevention in men who have sex with men. *New England Journal of Medicine*, *363*(27), 2587–2599.

Internet Resources

Association for Professionals in Infection Control, www.apic.org

Centers for Disease Control and Prevention, www.cdc.gov

National Center for Infectious Disease, www.cdc.gov/ncidod/nicid.htm

Risk for Injury

Alcee, D. (2000). The experience of a community hospital in quantifying and reducing patient falls. *Journal of Nursing Care Quality*, 14(3), 43–53.

American Academy of Orthopedic Surgeons. (2012). *Lawn mower safety*. Retrieved from www.orthoinfo.org/topic.cfm?topic=A00670

American Academy of Orthopedic Surgeons. (2016). *Bicycle safety* Retrieved from http://orthoinfo.aaos.org/topic.cfm?topic=A00711

Annweiler, C., Montero-Odasso, M., Schott, A. M., Berrut, G., Fantino, B., & Beauchet, O. (2010). Fall prevention and vitamin D in the elderly: An overview of the key role of the non-bone effects. *Journal of Neuroengineering and Rehabilitation*, 7(1), 1.

*Baumann, S. L. (1999). Defying gravity and fears: The prevention of falls in community-dwelling older adults. *Clinical Excellence for Nurse Practitioners*, *3*(5), 254–261.

Beling, J., & Roller, M. (2009). Multifactorial intervention with balance training as a core component among fall-prone older adults. *Journal of Geriatric Physical Therapy*, *32*(3), 125–133.

Centers for Disease Control and Prevention (CDC). (2001). *Smoking and tobacco use*. Retrieved from www.cdc.gov/tobacco/data_statistics/

CDC. (2012). *Protect the ones you love: Child injuries are preventable. Journal of the American Geriatrics Society*, *60*(1), 124–129. doi:10.1111/j.1532.5415.2011.03767.x. Retrieved from www.cdc.gov/safechild/Child_Injury_Data.html

CDC. (2015). Growing stronger: Strength training for older ADULTS. Retrieved from http://www.cdc.gov/physicalactivity/growingstronger/

CDC. (2016). Deaths: Final data for 2013. Retrieved from www.cdc.gov/nchs/data/nvsr/nvsr64/nvsr64_02.pdf

*Clemen-Stone, E., Eigasti, D. G., & McGuire, S. L. (2001). *Comprehensive family and community health nursing* (6th ed.). St. Louis, MO: Mosby-Year Book.

Gray-Miceli, D., Ratcliffe, S. J., & Johnson, J. (2010). Use of a postfall assessment tool to prevent falls. *Western Journal of Nursing Research*, *32*(7):932–948.

Grossman, S., & Porth, C. A. (2014). *Porth's pathophysiology: Concepts of altered health states* (9th ed.). Philadelphia: Wolters Kluwer.

Himes, C. L., & Reynolds, S. L. (2012). Effect of obesity on falls, injury, and disability. *Journal of the American Geriatrics Society*, *60*(1), 124–129. doi:10.1111/j.1532-5415.2011.03767.x

Hockenberry, M. J., & Wilson, D. (2015). *Wong's essentials of pediatric nursing* (10th ed.). New York: Elsevier.

Jefferis, B. J., Iliffe, S., Kendrick, D., Kerse, N., Trost, S., Lennon, L. T., . . . & Whincup, P. H. (2014). How are falls and fear of falling associated with objectively measured physical activity in a cohort of community-dwelling older men? *BMC geriatrics*, *14*(1), 114. Retrieved from www.biomedcentral.com/1471-2318/14/114

Kaufmann, H., Freeman, R., & Kaplan, N. M. (2010). Treatment of orthostatic and postprandial hypotension. In *UpToDate*. Retrieved from www.uptodate.com/patients/content/topic.do?topicKey=~tbbgIjyWVqqVE5

Kaufman, H., & Kaplan, N. M. (2015a). Mechanisms, causes, and evaluation of orthostatic hypotension. In *UpToDate*. Retrieved from www.uptodate.com/contents/mechanisms-causes-and-evaluation-of-orthostatic- hypotension.

Kaufman H., & Kaplan, N. M. (2015b). Treatment of orthostatic and postprandial hypotension. In *UpToDate*. Retrieved from www.uptodate.com/contents/treatment-of-orthostatic-and-postprandial-hypotension.

Lancaster, A. D., Ayers, A., Belbot, B., Goldner, V., Kress, L., Stanton, D., . . . Sparkman, L. (2007). Preventing falls and eliminating injury at Ascension Health. *Joint Commission Journal on Quality and Patient Safety*, *33*(7), 367–375.

Miller, C. (2015). *Nursing for wellness in older adults* (7th ed.). Philadelphia: Wolters Kluwer.

Misra, A. (2014). *Common sports injuries: Incidence and average charges*. Washington, DC: Department of Health and Human Services. Retrieved from http://aspe.hhs.gov/health/reports/2014/SportsInjuries/ib_SportsInjuries.pdf

Morse, J. (2009). *Preventing patient falls: Establishing a fall intervention program* (2nd ed.). New York. Springer Publishing Company.

National Safety Council. (2014). Injury and fatality statistics and trends. Retrieved from www.nsc.org/newsdocuments/2014-press-release-archive/3-25-2014-injury-facts-release.pdf

*Podsiadlo, D., & Richardson, S. (1991). The timed 'Up and Go' test: A test of basic functional mobility for frail elderly

persons. *Journal of American Geriatric Society*, *39*, 142–148. Retrieved August 2, 2012, from www.fallrventiontaskforce.org-pdf.Timed UpandGoTest.pdf

Perlmuter, L. C., Sarda, G., Casavant, V., & Mosnaim, A. D. (2013). A review of the etiology, asssociated comorbidities, and treatment of orthostatic hypotension. *American journal of therapeutics*, *20*(3), 279–291.

*Riefkohl, E. Z., Bieber, H. L., Burlingame, M. B., & Lowenthal, D. T. (2003). Medications and falls in the elderly: A review of the evidence and practical considerations. *Pharmacy&Therapeutics*, *28*(11), 724–733.

*Schoenfelder, D. P. (2000). A fall prevention program for elderly individuals. *Journal of Gerontological Nursing*, *26*(3), 43–45.

*Shields, B. J., & Smith, G. A. (2006). Success in the prevention of infant walker-related injuries: An analysis of national data, 1990–2001. *Pediatrics*, *117*(3), e452–e459.

Risk for Aspiration

American Association of Critical Care Nurses. (2011). *Prevention of aspiration*. Aliso Viejo, CA: Author. Retrieved from www.aacn.org/wd/practice/docs/practicealerts/prevention-aspiration-practice-alert.pdf?menu=aboutus

Goldsmith, T., & Cohen, A. K. (2014). Swallowing disorders and aspiration in palliative care: Assessment and strategies for management. In *UpToDate*. Retrieved from www.uptodate.com/contents/swallowing-disorders-and-aspiration-in-palliative-care-assessment-and-strategies-for-management

Risk for Perioperative Positioning Injury

Conner, R. L. (2006). Preventing intraoperative positioning injuries. *Nursing Management*, *37*(7, Suppl), 9–10. Retrieved from www.nursingcenter.com/journalarticle?Article_ID=655629

*Martin, J. T. (2000). Positioning aged patients. *Geriatric Anesthesia*, *18*, 1.

*Rothrock, J. C. (2003). *Alexander's care of the patient in surgery* (12th ed.). St. Louis: Mosby.

Webster, K. (2012). *Peripheral nerve injuries and positioning for general anesthesia*. London: World Federation of Societies of Anesthesiologists. Retrieved from www.frca.co.uk/Documents/258 Peripheral Nerve Injuries and Positioning for Anaesthesia.pdf

Risk for Falls

Himes, C. L., & Reynolds, S. L. (2014). *NSC releases latest injury and fatality statistics and trends*. Itasca, IL: National Safety Council. Retrieved from www.nsc.org/newsdocument/2014-press-release-archive/3-25-2014-injury- facts-release.pdf

Jefferis, B. J., Iliffe, S., Kendrick, D., Kerse, N., Trost, S., Lennon, L. T., . . . Whincup, P. H. (2014). How are falls and fear of falling associated with objectively measured physical activity in a cohort of community-dwelling older men? *BMC geriatrics*, *14*(1), 114.

Kaufman, H., & Kaplan, N. M. (2015a). Mechanisms, causes, and evaluation of orthostatic hypotension. In *UpToDate*. Retrieved from www.uptodate.com/contents/mechanisms-causes-and-evaluation-of-orthostatic- hypotension.

Kaufman H., & Kaplan, N. M. (2015b). Treatment of orthostatic and postprandial hypotension. In *UpToDate*. Retrieved from www.uptodate.com/contents/treatment-of-orthostatic-and-postprandial-hypotension.

Lancaster, A. D., Ayers, A., Belbot, B., Goldner, V., Kress, L., Stanton, D., . . . Sparkman, L. (2007). Preventing falls and eliminating injury at Ascension Health. *Joint Commission journal on quality and patient safety*, *33*(7), 367–375.

Perlmuter, L. C., Sarda, G., Casavant, V., & Mosnaim, A.D. (2013). A review of the etiology associated comorbidities and treatment of orthostatic hypotension. *American Journal of Therapeutics*, *20*, 279.

*Shields, B. J., & Smith, G. A. (2006). Success in the prevention of infant walker-related injuries: An analysis of national data. *Pediatrics*, *117*(3), e452–459.

Internet Sources

Centers for Disease Control and Prevention. (2011). Retrieved August 8, 2011 from www.cdc.gov/tobacco/data

Professional Assisted Cessation Therapy (PACT), www.endsmoking.org

Tobacco.org, www.tobacco.org

Osteoporosis

*Eastell, R., Boyle, I., Compston, J., Cooper, C., Fogelman, I., Francis, R. M., . . . Stevenson, J. C. (1998). Management of male osteoporosis: Report of the UK Consensus Group. *Quarterly Journal of Medicine*, *91*(2), 71–92.

*Hansen, L. B., & Vondracek, S. F. (2004). Prevention and treatment of nonpostmenopausal osteoporosis. *American Journal of Health System Pharmacy*, *61*(24), 2637–2654.

*Lindsay, R. (1989). Osteoporosis: An updated approach to prevention and management. *Geriatrics*, *44*(1), 45–54.

Sommers, M. S., Johnson, S. A., & Berry, T. A. (2007). *Diseases and disorders: A nursing therapeutic manual* (3rd ed.). Philadelphia: F. A. Davis.

*Woodhead, G., & Moss, M. (1998). Osteoporosis: Diagnosis and prevention. *Nursing Practitioner*, *23*(11), 18, 23–24, 26–27, 31–32, 34–35.

Internet Resources

American Society of Aging. *The live well, live long: Health promotion and disease prevention for older adults*. www.cdc.gov/agency.htm

Centers for Disease Control and Prevention, www.cdc.gov/aging.htm.

Mayo Clinic, www.mayo.edu

Latex Allergy Response

American Association of Nurse Anesthetists. (2014). Latex allergy management (Guidelines). Retrieved from www.aana.com/resources2/professionalpractice/Pages/Latex-Allergy-Protocol.aspx

American Latex Allergy Association. (2010). Statistics. Retrieved from http://latexallergyresources.org/statisticsLatex allergy response

DeJong, N. W., Patiwael, J. A., de Groot, H., Burdorf, A., & Gerth van Wijk, R. (2011). Natural rubber latex allergy among healthcare workers: Significant reduction of sensitization and clinical relevant latex allergy after introduction of powder-free latex gloves. *Journal of Allergy and Clinical Immunology*, *127*(2), AB70.

*Kleinbeck, S., English, L., Sherley, M. A., & Howes, J. (1998). A criterion-referenced measure of latex allergy knowledge. *Association of Perioperative Registered Nurses Journal*, *68*(3), 384–392.

*Reddy, S. (1998). Latex allergy. *American Family Physician*, *57*(1), 93–100.

Sedentary Lifestyle

*Allison, M., & Keller, C. (1997). Physical activity in the elderly: Benefits and intervention strategies. *Nursing Practice*, *22*(8), 53–54.

Haskell, W. L., Lee, I. M., & Pate, R. R. (2007). Physical activity and public health: Updated recommendation for adults. *The American College of Sports Medicine and the American Heart Association Circulation*, *116*(9), 1081–1093.

Lacharité-Lemieux, M., Brunelle, J. P., & Dionne, I. J. (2015). Adherence to exercise and affective responses: Comparison between outdoor and indoor training. *Menopause*, *22*(7), 731–740.

*Lee, K. A. (2001). Sleep and fatigue. *Annual Review of Nursing Research*, *19*, 249–273.

Liu, C. J., & Latham, N. K. (2009). Progressive resistance strength training for improving physical function in older adults. *Cochrane Database Systematics Review*, *8*(3), CD002759. doi:10.1002/14651858.CD002759.pub2

McMahon, S., & Fleury, J. (2012, January). Wellness in older adults: A concept analysis. *Nursing forum*, *47*(1), 39–51.

*Moore, S. M., & Charvat, J. M. (2002). Using the CHANGE intervention to enhance long-term exercise. *Nursing Clinics of North America*, *37*(2), 273–283.

*Nies, M. A., & Chruscial, H. L. (2002). Neighborhood and physical activity outcomes in women: Regional comparisons. *Nursing Clinics of North America*, *37*(2), 295–301.

*Resnick, B., Orwig, D., & Magaziner, J. (2002). The effect of social support on exercise behavior in older adults. *Clinical Nursing Research*, *11*(1), 52.

*Schoenfelder, D. P. (2000). A fall prevention program for elderly individuals: Exercise in long-term care settings. *Journal of gerontological nursing*, *26*(3), 43

*Taggart, H. M. (2002). Effects of Tai Chi exercise on balance, functional mobility, and fear of falling among older women. *Applied Nursing Research*, *15*(4), 235–242.

Thompson, P. (2014). *ACSM's guidelines for exercise testing and prescription*. American College of Sports Medicine. Philadelphia: Wolters Kluwer.

*Young, H. M., & Cochrane, B. B. (2004). Healthy aging for older women. *Nursing Clinics of North America*, *39*(1), 131–143.

Risk for Loneliness

*Bidwell, R. J., & Deisher, R. W. (1991). Adolescent sexuality: Current issues. *Pediatric Annals*, *20*, 293–302.

ElSadr, C. B., Noureddine, S., & Kelley, J. (2009). Concept analysis of loneliness with implications for nursing diagnosis. *International Journal of Nursing Terminologies and Classifications*, *20*(1), 25–33.

*Elsen, J., & Blegen, M. (1991). Social isolation. In M. Maas, K. Buckwalter, & M. Hardy (Eds.), *Nursing diagnoses and interventions for the elderly*. Redwood City, CA: Addison-Wesley Nursing.

Hawkley, L. C., & Cacioppo, J. C. (2010). Loneliness matters: A theoretical and empirical review of consequences and mechanisms. *Annals of Behavioral Medicine*, *40*, 218–227. Retrieved at http://psychology.uchicago.ecu/people/faculty/cacioppo/abm218.pdf

*Hillestad, E. A. (1984). Toward understanding of loneliness. In *Proceedings of conference on spirituality*. Milwaukee, WI: Marquette University.

Holt-Lunstad, J., Smith, T. B., & Layton, J. B. (2010). Social relationships and mortality risk: A meta-analytic review. *PLoS Medicine*, 7(7), 859.

Holt-Lunstad, J., Smith, T. B., Baker, M., Harris, T., & Stephenson, D. (2015). Loneliness and social isolation as risk factors for mortality: A meta-analytic review. *Perspectives on Psychological Science*, *10*(2), 227–237.

*Longino, C. F., & Karl, C. S. (1982). Explicating activity theory: A formal replication. *Journal of Gerontology*, *37*, 713–722.

Miller, C. (2015). *Nursing for wellness in older adults* (7th ed.). Philadelphia: Wolters Kluwer.

Osborne, J. W. (2012). Psychological effects of the transition to retirement. *Canadian Journal of Counseling and Psychotherapy*, *46*(1), 45–58.

Singh, A., & Misra, N. (2009). Loneliness, depression and sociability in old age. *Industrial Psychiatry Journal*, *18*(1), 51–55.

Uchino, B. N. (2006). Social support and health: a review of physiological processes potentially underlying links to disease outcomes. *Journal of Behavioral Medicine*, *29*(4):377–387.

Wang, M., & Hesketh, B. (2012). *Achieving well-being in retirement: Recommendations from 20 years' society for industrial and organizational psychology*. Bowling Green, OH: Society for Industrial and Organizational Psychology, Older Work Employment, Retirement.

*Warnick, J. (1993). *Listening with different ears: Counseling people over sixty*. Ft. Bragg CA: QED Press.

Impaired Memory

*Maier-Lorentz, M. (2000). Effective nursing interventions for the management of Alzheimer's disease. *Journal of Neuroscience Nursing*, *32*(3), 153–157.

Impaired Physical Mobility

*Addams, S., & Clough, J. A. (1998). Modalities for mobilization. In A. B. Mahler, S. Salmond, & T. Pellino (Eds.), *Orthopedic nursing*. Philadelphia: W. B. Saunders.

Adler, J., & Malone, D. (2012). Early mobilization in the intensive care unit: A systematic review. *Cardiopulmonary Physical Therapy Journal*, *23*(1), 5. Accessed at www.ncbi.nlm.nih.gov/pmc/articles/PMC3286494/table/T3/

American Association of Critical Care Nurses . (2012). *Early progressive mobility protocol*. ACCNPearl. Retrieved from www.aacn.org/wd/practice/docs/tool%20kits/early-progressive-mobility-protocol.pdf

American Hospital Association, & USDHHS. (2014). Health Research & Educational Trust, American Hospital Association, partnership for patients ventilator associated events (VAE) change package: Preventing harm from VAE 2014 Update. Retrieved from www.hret-hen.org/index.php?option=com_content&view=article&id=10&Itemid=134

*Convertino, V. A., Previc, F. H., Ludwig, D. A., & Engelken, E. J. (1997). Effects of vestibular and oculomotor stimulation on responsiveness of the carotid-cardiac baroreflex. *American Journal of Physiology-Regulatory, Integrative and Comparative Physiology*, *273*(2), R615–R622.

De Jonghe, B., Bastuji-Garin, S., Durand, M. C., Malissin, I., Rodrigues, P., Cerf, C., . . . Sharshar, T. (2007). Respiratory weakness is associated with limb weakness and delayed weaning in critical illness. *Critical Care Medicine*, *35*(9), 2007–2015.

Gillis, A., MacDonald, B., & MacIssac, A. (2008). Nurses' knowledge, attitudes, and confidence regarding preventing and treating deconditioning in older adults. *The Journal of Continuing Education in Nursing*, *39*(12), 547–554.

Halsstead, J., & Stoten, S. (2010). Orthopedic nursing: Caring for patients with musculoskeletal disorders. Brockton, MA : Western Schools.

Hopkins, R. O., & Spuhler, V. J. (2009). Strategies for promoting early activity in critically ill mechanically ventilated patients. *AACN Advanced Critical Care*, *20*(3), 277–289.

*Killey, B., & Watt, E. (2006). The effect of extra walking on the mobility, independence and exercise self-efficacy of elderly hospital in-patients: A pilot study. *Contemporary Nurse*, *22*(1), 120–133.

King, L. (2012). Developing a progressive mobility activity protocol. *Orthopaedic Nursing, 31*(5), 253–262.

Miller, C. (2015). *Nursing for wellness in older adults* (7th ed.). Philadelphia: Wolters Kluwer.

Rantanen, T. (2013). Promoting mobility in older people. *Journal of Preventive Medicine and Public Health, 46*(Suppl 1), S50–S54. Retrieved from www.ncbi.nlm.nih.gov/pmc/articles/PMC3567319/

Timmerman, R. A. (2007). A mobility protocol for critically ill adults. *Dimensions of Critical Care Nursing, 26*(5), 175–179. Retrieved from www0.sun.ac.za/Physiotherapy_ICU_algorithm/Documentation/Rehabilitation/References/Timmerman_2007.pdf

Vollman, K. M. (2012). Hemodynamic instability: Is it really a barrier to turning critically ill patients? *Critical care nurse, 32*(1), 70–75.

Winkelman, C., & Peereboom, K. (2010). Staff-perceived barriers and facilitators. *Critical Care Nurse, 30*(2), S13–S16.

Zomorodi, M., Topley, D., & McAnaw, M. (2012). Developing a mobility protocol for early mobilization of patients in a surgical/trauma ICU. *Critical Care Research and Practice*. Article ID 964547. doi:10.1155/2012/964547

Moral Distress

*American Association of Critical Care Nurses. (2004). *The 4 A's to rise above moral distress.* AACN Ethics Work Group. Aliso Viejo, CA: AACN.

*American Nurse's Association. (2003). *Nursing's social policy statement* (2nd ed.). Silver Spring, MD: Author.

American Nurse's Association. (2010a). *Just culture*. Retrieved from www.justculture.org/Downloads/ANA_Just_Culture.pdf

American Nurses Association. (2010b). *Nursing: Scope and standards of practice* (2nd ed.). Silver Springs, MD: Author.

American Association of Colleges of Nursing. (2010). *Nursing shortage fact sheet.* Washington, DC: Author. Retrieved from www.aacn.nche.edu/Media/pdf/NrsgShortageFS.pdf

Bamsteiner, J., Disch, J., & Walton, M. L. (2014). *Person and family centered care.* Indianapolis, IN: Sigma Theta Tau International.

Baxter, M. L. (2012). *Being certain: Moral distress in critical care nurses* (Doctoral Dissertation). VCU Scholars Compass. Retrieved from scholarscompass.vcu.edu/cgi/viewcontent.cgi?article=3938&context=etd

*Beckstrand, R. L., Callsiter, L. C., & Kirchhoff, K. T. (2006). Providing a "Good Death": Critical care nurse's suggestions for improving end-of-life care. *American Journal of Critical Care, 15*(1), 38–45.

*Caswell, D., & Cryer, H. G. (1995). Case study: When the nurse and physician don't agree. *Journal of Cardiovascular Nursing, 9*, 30–42.

*Cipriano, P. F. (2006). Retaining our talent. *American Nurse Today*, 1(2), 10.

*Corley, M., Minick, P., Elswick, R., & Jacobs, M. (2005). Nurse moral distress and ethical work environments. *Nursing Ethics, 12*(4), 381–389.

Coverston C. R., & Lassetter, J. (2010). Potential erosion of ethical sentiments: When nurse, patient, and institution collide. *Forum on Public Policy Online, 9*(3). Electronic version.

*Cowin, L. S., & Hengstberger-Sims, C. (2006). New graduate nurse self-concept and retention: A longitudinal survey. *International Journal of Nursing Studies, 43*(1), 59–70.

Edmonson, C. (2015). Strengthening moral courage among nurse leaders. *The Online Journal of Issues in Nursing, 20*(2). Retrieved from www.nursingworld.org/MainMenuCategories/ANAMarketplace/ANAPeriodical s/OJIN/TableofContents/Vol-20-2015/No2-May-2015/Articles-Previous- Topics/Strengthening-Moral-Courage.html

*Elpern, E., Covert, B., & Kleinpell, R. (2005). Moral distress of staff nurses in a medical intensive care unit. *American Journal of Critical Care, 14*(6), 523–530.

Frank, A. (2007). *Practical generosity: The professions and the recovering caregiver.* Washington, DC: U.S. President's Council on Bioethics. Retrieved from http://bioethics.georgetown.edu/pcbe/transcripts/nov07/session1.html.

*Gallagher, A. (2010). Moral distress and moral courage in everyday nursing practice. *The Online Journal of Issues in Nursing, 16*(2), 1–8. Retrieved from www.nursingworld.org/OJIN

Gallup Poll. (2009). *Honesty and ethics poll finds congress' image tarnished.* Retrieved from www.gallup/poll124625/honesty-ethics-pol

Gallup Poll. (2014). *Honesty/ethics in professions.* Washington, DC: Gallup. Retrieved from www.gallup.com/poll/1654/honesty-ethics-professions.aspx

*Gert, B., Culver, C., & Clouser, K. (2006). *Bioethics: A systematic approach* (2nd ed.). New York: Oxford University Press.

*Gordon, E., & Hamric, A. B. (2006). The courage to stand up: The cultural politics of nurses' access to ethics consultation. *Journal of Clinical Ethics, 17*(3), 231–254.

*Gutierrez, K. M. (2005). Critical care nurses' perceptions of and responses to moral distress. *Dimensions of Critical Care Nursing, 24*(5), 229–241.

Hall, M. J., Levant, S., Carold, J., & DeFrances, C. J. (2013). *Trends in inpatient hospital deaths: National hospital discharge survey, 2000–2010.* Atlanta, GA: Centers for Disease Control and Prevention (CDC). Retrieved from www.cdc.gov/nchs/data/databriefs/db118.htm.

Hamric, A. B., Borchers, C. T., & Epstein, E. G. (2012). Development and testing of an instrument to measure moral distress in healthcare professionals. *AJOB Primary Research, 3*(2), 1–9.

*Jameton, A. (1984). *Nursing practice: The ethical issues*. London: Prentice-Hall.

Jones, A., Moss, A. J., & Harris-Kojetin, L. D. (2011). *Use of advance directive in long-term care populations.* National Center for Health Statistics. NCHS Data Brief, No. 54. Atlanta, GA: CDC. Retrieved from www.cdc.gov/nchs/data/databriefs/db54.pdf.

*Jormsri, P., Kunaviktikul, W., Ketefian, S., & Chaowalit, A. (2005). Moral competence in nursing practice. *Nursing Ethics*, 12(6), 582–594.

*Kass-Bartelmes, B. L., Hughes, R., & Rutherford, M. K. (2003). *Advance Care Planning: Preferences for Care at the End of Life*. Rockville, MD: Agency for Healthcare Research and Quality. Research in Action Issue #12. AHRQ Pub No. 03-0018. Retrieved from www.ahrq.gov/research/endliferia/endria.pdf

Kupperschmidt, B., Kientz, E., Ward, J., & Reinholz, B. (2010). A healthy work environment: It begins with you. *The Online Journal of Issues in Nursing, 15*(1). doi:10.3912/OJIN.Vol15No1Man03.

*Lachman, V. D. (2010). Strategies necessary for moral courage. *The Online Journal of Issues in Nursing, 15*(3). Retrieved from www.nursingworld.org/MainMenuCategories/EthicsStandards/Courage-and-Distress/Strategies-and-Moral-Courage.html

LaSala, C. A., & Bjarnason, D. (2010). Creating workplace environments that support moral courage. *The Online Journal of Issues in Nursing, 15*(3), 1–11. Retrieved from www.nursingworld.org/OJIN

Lusardi P., Jodka, P., Stambovsky, M., Stadnicki, B., Babb, B., Plouffe, D., . . . Montonye, M. (2011). The going home initiative: Getting critical care patients home with hospice. *Critical Care Nurse*, 31(5), 46–57.

MacKusick, C. I., & Minick, P. (2010). Why are nurses leaving? Findings from an initial qualitative study on nursing attrition. *Medsurg Nursing, 19*(6), 335–340.

Mathieu, F. (2012). *The compassion fatigue workbook: Creative tools for transforming compassion fatigue and vicarious traumatization* (Psychosocial Stress Series, 1st ed.). East Sussex: Routledge. Retrieved from http://tandfbis.s3.amazonaws.com/rt-media/pp/common/sample-chapters/9780415897907.pdf

*Murray, J. S. (2010). Moral courage in healthcare: Acting ethically even in the presence of risk. *The Online Journal of Issues in Nursing, 15*(3). Retrieved from www.nursingworld.org/MainMenuCategories/EthicsStandards/Courage-and-Distress/Moral-Courage-and-Risk.html#Gert

*Rodney, P., Varcoe, C., Storch, J., McPherson, G., Mahoney, K., Brown, H., . . . Starzomski, R. (2002). Navigating towards a moral horizon: A multisite qualitative study of ethical practice in nursing. *Canadian Journal of Nursing Research, 34*(3), 75–102.

*Scanlon, C., & Fleming, C. (1989). *Ethical issues in caring for the patient with advanced cancer. Nursing Clinics of North America, 24*, 977–986.

*Söderberg, A., Gilje, F., & Norberg, A. (1997). Dignity in situations of ethical difficulty in intensive care. *Intensive and Critical Care Nursing, 13*(3), 135–144.

Stanford Encyclopedia of Philosophy. (2007). *Plato's ethics: An overview.* Stanford: Center for the Study of Language and Information. Retrieved from plato.stanford.edu/entries/plato-ethics/

*Tiedje, L. B. (2000). Moral distress in perinatal nursing. *Journal of Perinatal & Neonatal Nursing, 14*(2), 36–43.

*Wilkinson, J. M. (1988). Moral distress in nursing practice: Experience and effect. *Kansas Nurse, 63*(11), 8.

Zomorodi, M., & Lynn, M. R. (2010). Instrument development measuring critical care nurses' attitudes and behaviors with end-of-life care. *Nursing Research, 59*(4), 234–240.

Zuzelo, P. R. (2007). Exploring the moral distress of registered nurses. *Nursing Ethics, 14*(3), 344–359.

Unilateral Neglect

*Bailey, M. J., Riddoch, M. J., & Crome, P. (2002). Treatment of visual neglect in elderly patients with stroke: A single-subject series using either a scanning and cueing strategy or a left-limb activation strategy. *Physical Therapy, 82*(8), 782–797.

*Barrett, A. M. (2014). Spatial neglect. In *Medscape*. Retrieved from http://emedicine.medscape.com/article/1136474-overview

Becker, E., & Kamath, H. O. (2010). Neuroimaging of eye position reveals spatial neglect. *Brain, 133*, 909–914. Retrieved from http://brain.oxfordjournals.org/content/133/3/909

*Berger, M. F., Pross, R. D., Ilg, U. J., & Karnath, H. O. (2006). Deviation of eyes and head in acute cerebral stroke. *BMC Neurology, 6*(23), 1–8.

Chan, D., & Man, D. (2013). Unilateral neglect in stroke: A comparative study. *Topics in Geriatric Rehabilitation, 29*(2), 126–134.

Davis, J. (2013). *One-side neglect: Improving awareness to speed recovery.* Dallas, TX: American Heart Association/American Strokes Association.

Ferreira, H. P., Leite Lopes, M. A., Luiz, R. R., Cardoso, L., & André, C. (2011). Is visual scanning better than mental practice in hemispatial neglect? Results from a pilot study. *Topics in Stroke Rehabilitation, 18*(2), 155–161.

Hibbard, J. H., & Greene, J. (2013). What the evidence shows about patient activation: Better health outcomes and care experiences; fewer data on costs. *Health affairs, 32*(2), 207–214.

Jehkonen, M., Ahonen, J. P., Dastidar, P., Koivisto, A. M., Laippala, P., Vilkki, J., & Molnar, G. (2000). Visual neglect as a predictor of functional outcome one year after stroke. *Acta Neurologica Scandinavica, 101*(3), 195–201.

Mizuno, K., Tsuji, T., Takebavashi, T., Fujiwara, T., Hase, K., & Liu, M. (2011). Prism adaptation therapy enhances rehabilitation of stroke patients with unilateral spatial neglect: A randomized, controlled trial. *Neurorehabilitation Nueral Repair, 25*(8), 711–720. doi:10.3389/fnhum.2013.00137

Newport, R., & Schenk, T. (2012). Prisms and neglect: What have we learned? *Neuropsychologia, 50*(6), 1080–1091.

*Plummer, P., Morris, M. E., & Dunai, J. (2003). Assessment of unilateral neglect. *Physics Therapy*, 83, 732–740.

Priftis, K., Passarini, L., Pilosio, C., Meneghello, F., & Pitteri, M. (2013). Visual scanning training, limb activation treatment, and prism adaptation for rehabilitation left neglect: Who is the winner? *Frontiers in Human Neuroscience*, 7, 360.

Riestra, A. R., & Barrett, A. M. (2013). Rehabilitation of spatial neglect. *Handbook of Clinical Neurology, 110*, 347–355. Retrieved from www.ncbi.nlm.nih/gov/entrez/eutils/elink.fcgi?dbfrom=pubmed&retmode=ref&cmd=prlinks&id=23312654

*Sireteanu, R., Goertz, R., Bachert, U., & Wander, T. (2006). Children with developmental dyslexia show a left visual "Minineglect." *Vision Research*,. 45(25/26), 3075–3082.

Yang, N. Y., Zhou, D. R., Li-Tsang, C., & Fong, K. (2013). Rehabilitation interventions for unilateral neglect after stroke: A systematic review from 1997 through 2012. *Frontiers in Human Neuroscience*, 7, 187.

Noncompliance

Refer to *Compromised Engagement*.

Imbalanced Nutrition

American Association for Clinical Chemistry. (2013). Malnutrition. *Labs Tests on Line*. Retrieved from https://labtestsonline.org/understanding/conditions/malnutrition/start/2/

American Nurses Association (2013). *Artificial feeding ethics*. Retrieved from www.nursingworld.org/codeofethics

American Pediatric Association (APA). (2008). Vitamin D supplementation. *Pediatrics*, *122*(4):908–910. Retrieved from http://pediatrics.aappublications.org/content/122/5/1142.short

American Academy Of Pediatrics (APA); Meek, J. Y., & Yu, W. (2011). The American Academy of Pediatrics new mother's guide to breastfeeding [Paperback]. Media, PA: APArition.

Andrews, M., & Boyle, J. (2012). *Transcultural concepts in nursing* (8th ed.). Philadelphia: Lippincott Williams & Wilkins.

Association of Women's Health, Obstetrics, and Neonatal Nurses (AWHONN). (2007). *Breastfeeding support: prenatal care through the first year* (1st ed.). Washington, DC: Author.

Beier, J., Landes, S., Mohammad, M., & McClain, C. (2014). Nutrition in liver disorders and the role of alcohol. In M. E. Shils, M. Shike, A. Catherine Ross, B. Caballero, & R. J. Cousins (Eds.), *Modern nutrition in health and disease*. Philadelphia: Wolters Kluwer.

*Bowman, S. A., Gortmaker, S. L., Ebbeling, C. B., Pereira, M. A., & Ludwig, D. S. (2004). Effects of fast-food consumption on energy intake and diet quality among children in a national household survey. *Pediatrics*, *113*(1), 112–118.

Chang, C. Y., Cheng, T. J., Lin, C. Y., Chen, J. Y., Lu, T. H., & Kawachi, I. (2013). Reporting of aspiration pneumonia or choking as a cause of death in patients who died with stroke. *Stroke*, *44*(4), 1182–1185.

*Chima, C. (2004). *The nutrition care process: Driving effective intervention and outcomes*. Retrieved from www3.uakron.edu/.../Screening%20Nutrition%20Ca

Coleman-Jensen, A., Gregory, C., & Singh, A. (2013). Household food security in the United States. Washington, DC: U.S. Department of Agriculture/Economic Research Service.

Demory-Luce, D., & Moti, K. (2014). Fast food for children and adolescents. In *UpToDate*. Retrieved from www.uptodate.com/contents/fast-food-for-children-and-adolescents

Dudek, S. (2014). *Nutrition essentials for nursing practice* (7th ed.). Philadelphia: Wolters Kluwer.

Fass, R. (2014). Overview of dysphagia in adults. In *UpToDate*. Retrieved from www.uptodate.com/contents/overview-of-dysphagia-in-adults

Goldstein, J. E., Roque, H., & Ruvel, J. (2015). Nutrition in pregnancy. In *UpToDate*. Retrieved from www.uptodate.com/contents/nutrition-in-pregnancy

Gröber, U., & Kisters, K., (2007). Influence of drugs on vitamin D and calcium metabolism. *Dermatoendocrinology*, *4*(2), 158–166

*Hammond, K. A. (2011). Assessment: Dietary and clinical data. In L. Kathleen Mahan, J. L Raymond, & S. Escott-Stump (Eds.), Krause's food & the nutrition care process (13th ed.). St. Louis: Elsevier.

Hickey, J. (2014). *The clinical practice of neurological and neurosurgical nursing* (5th ed.). Philadelphia: Wolters Kluwer.

Hockenberry, M. J., & Wilson, D. (2015). *Wong's essentials of pediatric nursing* (10th ed.). New York: Elsevier.

Humbert, I. A., & Robbins, J. (2008). Dysphagia in the elderly. *Physical Medicine and Rehabilitation Clinics of North America*, *19*(4), 853–866.

*Hunter, J. H. & Cason, K. L. (2006). Nutrient density clemson university cooperative extension service. Retrieved from www.clemson.edu/extension/hgic/food/nutrition/nutrition/dietary_guide/hgic40 62.html

*Institute of Medicine. (2009). Weight gain during pregnancy: Reexamining the guidelines. Retrieved from www.nap.edu

Janssen, H. C., Samson, M. M., & Verhaar, H. J. (2002). Vitamin D deficiency, muscle function, and falls in elderly people. *The American Journal of Clinical Nutrition*, *75*(4), 611–615.

MacFie, J., Woodcock, N. P., Palmer, M. D., Walker, A., Townsend, S., & Mitchell, C. J. (2000). Oral dietary supplements in pre-and postoperative surgical patients: A prospective and randomized clinical trial. *Nutrition*, *16*(9), 723–728.

*Mahan, L. K., & Arlin, M. T. (1996). *Food, nutrition, and diet therapy* (9th ed.). Philadelphia: W. B. Saunders.

Miller, C. (2015). *Nursing for wellness in older adults* (7th ed.). Philadelphia: Wolters Kluwer.

National Research Council. (1989). *Recommended dietary allowances*. Retrieved from www.nap.edu/read/1349/chapter/1

Ogden, C. L., Carroll, M. D., Kit, B. K., & Flegal, K. M. (2014). Prevalence of childhood and adult obesity in the United States, 2011–2012. *JAMA*, *311*(8), 806–814.

*Park, Y., Neckerman, K. M., Quinn, J., Weiss, C., & Rundle, A. (2008). Significance of place of birth and place of residence and their relationship to BMI among immigrant groups in New York City. *International Journal of Behavioral Nutrition and Physical Activity*, *5*(19), 1–35.

Pillitteri, A. (2014). *Maternal and child health nursing* (7th ed.). Philadelphia: Wolters Kluwer.

Posthauer, M. E., Collins, N., Dorner, B., & Sloan, C. (2013). Nutritional strategies for frail older adults. *National Center for Biotechnology Information*, *26*(3), 128–140; quiz 141–142.

*Roy, P. (2011). *Lactose intolerance*. Retrieved from http://emedicine.medscape.com/article/187249-overview/a0199

Smith-Hammond, C. A., & Goldstein, L. B. (2006). Cough and aspiration of food and liquids due to oral-pharyngeal dysphagia: ACCP evidence-based clinical practice guidelines. *CHEST Journal*, *129*(1, Suppl), 154S–168S.

Sura, L., Madhavan, A., Carnaby, G., & Crary M. A. (2012). Dysphagia in the elderly: management and nutritional considerations. *Clinical Interventions in Aging*, 7, 287–298.

Tanner, D., & Culbertson, W. (2014). Avoiding negative dysphagia outcomes. *Online Journal of Issues in Nursing* 19(3). Retrieved from www.nursingworld.org/MainMenuCategories/ANAMarketplace/ANAPeriodicals/OJIN/TableofContents/Vol-19-2014/No2-May-2014/Articles-Previous-Topics/Avoiding-Negative-Dysphagia-Outcomes.html

Tisdale, M. J. (2003). Pathogenesis of cancer cachexia. *Journal Support Oncology*, 21, 159–168.

U.S. Department of Agriculture; & U.S. Department of Health and Human Services. (2010). *Dietary guidelines for Americans* (7th ed.). Washington, DC: U.S. Government Printing Office, The U.S. Departments of Agriculture (USDA).

U.S. Department of Agriculture. (2011). *Food groups*. Retrieved at www.choosemyplate.gov/food-groups/.

U.S. Department of Agriculture. (2016). *Choose my plate*. Retrieved from www.choosemyplate.gov/MyPlate

World Health Organization (WHO) (2012) Infant and young child feeding. Retrieved from www.who.int/mediacentre/factsheets/fs342/en/

Impaired Swallowing

*Emick-Herring, B., & Wood, P. (1990). A team approach to neurologically based swallowing disorders. *Rehabilitation Nursing, 15*, 126–132.

Obesity & Overweight

*Barner, C., Wylie-Rosett, J., & Gans, K. (2001). WAVE: a pocket guide for a brief nutrition dialogue in primary care. *The Diabetes Educator*, *27*(3), 352–362.

Barlow, S. E. (2007). Expert Committee Recommendations regarding the prevention, assessment, and treatment of child and adolescent overweight and obesity: Summary report. *Pediatrics, 120*(Suppl 4), S164–S192.

*Buiten, C., & Metzger, B. (2000). Childhood obesity and risk of cardiovascular disease: A review of the science. *Pediatric Nursing, 26*(1), 13–18.

Dennis, K. (2004). Weight management in women. *Nursing Clinics of North America, 39*(14), 231–241.

Dudek, S. G. (2014). *Nutrition essentials for nursing practice* (7th ed.). Philadelphia: Wolters Kluwer.

Gans, K. M., Ross, E., Barner, C. W., Wylie-Rosett, J., McMurray, J., & Eaton, C. (2003). REAP and WAVE: New tools to rapidly assess/discuss nutrition with patients. *The Journal of nutrition, 133*(2), 556S–562S.

Harsha, G.A., & Bray, G. A. (2008). Controversies in hypertension weight loss and blood pressure control (Pro). *Hypertension, 51*, 1420–1425

Hockenberry, M. J., & Wilson, D. (2015). *Wong's essentials of pediatric nursing* (10th ed.). New York: Elsevier.

Hibbard, J. H., & Cunningham, P. J. (2008). How engaged are consumers in their health and health care, and why does it matter? Findings from HSC No. 8: Providing insights that contribute to better health policy. Washington, DC: HSC.

*Hunter, J. H., & Cason, K. L. (2006). *Nutrient density*. Clemson University Cooperative Extension Service. Retrieved at www.clemson.edu/extension/hgic/food/nutrition/nutrition/dietary_guide/hgic40 62.html

Institute of Medicine. (2009). *Weight gain during pregnancy: Reexamining the guidelines*. Retrieved from www.nap.edu

*Martin, L. R., Williams, S. L., Haskard, K. B. & DiMatteo, M. R. (2005). The challenge of patient adherence. *Therapeutic Clininical Risk Management, 1*(3), 189–199.

Martin, L. R., Haskard Zolnierek, K. B., & DiMatteo, M. R. (2010). *Health behavior change and treatment adherence: Evidence-based guidelines for improving healthcare*. New York: Oxford University.

*Myers, S., & Vargas, Z. (2000). Parental perceptions of the preschool obese child. *Pediatric Nursing, 26*(1), 23.

National Center for Health Statistics. (2011). *Health, United States, 2011: With special features on socioeconomic status and health*. Hyattsville, MD: U.S. Department of Health and Human Services.

*Nead, K. G., Halterman, J. S., Kaczorowski, J. M., Auinger, P., & Weitzman, M. (2004). Overweight children and adolescents: A risk group for iron deficiency. *Pediatrics, 114*(1), 104–108.

Ogden, C. L., Carroll, M. D., Kit, B. K., & Flegal, K. M. (2014). Prevalence of childhood and adult obesity in the United States 2011–2012. *JAMA, 311*(8), 806–814.

Pelzang, R. (2010). Time to learn: understanding patient-centered care. *British Journal of Nursing, 19*(14), 912–917.

Pillitteri, A. (2014). *Maternal and child health nursing* (7th ed.). Philadelphia: Wolters Kluwer.

Reedy, J., & Krebs-Smith, S. M. (2010). Dietary sources of energy, solid fats, and added sugars among children and adolescents in the United States. *Journal of the American Dietetic Association, 110*, 1477–1484. Retrieved from www.nccor.org/downloads/jada2010.pdf

U.S. Department of Agriculture; & U.S. Department of Health and Human Services. (2010). *Dietary guidelines for Americans* (7th ed.). Washington, DC: U.S. Government Printing Office, The U.S. Departments of Agriculture (USDA).

*Wiereng, M. E., & Oldham, K. K. (2002). Weight control: A lifestyle-modification model for improving health. *Nursing Clinics of North America, 37*(2), 303–311.

Post-Trauma/Rape-Trauma Syndrome

Acierno, R., Hernandez, M. A., Amstadter, A. B., Resnick, H. S., Steve, K., Muzzy, W., & Kilpatrick, D. G. (2010). Prevalence and correlates of emotional, physical, sexual, and financial abuse and potential neglect in the United States: The National Elder Mistreatment Study. *American Journal of Public, 100*(2), 292–297.

Bernardy, N., Lund, B., Alexander, B., & Friedman, M. (2013). Increased polysedative use in veterans with posttraumatic stress disorder. Pain Medicine. doi: 10.1111/pme.12321

Boyd, M. A. (2012). Psychiatric nursing: Contemporary practice (5th ed.). Philadelphia: Lippincott Williams & Wilkins.

*Burgess, A. W. (1995). Rape-trauma syndrome: A nursing diagnosis. *Occupational Health Nursing, 33*(8), 405–410.

*Burgess, A. W., Dowdell, R. N., & Prentley, R. (2000). Sexual abuse of nursing home residents. *Journal of Psychosocial Nursing, 38*(6), 10–18.

*Carson V. M., & Smith-DiJulio, K. (2006). Sexual assault. In E. Varcarolis, V. M. Carson, & N. C. Shoemaker (Eds.), *Foundations of psychiatric-mental health nursing* (5th ed.). Philadelphia: W. B. Saunders.

Centers for Disease Control and Prevention. (2013). *Sexually transmitted disease surveillance*. Retrieved from www.cdc.gov/std/stats13/surv2013-print.pdf

Ciechanowski, P. (2014). Posttraumatic stress disorder: epidemiology, pathophysiology, clinical manifestations, course, and diagnosis. In *UpToDate*. Retrieved from www.uptodate.com/contents/posttraumatic-stress-disorder-in-adults-epidemiology-pathophysiology-clinical-manifestations-course-and-diagnosis

Department of Health and Human Services. (2013). *Administration for children and families, administration on children, youth and families, children's bureau child maltreatment*. Retrieved from www.acf.hhs.gov/programs/cb/research-data-technology/statistics-research/child-maltreatment

Dube, S. R., Anda, R. F., Whitfield, C. L., Brown, D. W., Felitti, V. J., Dong, M., & Giles, W. H. (2005). Long-term consequences of childhood sexual abuse by gender of victim. *American Journal of Preventive Medicine, 28*(5), 430–438.

Fourth National Incidence Study of Child Abuse and Neglect (NIS-4). (2010). Retrieved from www.acf.hhs.gov/programs/opre/resource/fourth-national-incidence-study-of-child-abuse-and-neglect-nis-4-report-to-congress

Friedman, M. J. (2016). PTSD history and overview. Retrieved from www.ptsd.va.gov/professional/PTSD-overview/ptsd-overview.asp

*Gabbay, V., Oatis, M. D., Silva, R. R., & Hirsch, G. S. (2004). Epidemiological aspects of PTSD in children and adolescents. In R. R. Silva (ed.), *Posttraumatic stress disorder in children and adolescents: Handbook* (pp. 1–17). New York: Norton.

*Goldstein, M. Z. (2005). *Comprehensive textbook of psychiatry* (Vol. 2, 8th ed., pp. 3828–3834). Philadelphia: Lippincott Williams & Wilkins.

Health Research Funding.org. (2015). *Engrossing PTSD suicide statistics*. Retrieved from http://healthresearchfunding.org/engrossing-ptsd-suicide-statistics/

*Heinrich, L. (1987). Care of the female rape victim. *Nursing Practitioner, 12*(11), 9.

Hockenberry, M. J., & Wilson, D. (2015). Wong's essentials of pediatric nursing (10th ed.). New York: Elsevier.

*Horowitz, M. J. (1986). Stress response syndromes: A review of posttraumatic and adjustment disorders. *Hospital and Community Psychiatry, 37*, 241–248.

*Jacobsen, L. K., Southwick, S. M., & Kosten, T. R. (2001). Substance use disorders in patients with posttraumatic stress disorder: a review of the literature. *American Journal of Psychiatry, 158*(8), 1184–1190.

*Kilpatrick, D. G., Ruggiero, K. J., Acierno, R., Saunders, B. E., Resnick, H. S., & Best, C. L. (2003). Violence and risk of PTSD, major depression, substance abuse/dependence, and comorbidity: results from the National Survey of Adolescents. *Journal of Consulting and clinical Psychology, 71*(4), 692–700.

*Ledray, L. E. (2001). Evidence collection and care of the sexually assault survivor: SANE-SART response. Retrieved from www.vaw.umn.edu/documents/commissioned/2forensicvidence.htlm

Lifespan of Greater Rochester, Inc. (2011). *Under the radar: New York state elder abuse prevalence study*. Retrieved from http://ocfs.ny.gov/main/reports/Under%20the%20Radar%2005%2012%2011%20final%20report.pdf

Masho, S. W., & Anderson, L. (2009). Sexual assault in men: A population-based study of Virginia. *Violence and Victims, 24*(1), 98–110.

*Petter, L. M., & Whitehill, D. L. (1998). Management of female sexual assault. *American Family Physician, 58*(4), 920–926.

*Pfefferbaum, B., Gurwich, R. H., McDonald, N. B., Leftwich, M. J. T., Sconzo, G. M., Messenbaugh, A. K., & Schultz, R. A. (2000). Posttraumatic stress among young children after the death of a friend or acquaintance in a terrorist bombing. *Psychiatric Services, 51*(3), 386–388.

*Rape, Abuse and Incest National Network (RAINN). (2002). *RAINN News*. Retrieved from www.ncdsv.org/RAINN_NEWS.doc

*RAINN. (2009). Retrieved from www.rainn.org/news/ncvs2009

Stokowski, L. A. (2008). Forensic nursing: Part 2. Inside forensic nursing. In Medscape. Retrieved from www.medscape.com/viewarticle/571555_3

Teaster, P. B., Dugar, T. D., Mendiondo, M. S., Abner, E. L., & Cecil, K. A.(2006). *The 2004 survey of state Adult Protective Services: Abuse of adults 60 years of age and older*. Report to the National Center on Elder Abuse, Administration on Aging, Washington, DC.

U.S. Department of Justice. (2014). *Rape and sexual assault*. Retrieved from www.bjs.gov/index.cfm?ty=tp&tid=317

Woman's Health.org. (2012). *Sexual assault*. Retrieved from www.womenshealth.gov/publications/our-publications/fact-sheet/sexual-assault.html

Powerlessness

Abad-Corpa, E., Gonzalez-Gil, T., Martínez-Hernández, A., Barderas-Manchado, A. M., De la Cuesta-Benjumea, C., Monistrol-Ruano, O., & Mahtani-Chugani, V. (2012). Caring to achieve the maximum independence possible: A synthesis of qualitative evidence on older adults' adaptation to dependency. *Journal of Clinical Nursing, 21*(21/22), 3153–3169. doi:10.1111/j.1365-2702.2012.04207

Andrews, M., & Boyle, J. (2012). *Transcultural concepts in nursing* (8th ed.). Philadelphia: Lippincott Williams & Wilkins.

*Burkhart, P. V, & Rayens, M. K. (2005). Self-concept and health focus of control: Factors related to children's adherence to recommended asthma regimen. *Pediatric Nursing, 31*(5), 404–409.

*Garrett, P. W., Dickson, H. G., Young, L., & Whelan, A. K. (2008). "The Happy Migrant Effect": Perceptions of negative experiences of healthcare by patients with little or no English: A qualitative study across seven language groups. *Quality and Safety in Health Care, 17*(2), 101–103.

Giger, J. (2013). *Transcultural nursing: Assessment and intervention* (6th ed.). St. Louis, MO: Mosby-Year Book.

Haugan, G., Innstrand, S. T., & Moksnes, U. K. (2013). The effect of nurse-patient interaction on anxiety and depression in cognitively intact nursing home patients. *Journal of Clinical Nursing*, 22(15/16), 2192–2205. doi:10.1111/jocn.12072

Hinton, R., & Earnest, J. (2010). 'I worry so much I think it will kill me': Psychosocial health and the links to the conditions of women's lives in Papau New Guinea. *Health Sociology Review, 19*(1), 5–17.

Hockenberry, M. J., & Wilson, D. (2015). Wong's essentials of pediatric nursing (10th ed.). New York: Elsevier.

*Johansson, K., Salantera, S., & Katajisto, J. (2007). Empowering orthopaedic patients through preadmission education: Results from a clinical study. *Patient Education and Counseling, 66*(1), 84–91.

Meeker, M.A., Waldrop, D. P., Schneider, J., Case, A. A. (2013). Contending with advanced illness: Patient and caregiver perspectives. *Journal of Pain & Symptom Management*, 47(5), 887–895. doi:10.1016/j.jpainsymman.2013.06.009

*Nápoles-Springer, A., Ortíz, C., O'Brien, H., & Díaz-Méndez, M. (2009). Developing a culturally competent peer support intervention for Spanish-speaking Latinas with breast cancer. *Journal of Immigrant & Minority Health, 11*(4), 268–280. doi:10.1007/s10903-008-9128-4

Orzeck, T., Rokach, A., & Chin, J. (2010). The effects of traumatic and abusive relationships. *Journal of Loss & Trauma, 15*(3), 167–192. doi:10.1080/15325020903375792

*Stang, I., & Mittelmark, M. B. (2008). Learning as an empowerment process in breast cancer self-help groups. *Journal of Clinical Nursing, 18*(14), 2049–2057.

*Stephenson, C. A. (1979). Powerless and chronic illness: Implications for nursing. *Baylor Nursing Educator, 1*(1), 17–23.

*Thomas, S. A., & Gonzalez-Prendes, A. (2009). Powerless, anger, and stress in African American women: Implications for physical and emotional health. *Health Care for Women International, 30*(1/2), 93–113. doi:10.1080/07399330802523709

Ineffective Protection

Agency for Healthcare Research and Quality. (2011). *Are we ready for this change? Preventing pressure ulcers in hospitals: A toolkit for improving quality of care*. Rockville, MD: Author. Retrieved from www.ahrq.gov/professionals/systems/long-term-care/resources/pressure-ulcers/pressureulcertoolkit/putool1.html

Baumgarten, M., Margolis, D. J., Orwig, D. L., Shardell, M. D., Hawkes, W. G., Langenberg, P., . . . Kinosian, B. P. (2009). Pressure ulcers in elderly patients with hip fracture across the continuum of care. *Journal of the American Geriatrics Society*, *57*(5), 863–870.

*Bergstrom, N., Allman, R., Alvarez, O., Bennett, M., Carlson, C., Frantz, R., . . . Yarkony, G. (1994). *Treatment of pressure ulcers*. Clinical practice guideline (No. 15). Rockville, MD: Agency for Health Care Policy and Research, AHCPR Publication No. 95-0652.

Berlowitz, D. (2015). Clinical staging and management of pressure ulcers. In *UpToDate*. Retrieved from www.uptodate.com/contents/clinical-staging-and-management-of-pressure-ulcers?

Brem, H., Maggi, J., Nierman, D., Rolnitzky, L., Bell, D., Rennert, R., . . . Vladeck, B. (2010). High cost of stage IV pressure ulcers. *American Journal of Surgery*, *200*(4), 473–477. Retrieved from www.ncbi.nlm.nih.gov/pmc/articles/PMC2950802/

Coleman, S., Gorecki, C., Nelson, E. A., Closs, S. J., Defloor, T., Halfens, R., . . . Nixon, J. (2013). Patient risk factors for pressure ulcer development: Systematic review. *International Journal of Nursing Studies*, *50*(7), 974–1003. Retrieved from www.ncbi.nlm.nih.gov/pubmed/23375662

Dudek, S. G. (2014). *Nutrition essentials for nursing practice* (7th ed.). Philadelphia: Wolters Kluwer.

Grossman, S., & Porth, C. A. (2014). *Porth's pathophysiology: Concepts of altered health states* (9th ed.). Philadelphia: Wolters Kluwer.

Lin, J. B., Tsubota, K., & Apte, R. S. (2016). *A glimpse at the aging eye. Aging and mechanisms of disease*. Retrieved from www.nature.com/articles/npjamd20163

Ling, S. M., & Mandl, S. (2013). Pressure Ulcers: CMS update and perspectives. Retrieved from www.npuap.org/wp-content/uploads/2012/01/NPUAP2013-LingMandl-FINAL2-25-131.pdf

*Maklebust, J., & Sieggreen, M. (2006). *Pressure ulcers: Guidelines for prevention and nursing management* (3rd ed.). Springhouse, PA: Springhouse.

*Meurman, J. H., Sorvari, R., Pelttari, A., Rytömaa, I., Franssila, S., & Kroon, L. (1996). Hospital mouth-cleaning aids may cause dental erosion, *Special Care in Dentistry*, *16*(6), 247–250.

The National Pressure Ulcer Advisory Panel, European Pressure Ulcer Advisory Panel. (2014). *Clinical practice guideline*. Retrieved from www.npuap.org/resources/educational-and-clinical-resources/prevention-and-treatment-of-pressure-ulcers-clinical-practice-guideline/

Pillitteri, A. (2014). *Maternal and child health nursing* (7th ed.). Philadelphia: Wolters Kluwer.

*Rosen, J., Mittal, V., Degenholtz, H., Castle, N., Mulsant, B. H., Hulland, S., . . . Rubin, F. (2006). Ability, incentives, and management feedback: organizational change to reduce pressure ulcers in a nursing home. *Journal of the American Medical Directors Association*, 7(3), 141–146.

Rosenberg, J. B., & Eisen, L. A. (2008). Eye care in the intensive care unit: narrative review and meta-analysis. *Critical care medicine*, *36*(12), 3151–3155.

Weber, J. R., & Kelley, J. H. (2014). *Health assessment in nursing* (5th ed.). Philadelphia: Lippincott Wiliams and Wilkins.

*Wound Ostomy Continence Nursing (WOCN). (2003). *Guideline for prevention and management of pressure ulcers*. Glenview, IL: Author.

Risk for Corneal Injury/Risk for Red Eye

Azfar, M. F., Khan, M. F., & Alzeer, A. H. (2013). Protocolized eye care prevents corneal complications in ventilated patients in a medical intensive care unit. *Saudi Journal of Anaesthesia*, 7(1), 33–36.

*Ezra, D. G., Lewis, G., Healy, M., & Coombes, A. (2005). Preventing exposure keratopathy in the critically ill: A prospective study comparing eye care regimes. *The British Journal of Ophthalmology*, *89*(8), 1068–1069.

*Joyce, N. (2002). *Eye care for the intensive care patients. A systematic review* (No. 21). Adelaide: The Joanna Briggs Institute for Evidence Based Nursing and Midwifery.

Lawrence, S. L., & Morris, C. (2008). Ophthalmic Pearls: Lagophthalmos evaluation and treatment. In *EyeNet*. Retrieved from www.aao.org/eyenet/article/lagophthalmos-evaluation-treatment?april-2008

Leadingham, C. (2014). *Maintaining the vision in the intensive care unit* (Doctoral dissertation). Retrieved from http://corescholar.libraries.wright.edu/nursing_dnp/1

Mayo Clinic. (2010). *Red eye*. Retrieved from www.mayoclinic.org/symptoms/red-eye/basics/definition/sym-20050748

*Mercieca, F., Suresh, P., Morton, A., & Tullo, A. (1999). Ocular surface disease in intensive care unit patients. *Eye*, *13*, 231–236.

Rosenberg, J. B., & Eisen, L. A. (2008). Eye care in the intensive care unit: Narrative review and meta-analysis. *Critical Care Medicine*, *36*, 3151–3155.

Yanoff, M., & Duker, J. (2009). *Ophthalmology*. New York: Elsevier.

Risk for Impaired Tissue Integrity/Pressure Ulcer

Armstrong, A., & Meyr, D. (2014). Clinical assessment of wounds. In *UpToDate*. Retrieved from www.uptodate.com/contents/clinical-assessment-of-wounds

*Bennett, M. A. (1995). Report of the task force on the implications for darkly pigmented intact skin in the prediction and prevention of pressure ulcers. *Advances in Skin & Wound Care*, *8*(6), 34–35.

Berlowitz, D. (2015). Clinical staging and management of pressure ulcers. In *UpToDate*. Retrieved from www.uptodate.com/contents/clinical-staging-and-management-of-pressure-ulcers?

Clark, M. (2010). Skin assessment in dark pigmented skin: A challenge in pressure ulcer prevention. *Nursing Times*, *106*(30), 16–17.

de Souza, D. M. S. T., & de Gouveia Santos, V. L. C. (2010). Incidence of pressure ulcers in the institutionalized elderly. *Journal of Wound Ostomy & Continence Nursing*, *37*(3), 272–276.

Doley, J. (2010). Nutrition management of pressure ulcers. *Nutrition in clinical practice*, *25*(1), 50–60.

Dorner, B., Posthauer, M. E., & Thomas, D. (2009). The role of nutrition in pressure ulcer prevention and treatment: National Pressure Ulcer Advisory Panel white paper. *Advances in Skin & Wound Care*, *22*(5), 212–221.

*Fore, J. (2006). A review of skin and the effects of aging on skin structure and function. *Ostomy Wound Manage*, 52(9), 24–35.

Guo, S., & DiPietro, L. A. (2010). Factors affecting wound healing. *Journal of dental research*, *89*(3), 219–229.

*Maklebust, J., & Sieggreen, M. (2006). *Pressure ulcers: Guidelines for prevention and nursing management* (3rd ed.). Springhouse, PA: Springhouse.

National Pressure Ulcer Advisory Panel, European Pressure Ulcer Advisory Panel. (2014). *Clinical practice guideline*. Retrieved from www.npuap.org/resources/educational-and-clinical-resources/prevention-and-treatment-of-pressure-ulcers-clinical-practice-guideline/

Peterson, M. J., Gravenstein, N., Schwab, W. K., van Oostrom, J. H., & Caruso, L. J. (2013). Patient repositioning and pressure ulcer risk—monitoring interface pressures of at-risk patients. *Journal of Rehabilitation Research and Development*, *50*(4), 477–488.

Impaired Oral Mucous Membrane

American Dental Association. (2014). *Learn more about flossing and interdental cleaners*. Retrieved February 2, 2015, from www.ada.org/en/science-research/ada-seal-of-acceptance/product-category-information/floss-and-other-interdental-cleaners

Carlotto, A., Hogsett, V. L., Maiorini, E. M., Razulis, J. G., & Sonis, S. T. (2013). The economic burden of toxicities associated with cancer treatment: Review of the literature and analysis of nausea, vomiting, diarrhea, oral mucositis and fatigue. *Pharmacoeconomics*, *31*, 753–766. doi:10.1007/540273-013-0081-2

Chan, E. Y., Lee, Y. K., Poh, T. H., & Prabhakaran, L. (2011). Translating evidence into nursing practice: Oral hygiene for care dependent adults. *International Journal of Evidenced-Based Healthcare*, 9, 172–183.

Clocheret, K., Dekeyser, C., Carels, C., & Willems, G. (2014). Idiopathic gingival hyperplasia and orthodontic treatment: A case report. *Journal of Orthodontics*, *30*(1), 13–19.

*Cutler, C. J., & Davis, N. (2005). Improving oral care in patients receiving mechanical ventilation. *American Journal of Care*, *14*(5), 389–394.

Eilers, J., Harris, D., Henry, K., & Johnson, L. A. (2014). Evidence-based interventions for cancer treatment-related mucositis: Putting evidence into practice. *Clinical Journal of Oncology Nursing*, *18*, 80–96.

Fieder, L. I., Mitchell, P., Bridges, E. (2010). Oral care practices for orally intubated critically ill adults. *American Journal of Critical Care*, *19*(2), 175–183.

Fields, L. (2008). Oral care intervention to reduce incidence of ventilator-associated pneumonia in the neurological intensive care unit. *American Association of Neuroscience Nurses*, *40*(5), 291–298.

Freifeld, A. G., Bow, E. J., Sepkowitz, K. A., Boeckh, M. J., Ito, J. I., Mullen, C. A., . . . Wingard, J. R. (2011). Clinical practice guideline for the use of antimicrobial agents in neutropenic patients with cancer: 2010 update by the Infectious Diseases Society of America. *Clinical Infectious Diseases*, *52*(4), e56–e93. doi:10.1093/cid/cir073

Gibson, R. J., Keefe, D. M., Lalla, R.V., Bateman, E., Blijlevens, N., Fijlstra, M., . . . Bowen, J. M. (2013). Systemic review of agents for the management of gastrointestinal mucositis in cancer patients. *Supportive Care in Cancer*, 21, 313–326. doi:10-1007/s00520-012-1644z

Goss, L. K., Coty, M. B., & Myers, J. A. (2011). A review of documented oral care practices in an intensive care unit. *Clinical Nursing Research*, *20*(2), 181–196. doi:10.1177/1054773810392368

National Cancer Institute. (2014). *Oral complications of chemotherapy and head/neck radiation*. Retrieved January 31, 2015, from www.cancer.gov/cancertopics/pdq/supportivecare/oralcomplications/HealthProfessional/page5

National Comprehensive Cancer Network. (2008). *Oral mucositis is often underrecognized and undertreated*. Retrieved from www.nccn.org/professionals/meetings/13thannual/highlights

Needleman, I., Hyun-Ryu, J., Brealey, D., Sachdev, M., Moskal-Fitzpatrick, D., Bercades, G., . . . Suvan, J. (2012). The impact of hospitalization on dental plaque accumulation: An observational study. *Journal of clinical periodontology*, *39*(11), 1011–1016.

Oncology Nursing Society. (2007). Mucositis: What interventions are effective for managing oral mucositis in people receiving treatment for cancer, ONS PEP Cards.

Perry, S. E., Hockenberry, M. J., Lowdermilk, D. L., & Wilson, D. (2014). *Maternal child nursing care* (5th ed.). St. Louis, MO: Elsevier.

Quinn, B., Baker, D. L., Cohen, S., Stewart, J. L., Lima, C. A., & Parise, C. (2014). Basic nursing care to prevent nonventilator hospital-acquired pneumonia. *Journal of Nursing Scholarship*, 46 (1), 11–17.

Shi, Z., Xie, H., Wang, P., Zhang, Q., Wu, Y., Chen, E., . . . Furness, S. (2013). Oral hygiene care for critically ill patients to prevent ventilator-associated pneumonia. *Cochrane Database Systematic Review*, 8, doi:10.1002/14651858.CD008367.pub2

Relocation Stress

*Armer, J. M. (1996). An exploration of factors influencing adjustment among relocating rural elders. *Image*, *28*(1), 35–39.

*Barnhouse, A. H., Brugler, C. J., & Harkulich, J. T. (1992). Relocation stress syndrome. *International Journal* of *Nursing Terminologies and Classifications*, *3*(4), 166–168.

Beck, K. D., & Luine, V. N. (2002). Sex differences in behavioral and neurochemical profiles after chronic stress: Role of housing conditions. *Physiology & Behavior*, *75*(5), 661–673.

*Beirne, N. F., Patterson, M. N., Galie, M., & Goodman, P. (1995). Effects of a fast-track closing on a nursing facility population. *Health and Social Work*, *20*, 117–123.

Buhs, E. S., Ladd, G. W., & Herald, S. L. (2006). Peer exclusion and victimization: Processes that mediate the relation between peer group rejection and children's classroom engagement and achievement?. *Journal of Educational Psychology*, *98*(1), 1–13

*Chaboyer, W., Thalib, L., Foster, M., Ball, C., & Richards, B. (2008). Predictors of adverse events in patients after

discharge from the intensive care unit. *American Journal of Critical Care, 17*(3), 255–263.

Chrisitie, L. (2014). *Foreclosures hit six-year low in 2013*. Retrieved from http://money.cnn.com/2014/01/16/real_estate/foreclosure-crisis/

*Davies, S., & Nolan, M. (2004). Making the move: Relatives' experiences of the transition to a new home. *Health and Social Care in the Community, 12*(6), 517–523.

Droogh, J. M., Smit, M., Absalom, A. R., Ligtenberg, J. J., & Zijlstra, J. G. (2015). Transferring the critically ill patient: are we there yet?. *Critical Care, 19*, 62.

*Flanagan, V., Slattery, M. J., Chase, N. S., Meade, S. K., & Cronenwett, L. R. (1996). Mothers' perceptions of the quality of their infants' back transfer: Pilot study results. *Neonatal Network, 15*(2), 27–33.

Goldfrad, C., & Rowan, K. (2000). Consequences of discharges from intensive care at night. *The Lancet, 355*(9210), 1138–1142.

Häggström, M., & Bäckström, B. (2014). Organizing safe transitions from intensive care. *Nursing Research and Practice* Article ID 175314

Harris-Kojetin, L., Sengupta, Park-Lee, E., & Valverde, R. (2013). Long-term care services in the United States: 2013 overview. *National Centerfor Health Statistics. Vital Health Statistics 3*(37), 1–107.

Hockenberry, M. J., & Wilson, D. (2015). *Wong's essentials of pediatric nursing* (10th ed.). New York: Elsevier.

*Houser, D. (1974). Safer care of MI patient. *Nursing 74, 4*(7), 42–47.

Jacobsen, M. A. (2011). *Reducing relocation stress senior care coalition*. Retrieved from www.seniorcarecoalition.org/articles/reducing-relocation-stress

*Johnson, R. A., & Tripp-Reimer, T. (2001). Relocation among ethnic elders. *Journal of Gerontological Nursing, 27*(6), 22–27.

Kaplan, D. B., Barbara, J., Berkman, B. B. (2013). *Effects of life transitions on the elderly*. Retrieved from www.merckmanuals.com/professional/geriatrics/social-issues-in-the-elderly/effects-of-life-transitions-on-the-elderly

Laupland, K. B., Zahar, J. R., Adrie, C., Minet, C., Vésin, A., Goldgran-Toledano, D., . . . & Jamali, S. (2012). Severe hypothermia increases the risk for intensive care unit–acquired infection. *Clinical infectious diseases*, 54:1064–1070.

*Longino, C. F., & Bradley, D. E. (2006). Internal and international migration. In R. H. Binstock & L. K. George (Eds.), *Handbook of aging and social services* (6th ed., pp. 76–93). San Diego: Academic Press.

*Lutgendorf, S. K., Reimer, T. T., Harvey, J. H., Marks, G., Hong, S. Y., Hillis, S. L., & Lubaroff, D. M. (2001). Effects of housing relocation on immunocompetence and psychosocial functioning in older adults. Journal of Gerontology Series A: Biological Sciences and Medical Sciences, 56(2), M97–M105.

*Meacham, C. L., & Brandriet, L. M. (1997). The response of family and residents to long-term care placement. *Clinical Gerontologist, 18*(1), 63–66.

*Mitchell, M. G. (1999). The effects of relocation of elderly. *Perspectives in Gerontological Nursing, 23*(1), 2–7.

*Mitchell, M. L., Courtney, M., & Coyer, F. (2003). Understanding uncertainty and minimizing families' anxiety at the time of transfer from intensive care. *Nursing Health Science, 5*(3), 207–211.

O'Riley, A., Nadorff, M. R., Conwell, Y., & Edelstein, B. (2013). Challenges associated with managing suicide risk in long-term care facilities. *Annals of Long-Term Care, 21*(6), 28–34.

*Priestap, F. A., & Martin, C. M. (2006). Impact of intensive care unit discharge time on patient outcome. *Critical care medicine, 34*(12), 2946–2951.

*Puskar, K. R. (1986). The usefulness of Mahler's phases of the separation-individuation process in providing a theoretical framework for understanding relocation. *Maternal-Child Nursing Journal, 15*(1), 15–22.

*Puskar, K. R. (1990). Relocation support groups for corporate wives. *American Association of Occupational Health Nurses Journal, 38*(1), 25–31.

*Puskar, K. R., & Dvorsak, K. G. (1991). Relocation stress in adolescents: Helping teenagers cope with a moving dilemma. *Pediatric Nursing, 17*, 295–298.

*Puskar, K. R., & Rohay, J. M. (1999). School relocation and stress in teens. *Journal of School Nursing, 15*(1), 16–22.

*Reinardy, J. R. (1995). Relocation to a new environment: Decisional control and the move to a nursing home. *Health and Social Work, 20*(1), 31–38.

*Rodgers, W. L. (1986). Comparisons of two sampling frames for surveys of the oldest old. In R. B. Warnecke, (Ed.), *Health survey research methods*. DHHS Publication No. (PHS)96-1013. Centers for Disease Control, National Center for Health Statistics, Public Health Service, U.S. Department of Health and Human Services.

Singh, S. P., Winsper, C., Wolke, D., & Bryson, A. (2014). School mobility and prospective pathways to psychotic-like symptoms in early adolescence: A prospective birth cohort study. *Journal of the American Academy of Child & Adolescent Psychiatry, 53*(5), 518–527.e1.

Substance Abuse and Mental Health Services Administration. (2011). *Results from the 2011 National Survey on drug use and health: Summary of national findings*. Retrieved from http://archive.samhsa.gov/data/NSDUH/2k11results/nsduhresults2011.pdf

*Wilson, S. A. (1997). The transition to nursing home life: A comparison of planned and unplanned admissions. *Journal of Advanced Nursing, 26*(5), 864–871.

Risk for Ineffective Respiratory Function

*Chan, L. (1998). Effectiveness of a music therapy intervention on relaxation and anxiety for patients receiving ventilation assistance. *Heart and Lung, 27*(3), 169–176.

Chen, C. J., Lin, C. J., Tzeng, Y. L., Hsu, L. N. (2009). Successful mechanical ventilation weaning experiences at respiratory care centers. *Journal of Nursing Research, 17*(2), 93–101.

Dudek, S. G. (2014). *Nutrition essentials for nursing practice* (7th ed.). Philadelphia: Wolters Kluwer.

Engström, Å., Nyström, N., Sundelin, G., Rattray, J. (2013). People's experiences of being mechanically ventilated in an ICU: A qualitative study. Intensive and Critical Care Nursing, *29*(2), 88–95.

Epstien, S. (2015). Weaning from mechanical ventilation: Readiness testing. In *UpToDate*. Retrieved from www.uptodate.com/contents/weaning-from-mechanical-ventilation-readiness-testing

Halm, M. A., & Krisko-Hagel, K. (2008). Instilling normal saline with suctioning: Beneficial technique or potentially harmful sacred cow? *American Journal of Critical Care, 17*(5), 469–472.

Grossman, S., & Porth, C. A. (2014). *Porth's pathophysiology: Concepts of altered health states* (9th ed.). Philadelphia: Wolters Kluwer.

*Henneman, E. A. (2001). Liberating patients from mechanical ventilation, a team approach. *Critical Care Nursing, 21*(3), 25.

Hockenberry, M. J., & Wilson, D. (2015). *Wong's essentials of pediatric nursing* (10th ed.). New York: Elsevier.

*Huckabay, L., & Daderian, A. (1989). Effect of choices on breathing exercises post open heart surgery. *Dimensions of Critical Care Nursing, 9*, 190–201.

Institute for Healthcare Improvement. (2008). Implement the ventilator bundle: Elevation of the head of the bed. Retrieved from www.ihi.org/IHI/Topics/CriticalCare/IntensiveCare/Changes/IndividualChanges/Elevationoftheheadofthebed.htm

*Jenny, J., & Logan, J. (1991). Analyzing expert nursing practice to develop a new nursing diagnosis: Dysfunctional ventilatory weaning response. In R. M. Carroll-Johnson (Ed.), *Classification of nursing diagnoses: Proceedings of the ninth conference*. Philadelphia: J. B. Lippincott.

*Jenny, J., & Logan, J. (1994). Promoting ventilator independence. *Dimensions of Critical Care Nursing, 13*, 29–37.

*Jenny, J., & Logan, J. (1998). Caring and comfort metaphors used by critical care patients. *Image, 30*(2), 197–208.

*Krieger, B. P., Ershowsky, P. F., Becker, D. A., & Gazeroglu. H. B. (1989). Evaluation of conventional criteria for predicting successful weaning from mechanical ventilatory support in elderly patients. *Critical Care Medicine, 17*:858.

*Logan, J., & Jenny, J. (1990). Deriving a new nursing diagnosis through qualitative research: Dysfunctional ventilatory weaning response. *Nursing Diagnosis, 1*(1), 37–43.

*Logan, J., & Jenny, J. (1991). Interventions for the nursing diagnosis: Dysfunctional Ventilatory Weaning Response: A qualitative study. In R. M. Carroll-Johnson (Ed.), *Classification of nursing diagnosis: Proceedings of the ninth conference*. Philadelphia: J. B. Lippincott.

*MacIntyre, N. R., Cook, D. J., Ely, E. W. Jr., Epstein, S. K., Fink, J. B., Heffner, J. E., . . . American College of Chest Physicians; American Association for Respiratory Care; American College of Critical Care Medicine. (2001). Evidence-based guidelines for weaning and discontinuing ventilatory support: A collective task force facilitated by the American College of Chest Physicians; the American Association for Respiratory Care; and the American College of Critical Care Medicine. *Chest, 120*, 375S.

*Marini, J. J. (1991). Editorials. *New England Journal of Medicine, 324*, 1496–1498.

*Meade, M., Guyatt, G., Cook, D., Griffith, L., Sinuff, T., Kergl, C., . . . Epstein, S. (2001). Predicting success in weaning from mechanical ventilation. *Chest Journal, 120*(6_suppl), 400S–424S.

Miller, C. (2015). *Nursing for wellness in older adults* (7th ed.). Philadelphia: Wolters Kluwer.

*Munro, C. L., & Grap, M. J. (2004). Oral health and care in the intensive care unit: State of the science. *American Journal of Critical Care, 13*(1), 25–34.

Nance-Floyd, B. (2011). Tracheostomy care: An evidence-based guide to suctioning and dressing changes. *American Nurses Today, 6*(7), 14–16.

*Rose, L., Nelson, S., Johnston, L., & Presneill, J. J. (2007). Decisions made by critical care nurses during mechanical ventilation and weaning in an Australian intensive care unit. *American Journal of Critical Care, 16*(5), 434–443.

*Rose, R., Dainty, K. N., Jordan, J., & Blackwood. (2014). Weaning from mechanical ventilation: A scoping review of qualitative studies. *American Journal of Critical Care, 23*(5), e54–e70.

Schwartzstein, R. M., & Richards, J. (2014). *Hyperventilation syndrome*. Retrieved from www.uptodate.com/contents/hyperventilation-syndrome

Sedwick, M. B., Lance-Smith, M., Reeder, S. J., & Nardi, J. (2012). Using evidence-based practice to prevent ventilator-associated pneumonia. *Critical Care Nurse, 32*(4), 41–51.

Sharma, S., Sarin, J., & Bala, G. K. (2014). Effectiveness of endotracheal suctioning protocol, In terms of knowledge and practices of nursing personnel. *Nursing and Midwifery Research Journal, 10*(2), 47–60.

WebMD. (2012). *Hyperventilation*. Retrieved from www.webmd.com/a-to-z-guides/hyperventilation-credits

Internet Resources

Agency for Healthcare Research and Quality, www.ahrq.gov/

Asthma and Allergy Foundation of America, www.aafa.org/

Asthma Management Model, www.nhlbi.nih.gov/health/public/lung/index.htm

Global Initiative for Chronic Obstructive Lung Disease, www.goldcopd.org

Joint Council of Asthma, Allergy, and Immunology, www.jcaai.org/

Quitting Smoking Guidelines, www.surgeongeneral.gov/tobacco/default.htm

QuitNet, www.quitnet.com

Self-Care Deficit Syndrome

Gulic, D. (2013). *Ortho notes: Clinical examination pocket guide (Davis's Notes)* (3rd ed.). Philadelphia: FA Davis.

*Mosher, R. B., & Moore, J. B. (1998). The relationship of self-concept & self-care in children with cancer. *Nursing Science Quarterly, 11*(3), 116–122.

Disturbed Self-Concept

*Atherton, R., & Robertson, N. (2006). Psychological adjustment to lower limb amputation amongst prosthesis users. *Disability and Rehabilitation, 28*(9), 1201–1209.

Boyd, M. A. (2012). *Psychiatric nursing: Contemporary practice* (5th ed.). Philadelphia: Lippincott Williams & Wilkins.

*Camp-Sorrell, D. (2007). Chemotherapy: Toxicity management. In C. Yarbro, M. H. Frogge, M. Goodman, & S. Groenwald, *Career nursing* (6th ed.). Boston: Jones and Bartlett.

Candela, F., Zucchetti, G., Magistro, D., Ortega, E., & Rabaglietti, E. (2014). Real and perceived physical functioning in Italian elderly population: associations with BADL and IADL. *Advances in Aging Research, 3*(05), 349.

Froggart, T., & Liersch-Sumkis, S. (2014). Assessment of mental health and mental illness. In N. Proctor, H. Hamer, D. McGarry, R. I. Wilson, & T. Froggat (Eds.), *Mental Health: A person—centered approach*. Sydney: Cambridge.

Halter, M. J. (2014). *Varcolaris Foundations of psychiatric mental health nursing* (7th ed.). Philadelphia: W. B. Saunders.

Hockenberry, M. J., & Wilson, D. (2015). *Wong's essentials of pediatric nursing* (10th ed.). New York: Elsevier.

Holzer, L. A., Sevelda, F., Fraberger, G., Bluder, O., Kickinger, W., & Holzer, G. (2014). Body image and self-esteem in lower-limb amputees. *PLoS One*, *9*(3): e92943. Retrieved from www.ncbi.nlm.nih.gov/pmc/articles/PMC3963966/

*Johnson, B. S. (1995). *Child, adolescent and family psychiatric nursing*. Philadelphia: J. B. Lippincott.

*Leuner, J., Coler, M., & Norris, J. (1994). Self-esteem. In M. Rantz & P. LeMone (Eds.), *Classification of nursing diagnosis: Proceedings of the eleventh conference*. Glendale, CA: CINAHL.

Lobato, E. P. (2013). Self-esteem and ageing. In *Cordoba Translation*. Retrieved from www.healthyolderpersons.org/news/self-esteem-and-ageing

Martin, B. (2013). Challenging negative self-talk. In *Psych Central*. Retrieved on August 26, 2015, from psychcentral.com/lib/challenging-negative-self-talk/

McCormack, J. (2007). Recover and strengths based practice. In Scottish Recovery Network (ed.), *SRN Discussion series, Report No .6*. Glasgow: Glasgow Association for Mental Health.

Mohr, D. C., Spring, B., Freedland, K. E., Beckner, V., Arean, P., Hollon, S. D., . . . Kaplan, R. (2009). The selection and design of control conditions for randomized controlled trials of psychological interventions. *Psychotherapy and psychosomatics*, *78*(5), 275–284.

Mulla, N. M. (2010). Healthy personalities. *Homeopathic Journal*, *3*(12), Retrieved from www.homeorizon.com/homeopathic-articles/healthy-living/healthy-personalities

*Murray, M. F. (2000). Coping with change: Self-talk. *Hospital Practice*, *31*(5), 118–120.

*Norris, J., & Kunes-Connell, M. (1985). Self-esteem disturbance. *Nursing Clinics of North America*, *20*, 745–761.

*Pierce, J., & Wardle, J. (1997). Cause and effect beliefs and self-esteem of overweight children. *Journal of Child Psychology and Psychiatry and Allied Disciplines*, *38*(6), 645–650.

Pillitteri, A. (2014). *Maternal and child health nursing* (7th ed.). Philadelphia: Wolters Kluwer.

*Winkelstein, M. L. (1989). Fostering positive self-concept in the schoolage child. *Pediatric Nursing*, *15*, 229–233.

Risk for Self-Harm

American Foundation for Suicide Prevention. (2015). *Facts and figures*. Retrieved from www.afsp.org/understanding-suicide/facts-and-figures

Boyd, M. A. (2012). *Psychiatric nursing: Contemporary practice* (5th ed.). Philadelphia: Lippincott Williams & Wilkins.

*Carscadden, J. S. (1993a). *On the cutting edge: A guide for working with people who self injure*. London, Ontario: London Psychiatric Hospital.

*Carscadden, J. S. (1997). *Beyond the cutting edge: A survival kit for families of self-injurers*. London, Ontario: London Psychiatric Hospital.

*Carscadden, J. S. (1998). *Premise for practice (relationship management team)*. London, Ontario: London Psychiatric Hospital.

Centers for Disease Control and Prevention (CDC). (2012). *Suicide Facts*. Retrieved from www.cdc.gov/violenceprevention/pdf/Suicide- DataSheet-a.pdf

CDC. (2014). *National suicide statistics*. Retrieved from www.cdc.gov/violenceprevention/suicide/riskprotectivefactors.html

Fowler, J. C. (2012). Suicide risk assessment in clinical practice: Pragmatic guidelines for imperfect assessment. *Psychotherapy*, *49*(1), 81–90.

*Mallinson, R. K. (1999). The lived experiences of AIDS-related multiple losses by HIV-negative gay men. *Journal of the Association of Nurses in AIDS Care*, *10*(5), 22–31.

Morbidity and Mortality Weekly Report (MMWR). (2013). Suicide among adults aged 35–64 years—United States, 1999–2010. Retrieved from www.cdc.gov/mmwr/preview/mmwrhtml/mm6217a1.htm

Saewyc, E. M., Skay, C. L., Hynds, P., Pettingell, S., Bearinger L. H., Resnick, M. D., Reis, E. (2007). Suicidal ideation and attempts among adolescents in North American school-based surveys: Are bisexual youth at increasing risk? *Journal of LGBT Health Research*, *3*(2), 25–36.

Tofthagen, R., Talsethand, A. G., & Fagerström, L. (2014). Mental health nurses' experiences of caring for patients suffering from self-harm. *Nursing Research and Practice*. doi:10.1155/2014/905741

*U.S. Public Health Service. (1999). *The surgeon general's call to action to prevent suicide*. Washington, DC: U.S. Department of Health and Human Services.

*Wheatley, M. & Austin-Payne, H. (2009). Nursing staff knowledge and attitudes towards deliberate self-harm in adults and adolescents in an inpatient setsing. *Behavioural and Cognitive Psychotherapy*, *37*(3), 293–309.

*Ystgaard, M. (2003). Deliberate self-harm among young people. New research results and consequences for preventive work. *Suicidologi*, *8*(2), 7–10.

Ineffective Sexuality Patterns

*Annon, J. S. (1976). The PLISST model: A proposed conceptual scheme for the behavioral treatment of sexual problems. *Journal of Sex Education and Therapy*, *2*, 211–215.

Bauer, M., Fetherstonhaugh, D., Tarzia, L., Nay, R., & Beattie, E. (2014). Supporting residents' expression of sexuality: The initial construction of a sexuality assessment tool for residential aged care facilities *BMC Geriatrics*, *14*, 82. Retrieved from www.biomedcentral.com/1471-2318/14/82

Centers for Disease Prevention and Control. (2015). *Sexually trtansmitted diseases* (STDS). Retrived from www.cdc.gov/std/

*Gilbert, E., & Harmon, J. (1998). *Manual of high risk pregnancy and delivery* (2nd ed.). St. Louis: Mosby-Year Book.

Ginsburg, K. R. (2015). *Talking to your child about sex*. Retrieved from www.healthychildren.org/English/ages-stages/

gradeschool/puberty/Pages/Talking-to-Your-Child-About-Sex.aspx.

*Gray, J. (1995). *Mars and Venus in the bedroom: A guide to lasting romance and passion*. New York: HarperCollins.

Hockenberry, M. J., & Wilson, D. (2015). *Wong's essentials of pediatric nursing* (10th ed.). New York: Elsevier.

Katsufrakis, P. J., & Nusbaum, M. R. (2011). Chapter 12. Adolescent sexuality. In J. E. South-Paul, S. C. Matheny, &. E. L. Lewis (Eds.), *Current diagnosis and treatment in family medicine* (3rd ed.). New York: Lange Medical Books, McGraw-Hill.

Kazer, M. W. (2012a). Issues regarding sexuality. In: M. Boltz, E. Capezuti, T. Fulmer, & D. Zwicker (Eds.), *Evidence-based geriatric nursing protocols for best practice* (4th ed., pp. 500–515). New York: Springer.

Kazer, M. W. (2012b). *Sexuality assessment for older adults best practices in nursing care to older adults*. Retrieved from http://consultgerirn.org/uploads/File/trythis/try_this_10.pdf

*Lindau, S. T., Schumm, L. P., Laumann, E. O., Levinson, W., O'Muircheartaigh, C. A., & Waite, L. J. (2007). A study of sexuality and health among older adults in the United States. *The New England Journal of Medicine*, *357*, 762–744. Evidence Level IV: Non-experimental Study.

Miller, C. (2015). *Nursing for wellness in older adults* (7th ed.). Philadelphia: Wolters Kluwer.

*Polomeno, V. (1999). Sex and babies: Pregnant couples' postnatal sexual concerns. *Journal of Prenatal Education*, *8*(4), 9–18.

Smith, M. (1993). Pediatric sexuality: Promoting normal sexual development in children. *Nurse Practitioner*, *18*, 37–44.

*Wilmoth, M. C. (1994). Strategies for becoming comfortable with sexual assessment. *Oncology Nursing News*, *12*(2), 6–7.

Disturbed Sleep Pattern

Arthritis Foundation. (2012). *Sleep problems with arthritis*. Retrieved from www.arthritis.org/living-with-arthritis/comorbidities/sleep-insomnia/

Bartick, M. C., Thai, X., Schmidt, T., Altaye, A., & Solet, J. M. (2010). Decrease in as-needed sedative use by limiting nighttime sleep disruptions from hospital staff. *Journal of Hospital Medicine*, *5*(3), E20–E24.

Blissit, P. (2001). Sleep, memory, and learning. *Journal of Neurosurgical Nursing*, *33*(4), 208–215.

Boyd, J. (2004). Daytime consequences of sleep apnea in REM and NREM sleep. *The New School Psychology Bulletin*, *2*(1), 45–49.

Chasens, E. R., & Umlauf, M. G. (2012). Nursing standard practice protocol: Excessive sleepiness. Retrieved from http://consultgerirn.org/topics/sleep/want_to_know_more

Cirelli, C., & Tononi, G. (2015). Sleep and synaptic homeostasis. *Sleep*, *38*(1), 161–162.

Cole, C., & Richards, K. (2007). Sleep disruption in older adults: Harmful and by no means inevitable, it should be assessed for and treated. *The American Journal of Nursing*, *107*(5), 40–49.

Colten, H. E., & Altevogt, B. M. (Eds.). (2006). *Sleep Disorders and sleep deprivation: An Unmet Public Health Problem*. Washington, DC: Institute of Medicine of the National Academies, The National Academies Press. Retrieved from www.nap.edu

Faraklas, I., Holt, B., Tran, S., Lin, H., Saffle, J., & Cochran, A. (2013). Impact of a nursing-driven sleep hygiene protocol on sleep quality. *Journal of Burn Care & Research*, *34*(2), 249–254.

Hammer, B. (1991). Sleep pattern disturbance. In M. Maas, K. Buckwalter, & M. Hardy (Eds.), *Nursing diagnoses and interventions for the elderly*. Redwood City, CA: Addison-Wesley Nursing.

Hickey, J. (2014). *The clinical practice of neurological and neurosurgical nursing* (5th ed.). Philadelphia: Wolters Kluwer.

Hayashi, Y., & Endo, S. (1982). All-night sleep polygraphic recordings of healthy aged persons: REM and slow-wave sleep. *Sleep*, *5*, 277–283.

Landis, C., & Moe, K. (2004). Sleep and menopause. *Nursing Clinics of North America*, *39*(1), 97–115.

LaReau, R., Benson, L., Watcharotone, K., & Manguba, G. (2008). Examining the feasibility of implementing specific nursing interventions to promote sleep in hospitalized elderly patients. *Geriatric Nursing*, *29*(3), 197–206.

Larkin, V., & Butler, M. (2000). The implications of rest and sleep following childbirth. *British Journal of Midwifery*, *8*(7), 438–442.

Miller, C. (2015). *Nursing for wellness in older adults* (7th ed.). Philadelphia: Wolters Kluwer.

National Sleep Foundation. (2015). *Sleep disorders problems*. Retrieved from https://sleepfoundation.org/sleep-disorders-problems

Impaired Social Interaction

*Blumer, H. (1969). *Symbolic interactionism*. Englewood Cliffs, NJ: Prentice-Hall.

Corrigan, P. W., Larson, J. E., Hautamaki, J., Matthews, A., Kuwabara, S., Rafacz, J., . . . O'Shaughnessy, J. (2009). What lessons do coming out as gay men or lesbians have for people stigmatized by mental illness? *Community Mental Health Journal*, *45*(5), 366–374.

Hasson-Ohayon, I., Or, S. E. B., Vahab, K., Amiaz, R., Weiser, M., & Roe, D. (2012). Insight into mental illness and self-stigma: The mediating role of shame proneness. *Psychiatry Research*, *200*(2), 802–806.

Johnson, B. S. (1995). *Child, adolescent and family psychiatric nursing*. Philadelphia: J. B. Lippincott.

*Maroni, J. (1989). Impaired social interactions. In G. McFarland, & E. McFarlane (Eds.), *Nursing diagnosis and interventions*. St. Louis: C. V. Mosby.

*McFarland, G., Wasli, E., & Gerety, E. (1996). *Nursing diagnoses and process in psychiatric mental health nursing* (5th ed.). Philadelphia: J. B. Lippincott.

Miller, C. (2015). *Nursing for wellness in older adults* (7th ed.). Philadelphia: Wolters Kluwer.

Mashiach-Eizenberg, M., Hasson-Ohayon, I., Yanos, P. T., Lysaker, P. H., & Roe, D. (2013). Internalized stigma and quality of life among persons with severe mental illness: The mediating roles of self-esteem and hope. *Psychiatry research*, *208*(1), 15–20.

Stuart, G. W., & Sundeen, S. (2002). *Principles and practice of psychiatric nursing* (6th ed.). St. Louis: Mosby-Year Book.

Chronic Sorrow

*Burke, M. L., Hainsworth, M. A., Eakes, G. G., & Lindgren, C. L. (1992). Current knowledge and research on chronic

sorrow: A foundation for inquiry. *Death Studies, 16*(3), 231–245.

*Damrosch, S. P., & Perry, L. A. (1989). Self-reported adjustment, chronic sorrow, and coping of parents of children with down syndrome. *Nursing Research, 38*(1), 25–30.

*Eakes, G. G., Burke, M. L., & Hainsworth, M. A. (1998). Middle-range theory of chronic sorrow. *Image: Journal of Nursing Scholarship, 30,* 179.

*Eakes, G. G. (1995). Chronic sorrow: The lived experience of parents of chronically mentally ill individuals. *Archives of Psychiatric Nursing, 9*(2), 77–84.

*Gamino, L. A., Hogan, N. S., & Sewell, K. W. (2002). Feeling the absence: A content analysis from the Scott and White grief study. *Death Studies, 26*(10), 793.

Gordon, J. (2009). An evidence-based approach for supporting parents experiencing chronic sorrow. *Pediatric Nursing, 35*(2), 115–119.

Hobdell, E. F., Grant, M. L., Valencia, I., Mare, J., Kothare, S. V., Legido, A., & Khurana, D. S. (2007). Chronic sorrow and coping in families of children with epilepsy. *Journal of Neuroscience Nursing, 39*(2), 76–82.

Hockenberry, M. J., & Wilson, D. (2015). *Wong's essentials of pediatric nursing* (10th ed.). New York: Elsevier.

*Kearney, P. M., & Griffin, T. (2001). Between joy and sorrow: Being a parent of a child with developmental disability. *Journal of Advanced Nursing, 34*(5), 582–592.

*Lindgren, C. L., Burke, M. L., Hainsworth, M. A., & Eakes, G. G. (1992). Chronic sorrow: A lifespan concept. *Scholarly Inquiry for Nursing Practice, 24*(6), 27–42.

*Mallow, G. E., & Bechtel, G. (1999). Chronic sorrow: The experience of parents with children who are developmentally disabled. *Journal of Psychosocial Nursing, 37*(7), 31–35.

*Melnyk, B., Feinstein, N., Moldenhouer, Z., & Small, L. (2001). Coping of parents of children who are chronically ill. *Pediatric Nursing, 27*(6), 548–558.

*Monsen, R. B. (1999). Mothers' experiences of living worried when parenting children with spina bifida. *Journal of Pediatric Nursing, 14*(3), 157–163.

Nikfarid, L., Rassouli, M., Borimnejad, L., & Alavimajd, H. (2015). Chronic sorrow in mothers of children with cancer. *Journal of Pediatric Oncology Nursing, 32*(5), 314–319.

*Olshansky, S. (1962). Chronic sorrow: A response to having a mentally defective child. Social Casework, 43, 190–193.

Rassouli, M., & Sajjadi, M. (2014). Palliative care in Iran moving toward the development of palliative care for cancer. *American Journal of Hospice and Palliative Medicine*. doi:10.1177/1049909114561856

Rhode Island Department of Health. (2011). *Resource guide for families of children with autism spectrum*. Retrieved from www.health.ri.gov/publications/guidebooks/2011ForFamiliesOfChildrenWithAutismSpectrumDisorders.pdf

*Roos, S. (2002). *Chronic sorrow: A living loss*. New York: Brunner-Routledge.

*Teel, C. (1991). Chronic sorrow: Analysis of the concept. *Journal of Advanced Nursing, 16*(11), 1311–1319.

Spiritual Distress

Andrews, M., & Boyle, J. (2012). *Transcultural concepts in nursing* (8th ed.). Philadelphia: Lippincott Williams & Wilkins.

*Burkhart, M. A. (1994). Becoming and connecting: Elements of spirituality for women. *Holistic Nursing Practice, 8,* 12–21.

*Burkhart, L., & Solari-Twadell, A. (2001). Spirituality and religiousness: Differentiating the diagnoses through a review of the nursing diagnosis. *12*(2), 44–54.

*Carson, V. B. (1999). *Mental health nursing: The nurse-patient journey* (2nd ed.). Philadelphia: W. B. Saunders.

*Fowler, J. W. (1995). Stages of faith: The psychology of human development and the quest for meaning. San Francisco: Harper & Row.

*Halstead, H. L. (2004). Spirituality in the elderly. In M. Stanley & P. G. Beare (Eds.), *Gerontological nursing* (3rd ed., pp. 415–425). Philadelphia: F. A. Davis.

*Kelcourse, F. B. (2004). Human development and faith: Life-cycle stages of body, mind, and soul. St. Louis: Chalice Press.

*Kemp, C. (2006). Spiritual care interventions. In B. Ferrell & N. Coyle (Eds.), *Textbook of palliative nursing* (2nd ed., pp. 440–455). New York: Oxford.

*Kendrick, K. D., & Robinson, S. (2000). Spirituality: Its relevance and purpose for clinical nursing in the new millennium. *Journal of Clinical Nursing, 9*(5), 701–705.

*Lipson, J. G., & Dibble, S. L. (2006). *Culture & clinical care*. San Francisco: UCSF Nursing Press.

*Mauk, K. L., & Schmidt, N. A. (2004). Spiritual care in nursing practice. Philadelphia, PA: Lippincott Williams & Wilkins.

*Moberg, D. O. (1984). Subjective measures of spiritual well-being. *Review of Religious Research, 25,* 351–364.

*Nelson-Becker, H. (2004). Spiritul, religious, nonspiritual, nonreligious narratives in marginalized older adults: A typology of coping styles. *Journal of Religion, Spirituality, and Aging, 17*(1/2), 85–99.

Nelson-Becker, H., Nakashima, M., & Canda, E. R. (2008). Research on religions, spirituality, and aging: A social work perspective on the state of the art. *Journal of Religion, Spirituality & Aging, 20*(3), 77.

*O'Brien, M. E. (2010). *Spirituality in nursing: Standing on holy ground* (4th ed.). Boston: Jones and Bartlett.

*Piles, C. L. (1990). Providing spiritual care. *Nurse Educator, 15*(1), 36–41.

Puchalski, C. M., & Ferrell, B. (2010). *Making Health Care Whole: Integrating Spirituality into Patient Care.* West Conshohocken, PA: Templeton Press.

*Thorson, J. E., & Cook, T. C. (1980) *Spiritual well-being of the elderly*. Springfield IL.: Charles C., Thomas Publishers.

*Tinoco, L. (2006). *Providing culturally and linguistically competent health care*. Oakbrook Terrace, IL: Joint Commission Resources.

*Wright, L. M. (2004). *Spirituality, suffering, and illness: Ideas for healing*. Philadelphia: F.A. Davis Co.

Stress Overload

*Bodenheimer, T., MacGregor, K., & Sharifi, C. (2005). *Helping patients manage their chronic conditions*. Retrieved from www.chef.org/publications

*Cahill, L., Gorski, L., & Le, K. (2003). Enhanced human memory consolidation with post-learning stress: Interaction with the degree of arousal at encoding. *Learning & Memory, 10*(4), 270–274.

Edelman, C. L., Kudzma, E. C., & Mandle, C. L. (2014). *Health promotion throughout the life span* (8th ed.). CV Mosby: St. Louis.

Edelman, C. L., & Mandle, C. L. (2010). *Health promotion throughout the life span* (7th ed.). St. Louis, MO: Mosby-Year Book.

Peaceful Parenting Institute. (2015). *Avoiding stress overload.* Retrieved from www.peacefulparent.com/avoiding-stress-overload/

*Ridner, S. H. (2004). Psychological distress: Concept analysis. *Journal of Advanced Nursing, 45*(5), 536–545.

U.S. Department of Health and Human Service. (2015). *Healthy people 2020.* Retrieved from www.healthypeople.gov/2020/topics-objectives

Risk for Sudden Infant Death Syndrome

American Academy of Pediatrics. (2000). Task force on infant sleep position and Sudden Infant Death Syndrome: Changing concepts of Sudden Infant Death Syndrome; Implications for infants' sleeping environment and sleep position. *Pediatrics, 105*(3), 650–656.

American Association of Pediatrics. (2011). Task Force on sudden infant death syndrome (SIDS) and other sleep-related infant deaths: Expansion of recommendations for a safe infant sleeping environment. *Pediatrics*; 128, 1030.

Anderson, J. E. (2000). Co-sleeping: Can we ever put the issue to rest? *Contemporary Pediatrics, 17*(6), 98–102, 109–110, 113–114.

Centers for Disease Control and Prevention. (2015). Sudden unexpected infant death and sudden infant death syndrome. Retrieved from www.cdc.gov/sids/data.html

Corwin, M. J. (2015). Sudden infant death syndrome. In *UpToDate.* Retrieved from www.uptodate.com/contents/sudden-infant-death-syndrome-risk-factors- and-risk-reduction-strategies

*Sherratt, S. (1999). The pros & cons of movement monitors. *British Journal of Midwifery,* 7(9), 569–572.

Risk for Delayed Surgical Recovery

*Akbari, C. M., Saouaf, R., Barnhill, D. F., Newman, P. A., LoGerfo, F. W., & Veves, A. (1998). Endothelium-dependent vasodilatation is impaired in both microcirculation and macrocirculation during acute hyperglycemia. *Journal of Vascular Surgery, 28*(4), 687–694.

Armstrong, D. O., & Meyt, A. J. (2014). Wound healing and risk factors for non-healing. In *UpToDate.* Retrieved from www.uptodate.com/contents/wound-healing-and-risk-factors-for-non-healing

Centers for Disease Prevention and Control. (2015). *Surgical site infection (SSI) event.* Retrieved from www.cdc.gov/nhsn/PDFs/pscManual/9pscSSIcurrent.pdf

*Cheadle, W. G. (2006). Risk factors for surgical site infection. *Surgical Infections,* 7(Suppl 1), S7–S11.

Franz, M. G., Robson, M. C., Steed, D. L., Barbul, A., Brem, H., Cooper, D. M., . . . Wiersema-Bryant, L. (2008). Guidelines to aid healing of acute wounds by decreasing impediments of healing. *Wound Repair and Regeneration, 16*(6), 723–748.

*Geerlings, M. I., Deeg, D. J. H., Penninx, B. W. J. H., Schmand, B., Jonker, C., Bouter, L. M., & Van Tilburg, W. (1999). Cognitive reserve and mortality in dementia: the role of cognition, functional ability and depression. *Psychological Medicine, 29*(5), 1219–1226.

Giardina, E. G. (2015). Cardiovascular effects of nicotine. In *UpToDate.* Retrieved from www.uptodate.com/contents/cardiovascular-effects-of-nicotine

Guo, S., & DiPietro, L. A. (2010). Factors affecting wound healing. *Journal of Dental Research, 89*(3), 219–229.

Hart, S. R., Bordes, B., Hart, J., Corsino, D., & Harmon, D. (2011). Unintended perioperative hypothermia. *The Ochsner Journal, 11*(3), 259–270.

Pear, S. M. (2007). *Managing infection control: Patients risk factors and best practices for surgical site infection prevention* (pp. 56–63). Tucson, AZ: University of Arizona.

Price, C. S., Williams, A., Philips, G., Dayton, M., Smith, W., & Morgan, S. (2008). *Staphylococcus aureus* nasal colonization in preoperative orthopaedic outpatients. *Clinical Orthopaedics and Related Research, 466*(11), 2842–2847.

Sørensen, L. T. (2012). Wound healing and infection in surgery: The pathophysiological impact of smoking, smoking cessation, and nicotine replacement therapy: A systematic review. *Annals of Surgery, 255*(6), 1069–1079. Retrieved from http://archsurg.jamanetwork.com/article.aspx?articleid=1151013

Speaar, M. (2008). Wound care management: Risk factors for surgical site infections. *Plastic Surgical Nursing, 28*(4), 201–204.

Ineffective Tissue Perfusion

Grossman, S., & Porth, C. A. (2014). *Porth's pathophysiology: Concepts of altered health states* (9th ed.). Philadelphia: Wolters Kluwer.

*Miller, C. (2015). *Nursing for wellness in older adults* (7th ed.). Philadelphia: Wolters Kluwer.

Impaired Urinary Elimination

The American College of Obstetricians and Gynecologists. (2014). *Evaluation of uncomplicated stress urinary incontinence in women before surgical treatment.* Committee Opinion No. 603. Obstetrics and Gynecology; 123:1403–7. Retrieved from www.acog.org/Resources-And-Publications/Committee-Opinions/Committee-on-Gynecologic-Practice/Evaluation-of-Uncomplicated-Stress-Urinary-Incontinence-in-Women-Before-Surgical-Treatment

*Ball, J., & Bindler, R. (2008). *Pediatric nursing: Caring for children* (4th ed.). Upper Saddle River, NJ: Pearson Prentice Hall.

Beeckman, D., Bliss, D. Z., Doughty, D., Fader, M., Gray, M., Junkin, J., . . . Selekof, J. (2012). Incontinence associated dermatitis; A comprehensive review and update. *Journal of Wound, Ostomy and Continence Nursing,* 39, 61–74.

Beeckman, D., Verhaeghe, S., Defloor, T., Schoonhoven, L, & Vanderwee K. (2011). A 3-in-1 perineal care washcloth impregnated with dimethicone 3% versus water and pH neutral soap to prevent and treat incontinence-associated dermatitis: A randomized, controlled clinical trial. *Journal of Wound Ostomy and Continence Nursing, 38*(6), 627–634.

Buckley, B. S., & Lapitan, M. C. M. (2010). Prevalence of urinary incontinence in men, women, and children—current evidence: Findings of the Fourth International Consultation on Incontinence. *Urology, 76*(2), 265–270.

*Carpenter, R. O. (1999). Disorders of elimination. In J. McMillan, C. D. DeAngelis, R. Feigin, & J. B. Warshaw (Eds.), *Oski's pediatrics: Principles and practice* (3rd ed.). Philadelphia: Lippincott Williams & Wilkins.

Chatham, N., & Carls, C. (2012). How to manage incontinence-associated dermatitis. *Wound Care Advisor*, 1, 7–10. Retrieved June 27, 2015, from http://woundcareadvisor.com/wp-content/uploads/2012/05/WCA_M-J-2012_Dermatitis.pdf

Choi, H., Palmer M., & Parker, J. (2007). Meta-analyses of pelvic floor muscle training: Randomized controlled trials in incontinent women. *Nursing Research*, 56, 226–234.

Chatham, N., & Carls, C. (2012). How to manage incontinence-associated dermatitis. *Wound Care Advisor*, 1, 7–10. Retrieved June 27, 2015, from http://woundcareadvisor.com/wp-content/uploads/2012/05/WCA_M-J-2012_Dermatitis.pdf

Choi, H., Palmer M., & Parker, J. (2007). Meta-analyses of pelvic floor muscle training: Randomized controlled trials in incontinent women. *Nursing Research*, 56, 226–234.

Coyne, K., Sexton, C., Irwin, D., Kopp, Z., Kelleher, C., & Milsom, I. (2008). The impact of overactive bladder, incontinence and other lower urinary tract symptoms on quality of life, work productivity, sexuality and emotional well-being in men and women: Results from the EPIC study. *British Journal of Urology International*, *101*(11), 1388–1395.

*Dallosso, H., McGrother, C., Matthews, R., & Donaldson, M. (2003). The association of diet and other lifestyle factors with overactive bladder and stress incontinence: A longitudinal study in women. *British Journal of Urology International*, *92*, 69–77.

Davis, N. J., Vaughan, C. P., Johnson, T. M., Goode, P. S., Burgio, K. L., Redden, D. T., & Markland, A. D. (2013). Caffeine intake and its association with urinary incontinence in United States men: Results from National Health and Nutrition Examination Surveys 2005–2006 and 2007–2008. *The Journal of Urology*, *189*(6), 2170–2174.

DeMaagd, G. A., & Davenport, T. C. (2012). Management of urinary incontinence. *Pharmacy & Therapeutics*, *37*(6), 345–361, 361B–361H.

Derrer, D. (2014). Diet, drugs and urinary incontinence. WebMD. Retrieved from www.webmd.com/urinary-incontinence-oab/urinary-incontinence-diet-medications-chart?page=2

Devore, E., Minassian V., & Grodstein, F. (2013). Factors associated with persistent urinary incontinence. *American Journal of Obstetrics and Gynecology*, 209, 1–6.

Dumoulin, C., Hay-Smith, E., & Mac Habee-Segui, G. (2014). Pelvic floor muscle training versus no treatment, or inactive control treatments, for urinary incontinence in women. *Cochrane Database System Review*, *5*, CD005654.

DuBeau, C. E. (2014). Treatment and prevention of urinary incontinence in women. In *UpToDate*. Retrieved from www.uptodate.com/home

DuBeau, C. (2015). Epidemiology, risk factors, and pathogenesis of urinary incontinence in women. In *UpToDate*. Retrieved from www.uptodate.com/contents/epidemiology-risk-factors-and-pathogenesis-of-urinary-incontinence-in-women

Ganio, M. S., Armstrong, L. E., Casa, D. J., McDermott, B. P., Lee, E. C., Yamamoto, L. M., . . . Chevillotte, E. (2011). Mild dehydration impairs cognitive performance and mood of men. *British Journal of Nutrition*, *106*(10), 1535–1543. Retrieved June 27, 2015, from http://journals.cambridge.org/action/displayAbstract?fromPage=online&aid=8425835&fileId=S0007114511002005

Gleason, J. L., Richter, H. E., Redden, D. T., Goode, P. S., Burgio, K. L., & Markland, A. D. (2013). Caffeine and urinary incontinence in US women. *International Urogynecology Journal*, *24*(2), 295–302.

Gorina, Y., Schappert, S., Bercovitz, A., Elgaddal, N., & Kramarow, E. (2014). Prevalence of incontinence among older americans. *Vital & Health Statistics*, *3*(36), 1–33.

Gray, M., Bliss D., Doughty, D., Ermer-Seltun, J., Kennedy-Evans, K., & Palmer M. (2007). Incontinence-associated dermatitis: A consensus. *Journal of Wound Ostomy Continence Nursing*, *34*(1), 45–54.

Griebling, T. L. (2009). Urinary incontinence in the elderly. *Clinics in Geriatric Medicine*, *25*(3), 445–457.

Hickey, J. (2014). *The clinical practice of neurological and neurosurgical nursing* (7th ed.). Philadelphia: Lippincott Williams & Wilkins.

Holroyd-Leduc, J., Tannenbaum, C., Thorpe, K., & Straus, S. (2008). What type of urinary incontinence does this woman have? *Journal of the American Medical Association*, *299*, 1446–1456.

Irwin, D, Kopp, Z., Agatep, B., Milsom, I., & Abrams, P. (2011). Worldwide prevalence estimates of lower urinary tract symptoms, overactive bladder, urinary incontinence and bladder outlet obstruction. *BJU International*, *108*, 1132–1138.

Jackson, S., Boyko, E., Scholes, D., Abraham, L., Gupta, K., & Fihn, S. (2004). Predictors of urinary tract infection after menopause: A prospective study. *American Journal of Medicine*, 117, 903–911.

Junkin, J., & Selekof, J. (2007). Prevalence of incontinence and associated skin injury in the acute care inpatient. *Journal of Wound Ostomy Continence Nursing*, *34*(3), 260–269.

*Kelleher, R. (1997). Daytime and nighttime wetting in children: A review of management. *Journal of the Society of Pediatric Nurses*, *2*(2), 73–82.

Khandelwal, C., & Kistler, C. (2013). Diagnosis of urinary incontinence. *American Family Physician*, 87, 543–550.

Lawrence, J. M., Lukacz, E. S., Nager, C. W., Hsu, J. W. Y., & Luber, K. M. (2008). Prevalence and co-occurrence of pelvic floor disorders in community-dwelling women. *Obstetrics & Gynecology*, *111*(3), 678–685.

Long, M., Reed, L., Dynning, K., & Ying, J. (2012). Incontinence-associated dermatitis in a long-term acute care facility. *Journal of Wound Ostomy Continence Nursing*, *39*, 318–327.

Lukacz, E. (2015). Treatment of urinary incontinence in women. In *UpToDate*. Retrieved from www.uptodate.com/contents/treatment-of-urinary-incontinence-in-women

Mayo Clinic. (2012). Kegel exercises: A how-to guide for women. In *Healthy lifestyle/women's health*. Retrieved from www.mayoclinic.org/healthy-lifestyle/womens-health/in-depth/kegel-exercises/art-20045283?pg=1

Medina-Bombardo, D., & Jover-Palmer, A. (2011). Does clinical examination aid in the diagnosis of urinary tract infections in women? A systematic review and meta-analysis. *BMC Family Practice*, *12*, 111 Retrieved June 27, 2015, from www.ncbi.nlm.nih.gov/pmc/articles/PMC3140406/

Miller, J., Guo, Y., & Rodseth, S. (2011). Cluster analysis of intake, output, and voiding habits collected from diary data. *Nursing Research*, *60*(2), 115–123. Retrieved June 27, 2015, from www.ncbi.nlm.nih.gov/pmc/articles/PMC3140406/

*Morant, C. A. (2005). ACOG guidelines on urinary incontinence in women. *American Family Physician*, 72(1), 175–178.

National Clinical Guideline Centre. (2010). *Nocturnal enuresis: the management of bedwetting in children and young people*. London, UK: National Institute for Health and Clinical Excellence (NICE) (Clinical Guideline No. 111). Retrieved from www.guideline.gov/content.aspx?id=25680

Newman, D., & Willson, M. (2011). Review of intermittent catheterization and current best practices. *Urological Nursing, 31*, 12–29.

*Nygaard, I. E., Thompson, F. L., Svengalis, S. L., & Albright, J. P. (1994). Urinary incontinence in elite nulliparous athletes. *Obstetrics & Gynecology, 84*(2), 183–187.

*Peterson, J. (2008). Minimize urinary incontinence: Maximize physical activity in women. *Urological Nursing*, 28:351–356.

Pierce, H., Perry, L., Gallagher, R., & Chiarelli, P. (2015). Pelvic floor health: A concept analysis. *Journal of Advanced Nursing, 71*(5), 991–1004.

Rittig, S., Kamperis, K., Siggaard, C., Hagstroem, S., & Djurhuus, J. C. (2010). Age related nocturnal urine volume and maximum voided volume in healthy children: Reappraisal of International Children's Continence Society definitions. *The Journal of Urology, 183*(4), 1561–1567.

Rittig, N., Hagstroem, S., Mahler, B., Kamperis, K., Siggaard, C., Mikkelsen, M. M., ... & Rittig, S. (2013). Outcome of a standardized approach to childhood urinary symptoms—Long-term follow-up of 720 patients. *Neurourology and urodynamics, 33*(5), 475–481.

Sampselle, C., & DeLancey, J. (1998). Anatomy of female continence. *Journal of Wound, Ostomy and Continence Nursing, 25*(3), 63–74.

*Smith, D. B. (2004). Female pelvic floor health: a developmental review. *Journal of Wound Ostomy & Continence Nursing, 31*(3), 130–137.

Testa, A. (2015). Understanding urinary incontinence in adults. *Society of Urologic Nurses and Associates, 35*, 82–86.

Townsennd, M., Curhan, G., Resnick, N., & Grodstein, F. (2010). The inidence of urinary incontinence across Asian, black and white women in the United States. *American Journal of Obstetrics and Gyenecology, 202*, 378 e1–378e7.

*Townsend, M., Danforth, K., Curhan, G., Resnick, N., & Grodstein, F. (2007). Body mass index, weight gain, and incident urinary incontinence in middle-aged women. *Obstetrics and Gynecology, 110*, 346–353.

Tu, N. D., & Baskin, L. S. (2014). Nocturnal enuresis in children: Management. In *UpToDate*. Retrieved from www.uptodate.com/contents/nocturnal-enuresis-in-children-management?source=see_link

Tu, N. D., Baskin, L. S., & Amhym, A. M. (2014). Nocturnal enuresis in children: Etiology and evaluation. In *UpToDate*. Retrieved from www.uptodate.com/contents/nocturnal-enuresis-in-children-etiology-and-evaluation

University of Texas at Austin, School of Nursing. (2010). *Family nurse practitioner program. recommendations for the management of urge urinary incontinence in women* (p. 9). Austin, TX: University of Texas at Austin, School of Nursing. Retrieved from www.guideline.gov/content.aspx?id=16322

Wilkinson, J., & Van Leuven, K. (2007). *Fundamentals of nursing: Theory, concepts & applications*. Philadelphia: F. A. Davis Company.

Wilson, P., Berghmans, B., Hagen, S., Hay-Smith, J., Moore, K., Nygaard, I., . . . Wyman, J. (2005) Adult conservative management in incontinence. In: *Incontinence Volume 2: Management*. Paris: International Continence Society Health Publication.

Wolin, K., Luly, J., Sutcliffe, S., Andriole, G., & Kibel, A. (2010). Risk of urinary incontinence following prostatectomy: The role of physical activity and obesity. *The Journal of Urology. 183*, 629–633 Retrieved June 27, 2015, from www.ncbi.nlm.nih.gov/pmc/articles/PMC3034651/

Wood, L., & Anger, J. (2014). Urinary incontinence in women. *British Medical Journal. 349*, g4531. Retrieved June 27, 2015, from www.ncbi.nlm.nih.gov/pubmed/25225003

*Yap, P., & Tan, D. (2006). Urinary incontinence in dementia: A practical approach. *Australian Family Physician, 35*(4), 237.

Zaccardi, J. E., Wilson, L., & Mokrzycki, M. L. (2010). The effect of pelvic floor re-education on comfort in women having surgery for stress urinary incontinence. *Urologic nursing, 30*(2), 137–146, 148.

Risk for Vascular Trauma

Al-Benna, S., O'Boyle, C., & Holley, J. (2013). Extravasation injuries in adults. *ISRN Dermatology, 2013*, 8. Retrieved from www.ncbi.nlm.nih.gov/pmc/articles/PMC3664495/

Hayden, B. K., & Goodman, M. (2005).Chemotherapy: principles of administration. In C. H. Yarbro, M. H. Frogge, & M. Goodman (Eds.), *Cancer nursing principles and practice* (6th ed., pp 361–364). Boston: Jones and Bartlett Publishers.

Payne, A. S., & Savares, D. M. (2015). Extravasation injury from chemotherapy and other non-antineoplastic vesicants. In *UpToDate*. Retreived from www.uptodate.com/contents/extravasation-injury-from-chemotherapy-and-other-non-antineoplastic-v

Risk for Violence

Centers for Disease Control and Prevention. (2013). 10 leading causes of death by age group, United States—2013. Retrieved from www.cdc.gov/injury/wisqars/pdf/leading_causes_of_death_by_age_group_2013-a.pdf

Child Trends DataBank. (2015). *Child maltreatment*. Retrieved from www.childtrends.org/?indicators=child-maltreatment

*Del Vecchio, T., & O'Leary, K. D. (2004). The effectiveness of anger treatments for specific anger problems: A meta-analytic review. *Clinical Psychology Review, 24*, 15–34.

*Edari, R., & McManus, P. (1998). Risk and resiliency factors for violence. *Pediatric Clinics of North America, 45*(2), 293–303.

Farrell, S., Harmon, R., & Hastings, S. (1998). Nursing management of acute psychotic episodes. *Nursing Clinics of North America, 33*(1), 187–200.

Gun Violence Archive. (2015). Retrieved from www.gunviolencearchive.org/past-tolls

Kochanek, K. D., Xu, J., Murphy, S. L., Miniño, A. M., & Kung, H. C. (2011). Deaths: Final data for 2009. *National vital statistics reports. Centers for Disease Control and Prevention, National Center for Health Statistics, National Vital Statistics System, 60*(3), 1–116.

*Norris, M., & Kennedy, C. (1992). How patients perceive the seclusion process. *Journal of Psychosocial Nursing. 23*(6), 7–13.

Roche, M., Diers, D., Duffield, C., & Catling-Paull, C. (2010). Violence toward nurses, the work environment, and patient outcomes. *Journal of Nursing Scholarship, 42*(1), 13–22.

*Veenema, G. (2006). Children's exposure to community violence. *Journal of Nursing Scholarship, 33*(2), 167–173.

*Willis, E., & Strasburger, V. (1998). Media violence. *Pediatric Clinics of North America, 45*(2), 319–331.

Wandering

Alzheimer's Association. (2015). *Wandering and getting lost.* Retrieved from www.alz.org/care/alzheimers-dementia-wandering.asp

*Cohen-Mansfield, J. (1998). The effects of an enhanced environment on nursing home residents who pace. *Gerontologist, 38*(2), 199–208.

*Lai, C. K., & Arthur, D. G. (2003). Wandering behaviour in people with dementia. *Journal of Advanced Nursing, 44*(2), 173–182.

Lester, P., Garite, A., & Kohen, I. (2012). Wandering and elopement in nursing homes. *Annuals of Long Term Care, 20*(3), 32–36.

*Logsdon, R. G., McCurry, T. L., Gibbons, L. E., Kukuli, W. A., & Larson, E. B. (1998). Wandering: A significant problem among community-residing individuals with Alzheimer's disease. *Journal of Gerontological Behavioral, Psychological, and Social Science, 53B*(5), 294–299.

SECTION 2, PART 2: FAMILY/HOME NURSING DIAGNOSES

Acierno, R., Hernandez, M. A., Amstadter, A. B., Resnick, H. S., Steve, K., Muzzy, W., & Kilpatrick, D. G. (2010). Prevalence and correlates of emotional, physical, sexual, and financial abuse and potential neglect in the United States: The National Elder Mistreatment Study. *American Journal of Public, 100*(2), 292–297.

American Academy of Family Physicians. (2015). *Intimate partner violence*. Retrieved from www.aafp.org/about/policies/all/intimatepartner-violence.html

American Psychological Association. (2015a). *Elder abuse and neglect*. Retrieved from www.apa.org/pi/aging/resources/guides/elder-abuse.aspx

American Psychological Association. (2015b). *Intimate partner violence; facts and resources*. Retrieved from www.apa.org/topics/violence/partner.aspx

Aronson, M. (2015). Patient information: Alcohol use—When is drinking a problem? In *UpToDate*. Retrieved from www.uptodate.com/contents/alcohol-use-when-is-drinking-a-problem-beyond-the-basics

Ball, J., Bindler, R., & Cowen, K. (2015). *Principles of pediatric nursing: Caring for Children* (6th ed.). Upper Saddle River, NJ: Pearson.

Barnsteiner, J., Disch, J., & Walton, M. K. (2014). *Person and family-centered care*. Indianapolis, IN: Sigma Theta Tau International.

Brandl, B., & Raymond, J. A. (2012). Policy implications of recognizing that caregiver stress is not the primary cause of elder abuse. *Journal of the American Society on Aging, 36*(3), 32–39.

Campinha-Bacote, J. (2011). Delivering patient-centered care in the midst of a cultural conflict: The role of cultural competence. *The Online Journal of Issues in Nursing, 16*(2), 5.

*Carson, V. B., & Smith-DiJulio, K. (2006). Family violence. In E. M. Varcarolis, V. M. Carson, & N. C. Shoemaker (Eds.), *Foundations of psychiatric mental health nursing* (5th ed.). Philadelphia: W. B. Saunders.

Centers for Disease Control and Prevention. (2013). *Intimate partner violence during pregnancy*. Atlanta, GA: Author. Retrieved from www.cdc.gov/reproductivehealth/violence/intimatepartnerviolence/sld001.htm

*Collins, R. L. Leonard, K. E. & Searles, J. S. (Eds.). (1990). Alcohol and the family research and clinical perspectives. New York: Guilford Press.

Department of Health and Human Services: Administration for Children & Families. (2013). *Child Maltreatment 2013*. Retrieved from www.acf.hhs.gov/programs/cb/resource/child-maltreatment-2013

Department of Justice. (2014). *Domestic violence*. Retrieved from www.justice.gov/ovw/domestic-violence

Durham, R., & Chapman, L. (2014). *Maternal-newborn nursing* (2nd ed.). Philadelphia, PA: FA Davis.

*Duvall, E. R. (1977). *Marriage and family development*. Philadelphia: Lippincott Williams Wilkins.

Edelman, C., Kudzma, E. C., & Mandle, C. L. (2014). Health promotion throughout the life span (8 ed.). New York: Elsevier.

Gage, J., Everett, K., & Bullock, L. (2006). Integrative review of parenting in nursing research. *Journal of Nursing Scholarship, 38*(1), 56–62. Retrieved from CINAHL Plus with Full Text database.

*Grishman, K., & Estes, N. (1982). Dynamics of alcoholic families. In N. Estes & M. E. Heinemann (Eds.), *Alcoholism: Development, consequences and interventions*. St. Louis, MO: Mosby-Year Book.

Harris, R. J., Firestone, J. M., & Vega, W. A. (2005). The interaction of country of origin, acculturation, and gender role ideology on wife abuse*. *Social Science Quarterly, 86*(2), 463–483.

Hockenberry, M. J., & Wilson, D. (2015). *Wong's essentials of pediatric nursing* (10th ed.). New York: Elsevier.

Kaakinen, J. R., Coehlo, D. P., Steele, R., Tabacco, A., Hanson, S. M. H. (2015). *Family health care nursing: Theory, practice, and research* (5th ed.) Philadelphia: FA Davis.

Kalmakis, K. (2010). Cycle of sexual assault and women's alcohol misuse. *Journal of the American Academy of Nurse Practitioners, 22(12)*, 661–667.

*Kaufman, K., & Straus, M. (1987). The "drunken Bum "theory of wife beating. *Social Problems, 34*, 213–230.

*Kelly, S. J., Day, N., & Streissguth, A. P. (2000). Effects of prenatal alcohol exposure on social behavior in humans and other species. *Neurotoxicology and teratology, 22*(2), 143–149.

*Lindeman, M., Hawks, J. H., & Bartek, J. K. (1994). The alcoholic family: A nursing diagnosis validation study. *International Journal of Nursing Terminologies and Classifications, 5*(2), 65–73.

Miller, C. (2015). *Nursing for wellness in older adults* (7th ed.). Philadelphia, PA: Wolters Kluwer.

Montalvo-Liendo, N., Koci, A., McFarlane, J., Nava, A., Gilroy, H., & Maddoux, J. (2013). Abused women US-born compared to non-US-born women: 7-year prospective study. *Hispanic Healthcare International* (in press).

*National Association for Children of Alcoholics. (2001). *Children of alcoholics: A kit for educators*. Kensington, MD: Author. Retrieved from htttp://www.nacoa.org/pdfs/EDkit_web_06.pdf

National Center for Elder Abuse. (2015). *Elder abuse*. Alhambra, CA: Author. Retrieved from www.ncea.aoa.gov/library/data/#problem

The National Coalition for the Homeless. (2015). Retrieved from www.nationalhomeless.org

National Institute of Alcohol Abuse and Addiction. (2013). *Alcohol use disorder*. Bethesda, MD: Author. Retrieved from www.niaaa.nih.gov/alcohol-health/overview-alcohol-consumption/alcohol-use-disorders

National Transitions of Care Coalition. (2009). *Improving transitions of care: Hospital to home*. Retrieved from www.ntocc.org/portals/0/pdf/resources/implementationplan_hospitaltohome.pdf

*Needell, B., & Barth, R. P. (1998). Infants entering foster care compared with other infants using birth status indicators. *Child Abuse & Neglect, 22*(12), 1179–1187.

NIH. (2012). *A family history of alcoholism*. Retrieved from pubs.niaaa.nih.gov/publications/FamilyHistory/famhist.htm

*Ramsey-Klawsnik, H. (2000). Elder abuse offenders: A typology. *Generations, 24*(11), 17–22.

Siqueira, L., Smith, V. C., & Committee on Substance Abuse. (2015). Binge drinking. *Pediatrics, 136*(3), e718–e726.

*Smith-DiJulio, K., & Holzapfel, S. K. (1998). Families in crises: Family violence. In E. M. Varcarolis (Ed.), *Foundations of psychiatric mental health nursing: A clinical approach* (3rd ed). St. Louis: Saunders/Elsevier

*Spencer, N., Wallace, A., Sundrum, R., Bacchus, C., & Logan, S. (2006). Child abuse registration, fetal growth, and preterm birth: A population based study. *Journal of Epidemiology and Community Health, 60*(4), 337–340.

*Starling, B. P., & Martin, A.C. (1990). Adult survivors of parental alcoholism: implications for primary care. *The Nurse Practitioner, 15*(7), 16, 19–20, 22–24.

Tetrault, J. M., & O'Connor, P. G. (2015). *Risky drinking and alcohol use disorder: Epidemiology, pathogenesis, clinical manifestations, course, assessment, and diagnosis*. In *UpToDate*. Retrieved from www.uptodate.com/contents/risky-drinking-and-alcohol-use-disorder-epidemiology-pathogenesis-clinical-manifestations-course-assessment-and-diagnosis

*Ullman, S. E., & Brecklin, L. R. (2003). Sexual assault history and health-related outcomes in a national sample of women. *Psychology of* Women *Quarterly*, 27(1), 46–57.

Vagianos, A. (2014). 30 shocking domestic violence statistics that remind us it's an epidemic. *The Huffington Post*. Retrieved from www.huffingtonpost.com/2014/10/23/domestic-violence-statistics_n_5959776.html

Varcarolis, E. M. (2011). *Manual of psychiatric nursing care planning* (4th ed.). St. Louis, MO: Saunders.

*Varcarolis, E. M., Carson, V. B., & Shoemaker, N. C. (2006). *Foundations of psychiatric mental health nursing: A clinical approach* (5th ed.). St. Louis (MO): Elsevier.

Vespa, J., Lewis, J. M., & Kreider, R. M. (2013). America's families and living arrangements: 2012. In *Current population reports* (pp. 20–570). Washington. DC: U.S. Census Bureau.

Wegscheider-Cruse S., & Cruse, J. (2012). Understanding codependency, updated and expanded: The science behind it and deerfield. Florida: Health Communications.

*Wing D. (1995). Transcending alcoholic denial. *Image, 27*, 121–126.

Disabled Family Coping

*Blair, K. (1986). The battered woman: Is she a silent partner? *Nurse Practitioner, 11*(6), 38.

*Browne, K. (1989). The health visitor's role in screening for child abuse. *Health Visitor, 62*(3), 275–277.

*Carlson-Catalano, J. (1998). Nursing diagnoses and interventions for post-acute phase battered women. *Nursing Diagnosis, 9*(3), 101–109.

*Cowen, P. S. (1999). Child neglect: Injuries of omission. *Pediatric Nursing, 25*(4), 401–418.

*Fulmer, T., & Paveza, G. (1998). Neglect in the elderly. *Nursing Clinics of North America, 3*(3), 457–466.

Kaakinen, J. R., Gedaly-Duff, V., Coehlo, D., & Hanson, S. (2010). *Family health care nursing, theory, practice, and research* (4th ed.). Philadelphia: F.A. Davis.

*Sammons, L. (1981). Battered and pregnant. *Maternal-Child Nursing Journal, 6*, 246–250.

*Smith-DiJulio, K., & Holzapfel, S. K. (2006). Families in crises: Family violence. In E. M. Varcarolis, V. M. Carson, & N. C. Shoemaker (Eds.), *Foundations of psychiatric mental health nursing* (5th ed.). Philadelphia: W. B. Saunders.

Impaired Home Maintenance

*Green, K. (1998). *Home care survival guide*. Philadelphia: Lippincott.

*Holzapfil, S. (1998). The elderly. In E. Varcarolis (Ed.). *Foundations of psychiatric mental health nursing* (3rd ed.). Philadelphia: W. B. Saunders.

Impaired Parenting

Parent-Infant Attachment

*Goulet, C., Bell, L., & Tribble, D. (1998). A concept analysis of parent–infant attachment. *Journal of Advanced Nursing, 28*(5), 1071–1081.

*Mercer, R., & Ferketich S. (1990). Predictors of parental attachment during early parenthood. *Journal of Advanced Nursing, 15*(3), 268–280.

Parental Role Conflict

*Clements, D., Copeland, L., & Loftus, M. (1990). Critical times for families with a chronically ill child. *Pediatric Nursing, 16*(2), 157–161.

*Melnyk, B., Feinstein, N., Moldenhouer, Z., & Small, L. (2001). Coping in parents of children who are chronically ill. *Pediatrics, 27*(6), 548–558.

*Schepp, K. (1991). Factors influencing the coping effort of mothers of hospitalized children. *Nursing Research, 40*, 42–45.

SECTION 2, PART 3: COMMUNITY NURSING DIAGNOSES

Agency for Healthcare Research and Quality. (2014). *Vulnerable populations*. Retrieved from https://innovations.ahrq.gov/taxonomy-terms/vulnerable-populations

Agency for Toxic Substances and Disease Registry (ATSDR). (2014). *Toxic substances*. Retrieved from www.atsdr.cdc.gov/toxprofiles/index.asp

Allender, J. A., Rector, C., & Warner, K. (2010). *Community health nursing: Promoting and protecting the public* (7th ed.). Philadelphia, PA: Lippincott Williams & Wilkins.

Allender, J. A., Rector, C., & Warner, K. (2014). *Community health nursing* (8th ed.). Philadelphia, PA: Wolters Kluwer.

Boscarino, J. A. (2015). Community disasters, psychological trauma, and crisis intervention. *International Journal of Emergency Mental Health, 17*(1), 369.

*Bushy, A. (1990). Rural United Sates women: Traditions and transitions affecting health care. *Health Care for Women International, 11*, 503–513.

Clark, L. (2009). Focus group research with children and youth. *Journal for Specialists in Pediatric Nursing*, 14(2), 152–154.

Clark, J. S., & Bujnowski, A. (2014). Nursing and the science of prevention for population health. *Nursing Administration Quarterly*, *38*(2), 147–154.

*Clemen-Stone, E., Eigasti, D. G., & McGuire, S. L. (2001). *Comprehensive family and community health nursing* (6th ed.). St. Louis, MO: Mosby-Year Book.

Edelman, C., Kudzma, E. C., & Mandle, C. L. (2014). *Health promotion throughout the life span* (8th ed.). New York: Elsiever.

Ferguson, C. (2007). Barriers to serving the vulnerable: Thoughts of a former public. Retrieved from http://content.healthaffairs.org/content/26/5/1358.fullOfficial Health Affairs

*Gordon, M. (1994). *Nursing diagnosis: Process and application*. St. Louis, MO: Mosby-Year Book.

Hobfoll, S. E., Watson, P., Bell, C. C., Bryant,R. A., Brymer, M. J., Friedman, M. J. & Ursano, R. J. (2007). Five essential elements of immediate and mid-term mass trauma intervention: Empirical evidence. *Psychiatry: Biological and Interpersonal Issues*, *70*(4), 283–315; discussion 316–369. doi:10.1521/psyc.2007.70.4.283

*Kindig, D., & Stoddart, G. (2003). What is population health? *American Journal of Public Health*, *93*(3), 380–383.

Loue, S., & Quill, B. E. (Eds.). (2013). *Handbook of rural health*. New York: Springer.

*Maslow, A. (1971). *The farther reaches of human nature*. New York: Penguin/Arkana.

*McLeroy, K. R., Norton, B. L., Kegler, M. C., Burdine, J. N., & Sumaya, C. V. (2003). Community-based interventions. *American Journal of Public Health*, *93*(4), 529–533.

Shinkus Clark, J. , & Bujnowski, A. (2014). Nursing and the science of prevention for population health. *Nursing Administration Quarterly*, *38*(2), 147–154.

Siegel, J. D., Rhinehart, E., Jackson, M., Chiarello, L., & The Healthcare Infection Control Practices Advisory Committee. (2007, June). *2007 guideline for isolation precautions: Preventing transmission of infectious agents in healthcare settings*. Retrieved August 12, 2008, from www.cdc.gov/ncidod/dhqp/pdf/isolation2007.pdf

*Thornton, J. W., McCally, M., Houlihan, J. (2002). Biomonitoring of industrial pollutants: Health and policy implications of the chemical body burden. *Public Health Report*, *117*(4), 315–323.

*Veenema, T. G. (2013). *Disaster nursing and emergency preparedness for chemical, biological, and radiological terrorism and other hazards*. New York: Springer.

Winters, C. A., & Lee, H. (2009). *Rural nursing: Concepts, theory, & practice* (3rd ed.). New York, NY: Springer.

Contamination: Community

Agency for Toxic Substances and Disease Registry (ATSDR). (2014). *Medical management guidelines*. Retrieved from www.atsdr.cdc.gov/MMG/index.asp

*Children's Environmental Health Network. (2004). *Resource guide on children's environmental health*. Retrieved from www.cehn.org

*Thornton, J. W., McCally, M., & Houlihan, J. (2002). Biomonitoring of industrial pollutants: Health and policy implications of the chemical body burden. *Public Health Reports*, *117*, 315–323.

Veenema, T. G. (2003). *Disaster nursing and emergency preparedness for chemical, biological and radiological terrorism and other hazards*. New York: Springer.

Ineffective Community Coping

Edelman, C. L., Kudzma, E. C. & Mandle, C. L. (2014). *Health promotion throughout the Life span* (8th ed.). St. Louis: CV Mosby.

Allender, J. A., Rector, C., & Warner, K. (2014). *Community & public health nursing* (8th ed.). Philadelphia, PA: Wolters Kluwer.

Readiness for Enhanced Community Coping

Allender, J. A., Rector, C., & Warner, K. (2014). *Community & public health nursing* (8th ed.). Philadelphia, PA: Wolters Kluwer.

Edelman, C. L., Kudzma, E. C., & Mandle, C. L. (2014). *Health promotion throughout the Life span* (8th ed.). St. Louis: CV Mosby.

*Bushy, A. (1990). Rural determinants in family health: Considerations for community nurse. *Family and Community Health*, *12*(4), 89–94.

SECTION 2, PART 4: HEALTH PROMOTION/ NURSING DIAGNOSES

*Bodenheimer, T., MacGregor, K., & Sharifi, C. (2005). *Helping patients manage their chronic conditions*. Retrieved January 10, 2007, from www.chef.org/publications

*Blackburn, S. (1993). Assessment and management of neuralgic dysfunction. In C. Kenner, A. Brueggemeyer, & L. Gunderson (Eds.), *Comprehensive neonatal nursing*. Philadelphia: W. B. Saunders.

*Blackburn, S., & Vandenberg, K. (1993). Assessment and management of neonatal neurobehavioral development. In C. Kenner, A. Brueggemeyer, & L. Gunderson (Eds.), *Comprehensive neonatal nursing*. Philadelphia: W. B. Saunders.

*Breslow, D., & Hron, B. G. (2004). Time-extended family interviewing. *Family Process*, *16(1)*, 97–103 (reprint, March 1977).

*Carson, V. B. (1989). *Spiritual dimensions of nursing practice*. Philadelphia: W. B. Saunders.

*Carson, V. B., Green, H. (1992). Spiritual well-being: A predictor of hardiness in patients with acquired immunodeficiency syndrome. *Journal of Professional Nursing*, *8*(4):209–320.

Edelman, C. L., Kudzma, E. C. & Mandle, C. L. (2014). *Health promotion throughout the Life span* (8th ed.). St. Louis: CV Mosby.

*Gordon, M. (2002). *Manual of nursing diagnosis*. St. Louis: Mosby-Year Book.

*Kalichman, S. C., Cain, D., Fuhrel, A., Eaton, L., Di Fonzo, K., & Ertl, T. (2005). Assessing medication adherence self-efficacy among low-literacy patients: Development of a pictographic visual analogue scale. *Health Education Research*, *20*(1), 24–35.

Lawhon, G. (2002). Integrated nursing care: Vital issues important in the humane care of the newborn. *Seminars in Neonatology*, 7, 1441.

Merenstein, G., & Gardner, S. (1998). *Handbook of neonatal intensive care* (4th ed.). St. Louis, MO: Mosby-Year Book.

*Piette, J. D. (2005). *Using telephone support to manage chronic disease*. Oakland, CA: California Healthcare Foundation. Retrieved from www.chef.org/topics/chronicdisease/index.cfm

*Vandenberg, K. (1990). The management of oral nippling in the sick neonate, the disorganized feeder. *Neonatal Network*, *9*(1), 9–16.

Varcarolis, E.M. (2011). *Manual of psychiatric nursing care planning* (4th ed.). St. Louis, MO: Saunders.

Varcarolis, E. M., Carson, V. B., & Shoemaker, N. C. (2006). *Foundations of psychiatric mental health nursing: a clinical approach* (5th ed.). St. Louis, MO: Elsevier.

Waryasz, G. R., & McDermott, A. Y. (2010). Exercise prescription and the patient with type 2 diabetes: A *clinical* approach to optimizing patient outcomes. *Journal of the American Academy of Nurse Practitioners*, *22*(4), 217–227.

SECTION 3: MANUAL OF COLLABORATIVE PROBLEMS

*American Academy of Pediatrics (AAP) Subcommittee on Hyperbilirubinemia. (2004). Clinical practice guidelines: Management of hyperbilirubinemia in the newborn infant 35 weeks or more of gestation. *Pediatrics*, *114*(1), 297–316.

American Academy of Pediatrics (AAP) Subcommittee on Fetus & Newborn. (2011). Phototherapy to prevent severe neonatal hyperbilirubinemia in the newborn infant 35 or more weeks of gestation. *Pediatrics*, *128*(4), e1046–e1052.

Aisiku, I. P., Smith, W. R., McClish, D. K., Levenson, J. L., Penberthy, L. T., Roseff, S. D., ... & Roberts, J. D. (2009). Comparisons of high versus low emergency department utilizers in sickle cell disease. *Annals of Emergency Medicine*, *53*(5), 587–593.

Atkinson, J., Cicardi, J., & Zuraw, B. (2014). Hereditary angioedema: Treatment of acute attacks. In *UpToDate*. Retrieved from www.uptodate.com/contents/hereditary angioedema-treatment-of-acute-attacks

Auckland Allergy Clinic. (2012). Food allergies and intolerance. Retrieved from www.allergyclinic.co.nz/fa_intolerance.aspx

Association of Women's Health, Obstetric & Neonatal Nurses (AWHONN). (2006). *Hyperbilirubinemia: Identification and management in the healthy term and near-term newborn* (2nd ed.). Washington, DC: Author.

Balach, T., & Peabody, T. (2011). *Management* of *skeletal metastases*. In W. M. Stadler (Ed.), *Renal cancer*. New York, NY: Demos Medical.

Ball, C., deBeer, K., Gomm, A., Hickman, B., & Collins, P. (2007). Achieving tight glycaemic control. *Intensive and Critical Care Nursing*, *23*(3), 137–144.

Barbar, S., Noventa, F., Rossetto, V., Ferrari, A., Brandolin, B., Perlati, M., . . . Prandoni, P. (2010). A risk assessment model for the identification of hospitalized medical patients at risk for venous thromboembolism: The Padua Prediction Score. *Journal of Thrombosis and Haemostasis*, *8*(11), 2450–2457.

Barrisford, G., & Steele, G. S. (2014). Acute urinary retention. In *UpToDate*. Retrieved from www.uptodate.com/contents/acute-urinary-retention

Bartlett, J. (2014). Diagnostic approach to community-acquired pneumonia in adults. In *UpToDate*. Retrieved from www.uptodate.com/contents/diagnostic-approach-to-community-acquired-pneumonia-in-adults

Beretta, L., Rocchetti, S., & Braga, M. (2010). What's new in emergencies, trauma, and shock? Nitrogen balance in critical patients on enteral nutrition. *Journal of Emergencies, Trauma, and Shock*, *3*(2), 105–108. Retrieved from www.onlinejets.org/text.asp?2010/3/2/105/62099

*Bhutani, V. K., Johnson, L., & Sivieri, E. M. (1999). Predictive ability of a predischarge hour-specific serum bilirubin for subsequent significant hyperbilirubinemia in healthy term and near-term newborns. *Pediatrics*, 103(1), 6–14.

Blackburn, S. T. (2013). *Maternal, fetal & neonatal physiology: A clinical perspective* (3rd ed., pp. 512–515). St. Louis: Saunders Elsevier.

Boggs, J. G. (2015). Seizures and epilepsy in the elderly patient: Etiology, clinical presentation, and diagnosis. In *UptoDate*. Retrieved from //www.uptodate.com/contents/seizures-and-epilepsy-in-the-elderly-patient-etiology-clinical-presentation-and-diagnosis?source=see_link

Bordeianou, L., & Yeh, D. D. (2015). Epidemiology, clinical features, and diagnosis of mechanical small bowel obstruction in adults. In *UpToDate*. Retrieved from http://www.uptodate.com/contents/epidemiology-clinical-features-and-diagnosis-of-mechanical-small-bowel-obstruction-in-adults

Byrd, R. (2014). *Respiratory alkalosis clinical presentation*. In *Medscape*. Retrieved from http://emedicine.medscape.com/article/301680-clinical#a0218

Carbone, J. W., McClung, J. P., & Pasiakos, S. M. (2012). Skeletal muscle responses to negative energy balance: Effects of dietary protein. *Advances in Nutrition*, *3*(2), 119–126. Retrieved from http://advances.nutrition.org/content/3/2/119.full

Centers for Disease Control and Prevention. (2014). *Opportunistic infections*. Atlanta, GA: Author. Retrieved from www.cdc.gov/hiv/living/opportunisticinfections.html

Chow, E., Bernjak, A., Williams, S., Fawdry, R. A., Hibbert, S., Freeman, J., … Heller, S. R. (2014). Risk of cardiac arrhythmias during hypoglycemia in patients with type 2 diabetes and cardiovascular risk. *Diabetes*, 63(5), 1738–1747.

Chu, Y. F., Jiang, Y., Meng, M., Jiang, J. J., Zhang, J. C., Ren, H. S., & Wang, C. T. (2010). Incidence and risk factors of gastrointestinal bleeding in mechanically ventilated patients. *World J Emergency Medicine*, *1*(1), 32–36.

Curhan, G. C., Aronson, M. D., & Preminger, G. M. (2014). Diagnosis and acute management of suspected nephrolithiasis in adults. In *UpToDate*. Retrieved from www.uptodate.com/contents/diagnosis-and-acute-management-of-suspected-nephrolithiasis-in-adults

DeBaun, M. R., & Vichinsky, E. P. (2014). Acute pain management in adults with sickle cell disease. In *UpToDate*. Retrieved from www.uptodate.com/contents/acute-pain-management-in-adults-with-sickle-cell-disease?source-see_link

Deegens, J. K., & Wetzels, J. F. (2011). Nephrotic range proteinuria. In John T. Daugirdas (Ed.), *Handbook of chronic kidney disease management* (pp. 313–332). Philadelphia: Lippincott Williams & Wilkins.

de Jong, J. S. S. G. (2014). *Electrolytes disorders*. In *Ecgpedia*. Creative Commons Attribution Non-Commercial Share Alike. Retrieved from http://en.ecgpedia.org/wiki/Electrolyte_Disorders

Emmett, M. (2013). Approach to the adult with metabolic acidosis. In *UpToDate*. Retrieved from www.uptodate.com/contents/approach-to-the-adult-with-metabolic-acidosis

Eriksson, E. A., Schultz, S. E., Cohle, S. D., & Post, K. W. (2011). Cerebral fat embolism without intracardiac shunt: A novel presentation. *Journal of Emergencies, Trauma, and Shock*, *4*(2), 309–312.

Fazia, A., Lin, J., & Staros, E. (2012). *Urine sodium*. Retrieved December 28, 2012, from http://emedicine.medscape.com/article/2088449-overview#showall

Field, J. J., & Debaun, M. R. (2014). Acute chest syndrome in adults with sickle cell disease. In *UpToDate*. Retrieved from www.uptodate.com/contents/acute-chest-syndrome-in-adults-with-sickle-cell-disease

Field, J. J., Vichinsky, E. P., & DeBaun, M. R. (2011). *Overview of the management of sickle cell disease.* Retrieved from www.uptodate.com

Fisher, R. S., Acevedo, C., Arzimanoglou, A., Bogacz, A., Cross, J. H., Elger, C. E., . . . Hesdorffer, D. C. (2014). ILAE official report: a practical clinical definition of epilepsy. *Epilepsia*, *55*(4), 475–482.

Garzon, D. L., Kempker, T., & Piel, T. (2011). Primary care management of food allergy and food intolerance. *The Nurse Practitioner*, *36*(12), 34–40.

Gauer, R., & Braun, M. (2012). Thrombocytopenia. *American Family Physician*, *85*(6), 612–622.

George, J., & Arnold, D. (2014). Approach to the adult with unexplained thrombocytopenia. In *UpToDate*. Retrieved from www.uptodate.com/contents/approach-to-the-adult-with-unexplained-thrombocytopenia

Gestring, M. (2015). Abdominal compartment syndrome. In *UpToDate*. retrieved from http://www.uptodate.com/contents/abdominal-compartment-syndrome

Givertz, M. (2015). Noncardiogenic pulmonary edema. In *UpToDate*. Retrieved from http://www.uptodate.com/contents/noncardiogenic-pulmonary-edema

Goldberg, E., & Chopra, S. (2015). Acute liver failure in adults: Etiology, clinical manifestations, and diagnosis. In *UpToDate*. Retrieved from http://www.uptodate.com/contents/acute-liver-failure-in-adults-etiology-clinical-manifestations-and-diagnosis

Goltzman, D. (2014). Treatment of hypocalcemia. In *UpToDate*. Retrieved from www.uptodate.com/contents/treatment-of-hypocalcemia

Greenberger, E., Lessard, J., Chen, C., & Farruggia, S. P. (2008). Self-entitled college students: Contributions of personality, parenting, and motivational factors. *Journal of Youth Adolescence*, *37*, 1193–1204.

Grober, U., & Kister, K. (2012). Influence of drugs on vitamin D and calcium metabolism. *Dermatoendocrinology*, *4*(2), 158–166. Retrieved from www.ncbi.nlm.nih.gov/pmc/articles/PMC3427195/

Grossman, S., & Porth, C. A. (2014). *Porth's pathophysiology: Concepts of altered health states* (9th ed.). Philadelphia: Wolters Kluwer.

Gysels, M. H., & Higginson, I. J. (2011). The lived experience of breathlessness and its implications for care: A qualitative comparison in cancer, COPD, heart failure and MND. *BMC Palliative Care*, *10*(15), 1.

Halloran, R. S. (2009). Caring for the patient with inflammatory response, shock, and severe sepsis caring for the patient with inflammatory response, shock, and severe sepsis (Chap. 61). In Osborn, K. (Ed.), *Medical surgical nursing: preparation for practice* (Vol. 1). Upper Saddle River, NJ: Prentice Hall.

Hamdy, O. (2012). *Hypoglycemia*. Retrieved from http://emedicine.medscape.com/article/122122-overview

Heist, E. K., & Ruskin, J. N. (2010). Drug-induced arrhythmia. *Circulation*, 122(14), 1426-1435.

Hoffman, R. S., & Weinhouse, G. L. (2015). Management of moderate and severe alcohol withdrawal syndromes. In *UpToDate*. Retrieved from www.uptodate.com/contents/management-of-moderate-and-severe-alcohol-withdrawal-syndromes

Holodinsky, J. K., Roberts, D. J., Ball, C. G., Blaser, A. R., Starkopf, J., Zygun, D. A., ... Kirkpatrick, A. W. (2013). Risk factors for intra-abdominal hypertension and abdominal compartment syndrome among adult intensive care unit patients: A systematic review and meta-analysis. *Critical Care*, *17*(5), R249.

Institute for Clinical System Improvement [ICSI]. (2008). *Health care guideline: Venous thromboembolism prophylaxis* (5th ed.). Bloomington, MN: Author. Retrieved from www.icsi.org

Inzucchi, S., Bergenstal, R., Buse, J., Diamant, M., Ferrannini, E., Nauck, M., . . . Mathews, D. (2012). *Position statement of the American Diabetes Association (ADA) and the European Association for the Study of Diabetes (EASD)*. Retrieved from http://care.diabetesjournals.org/content/early/2012/04/17/dc12-041.full.pdf+html

Kibel, S., Adams, K., & Barlow, G. (2011). Diagnostic and prognostic biomarkers of sepsis in critical care. *Journal of Antimicrobial Chemotherapy, 66*(Suppl 2), ii33–ii40.

Kovesdy, C. P., Kopple, J. D., & Kalantar-Zadeh, K. (2015). Inflammation in renal insufficiency. In *UpToDate*. Retrieved from http://www.uptodate.com/contents/inflammation-in-renal-insufficiency

Labbé, E., Herbert, D., & Haynes, J. (2005). Physicians' attitudes and practices in sickle cell disease pain management. *Journal of Palliative Care*, *21*, 246–251.

Labs on Line. (2014). Retrieved from https://labtestsonline.org/

Lawn, N., Kelly, A., Dunne, J., Lee, J., & Wesseldine, A. (2013). First seizure in the older patient: Clinical features and prognosis. *Epilepsy research*, *107*(1), 109–114.

Lee, R. K. (2012). Intra-abdominal hypertension and abdominal compartment syndrome: A comprehensive overview. *Critical Care Nurse*, 32(1), 19–31.

Lim, W. S., Van der Eerden, M. M., Laing, R., Boersma, W. G., Karalus, N., Town, G. I., . . . Macfarlane, J. T. (2003). Defining community acquired pneumonia severity on presentation to hospital: An international derivation and validation study. *Thorax*, *58*, 377–382.

*Lynn-McHale Wiegand, D. J., & Carlson, K. K. (2005). *AACN procedure manual for critical care*. St. Louis, MO: Elsevier.

Mabvuure, N. T., Malahias, M., Hindocha, S., Khan, W., & Juma, A. (2012). Acute compartment syndrome of the limbs: current concepts and management. *The Open Orthopaedics Journal*, *6*(1), 535–543.

Martin, G. M., Thornhill, T. S., & Katz, J. N. (2015). Total knee arthroplasty. In *UpToDate*. Retrieved from http://www.uptodate.com/contents/total-knee-arthroplasty

Mayo. (2014). *DLMP critical values/critical results list summary*. Retrieved from www.mayomedicallaboratories.com/articles/criticalvalues/view.php?name=Critical+Values%2FCritical+Results+List

Methven, S., MacGregor, M. S., Traynor, J. P., O'Reilly, D. S. J., & Deighan, C. J. (2010). Assessing proteinuria in chronic kidney disease: protein–creatinine ratio versus albumin–creatinine ratio. *Nephrology Dialysis Transplantation, 25*, 2991–2996

McCutcheon, T. (2013). The Ileus and Oddities After Colorectal Surgery. *Gastroenterology Nursing, 36*(5), 368–375.

McGrath, J. M., & Hardy, W. (2011). The infant at risk. In S. Mattson & J. E. Smith (Eds.), *Core curriculum for maternal-newborn nursing* (4th ed., pp. 362–414). St. Louis: Saunders.

Monczewski, L. (2013). Managing Bone Metastasis in the Patient With Advanced Cancer. *Orthopaedic Nursing, 32*(4), 209–214.

National Cancer Institute. (2012). *HPV and cancer*. Retrieved from www.cancer.gov/cancertopics/factsheet/Risk/HPV

National Diabetes Statisitcs Report. (2014). Retrieved from http://www.cdc.gov/diabetes/pubs/statsreport14/national-diabetes-report-web.pdf

National Qualitty Forum. (2011). *Serious reportable events in healthcare—2011 update: A consensus report*. Retrieved from http://www.qualityforum.org/projects/hacs_and_sres.aspx

Neviere, R. (2015). Sepsis and the systemic inflammatory response syndrome: Definitions, epidemiology, and prognosis. In *UpToDate*. Retrieved from www.uptodate.com/contents/sepsis-and-the-systemic-inflammatory-response-syndrome-definitions-epidemiology-and-prognosis

O'Donnell, P. (2012). *Impending fracture & prophylactic fixation ortho bullets*. Retrieved January 26, 2013, from www.orthobullets.com/pathology/8002/impending-fracture-and-prophylactic-fixation

O'Dowd, L. C., & Kelle, M. A. (2015). Air embolism. In *UpToDate*. Retrieved from http://www.uptodate.com/contents/air-embolism

*Pack-Mabien, A., Labbe, E., Herbert, D., & Haynes, J., Jr. (2001). *Nurses' attitudes and practices in sickle cell pain management. Applied Nursing Research, 14*, 187–192.

Pasero, C., & McCaffery, M. (2011). *Pain assessment and pharmacologic management*. St. Louis: Mosby.

Payne, A. B., Miller, C. H., Hooper, W. C., Lally, C., & Austin, H. D. (2014). High factor VIII, von Willebrand factor, and fibrinogen levels and risk of venous thromboembolism in blacks and whites. *Ethnicity & Disease, 24*(2), 169–174.

Pereira de Melo, R., Venícios de Oliveira Lopes, M., Leite de Araujo, T., de Fatima da Silva, L., Aline Arrais Sampaio Santos, F., & Moorhead, S. (2011). Risk for decreased cardiac output: validation of a proposal for nursing diagnosis. *Nursing in Critical Care, 16*(6), 287–294.

Pillai, B. P., Unnikrishnan, A. G., & Pavithran, P. V. (2011). Syndrome of inappropriate antidiuretic hormone secretion: Revisiting a classical endocrine disorder. *Indian Journal of Endocrinology and Metabolism*, S208–S215. Retrieved from www.ncbi.nlm.nih.gov/pmc/articles/PMC3183532/

Rangel-Castillo, L., Gopinath, S., & Robertson, C. S. (2008). Management of intracranial hypertension. *Neurologic Clinics*, 26(2), 521–541.

The Renal Association. (2013). *Clinical practice guidelines*. Retrieved at www.renal.org/information-resources/the-uk-eckd-guide/ckd-stages#sthash.B1UX7gPz.3q8WiJDw.dpbs

Schachter, S. C. (2015). Evaluation of the first seizure in adults. In *UpToDate*. Retrieved from www.uptodate.com/contents/evaluation-of-the-first-seizure-in-adult

Schmidt, A., & Mandel, J. (2012). Management of severe sepsis and septic shock in adults. In *UpToDate*. Retrieved January 19, 2013, from www.uptodate.com/contents/management-of-severe-sepsis-and-septic-shock-in-adults

Schneidman, A., Reinke, L., Donesky, D., & Carrieri-Kohlman, V. (2014). Patient information series. Sudden breathlessness crisis. *American Journal of Respiratory and Critical Care Medicine*, 189(5), P9–P10.

Shadgan, B., Menon, M., Sanders, D., Berry, G., Martin, C., Duffy, P., Stephen, D., O'Brien, P. J. (2010). Current thinking about acute compartment syndrome of the lower extremity. *Canadian Journal of Surgery, 53*(5), 329–334.

*Shapiro, B. S., Benjamin, L. J., Payne, R., Heidrich, G. (1997). Sickle cell-related pain: Perceptions of medical practitioners. *Journal of Pain & Symptom Management, 14*, 168–174.

Shaughnessy, K. (2007). Massive pulmonary embolism. *Critical Care Nurse*, 27(1), 39–51.

Singer, P., Berger, M. M., Van den Berghe, G., Biolo, G., Calder, P., Forbes, A., . . . Pichard, C. (2009). ESPEN guidelines on parenteral nutrition: intensive care. *Clinical nutrition, 28*(4), 387–400.

Smith, E. R., & Amin-Hanjani, S. (2013). Evaluation and management of elevated intracranial pressure in adults. In *UpToDate*. Retrieved from www.uptodate.com/contents/evaluation-and-management-of-elevated-intracranial-pressure-in-adults

Smith, J. R. & Carley, A. (2014). Common neonatal complications. In K.R. Simpson & P.A. Creehan (Eds.), *Perinatal Nursing* (4th ed., pp. 662–698). Philadelphia: Lippincott Williams & Wilkins.

Solomon, L. R. (2010). Pain management in adults with sickle cell disease in a medical center emergency department. *Journal of the National Medical Association, 102*(11), 1025.

Stanford Medicine: Pathology & Laboratory Medicine. (2009). *Laboratory Critical/Panic Value List*. Retrieved at www.stanfordlab.com/pages/panicvalues.htm

Stracciolini, A., & Hammerberg, E. M. (2014). Acute compartment syndrome of the extremities. In *UpToDate*. Retrieved from http://www.uptodate.com/contents/acute-compartment-syndrome-of-the-extremities

Szucs, K. A., & Rosenman, M. B. (2013). Family-centered, evidence-based phototherapy delivery. *Pediatrics, 131*(6), e1982–e1985.

Trinka, E., Cock, H., Hesdorffer, D., Rossetti, A. O., Scheffer, I. E., Shinnar, S., . . . Lowenstein, D. H. (2015). A definition and classification of status epilepticus–Report of the ILAE Task Force on Classification of Status Epilepticus. *Epilepsia, 56*(10), 1515–1523.

Urinary Retention. (2012,). Retrieved from http://kidney.niddk.nih.gov/kudiseases/pubs/UrinaryRetention/

Volpin, G., Gorski, A., Shtarker, H., & Makhoul, N. (2010). Fat embolism syndrome following injuries and limb fractures. *Harefuah, 149*(5), 304–308.

Weinhouse, G. L. (2016). Fat embolism syndrome. In *UpToDate*. Retrieved from http://www.uptodate.com/contents/fat-embolism-syndrome

Williamson, M. A., & Snyder, L. M. (2014). *Wallach's interpretation of diagnostic tests: Pathways to arriving at a clinical diagnosis (interpretation of diagnostic tests)*. Philadelphia: Wolters Kluwer.

Yu, A. (2013). Causes of Hypomagnesemia. In *UpToDate*. Retrieved at www.uptodate.com/contents/causes-of-hypomagnesemia.

Zafren, K., & Mechem, C. (2014). Accidental hypothermia in adults. In *UpToDate*. Retrieved from http://www.uptodate.com/contents/accidental-hypothermia-in-adults

Zisman, A. L., Worcester, E. M., Coe, F. L. (2011). Evaluation and management of stone disease. In J. T. Daugirdas (Ed.), *Handbook of chronic kidney disease management* (pp. 482–492). Philadelphia, PA: Lippincott Williams & Wilkins.

Appendices

*Cornish, P. L., Knowles, S. R., Marchesano, R., Tam, V., Shadowitz, S., Juurlink, D. N., & Etchells, E. E. (2005). Unintended medication discrepancies at the time of hospital admission. *Archives of Internal Medicine*, *165*(4), 424–429.

DeWalt, D. A., Callahan, L., Hawk, V. H,. Broucksou, K. A., & Hink, A. (2010). *Health literacy universal precautions tool kit*. Rockville, MD: Agency for Healthcare Research and Quality. Retrieved from www.ahrq.gov/professionals/quality-patient-safety/quality-resources/tools/literacy-toolkit/healthliteracytoolkit.pdf

Entwistle, V. A., McCaughan, D., Watt, I. S., Birks, Y., Hall, J., Peat, M., . . . Wright, J. (2010). Speaking up about safety concerns: multi-setting qualitative study of patients' views and experiences. *Quality and Safety in Health Care*, *19*(6), e33–e33.

Franz, M. G., Robson, M. C., Steed, D. L., Barbul, A., Brem, H., Cooper, D. M., . . . Wiersema-Bryant, L. (2008). Guidelines to aid healing of acute wounds by decreasing impediments of healing. *Wound Repair and Regeneration*, *16*(6), 723–748.

Frosch, D. L., & Elwyn, G. (2014). Don't blame patients, engage them: transforming health systems to address health literacy. *Journal of Health Communication*, *19*(Suppl 2), 10–14.

Frosch, D. L., May, S. G., Rendle, K. A., Tietbohl, C., & Elwyn, G. (2012). Authoritarian physicians and patients' fear of being labeled 'difficult'among key obstacles to shared decision making. *Health Affairs*, *31*(5), 1030–1038.

*Hibbard, J. H., & Cunningham, P. J. (2008). How engaged are consumers in their health and health care, and why does it matter? Findings from HSC No. 8: Providing insights that contribute to better health policy. Washington, DC: HSC

*Kutner, M., Greenberg, E., Jin, Y., & Paulsen, C. (2006). *The health literacy of America's adults: Results from the 2003 National Assessment of Adult Literacy*. U.S. Dept. of Education. Washington, DC: National Center for Education Statistics. Retrieved from http://nces.ed.gov/pubs2006/2006483.pdf

Morse, J. M. (1997). *Preventing patient falls*. Thousand Oaks: Sage Broda

*National Association of Adult Literacy. (2003). Health Literacy of America's Adults: Results of the National Assessment of Adult Literacy (NAAL). Retrieved from https://nces.ed.gov/naal/

Pear, S. M. (2007). *Managing infection control: Patients risk factors and best practices for surgical site infection prevention* (pp. 56–63). Tucson, AZ: University of Arizona.

*Podsiadlo, D., & Richardson, S. (1991). The timed 'Up and Go' test: A test of basic functional mobility for frail elderly persons. *Journal of American Geriatric Society*, *39*, 142–148. Retrieved August 2, 2012, www.fallrventiontaskforce.orgpdf.Timed UpandGoTest.pdf

Price, C. S., Williams, A., Philips, G., Dayton, M., Smith, W., & Morgan, S. (2008). *Staphylococcus aureus* nasal colonization in preoperative orthopaedic outpatients. *Clinical Orthopaedics and Related Research*, *466*(11), 2842–2847.

*Ratzan, S. C. (2001). Health literacy: Communication for the public good. *Health Promotion International*, *16*(2), 207–214.

*Roter, D. L., Rune, R. E., & Comings, J. (1998). Patient literacy: A barrier to quality of care. *Journal General Internal Medicine*, *13*(12), 850–851.

Sofaer, S., & Schumann, M. J. (2013). *Fostering successful patient and family engagement*. This White Paper was prepared for the Nursing Alliance for Quality Care with grant support from the Agency for Healthcare Research and Quality (AHRQ); Approved. Retrieved from www.naqc.org/WhitePaper-PatientEngagement

Sørensen, L. T. (2012). Wound healing and infection in surgery: The pathophysiological impact of smoking, smoking cessation, and nicotine replacement therapy: A systematic review. *Annals of Surgery*, *255*(6), 1069–1079. Retrieved from http://archsurg.jamanetwork.com/article.aspx?articleid=1151013

Weiss, B. D. (2007). *Health literacy and patient safety: Help patients understand*. American Medical Association. Retrieved from http://med.fsu.edu/userFiles/file/ahec_health_clinicians_manual.pdf

*White, S., & Dillow, S. (2005). Key concepts and features of the 2003 National Assessment of Adult Literacy. National Center for Education Statistics. Retrieved from http://nces.ed.gov/NAAL/PDF/2006471.PDF

*Williams, M. V., Parker, R. M., Baker, D. W., Parikh, N. S., Pitkin, K., Coates, W. C., & Nurss, J. R. (1995). Inadequate functional health literacy among patients at two public hospitals. *JAMA*, *274*(21), 1677–1682.

Index

Note: Page numbers followed by *b*, *f*, and *t* indicate boxes, figures, and tables, respectively. Nursing diagnoses are indicated by initial capitals.

B

D

E

F

I

N

Q

R

CCS0616